Avidya ksetram uttaresam prasupta tanu vicchinna udaranam.
*The lack of true knowledge is the source of all pain and sorrows,
whether dormant, interrupted, or fully active.*

Patanjali, Yoga Sutra II.4 (200–800 BC)

. . . .

What a piece of work is man.

William Shakespeare, *Hamlet* (1603)

. . . .

*Exercise and recreation are as necessary as reading; I would say
rather more necessary, because health is more important than
learning.*

Thomas Jefferson (1743–1826)

. . . .

*A man thinks as well through his legs and arms as his brain. We
exaggerate the importance of the headquarters.*

Henry David Thoreau (1817–1862)

. . . .

*The great phase in man's advancement is that in which he passes
from subconscious to conscious control of his own mind and body.*

F. M. Alexander (1869–1955)

. . . .

*Knowledge comes in two forms: lifeless, stored in books, and alive in
the consciousness of men. The second form ... is the essential one.*

Albert Einstein (1939)

. . . .

I don't know anything, but I do know that everything is interesting
if you go into it deeply enough.

Richard P. Feynman, Nobel laureate (1965)

. . . .

*When I practice, I am a philosopher.
When I teach, I am a scientist.
When I demonstrate, I am an artist.*

B. K. S. Iyengar (2008)

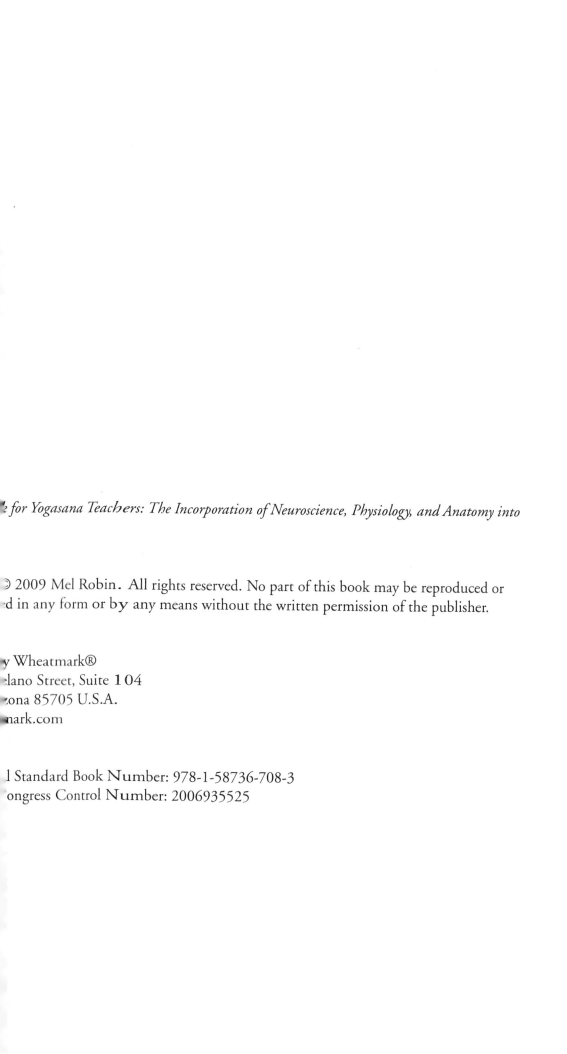

for Yogasana Teachers: The Incorporation of Neuroscience, Physiology, and Anatomy into

y Wheatmark®
·lano Street, Suite 104
·ona 85705 U.S.A.
·nark.com

·l Standard Book Number: 978-1-58736-708-3
·ongress Control Number: 2006935525

A Handbool

Yogasana Tea

The Incorporation of Neuroscien(
and Anatomy into the Pr

A Handbo(
the Practic(

Published b
610 East D
Tucson, Ar
www.whea

Internation
Library of (

rev201101

MEL ROBIN

A Handbook for Yogasana Teachers

Yogasana Teachers

The Incorporation of Neuroscience, Physiology, and Anatomy into the Practice

MEL ROBIN

A Handbook for Yogasana Teachers: The Incorporation of Neuroscience, Physiology, and Anatomy into the Practice

Published by Wheatmark®
610 East Delano Street, Suite 104
Tucson, Arizona 85705 U.S.A.
www.wheatmark.com

International Standard Book Number: 978-1-58736-708-3
Library of Congress Control Number: 2006935525

rev201101

Contents

Prologue

In the Beginning

The possibility of writing a handbook connecting the sciences of *yogasana* practice and Western medicine was born in my mind ten years ago. To this end, I combed the literatures of *yogasana* and medical science as completely as I could, and in an earlier edition of this handbook [709], published in 2002, I laid before readers the juxtaposed pictures of the two sciences as I found them. Inasmuch as the sciences of *yogasana* and Western medicine have evolved independently of one another, it is no surprise that direct comparisons of the two occur only infrequently so that one is working to assemble a puzzle for which many key pieces are still missing. However, considering the pieces of the puzzle that could be connected, with a little imagination one can then guess the shape and coloring of the missing pieces with some confidence. I did this in several places, being careful to point out that this "missing information" was only my best guess as to what is going on and may well be incomplete, or even incorrect.

Initially, the intended audience for the handbook consisted of *yogasana* teachers with perhaps five to ten years' experience (but not necessarily in the Iyengar approach [388]), who have not otherwise been trained in science, but who probably have been exposed to the medical side of yoga without understanding much of that aspect. It was assumed in turn that these teachers were working with beginning students, practicing those *yogasanas* with which beginners most often work. It appears now that the handbook additionally has found an audience among those doing bodywork outside of yoga, and among *yogasana* students who are not presently teaching. As I worked on the earlier edition of this handbook, my feeling was that it would be the first and only one of its kind to meld *yogasana* and Western medicine in aid to both *yogasana* teachers and medical experts. And at the same time, I estimated that I would be lucky if more than a hundred copies of such a specialized book would be sold, filled with so many ideas that would seem so foreign to most yoga teachers and to most medical doctors. Still, I persevered with the thought that in my way and from my position at the bottom of the *yogasana* hierarchy, this nonetheless could be a meaningful contribution to yoga. Indeed, how lucky one would be to make any contribution to yoga after its illustrious history of 5,000 years!

The past few years have proved me wrong quantitatively. In the intervening years, other books on the subject have come to my attention, most especially those of Coulter [167], Raman [694], Stiles [832], and Telang [851], the first three of which preceded my publication by several months, and the fourth by several years. Though differing in several respects from this handbook, Dr. Coulter's book does cover much of the same territory and thus is very useful to the student and teacher. In fact, had I known that his book was on the horizon, I am not sure that I would have continued work on mine! Rather than acknowledge in detail the many points on which he and I agree, I recommend his book to you, with the thought that in spite of the differing accents put on the common material, having our two books in hand gives the student a more evenhanded picture of the field than either does alone. The books by Drs. Telang and Raman are recommended, as they present views of the subject that are more Eastern in their approaches than are those books published by us Western authors. Taken in combination, these books give both the Eastern and Western readers a more rounded picture of this developing field.

Anatomy and Physiology

Recently I have seen that more and more of the articles in yoga journals discuss the anatomy and physiology of the postures, that a much larger percentage of the classes given at *yogasana* workshops today are focused on anatomy and physiology, and that all yoga teacher-training courses now appear to offer anatomy and physiology as distinct parts of the coursework. I think it is not an illusion to say that interest in these subjects is quickly gaining ground in the yoga community. It is my hope that this interest will expand to include the newly burgeoning field of neuroscience as well.

A Second Chance

The publication of the earlier edition of this handbook and its positive reception by some *yogasana* and bodywork enthusiasts has given me the time and stimulus to consider a major revision of the earlier work, differing from it in being organized along different lines while introducing many new topics of great scientific interest (current to February 2007), along with their relevance to *yogasana* practice.

In order to hold the revised edition of this work to manageable proportions, certain parts of the earlier work have been omitted and many of the figures have been redrawn in the interest of improved clarity and accuracy. In this process, a certain amount of repetition has been removed from the text while other explanations have been expanded to make them more understandable. Additionally, a few other discussions have been omitted entirely from the revised edition, because they were felt, in hindsight, to be of only minimal interest to the reader. On the other hand, the volume of revised text has been greatly enlarged by the addition of totally new material, for we have

been in the midst of an explosive increase of our understanding of the functions of various brain centers over the past few years, almost all of which I find relevant to *yogasana* practice. Thus, the revised edition contains significantly more meaningful material of high current interest, hopefully justifying its 100-percent increase in bulk.

Most of the subsections in this new version of the handbook have been further subdivided, using italicized subtopic headings ("*A Second Chance*," for example), whose key phrases make browsing the handbook faster and more interesting. Within the text, whenever a particular item in one place has relevance to material in another place, it will reference that related material parenthetically as "(see also Subsection X.Y, page xxx)." These "hyperlinks" have been inserted in the text to allow the reader rapid access to closely related material without having to search the index. On the other hand, for those who choose to go deeper/further, the index has been internally cross-referenced with great detail so as to maximize the number of such associations.

The appearance of this revised edition seven years after the initial effort is embarrassing on one score: it really isn't right that one pays so much for a book, and then, in a few years, finds that it is out of date and so is forced to buy a revised edition. All I can say in defense of this is that I have worked on the revised edition so as to make a significant improvement in the text and to incorporate a very large amount of genuinely new material (so new, in fact, that it is just now appearing in the scientific technical literature). Hopefully, the reader will find that this augmented and revised edition is well worth having over and above whatever merits the earlier edition had to offer.

What's Old, What's New?

If asked what the key phrase or idea was in the earlier edition of this handbook, I would say, in hindsight, that it was the largely unsuspected importance of the autonomic nervous system to our practice of *yogasana*. I choose to say "autonomic nervous system" because other textbooks on yoga rarely (if ever) mention it at all, yet it is a substantial component of the earlier edition. Applying the same question to the present work, I would have to say the key word in my mind is now "flexibility." As students of yoga, I know that on reading this, your mind has skipped automatically to the flexibility of the muscles and joints in the body; however, I remind you of how tightly this body is connected by yoga to the mind, to the emotions, and to the spirit. In this case, by "flexibility" I refer not only to the muscles and joints, but just as well to the flexibility and mutual connectivities of the emotions, of the hormonal systems, of the peripheral nervous systems, of the gross and subtle structures of the brain, of the myofascial tissues, of the levels of consciousness, of the modes of learning and remembering, and of our attitudes toward accepting or rejecting both new and old ideas. In all of these areas, one can find not only flexibility among students and teachers, but also hyperflexibility, as well as a lack of flexibility.

To the more traditional aspects of Western medicine must be added the recent advances in the field of neuroscience; suffice it to say here that advances in the last few years have greatly expanded our understanding of how the brain is connected to the body, mind, and emotions, and this new understanding has made the study of Western medical science vastly more relevant to the study of *yogasana*. This subject now occupies a much larger fraction of the text in the revised handbook than it did in the earlier volume, and its discoveries not only illuminate the discussion of the autonomic nervous system for *yogasana* students, but may also soon overtake it in importance.

Definitions

Let us take a moment, then, to define our terms. By *"yogasana"* is meant the scientific study and practice of the traditional Indian postures, performed with alignment, strength, and grace as per the directives of B. K. S. Iyengar [388, 393]. By stabilizing the body through this practice, one can then stabilize and quiet the mind. *"Pranayama"* is the science of the control of the breath while in a stable body posture; when the breath is controlled, it is refined, with the mind being quiet but inwardly alert. Traditionally, by "Western medicine" we mean the scientific study of body systems and their understanding in terms of anatomy and physiological processes such as heart rate, blood pressure, autonomic stimulation, muscle-spindle response, motor units, hormones, learning, memory, etc. [196]. Note that a large amount of high-quality "Western medical science" focused on yoga processes has begun to surface recently in the Indian medical journals (see, for example, the work of Telles et al. in this regard).

The largest overlap of Eastern *yogasana* practice and Western medical practice centers on the autonomic nervous system and its branches, the sympathetic, parasympathetic, and enteric nervous systems; in anticipation of newer advances in both medicine and the *yogasanas,* the handbook mentions many aspects of the autonomic nervous system that are presently relevant to *yogasana* work or could be so in the future. Of course, a full discussion of the autonomic effects with respect to *yogasana* practice entails descriptions of many other subjects—muscles, nerves, reflexes, the brain, bones, the breath, vision, etc.—and all of these have been included at the relevant levels. An Eastern version of medicine, Ayurveda, also exists with a wide following [473]; however, this handbook deals exclusively with the relation between *yogasana* practice [388] and the concepts of Western medicine.

Though there are eight limbs to the yoga tree of Patanjali [391], the present work deals almost totally with the third limb, the *yogasanas* or postures, only tangentially with the fourth limb, *pranayama,* and not at all with the others. This is not to say that they are not all equally important, but it is at the levels of *yogasana* and *pranayama* that Western medicine and the eight limbs of yoga have their largest common ground. Hence it is at this level that the integration of *yogasana* and medical understanding makes the most sense, especially in the context of teaching beginning and intermediate students.

A Rational Approach

This handbook deals with those aspects of *yogasana* that are amenable to rational thought and experiment. Such a mechanistic approach, I feel, is undeniably relevant to *yogasana* practice for beginners. It is equally undeniable that the mechanistic approach is less relevant for the more advanced practitioner, for whom *yogasana* and its effects go far beyond our Western powers to quantify, measure, or understand. Perhaps we can think of the mechanistic approach employed here as equivalent to the use of props, a practice that helps beginning students and their teachers in the performance of the *yogasanas* but which is not intended necessarily to be used at higher levels of the yoga tree.

Scope

The present scope of this handbook can be set out in more detail:

1) Though this handbook is meant to be a bridge between Western medicine and Eastern *yogasana,* is not a description of a mature field, although its component parts, medicine and *yogasana,* each have long histories and deal with very sophisticated subjects.

2) This handbook is centered upon the practice of *yogasana;* rather than being a "How-do-you-do-it?" book concerning the basic and intermediate-level *yogasanas,* it deals instead with "What-happens-when-you-do-it?" The answers to these yogic questions are framed within the neuroscientific, physiological, and anatomic explanations of the body as given largely by Western medical science. For teachers and intermediate-level students of *yogasana,* a goal of the handbook is to help you understand rationally what you already "know" intuitively or have been told *ex cathedra*. In this work, I attempt to honor aspects of the traditional hatha yoga approach while focusing on the scientifically documented, objective effects of *yogasana* practice on the body and mind, and applying these proven concepts to the more subjective but unquantifiable feelings often attendant to this practice.

3) This handbook offers discussions of several scientific topics in appendices that are somewhat off the main track (for example, Section IV.D, page 856, concerning gravitational effects on *yogasana* postures). Shorter expositions of materials that are somewhat off the general theme of the text are also appended as highlighted text boxes and/or as footnotes.

4) Though the subject is *yogasana* and medicine, it is not specifically about *yogasana* as therapy. Still, where the discussion unavoidably bears on *yogasana* as therapy, this aspect is noted.

5) This handbook's approach is most strongly focused on the yogic approach of B. K. S. Iyengar [388, 393] and his family, as this is the most scientific of the various approaches to *yogasana* (and apparently among the most popular, as it is estimated to account for 30 percent of the fifteen million yoga practitioners in the United States [781]) and so is closest to the Western medical explanations of how the body functions.

6) Because this handbook offers rational discussion of the reasons why we work the *yogasanas* as we do and why we feel as we do while doing them, it can make *yogasana* more interesting to students and so bind them more firmly to their practice.

7) This handbook does not consider the great mass of medical data and understanding derived from experiments on invertebrates or nonhuman vertebrates.

8) In the past five years, many of those who have read preliminary drafts of the revised manuscript independently have written the same phrase in the margin: "Interesting, but what does this have to do with yoga?" Thus sensitized, I have worked diligently in the present work to make this connection as concrete as I can, within the bounds of reason. Thus, esoteric subtopics do appear in the text that seemingly may have no relation to your *yogasana* practice; in these cases, they are included because I feel that they are at least tangentially related, and that with further thought, they may well become important to us in the yoga world as our understanding broadens. (This point of view is discussed further in the epilogue, page 821.)

9) A special effort has been made to make

the index multidimensional. As explained there (page 999), the multidimensional aspect means that one can use the index not only to find a particular topic in the handbook, but due to the extensive cross-referencing within the index, one also can uncover unique relations between any two topics. The index's formatting is somewhat nonstandard so as to accommodate the breadth of its information while keeping it to a reasonable length; please read the introduction on p. 999 before looking up a topic. The text of the handbook also can be searched electronically using Amazon's "Search Inside" feature.

Refreshing One's Practice

My own experience (twenty-five years as student, twenty-one years as teacher) is that one can more easily keep the experience of *yogasana* practice fresh and bright in one's awareness if one can make the connections between what is being experienced in the *yogasana* and what one understands of the functions of the body, mind, and emotions as put forth by Western medicine. At the same time, I am well aware of how disjointed this medically intense approach appears to be with most of yogic history; I ask that you approach it with an open mind and see if it does not add something fresh to your practice and teaching.

I have found this attempt at bringing Western medicine and *yogasana* into a rational relationship to be satisfying, and though there are many loose ends, the new awareness of the connections has led me to yet more avenues to explore. Each of the hours that one practices and each of the hours that one teaches can be energized by un-

derstanding how these two sciences, which have developed so independently of one another, have come to dovetail as nicely as they do. Because the new avenues opened by simultaneously considering Western medicine and *yogasanas* serve to refresh and invigorate one's practice and teaching, it has been my intention in writing the present edition to extend the number of such connections to the maximum. In doing so, it has become a goal in this handbook to take the mystery out of Western medicine and out of *yogasana* practice but not the wonder of the connections within each of them, and especially those between them.

Who Does Yoga Today?

Information is limited in regard to this question, but data gathered in 1998 in the United States and published in 2003 is available [737]. In this study, it was found that approximately 15.0 million Americans had tried yoga at least once and 7.4 million had done so in the year 1997, the total population being approximately 200 million at that time. Among those who tried yoga more than once in 1997, the male to female ratio was 32 percent to 68 percent; 68 percent of such practitioners were college educated, and 93 percent were urban dwellers. These students also reported that 64 percent used yoga for general wellness, 48 percent for specific health conditions, and 21 percent for the relief of back or neck pain. From these numbers, one can see that yoga already has a strong medical flavor in the minds of Westerners, and it is a goal of this work to strengthen it even more.

Acknowledgments

It has been my experience as a solo beginner that performing a *yogasana* opened the door to many sensations and feelings, some pleasant and some painful, but with little understanding as to which were appropriate to the practice and which should have been avoided. Only after working with a teacher was there some light shed on which sensations to encourage and which to discourage. I find that this initial lack of direction also appears for me when writing a book about *yogasanas* and Western medicine. The field is ripe for many new ideas; however, in the beginning, one has no firm understanding of which ideas are sensible and which are nonsense, and so one must turn to dispassionate observers on the outside for critical input. It is for this reason that I am pleased to acknowledge that this handbook has been road tested by several *yogasana* teachers who were willing to read the text and give feedback on what needed to be changed. I especially am happy to acknowledge Carol Wipf, Karen Wachsmuth, Eliza Childs, Mary Dalziel, Susan Ahlstrom, Karin Eisen, Ellen Kiley, and Elaine Patterson for their valuable help in this important aspect of putting the initial and present versions of the handbook together. Special thanks go to Dr. Arlene Thoma, who diligently proofread Chapter 4 of the earlier edition, and to William Egbert, who was so generous with his time in regard to Chapter 18 in the present edition. Similarly, I am indebted to Wendy Rasmussen, Royane Mosley, and Nancy Barr for their skill and patience in regard to drawing and redrawing many of the figures. The mandala decorating the front cover of this volume is the artwork of Nancy Lee Schnabel, who generously donated it to this project.

Finally, I thank Roger Cole and Fernando Pages Ruiz, for several helpful technical discussions, and Jean Fisher, for help in searching various databases. Special thanks again to Roger Cole for permission to mention his unpublished thoughts on vascular processes and on the bones of the lower leg.

Tom and Susan Parrish of the Quakertown Kung Fu Center and Dr. Brian Trachtenberg have been especially helpful in support of this project, and it is a pleasure to acknowledge publicly the time and energy they have volunteered in aid of the completion of this work.

I owe more than I can say to my day-to-day *yogasana* teachers, Theresa Rowland, Gabriella Giubilaro, Nancy Stechert, and Judy Freedman, each of whom has been an inspiration to me in their depth of knowledge and their dedication to both their art and their students. In this regard, special thanks go as well to Aadil Palkhivala, Kofi Busia, Patricia Walden, and Rodney Yee, who helped to mold my yogic thinking in past years. Of course, none of the above is responsible in any way for whatever mistakes or omissions I may have committed in this work.

Many of the connections presented in the handbook between medicine and *yogasana* are not newly discovered by me. Others have considered these two sciences and written briefly on the connections they have found. I have gathered all of their wisdom as best I could into one place, so that the reader can easily find in a handbook format what they have to say. In particular, I thank *yogasana* teachers such as Judith Lasater, Arthur Kilmurray, Mary Schatz, and Roger Cole, who have put so much into the literature on how physiological processes and anatomy relate to *yogasana* practice. I have incorporated much of their published work into this handbook, and I thank them for all they have explained to me (and you) in regard to how *yogasana* and Western medicine interrelate. A more complete list of my indebtedness can be found on pages 971–97.

Following the publication of the earlier edition, I have been fortunate in making contact with Dr. Ruth Gilmore, who is both a professional yoga therapist and an anatomist, and who has read the earlier text, commenting on errors of commission and omission. I am grateful for her highly erudite reading of and comments on the earlier edition and especially so for her complete answers to many of the questions I have raised since that edition appeared. Thanks as well to those who, by word of mouth, have promoted the distribution of this handbook via their students and other teachers.

As with any project of the size of this handbook, successful completion rests largely in the hands of an editor willing and able to add her skills, patience, and hard work to the mix. It has been my good fortune to have Ms. Susan Wenger play this role in the production of the handbook,

and I am pleased to acknowledge her substantial contribution to this effort. Many thanks, Susan, for all the polish you have added to a book sorely in need of same.

By necessity, one important reference has been omitted from the reference list, for if I were to specifically acknowledge each item my day-to-day teacher, Theresa Rowland, has taught me in the past twenty years, it would swell the size of this handbook to unmanageable proportions. Neither *A Physiological Handbook for Teachers of Yogasana* nor *A Handbook for Yogasana Teachers: The Incorporation of Neuroscience, Physiology, and Anatomy into the Practice* would have materialized without the inspiration and understanding I have drawn from her. Of course, eventually all such credit and thanks must be placed at the feet of our guru, B. K. S. Iyengar and his family, whose systematic study of the *yogasanas* forms the basis of any work seeking to relate *yogasana* and medical principles to one another.

Mel Robin
Upper Black Eddy, Pennsylvania 18972
AandMRobin@aol.com
April 20, 2009

Eastern Yoga and Western Medicine

Section 1.A: Differences and Similarities

Historical Perspective

The ancient Chinese art of *cong fou,* which existed before 1000 BC, is the oldest known form of therapeutic exercise; it is concerned with body positions and breathing routines for the relief of pain and other symptoms. The ancient therapeutic use of body positions by Hindu Brahmans dates back to about 800 BC; however, this was derived from the practice of yoga postures in the Indus Valley culture of India dating as far back as 2500–2000 BC [222].

Patanjali and Eastern Yoga

Though yoga was first mentioned in the ancient Vedic texts of India approximately 3,000 years ago, it is thought to have existed for millennia before that as an oral tradition. Various references to yoga in these ancient texts were drawn together and codified by Patanjali in the Yoga Sutras sometime in the period 200–800 BC [196, 559]. In this work, Patanjali laid out the basic philosophy behind the actions one must take in order to bring the mind to a steady, unwavering single focus, opening the doorway to higher states of consciousness and ultimately to liberation from the pains of ordinary life.

Many variations on Patanjali's basic theme have taken shape, including the hatha yoga ap-proach, which employs the yoga postures as focal points for increasing one's strength and sharpening one's self-awareness and concentration. The *hatha* form of yoga based upon the *yogasanas* is relatively young, possibly having been introduced in the fifteenth century [797]. Patanjali says of the yoga postures *(yogasanas)* that they are to be done in such a way that one is steady, alert, graceful, and with the mind at ease. Though Patanjali's Yoga Sutras mention no specific *yogasana* by name, they have survived as one of the cornerstones of hatha yoga practice to the present day.

The *yogasanas* of hatha yoga number approximately 750,000 and are performed with the intention of manipulating the body's inherent energy upward (through willpower and awareness) or downward (through relaxation). It is only relatively recently that such yogic exercises have come to be important as therapeutic aids for curing or preventing illness and disease, rather than as points on which to focus one's mental powers in an effort to gain liberation. That is not to say that in the earliest days of yoga, postures were not recognized for their therapeutic value.

As the dissection of cadavers historically was forbidden in Eastern traditions, doctors obtained their understanding of the body by the observation of living human beings and the energy patterns within them [150, 507]. Lad [473] explains that the Eastern perspective, as practiced by Ayurvedic and yogic doctors past and present, requires acceptance, observation, and experience, whereas the Western perspective has been based on questioning, analysis, and logical deduction.

Operating in their way, yogis of the Eastern world divided the body into physical zones, hav-

Table 1.A-1: Relation of the *Chakras* to Specific Endocrine Glands and Their Psychological Attributes [507]

Chakras	Neuroendocrine Plexus	Psychological Attribute
Genital	Gonads	Sexuality
Sacral	Adrenal	Fear
Solar plexus	Pancreas	Power
Heart	Thymus	Love
Throat	Thyroid	Creativity
Brow	Pituitary	Intuition
Crown	Pineal	Bliss

ing intuited the seven major psychic centers of the body, the *chakras*, as listed in table 1.A-1. Though it was not their original intention to attribute the *chakras* to physical structures, it is amazing to see how closely they do correspond to known specific neuroendocrine plexuses in the body. The possible relationships of the *chakras* and their subunits to physical structures in the human body are discussed further in Subsection 5.G, page 201. Additionally, it is a part of Eastern wisdom that the body consists of five concentric sheaths, the two outermost sheaths being the *annamaya kosha* and the *pranamaya kosha*, referring to the anatomy and the physiology of the body respectively [401]. It is within these outermost two sheaths of the Eastern point of view that we hope to find the largest areas of agreement when compared with the concepts of Western medicine.

Western Medical Science

The modern occidental practice of exercise is Greek in origin. The first Greek to write on the subject was Herodius in approximately 480 BC. At that time, Hippocrates said of his teacher Herodius that he killed the weak with walking, too much wrestling, and fomentation. Quoting Hippocrates, "There is nothing more pernicious for the febrile than wrestling, walking, and massage. It is like treating a disturbance with a disturbance." Plato also condemned Herodius for excessive use of exercise, saying that a twenty-mile walk without rest was too much for patients; however, he later reversed his opinion.

The present chasm between Western medical science and Eastern yogic science is based largely on the early differences between Eastern and Western modes of medical experimentation: in contrast to the situation in regard to Eastern yoga, Western medicine was founded upon facts first learned by dissection of the cadavers of criminals beginning in the fifteenth century, i.e., in bodies lacking all energy.[1] Today, the Western focus remains on the use of inanimate instrumentation to probe the intimate aspects of the physical, mental, and emotional states of live and willing subjects.

Though Hippocrates, in the early days of Western medicine, stressed the importance of the physician understanding both the body and the mind, this admonition largely has been bypassed today by Western doctors in favor of the separate study of these two spheres. It was only in the early 1800s that Western medicine broke away from religion and superstition, leaving behind the influences of the medicine woman, myth, and magic and adopting attitudes based instead on medical science, experimentation, and logical reasoning. Since that time, it has succeeded, in its own way, in inventing, discovering, and pushing ahead the frontiers of knowledge about the body and about the mind, although the push has been largely in only one direction (Subsection 1.A, page 6).

Because the success of Western science has been almost totally in the observation of physical

---

1   Actually, the dissection of cadavers for religious reasons can be traced back to 300 BC in Alexandria, Egypt, where bodies were prepared for mummification.

phenomena, it has been associated historically with a philosophy of the physical world that is based on the belief that everything observable can be reduced to an understanding of basic physical processes. This philosophy occasionally leads Western scientists to label phenomena that cannot be understood within the bounds of the purely physical as being the work of observers who are not sufficiently "detached" and to say that their observations are "unreliable," "unscientific," or just "too difficult to understand." Yet another factor is that the observations of the Eastern practitioners often are "ineffable" to Westerners, meaning that they are best communicated using right-hemisphere nonverbal modes (Subsection 4.D, page 99) and least easily in terms of the left-hemisphere principles appropriate to the physical world [848].

From the Western perspective, the functions of the body can be divided into eleven subsystems: the integumentary system (the external skin), the skeletal system (the bones and joints), the muscular system (skeletal, cardiac, and smooth muscles), the nervous system (central and peripheral nervous systems), the endocrine system (hormones), the cardiovascular system (the heart and blood vessels), the lymphatic system, the respiratory system (lungs and the breath), the digestive system (the gastrointestinal tract), the urinary system, and the reproductive system (the gonads). The chapters in this handbook are based largely on this eleven-part Western division of the body.

The Two World Views

Given the huge number of books on Western medicine at all levels of sophistication and similarly the huge number of books on *yogasana* (for example, see [388 and 559]), it is something of a mystery why in-depth books have appeared only very recently on the relation between the two [167, 694, 832, 851]. Of course, one also could ask why there are so few books relating ballroom dancing to architecture, for example; but clearly, in this case, there is no reason to expect much overlap of understanding between the two fields, whereas with medicine and *yogasana,* the situation is just the opposite. One can reasonably expect that the truths of *yogasana* will stand in one-to-one correspondence with the truths of Western medicine, if indeed they are truths after all.

In regard to this question, perhaps the relative lack of books relating *yogasana* to Western medicine may be due to the two world views that pervade human thinking. As shown in table 1.A-2, there are two world views about most subjects, *yogasana* and Western medicine included. "World View I" has been developed intuitively in the Eastern world, then refined and sharpened by the test of time and out of respect for the sages of the past; whereas "World View II" has been developed in the Western world and refined by experiment and observation using modern scientific tools and methods. The separate and unquestioned existence of these two world views implies, more or less, that they are antithetical: one must subscribe either to one of the views or the other. Undoubtedly, the list in table 1.A-2 could be expanded by adding "Yoga" to the list for World View I and "Medical Science" to the list for World View II.

Table 1.A-2: Comparison of the Two World Views

World View I	World View II
Ancient	Modern
Traditional	Non-traditional
Intuitive	Demonstrative
Subjective	Objective
Irrational	Rational
Faith	Reason
Spiritual	Materialistic
Magical/mystical	Real world
Feeling	Knowing
Sensations	Facts
Right brain	Left brain
Yin	Yang
Soft	Hard
Vague	Specific
Nonlinear	Linear
East	West
Moon	Sun

World View I	World View II
Feminine	Masculine
Shakti	Shiva

Inherent Dissonance

Unfortunately, the qualities of the two lists in the table are so opposite that combining them would appear to lead to laughable oxymorons ("Vague Facts," "Subjective Real World," "Rational Faith," etc.).[2] Among the better oxymorons within this framework would be "Yogic Science" or "Scientific Yoga." One's first thought might be that the two categories of yoga and science might be held in one's mind sequentially but not simultaneously, as the dissonance would be too great for that! In fact, it is an aim of this handbook to demonstrate that the fields of yoga and medical science actually have a much closer and more rational relation than the two world views would suggest and that their apparent conflict can be the source of many new and useful ideas.

In a different context, Ornstein [635] discusses a dichotomy of attitude much like that presented here as the two world views. He correlates this separation of attitude with the two cerebral hemispheres of the brain (Section 4.D, page 98), where World-View-I type thinking is favored by the right cerebral hemisphere and World-View-II type thinking is favored by the left cerebral hemisphere. As is discussed in Subsection 4.D, page 105, there is abundant evidence that, when healthy, our mental processes

oscillate between right and left hemispherical dominance once every few hours, so that we tend to swing between the two world views several times a day!

Lacking any reconciliation of the apparent conflict between science and yoga, and with the ascendancy of World View II in Western society, we have come to a situation in which many Western medical doctors, who hold science in the highest regard, hold yoga's understanding of the body in low regard because it has not been proved in the accepted Western way. At the same time, many yogis hold Western medicine in low regard because it has no historic precedence in that Eastern world in which yoga was born and developed [314].

Opposing Views

To see examples of the recent animosity between the adherents of the Eastern yogic and Western medical philosophies, turn to the letters of Seibert [768] and Frawley [254], each arguing one of the two sides of the yoga-versus-medicine question, and to the traditional Western medical view of craniosacral therapy, as mentioned in Subsection 4.E, page 107. A somewhat more optimistic view is evident in Lipson's review of Western medicine's acceptance of Ornish's work on the efficacy of *yogasana* training in battling cardiovascular disease [516]. It is clear as well that some practitioners of *yogasana* are reluctant to give credit to the substantial improvement in the quality of life that Western medicine has given all of us through the basic ideas of germs, sanitation, and vaccination. On the other hand, Western medicine fails to understand that yoga too is a highly experimental and empirical science that is based upon observations of a most discriminating kind and subject to verification by others [625]. It is only with the utmost concentration, self-awareness, and effort that yogis are able to perform their amazing physical and mental feats, and the yogic science that has led to these accomplishments should not be so easily discounted by Westerners.

Ignoring the more esoteric aspects of yogic science, not everyone on the Western side of the

---

2   Note the recent publication of the book entitled *Rational Mysticism* and the reviewer's first two sentences: "Can there be such a thing as *Rational Mysticism?* Apart from the difficulty of reconciling the two words ..." [364]. In regard to holding two conflicting ideas simultaneously in one's mind, Tom Ward, editor of the *Journal of Creative Behavior,* advises: "Merge two previously separate concepts that are in conflict with one another. For example, combinations such as 'friendly enemy' and 'healthful illness.' The more discrepant the concepts, the more likely they are to result in novel properties." See a similar statement by C. P. Snow quoted in Subsection 1.A, page 6.

Box 1.A-1: Eastern *Yogasana*, Western Medicine, and the Tomato Effect

The Tomato Effect refers to the belief in eighteenth-century America that tomatoes were poisonous because they are members of the nightshade family of plants. However, though they had good reasons to avoid eating poisonous tomatoes, eighteenth-century Americans also knew that in Europe, people had been eating tomatoes for 200 years without ill effects. In spite of the European experience, American "common sense" demanded that tomatoes not be eaten! This World-View-I denial of an experience because it does not correspond with a previously held theory or understanding, in spite of strong evidence to the contrary, is known as the "Tomato Effect" in the medical literature [64]. A somewhat related World-View-I phenomenon can be found in Tasmania, where for almost 4,000 years, large parts of the population starved to death despite the fact that their island was surrounded by seas rich in fish [66]; unfortunately, certain tribal cultures did not define fish as food!

In more recent times, aspirin and gold emulsions were known to relieve the pain of arthritis; however, as more was learned about this disease, the use of aspirin and gold emulsions made less and less sense, until finally, medical students were no longer taught about their use in treating arthritis pain. Though no one challenged the efficacy of the treatments, the use of aspirin and gold emulsions was discontinued on the basis that their beneficial effects could not be understood—again, the Tomato Effect, updated to our own time.

Yet another tomato on the medical vine today is the question of hormesis (Subsection 16.F, page 654), wherein experiments by the thousands have shown that low levels of physiological stress (radiation exposure, toxins, exercise, heat, carcinogens such as dioxin, etc.) can be beneficial to the organism, whereas high levels clearly are not [130, 370, 906a]. Disbelievers in hormesis argue logically that **all** levels of stress are harmful, in spite of abundant experimental evidence to the contrary; they are simply unable to accept the positive effects of hormesis as real, because no one understands how hormesis functions.

Western medicine has made strides in opening its collective mind to alternative therapies, both to its benefit and to that of the patients it treats. This is not to say that there are still no tomatoes hanging on the medical vines. For example, the medical treatment of sciatica as strictly a herniated intervertebral disc requiring lower-back surgery is solidly in the World-View-II column but ignores the many successes *yogasana* therapy has had with this problem by releasing the compression on the sciatic nerve caused by the tightness of the piriformis muscle within the buttocks. On the other side of the coin, *yogasana* students should understand that a torn meniscus in the knee may require fifteen or more years to heal by itself but that by arthroscopic surgery on an outpatient basis, the same knee problem can be cleared up in ten days [712]!

divide agrees as to the benefits of stretching in the *yogasana* way. This negative attitude among sports doctors and trainers is largely due to the negative consequences of inappropriate stretching by non-yogic practitioners; *e.g.*, stretching while misaligned, overstretching, or lack of proper warm-up, as so eloquently pointed out by Couch [163]. Hopefully, this negative attitude among sports doctors and trainers will change as more and more of their patients and athletes are referred to *yogasana* teachers for treatment.

If one is committed wholly to one of the two world views, it can be difficult to accept the other side, as for example in the "Tomato Effect" of Western medicine, discussed in Box 1.A-1.

Reconciling the Rationality of Medicine with the Sublimity of *Yogasana*

Mixing of Medicine and Yoga

In 1959, C. P. Snow delivered a much-quoted lecture entitled "The Two Cultures," in which he made the point that society is polarized into two groups: on one hand, the world of human-ism (here called World View I), and on the other, the world of science (here called World View II). "Between the two," he said, "a gulf of mutual in-comprehension, sometimes (particularly among the young) hostility and dislike but most of all a lack of understanding." Continuing, he said, "At the heart of thought and creation, we are letting some of our best chances go by default. The clash-ing point of two subjects, two disciplines, two cultures ought to produce creative chances. In the history of mental activity that has been where some of the breakthroughs come." By not trying to reconcile Western medicine and the science of *yogasana,* we forfeit the chance to experience the clashing point, the chance to make discover-ies that will advance both. Hopefully, rubbing Western medicine and yoga science against one another can produce not only heat, but light.

Medicine Changes Direction

The dissonance between Western medicine and *yogasana* practice seems to be declining at the present moment, due in part to the fact that the nature of medical challenges has changed precipitously in the past few decades. Until the 1970s, the primary concern of medicine was to fight infectious agents such as smallpox, diphthe-ria, influenza, tuberculosis, polio, etc. Using sci-entific techniques to identify the disease-causing agents and to then conquer them with drugs or surgery, Western medicine has been so success-ful that many scourges are now only of historical interest. The medical community is commit-ted to this scenario, and indeed, it is very much relevant today in third-world countries. On the other hand, the current medical crises in many first-world countries now involve chronic de-generative diseases such as cancer, cardiovascular

conditions, arthritis, obesity, dietary ailments, and drug abuse [280, 605, 611], with only lesser threats from pathogenic organisms. As Western medicine slowly takes a turn in the new direction, it comes face to face with medical conditions that *yogasana* practitioners and teachers have been wrestling with for millennia. How fortunate we are that many of these "new" conditions can be ameliorated or avoided by *yogasana* practice! This particular situation is in part responsible for the general public's turning more and more to alter-native medicine for treatment, one significant part of which is *yogasana,* practiced for its own sake and practiced as both prevention and as therapy (see Prologue, page xix).

Yoga Changes Direction

McCall gives an interesting overview of the interactions between medical science and yoga as of 2002 [547], and B. K. S. Iyengar, in a lecture in 1996, stresses the need for cooperation between the scientific research and yoga communities in minimizing suffering and promoting worldwide good health [399]. The close relation between the science of the body, as represented by Western medicine, and the refined art of yoga, as repre-sented by B. K. S. Iyengar [393] in the *yogasanas,* is clearly stated by Iyengar: "Art and science are in-terrelated and interconnected. Both require study, imagination, discipline and an orderly method. Both depend on technique. All art is science and all science an art. Hence it is hard to compare or differentiate between the two." In this handbook, we endeavor to forge even stronger links between the medical and *yogasana* sciences.

Perusal of the references on pages 971–97 and especially reference [26a], listing the physiological and psychological ramifications of yoga practice, reveals the significant contribution Eastern scien-tists have made to today's understanding of the physiological effects of yoga practice on the body from the Western point of view. However, this meeting of East and West is less obvious among those yoga practitioners who do not operate on the scientific plane and among those Western doctors who are unaware of the yogic plane. Nonetheless, the high quality and quantity of scientific work coming out of India and the burgeoning study of alternative medicine in the Western world both are working to bring the two sides together, speaking a common language.

That there can be common ground between yoga science and medical science is more than just a wish. Looking back at what has been said in the past, consider that "when the brain is abnormally moist, of necessity it moves and when it moves neither sight nor hearing are still, but we see or hear now one thing and now another and the tongue speaks in accordance with the things seen and heard on any occasion. But all the time the brain is still, a man is intelligent." The author of these thoughts is not a disciple of Patanjali or B. K. S. Iyengar, as one might think, but Hippocrates, the father of Western medicine, who wrote these words in the fifth century BC [427].

Unavoidable Conflict for the Student

In addition to Hippocrates, many others have spoken of the detachment of the mind that is necessary to reach the highest levels of yogic mental transformation, and I have no reason to doubt what others have said about this for thousands of years. With this idea in mind, it would seem fruitless to try to graft Western medicine and Eastern yoga onto one another, for the mind cannot be both engaged in rational analysis (in the Western way) and totally detached (in the Eastern way) at the same time. My view is that, because yoga itself is a multilevel structure, it is not unreasonable that the apparent goals of yoga are dependent upon which level is being addressed and how long a student has been at that level. Furthermore, even at a particular level, there will be many goals, all valid but with relative priorities depending upon an individual's situation. Therefore, it is neither necessary nor appropriate to have these contrary world views operating in the mind simultaneously; rather, they should be present sequentially, as discussed below. Approached in this way, the marriage of *yogasana* and Western medicine in the student's mind does make sense.

Making Progress

Because the eight levels of Patanjali's yoga are hierarchical, the Western-style rational analysis that is inappropriate for achieving the levels from *pratyahara* through *samadhi* still may be of great utility to those working at the levels of *yogasana* and *pranayama*. This, then, is the philosophy of this handbook: at the level of the student working to master the *yogasanas*, there is much to be gained by understanding the anatomy and physiology that lie behind the manifold effects that *yogasanas* bring into our awareness. However, this rational approach is less appropriate at the higher levels of yoga, in which the more meditative aspects are incorporated into the postures. At these higher levels, the Western scientist who remains interested in the rational approach must turn from physiology and anatomy to neuroscience, an increasingly important subject also discussed in this handbook.

As with everything, we aim to arrive at some balanced *(sattvic)* position on the seemingly opposite points of view on how the body/mind functions. From the *sattvic* perspective, both the denial of the importance of the physiology and anatomy attendant to *yogasana* practice and the slavish focusing on the Western rationale of the functionality of the body are barriers to further growth, and so should be avoided. Instead, the *sattvic* position is to be intensely aware of both the Eastern yogic and the Western medical aspects of *yogasana* practice and to apply them both without prejudice, in order to increase both awareness and understanding, especially at the lower levels of the practice. An encouraging report of the successful marriage of yoga and Western medicine is given by Michael Cheiken [113a], a physician who has incorporated all aspects of yoga science into his medical practice.

Section 1.B: The Goals of Yogasana Practice

The goals of *yogasana* can be stated at many different levels. At the highest level, one has

Patanjali's sutras in regard to stilling the fluctuations of the mind and achieving *samadhi*; however, at the lower level of *yogasana* considered in this handbook, the goals are more modest, as listed below.

Avoiding the Ruts

As Patanjali teaches, the primary goal of *yogasana* practice is to still the fluctuations of the mind, and the practice of the *yogasanas* provides an excellent laboratory for developing this talent. Furthermore, there are other, lesser goals to be realized. Thus, for example, Juhan [422] states a practical truth that underlies our practice of the *yogasanas*:

The system of sensorimotor integration is marvelously adaptive and its simple elements can be manipulated to produce the entire range of complex human skills. Unfortunately, the sense of "rightness" which comes about through repetition may not necessarily correspond to movements and habits that are "optimal" in their efficiency. "Rightness" in this context only means "familiarity"; *i.e.*, grooves that are well-worn. It is often strongly associated with movements and habits that are merely "satisfactory" in some limited way, or "normal" in the sense of "like before." Astonishingly enough, once a sense of normalcy has been established in connection with a way of doing something, perceived inefficiency or even pain are usually not enough to alter our behavior. We will tend to continue to do a thing the way we learned it, the way in which we first established our "feel" for it, in spite of the fact that subsequent problems develop as a result.

To this I would add that the more pain we have endured and the more effort we have expended in learning a particular aspect of *yogasana*, the more we are wed to this way of doing it, especially if our performance is automatic and unthinking.

This, in a nutshell, is the way many of us are going through life: trapped in ruts that make every day the same as the one before and in ways that reduce our responses to life's situations to formulaic, unthinking, mechanical motions. That is, we surrender our awareness—and the opportunity to solve a problem in a new and more efficient way—to the "old, tried and true" methods that seemingly have worked so well for us in the past. As we repeat our actions, our options for response become fewer and fewer, and we become more like the man who has a hammer and sees everything as a nail. His perspective may fix a few things but will leave many more things in ruins. In this regard, also see Subsection 4.E, page 124, on convergent versus divergent thinking and their effects on creativity.

As discussed so clearly by Desikachar [194], setting our brains on automatic pilot leads to too many accidents when circumstances change but our methods of handling them do not. We are speaking now in the broadest terms.[3] If we are to navigate successfully through life, we must be flexible in every sense, be aware of what is going on around us, and understand what is the optimal response, rather than the easiest response, to each situation. Further, in finding new ways to approach problems, we grow. If our approach is always the same, we have ceased to grow and will therefore stagnate. Stagnation is the enemy of *yogasana*, and attentive *yogasana* practice can be the medicine that banishes stagnation. Note too

---

3   A very interesting but indirect approach to dieting (based on the Framework for Internal Transformation [186a]) encourages people to deliberately change their daily routines so that they think more deeply about the decisions that they otherwise make with little or no forethought. Though the participants were not given any incentive for altering their diets or exercise routines, the result of being more thoughtful more often about their day-to-day choices of behavior led to a natural turn toward positive long-term dietary and exercise changes as well as decreases in the levels of depression and anxiety. This modern psychological approach to changing behavior shares considerable ground with the ancient goal of yoga in regard to being mindful in the moment.

that the establishment of habitual mental patterns works to strengthen self-absorption and the ego, whereas it is one of the goals of *yogasana* practice to overcome the ego, not to encourage it. At the same time, such reinforced mental patterns work to confine not only the mind but the body, making the introduction of new thoughts or new body positions frightening [518].

Another of the goals of *yogasana* practice is to make our intentions and the subsequent actions correspond as closely as possible. This is discussed further from the Western point of view in Subsection 4.G, page 148.

Awareness

Through the practice of *yogasana*, we have a tool with which we can raise our level of self-awareness and experiment with new types of strategies for solving life's problems. If we are aware as we work in *yogasana*, we will come to see the common threads of how we approach the solution to all yogic problems, and we will see that a yogic problem is neither more nor less than a metaphor for life's problems in general and how we go about solving them [255]. If we can, through heightened awareness, find a new way to approach a problem in *yogasana,* then that approach may well be a new and useful strategy in broader life situations. Moreover, with a higher degree of awareness comes the chance to make one's actions more congruent with one's intentions, an essential aspect of reducing tension in the mind and body (Subsection 4.G, page 148). Finally, it appears that focusing the mind on inner aspects of our being has the effect of bringing subconscious sensations into the conscious realm (Subsection 1.B, page 12, and Section V.H, page 930).

As we practice *yogasana* with awareness, we will find unthought-of avenues of attitude and action, some of which are dead ends and some of which lead to unexpectedly beautiful and exotic places that we never would have come across if we had remained with the Western scientist's narrow approach. However, the practice of *yogasana* is a two-edged sword; *yogasana* presents its own dangers, because it too can be practiced in a rote,

mechanical way. If it is practiced in this way, it is no less instructive to the body and mind; it is just that the lesson now acts to reinforce old ideas and ways of reacting, rather than opening up new avenues of thought and behavior. It is from this point of view that we can understand B. K. S. Iyengar's comments on practice quoted in Subsection 11.C (page 445) in which he encourages the student to constantly seek new understanding of the *yogasanas* by observation and questioning of what is being felt, by analyzing the posture and experimenting so as to refine it, always being aware of the feeling and trying today to extend the feeling beyond what it was yesterday. These generalizations in regard to learning and practice are supported by recent brain-imaging studies, as discussed in Subsection 4.G, (page 135).

For those students and teachers for whom *yogasana* practice has become monotonous and consequently whose bodies have become dull and unresponsive, it may be that the added dimension of a rational understanding of the anatomic, physiological, and neuroscientific effects of the *yogasanas* will brighten their practice again. As I have repeatedly found in my own work, the stimulation that comes from an attempt at understanding the *yogasanas* from a Western perspective can invigorate one and renew one's zest for practice. The neuroscience lying behind this all-too-common situation of *yogasanas* becoming progressively subconscious with practice is discussed in the following subsection.

What is one to do once one can "do" the postures? According to Prashant Iyengar, one then works to maximize the grace and mental ease in the posture while minimizing the effort involved in its execution, as per Patanjali's prescription. Even in this situation, one is nonetheless advised to strive to sense the novel aspects of the posture, so as not to fall into the trap of the mundane.

Levels of Consciousness

According to Western thought, there are agreed to be at least three levels of consciousness in human beings: the conscious, the subconscious, and the unconscious [742]. According to Eastern thought, we must add the level called the "super-conscious" to this list of levels. The conscious level involves the knowing and thinking parts of the mind and is active in awareness. However, only a small fraction of the brain is used in conscious thought at any one time, and only some of the remainder is involved in subconscious action (as in controlling the autonomic nervous system) and in unconscious modes during that time. Though it is the aim of some people to "use the brain fully," the state of the brain in which all circuits are simultaneously activated is that of the grand mal epileptic seizure! We work in the *yogasanas* to heighten the presence of bodily sensations at the conscious level, but with no need to use simultaneously all of the elements of the brain.[4]

Western Consciousness

In his *Dictionary of Psychology*, Stuart Sutherland states, "Consciousness is a fascinating but elusive phenomenon; it is impossible to specify what it is, what it does, or why it evolved. Nothing worth reading has ever been written about it." In the hands of modern neuroscientists, the slippery philosophic concept of "consciousness" has been reframed into a determination of which specific centers of the brain are involved in specific brain functions. From studies involving brain-imaging techniques such as functional magnetic resonance imaging (fMRI),[5] it has become clear that attention is a key aspect of con-

sciousness; events that are so mundane that they do not merit our attention hardly seem to exist for us, for they reside instead in the subcortical levels of the subconscious.

Neurologically, conscious sensations and actions are centered in the cortex, its association regions, and possibly in the thalamus of the brain (Subsection 4.C, page 94), whereas subconscious actions are localized in the lower regions of the central nervous system; i.e., the limbic system (Subsection 4.C, page 80), the brainstem (Section 4.B, page 72), and even within the spinal cord (Section 4.A, page 67). Thus, various mental functions may be said to be high or low, both in terms of their relative vertical positions in the central nervous system and in terms of their degree of mental, conscious awareness.

Sensations of events that are so new that they are successful in garnering our attention are quickly brought to the cortical centers at the conscious level. The newness of an event is aided by the use of various memories. If an event is important but already known, it will attain a minimal subcortical level of consciousness; but if it is "important to know," then it appears in the full consciousness.

In general, "consciousness" is not a single state but a spectrum that stretches from hypervigilance at one end, through attentiveness and drowsiness, to coma and death at the opposite end, with those states at the further ends of the spectrum corresponding to highly altered states of consciousness (see also Subsection 1.B, page 16). An operational definition of "conscious," in terms of activation of the reticular formation in the brainstem, is given in Section 4.B, page 76.

Association Regions

To be aware consciously of a particular event means that the relevant sensory signal rises to or above the thalamic level and is processed in the association regions of the cerebral cortex; i.e., in those regions of the cortex lying between the outermost cortical layer and the thalamus (see Subsection 4.C, page 94, for further description of the association region). Should a signal corresponding to a new sensation or motor function

---

4   Actually, there is a neural state of the brain, bordering on the grand mal seizure, in which EEG gamma waves of high frequency (40 hertz) are generated simultaneously throughout the brain (Subsection 4.H, page 153). This state is prominent in the EEGs of adepts deep in meditation and possibly in *yogasana* practitioners at the higher levels of the yoga tree.

5   In this technique, blood flowing through the many nuclei within the brain is monitored through the use of magnetic resonance, and shifts of the blood flow are easily noted when the brain is stimulated to perform certain tasks or experience certain emotions. Resolution of this technique in both space and time is high, so that subtle shifts of flow in both space and time are discernible. See Subsection 23.D, page 802, for an example of fMRI at work.

reach the association region of the cortex, there is an immediate rewiring of a specific area of its neural net, with some synapses reinforced and others weakened. This results in the formation of a new neural unit to be associated with the newly learned act; i.e., a memory of the event has been formed. If the novel event is repeated, the individuality and integrity of the new unit increases up to a point, and the synapses strengthen and so function with less mental effort. However, if the event repeats itself too often, the new sensation becomes old news, and the relevant pattern in the association region begins to shrink in size and complexity and to shift both upward to the motor cortex and downward toward subconscious centers, such as the cerebellum and the basal ganglia [722].[6] This sequence of neural events mirrors closely the *yogasana* student's experience of being conscious of the new feelings when performing a new *yogasana* (or an old one in a new way) and the tendency to grow dull and unthinking with repetition of the actions. One must constantly work to find new aspects of the *yogasana,* if it is to be kept bright and shiny in the consciousness.

Level Shifting

The shifting of an event from the conscious to the subconscious with practice is understandable if one recognizes that, though the action at a synapse between neurons in the brain lasts only a millisecond in both the conscious and subconscious spheres, the neural processes that follow in the conscious sphere are of the order of one second or even longer. Because neural processes in the conscious sphere develop more slowly compared to those in the subconscious sphere, they are more subject to error and require more energy, as compared to handling the same task with the high-speed subconscious. It appears that the brain is working constantly to remove sensations from the conscious sphere

and to press them into the subconscious, thereby making the neural response more automatic, faster, and more economical metabolically. Most information processing in the brain is at the subconscious level, with the conscious levels serving more as advisors than as decision makers in shaping our actions.

Information Theory

The basic qualitative idea of information theory is that the more improbable an event or observation, the higher its informational content; i.e., the more likely it is to be a factor in arousing the senses (Subsection 4.B, page 74). Thus, as mentioned above, when our existence is filled repeatedly with the ordinary and humdrum, the tendency is to lower one's consciousness to the level of the subconscious and put the mind to sleep without a corresponding lifting of subconscious actions into the conscious realm. Because consciousness and the mind thrive on information, "the mind is nature's supreme design for receiving, generating and transducing information" [721]. As students of *yogasana*, then, it is incumbent upon us to make each *yogasana* practice interesting and open to new sensations, invention, and creativity, for only in this way do we resist sinking into the subconscious.

The Subconscious

The subconscious is a subtle area lying just beneath consciousness; virtually all of the actions of the autonomic nervous system (Chapter 5, page 160) take place in the subconscious sphere, a buffer area between the conscious level and the forces of the unconscious. Subconscious signals in the brain can originate in the spinal cord and travel as high as the thalamus, where they are but dimly sensed consciously. One usually has a blurry impression of thoughts lying just below consciousness, but during meditation, such thoughts can be more distinct. Paradoxically, though we remain more or less unaware of the processes going on within our own subconscious, others may be more or less aware of what is going on in our subconscious by observing our actions and body language.

---

6   This appears to be very much like the process of neural habituation (Subsection 4.F, page 129), in which the repetition of a nonthreatening action results in a successive lowering of the neural response to the stimulus with each repetition.

When viewed neurologically, recent Western experiments show that subconscious recognition of an external visual stimulus involves a low neural current in the primary visual cortex, whereas conscious recognition differs only in showing a stronger neural current in the same area [295]; when the size of the neural current rises above a certain threshold value, the awareness switches from the subconscious to the conscious level. If this finding is true of all sensations generally, then we see that a practice that intensifies a certain subconscious neural signal lifts the awareness of that sensation into consciousness, and presumably the reverse can happen as well. In the same way, practice of the *yogasanas* can shift many bodily sensations and controlling actions from the subconscious level to consciousness. This also implies that if the signal strength of a conscious sensation adapts toward zero strength with time (Subsection 13.B, page 506), conscious awareness of it retreats into the subconscious.

The subconscious is the place where we hide the greedy, fearful, ambitious aspects of our being, hiding them from others and from ourselves [467]. Once the barrier between the conscious and subconscious becomes more porous through the agency of *yogasana* practice, one comes more readily to consciously see these hidden faults, at which point one can choose either to confront them or suppress them. Our *yogasana* practice, though outwardly physical, holds the keys to unimagined doorways into deeper levels of our psyche, through the yoga-driven mixing of conscious, subconscious, and unconscious levels of being.

Other Levels

Forces originating in the unconscious are extremely powerful. This realm contains the archetypes, which are the foundations of our basic drives and instincts. The three lower areas considered here can interact strongly, so that the unconscious can indirectly influence the subconscious and conscious levels. For example, if negativity is preponderant in the unconscious, then this may influence the subconscious in a way that leads to real-time vascular hypertension, which is readily sensed in the conscious sphere.

Eastern Consciousness

Yogis recognize a higher level of consciousness: the level of the superconscious. It is the ultimate goal of the yogic practitioner to join the individual consciousness to the universal consciousness and so to reach a blissful state of superconsciousness, that of *samadhi*. The state of *samadhi* is the highest of the eight limbs of yoga, each of which may be considered as a progressively higher state of consciousness or awareness than the one preceding it. The eight levels of consciousness, in ascending order in the *Ashtanga* (eight-limb) hierarchy, are *yama, niyama, asana, pranayama, pratyahara, dharana, dhyana,* and *samadhi*. The first three of these are the basis of the yoga of action (*karmayoga*), whereas *pranayama, pratyahara,* and *dharana* are the yoga of knowledge (*jnanayoga*), and *dhyana* and *samadhi* are the yoga of devotion and love (*bhaktiyoga*) [394].

From the Ayurvedic point of view, the levels of consciousness are represented by the *chakras*, ascending from the *muladhara* at the base of the spine to the *sahasrara* at the crown of the head (table 5.G-1). This ascension of the *chakras* from *muladhara* to *sahasrara* parallels that of the hierarchy from *yama* to *samadhi* in *Ashtanga yoga*. The characteristics of these levels are discussed further in Section 5.G, page 201.

Yoga-Driven Level Mixing

In One Dimension

In regard to the situation of the levels of Western consciousness and their interactions in the neophyte student of *yogasana*, consider figure 1.B-1. Before a beginner commences *yogasana* practice, the mind is structured as in figure 1.B-1a, with sharp divisions between the conscious, subconscious, and unconscious levels of the mind; the unconscious and superconscious levels are irrelevant for the case of the beginning student. Within the conscious realm (o o o), there exists a spectrum of altered states of consciousness, stretching from near-coma at the lowest level to hypervigilance at the uppermost level. Conscious awareness and volition involve the cortex of the brain and can extend downward to as low as the thalamus (Section 4.C, page 85).

As applied to a beginning *yogasana* student (figure 1.B-1a), the straightening of the legs in *paschimottanasana*, for example, will be a deliberate effort of the conscious mind involving the contraction of the quadriceps muscles; at the same time, there will be subconscious reflex actions that change the breathing pattern and relax the antagonist muscles at the back of the legs—in this case, the hamstrings (Subsection 11.A, page 420).

As shown in figure 1.B-1b, with an extended

practice of the *yogasanas* in which close attention is paid to specific details of the activity, certain of the conscious, deliberate actions of the beginner can become more intuitive and reflexive; e.g., the legs automatically straighten as they should in *ardha chandrasana*, without conscious thought, whereas on the other hand, the previously automatic mode of breathing is now deliberately controlled so as to move in a smooth, slow, and rhythmic way while the muscles of the jaw remain relaxed. Through the practice of the *yogasanas*, certain subconscious reflexive actions come under the control of the conscious sphere, while

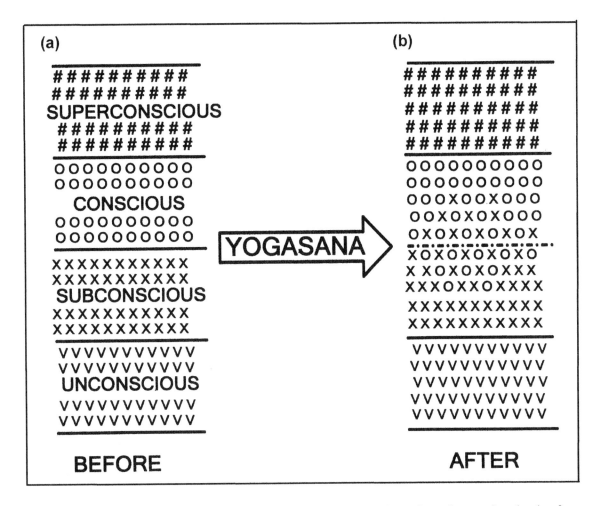

Figure 1.B-1. (a) Without *yogasana* practice, the human mind is divided neatly into four levels of consciousness. Within the conscious realm (o o o), there exists a spectrum of altered states of consciousness and, similarly, within the subconscious realm (x x x), the highest level corresponds to a fuzzy, slight awareness and at the lowest, to total unawareness. Also shown are the unconscious (v v v) and superconscious (# # #) levels. (b) Once *yogasana* practice has commenced, the boundary between conscious and subconscious levels becomes indistinct and porous, with practice making some conscious actions more subconscious (intuitive and automatic) and some subconscious actions more conscious (deliberate and with forethought).

at the same time, certain other conscious actions become more reflexive, as if under the control of the subconscious (Subsection 4.C, page 78). The result is that the previous sharp line dividing the conscious and subconscious levels is now blurred; the configuration of figure 1.B-1**b** may be taken as a state of altered consciousness with respect to the "normal state" shown in figure 1.B-1**a**.

Making It Happen

The arrow in figure 1.B-1 labeled "YOGASANA," which mixes the conscious and subconscious levels, is deceptively simple. Just what does one do while doing "YOGASANA" that will lead to this mixing? The answer to this has been given to us by the American philosopher William James, who points out that the surfacing of the contents of the subconscious into the conscious realm is the result of unwavering concentration and attentiveness (see footnote, page 81). When we practice the *yogasanas* and at the same time "turn our awareness inward," we are focusing our mental effort to blur the line between the conscious and subconscious, trying to make the ordinarily subconscious sensations of ordinary awareness surface into the realm of the conscious, much as in figure 1.B-1**b**. Neurologically, this means that neural signals that ordinarily ascend only to the thalamus become strengthened and elevated instead to the level of the cortex (Subsection 4.C, page 94).

B. K. S. Iyengar recently has spoken of the "two I's," one of which is the conscious *I* (the conscious Self) and the other the intuitive *I* (the intuitive Self) [4a, 4b]. He points out that, as we repeatedly practice the *yogasanas* with focus and intensity, we come to see that the conscious Self normally has hidden the intuitive Self; the intuitive Self is revealed to us by this practice, and it eventually comes to dominate the conscious Self in our awareness (Section VI.A, page 934). The practice lifts our subconscious sensations into the conscious sphere.

Speaking generally, Jung states, "The unconscious is the matrix out of which consciousness grows, for consciousness does not enter the world as a finished product but is the end result of small

beginnings. The conscious rises out of the unconscious as an island newly risen from the sea" [423]. From this perspective, if we are to understand our *yogasana* totally, we must understand the intuitive, subconscious foundation, which is generally out of sight but supports the conscious part that is so visible and accessible, much as does the conscious understanding with which we work to develop the more physical aspects of building our *yogasana*.

Reflex Actions

One goal of *yogasana* practice for beginners is to bring sensations and the control of subconscious functions (reflexes) into the realm of the conscious and the deliberate, and at the same time, to bring deliberate, conscious actions, through practice, into the realm of reflex. For example, whenever the feet are deliberately set for *trikonasana*, there is an automatic increase in the muscle tone of the quadriceps; i.e., the action becomes reflexive. Thus, by *yogasana* practice, we can forge a link between reflexive and deliberate actions, and this link can be a bridge that can be crossed from either direction. That is to say, the intuitive and reflexive can be made voluntary, and the voluntary can be made intuitive or reflexive through practice. Very much the same idea is implicit in Iyengar's dictum in regard to *yogasana* practice: "Bring the unknown into the sphere of the known," (Section VI.F, page 944). For the very adept yoga practitioner, one can imagine that the mixing of the levels of consciousness involves not only the conscious and subconscious levels but the conscious and the superconscious levels as well.

Neural Maturation

Looked at in another way, as infants, our consciousness is minimal and all of our actions are reflexive; i.e., in the subconscious realm. As our nervous system matures, some but not all of the reflexes more and more come under the conscious control of higher brain centers. The goal of *yogasana* practice in the adult is to lift the remaining subconscious or reflexive actions into the region of the conscious and to thereby control them through the conscious action of the higher mental centers. At the same time, certain conscious actions in *yogasana* are practiced so often that they become more or less reflexive in nature, in that they receive minimal conscious attention; i.e., they are placed on "second attention." Such internalization of the *yogasana* principles leads to a continual awareness of the Self, regardless of whether or not one is in *yogasana* practice at the moment. A nice example of conscious and subconscious mixing is presented in Chapter 5, page 157, where the larger subject of the fight-or-flight response to danger is considered.

Certain of the autonomic responses that *yogasana* exercises bring about are not necessarily those sought in our practice, for the body's response to stress is one appropriate to a former way of life, which is different from the one we live today. We must learn in *yogasana* practice to encourage some of these responses and moderate or reduce others. This is one of the challenges of yoga: i.e., not preparing to fight when stressed and not allowing the blood pressure to rise when frightened or working hard. At the same time, the purely physical benefits of *yogasana* practiced as exercise are manifold and well known [388, 404, 559].

Because we are less than perfect, even with extensive practice, we flutter from one moment to the next between different states within the conscious and subconscious manifolds. Thus, Patanjali instructs us in Sutra I.2 to direct our yoga practice toward stilling these fluctuations within the mind [401].

The Tripartite Nature of Yoga

Mixing in Three Dimensions

Though there are many exercise regimens that offer the participant undreamed-of health benefits, and there are many other relaxation regimens that offer the participant undreamed-of levels of altered consciousness, the practice of the *yogasanas* is unique in offering both. By the study of the *yogasanas*, we come to a state of physical strength and mental tranquility, which then allows one to enter into states of meditation;

practice of the *yogasanas* prepares the body, the mind, and the spirit for entering the doorway to meditation [121]. However, due to the tripartite nature of yoga, a more complete picture of the mixing of Western levels of mental consciousness (depicted in figure 1.B-1) also must include the mixing effects of physical states as appropriate to Eastern thinking. As B. K. S. Iyengar said [390], not only does *yogasana* practice offer the possibility of exerting "mind over matter but also matter over mind," implying the mutual interaction and alteration of both the body and the mind as their states interact and are mixed to form body/mind states of being and awareness. In addition to the body/mind states, the emotions and moods also should be factored into figure 1.B-1.

An effort to graphically combine the tripartite aspects of *yogasana* practice is shown in figure 1.B-2. In this three-dimensional plot, the "ranges of motion" for the body, for the mind's consciousness, and for the emotions or moods are plotted on the three axes. Any point within the pyramid signifies a particular state of the body/mind/spirit; the measures of the three quantities characterizing this state are represented by lines from the point in question to the three axes, with each line perpendicular to its relevant axis. For example, a student at point 1 is physically in the relaxed state of *sarvangasana*, in a detached emotional state, and, as regards consciousness, tending toward subconscious or reflexive awareness.

Each of the three axes in the figure above shows an extreme range of motion, going from "superconscious" to "unconscious" on the mental axis, from "hyperactive" to "dead" on the physical axis, and from "manic" to "depressed" on the emotional axis. The midpoint of the mental axis is labeled "meditative," meaning the state of mixed subconscious and conscious character shown in figure 1.B-1; whereas the midpoint on the physical axis is labeled "Patanjalic," meaning that physical state defined by Patanjali in which the body shows strength, grace, and steadiness of effort. The midpoint of the emotional axis is a state of emotional detachment, somewhere between "happy" and "sad." The axes purposely have been drawn nonorthogonally so that motion of the body, mind, or spirit parallel to one of the axes requires appropriate changes on the other two axes as well.

Ideally, the student starting at point **1** should move through *yogasana* practice toward the *sattvic* "yoga zone," defined by the area between the dashed lines in the diagram. Because the student's state at point **1** has right-angle projections onto the three axes marked by intercepts "a," it is a state in which the mental component is "subconscious," the physical is close to that of *savasana,* and the emotional component is close to "detached." If the mental state can be changed from "subconscious" to "meditative," bringing the student to point **2** with intercepts marked

"b," the emotions are only slightly lifted toward "sad," and the physical state of the body moves slightly toward *sarvangasana* as it works with increased energy. However, the student is not yet in the *sattvic* yoga zone. A final introduction of supported standing postures into the practice on the physical axis (point **3** with intercepts marked "c") brings one to a Patanjalic physical state and to a detached emotional state, with a shift toward a more conscious, meditative mental state. Of course, there will be many distinct paths from outlying points to the yoga zone depending upon the number of steps to be taken and the variable (mental level, physical level, or emotional level) to be changed at each step.

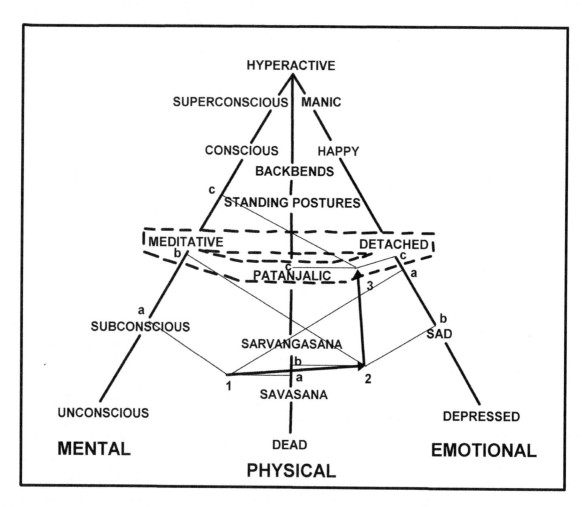

Figure 1.B-2. Variation of the qualities of the body ("physical"), mind ("mental"), and emotion ("emotional"), each over wide ranges. The midpoints of these aspects of our being, labeled "Patanjalic," "meditative," and "detached," respectively, define the "yoga zone" in which the system is in a *sattvic* state in all three variables. Points 1, 2, and 3 in the diagram have intercepts labeled "a", "b" and "c," respectively, on each of the three axes. This is a two-dimensional representation of a three-dimensional figure.

Table 1.C-1: Genetic and Environmental Influences on Body Functions [630]

Trait	% Genetic	% Environmental
Sense of humor	0	100
Breast cancer	28	72
Nightmares	38	62
Depression	38	62
Homosexuality	45	55
Blood pressure	55	45
Obesity	70	30
Type 1 diabetes	70	30
Earache in children	73	27
Perfect pitch	77	23
Autism	90	10
Blood group	100	0

Section 1.C: *Yogasana, Transformation, and Heritability*

One of the very attractive aspects of *yogasana* practice is how transformative it can be in regard to body, mind, and spirit. With that in mind, it is relevant to ask just which aspects of the body, mind, and spirit are amenable to transformation and which are inherited conditions and so are either more resistant to change or are unchangeable. At first, it may be thought that many properties within us are strictly controlled by our heredity; however, there is more latitude here than normally thought. In studies of identical twins, the genetic makeup is near identical at birth; however, with time, various events in the lives of the twins will act to turn on certain genes and turn off others. Thus, given different life events, the two members of an identical twin set diverge with respect to their epigenetic makeup. Such life events may include diet, exercise habits, and alcohol or tobacco use. Thus, environment makes itself felt in respect to which genes are turned on and which are turned off, and thus how cells operate. In this way, how one has been nurtured may have a heavy impact on one's nature [97, 884a].

The DNA within our cells is fixed and unalterable; however, a chromosome is only about 50 percent DNA, the remainder being a mix of markers and switches which parallel the DNA strands and influence the activities of the genes encoded within the DNA. The DNA contains a cell's genome whereas the markers and switches comprise the epigenome. Our patterns of disease, heredity, identity, and gender response to various external factors will depend upon what we eat, smoke, and think, how we exercise, how we behave, etc. Moreover, these epigenetic tendencies are transmissible to our progeny [884a], i.e., they will receive not only the appropriate genome, but also will inherit our epigenome as altered by the lifestyle histories of our parents, grandparents, etc. This new point of view offered by epigenetics leads to semiquantitative estimates of the average relative significance of nature (genome) and nurture (epigenome) operating in various body functions.

Nature versus Nurture

Estimates of the extent of the nature versus nurture (genetic versus environmental) balance for various aspects of body function are presented in table 1.C-1, above, as determined from studies of identical twins. Numbers are approximate for an average genetic composition in an average population, and the possible variability in these numbers is not shown. At the extremes, it is seen that your blood group will be very difficult to change, but the breadth of your sense of humor will depend totally on those that you find in your environment, whereas your blood pressure and your sexual orientation are about equally defined by your genetics and by your lifestyle. One might expect that *yogasana* practice will have the largest impact on those conditions toward the top of this list; i.e., those that are not strongly predetermined by one's genetics.

Nervous Systems of the Body 2

Section 2.A: Nervous-System Function

Reflex

For every cellular organism, regardless of size, there exists a signaling system of some sort that allows it to sense its environment and a second system that then reacts to that sensation in some way that is beneficial to the organism. For example, some unicellular organisms can sense the surrounding temperature and then can move by activation of their cilia in directions that are either hotter or colder, as best serves them thermally. Similarly, many bacteria navigate spatially by sensing the direction of the local magnetic field. On a much larger scale, when evergreen trees within a grove are under insect attack, they are known to transmit chemical signals diffusively through the air to their neighbors, which neighbors then react to produce repellent substances in their needles and bark. Needless to say, these purely reflexive responses to stimuli do not involve any element of thought, and whereas the response time in a single cell may be short, that in a large organism, such as a forest, is necessarily much longer.

For large and mobile organisms, the need for speed and accuracy of signaling from one specific site in the organism to another has led to the development of signaling systems that operate not on the basis of diffusion but instead on bioelectrochemical principles (Section 3.B, page 39). In such multicellular systems, a central nerve center is bidirectionally and instantaneously connected by neurons with all outlying parts of the organism, both for gathering sensory information about the environment and for initiating physiological action in response to what is sensed.

Free Will

There is yet another dimension to the signaling and response interactions possible in these bioelectrochemical neural systems. Though the reflexive signaling systems of the sort mentioned above have been fine-tuned to a high degree in many animals, the responses are largely hardwired in such animals, so that given a particular set of circumstances, the response is always the same. Only in human beings (and possibly other primates [49]) have the dimensions of free will, volition, imagination, reason, creativity, intellect, passion, and appreciation of beauty been added. The incorporation of these aspects into the neural systems of human beings places us at the pinnacle of nervous-system development. Nonetheless, even in human beings, the neural response to a given situation also may become hardwired through habit or reflex. It is for this reason that we must practice our *yogasanas* with creativity and awareness so as not to reinforce old patterns of thought and behavior (see Section 1.B, page 8 and Subsection 4.E, page 123). Nonetheless, there is an automatic aspect to our free will, which implies that it is not so free; see Subsection 4.C, page 80.

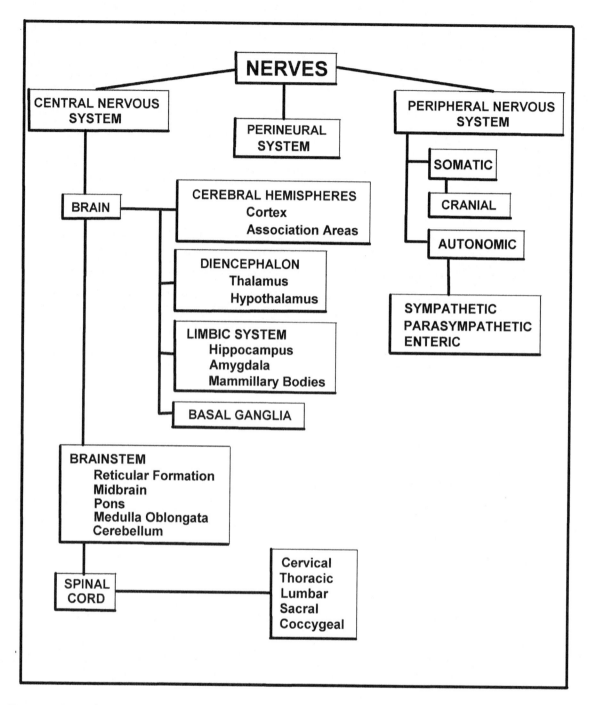

Figure 2.A-1. Classification scheme for the nervous systems of the human body

What Is a Nerve?

The messages of the body are carried most quickly from one place to another via specific cells called neurons (Section 3.A, page 30) on a time scale of tens of milliseconds. Should there be large numbers of neurons with approximately the same origin (A) and approximately the same destination (B), then these neurons, together with

vascular components, will be bundled as a single larger unit over much of the traversal from A to B. Within the human body, those neurons that are bundled into larger structures are called nerves.

Three Nervous Systems

Though the human nervous system is integral and whole, for the purposes of discussion, it can be artificially divided using two criteria, based either on function or on structure. Figure 2.A-1 is a hybrid division of the human nervous system, in that the primary division into the central nervous system, the peripheral nervous system, and the perineural system is based on structure; the peripheral system also has been bisected into the autonomic and somatic subsystems on the basis of function.

At the highest level, nerves belong to either a central nervous system (concentrated most strongly on the central axis of the body) or the peripheral nervous system radiating from the central axis toward the more distant parts of the body. The perineural system is a very new entry in this chart, having both central and peripheral properties that have not been widely studied as yet but which could be of great possible interest to *yogasana* students.

The central nervous system, consisting of the brain, the spinal cord, and all parts in between, is involved largely with the coordination and control of body functions such as homeostasis, memory, mentation, and learning, whereas the peripheral nervous system represents the lines of communication between the central nervous system and the outlying muscles, glands, and organs. The brain centers of the central nervous system that are most significant for *yogasana* study are discussed in Section 2.B, page 21.

The dissection of the human nervous system (as shown in figure 2.A-1) is deceptive, in that each category sits neatly within the borders of its box; in fact, the interaction between systems on the right and those on the left can be so strong that the separateness implied by the boxes simply cannot be supported. Strong interactions are common not only left-to-right but also top-to-bottom in this diagram, and some nerves belong logically to more than one box. Thus, for example, several of the cranial nerves are also part of the parasympathetic nervous system. Though we will use the hierarchy given in figure 2.A-1, it is to be understood that the elements shown there are not as independent as the drawing implies.

Afferents and Efferents

Though the central and peripheral nervous systems are separate anatomically, they are intimately connected functionally through intervening neural junctions called synapses (Section 3.C, page 48). In both the peripheral and central nervous systems, the nerves that carry sensory information (temperature, pH, blood pressure, muscle tension, etc.) from receptors in the peripheral regions to the central region are called afferents, whereas those that carry excitatory neural signals from the central region toward the muscles, organs, and glands at the periphery are called efferents. The cell bodies of the afferent nerves lie outside the central nervous system, whereas those of the efferent nerves lie within the central nervous system. Afferents are a part of ascending pathways (figure 4.C-7**a**), whereas efferents are a part of descending pathways (figure 4.C-7**b**).

Section 2.B: The Central Nervous System

The Brain

Brain Centers

The central nervous system is composed of the brain, the spinal cord, and those brainstem structures that stand between them (figure 2.B-1). The brain itself can be further divided geographically top-to-bottom into the cortical brain and association areas covering the cerebral hemispheres (phylogenetically very new), the diencephalon (within which are the thalamus and hypothalamus), the limbic brain (strongly involved in emotion and memory and containing the hippocampus, amygdala, and mammillary bodies), the basal ganglia (involved in posture and movement), and the brainstem (very old and very subconscious). The brain itself is contained within the neurocranium, and its subcomponents are more completely described in Section 4.C, page 78, whereas the

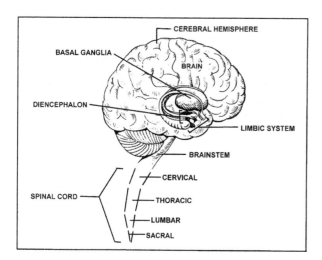

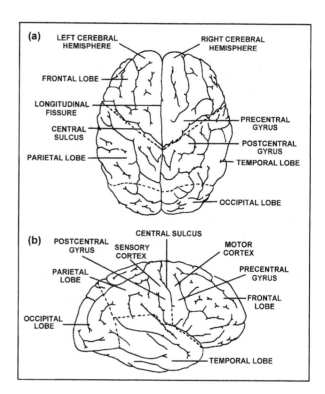

Figure 2.B-1. The central nervous system and its division into components, the spinal cord, the brainstem, and the brain. The brain in turn is further divided into the cerebral hemispheres, the diencephalon, the limbic system, and the basal ganglia. Not shown are the various associative connections within and between the two cerebral hemispheres. The view is that of the right cerebral hemisphere as seen facing right.

Figure 2.B-2. (a) Superior view of the cerebral hemispheres and (b) lateral view of the right cerebral hemisphere showing major topographical features (sulci and gyri) and the division into hemispheric lobes.

internal structures of the spinal cord within the spinal column and of the brainstem are described in detail in Section 4.A, page 67, and Section 4.B, page 72, respectively; these two components of the central nervous system are only briefly described here.

Most important in the brain are the cerebral hemispheres, each of which is covered by the cerebral cortex (Subsection 4.C, page 94). The cortex contains many of the elements of our rational intelligence and is the source of our direct and deliberate actions and the uppermost terminus for the reception and awareness of our sensations. The conscious awareness of sensations (temperature, body posture, hunger, etc.) is delivered to the sensory cortex in each hemisphere, whereas the motor neurons that consciously drive the muscles are found in the adjacent motor cortex (figure 2.B-2**b**). The sensory and motor functions are components of the somatic nervous system.

Elements of the diencephalon deep within the brain (figure 2.B-1) are important both to the regulation of bodily processes (the hypothalamus, Section 5.B, page 165) and as a gateway into and out of the cortex (the thalamus, Subsection 4.C, page 84). The brainstem contains several specific but subconscious centers along its length.

Though formally not considered to be parts of the central nervous system, it is appropriate here to mention the fibrous sac (the dura mater) in which the central nervous system is contained and the fluid within the sac, in which the central nervous system is suspended (Subsection 4.E, page 107). These two non-neural elements are essential to maintaining the health and function of the central nervous system. The dura mater is the outermost of a three-layered sac in which the central nervous system is suspended, the inner two being the pia mater and the arachnoid mater.

Decussation

The approximate left-right symmetry of the body parts is reflected in the approximate left-right symmetry of the brain (figure 2.B-2**a**). However, both the sensory and motor systems of the central nervous system show a peculiar crossing-over of the nerves, such that sensory and motor signals appropriate to one side of the body are connected neurally to the cerebral hemisphere on the **opposite** side of the brain. In some neurons, the left-right crossings of the neural sensory and motor pathways (called decussation) occur at the level of the spinal cord; in others, the decussation is found in the brainstem. A partial decussation of sorts also occurs in the visual and auditory systems in the higher centers of the brain, as discussed in Section 17.D, page 676, and Section 18.A, page 689.

The Brainstem

The brainstem is an integrated structure that deals with sensory information from the head, neck, and face and in turn, controls the muscles in these areas via the cranial nerves (Subsection 2.C, page 24); it is also responsible for many other subconscious functions. Neural information from the spinal cord passes through the brainstem on its way upward to higher centers in the brain, and processed information from these higher centers similarly passes downward through the brainstem. Interestingly, there is a mutual neural communication and modulation of the ascending and descending information streams, with selective reinforcement of some signals in both streams and inhibition of others. For example, see Subsection 13.C, page 525, for the mechanism whereby upward-moving pain signals are intercepted in the brainstem, where they can be negated by downward-moving neural signals.

The reticular formation passes lengthwise through the brainstem and is involved in the arousal of awareness, among other things. All of the significant centers in the central nervous system are discussed further in Chapter 4, page 67.

The Spinal Cord

The bundle of neural bodies that form the spinal cord extends from the base of the skull into the region of the lumbar vertebrae, occupying the channel within the bony structure of the spinal column. Indeed, the entire central nervous system is encased within the bones of the skull and the spinal column for reasons of protection.

The spinal cord serves the trunk and the limbs of the body, receiving sensory information from the skin, glands, joints, and muscles in these areas and in turn activating muscles, glands, and organs in the same areas via both voluntary and reflex mechanisms.

Spinal Neurons

The neural fibers of the spinal cord are segmented into thirty-one sectors in registration with the vertebral structure of the spinal column and are divided in the following way:

» Eight cervical branches, serving the diaphragm and the muscles of the neck, arms, and hands
» Twelve thoracic branches, serving the trunk and intercostal muscles
» Five lumbar and upper sacral branches, serving the muscles of the abdomen, legs, and feet
» Five lower sacral branches, serving the anal and perineal muscles

Within the spinal nerves, sensory signals may go only as high as the spinal cord and lower brainstem, where they trigger muscular or glandular responses; however, these will be reflexive or automatic in nature and totally subconscious. Should the sensation travel as high as the thalamus in the diencephalon, then the sensation will be crudely identified as to modality and location, but it is only when it reaches the cerebral cortex that it is clearly identified as to type and precise location and given total recognition by the conscious Self. Thus it is seen that there are many levels at which the upward-moving afferent and downward-moving efferent signals can interface with one another, each with its own level of conscious awareness.

Section 2.C: The Peripheral Nervous System

The Somatic Branch

The somatic branch of the peripheral system is concerned with muscles, joints, and organs and their embedded sensors; it consists of those afferent nerves that carry sensory signals from the muscles, joints, and organs via synapses to the central nervous system and those efferent nerves that carry excitatory signals via synapses from the central nervous system to the muscles, joints, and organs.

In accord with the strong left-right symmetry of the muscles of the body, the efferent nerves innervating the muscles are found to exit the spinal cord ventrally in thirty left-right pairs; correspondingly, there are thirty pairs of peripheral somatic nerve bundles carrying afferent signals; these converge upon the set of thirty dorsal spinal nerve roots radiating from the spinal cord (figure 4.A-2). The points of juncture between the nerves of the central nervous system and those of the peripheral nervous system are called synapses. The length of the peripheral somatic nerve connecting a sensor with the central nervous system can be as short as 0.1 centimeters (0.04 inch) as it is for olfaction, as long as 10 centimeters (3.9 inches) for vision, and longer than 100 centimeters (39 inches), as with the mechanoreceptors in the feet [427]. The efferent part of the somatic branch of the peripheral nervous system is activated by centers in the central nervous system at both the conscious (cortical) and subconscious (spinal cord) levels and at points in between (the brainstem and diencephalon). Similarly, the afferent part of the peripheral nervous system terminates in the central nervous system at both the conscious and subconscious levels. As suggested in figures 1.B-1 and 1.B-2, actions originating at the lower, more

subconscious levels can be brought into the higher, more conscious levels through the practice of the *yogasanas*.

The Cranial Nerves

The cranial nerves are a subset of the somatic system. Many of the nerves that serve the head, face, and neck areas of the body are essentially at or above the cervical vertebrae in the neck and so synapse directly with centers in the forebrain or the brainstem, passing directly through the dura mater at the base of the skull without passing through the spinal cord. Though one of the cranial nerves travels as far south as the lower abdomen (cranial nerve X), it too synapses directly with the brainstem without passing through the spinal cord. The cranial nerve bundles may contain both motor neurons and sensory neurons, and they have the brainstem as the terminus in either case. Some of the cranial nerves play a role in the parasympathetic autonomic system; however, all of the components of the sympathetic nervous system have spinal connections rather than cranial connections. Some of the cranial nerve bundles consist only of sensory afferents, whereas others have mixed proprioceptive sensory-afferent/motor-efferent character [107, 295, 621]. Ten of the twelve cranial-nerve pairs pass through the reticular formation within the brainstem (Subsection 4.B, page 74).

There are twelve pairs of cranial nerve bundles in the body (I–XII), with each member of a pair serving one side of the body; the names and functions of the cranial nerves are listed below. Unlike the spinal nerves, the cranial nerves generally do not decussate, so that if one were to have a stroke in the left cerebral hemisphere, for example, the muscles of the right arm might be paralyzed along with the facial muscles of the left cheek. More information on the roles played by the cranial nerves in the body can be found in the relevant sections in which the various affected organs, sensors and muscles are described.

» **Cranial Nerve I.** The olfactory sensory nerves carry the sensations of odor from the roof of the nasal cavity to the limbic system and to the cortex; afferent only.

» **Cranial Nerve II.** These are the sensory optic nerves (figure 17.A-2), carrying the sensory signals from the retinas of the two eyes to the visual areas in the occipital lobes at the back of the skull. This nerve is enclosed by the three meninges of the brain [671a]; afferent only.

» **Cranial Nerve III.** As their name implies, the oculomotor nerves are involved with the intrinsic muscles that adjust the sizes of the pupils according to the light level (oculo-) and the extrinsic muscles that move the eyeballs in their sockets (-motor). Certain of the fibers in the oculomotor nerve bundle are part of the parasympathetic nervous system as well, and certain of the fibers in this nerve bundle decussate; efferent only.

» **Cranial Nerve IV.** The trochlear nerves innervate the extrinsic superior oblique muscles of the eyes, acting to pull the eyeball down and toward the nose (figure 17.A-1c). If the trochlear nerve on one side is paralyzed, the head tilts in that direction, demonstrating the proprioceptive role played by these nerves; efferent only.

» **Cranial Nerve V.** The trigeminal nerves are active in various areas of the face: their afferents originate at the skin of the face, the corneas of the eyes, and at the teeth, whereas their efferents control the muscles of the jaw when chewing.

» **Cranial Nerve VI.** The abducens nerve is used in the movement of the eyeball through the lateral rectus muscle (figure 17.A-1c); efferent only.

» **Cranial Nerve VII.** The facial nerves innervate the muscles of the face and so make the face expressive. Additionally, they are involved with the sense of taste and control saliva and tears production; both afferent and efferent.

» **Cranial Nerve VIII.** The sensory acoustic nerves serve two distinct purposes: they carry acoustic signals from the middle ears to the brain and also connect the balancing apparatus of the inner ears to brain centers concerned with posture and balance; afferent only.

» **Cranial Nerve IX.** Taste sensations from the back of the tongue and sensations of pressure and pain in the throat are transmitted to the brain by the glossopharyngeal nerves. Additionally, these parasympathetic nerves activate saliva glands and also help regulate the breathing rate; both afferent and efferent.

» **Cranial Nerve X.** These are the very important left and right branches of the vagus nerve; they allow the control of many important processes such as breathing, digestion, and heart rate, as well as tension in the vocal cords. More details on the roles that the parasympathetic vagus nerves play in the body are listed in Subsection 5.D, page 180; both afferent and efferent.

» **Cranial Nerve XI.** The spinal-accessory nerves primarily activate the trapezius and sternocleidomastoid muscles in the neck; these turn the head from side to side and also help to lift the rib cage when one inhales deeply; efferent only.

» **Cranial Nerve XII.** The hypoglossal nerves control the muscles of the tongue and throat and hence are important in the speech process; efferent only.

As the cranial nerves often synapse to the subconscious centers of the brainstem, they can readily participate in reflex actions such as coughing, vomiting, blinking, and swallowing. However, as these lower centers are connected within the brain to higher, more conscious centers, their reflexive nature can be controlled in a deliberate way by the conscious brain.

With respect to our practice of the *yogasanas*, the most important of the cranial nerves are the second (optic), which carries the visual signals that are of such great importance when attempting to balance (appendix V, page 865); the eighth (vestibular), which also is an important aid in balancing (Section 18.B, page 696); and the tenth (vagus), which is extremely important as a regulator of the heartbeat and so controls blood pressure, etc. (Subsection 5.D, page 180 and Subsection 14.A, page 543).

The Autonomic Nervous System

Certain of the nerves of the peripheral nervous system have special functions in regard to the glands and visceral organs and are grouped together as the autonomic nervous system, within which there are three subgroupings: the sympathetic, the parasympathetic, and the enteric nervous systems. The autonomic systems work in an essentially automatic fashion at the subconscious level. As discussed in many places throughout this handbook, the autonomic nervous system is of great relevance to the understanding of the effects of *yogasana* practice on the body, mind, and emotions. The autonomic branches of the peripheral nervous system are discussed in detail in Chapters 5 and 19.

As its name implies, the autonomic nervous system (Chapter 5, page 157) works normally in an automatic way, silently adjusting the various parameters of the body so as to keep its operating parameters within certain bounds. In doing this, the autonomic system works largely on the internal organs and viscera of the body, adjusting the levels of their functioning as appropriate for self-defense (the sympathetic branch), for relaxation (the parasympathetic branch), or for digestion (the enteric branch). The subconscious actions of the autonomic nervous system are protective in another sense, for were they in the conscious realm, they would flood the consciousness with a mass of data (estimated at 10–100 million bits per second) that would make further conscious action difficult. However, as with the somatic branch of the peripheral nervous system, so too can certain actions of the autonomic system be brought to the level of consciousness by the practice of the *yogasanas* (Section 5.E, page 182).

The Perineural Nervous System

The perineural nervous system is associated largely with the connective tissue of the body, both at the level of muscle, tendon, and ligament at one extreme and with the internal mechanical scaffolding within each cell of the body (called the cytoskeleton) at the other; this is discussed further in Subsection 12.B, page 492.

The electrical nature of the signals in the central and peripheral nervous systems is well known, these being essentially digital (on or off) in nature. However, the perineural nervous system, perhaps much more ancient in origin, functions not on the basis of synapses, digital signals, and neural electric currents but instead operates on the basis of mechanical signaling (push and pull) and static electrical charging within the connective tissues. The mechanical stresses on the perineural system must be distinguished from those generally thought to be functional in the neurological proprioceptive sphere (Section 11.C, page 441).

This simpler nervous system is called the perineural system because its constituent cells lie just outside those of the central and peripheral nervous systems and generally were thought to serve only as housekeepers for these more modern systems. Indeed, they do serve as such, but they also directly connect every cell and its cytoskeleton with every other cell in the body and so are able to register the levels of compressive and tensile stress in and between the cells of the body.

It is thought that the perineural system functions in some way to assist healing in the body [603, 637]. Details of the cytoskeletons within cells and their connections to other components of the perineural nervous system are presented in Subsection 12.B, page 492.

Section 2.D: The Nervous Systems and *Yogasana* Action

With the sketchy outline of the various nervous systems given in the sections above, how would they interact among themselves within a student being guided in the execution of a *yogasana*, say, *virabhadrasana I*? In answer to this, the inputs and outputs of the central nervous system and the autonomic nervous system are shown schematically in Box 2.D-1 as they would function during the teaching and performance of *virabhadrasana I*.

Box 2.D-1. Interactions of the Central and Autonomic Nervous Systems in the Teaching and Performance of *Virabhadrasana I*

Let us see just how the sensory, motor, and limbic systems of the brain might interact in a student being adjusted while in *virabhadrasana I* (figure 2.D-1). Before adjustment, the various peripheral proprioceptors in the student's skin, muscles, and joints (Section 11.C, page 441) report on the various joint angles and levels of muscle tension, using sensory afferents. From this, the cerebellum synthesizes a picture of the current posture of the body; this will be only partially in the student's consciousness, if at all. At the same time, the teacher's spoken instructions are converted into neural signals that are sent from the ears to the auditory cortex over decussated afferent pathways (Subsection 18.A, page 691). Postural information from the proprioceptors will serve eventually as input to the motor cortex, whereas the spoken information will serve to activate the auditory cortex in accord with the teacher's instructions.

Signals from both sensory systems can be applied to the posture if and when they act on the motivational system within the limbic system. That is to say, there must be some part of the brain that serves as a motivational system with input to the somatic motor cortex. Such a motivational system resides within the limbic system of the brain, deep within the cerebral hemispheres [427] (figure 2.D-1). The outputs of both the sensory and the motivational systems serve as inputs to both the spinal cord directly (producing reflex reactions) and to the motor cortex. As discussed in Subsection 4.C, page 91, simultaneous with the activation of the motivational system, there is an activation of the premotor cortex in preparation for the coming actions appropriate to the performance of the *yogasana*, all of which are orchestrated by processes in the basal ganglia and the cerebellum, ensuring a smooth and successful attempt at the posture.

Using both direct and indirect (reflexive) activation of the relevant muscles, each side of the body is coaxed by the motor nerves into the position appropriate to *virabhadrasana I*. This will involve the contraction of certain muscles and the relaxation of others. With luck, the end result of these ascending and descending neural stimuli will be a posture resembling that in the figure. As the posture is practiced time after time [632], the muscular actions are smoothed by the basal ganglia (Subsection 4.C, page 83) and then further refined and coordinated by the cerebellum (Section 4.B, page 73).

As the posture is practiced repeatedly, a muscular learning process comes into being (Section 4.G, page 137), with certain neural pathways being reinforced so that the mechanics of the posture become more intuitive and less deliberate, but in either case, becoming part of our memory. Note, however, that figure 2.D-1 accompanying this box is quite schematic and bypasses many functionally important brain centers that are here only represented by arrows.

The change of shape of the body as viewed externally is accompanied by significant changes in the body's operating parameters. The effort expended in coming into and holding the posture results in a general activation of the sympathetic/cranial nervous system, with attendant rises of blood pressure, heart rate, and respiration rate, heightened levels of catecholamines in the bloodstream, and a decrease in digestion (see Subsection 4.C, page 84 for a discussion of the role of the hypothalamus in this situation). Moving from *virabhadrasana I* to *savasana*, the nervous system switches from sympathetic to parasympathetic activation and relaxation follows.

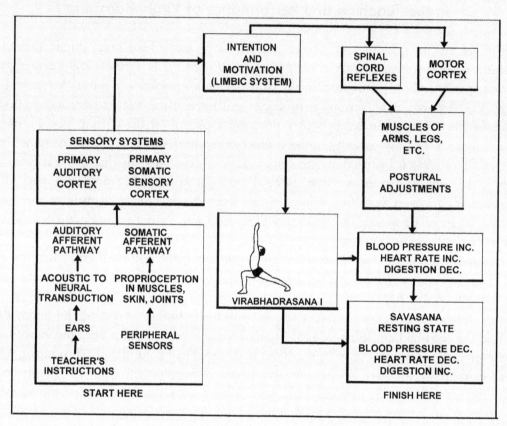

Fig. 2.D-1. The three subsystems of the central nervous system, the sensory, the motor, and the limbic, interact as shown when the student in *virabhadrasana I* is adjusted according to the teacher's instructions. With practice, learning takes place, with its reinforcing effects on the motor and sensory cortices. Other anatomic, physiological, and emotional changes also occur during the performance of this *yogasana*, for the sympathetic nervous system has been activated; however, these sympathetically driven changes induced by the performance of the *yogasana* are reversed by the parasympathetic excitation associated with releasing from *virabhadrasana I* and entering into *savasana*.

Neural Mechanisms 3

All of the sensory organs of the body report the levels of their sensations (signals referring to pain, temperature, vision, blood pressure, stomach acidity, the level of oxygen in the blood, etc.) to a central site in the body (the central nervous system), where they are evaluated and acted upon. A second set of signals is then sent from this central site to effector organs, internal and external (the muscles of the upper arm, nuclei within the hypothalamus, the blood vessels of the spleen, the muscles of the middle ear, etc.), directing how their states are to be adjusted in order to maintain or change conditions in the body at that moment. The incoming afferent signals representing the levels of sensation may be either in the conscious realm or in the subconscious, with the received information either integrated or not with that from other sensors of the same or different types. Once an incoming signal is held to be a cause for action, the body's response, in the form of outgoing signals to muscles and organs, may be instantaneous or may be drawn out over a lifetime. Many of the incoming and outgoing signals travel through the body by way of the nervous systems outlined in Chapter 2.

If there is any doubt in the minds of readers as to the relevance of such neural pathways to *yogasana* practice, consider B. K. S. Iyengar's recent comment [403] on this: "All the props are meant for neurological control, which is the hub for higher and lower action. Neurological body is the medium between psychology and organic body. That is why you have to work on neurology. Yoga is completely a neurological science. It is hundred percent a neurological science."

For coordination and communication be-tween distant cells in the body, there are several systems available: (1) the endocrine system, a chemical-transport system using the bloodstream to transfer a specific hormone from an endocrine gland to cells, muscles, glands, and sensors; this is dealt with in Chapter 6; (2) the immune system, in which considerable information is transferred between mobile cells in regard to invasion by foreign cells; (3) the perineural and cytoskeleton systems; and (4) the nervous system, a bioelectrochemical network using neurons to transfer electrochemical signals between cells, muscles, glands, and sensors; this mode is the subject of the present chapter.

Two aspects of neural tissue are worth noting: neural signaling is faster and more localized than are endocrine, perineural, or immunological signaling, and so it can be more highly resolved in both space and time. Though neurons are rapidly conductive of information within the body, their regenerative powers in adults are slight to nonexistent, should they be badly injured. Just as with muscle cells, mature neurons have become highly specialized in their function, and in the process, they have lost the ability to reproduce; they have a finite lifetime and are incapable of mitotic reproduction.

The Nervous Systems

The neurons of the body are organized into systems and subsystems depending upon function or geography [175, 632]. Often the neurons retain their individuality, but they nonetheless exist side by side, forming neural bundles called nerves. Most nerve bundles are of mixed character, carrying both sensory and motor neurons. Of highest importance are the nerves of the brain, the brainstem, and the spinal cord, which together form the central nervous system (figure 2.A-1); whereas those nerves outside the central nervous system (but connected to it) form the peripheral nervous system (Section 2.C, page 24). The central nervous system is the terminus for information coming from the sensory organs and also is the site of information integration and decision making; it also is the origin of nerve signals deemed appropriate for activating the effector organs. Those nerves of the peripheral system that radiate directly from the brain and bypass the spinal cord are called cranial nerves (Section 2.C, page 24), whereas those that radiate from the spinal cord are called spinal nerves. All aspects of the gathering of information, its integration and evaluation, and deciding courses of action and setting them in motion are under the control of the nervous systems of the body and their component parts: the neurons, the gaps between them, and the myriad cells that support the neurons by performing housekeeping tasks. Obviously, there are many decisions that have to be made quickly among an infinity of neural choices. Were all of the factors that enter into such a decision to be weighed simultaneously in the conscious realm, we would be perpetually overwhelmed.

The Neural Railroad

If one imagines the nervous system to be like a railroad, then the nerves are the rails going from a Grand Central Station out to peripheral ones, and the trains are the bioelectrochemical depolarization waves passing along the nerve fibers (see below), some moving rapidly and some much more slowly, depending upon the urgency of their cargo. The gaps between communicating nerves, called synapses, are switching centers redirecting or stopping further movement, and the central nervous system is the engineer making the decisions about scheduling, course, speed, etc. The ganglia of the nervous system are the large urban centers toward which many rail lines converge and where many passengers change trains.

The trip may be one way or it may be a round trip, but either way, the train always makes a stop at the central nervous system, except possibly for the local trains within the enteric nervous system (Chapter 19, page 703).

As passengers on this train, we may view all aspects of the trip with curiosity and take pleasure in what we see, or we may sleep through the entire adventure, unaware of the interesting territory through which we pass. Perhaps we no longer pay attention because we have been there so many times before, and we do not make the effort to find what is new about what can be seen from the train.

Our goal in this chapter is to discuss the nature of the incoming (afferent) signals from the senses, their transport over a distance of over one meter (39 inches) to the central nervous system, the nature of the outgoing (efferent) signals from the central nervous system to the effector organs, and how these signals interact among themselves to prompt a decision for action or inhibition. Key elements of the discussion define just what is meant by "signal," determine how this signal is moved from place to place, how it is turned on and off, and what the consequences of this understanding are for the *yogasana* teacher. In a word, the key to the understanding of these phenomena lies in the area of bioelectrochemistry, an area of science lying at the intersection of the fields of biology, electricity, and chemistry.

Section 3.A: The Neuron, Basic Unit of the Nervous System

Neural Function

The signal-carrying neurons in our bodies perform two distinct functions. The sensory neurons are afferents, carrying electrical signals from the sensory organs (eyes, ears, skin, muscle spindles, viscera, etc.) of the body to the spinal cord; as cells, they have shapes that are typically pseudo-unipolar (figure 3.A-1**b**) or bipolar (figure

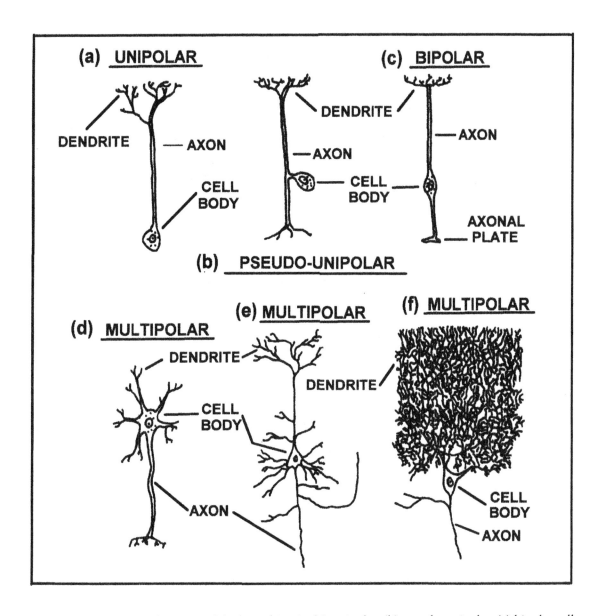

Figure 3.A-1. Schematic drawings of the branching in (**a**) unipolar, (**b**) pseudo-unipolar, (**c**) bipolar cells, and (**d, e, f**) three types of multipolar cells. The Purkinje cell (**f**) is flat and fan-like, with a huge number of dendrites.

3.A-1**c**). Motor neurons are efferents in the somatic nervous system that carry signals from the brain and spinal cord to the muscles (skeletal and smooth) and glands; they are generally multipolar (figures 3.A-1**d**, 3.A-1**e**, and 3.A-1**f**). The simplest cell shape, unipolar (figure 3.A-1**a**), is found among the invertebrates.

Though the shapes of the neurons in figure 3.A-1 vary widely, there are certain constants of their structures that can be pointed out. Being cells that serve as signal-carrying components of a larger system, neurons both receive signals from other neurons via their relatively short but highly branched dendrites (afferent structures conducting signals toward the cell body) and send signals to other neurons, muscles, or organs via their axons (efferent structures conducting signals away from the cell body); axons are longer structures, over one meter (39 inches) in length (figure 3.A-1), as they may have to carry the neural signal to far-distant cells. Because the dendrites function as incoming pathways in the neuron, they have a sensory function and so are known to yogic scientists as *dnyanendriya;* whereas the axons function as outgoing pathways in the neuron, having a motor-like function, and so are called *karmendriya* [851]. The thicker part of the neuron in all cases is the cell body, which is filled with a fluid cytoplasm, the cell's nucleus, and several solid bodies called organelles, whereas the longest part of the neuron is the axon.

Neural Types

The general types of signal-carrying neuron in humans are among those depicted in figure 3.A-1. In a pseudo-unipolar cell (figure 3.A-1**b**), there are two axonal appendages, each ending in a web of dendrites. One of the two dendritic trees (the receptor) ends peripherally at skin or muscle, while the other (the transmitter) terminates in the spinal cord. A closely related cell type is the bipolar cell (figure 3.A-1**c**), in which there again are two processes emerging from the cell body, with the receptor process ending in a dendritic tree and the other being a transmitting axon ending with an axonal plate affixed to a muscle fiber. Bipolar nerve cells are also prominent in the sensory systems, being most often used in the visual, auditory, and vestibular systems [107]. Finally, there is the class of multipolar cells, in which there is a single axon but a large and variable number of dendrites, as shown in figures 3.A-1**d**, 3.A-1**e**, and 3.A-1**f**. In the extreme case, the Purkinje cell of the cerebellum (figure 3.A-1**f**) has approximately 150,000 dendrites at the receptor end, implying that 150,000 input signals are summed algebraically within this cell and the result is then sent along the single axon for transmission to an adjacent cell. Multipolar cells are the most common type of cell in the central nervous system. In the human body, there are approximately 220 unique cell types (neural, muscle fiber, adipose tissue, liver, etc.); the growth of each corresponding tissue type, mitotic or not, can be promoted by stem cells.

In addition to the cell types of figure 3.A-1 that are actively involved in signal transmission, several other neural-cell types (three of them called neuroglia) also play important roles (see below). In addition to the neuroglia and the afferent and efferent neurons, a class of neurons called association neurons, comprising 90 percent of all neurons in the body, facilitate communication between afferent and efferent nerve centers in the brain.

Bundles of nerves within the brain and spinal cord having approximately the same origin and destination are called tracts. There are tracts within the cranial lobes and between lobes, all using the white matter underlying the gray matter of the cerebrum; and there are also tracts that connect the higher brain centers with the lower ones in the spinal cord. Neural cells with similar functions tend to aggregate into structures called ganglia, forming bundles of their neural processes or peripheral nerves.

Neural Pruning

As is the case with muscle fibers, so too are the neurons a part of the same "use it or lose it" scenario. Thus an often-used neuron can function for a lifetime, and it will have to, because neurons do not divide and reproduce once sexual maturity has been reached [574]. On the other hand, nerves and nerve circuits that are not used eventually wither away in a process called apoptosis (Subsection 11.A, page 377, and Subsection 16.F, page 653). The apoptosis (planned liquidation) of neurons can be driven by their exposure to excessive amounts of the neurotransmitter GABA, which is a neurotoxin in sufficiently high concentrations. With neural pruning by apoptosis operating in this way, one's nervous system tends to become more highly refined, preserving circuits that are used most often, which thereby require more space while becoming more narrow in scope as unused circuits die off from neglect [878]. An endless variety of *yogasana* practice works to keep the scope of our neural circuitry as broad as possible; in this regard, see Section 4.G, page 137, for a discussion of how neural structures change as they are used repeatedly when practicing *yogasana*.

Plasticity and Flexibility

Whereas certain aspects of the central nervous system appear fixed, others are capable of reorganization, thanks to the plasticity of the neural circuits in the brain (Subsection 4.G, page 137). By plasticity, I mean not only the ease with which connections between neurons are made or broken, but also the action of neural pruning by apoptosis mentioned above, each of which allows a reconfiguration of overall neural function.

By changing the patterns of connection within the nervous system through its plasticity, we can develop, we can learn, and we can grow as individuals in our own unique way. With plasticity, we not only can perform the stereotypical, hard-wired tasks such as walking, but we can also learn how to perform new tasks, such as standing on our head without falling [192]. Not only can we develop new neural patterns working either alone or with others, but we also can learn how to teach our new patterns to others. In this context, it is interesting to note that with increasing age, mental abilities generally shrink, but at the same time, new connections are made within the brain that can work in beneficial ways to compensate, at least in part, for losses in other areas [83a, 362].

Structure of the Neuron

Fetal Development

Beginning at the beginning, four weeks after conception, the embryo's muscles show a spontaneous rhythmic contraction, even though there are no nerves, bones, or joints. In this mesoderm phase, α-motor neurons then form in the soft, jelly-like tissue, followed by afferent fibers and γ-neurons, which are the last to develop. True nerve-stimulated movement occurs only after the seventh week of gestation, and by the fourteenth week, all basic movements are active. In the fetus, flexor musculature is paramount, so as to allow taking the fetal posture (Box 8.A-1, page 270), and in utero, stimulation of the soles of the fetal feet triggers walking-like leg movements.

Infant Development

The course of neural development, during the first year following birth, progresses from the head to the foot (cranial to caudal) and from near to far (proximal to distal) in the limbs; refinement is proximal to distal and coarse to fine in regard to motor control [288]. Thus the one-year-old child draws with a sweeping arm movement pivoting about the shoulder and later brings elbow motion into play, followed finally by thumb and forefinger action by age three. Myelination of the neurons (see below) continues until one matures, at which time, one's control of the muscles then should be optimal for the tasks undertaken at that point in life. If we as adults are in any way less than fully developed neurally, then we will have too little control over the more caudal or distal parts. This correlates with Iyengar's dictum that our muscular control and awareness lessen as the muscles are more distant from the head (see Section VI.A, page 937).

Cell Membranes

All neurons distinguish themselves from the surrounding fluids by a thin but selectively permeable wall known as the cell membrane. As shown in figure 3.A-2, the cell membrane has a unique molecular structure, the lipid bilayer. The component phospholipid molecules of the bilayer each have a polar (electrically charged) head that is strongly attracted to water (hydrophilic) and a nonpolar hydrocarbon tail that, by its hydrophobic nature, instead is strongly attracted to other hydrophobic, oily molecules such as the tail of another phospholipid molecule. Due to these preferences for the types of molecule with which the two ends of a phospholipid molecule choose to associate, the bilayer is formed from a tail-to-tail alignment, with the polar heads of the phospholipids presented to the aqueous phases on each side of the membrane and the nonpolar tails presented to one another in the inner layer of the sandwich structure. The bilayer membranes are penetrated by protein channels, which act as gates, allowing or blocking the passage of certain ionic (electrically charged) substances (Na^+, for example) from one side of the bilayer to the other. All neural and muscle-cell membranes are constructed of such lipid bilayers, though the proteins enclosed within the bilayer may be dif-

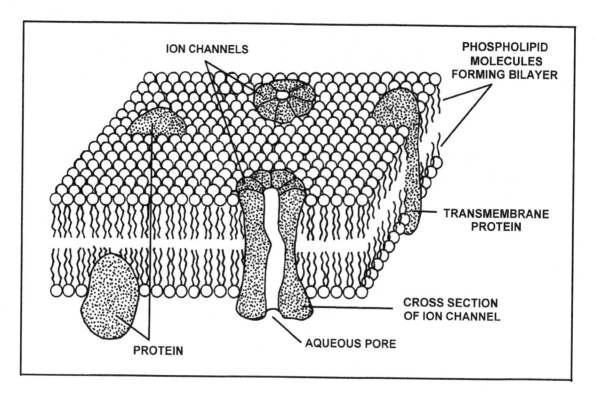

Figure 3.A-2. The molecular structure of the lipid bilayer membrane that encapsulates all cells in the human body. Shown are the two layers of phospholipid molecules, tail to tail, with the heads (O) hydrophilic and the tails (VVV) hydrophobic, interspersed with various protein molecules, some of which act as ion channels, some of which completely penetrate the lipid bilayer, and some of which only partially penetrate the bilayer. In actuality, the lipid bilayer is a rather fluid affair, with easy mobility of the embedded proteins and of the bilayer molecules themselves.

ferent, as may the protein coats surrounding the bilayers [426, 544].[1]

_____

1   In general, the larger an animal is, the slower is its metabolic rate and the longer is its longevity. Interestingly, this metabolic rate that is so determinative of our longevity is dependent upon the chemical makeup of the phospholipids forming our cell membranes; if the fatty-acid tails of the membrane phospholipids are chemically saturated (only 0.2% unsaturated in elephants), then metabolism is slow and life is prolonged; whereas if the fatty acids are unsaturated (up to 20% unsaturated in mice), the metabolism is rapid and life is short! Chemical saturation means that all carbon-carbon bonds are single bonds, whereas in unsaturated molecules, there are one or more carbon-carbon double bonds in addition to the single bonds. The key to understanding how saturation or unsaturation of the carbon-carbon bonds controls longevity appears to be that saturated fatty-acid tails inhibit functioning of the ion channels that pump ions across the mem-

All of the cell membranes of the body are bathed by an extracellular fluid that is in constant motion and acts to transport materials between cells that are not otherwise in contact. Thus, for example, cells not in direct contact with the oxygen-carrying capillaries still are oxygenated by the diffusion of the oxygen through the capillary walls into the extracellular fluid, through which it then diffuses rapidly to serve nearby cells. In addition to oxygen and carbon dioxide, the extracellular fluid may transport other metabolites, hormones, enzymes, ions, and heat to and from neighboring cells.

The proteins that penetrate the lipid bilayer but do not form channels for the passage of ions through the membrane are nonetheless of great

_____

brane and so can slow the metabolism, whereas there is not as strong an inhibition in membranes built from unsaturated fatty acids [248].

importance. These molecules bear receptors for hormones in the extracellular fluid; when so contacted, they are able to pass a signal to a molecule (called the second messenger) in the intracellular fluid, which then initiates the appropriate chemical reaction within the cell. It is through a mechanism of this sort that serotonin, for example, is able to influence the intracellular chemistry of cells via the bloodstream, even though it cannot enter the cell.

Microtubules

Though the axons of neurons can be quite long (approximately one meter, or three feet, in humans and five meters, or fifteen feet, in the giraffe), the cell body of the neuron is only 10–20 µ in diameter and that of the axon can be smaller than 0.5 µ. Because there are many substances produced in the cell body that are required by the axon for its own welfare, there must exist an active transport system carrying materials from the cell body to the distant axonal tip and returning. This miniature railway is built upon filamentous structures known as microtubules that span the axon from end to end. Microtubules, in turn, are constructed of a material known as microtubulin. Motor proteins attach both to the microtubulin tracks and to cargo molecules such as polypeptides, structural proteins, whole mitochondria, and vesicles filled with neurotransmitters, all of which can be transported from the cell body to the axonal tip; worn-out neural components bound for recycling are transported in the axonal-tip-to-cell-body direction.

By changing their molecular configurations in a way reminiscent of the actin-myosin action (Subsection 11.A, page 385), the motor proteins of the microtubules work their way along the track filaments, carrying their cargo from one end of the axon to the other. A specific motor protein will carry only specific cargo, and a one-way trip from the cell body to the axonal tip may require between a few days and eight months, depending upon the cargo and its motor protein. Though the axon contains up to 95 percent of the fluid content of the neuron, all of the protein-synthesis, mitochondrial, and genetic-control functions of the cell lie within the cell body.

In the past, many neural diseases were thought to be the end results of neural apoptosis, a programmed neural suicide (Subsection 11.A, page 377, and Subsection 16.F, page 653); however, that view has changed. It recently has been suggested that certain neural diseases result from a defect in the structure or function of the microtubule machinery, which fails to deliver its cargo for whatever reason, leading to swollen axons and eventual neural death. This has proved to be the case with amyotrophic lateral sclerosis (Lou Gehrig's disease), in which the α-motor neurons fail to function; it is also a strong suspect in diabetic nerve damage, stroke, HIV-associated dementia, muscular dystrophy, and Alzheimer's disease [148]. Considering that we cannot move, sense, or think unless the microtubule machinery of our neurons is in good working order, one can only wonder about the possible dangers of *yogasana* overstretching (see Subsection 3.E, page 63) on the microtubule machinery.

Myelination

Neurons also may be classified on the basis of their signal-conducting properties, rather than on the basis of their shapes. This involves determining their axonal diameters and the velocities of the nerve impulses as they rocket down the axons. This classification scheme is described more fully in Section 3.B (page 44). The nerves having the fastest conduction velocities are coated with a fatty substance called myelin and so are said to be myelinated; 60 percent of the brain consists of fatty substances. The myelination of the axons is somewhat different depending upon whether the axon is within or outside the central nervous system; in the former case, it is oligodendrocytes that perform the myelination, whereas in the latter case, it is Schwann cells that perform this function. All of the nerves of the peripheral nervous system are myelinated by Schwann cells [884]; all of the Schwann cells in turn are integral parts of the perineural nervous system (Subsection 2.C, page 26). Only axons with a diameter larger than 0.5 µ are myelinated.

In both cases, myelinated neurons are wrapped by protective cells in a pattern looking like a string of sausages (figure 3.A-3). Each spiral wrap of a myelinating cell protects that portion of the axonal membrane from contact with the extracellular fluids; however, at the nodes between the protective cells, there is exposure of the cell membrane and its unusually high number of Na$^+$ and K$^+$ transmembrane channels.

Myelination of the peripheral nervous system is minimal in the newborn; in infancy, muscular actions are coarse and uncoordinated, because the associated motor neurons are slow and their patterns of activation are slow, inefficient, and

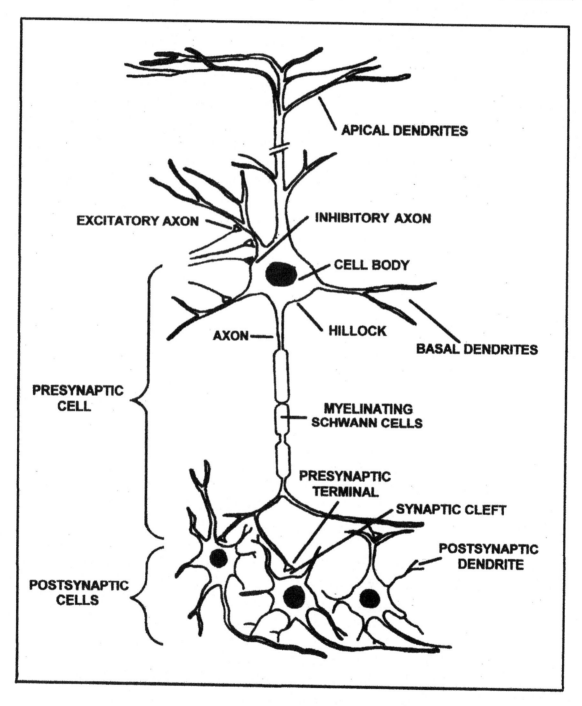

Figure 3.A-3. The anatomic relationship between the presynaptic neuron (*top*) and the postsynaptic neuron (*bottom*) and the intervening presynaptic axon in the peripheral nervous system, myelinated with Schwann cells (*middle*). The neural conduction is from top to bottom, presynaptic to postsynaptic.

seemingly random. As an infant's central nervous system is myelinated only in the lower, subcortical regions of the brain (Subsection 4.E, page 119), all of its actions are reflexive. With time, myelination proceeds upward toward the cortex, and deliberate muscle actions assert themselves as reflexive actions fall away [387]. On the other hand, the neurons of the newborn remain mitotic for about six months and so are able to divide and reproduce. However, once myelinated, the neurons are susceptible to irreversible damage and death, as reproduction is no longer possible. This is especially so when the damage is to the cell body or to the myelin formed by the oligodendrocytes, whose damage transforms the nerve tissue into scar tissue. If, instead, the myelination by oligodendrocytes remains intact, then healing is actually accentuated by these cells, provided the healing is faster than the formation of scar tissue by the nearby glial cells. Axons of very short neurons, such as interneurons, are not myelinated; but almost all long neurons in adults are so myelinated by either oligodendrocytes or Schwann cells.

Ion Channels

The functioning of a neuron depends very much on the fact that the part of it that is not myelinated is wrapped in a membrane that normally is selectively impermeable in the resting state to certain electrically charged ions (Na^+, K^+, Cl^-, etc.). Due to this selective impermeability, concentration gradients of these ions can be maintained across the lipid membrane, as in figure 3.A-4a. The phrase "concentration gradient" refers to the difference in ion concentration at two points—in this case, the different concentrations within the extracellular and the intracellular fluids. A nonzero concentration gradient of an electrically charged ionic species in turn implies a voltage difference between the two points in question. This is called the transmembrane voltage, usually about -70 millivolts in the resting state and 0.0 millivolts when the ionic gradient is zero. The mechanism by which the transmembrane voltage is changed upon neural excitation is described in Subsection 3.B, page 39.

Neuroglia

Microglia

In the brain and in nerve bundles leading thereto and therefrom, several cell types called neuroglia are found, which in part support the information-carrying role of the neurons but are not themselves neurons. The first of the three types of neuroglia, the microglia, function much like connective tissue, are generally smaller than the neurons, can locally outnumber the neurons by about ten to one, and serve to physically support the nerve tissue. In this, they act like collagen (Subsection 12.A, page 483), gluing neighboring units together and so giving the brain its large-scale and small-scale shape and structure. The microglia are especially useful in helping to control the ionic concentrations in the extracellular fluid surrounding the nerve cells. In the developing brain, the microglia are known to guide migrating neurons and also to guide the formation of synapses [573].

Microglia also insulate nerves from one another and aid in the nerves' good health by providing nutrition and by cleaning up debris in their vicinity, acting in the brain as do macrophages in the rest of the body. Recent microscopy studies [241] show that the microglia are studded with long arms that are quite mobile, surrounding damaged sites in the brain and clearing them of the debris of dead and dying cells. They would appear to be the first line of defense against brain injury or the invasion of the brain by foreign pathogens. On the negative side, neuroglia are a common source of brain tumors, and when they start to die, the result can be a loss of myelination followed by multiple sclerosis.

Recent research [242] strongly suggests that the roles of the microglia in the central nervous system go far beyond passive housekeeping. In fact, they are now thought to influence the formation and apoptosis of neural cells and both the strengthening and the weakening of synaptic connections between cells. This ability to affect the synapses within the brain in turn directly affects our abilities to learn and remember. Moreover,

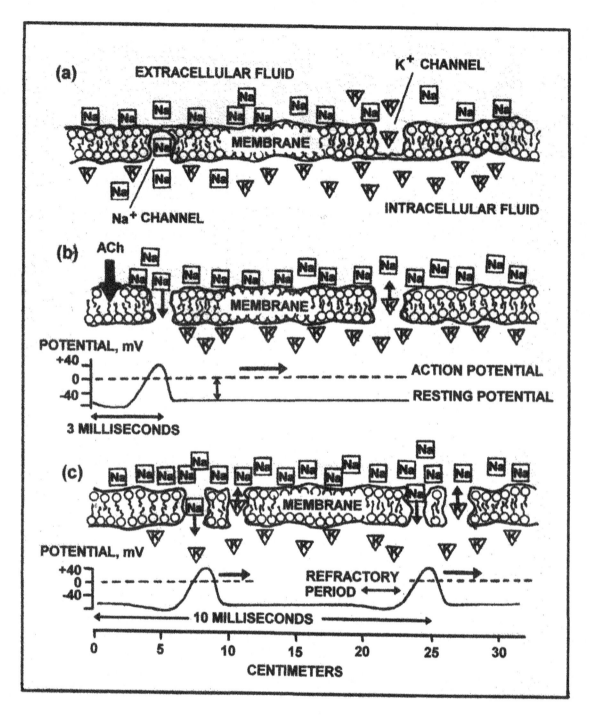

Figure 3.A-4. (a) The neural bilipid membrane in the resting state, with the concentration of Na⁺ much higher in the extracellular fluid than in the intracellular fluid and the Na⁺ ion channels closed. The reverse situation holds for the K⁺ ion concentrations, but to a lesser extent. The difference of the Na⁺ and K⁺ ion concentrations on the two sides of the membrane results in a transmembrane voltage potential of -70 millivolts. This is called the resting potential. (b) When the nerve is energized locally by acetylcholine (ACh), the ion channels in the membrane open and Na⁺ ions flood through them, moving from the extracellular side of the cell membrane to the intracellular side and locally reducing the transmembrane voltage potential to -60 millivolts or less; i.e., depolarizing it. (c) As the channels open sequentially from left to right on energizing the nerve, one or more depolarization-voltage pulses sweep from left to right [422].

the microglia are now known to communicate among themselves using chemical means rather than electrical. Not surprisingly, the ratio of microglial cells to neurons in the brains of mammals increases as one moves up the evolutionary scale (figure 4.C-4).[2]

Oligodendrocytes

The oligodendrocytes are a second type of neuroglial cell that has direct impact on nerve conduction and neural regeneration. It is thought that when the oligodendrocytes malfunction, the myelination of the neurons within the central nervous system is disrupted, and multiple sclerosis follows [573]. If the demyelination occurs instead in the peripheral nervous system, as when the myelinating Schwann cells malfunction, then neural diseases such as Guillain-Barre syndrome result.

Astrocytes

The third type of neuroglia are known as astrocytes. They function as important parts of each synapse, contributing substantially to the nutritional needs of the neurons. Interestingly, the concentrations of astrocytes are significantly below normal in persons who are depressed and who die young, often by suicide.

Section 3.B: Neural Conduction

Generation of an Action Potential

Most neurons, whether sensory neurons, motor neurons, interneurons, or neuroendocrine neurons, have in common four local regions that function sequentially in a similar way when the neuron is activated. As a concrete example, consider an afferent sensory neuron, myelinated,

in which the sensor is sensitive to the degree of muscle stretch (figure 3.B-1). The neural information flow begins with the transduction of a mechanical stretch into a voltage signal within the stretch sensor (called a muscle spindle; see Section 11.B, page 429) at the receptor end of the neuron. Three possible levels of stretch are shown in the figure: (1) a brief, gentle stretch, (2) a more intense stretch held for the same time, and (3) an intense stretch held for a much longer time.

The stretching profile (intensity and duration) at the transduction site (the muscle) in each case has been transformed from a mechanical stress into an electrical signal called the receptor potential (A). This transformation is initiated by changes in ionic concentration gradients and in the permeability to certain ions in the cell membrane of the muscle spindle. Further along the spindle axon, the receptor potential is transformed into an integration signal (B); as shown, this signal contains the profile of the receptor potential but is also decorated with voltage spikes of constant height but with a frequency[3] that increases with increasing amplitude of the receptor potential. It is the spiked part of this voltage profile that becomes the mobile action potential, arriving at the far end of the axon (C) with the duration and frequency of the spikes reflecting the duration and intensity, respectively, of the original stimulus in each of our three cases. Finally, the arrival of the action potential at the far end of the neuron acts to release a neurotransmitter at the synaptic terminal (D), with each spike of the action potential setting free a burst of neurotransmitter into the synapse.

When there is a constant input signal from a receptor for a long duration, as in example (3) of figure 3.B-1, the receptor potential tends to fall with time, due to a process called adaptation.

---

2   The overall ratios of neuroglial cells to neurons in the brains of the worm, rodent, and human are 0.17, 0.4, and 2.0 respectively; however, it is 3.0 in dolphins!

---

3   "Frequency" refers to how many pulse spikes occur in one second, usually given the unit of hertz or, equivalently, cycles per second (cps). The shorter the time between pulses, the higher the pulse frequency, and vice versa. By way of example, the time between pulse maxima in the alternating-current (AC) house voltage in the United States is 0.0167 seconds; therefore, its frequency is 1/0.0167 = 60 hertz.

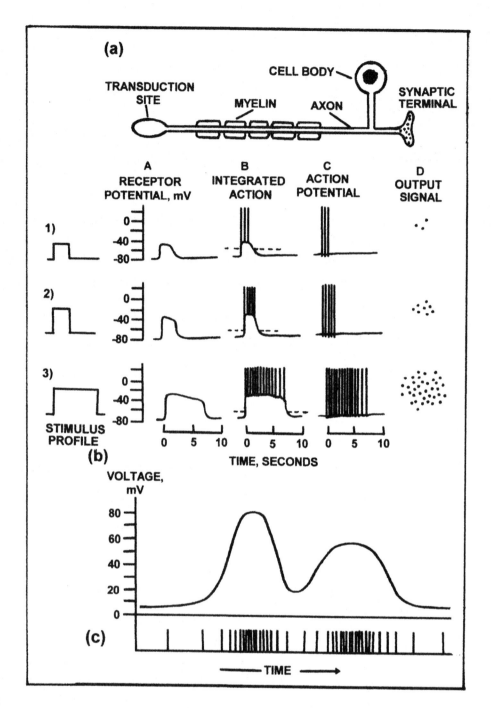

Figure 3.B-1. (a) The four stages A → B → C → D of action, transmitting a signal from the sensory bulb of a muscle spindle (left) to the synaptic terminal (right) along a myelinated afferent nerve. Three cases are shown: A weak stretch (1) excites the muscle spindle and generates a receptor potential (A) barely sufficient to reach the conduction threshold. This potential is transformed into the frequency realm (B) and then becomes the action potential (C) that travels to the opposite end of the neuron and there releases a small amount of acetylcholine into the synapse (D). (2) A more intense stretch results in a higher action-potential frequency and consequently more acetylcholine released into the synapse. (3) A stretch that is both more intense and of a longer duration shows adaptation (Section 13.B, page 506) and the release of a large amount of acetylcholine at the synapse. (b) The display of the time variation of a typical analog neural receptor signal displayed in the voltage mode in which the intensity of the signal is represented by its height in millivolts and (c) its conversion into the digital frequency mode, in which the intensity of the original signal is now represented by the number of voltage spikes of constant intensity appearing per second.

Table 3.B-1. Characteristics of the Various Electrical Potentials Relevant to Neural Conduction [427]

	Sensory Neuron Receptor Potential	Motor Neuron Synaptic Potential	Action Potential
Amplitude, millivolts	0.1 to 10	0.1 to 10	70 to 110
Duration, milliseconds	5 to 100	5 to 20	1 to 10
Summation	Graded	Graded	All or none
Polarity	Depolarizing or hyperpolarizing	Depolarizing or hyperpolarizing	Depolarizing
Propagation	Passive	Passive	Active

This is not due to any fatigue of the sensors involved but instead reflects the tendency of sensors in the body to respond preferentially to **changes** in sensory-signal stimulus rather than to constant sensory stimulus (Subsection 13.B, page 507).

The processes occurring within the spindle neuron in figure 3.B-1a can be interpreted in part in terms of the ionic processes depicted in figure 3.A-4. In the resting state (no signal at the transduction site, **A** in figure 3.B-1), the Na^+ ion concentration is fourteen times higher in the extracellular fluid than it is within the neuron (figure 3.A-4a), whereas an opposite but weaker concentration gradient holds for the K^+ ion. Additionally, both the Na^+ and K^+ ion channels in the resting state are closed. Because the transmembrane permeability for K^+ is much larger than it is for Na^+ and the negatively-charged ions are more numerous within the neural membrane than outside it, there is an imbalance of net charge in the resting state, making the inside of the membrane more negatively charged electrically than the outside. This difference of net charge across the membrane expresses itself as a transmembrane voltage or potential, typically -70 millivolts along the entire length of the neuron. As the transmembrane voltage is the same at all points along the length of the neuron in the resting state, no current flows in that direction.

The transmembrane voltage is maintained across the membrane by the expenditure of energy within the neuron, for such a nonzero voltage is the result of gradients (differences) in the concentrations of the various ions on the two sides of the membrane, which are maintained in spite of the tendency in inanimate situations for such gradients to reduce to zero with time. The energy required to develop and maintain the differences in ion concentration in the resting state of the membrane is supplied by the chemical adenosine triphosphate (ATP; see Subsection 11.A, page 391). Actually, the membrane has many channels through which Na^+ ions could flow in order to equilibrate the concentration of Na^+ on the two sides of the membrane, but these channels are more or less closed in the resting state, thanks to the ATP, and therefore the concentration gradient is maintained.

When a dendrite of the neuron is stimulated by the release of the appropriate neurotransmitter—acetylcholine, in our case—the permeability of the membrane to Na^+ and K^+ ions is altered drastically as certain ion channels formed by membrane proteins in the bilayers are opened (figure 3.A-4b). With this opening of the ion channels, there is a first-stage flow of ions across the membrane at the transduction site that changes the voltage by +/- 0.1 to 10 millivolts. The magnitude of the voltage change reflects the magnitude of the impinging stimulus, and the sign of the voltage change (+/-) determines whether the neural impulse will be excitatory (+, depolarizing) or inhibitory (-, hyperpolarizing). The formation of a depolarizing potential means that the ion flow acted to reduce the ion gradients, whereas the formation of a hyperpolarizing potential means that the ion flow acted to increase the gradients. The initiating event may be sensory (light, pressure, sound, proprioceptive, etc.) or chemical (acetylcholine, norepinephrine, etc.); most first-stage voltage changes are depolarizing, but not all of them are so. The first-stage induced voltages in sensory neurons are called receptor potentials, while those for motor neurons are called synaptic potentials. The properties of such potentials are summarized in table 3.B-1.

As can be seen in table 3.B-1 and figure 3.B-1, the time profile of the initial potential closely reflects that of the initial stimulus, except for a slight adaptation at longer times. The initial induced-potential change of +/- 0.1 to 10 millivolts passively extends only 2–3 millimeters (0.1–0.2 inches) along the neuron before it enters the region of integration (B in figure 3.B-1a). In this region, all parts of the initial potential that are more positive than a certain threshold (-65 millivolts, dashed line) are converted into pulses of constant voltage but with a pulse frequency that reflects the amount of voltage by which the signal at that point exceeds the threshold.

If the initial signal is too weak or the receptor potential is hyperpolarizing, all parts of the signal fail to reach threshold (-65 millivolts), no spikes are generated, and the signal transmission stops at the integration stage. The amplification of the receptor potentials at the integration stage occurs when the receptor (or synaptic) voltage reaches a value at which Na^+ channels open in an avalanche fashion and the inner Na^+ concentration soars until such a high voltage is reached that the Na^+ channels close and the K^+ channels then open to allow K^+ to stream out. This brings the membrane back to the resting potential. Because of the huge difference in the Na^+ ion concentrations on the two sides of the neural membrane in the resting state, thousands of action potentials can be launched before the Na^+ and K^+ ion pumps within the cell membrane must be activated by ATP in order to restore the Na^+ and K^+ concentration gradients.

The axon hillock at the root of the axon (figure 3.A-3) is unmyelinated and has no neural synapses on it but serves as a summing point for all of the neural potentials otherwise impressed upon the axon and is the potential site for the launching of an action potential [450].

Transport of the Action Potential

Conduction Velocity and Refraction

When the receptor potential is large and depolarizing, the initial polarization of the region at the transduction site (figure 3.B-1a) shows a refractory period of a few milliseconds, during which time that part of the membrane already excited is insensitive to further excitation. However, the strong receptor voltage does serve as a further source of electrical depolarization for the **adjacent** downstream region of the unmyelinated axon, and so the integration signal, now called the action potential, moves in that direction only (figure 3.A-4**b**); it cannot move upstream, since the refractory period of the already-depolarized transduction site is a roadblock for instantaneous motion in the right-to-left-direction (figure 3.A-4**d**). As the shortest refractory period is about one millisecond, the theoretical upper limit on the number of action potentials that can be generated in a second is approximately 1,000 and in practice, it is only about 200 [544].

Not only is the action potential mobile in the direction away from the initial stimulus, thanks to the refractory period, but it now consists a series of voltage spikes of constant amplitude. The profile of the spikes in toto matches that part of the time profile of the stimulus that is above the threshold (-65 millivolts), but the strength of the stimulus is now expressed in the **frequency** of the action-potential spikes rather than in their amplitude. The neural consequences of transporting the action potential to the axonal terminal are discussed in Section 3.C, page 48.

As discussed more fully in Section 5.G, page 201, there is a very suggestive correlation between the nervous system as modern-day anatomists know it and the paths of vital-energy flow as in-

---

Box 3.B-1. What Really Moves When an Action Potential Flows along an Unmyelinated Axon?

Note that though a neuron such as one in the sciatic bundle running from the buttock to the heel may conduct the action potential for a distance of one meter (39 inches), and though the action potential is initiated by the movement of charged ions through the neural membrane, **the ions themselves do not move along the axon**; only the changing voltage of the electrical depolarization moves as a wave along the length of the nerve (figure 3.A-4c).

This is much like the case of a boat in the water. As the wave energy moves from left to right on the water's surface, the boat rises and falls in place in response to the wave's crests and troughs, but it does not itself move from left to right. The wave may originate in San Francisco and travel 2,000 miles to Hawaii, but the boat only moves up and down by five feet as the energy of the wave passes. Similarly, the nerve impulse (action potential) can travel for one meter, but the ionic motions defining the wave only span a distance of 10 μ, the thickness of the neural membrane. It is the site of the microscopic transmembrane leakage of ions that moves down the length of the axon. Note also that the conduction of the ionic current in neural membranes involves far smaller velocities and far smaller distances than is the case for the conduction of an electric current through a metallic wire.

Yet another way to think about the neural current is to consider a pair of scissors held horizontally in the right hand. The top blade of the scissors moving toward the bottom one mimics the ions traversing the cell membrane; however, as the top blade moves toward the bottom one, it is the point of intersection of the blades that moves from right to left, essentially in a direction perpendicular to the motions of the blades. This motion of the intersection corresponds to the motion of the neural current along the axon as the ions (the blades of the scissors) move perpendicular to the axon [383].

---

tuited by the ancient yogis. To the extent that this apparent one-to-one correspondence is valid, the neural conduction of the transmembrane potential as described above corresponds to the flow of *prana,* the life force. The medium through which the action potential flows, the neural axon, corresponds to the *nadis* of the yogis.

What Moves?

But what is it that actually moves down the axon when the neuron is excited? All nerve conduction is based upon the fact that the neural membrane is able to selectively allow charged ions such as Na^+, K^+, Cl^-, and CH_3COO^- (acetate ion) to pass in and out of the cell through size-selective channels in the membrane (figure 3.A-1) that can be opened by both chemical and electrical means. The answer to the question "What

really moves in an excited neuron?" is revealed in Box 3.B-1, above.

Discharge at the Axon Terminal

Once the action potential reaches the far end of the axon, each of its spikes triggers the release of the neurotransmitter into the extracellular fluid surrounding the presynaptic terminal. The stronger the intensity of the stimulus at the receptor end, the more frequent is the burst of neurotransmitter at the far end of the axon.

Hopping Conduction

The conduction mechanism is somewhat more complicated in the case of myelinated neurons. In this case, the Schwann or oligodendrocyte cells partially cover the cell membrane and so partially block the flow of ions across it. However, there are

Table 3.B-2. Characteristics of General Neural-Fiber Groups
[7, 308, 360, 427, 562, 801, 884]

	A_α	A_β	A_γ	A_δ	B	C
Diameter, μ	12–20	5–15	2–8	1–5	3	0.3–1.5
Myelinated	Yes	Yes	Yes	Yes	-	No
Velocity, meters/second	65–120	40–80	20–50	6–30	4–25	0.2–2.0
Refractory period, milliseconds	0.4	-	1.0	-	1.2	2.0
Muscle type	Fast twitch	Slow twitch	-	-	-	-
Location	-	Spindles	Spindles	-	ANS	ANS

small nodal spaces between adjacent myelinating cells, at which points the transmembrane ion flow can occur. When the first node of the myelinated neuron is depolarized, the effect is so large that it reaches electrostatically to the next downstream node about 1 millimeter (0.04 inches) away, triggering depolarization there. Rather than propagate uniformly down the axon in a wave-like way, as in an unmyelinated fiber, there is a rapid hopping of the depolarization condition from one node to the next, with the motion again only in one direction due to the refractory-time effect. This hopping of the neural excitation is also known as saltatory conduction. Nerve conduction in myelinated fibers is faster than in the unmyelinated fibers by a factor of more than 100.

Classification of Neurons

A general classification scheme will be used here for neurons based on their diameters and conduction velocities (table 3.B-2). The largest myelinated neurons in the central nervous system have the highest conduction velocities and are placed in Group A. Neurons in Group B are lightly myelinated but serve the autonomic and ganglionic nervous system, while neurons in Group C are the thinnest and slowest fibers and serve as the afferent neurons in the autonomic nervous system. Neurons in Group A are somatic and myelinated and are further classified as α, β, γ, or δ fibers of decreasing diameter [360]. There are other

neural classification schemes in the literature, but that of table 3.B-2 will be used in this work.

In general, as the diameter of a nerve fiber increases, so does the conduction velocity; however, the fast, large-diameter bundles that would be needed for complex signaling would be too ungainly. A typical motor-nerve bundle in the human body has about 1,000 fibers, and were it unmyelinated, it would have a diameter of 38 millimeters (1.5 inches) in order to have the same conduction velocity that the myelinated fiber has with a diameter of only 1 millimeter (0.04 inches) [432]. The smallest-diameter motor neurons in the somatic system are myelinated so as to have rapid conduction and a speedy response, whereas the neurons serving the autonomic nervous system are not myelinated and so are not as rapidly conducting [582].

Physiologists in the sensory field use a second classification scheme to classify afferent neurons, and this is often encountered in reading the literature. This version is presented here in table 3.B-3. The afferent neurons in general are slower and are the oldest phylogenetically, whereas the larger and faster fibers (Ia and Ib) are the more recent ones. In the autoimmune diseases multiple sclerosis and Guillain-Barre syndrome, the nerves are demyelinated, so that nerve-conduction velocity is very low and muscle control thereby is degraded.

The Ia and Ib fibers are sensory fibers (for temperature and largely in the proprioceptive sys-

Table 3.B-3. Characteristics of Afferent Sensory Neurons
[7, 308, 360, 427, 562, 801, 884]

	Ia	Ib	II	III	IV
Afferent					
Myelinated	Yes	Yes	Yes	Yes	No
Diameter, μ	13–20	12–18	5–12	1–5	0.5-2
Sensory modes					
Sharp pain, thermal	-	-	-	Yes	Yes
Sharp pain, mechanical	-	-	-	Yes	-
Slow, dull pain	-	-	-	-	Yes
Vibration, skin indentation	-	Yes	Yes	-	Yes
Tickle	-	-	-	-	Yes
Muscle spindles	Yes[a]	Yes[b]	Yes	-	-
Joint capsule	Yes	Yes	-	-	-
Golgi tendon organ	-	Yes	-	-	-
Hair receptors	Yes	Yes	Yes	Yes	-
Vibration[c]	Yes	Yes	Yes	-	-
Crude touch	-	-	-	-	Yes
Fine touch[d]	-	Yes	Yes	-	-
Deep pressure	-	Yes	Yes	-	-

a primary ending
b secondary ending
c Pacinian corpuscle
d Meissner's corpuscle

tems; see Section 11.C, page 441) with conduction velocities of 40–120 meters/second, while the sensory II fibers (sharp pain and slow, dull pain), being much thinner, have conduction velocities of only 10–50 meters/second. The C and IV fibers of the somatic and autonomic systems are identical in the two classification schemes, and being unmyelinated, they show conduction velocities of only 2.5 meters/second or less and are used in situations that are not life-threatening and so do not require rapid action. The afferent neurons classified as being in Groups I, II, and III in table 3.B-3 would fall under Groups A_α, A_β, A_γ, and A_δ in the general classification scheme of table 3.B-2.

As the mature nervous system ages, neurons are lost but not replaced, while the neurons that remain suffer a loss of conduction velocity, leading in turn to a slowing of movement and a lengthening of reaction times. Receptors are similarly affected by aging, so that one slowly loses sensitivity with respect to seeing, hearing, tasting, smelling, and touching. It is no surprise, then, that conduction velocities can be affected by old age, disease, and temperature, as well as by other factors.

On a macroscopic scale, the strength of response of a neural signal to a stimulus will be reflected not only in the frequency of the action potential from a neuron but also upon the number of neurons so activated in a particular neighborhood. Thus the strength of muscle contraction, for example, will depend upon the frequencies of the action potentials in a particular motor unit and also upon the number of muscle fibers contained within the motor unit (Subsection 11.A, page 369). Correspondingly, the intensity of a pain signal radiating from a particular area of the body will depend upon the density of pain sensors in that area; this density map for sensors in the skin is shown in figure 13.B-2.

Intention and Reaction Times

When we receive a brief but sharp pinch of the skin and withdraw from it reflexively, it can take as little as twenty-five milliseconds to react to the pinch. This is the advantage of the reflexive spinal pathway; i.e., immediate response, thanks to a short reaction time. By contrast, the longer trip of the same signal via the conscious levels of the cortex, as when one voluntarily withdraws, will require approximately 200 to 300 milliseconds! When the response is cortical rather than spinal, it is the right cerebral hemisphere that is doing the work of preparing both sides of the body to act. During the 250 milliseconds spent in preparing the body for a voluntary action, one is exercising one's **intention**. This is of interest to us as *yogasana* students, because many of our actions in our practice are intentional, and a measure of our success in our practice is how closely our actions match our intentions. With more and more practice, our actions come more and more to resemble our intentions, implying that our actions become more meditative and less reflexive.[4]

It is even stranger that though the brain's clock is started when we first consciously decide or desire to move a certain muscle, and the muscle action then occurs 200 to 300 milliseconds later, subconscious premotor brain actions are set in motion 400 to 800 milliseconds **before** our conscious knowledge of the desire to make the move! That is, every conscious, voluntary action is preceded by a subconscious involuntary brain process occurring almost a second before the conscious action is initiated. This readiness delay occurs in the premotor cortex of the frontal lobes (more

---

4   The intention/action duality of our practice can be expressed in the cycles of the breath. Thus, the exhalation is a manifestation of our intention to move into the posture and the inhalation is a manifestation of our attaining the posture [859]. Aspects of the intention/action process are handled in the cerebellum (Section 4.B, page 73).

so in the right frontal lobe, even when preparing both sides of the body for motion) and may relate to the phenomenon of "mirror neuron" activation discussed in Subsection 4.G, page 142. The reality of the "premature" activation of the subconscious premotor neurons of the brain raises questions about the meaning of free will (Section 2.A, page 19, and Subsection 4.C, page 96).

The complex action of something like speech involves about 15,000 neuromuscular events per minute of speech, each of which involves many nerves of different lengths and conduction velocities activating dozens of different muscles; yet the brain is able to get all of the timing right, so that meaningful sounds result! The same timing is evident in the successful assimilation of the flood of sensory information coming into our brains from various afferent nerves of different length, diameter, and velocity as we move into and out of a *yogasana* posture.

For example, when we attempt to kick up into *adho mukha vrksasana*, the relevant muscles will be activated and deactivated at the appropriate times by the brain only after it accounts for the different lengths of the nerves involved and their different conduction velocities. That is to say, if two muscle fibers in different motor units are meant to be activated at the same time, but the efferent nerve to one is rapidly conducting and the other is slowly conducting, even with nerves of the same length, the initial signal on the slow one must be launched well before that on the fast one if the fibers are to contract simultaneously. The brain handles timing problems of this sort without any sign of conscious effort once the action has been practiced. It is no less a miracle than that of coherent speech that the timing of the muscle action in going up into *adho mukha vrksasana* is handled effortlessly by the brain. The clocks that adjust these relative timings are found in the cerebellum and basal ganglia (Chapter 4, page 67).

It is interesting that the life spans of adults first tested at age fifty-six years are longer the higher the tested IQ and the shorter the neurological reaction times. The measured reaction times have about as strong a link to survival to age seventy years as does smoking in the fourteen-year time interval between ages fifty-six and seventy years.

Mixed-Mode Sensations

Synesthesia

Once launched along the afferent fibers to the central nervous system, all nerve signals are identical; e.g., a series of -65 millivolt peaks differing only in their frequencies, a reflection of the intensities of their stimuli. It follows that if the electrical signals from the eyes could be rerouted to the adjacent auditory areas of the brain, for example, then we could hear colors through our eyes! In fact, there are people who have the gift of synesthesia; e.g., "seeing" pure colors when they hear pure acoustic tones [690a]. The synesthesia phenomenon can involve not only seeing and hearing, but also combinations of the senses of touch, taste, and smell.

The phenomenon of synesthesia appears to involve the partial leakage of one type of neural information, such as that representing the tone of a musical note, into another area of the brain responsible for handling different types of information, such as one of the visual centers. The result of such a transfer of neural signal would be the sensing of a specific color sensation along with the hearing of the tone. Indeed, during synesthetic processing, PET scans show increased blood flow to both of the sensory areas of the brain involved in the synesthesia, and in the more common types of synesthesia, the two sensations are recorded in neighboring brain centers [690a]. Some synesthetes also report the associations of specific olfactory sensations when they view specific shapes, and others hear sounds within tastes.[5]

In synesthetes oriented along the sound-color

axis, it has been observed that the visual cortex also becomes very active when certain words are heard. On the other hand, others hold that the synesthetic phenomenon is a manifestation of processes in the limbic system. Synesthesia is a one-way phenomenon in the sense that words may evoke the sensation of colors, but colors will not evoke the sensation of words. Experiments show that we all are synesthetes at a subconscious level, whereas some of us also experience this sensation at the conscious level.

As the synesthetic phenomenon is seven times more common among artists, authors, and poets, it is held to be related to the creative impulse, which is otherwise active in blending seemingly unrelated phenomena into a comprehensible whole. It is found most often in women, and there appears to be a genetic link within families. Synesthetes not only have an exceptional correlation of the senses, but in payment for this, they often have trouble with arithmetic, right-left orientation, and finding directions.

It is believed that the cross-wiring of different modes of sensory perception is a common situation among the newborn but that with normal development, these crossings are severed by apoptosis with the characteristic neural connections resolved into their usual modes. On the other hand, if this resolution of the infant's perceptual neural wiring does not occur in the adult, then synesthesia results.

A synesthesia-like effect can be simulated using simple electronics. For example, a blind person is outfitted with a properly pixelated signal from a video camera, and this signal is applied to the surface of the tongue, an organ having a high density of mechanoreceptors (figures 4.C-6 and 13.B-2). When the picture represents a simple motion, such as that of a ball rolling from left to right on a table top, the blind person can successfully interpret the shifting pattern of tingling on the tongue so as to catch the ball before it rolls off the table [3]! This is yet another example of the facile and ready plasticity of the brain's functions.

Yet another possible synesthetic effect present in almost all of us involves the hot taste of chili peppers. It is the molecule capsaicin that is the

---

5   In one case, a musician reports the following correlations of perceived auditory tone intervals with taste experiences: minor second = sour; major second = bitter; minor third = salty; fourth = mown grass; tritone = disgust; fifth = pure water; minor sixth = cream; major sixth = low-fat cream; minor seventh = bitter; major seventh = sour; octave = no taste [291].

active agent in chili peppers, and in the mouth, this molecule binds very strongly to the Ruffini corpuscles (Subsection 11.B, page 440) sensitive to heat. The result is a strong sense of heat on the tongue, though there is no increase of temperature.

Section 3.C: Neural Connections: Synapses

Synaptic Structure

Given that a sensory organ has successfully transduced its stimulus into an electrical action potential which then is transported to the tip of its axon, how does this signal within a peripheral nerve then enter the central nervous system? The mechanism for conducting a nerve impulse along the length of a neuron is discussed above (Section 3.B), with the impulse beginning at the receptor sites among the dendrites and propagating to the far end of the axon in the simplest case. In no case does the far end of the axon connect to its eventual destination without interruption. In fact, the neural paths between the brain and outlying sensors, muscles, and organs are always interrupted by small gaps called synapses. How such an electrical signal can then move from the axon tip of the presynaptic neuron to effector organs or to an adjacent receptor neuron via synapses is the subject of this section. As will be seen, the synapses allow the control of propagating action potentials, offering the opportunity to turn them on or off or otherwise moderate their effects either positively or negatively.

Gap Junctions

There are two general mechanisms for the transmission of the neural signal across the space (the synapse) that separates the axon of one neuron and the dendrite of an adjacent neuron: the electrical and the chemical. In the electrical synapse, the two adjacent nerve endings are connected by hollow tubes (gap junctions) that are capable of transmitting an ionic current from one neuron to the next, either depolarizing or hyperpolarizing it in the process. Signal conduction through a gap junction can be turned on or off by local changes in the H^+ or Ca^{2+} ion concentrations. The gap junctions are channels of 15 to 20 angstroms in width (the hydrogen atom is 1.2 angstroms in diameter) within the cell membranes and allow ions to move between adjacent cells. These gap junctions in the brain and heart allow rapid, near-synchronous activation of the muscle fibers in these organs. Also, in the uterus of a pregnant woman, gap junctions allow all of the motor units within the uterine walls to contract simultaneously during delivery so as to expel the fetus [450]. In the ventricles of the heart (figure 14.A-1), excitations across the gap junctions lead to simultaneous contraction of the muscle fibers.

The Chemical Synapse

The advantage of the gap junction is that it allows rapid and simultaneous excitation over a large collection of synapses. On the other hand, the chemical synapse, though much slower, is constructed so that it has a much higher plasticity, being able to change its characteristics under the stress of learning, and so forms the basis of both learning and memory [427a] (Subsection 4.G, page 135). In the chemical synapse, the only structural connective element between adjacent neurons is a ring of adhesion proteins keeping the presynaptic and postsynaptic partners of the synapse in position to influence one another. Within the ring of adhesion between the two interacting neurons, there is a cleft having a width of only 200 to 400 angstroms and filled with extracellular fluid (figure 3.C-1). When the presynaptic membrane at the axonal tip of the transmitter neuron reaches the action potential, it opens channels for the inward transport of Ca^{2+} ions, which in turn stimulate the release at that point of a chemical messenger (a neurotransmitter) into the volume of the synaptic cleft. Pending their release, the neurotransmitters are stored in small packets called vesicles located very close to the synaptic cleft, with each vesicle holding about 10,000 molecules of the neurotransmitter [544];

there can be thousands of vesicles in an axonal tip, carried there by the microtubules from the cell body. When called upon to do so, the vesicles move to the outer surface of the presynaptic neuron and then turn themselves inside out in order to launch their load of neurotransmitter into the synaptic cleft. The stronger the initial stimulus at the receptor end of the neuron, the more frequent are the bursts of neurotransmitter released from vesicles at the neural terminal (also called the axonal tip).

Any neurotransmitter released on the presynaptic side of the cleft diffuses across the cleft to the postsynaptic membrane 200 to 400 angstroms away, where it is recognized by receptors and is then bound to that membrane. Binding of

the neurotransmitter to the postsynaptic membrane initiates a receptor or synaptic potential in that neuron, and signal propagation begins again, possibly spreading simultaneously to widely separated target organs or brain centers.

The chemical synapse works somewhat like glandular secretion (Subsection 6.A, page 207), but it is faster and more directed; however, intermediate cases are known, in which the synaptic cleft spacing is relatively large and the release of neurotransmitter activates receptors on many neurons in its locale. It also happens that a nerve cell may release its neurotransmitter directly into the intercellular fluids; lacking a synapse, these molecules then diffuse for long distances before finding appropriate receptors. In this case, the

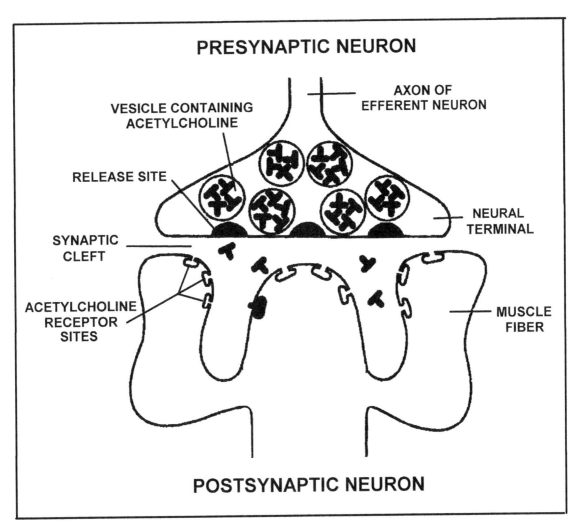

Figure 3.C-1. Elements of the chemical synapse between a neuron and a muscle fiber. In this case, the vesicles within the presynaptic half of the synapse are filled with acetylcholine, and the receptors on the postsynaptic side are shaped to absorb and respond to this neurotransmitter.

neurotransmitter is acting as a neurohormone. Indeed, many neurotransmitters play roles as neurohormones in the body [878].

The receptor sites on the postsynaptic membranes are activated by the specific molecule that is released into its synapse or by ones closely similar in their chemical shapes and reactions. A variety of small molecules and ions (approximately fifty) serve as the neurotransmitters in human synapses (see Section 3.D, page 53).

Once having entered the synaptic cleft and initiating a receptor potential, the neurotransmitter blocks all further action until it has been cleared from the volume of the cleft and removed from the postsynaptic surface. This is the phenomenon behind the inherent upper limit to the number of times per second a neuron can deliver a signal across a chemical synapse. During this refractory period in which no signal can be transported across the synapse, the neurotransmitter must be reabsorbed by the presynaptic membrane, unbound neurotransmitters must diffuse out of the cleft, and any neurotransmitter remaining within the cleft or on the receptor surface must be enzymatically degraded. Clearing of the neurotransmitter signal is very rapid in the case of the small-molecule neurotransmitters (with refractory times of approximately one millisecond) but can take a very long time in the case of the larger neurotransmitters (refractory times of tens of seconds to several minutes), leading to long-lasting activation of the receptors.

In order to get sustained action at a synapse with small-molecule neurotransmitters, it is necessary to provide the synapse with a sustained barrage of action potentials. Alternatively, circuits consisting of groups of neurons exist, in which a signal is sent sequentially from one neuron to the next, and then to the next, but eventually is relayed so as to excite the initial source of excitation. Called a reverberating circuit, such a circular arrangement results in the generation of a repetitive, oscillating neural signal extended in time from seconds to hours but initiated by a single instantaneous action potential. Such circuits are thought to control time-based reflexes such as the wake/sleep cycle, the breathing rate,

and the storage of short-term memories [426, 863].

Synapses within the Immune System

High-resolution microscopy recently has shown that when two species of the immune system meet or when one meets a foreign invader, the two parties are bound together by adhesion proteins for an hour or so. During this time, a synaptic structure forms at the point of contact that closely resembles the one involved in the chemical synapse between neurons. There then follows a transfer of either chemical-structural information or a chemical toxin, depending upon the goal of the immune system [186] (Subsection 16.B, page 642).

Convergent/Divergent Neural Nets

Looked at globally, many neural systems are found to be either convergent or divergent, there being an unequal number of terminal points at the two ends of the system in either case. Thus, in a divergent system, there are fewer originating points in the system than there are terminating points (figure 3.C-2**a**). This downward neural divergence characterizes the phenomenon of the "motor unit," in which one efferent neuron originating in the brain repeatedly branches so as to feed the identical neural signal to a number of individual muscle fibers (Subsection 11.A, page 369).

In a convergent neural net, there are more originating points in the system than there are terminating points (figure 3.C-2**b**), as is the case for the ganglia of the rods and cones in the retina of the eye. This convergence in the eye leads to the phenomenon of the "receptive field," in which the optical signals originating with many afferent neurons in the retina are combined into one signal carried upward by the optic nerve to the visual cortex (figure 17.B-1). Another example of an upwardly convergent system is found in the neural net of the skin sensors of the body, which leads to the phenomena of "dermatomes" and "referred pain" (Section 13.D, page 530).

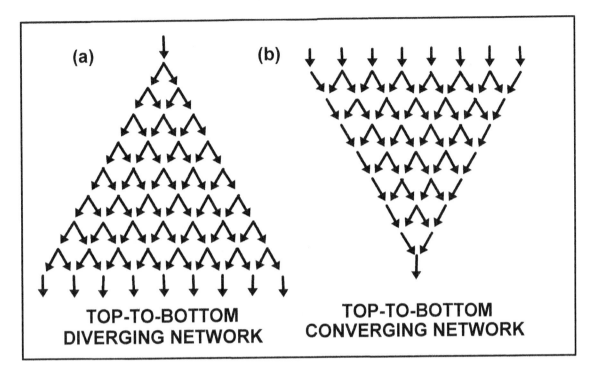

Figure 3.C-2. Schematic representations of (**a**) top-to-bottom divergent and (**b**) top-to-bottom convergent neural nets.

Excitation versus Inhibition

Interneurons

Once bound to the postsynaptic membrane, the neurotransmitter's function is then to open and close ion channels so as to change the electrical-charge state surrounding the membrane. If Na$^+$ gates are opened, the inner membrane will be flooded with this ion, and the membrane will tend to be depolarized. If the depolarization effect is large enough, then a depolarization action-potential wave will be propagated; i.e., the signal moves on.

On the other hand, the action of the neurotransmitter instead may be to open K$^+$ and Cl$^-$ channels, letting the first of these out and the second of these into the cell from outside the membrane. In this case, the transmembrane voltage becomes even more negative and so is discouraged from reaching the less-negative (-65 millivolt) threshold necessary for the formation of an action potential; this synaptic connection will be inhibitory, even if other synaptic connections to the same neuron are excitatory.

Depending upon the action and nature of the postsynaptic receptor site, the binding of a particular neurotransmitter can lead to either an excitatory or an inhibitory signal. Thus acetylcholine is an excitatory neurotransmitter in the synapse between motor neuron and skeletal-muscle fiber, as in figure 3.C-1, but is inhibitory when released in the synapses of cardiac muscle, where the result of the inhibiting action is to slow the heart rate.

Clearly, not all neurons are simply passive conduits for transmission of a signal from point A to point B. Were this the case, then it would be hard to see how competing points of view within the brain could be weighed and decided either for or against, or how a compromise ever could be reached. In fact, successful decision making requires the possibility of negative input as well as positive, and this negative input, called neural inhibition, is supplied by cells in the central nervous system called interneurons. The actions of interneurons are always inhibitory, meaning that their action on the transmembrane voltage is to lower it rather than to raise it (figure 3.A-3); due to the -65 millivolt threshold for propagation, in-

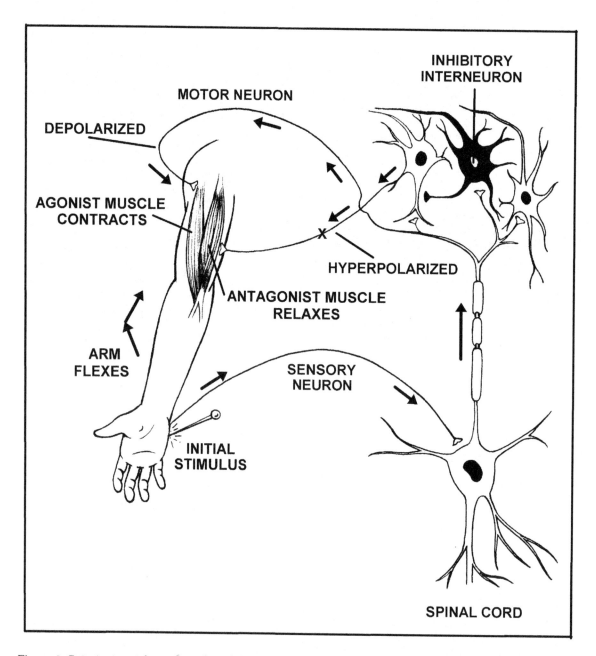

Figure 3.C-3. A pinprick on the palm of the right hand reflexively stimulates an afferent sensory neuron in the skin, which synapses with a neuron in the spinal cord. However, the efferent spinal neuron bifurcates, with one branch forming a depolarized neuromuscular synapse with the biceps muscle, and the other traveling to an interneuron, which then acts to hyperpolarize the motor neuron stimulating the antagonist triceps muscle. Consequently, the antagonist muscle is relaxed through the action of the interneuron, the agonist muscle is excited to contract, and the hand pulls away from the noxious stimulus.

terneurons act to block transmission of the neural signal by making it more negative. The blocking effect of the interneuron is felt at the axon hillock (figure 3.A-3), where its inhibitory strength is measured against that of the excitatory signals also incident on the neuron, and a decision is then made, on the basis of the relative strengths of the two types of excitation, to either launch an action potential along the neural axon or not.

Interneurons exert their influence by moderating the interplay between the sensory neurons and the motor neurons; in doing so, they control our response to the environment. See Section 11.A, page 420, for examples of interneurons at work. For other examples of the inhibiting effects of interneurons in action, see Subsection 4.C, page 95; Subsection 4.D, page 105; Section 11.A, page 420; and Subsection 11.D, page 448. The role of interneurons in the phenomenon of reciprocal inhibition following a sharp pinprick is shown in figure 3.C-3.

One readily sees the importance of interneurons in the human body, for the default setting of the muscles in the body is contraction; however, this contraction is inhibited by the net of interneurons. In the case of a tetanus infection, the toxin from this bacterial invasion acts only on interneurons, blocking their action. As a result, the body loses its muscular inhibitions in the spinal cord, and the body readily goes into muscular spasms, beginning at the jaw (lockjaw) and finally involving the entire body [213]. Once muscular inhibition has been shut down by the tetanus bacterium, the body is subject to muscular spasms when it is touched by something as inconsequential as a small breeze or a soft noise; from this, one can fully appreciate the important balancing roles interneurons otherwise must play in our *yogasana* practice. In fact, the primary action of the higher centers of the brain is the inhibition of global muscle contraction.

Changing the Synaptic Threshold

Nerve fibers either conduct a depolarization wave or they do not, depending in part on the magnitude of the threshold for the action potential. Through experience, this threshold can be raised or lowered to fine-tune the action. Adjustment of the action threshold is more easily accomplished in the chemical synapses. Though somewhat slower than the electrical synapses, the chemical synapses are much more easily modified by experience and so allow learning to occur through practice. As applied to the *yogasanas*, the reduction of the action potentials through practice means that less nervous energy and less neurotransmitter need be expended in order to achieve a particular muscular state of contraction. As a consequence, one can stay longer in a posture before nervous exhaustion becomes a factor. The neurochemical consequences of learning are discussed further in Section 4.G, page 137.

In general, a single motor neuron is able to generate a sufficient action potential at its synaptic junction with a single muscle fiber and so excite the fiber with almost total certainty. On the other hand, in the central nervous system, the single-neuron receptor potential is far below that necessary for propagation of an action potential. Note, however, that on such multipolar receptor neurons, there are receptor sites over the entire neuron, and so there can be hundreds of synaptic junctions, all in a position to add their signal in a communal way so as to exceed the action-potential threshold (figures 3.A-4 and 3.C-3). Often, synapses to the multipolar cell body are inhibitory, while those to the dendrites are excitatory, and those along the axon are modulatory. In any event, the various depolarizing and hyperpolarizing voltages are summed algebraically in both space and time at the hillock where the axon joins the multipolar cell body, and depending upon the size of the summed signal, the excitation will prove to be either excitatory and lead to a propagating action potential, or inhibitory, due to too-negative a net receptor potential. It is in this way that signals from many different organs and sensors from distant points can be integrated and prioritized so as to finally influence a neural action serving the greatest good. In this scheme, learning can occur both by changing the relative intensities of the component signals so as to excite or inhibit a potential signal in the receptor neuron, or by a change in the threshold potential of the receptor.

Section 3.D: Neurotransmitters and Neuromodulators

The message that is sent from the axonal terminal of a presynaptic neuron to the receptor sites in the neighboring postsynaptic neuron in a muscle or gland most often is a chemical one. Within the cell body of the presynaptic neuron, the particular chemical to be used in transmitting the message is manufactured in the cell body and packaged in the vesicles. Once filled with the appropriate neurotransmitter molecules, the vesicles are then propelled along the full length of the axon via the two-way axonal transport system (Subsection 3.A, page 35), to arrive and be stored finally at the axonal terminals. Whenever an action potential travels the length of the axon and arrives at the terminal, this potential triggers the opening of the vesicles and the release of the neurotransmitters contained within them. In turn, the released neurotransmitters flood the synaptic cleft, to be sensed by the receptors on the postsynaptic neuron. The axonal transport system then returns the empty vesicles to the cell body for repair or recycling. The neurotransmitters injected into the synaptic cleft may be either excitatory or inhibitory. In the former case, they depolarize the postsynaptic membrane, thereby initiating a propagating neural signal in the postsynaptic neuron or muscle fiber; whereas if they hyperpolarize this membrane, they inhibit the propagation of a neural signal beyond the synapse. There are four broad classes of neurotransmitters: (i) acetylcholine (in a class by itself), (ii) the small-molecule biogenic amines such as dopamine, norepinephrine, and serotonin, (iii) the amino acids such as gamma-aminobutyric acid (GABA) and glycine, and (iv) the large-molecule neuropeptides such as oxytocin, insulin, and β-endorphin. Prime among the small-molecule neurotransmitters are the following.

Acetylcholine

Acetylcholine is the neurotransmitter in all neuromuscular (cholinergic) synapses in the peripheral nervous system, in the paravertebral ganglia of the sympathetic trunk, and in the pre- and post-ganglia of the parasympathetic nervous system (figure 5.C-1); it also appears prominently in the central nervous system, where it influences psychological function [266].

Action in the Muscles and Viscera

Acetylcholine is almost always excitatory at the neuromuscular synapse of skeletal muscle (when there is no inhibitory signal), and though each acetylcholine release at a neuromuscular synapse results in an action potential, the signal may be either excitatory or inhibitory at the autonomic synapses to the heart and visceral organs. Acetylcholine's action at the neuromuscular junction generally is to depolarize the muscle fiber so that Ca^{2+} channels open, and these ions then initiate muscle contraction (Subsection 11.A, page 378). Should the acetylcholine receptors in the muscles be blocked by antibodies formed through an autoimmune reaction within the body, then the muscles will be prevented from contracting, and one has the muscle-wasting disease myastenia gravis, whereas if the body is infected with the tetanus bacterium, the consequence is lack of muscular inhibition followed by global muscular contraction.

The binding of acetylcholine at a receptor site opens ion channels for only one millisecond, after which the acetylcholine is enzymatically degraded or reabsorbed, and the channel closes. Given that the ion channels are open for about one millisecond or less, it is theoretically possible then to excite a muscle fiber at up to 1,000 times per second (1,000 hertz); however, in practice, the upper limit is more like 200 times per second (200 hertz).

Action in the Brain

Acetylcholine is also a very active neurotransmitter in the brain, working from the medulla oblongata up to the cortex, and at all points in between, to shape our consciousness. In this, it acts both as an excitatory neurotransmitter in some regions of the brain and as an inhibitory neurotransmitter in other regions. The primary role of acetylcholine in the cortex is largely inhibitory, promoting the excitation of the inhibitory interneurons in this region.

The Catecholamines

Neural excitation of the adrenal medulla gland results in the release of a mixture of epinephrine (80 percent) and norepinephrine (20 percent); this mixture is otherwise known as the catecholamines. Upon being stimulated by the sympathetic nervous system (Subsection 6.B, page 219), the catecholamines are released into the bloodstream as hormones by the adrenal medulla and are able to stimulate both alpha and beta cells in a variety of tissues.

Norepinephrine

Norepinephrine functions both as a neurotransmitter and as a hormone. In the former situation, it is active in the brainstem and hypothalamus, causing excitation at some centers and inhibition at others. Norepinephrine is found in high concentrations in the locus ceruleus of the brain, a center that affects levels of attention and arousal [266]. At high concentrations, it helps to focus attention; the negative effects of low levels of the catecholamines in the brain are discussed in Section 22.A, page 759.

The release of the catecholamines is triggered by acetylcholine's action in the neuroendocrine synapse. Because the receptors on a postsynaptic membrane can be of more than one type, the alpha and beta receptors for the catecholamines on each of the postsynaptic membranes throughout the body can be sensitive to both epinephrine and norepinephrine, though some synapses are more sensitive to the former, while others are more sensitive to the latter.

Epinephrine

Epinephrine binds to both alpha and beta receptors, but in the case of the small blood vessels, the alpha binding leads to constriction, whereas the beta binding leads to dilation of the vessels. Epinephrine prefers beta receptors, such as those found in the heart and gastrointestinal tract, where it dilates arterioles; norepinephrine prefers alpha receptors, as found in the vascular smooth muscle, the gut, bladder, spleen, and the sphincters.

Serotonin

Though serotonin functions as a neurotransmitter in the enteric branch of the autonomic nervous system within the gut, it is not found to function in either the sympathetic or parasympathetic branches of the autonomic nervous system

[268]. Within the brain, serotonin is generated in the brainstem. The consequence of low serotonin levels in the brain is depression (Chapter 22.A, page 760), along with disregulation of levels of anxiety, food intake, and impulsive violence [427a]; many antidepressants function by increasing the amount of serotonin in the synapses of the central nervous system, often leading to salutary effects on mood and behavior, blocking of pain signals in the spinal cord, and possibly to neurogenesis. Serotonin exerts its inhibitory action by opening K^+ channels, which tends to hyperpolarize the postsynaptic membrane. When serotonin is released by the platelets at the site of a wound, it acts as a constrictor of nearby blood vessels, thereby stanching the loss of blood in the area of the wound.

Gamma-Aminobutyric Acid

Gamma-aminobutyric acid (GABA) is found in large amounts in the central nervous system, where it acts as the major neurotransmitter for inhibitory synaptic potentials and is highly concentrated in the hypothalamus. It also is found in the heart, lungs, and kidneys of other animals and in certain plants as well. In all of these, it functions by opening channels for Cl^- ions. Its action is similar to that of glycine, the simplest amino acid, which depresses neural activity in the spinal cord by opening the Cl^- channels. GABA in the brain influences psychological function through inhibition, but its chemical precursor is glutamic acid, a potent excitatory neurotransmitter in the brain [30, 266].

Were it not for GABA's strongly hyperpolarizing/inhibitory effects and its high concentration in the brain, the body and mind would be in a constant state of muscular convulsion and hyperexcitability. A number of drugs enhance GABA binding to its receptor site and so increase the strength of neural inhibition and thereby lessen anxiety. This binding is enhanced by ingesting psychological and physiological depressors such as phenobarbital, ethyl alcohol, and Valium.

Dopamine

Dopamine in the brain is an important neurotransmitter, influencing not only the control of movement but also the brain's reward and motivation systems; thus, it is a chemical factor in addiction when active in the reward center (the nucleus accumbens) and in the motivation center (the dorsal striatum). Increases in the dopamine, β-endorphin, oxytocin, and prolactin levels in the blood plasma result in a happy, relaxed frame of mind, whereas dopamine deficiency is a factor in schizophrenia. The role of dopamine in the pain and pleasure centers of the brain and its role in addiction are discussed further in Subsection 13.C, page 521.

Because dopamine is integral to motivation and also is important to the release of the endorphins, it is no surprise that thrill-seekers are strongly addicted to intoxication by excess dopamine, possibly due to a deficiency of monamine oxidase, an enzyme which normally destroys dopamine in the synapses. These thrill-seekers not only seek dangerous situations but can easily imagine situations that are not really risky but nonetheless stimulate dopamine production.

Loss of dopamine in the substantia nigra (Subsection 4.C, page 84) can lead to Parkinson's-like motor problems; in this, the posture is shifted strongly toward flexion, and movement is glacial until levodopa is administered, its effects being the generation of dopamine, a strong shift of the posture toward extension, and the stimulation of freedom of movement. If dopamine is lacking on only one side of the brain, then the Parkinson's symptoms are localized to the contralateral side of the body due to decussation of the relevant neurons.

Anionic Neurotransmitters

Glutamate and aspartate anions are among the most common neurotransmitters in the brain's excitatory synapses, with glutamate being the major excitatory neurotransmitter. An excess of glutamate in a synapse leads to excessive excitation and nerve death by "excitotoxicity" [268]. It is hypothesized that there can be deliberate local over-excitation by glutamate in the brain, in order to both pare out unused neural circuits and to generate more room for rapidly growing tumors. It is further hypothesized that excess glutamate may be responsible for the neural degeneration that characterizes multiple sclerosis [887]. The excitatory functions of glutamate and aspartate ions in the brain are countered by the inhibitory neurotransmitters GABA and glycine.

The Neuropeptides

Specificity

Neuropeptides that function as neurotransmitters throughout the body number between fifty and one hundred. As a class, the neuropeptides are relatively short polymers of the various amino acids linked together in specific orders. For example, the neuropeptide oxytocin contains nine amino acids strung together end to end in the order cystine-tyrosine-isoleucine-glutamic acid-asparagine-cystine-proline-leucine-glycine, with the two cystine groups joined by a disulfide -S-S- linkage [660]; whereas the growth hormone GHRH consists of a chain of forty-four such amino acids strung together in a shoestring fashion [427]. Vasopressin (ADH), angiotensin II, cholecystokinin, substance P, and the enkephalins are all examples of neuropeptides.

The neuropeptides are concentrated in both the upward-going hypothalamic extensions to the thalamus and in the downward-going hypothalamic extensions to the pituitary gland. The nerves carrying pain signals (nociceptors) converge on the dorsal horns of the spinal cord (figure 4.A-2), which, appropriately, are the loci of neuropeptide receptors, and there are receptors for the neuropeptide angiotensin II in both the brain and in the kidneys.

Neuropeptide Global Consciousness

The action of a particular neurotransmitter at a particular site is guaranteed by the highly specific nature of the intimate interaction between the transmitter and the receptor sites. In contrast, for peptide neurotransmitters, there are no short-range synapses of the kind ordinarily met with as when acetylcholine is the transmitter. Because a neuropeptide receptor will only accept that one neuropeptide with the proper number and order of the appropriate amino acids, the neuropeptides are released into the circulatory system just as with hormones. Though these "neurohormones" are dispersed freely over the body via the circulatory system and are relatively slow to have an effect, they are able to activate distant sites with great specificity.

It would be difficult to overstate the importance of the neuropeptides as neurotransmitters. Thus certain short-chain neuropeptides are key players in the body's very successful efforts to erase pain sensations (see below). Because the neuropeptides were first identified in the brain, it was quite a shock to find so many sources of and receptors for the neuropeptides throughout the body. Consequently, the neuropeptides have come to be viewed as extending the body's intelligence to the furthest points [654].

Furthermore, the circulating cells of the immune system (Section 16.B, page 642) have receptors for all of the neuropeptides first found in the brain. In a sense, the neuropeptides, when coupled with the immune system, the gastrointestinal tract, and the central nervous system, form a global system of neural consciousness, allowing signals to be sent between any two points in the body, albeit somewhat slowly [635]. Once again, there is a resonance between such medical discoveries and Iyengar's repeated dictum to work the *yogasanas* so as to extend one's intelligence from the brain to the furthest parts of the body [391] (see Appendix VI, page 937).

Endogenous Opioids

The spinal cord, brainstem, thalamus, and hypothalamus are able to manufacture three main types of morphine-like opioid neuropeptides called endogenous opioids: β-endorphin, the enkephalins, and the dynorphins. In contrast, morphine itself is termed an exogenous opioid, as it is not a natural product of the human body. As the opioids travel a long distance in the body in order to find their receptor sites, the effects of the opioids are slow at first, but the effects can build after that. In general, the actions of the opioids are inhibitory and generally produce either sedation or analgesia by exciting neural subsystems that inhibit the transmission of pain signals. Whether endogenous or exogenous, the effects of a given dose of any of the opioids are strongly coupled to the situational setting, the attitudes of the subject, and the mood. When the level of exercise brings one to about 90 percent of $\dot{V}O_{2max}$, endorphins are released into the bloodstream from the pituitary [618]. Moreover, receptors for β-endorphins are found in the hypothalamus and within the limbic system. These neuropeptides act in the synapses of the brain to produce a euphoric feeling—the runner's high.

Levels of β-endorphin peak in the spinal fluid at 6:00 to 7:00 AM and in the blood plasma at about 9:30 AM, with minima occurring approximately twelve hours later, just as one would expect for a normal sleep/wake cycle. See Subsection 13.C, page 524, for further discussion of the analgesic actions of β-endorphin and Subsection 13.C, page 528, for a discussion of the pain relief associated with ingesting placebo pills.

Drug Action in the Synaptic Cleft

Arousal

The most widely ingested exogenous stimulants of the central nervous system are caffeine (the most widely used drug in the world, found in coffee, tea, and cola), nicotine (found in cigarettes and other tobacco products), and amphetamines, all of which promote stimulation of the sympathetic nervous system. In contrast to these stimulants, sedatives induce sleep; in fact, whereas ethyl alcohol at low concentrations is a stimulant, at sufficiently high concentrations, it depresses the reticular formation so as to make one totally unconscious. Alcohol and barbiturates bind to GABA receptors (see below) in a way that promotes the inhibitory action of the GABA neurotransmitter. Opioids also depress nerve action

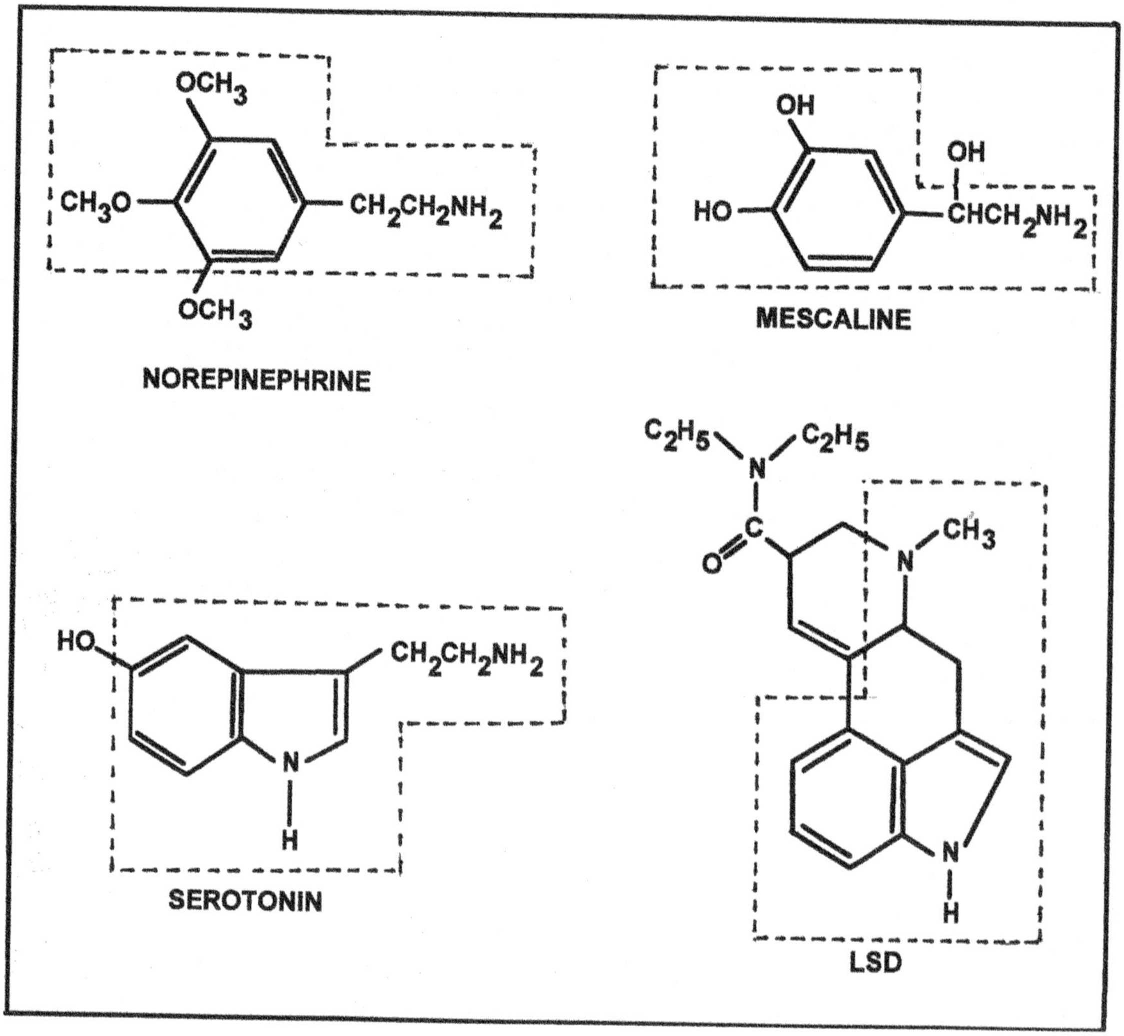

Figure 3.D-1. Chemical structures of the two neurotransmitters norepinephrine and serotonin, and the two drugs, mescaline and LSD, containing structures (within the dashed lines) that mimic them.

along the pathways that signal pain. Tranquilizers work by binding to receptors for dopamine, stimulating the receptors to increase their activity, possibly by blocking enzymatic degradation of the neurotransmitter.

Amphetamines and Norepinephrine

Because amphetamines increase the release of norepinephrine into the synaptic cleft and also block the re-uptake of the transmitter, they are powerful stimulants of the central nervous system. The resulting high concentration of norepinephrine in the synaptic cleft then leads to increased arousal, mood, excitability, and pleasure. If the concentrations of norepinephrine or serotonin are far below normal, as in depressed subjects (Section 22.A, page 759), amphetamines

can restore normal order and mood by raising neurotransmitter levels.

Norepinephrine and the drug mescaline have closely related molecular structures (figure 3.D-1). It appears that mescaline is tightly bound to the enzyme that otherwise degrades norepinephrine in the synaptic cleft. With this enzyme blocked, the norepinephrine has an unusually long lifetime in the cleft, and this leads to hallucinations [801]. Similarly, a drug such as LSD, which closely resembles serotonin in chemical structure (figure 3.D-1), can compete successfully with serotonin for receptor sites on neural membranes and degrading enzymes, and so it drastically alters the synaptic chemistry when ingested [801].

Anesthesia

Foreign substances such as mood-altering drugs and anesthetics can strongly influence synaptic chemistry when parts of their molecular structures closely mimic those of the natural neurotransmitters. Once within the area of the synapse, a neuroactive drug can act to stimulate a stronger release of neurotransmitter, can compete successfully with the natural substance for a position on the receptor membrane, and/or can block the enzymes that otherwise would destroy the natural transmitter within the synapse. Still others work their effect by blocking the channels otherwise used for transmembrane ion transport. Thus several local and general anesthetics work by blocking the opening of Na^+ channels in the pain axon, thwarting the formation of a depolarized pain wave [878]; the more potent natural plant and animal poisons, such as tetrodotoxin and tetanus toxin, also work in this way [549].

Receptors for the brain neurotransmitters glutamate, glycine, and GABA are controlling for neural excitation in the brain, with the first of these being excitatory and the second two being inhibitory. It is now argued that anesthetics work by either blocking glutamate receptors or activating receptors for GABA or glycine in the brain.

Acetylcholine

The acetylcholine receptors also bind nicotine, caffeine, and benzedrine, all of which facilitate neural action by reducing the transmembrane threshold for excitation by acetylcholine. The same receptors are blocked by curare, the paralyzing South American arrow poison. Once the neuromuscular junctions are blocked by curare, no muscle action is possible, and either relaxation or suffocation soon follows, depending on whether the application of the drug is local or global. Very strong effects on neural conduction are also observed when foreign chemicals interfere with the action of acetylcholinesterase, the enzyme that clears the synaptic cleft of its acetylcholine, thereby turning off the neural signal. The deadly phosphate nerve gases work in this way, whereas botulism toxin paralyzes by suppressing the release of acetylcholine from the presynaptic vesicles.

Caffeine

Caffeine functions as a central-nervous-system stimulant by interfering with the neural action of adenosine, a neurotransmitter that tends to constrict the bronchi, thereby reducing the ability to breathe. Caffeine works both by blocking the receptors for adenosine, which is generally inhibitory in its action, and promotes the release of epinephrine, thereby increasing alertness and energy levels, blood pressure, and heart and breathing rates, as well as stimulating the burning of calories. The stimulating effect of caffeine is apparent half an hour after ingestion and lasts for several hours thereafter. While under the influence of caffeine, one thinks quicker, reacts faster, and works more accurately in general.

Alcohol

Ethyl alcohol in low doses (one cocktail) **increases** neural activity and leaves one feeling comfortable; with a second drink, the reward system lights up, and one becomes chatty. After a third drink, alpha waves become significant in the EEG, and blood flow through the hippocampus and thalamus slows; a fourth drink slows blood flow through the cerebellum (motor control) and through the occipital region (vision). After drinking, sleep will be poor, as alcohol inhibits REM sleep; see Subsection 4.C, page 93, for a further discussion of the mental effects of imbibing alcohol.

A natural neuropeptide with the yoga-sounding name anandamide is found at very high levels in the CSF of schizophrenics, in whom it appears to act as an antipsychotic.

Neuromodulators

Learning

As discussed above, the neurotransmitters are transported between the presynaptic and postsynaptic membranes surrounding the synaptic cleft and function in either excitatory or inhibitory ways, generally over the course of several seconds' time. Yet another set of neuroactive substances function as "neuromodulators," wherein they act on the cell membranes of the presynaptic and postsynaptic membranes over much longer periods of time [708]. In this process, a neuromodulator in the extracellular fluid initially reacts with glycoprotein in the cell wall, which in turn releases an intracellular enzyme; this release is followed by a chemical chain reaction within and outside the cell's nucleus, all of which leads, over a span of several hours, to the formation and deposition of glycoprotein on both sides of the relevant synapse. In this process, the intracellular enzyme released by an extracellular reaction is known as a "second messenger." The end result of the neuromodulator's action is to strengthen the neural conductance across the synaptic cleft; when repeated a number of times, this offers a neurochemical mechanism for long-term learning by association.

According to Roberts [708], it is actions of the neuromodulators as described above that lead to those patterns of behavior described as "drives"; i.e., the appetites for food, sex, domination, understanding, etc., and moods such as gratification, satiety, aversion, despair, and the recognition of reward and punishment.

Section 3.E: Mechanical and Field Effects on Neurons

Because of the extreme physical postures that we assume in our *yogasana* practice, not only do the muscles show extreme flexibility, but so too must the nerves that accompany them; as the muscles stretch, so too must the nerves synapsed to them. Moreover, just as with the muscles, the nerves of the body are surrounded by connective tissues (with names like perinerium and epineurium), and just as with muscles, neural tissues, when traumatized, are subject to the cumulative injury cycle (figure 11.G-1). Thus, a nerve injured by compression or by muscular overstretching, for example, suffers intraneural

edema, chemical irritation, hypoxia, and microvascular stasis. The pain attending these changes promotes muscle spasms and altered movement patterns [117]. The eventual result of this train of cause and effect is a loss of neural-tissue elasticity.

Compression

Afferents

External pressure on the body is sensed by a variety of sensor organs called mechanoreceptors (Section 11.B, page 428), in which the sensor itself is found at the distal end of the receptor neuron. The pressure to which such sensors respond may be the result of an external object pressing into the body, or it may be a muscle action that inadvertently presses contracted or swollen muscle tissue or bone upon a pressure-sensitive mechanoreceptor. Moreover, pressure on the axon of the receptor neuron, rather than on the mechanoreceptor at the dendritic end of the neuron, also can result in secondary sensations. This is especially true for nerves that pass over bony knobs or through narrow channels of bone or fibrous tissue, as is the case with carpal-tunnel syndrome [264], for example, or for the ulnar nerve at the medial epicondyle of the elbow when in *sayanasana*. Compression of the neural axons can result in mechanical damage to the nerve by injury to its microtubule structure, neural edema, neural ischemia, inflammation, and delayed conduction.

When the axons of afferent nerves are under pressure, the feeling is one of "pins and needles," tingling, radiating pain, or numbness. As nerve fibers are rather fluid and relatively weak mechanically, it is tempting to imagine that the effect of pressure is to throttle the flow of the action potential along the axon, with the "pins and needles" sensation associated with intermittent transmission of the sensory signal and with numbness resulting when the flow of either the action potential along the neural membrane or of the vesicles along the microtubules within the axon (Subsection 3.A, page 35) is blocked totally.

With pressures of only 90 to 100 millimeters Hg, total blockage of the nerve signals ensues after just two hours (see Appendix II, page 835, for confirmation of this). The situation is worse if both the motor and sensory nerves are affected by compression, if the effect is felt on both sides of the body, or if the disturbance is farther from the spine [478]. In *yogasana* work, it can be a good sign to go from numbness to pain, as this signals a release of compression on the nerve in question. The most common sites for such compressive neuropathies among non-yogis are the wrist, elbow, and lower back, but this may not hold for *yogasana* practitioners.

Iyengar mentions that numbness in the feet is a common problem when spending long periods in postures for *pranayama* [394] and recommends *savasana*-like relaxation with legs alternately bent and stretched to restore feeling. This numbness involves compression of the afferent nerves from the foot, as well as a certain amount of ischemia due to compression of relevant vascular elements.

Peripheral nerves also are called upon to stretch in response to various muscle actions. If the ulnar nerve is struck at the point at which it passes the elbow, the pain signals will be sensed by the brain as coming from the sensors at the terminal ends of the nerves, and the hand will be felt to be in pain, though it has not been injured. This is much like the situation with the sciatic nerves in the leg sensing pain at a distance from the injury (Section 13.D, page 532).

Oscillating Pressure

It is known that rocking, which produces an oscillating pressure on the skin, is soothing to infants and children, and even aperiodic pressure, as delivered through massage, is relaxing.

Efferents

When it is an efferent nerve that is under pressure, the secondary effect of pressure on the nerve is one of weakness and tentative action (trembling) of the muscles so innervated, with seemingly low recruitment of motor units. This too is understandable if the action potential that drives muscle contraction is throttled by compression. Remember that intensity of muscular action depends both upon the frequency of the action potential transmitted along its axon and the number of motor units excited in a muscle; because compression can diminish both of these factors, the muscular response is noticeably weaker [478].

Nerves Surrounding Nerves

The connective-tissue sheaths that surround the peripheral nerves are innervated in turn by subsystems of yet smaller nerves called the nervi nervorum; i.e., the nerves themselves are self-innervated. Injury, compression, or inflammation of the nervi nervorum within the sheaths surrounding the peripheral nerves will be painful, as these subsystems are very reactive and easily transmit nociceptor pain signals. A pain signal originating from injury to a nerve itself is called neuropathic pain (Subsection 13.C, page 520).

Ischemia

Yet another possible mechanism working to thwart the transmission of the nerve signal is that the compression slows vascular circulation in the compressed area (ischemia) and as a consequence of this, the nerve does not receive sufficient oxygen for proper functioning (hypoxia).[6] If there is slight pressure on an afferent nerve, it can suffer ischemia, and this is sensed as pain [482]. As explained in Subsection 13.C (page 519), the decrease of oxygen to a nerve or muscle cell results in a release of arachidonic acid, a potent stimulator of pain receptors in the body. Thus in sciatica, pressure on the L4, L5, S1 nerve complex, as might be caused by a herniated disc (see Section 8.C, page 307), can result in symptoms of pain or even numbness [489].

Many of us experience the secondary effects

---

6 The nerves become exhausted if they do not receive an adequate supply of oxygen from the blood, because oxygen is needed by the mitochondria to produce ATP, which works to maintain the ionic gradients necessary for nerve action.

of pressure and ischemia on the nerves when going into *virasana* or *supta virasana* and staying there for a few minutes. On coming out of the posture, the legs are tingling and so weak that they can be straightened only with difficulty! The problem here would seem to be that one has a tourniquet effect at the knee, where extreme flexion at the knee and the pressure of the calf against the hamstring muscle not only restricts blood circulation but also compresses axons within the sciatic nerve. These effects can be avoided by sitting on a block in *virasana*, so as to open the angle at the knee, and by rolling the calf muscle laterally while rolling the back of the thigh medially as one sits, so as to avoid pressing one on the other. The lack of blood flow below the knees in these postures also can readily lead to foot cramps.

Interestingly, when a peripheral nerve passes through a joint, there is a preferred position within the joint for this. In most cases, the nerve chooses to pass on what is the inside of the joint when the joint is flexed. In this case, the nerve being on the inside results in less tensile stress than were it to take the outer path, which would be more stressful to the nerve whether the joint was flexed or extended. The only exceptions to this tendency to take the inner path are the ulnar nerve in the elbow and the sciatic nerve in the hip, both of which follow the outer paths, subject the nerves to tensile stress, and so become the loci of many neurological problems.

The ulnar nerve in the arm offers a good example of what can happen to both afferent and efferent nerves when the surrounding musculature and bone are involved in heavy exercise [53] and the nerve takes the outer route past the elbow joint. The ulnar-nerve bundle serves the inner aspect of the hand, traveling up the forearm and passing through a narrow channel (the cubital tunnel) in the elbow on its way to the upper arm [360]. The cubital tunnel is normally circular in cross section and open; however, when the arm is flexed at the elbow, as in *sirsasana I*, its shape changes to triangular, and the channel diameter decreases by more than 50 percent. Compression of this nerve by flexing the elbow can result in

severely reduced conduction velocities, as well as tingling, numbness, pain, and muscle weakness in the hands. An even more intense and immediate "paralysis" of the arm results if the arm is placed behind the back as in *paschima namaskarasana* and one then lies down on this facing upward. Placing both hands in *paschima namaskarasana* prayer position behind the back, as for *parsvottanasana*, also can aggravate nerves within the carpal tunnel at each wrist.

Active extension of the arm with the wrists flexed, as in *adho mukha vrksasana*, *urdhva dhanurasana*, or *purvottanasana*, acts as traction on the ulnar nerve and can extend it by almost 1.5 centimeters (0.5 inches).[7] Depending upon the mechanical actions at the elbow, the ulnar nerve in the cubital tunnel is subject to compression, friction, and traction with consequent symptoms when postures such as these are practiced. Carpal tunnel syndrome also can be mentioned here [264], wherein a swelling at the wrist impinges upon the nerves serving the fingers.

Tingling sensations in the arms are possibly due to the compression of nerves or blood vessels as these nerves or vessels pass between the thorax and the arms. Called thoracic outlet syndrome, it may be caused by over-developed muscles or poor posture, among other things. Numbness due to ulnar impingement is occasionally experienced by yoga students when resting in *savasana* with their elbows on the floor at their sides.

Nerve impingement can also occur when the vertebrae are misaligned but with discs not herniated, as discussed in Subsection 8.C, page 305. The weakened muscular response of a muscle when it is compressed externally is often met in the *yogasanas* and can be used to one's advantage. This is especially so when the compression is perpendicular to the long-axis direction of the muscle fibers being compressed. Thus the bent leg in

---

7   If you sleep with your wrist folded either forward or backward, you will wake up with the hand feeling numb from the pressure and the traction experienced by the ulnar nerve. Similarly, pressure on the sciatic nerve of the leg due to sitting too long without moving can make the leg "fall asleep."

ardha baddha padma paschimottanasana presses across the quadriceps muscle of the straight leg and so works to relax it in this posture. Similarly, *virasana* done with a rolled sticky mat set between the hamstrings and the calf muscles on each leg can relax the calf muscles and help them flatten (see also Subsection 11.D, page 448).

However, one must be careful not to overdo nerve compression, especially by either pressing too hard or by staying too long in those *yogasana* positions in which nerve compression may be a factor. For example, when meditators stay for hours in either *padmasana* or *muktasana,* the consequence can be a serious injury to the sciatic nerves in the legs at the points where one leg presses on the other (Subsection II.B, page 835). A similar statement holds for *paschimottanasana* performed for several hours at a time.

Neural Stretching

Because it is the longer afferent nerves going from the hands and feet to the spine that are most likely to be compressed at some point along their paths, tingling or numbness is not unusual in these parts when beginners first do their *yogasanas.* Nerve tissue is almost fluid in character, and though it is quite elastic and compressible, too sudden a stretch may overstretch it and so interfere with nerve conduction and/or microtubule transport, but slow and steady extension is easily accommodated [483]. Overstretching of the sciatic nerve can result in the phenomenon called "foot drop" (Subsection II.B, page 837).

When one moves from *tadasana* to *uttanasana,* not only are the hamstrings stretched but so too are the peripheral nerves that run along the back of the legs. This extension of the nerves is handled by the body in the following way [7]. As we stand with the back of the legs more or less relaxed in *tadasana,* the nerve bundles in the nerve bed are in a somewhat folded form (VVVVV), accordion style. On elongation of the surrounding muscle in *uttanasana,* such peripheral nerves can lengthen by up to 5 centimeters (2 inches) by just becoming straighter, with little or no stress being applied. Following this, the inherent elasticity of

the nerve fiber will allow another 20 percent extension; however, when the strain is between 20 and 30 percent, the extension becomes inelastic, and a certain amount of nerve damage is incurred; as the nerve is extended, its diameter decreases and its conduction velocity drops. At 30 percent extension, the nerve breaks.

Serious Injury to Nerves

Serious and long-lasting mechanical injuries to the nerves of the body can result from compression of the nerves, as when they are crushed when caught between two bones pressing on one another, from traction that overstretches and tears them, or from a combination of these situations. Extended pressure on a nerve first changes the properties of the nerve-blood barrier, followed by swelling, myelin thinning, and finally axonal degeneration. Nerves that are injured mechanically are slow to recover their functions, and if the nerve is completely severed, it will die, and so too will the muscle fibers innervated by it. Unlike simple creatures, mammals have nerves that do not mend themselves when severed. Mammals, with their large and complex brains, opt for stability rather than flexibility in this regard, trying to avoid the possible confusion of the neural miswiring that could occur if a bundle of severed nerves were reconnected [695].

Though there is no direct connection between the nerves that serve the two sides of the body, cases are reported in which a nerve on one arm is injured, for example, and the opposite arm sooner or later registers pain or numbness in a place that is the mirror image of the site of the initial injury [628]. This may be related to the phenomenon of "referral itch" (Section 13.D, page 532).

The functioning of neurons also is dependent on the acidity of the fluids in the vicinity of the nerves. In the pH range of 7.45 to 8.0, the extracellular fluid is basic, making the nerves hyperexcitable and possibly leading to cerebral convulsions. If the pH becomes more acidic, in the range 7.35 to 6.8, then the neurons become lethargic, and this can lead to a comatose state [863], as occurs when the carbon dioxide concentration rises too high in the air we breathe. Regarding body fluid, there is only a narrow basic range of pH, 7.35 to 7.45, within which the neurons of the body can operate optimally.

Degeneration of the efferent motor nerves in the brain and spinal cord leads to the muscle atrophy characteristic of amyotrophic lateral sclerosis (ALS), otherwise known as Lou Gehrig's disease. Though the glutamate ion is a neurotransmitter, it also is known to be toxic to motor neurons when in high concentrations and is present in excessive amounts in the spinal fluids of ALS patients. One wonders if the fatigue felt by *yogasana* students with multiple sclerosis is due to neural fatigue rather than to muscle fatigue.

Neurons Die

As with muscles, a neuron lasts a lifetime if used often (provided the microtubulin in its axon is not damaged); however, it withers away through apoptosis when it is not used at all. In this way, our signaling system tends to become more refined and more narrowed as our skills become more practiced and unused neural circuitry is discarded. This has the effect of making us better and better at skills that are more and more relevant to us, but at the same time, we become more and more narrow in what we can do physically, mentally, and emotionally. Practice of the endless variety of *yogasanas* certainly works to keep the largest possible number of neurons active and healthy.

Should the cell body of a neuron be destroyed by injury, then not only does the injured nerve die, but its synaptic neighbors also wither and die afterward (Subsection 11.A, page 377). The neural debris in the brain is cleared by the glial cells. In the adult, slight damage to axons in the peripheral nerves is self-repairing, but this generally is not so in the central nervous system [427, 553]. However, there is now intriguing evidence that certain of the neurons in the hippocampus are capable of regeneration and that rebirth of these neurons is stimulated by exercise [53]; however, the regeneration of the hippocampal cells is impeded by excess cortisol, as when stressed.

Should the spinal cord be severed at a particular point, then all axonal and dendritic features that are distal to the break will die if the features are those of efferent neurons in the cord, and all such features that are proximal to the break will die if the features are those of the afferent neurons in the cord. That is to say, all parts of the neurons severed from their cell bodies will die, whereas those parts that remain in contact with the cell body will survive.

Field Effects

The flow of electric charge along a neuron generates a magnetic field that can be easily sensed with modern medical equipment. The strongest such field arises from the beating of the heart [550, 637], which generates such an intense magnetic field that the entire body is enveloped by it and the heartbeat thereby becomes a synchronizing signal for many other body processes. Monitoring how this field changes with time yields a magnetocardiogram, much like an electrocardiogram (Section 14.A, page 548). One can take advantage of this coupling between magnetic field and electric current in the reverse way: the application of an external magnetic field focused on a particular area of the brain can either stimulate or inhibit it functionally and so allows one to understand the functions of the various brain nuclei by observing the consequences of turning them on or off (Subsection 4.D, page 105). This approach is known as transcranial magnetic stimulation. Evidence suggests that the laying on of hands for therapeutic purposes involves the radiation of intense magnetic fields from such hands [637].

Acoustic fields at frequencies far below the threshold for hearing also can have powerful effects on the body (Subsection 4.H, page 155, and Subsection 18.A, page 696), as can those that can be heard; for example, sounds at both acoustic and sub-acoustic frequencies can reduce pain sensations.

Section 3.F: Transduction of the Stimulus into the Sensory Signal

The Retina and Skin

Having discussed the important aspects of the formation of an action potential and how it might be conducted down the length of an axon and then chemically jump the synapse to an adjacent neuron, we turn briefly to the question of how a sensory organ can initiate such a process, given the wide diversity of sensors in the body. Unfortunately, there are answers to these questions for only a few of the receptor types, and even here, the explanation is sketchy. The best understood of these is the transduction of light at the retina into an action potential along the optic nerve [427].

When light is absorbed by the photopigment in the retina (Section 17.B, page 667), the pigment molecules first change their geometry in an act called "isomerization." The eventual result of this isomerization is the drastic reduction in the concentration of cyclic guanosine monophosphate (cGMP), a chemical within the retinal cell that effectively holds open the Na^+ channels in the cell's membrane. When the concentration of cGMP drops on exposure of the retina to light, the Na^+ channels close, while at the same time, the K^+ channels remain open to the outward flow of this ion. The net result of the blocking of the inward flow of Na^+ and the unrestricted outward flow of K^+ is the hyperpolarization of the retinal membrane when illuminated.

Remember now that a depolarized excitation wave can propagate for a long distance (over one meter) but hyperpolarization cannot (see Section 3.B, page 39). In the retina, the hyperpolarization upon illumination is able to travel passively for only 2 millimeters (0.1 inches), then connects to intermediate neurons (bipolar and multipolar) and then to the ganglion cells (figure 17.B-1). It is not yet clear how the hyperpolarization of the retinal cells eventually is transduced into depolarization of the ganglion cells, but it is relevant that in absolute darkness, there is an ongoing nonzero signal in the optic nerve called the "dark current." The effect of the hyperpolarization of the optical signal is to reduce the dark current, which is then sensed in the brain as proportional to the light intensity falling on the retina. In this way, the axons of the ganglion cells are depolarized and send their signals to higher centers in the brain via the optic nerves.

Transduction in the Pacinian corpuscles (Subsection 13.B, page 511), sensitive to deep pressure, is even less clear, involving in some way the mechanical deformation of the sensor bulb, the opening of specific ion channels, and the launching of a depolarizing action potential.

The Nature of Neural Information

Regardless of the nature of the sensory organ, if its stimulus is strong enough to result in an action potential, then a depolarization wave is launched toward its farther end. Depolarization waves traveling from different sensors are essentially the same: they are a series of voltage spikes, with frequencies proportional to their intensity of stimulation, but each traveling on its own unique highway, at first. The "signal" in nerve signaling is the depolarization wave (action potential) or its absence. Thus, every neuron in the body at any moment is either activated or not. The resulting pattern of activations and deactivations across all of the neural space—a pattern of ones and zeros, if you will—is the "information" contained within the nervous system. But now to add the aspect of stimulus intensity, one must consider a pattern of zeros, ones, twos, threes, etc., these representing the levels of excitation in a nerve fiber, ranging from none to very intense. As these signals move from the periphery to the central nervous system and return to the periphery, they are repeatedly fused together or separated into multiple branches, so that individual neural paths become more and more difficult to define the farther one moves away from the sensory source. Nonetheless, at any one instant, the patterns of zeros, ones, twos, threes, etc. represent a specific state of consciousness, but this is clearly shifting from moment to moment, if only because one is breathing, thinking, dreaming, acting, practicing *yogasana*, etc. The full spectrum of these neural states is represented schematically in figures 1.B-1 and 1.B-2.

This simplified picture of neural structure and states of consciousness appears in the work of Nobel Prize-winning scientist E. R. Kandel [427a], who points out that genetic and developmental processes control the pattern of connections within the brain, and though this is a constant of the brain within all of us, it offers a very wide spectrum of possibilities in the following way. Though we all are born with essentially the same pattern of neural connection in the brain, our learning experiences act to strengthen some synapses and weaken others; it is the control over the **strengths** of the synaptic connections in the brain, depending on our (learning) experiences, that leads to new patterns of behavior, differences in personality, varieties of interests, etc. Just how the strengths of synaptic connection are increased or decreased by learning is presented in Subsection 4.G, page 135.

Stochastic Resonance

Normally, noise is considered to be an interference when one is trying to sense a weak signal; however, it has been shown in several studies that the sensitivity of neural signals can be **increased** by the presence of noise, in a process known as stochastic resonance. In this phenomenon, the sensitivity of an organ increases when the sub-threshold, weak signal is superposed upon a background of subsensory random noise; the noise helps lift the signal into the realm of detectability by making some or all of it higher than the threshold value of the receptor potential. Because nerve cells fire spontaneously on a twenty-four-hour basis, leading to a certain amount of unavoidable noise in the neural channels, they generate the noise needed for stochastic resonance to function. Thus, for example, the pressure sensitivity of the Pacinian corpuscles in the soles of the feet, so useful for balancing, become even higher if the soles of the feet are vibrated randomly (Subsection V.C, page 895) [673, 675], and the sensitivity of the eye to detect an oscillation of the intensity of light increases when there is a random flickering of the light superposed upon a regular but weakly oscillating light source [375]. It has been demonstrated that stochastic resonance is not only an enhancing factor in balancing but is also a factor within the brain in problem solving and creativity, in tactile function, in stimulation of the muscle spindles, in the baroreflex, in the auditory system, and in aspects of brain function.

The Central Nervous System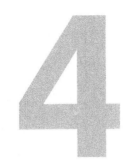

The central nervous system consists of the brain, the spinal cord, and the brainstem that connects them (figure 2.B-1); this division into three parts is a matter of topological convenience, as the spinal cord actually is able to perform several of the complex functions normally assumed to be under the brain's dominion. Each of these components of the central nervous system, from the lowest to the highest, is discussed in detail in Sections 4.A, page 67, 4.B, page 72, and 4.C, page 78.

The three distinct functional-geographic areas of the central nervous system (figures 2.A-1 and 2.B-1) are not only arranged geographically within the brain from the bottom to the top, but the levels of consciousness vary from nonexistent to high in the same order, and their appearance in the course of evolution of our species also followed in the same order; i.e., from lower to higher. The three levels, in order of (a) increasing height above the base of the spinal cord, (b) level of consciousness, and (c) evolutionary age, are the spinal cord, the brainstem, and the brain, the last of which includes the limbic system, the association areas, and the cerebral cortex.

Section 4.A: The Spinal Cord

Structure and Function

The spinal cord has three broad functions: (1) it is the pathway for ascending neural impulses from the body's sensors; (2) it is the pathway for the descending neural impulses that drive the body's muscles, organs and glands; and (3) it contains the relatively primitive neural circuitry that guides such reflexive actions as vomiting and repetitive actions such as breathing and walking [181]. All three functions of the spinal cord are integral to maintaining homeostasis.

Structure

Beginning at the foramen magnum at the base of the skull and passing through the canal within the vertebral column, the spinal cord is a half-meter-long (twenty-inch), one-centimeter-thick (0.4 inches) elongation of the central nervous system, terminating at the L1 vertebra, though the canal itself extends to S4, and individual nerves extend to S5 before exiting (figure 4.A-1a) [360, 427, 431, 432, 574]. The spinal cord is no thicker than 2.5 centimeters (one inch) at any point and is soft and jellylike, much like the tissue within the cranium [553]. Though some neurons in the spinal cord run its entire length, most are shorter, entering or leaving the cord at intermediate points. The spinal cord contains bundles of the axons of neurons called fascicles, which are surrounded by the perineural sheath. In turn, the fascicles are bound together by the epineural sheath.

The thickness of the spinal cord is largest at those places where it branches to begin its run to the limbs; i.e., at L1-S2 in the lumbar region, where it serves the legs, and at C3-T1, where it serves the arms. It is thinnest in the thoracic and lower sacral regions.

The weight of neural tissue in the spinal cord is only 4 percent that of the weight of the brain [68]; however, being tissue with an active metabolism, the spinal cord is well supplied with blood

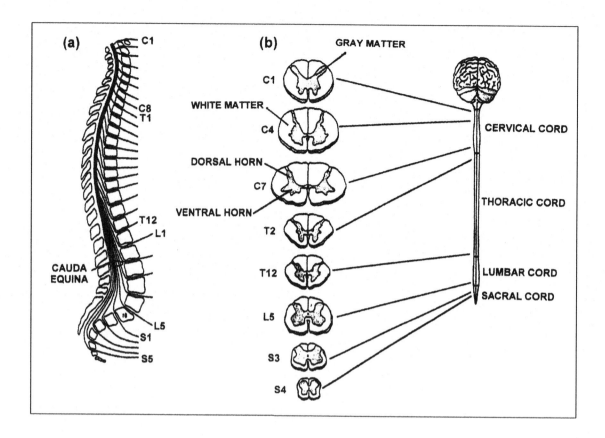

Figure 4.A-1. (a) The spinal cord within the spinal column as viewed with the posterior side to the left, showing the points at which the various spinal nerves exit through the intervertebral foramina between adjacent vertebrae. Note that the adult spinal cord proper extends only to L1, though the nerves exit as low as S5. The spinal nerves are numbered as one larger than the numbering of the vertebra above the nerve. (b) Selected cross sections of the spinal cord taken at the elevations as marked and with the demarcations between gray and white matter and between the dorsal and the ventral horns as indicated.

vessels lying within the tissue between the perineuria surrounding the neural fascicles. In this way, the tissue of the spinal cord differs from that of the vertebral discs. Surprisingly, nerves within the spinal cord can remain viable for up to thirty minutes without oxygen or glucose, whereas after only ten minutes under the same conditions, the neurons within the brain irreversibly cease to function. This difference probably relates to the fact that under normal conditions, the brain has a high-volume blood throughput, reflecting a strong need for oxygen, whereas that to the spinal cord is relatively meager, as evidenced by its much lower blood flow. The question of the proper oxygenation of nerve tissue is an important one, with many implications for those practicing *yogasana* (Subsection 3.E, page 61, and Subsection 11.B, page 437).

White and Gray Matter

Being the inferior section of the central nervous system, the spinal cord floats in the surrounding cerebrospinal fluid, just as does the brain itself (Subsection 4.E, page 107). Though floating, the spinal cord is anchored within the spinal canal by its connection to the brain at the top, by lateral ligaments to the surrounding dura mater at the sides, and by the connection to the coccyx at the bottom. As seen in radial cross section (figure 4.A-1b), the spinal cord shows a central region in the shape of the letter H (this material being called the gray matter), which is surrounded by a field of white matter. This pattern persists throughout the length of the spinal cord. Bundles of the white matter of the spinal cord (called ascending and descending tracts) appear so because the axons of each of the neurons within them are coated with a lipoprotein called myelin (Subsection 3.A, page 35). Whereas wearing a myelin coat insures a high velocity of nerve transmission along the fiber, when this coating is disrupted, the nerve signal within the axon too is blocked at the site of the disruption, rather than being transmitted [553]. Though the axons may be myelinated and appear as white tissue, the cell bodies themselves and the supporting neuroglia are not myelinated and so appear as gray tissue.

The gray matter in the cord is largely involved with the local transfer of neural signals at its particular level in the spinal cord, in contrast to the axons of the white matter, which run more or less the full length of the cord. Of course, there are interconnections between the white and gray matter, and there is branching of the white matter at different levels of the cord. Shorter intersegmental tracts connect the longer ascending and descending tracts of the white matter and are used in reflex reactions (Section 11.D, page 446). Nonetheless, if there were a severe injury to the gray matter at, say, T1, then ascending and descending nerve contact with the fingers and hands would be lost; however, the same injury to the white matter at T1 would mean paralysis not only of the functions particular to T1, but to all functions below that point as well (see tables 8.C-1, 8.C-2, 8.C-3, and 13.D-1 for listings of the correlation of vertebral roots with peripheral body parts).

Nerves that carry sensory information from the periphery to the central nervous system are called afferents, whereas those that carry neural impulses from the central nervous system to the muscles, glands, and viscera are known as efferents. The four prongs of the H-shaped gray matter (figure 4.A-2) are the dorsal (posterior, to the rear) and ventral (anterior, to the front) horns, the former of which is a reception point for afferent signals coming from the sensors on the left and right within the muscles, glands, and organs, whereas the latter is the point of departure for efferent motor neurons that will activate the viscera, the glands, and the left and right muscles [360, 553]. Neural axons within the gray region are not

myelinated, and consequently conduct signals at a much slower rate than do the myelinated axons.

Among the neural paths of the central nervous system at all levels of the spinal cord, there are both ascending and descending paths involving connections to the autonomic nervous system (Chapter 5, page 157). Nerve fibers originating in the spinal cord and ascending to the brain pass through the reticular formation (Subsection 4.B, page 74), where they may become relevant factors in the sleep/wake cycle, in arousal, attention, and in the inhibition of pain [432].

The white matter of the spinal cord consists of long tracts of afferent nerves transmitting sensory information upward to the higher centers and efferent motor-nerve impulses downward from those higher points to the relevant muscles and organs.[1] In both the white matter and the gray, there are many glial cells that help to keep the nerve fibers healthy by performing many housekeeping tasks (see also Subsection 3.A, page 37).

Decussation

Also shown in figure 4.A-2 is a decussation in which afferent neurons from the left side of the body synapse across the gray matter to ascend on the right side. In this case, an ascending neural signal coming from the left side of the body will be sent to the sensory cortex within the right cerebral hemisphere and vice versa (Section 4.D, page 98).

Each spinal nerve serves a specific body area or part. This segmentation of the nervous system is especially obvious in the dermatome map of the body's skin (Section 13.D, page 530) and can be traced backward in time to the segmentation of

---

1   It may be helpful to think of the neurons in the body as electrical wires connected in unique ways; however, it is equally important to realize that there are many breaks (synapses) in the "wires," which are chemically switched on and off in specific patterns by outside forces. Thus, brain function is dependent not only on which neurons are connected to one another, but also on which synapses at any one moment are conducting and which are not, and upon the relative signs of the effective electrical potentials being transferred across the synapses.

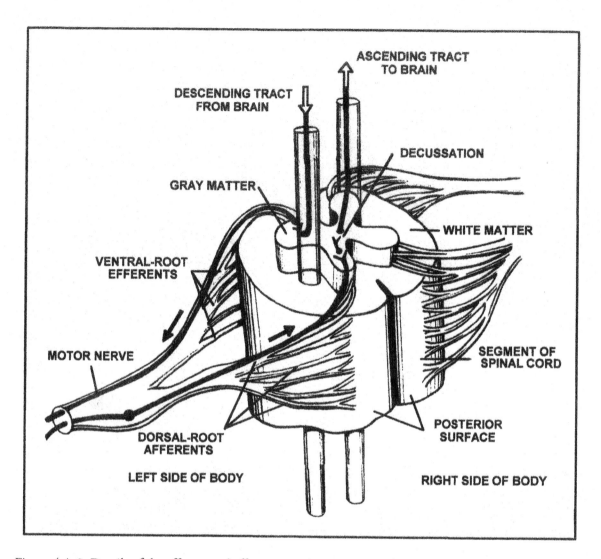

Figure 4.A-2. Details of the efferent and afferent neural roots in typical cross sections of the spinal cord. A left-to-right decussation is shown in the gray matter between the ascending and descending tracts. White matter also bears ascending and descending tracts of axons to and from the brain, which tracts also synapse to more local neurons.

the nervous system in an early ancestor of ours, the earthworm [574]!

Afferent and efferent nerves serving a particular peripheral location are bundled together between that location and the spinal cord. However, they are separate within the spinal cord, with the afferent nerves entering the dorsal surface of the spinal cord, whereas the efferent nerves leave at the ventral side of the spine and then join the nerve bundle (figure 4.A-2). Similarly, in the peripheral region, the bundle is again separated into those efferent neurons that will activate the muscles and organs and the afferent neurons that will carry the associated sensory signals. Once outside

the central nervous system, the cell bodies of the neural afferents tend to gather in loose groups of tissue called ganglia.

Neural Roots

Each of the vertebrae in the spinal column has left and right intervertebral foramina, through which openings the nerve bundles pass laterally to the outside (figure 4.A-1a); there are thirty such pairs of bundles (eight cervical, twelve thoracic, five lumbar, and five sacral). Each such bundle has dorsal and ventral components, the former for sensory neurons and the latter for motor neurons. Additionally, there are twelve pairs of nerve bundles that enter and leave the spinal cord at the level of the brainstem above the uppermost vertebra (C1); these are cranial nerves I through XII (Subsection 2.C, page 24). The fitting of the nerve bundles through the intervertebral foramina is not a tight one; for example, at L5, the nerve roots glide freely through the intervertebral foramina by up to 12 millimeters (0.5 inches), unless the sliding is restrained by intervertebral-disc pressure on the nerve root.

The nerve bundles exiting from the spinal cord are numbered according to the number of the vertebrae involved in forming their particular foramen. In the cervical region, each bundle has a number that is one larger than the number of the upper vertebra; thus, the lowest such nerve bundle is called C8, though there is no vertebra labeled as C8. However, in the remainder of the spine, the numbering is just that of the upper member of the vertebral joint; i.e., the bundles are called T1 to T11 as they issue from the foramina formed by the T1–T2 and T11–T12 joints in the spinal column, respectively.

Neural Connectivity

One sees that the spinal cord is an active intermediary in the flow of neural traffic signals, which signals flow from all parts of the body to the brain along sensory paths, and from the brain along somatic paths to the muscles (voluntary and involuntary), visceral organs, and glands in all parts of the body. However, the function of the spinal cord goes far beyond just being a conduit for two-way neural traffic, for there is considerable integration of nerve signals and processing of information involving interneurons that goes on within it. This integration is especially important for reflex reactions. Thus, for example, it is known that the neural circuitry that drives certain repetitive but unthinking actions such as breathing, swallowing, chewing, running, walking, and eye movements involves "central-pattern generators" located within the spinal cord itself [300]. Of course, the turning on and off of the central-pattern generators is a task for the higher brain centers, and bringing such repetitive, unthinking

actions under more conscious control is a goal for the *yogasana* student. Furthermore, fibers ascending to the sensory cortex have collateral excitatory and inhibitory synapses with descending signals from the thalamus in order to fine-tune sensory perceptions.

Not all of the sensory fibers synapse at the dorsal horns; those relaying information about pain, temperature, and crude tactile sensation use an extra-spinal pathway to the thalamus called the spinothalamic path. With its slow, unmyelinated type-C fibers (see table 3.B-2), the spinothalamic path is primitive but is found in all vertebrates, including man. A second afferent path to higher centers using swift type-A conductors (table 3.B-2) is found in humans and primates and carries the information concerning precise localization of touch sensations, pressure, vibration, and proprioception. The fibers of this more modern system run uninterrupted along the length of the spinal cord until they synapse in the medulla oblongata [432]. Of course, sensory and motor signals to and from the head and face do not move through the spinal cord, but use the cranial nerves instead.

The Foramen Magnum

The largest opening in the skull allowing access to the brain is the foramen magnum at the base of the occipital plate of the skull (figure 9.A-2b). It is at the foramen magnum that the pattern of white matter surrounding gray in the spinal cord is reversed, with the gray matter surrounding the white from this point upward. However, unlike the gray matter of the brain, that of the spinal cord does not "think," but is used instead for reflexive subconscious acts. It is also at the foramen magnum that many ascending and descending nerves decussate; which is to say, it is at this point that the sensations originating on the left side of the body cross over so as to register in the right cerebral hemisphere, and vice versa for those originating on the right side of the body. Similarly, the motor nerves from the cortex also decussate at the foramen magnum on their downward paths. The foramen magnum is also the portal through which the medulla oblongata and the vertebral and spinal arteries pass.

Injury

Unlike broken bones, which heal rapidly, and torn ligaments, which heal far more slowly, badly injured nerves in the spinal cord do not heal at all and do not regenerate spontaneously [553]; however, when injured only slightly, the more peripheral nerves can repair themselves somewhat more easily, provided the cell body is intact and scar tissue does not form too rapidly at the injury site. Stem-cell research offers hope for the growth of neurons to replace those in the spinal cord that are badly injured or dead.

Section 4.B: The Brainstem

Lying just above the spinal cord (figure 4.B-1), the vegetative/reflexive brainstem works to control various body functions, such as respiration and digestion, in an automatic way and also to integrate brain reflexes. The brainstem is continuous with the spinal cord, positioned between the upper end of the spinal cord and the base of the limbic system in the brain, and it passes from the skull to the spinal cord through the foramen magnum in the occipital bone of the skull. Also known as the reptilian brain, today's brainstem has survived for 200 million years in vertebrate animals. Given in top-to-bottom order, the brainstem is home to the midbrain, the pons, the medulla oblongata, and (also at the level of the medulla oblongata) the cerebellum. Yet another structure, the reticular formation, runs the length of the brainstem as a thin sheet.

The five major parts of the brainstem—the medulla oblongata, the pons, the cerebellum, the midbrain, and the reticular formation (figure 4.B-1)—are conduits for both ascending and descending information between the upper brain and the spinal cord. Of these, the reticular formation is an especially important area within the brainstem, for it regulates the levels of awareness and arousal by controlling which of the spinal signals are allowed to ascend to the higher cortical areas. The brainstem also is involved in receiving

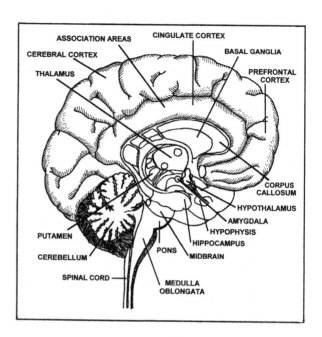

Figure 4.B-1. Cross section of the brain and brainstem in the parasagittal plane.

sensory information from the head and controlling muscle action in the face and neck via the cranial nerves.

Subconscious Action

In contrast to the high levels of awareness associated with neural excitations in the cerebral cortices, neural signals traversing the brainstem are largely below the level of our awareness but no less important to our being. Though the effects of the primitive vegetative brain rarely, if ever, impact on the conscious level,[2] the brainstem is essential for life, as it maintains the basic life processes, with damage to the brainstem being an immediate threat to life. In fact, the brainstem contains the one neurocranial structure (the reticular formation) without which life is impossible [199].

The Medulla Oblongata

The medulla oblongata within the brainstem (figure 4.B-1) is connected to and is continuous

---

2   However, see Subsection 11.C, page 441, for a contrary view.

with the spinal cord and is responsible for autonomic functions such as digestion, breathing, and heart rate (Section 14.A, page 550). In this region, the motor fibers for voluntary action connecting the cortex to the spinal cord decussate—i.e., cross over from side to side—so that muscle activation on the right-hand side of the body is controlled by the left cerebral hemisphere and vice versa [360]. When one is dreaming during sleep, the medial medulla is inactive, so that there is little or no muscle action, in spite of the action portrayed in the dream. In this regard, weakness of the hands on awakening is thought possibly to be the result of an inhibition of the central nervous system by the lateral medulla oblongata, which is active during sleep in order to keep the muscles passive while dreaming (but not while sleepwalking)!

The Cerebellum

As is the case with the cortex, the cerebellum (figure 4.B-1) is corrugated and has an outer layer of gray matter covering the white matter within; it is second only to the cerebral cortex in size. See figure 3.A-1f for a picture of the fan-like Purkinje neural cell of the cerebellum and the immense web of interconnection that such a neuron can provide. The cerebellum would have roughly the same surface area when laid flat as would one of the cortical hemispheres, and it actually is much more strongly folded than the cortex. Internally, the cerebellum is highly organized, appearing almost crystalline in the ordering of its parts.

As it is with the cerebrum, the cerebellum is divided into hemispheres; however, there is nothing to indicate any left-right hemispheric differences in the cerebellum. Thus, the cerebellum disobeys the general rule of contralaterality in the nervous system; i.e., each cerebellar hemisphere modulates motor activity (primarily through inhibition) of the limbs on its side of the body rather than on the opposite side. As appropriate for an organ of evolutionary importance in humans, the size of the cerebellum has increased over the past million years, yet the patterns of connectivity within the cerebellum have remained relatively constant for the past 200 million years in vertebrates. Though the cerebellum contributes only 10 percent of the brain's weight, it comprises 40 percent of the brain's surface area and contains more than 50 percent of the brain's neurons [85]. Five distinct types of neuron are found in the cerebellum, four of which are inhibitory in their actions and one of which is excitatory.

Proprioception and Yogasana

For the *yogasana* student, two of the major functions of the brain involve the receiving and weighing of sensory input from the proprioceptive sensors (Subsection 11.C, page 441) and then activating the appropriate muscles and organs at the appropriate times; this is carried out within the cerebellum. The cerebellum has no direct motor function but is the main center for the integration of proprioceptive information and thus is essential for the smooth subconscious control of the skeletal muscles and the learning of motor skills of the sort encountered in *yogasana* practice. The cerebellum also coordinates the proprioceptive signals from the muscles and joints with the afferent signals from the vestibular organs of the inner ears, the pressure sensors in the skin, and from the eyes and so is a key factor in keeping one's balance (Section V.C, page 886). The cerebellum not only communicates directly with the cortex in order to guide muscle action and to help maintain posture and balance, but it also actively inhibits postural reflexes (see Subsection 11.D, page 446).

In practicing a technique such as the *yogasanas*, the planning of the movements and the call for the activation of specific muscles originates at the motor cortex; however, the timing as to when these specific muscles are to be contracted or relaxed is the job of the cerebellum, which intercepts the cortical signals and delays them appropriately in time. Simultaneous with this motor control, the cerebellum is the destination for the proprioceptive afferents containing the information about muscle tension, joint angles, limb velocities, and general body posture. This ongoing stream of postural information is compared in the cerebellum with the planned movements, and any discrepancies are corrected as they are sensed. As mentioned in Section 1.B, page 9, it is one of the goals of *yogasana* practice to bring our actions into agreement with our intentions. To this end, the cerebellum is indispensable, for it functions as a comparator, measuring our muscular performance in real time against our intentions as dictated by the central commands for movement.

The subconscious functioning of the cerebellum in the performance of the *yogasanas* in both balancing and the timing of muscle actions cannot be overemphasized. As might be expected, disease or damage to the cerebellum leads directly to a loss of muscle coordination, balance, and muscle tone [528, 582, 621]. Diseases of the cerebellum can result in muscle tremors when the muscle action is intentional, unlike the tremor due to Parkinsonism, which occurs when the muscle is nominally at rest.

More modern experiments on the cerebellum show that it functions in a broader arena than just that of body movement [85], for not only is it involved intimately with the coordination of movements but also in the coordination of sensory input, largely involving finger touch in humans. This is especially interesting, for the application of finger-touch sensitivity to balancing on the foot as discussed in Subsection V.C, page 902, is otherwise quite remarkable and surprising, but now we see that the balancing actions on the foot and finger-touch sensitivity meet and interact in the cerebellum. For the role of the cerebellum in balance and dyslexia, see Subsection 18.B, page 699.

As with the cortex, there are also sensory maps within the cerebellum and within the hippocampus (Subsection 4.C, page 81); however, they are much more disjointed and fragmented than that within the cortex.

The Pons

The pons deals with information about body movement, carrying it from the cerebral hemisphere to the cerebellum. Together with the me-

dulla oblongata, the pons regulates the parameters of blood pressure and respiration. A most important function of the pons involves the reticular formation (see the relevant subsection beginning this page).

The Midbrain

The midbrain occupies the uppermost portion of the brainstem and not only controls reflex patterns associated with the visual and auditory systems (for example, the reflexive opening of the pupils of the eyes when in dim light is controlled by the midbrain) but also is a factor in controlling body movement.

Arousal within the Reticular Formation

The brain has evolved primarily as a pattern-recognition device with sensitivity toward those events that either enhance or threaten our survival in a world over-filled with neural signals that are largely irrelevant to our survival. This filtering and alerting action takes place in the brainstem in a narrow sheet of vertical tissue known as the reticular formation; almost all mammals have a reticular formation.

Structure

Being a column of diffuse neurons arranged in narrow, vertical sheets in the brainstem (figure 4.B-2), stretching from the medulla oblongata to the hypothalamus and beyond, the reticular formation regulates motor functions, sleep, consciousness, attention and concentration, respiration, and vascular functions [360, 432]. Fibers within the reticular formation are connected to the gray matter of the spinal cord at the lower end, pass through the hypothalamus and the thalamus (the gateway to the cortex), and terminate at the cortex at the upper end. Sensory signals from all of the sensory organs (proprioceptive, olfactory, taste, auditory, etc.) enter the reticular formation via the ascending reticular activating system for processing before being sent to the hypothalamus, except for visual information, which bypasses the reticular formation and goes directly

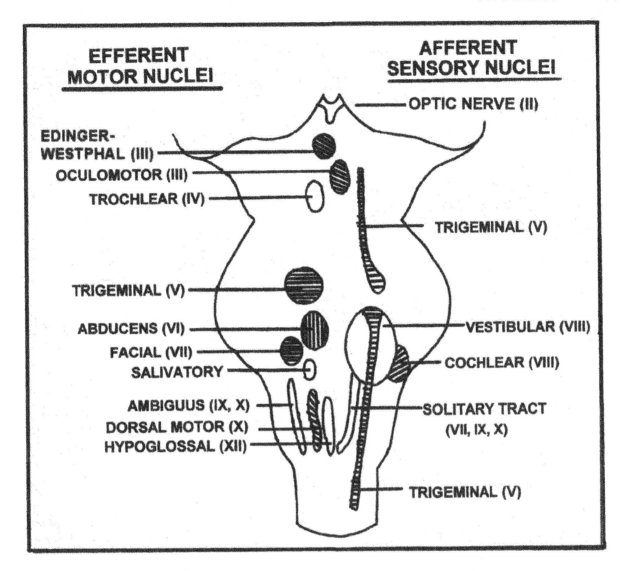

Figure 4.B-2. Anatomy of the reticular formation, showing several of the important brainstem nuclei, most connected to the cranial nerves in the motor and/or the sensory branches. The cranial nerves so involved (Subsection 2.C, page 24) are identified by the Roman numerals in parentheses.

to the hypothalamus. Norepinephrine acts as a neuromodulator within the synapses of the reticular formation.

Function

If the reticular formation deems the sensory message to be significant, it will pass that message upward to the cortex, alerting it to a possible relevant change in the status of one of the sensory receptors. It is estimated that between ten million and one hundred billion bits of information per second impinge on the sensors of the body and are then forwarded by afferent neurons to the reticular formation. If all of this sensory in-

formation sent to the reticular formation were to be transmitted upward to the higher centers in the brain, there would be an immediate overload. The function of the reticular formation is to filter this mass of data and then relay only that part that is of immediate importance. It does this on the basis of change: if signals from sensors or receptors are constant, then they safely can be ignored in favor of those few that are changing in time. Thus, any rapid change in the sensory field of the organism is immediately forwarded by the reticular formation for consideration by the higher faculties. This extreme filtering trims the number of information bits that exit the reticular formation to about sixteen to twenty bits per second.

Additionally, the reticular formation receives proprioceptive signals reflecting falling or loss of balance of the body and then reflexively stimulates the antigravity extensor muscles that support the body against falling or collapse. These proprioceptive signals arrive directly from balance sensors or indirectly via signals first sent to the cerebellum. In this regard, some of the most important proprioceptors are muscle spindles in the back of the neck (Section 11.C, page 441). The reticular formation is also the relevant terminus of many afferent cranial nerves (Subsection 2.C, page 24) from sensors to the central nervous system, and of efferent cranial nerves from the central nervous system to the muscles.

In addition to the motor functions that originate in the cerebral cortex, motor functions are also directed by the reticular formation. In general, motor functions are strongly interacting and widely dispersed in the brain, so that it is difficult to assign specific motor functions to specific locales in the brain, other than to the motor and premotor cortices [708].

Inhibition

The lowest part of the reticular formation is especially inhibitory. Yoga Sutra I.2 of Patanjali, which states, "The goal of yoga is to still the fluctuations of the mind," might be translated into modern medical language as "The goal of yoga practice is to repress virtually all of the afferent neural activations that impinge upon the reticular formation from below." This would be particularly relevant to the practice of *pratyahara,* during which one actively blocks out all external stimuli. The inhibition of such superfluous neural signals is accomplished through the use of interneurons (Subsection 3.C, page 51).

In an article describing the possible benefits and risks of performing *sirsasana,* Chandra [112a] mentions that the stimulation of the carotid baroreceptors in the arteries of the neck when in *sirsasana* results in an effective numbing of the reticular formation, thereby making it easier for one to fall asleep if the posture is performed at

bedtime, though it does not appear to be sleep-inducing when performed at other times. In fact, it is *sarvangasana,* which is traditionally the inversion used for relaxation of the body and the mind (Subsection 11.D, page 456).

Brain Waves

If one is totally relaxed, so that there are few or no external stimuli going beyond the reticular formation, then the EEG brain-wave pattern (Section 4.H, page 151) settles into the low-frequency, high-amplitude alpha-wave mode, signaling relaxed wakefulness and tranquility. On the other hand, any sensory input that successfully traverses the reticular formation brings one into a state of normal wakefulness, with the EEG pattern then shifting to that of high-frequency, low-amplitude beta waves.

Though it is generally true that any input signal from peripheral sensors (such as the pressure sensors in the sole of the foot) will arouse the reticular formation, as witnessed by the shift from the alpha to the beta brain-wave pattern, it is also to be noted that in the case of meditating adepts, there is no interruption of the alpha brain-wave pattern when the eyes are open, in a noisy room, etc. The brain waves of one meditator showed no change in alpha pattern when his hand was plunged into ice water and left there for forty-five minutes; another maintained a constant, unbroken pattern of alpha waves for nine hours [371]. According to B. K. S. Iyengar, it is possible to reach such deep states of alpha-wave inward directedness in the *yogasanas* [390]. The similarities between such deeply meditative yogic states and the hypnotic state have been pointed out repeatedly [178, 182, 371, 699]; however, the constancy of the alpha-wave pattern fluctuates when in the presence of distractions in the hypnotic state, whereas this is not the case when in the meditative yogic state [699].

Consciousness

Not only are there ascending sensory neurons from the both the muscles and the visceral organs passing through the reticular formation, but there are also descending signals from forebrain structures and the central nervous system. When functioning properly, the brain exhibits a high degree of coordination among the ascending and descending neural signals traversing the reticular formation. Not only does information move both upward and downward through the reticular formation, but their interactions within the reticular formation can also change our mental and physical states by stimulating both excitatory and inhibitory synapses in the brain. For example, ascending activity in the reticular formation leads to a change of consciousness from drowsy to attentive. This then leads (on the descending side) to increased muscle tone and stimulation of the sympathetic branch of the autonomic nervous system (Chapter 5, page 170); i.e., increased heart rate, blood pressure, etc.

In particular, the reticular formation and the cortex appear to be mutually activating, with a constant flow of neural signals between them. A similar mutual activation is ongoing between the reticular formation and the proprioceptors within the skeletal muscles. The simultaneous operation of the circuit between the cortical and reticular formation and the circuit between the reticular formation and the proprioceptors results in a mental state we know as "consciousness," whereas a temporary inactivation of the reticular formation is called "sleep." Should the reticular formation be damaged or otherwise nonfunctional, the result is eternal sleep (coma), as no cortical arousal is possible when the reticular formation is unresponsive [544].

Effects of Drugs

Activation and deactivation of the reticular formation is readily accomplished with the appropriate drugs. Thus, amphetamines stimulate the reticular formation, leading to a hyper-alert state of high consciousness and twitching muscles, whereas tranquilizers and depressants lower the level of excitation in the reticular formation, leading to states of relaxation or general anesthesia, depending upon the dose [422]. Drugs such as marijuana, LSD, and heroin have strong effects on the operation of the reticular formation [68], and even watching television for half an hour can lull the reticular formation into the alpha-state EEG characteristic of unfocused attention.

Relaxation in Savasana

Stimulation of any of the sensory organs leads to excitation of the reticular formation and consequently, an arousal of the sympathetic nervous system (Section 5.C, page 170). With this in mind, it is clear why a truly deep state of relaxation in *savasana* requires that the eyes be closed with the room lights off, no external sound, and the body being touched only by the floor, as these conditions strongly limit the sensations incident upon the reticular formation. Actually, even floor pressure gives a sensible signal for a few minutes, but if it is a comfortable contact, the sensory signal adapts downward, and the sense of pressure fades to zero (Subsection 13.B, page 506). Furthermore, any muscular movement beyond that of the breath and heart will be arousing to the reticular formation, and so has to be resisted in *savasana*. In contrast, when in the other *yogasanas,* one must constantly make micro-adjustments to the posture in order to keep the proprioceptive map from becoming static and so fading from consciousness (Subsection 11.C, page 441); in *savasana*, one does the opposite.

The oculomotor nucleus is one of over forty such nuclei in the reticular formation (figure 4.B-2) and is the termination of cranial nerve III. As this nerve and its reticular-formation center are prominently involved with all manner of eye motion [360], such eye motion can be taken as a rough measure of reticular-formation arousal. The eye movement so often seen in students while in *savasana* suggests that there is residual but random stimulation of the reticular formation in their "relaxed" state, rather like beta-wave activation or REM (rapid eye movement) sleep. As a truly deep state of *savasana* will be largely free of REM activity, the use of an eye bag (or any soft, opaque, and weighty material placed over the eyes) may be called for, as this acts to damp out extraneous motions of the eyes.[3]

---

3 Note that too heavy an eye bag can flatten the eyeball and that when it is removed, vision can be dis-

Note that as the proprioceptive signal fades while one is in *savasana,* one also experiences a loss of sense of Self (Subsection 13.B, page 506). *Yogasana* students suffering from depression or low blood pressure especially should be urged to keep their eyes open in all of the postures intended to energize them, for closing the eyes allows the reticular formation to relax, followed by a de-energized feeling and a loss of self-awareness.

When teaching *savasana,* one can talk the student toward a state of relaxation; however, in order for the student to achieve that state, the teacher must then be quiet, so that there is no further auditory stimulation of the reticular formation. When releasing into meditation or sleep, the last sense to disappear is that of sound, and it is the first to reappear when awakening. Thus, one sees how important it is for the teacher to remain as quiet as possible during the latter phase of this *yogasana.*

Section 4.C: Within the Brain

Brain Structure

Resting on top of the brainstem (figure 4.B-1), the brain is at the pinnacle of the central nervous system (figure 2.A-1). This marvelous human organ is even more astounding the more we learn of its abilities and the magnitude of problems it can solve with apparent ease. In this chapter, we will look at the basic components of the brain, their functions, and how these functions come into play when we practice the *yogasanas.* Needless to say, the subject of the brain, its structure, and function is endlessly complex; in this work, we will only scratch the surface as we connect the basic elements of brain function to

yogasana practice. As shown in figure 2.A-1, the brain can be dissected into a number of subsystems, which range in position from high (cerebral cortex) to low (the limbic system), but in decreasing degrees of awareness from high to low, and in increasing phylogenetic age from high to low position.

Size

The adult human brain weighs 1,350 grams (three pounds), has a volume of 1,400 cubic centimeters (1.4 liters) on average, and is thought to contain approximately 100 billion nerve cells (neurons). By comparison, the blowfly and the ant have brains weighing only 0.084 and 0.00001 grams, respectively, there being only ten to twenty thousand neurons in the brains of each of these. The neural count is about 250 thousand in the housefly, one million in the bee, and 700 million in the mouse. Considering the complex actions that insects such as the ant and the bee are capable only sets the stage for the amazing feats of a human brain more than a million times larger. Moreover, the human brain, with "new" hardware and software, is able to do things that the brains of lower beings could not dream of doing, even if their brains were magnified a million times. Though the size of the human brain is 700 percent larger than one might otherwise guess, given the size of the human body, both dolphins and whales have yet larger brains than man.

As if the sheer number of neurons in the human brain were not enough, be aware that many of these are connected to as many as 60,000 other neurons, averaging several thousand synapses per neuron. This leads to the numbers of synapses in the brain amounting to about one million billion. Furthermore, the strengths of these neural connections vary with our experiences. As a consequence, each of us has a unique pattern consisting of which neurons are connected to other neurons, with what strength of connection, and whether the signal passing from one neuron to the next supports or inhibits a particular action; these patterns literally have no limit in their variety.

---

torted temporarily. Extraneous movements, such as fluttering or darting eyes, also may occur when students are in other restorative postures, such as *supta baddha konasana,* and should be brought to the student's attention.

Surrounding Fluid

Though there is no collagen to bind the brain cells to one another, the overall texture of the brain is that of gelatin. This soft structure within the neurocranium is surrounded by cerebrospinal fluid (CSF), and because the brain has a density of 0.96 grams per milliliter (equal to 1,350 grams per 1,400 milliliters), somewhat less than that of the CSF surrounding it (density very close to 1.00 gram per milliliter), it tends to float in this cushioning fluid (Subsection 4.E, page 107).

Neurogenesis

Until recently, it was thought that neurons in the brain did not reproduce, so that the number of such cells could only decrease with time, and mental functioning could only degrade as one aged. With the recent discovery of stem cells and their amazing properties, this has changed. In particular, it is now known that stem cells can replace worn-out cells in their particular organs. Most amazing is the apparent plasticity of stem cells of one particular organ type that change their character to a second organ type when placed in contact with tissue of that second type [874]. At present, the general feeling is that there are few stem cells in the brain but that the brain is supplied with far too many cells at birth, and if we stay physically healthy and mentally active, the brain does not need replacement cells on a large scale [278]. Note too that the plasticity of the synaptic patterns allows rewiring of the brain to accommodate the loss of certain neurons with age.

Many recent experiments suggest that neurogenesis does occur within the brain, at least in the hippocampus, and that this process is aided significantly by the glial cells, which serve in part as housekeeper cells to the information-carrying neurons. On the other hand, it has been shown experimentally that the age of the cells in the cerebellum and the occipital cortices of subjects in their thirties equals the age of the brain since birth, implying that there has been very little or no neurogenesis in these areas for more than thirty years. In contrast, in the same subjects, the age of the gastrointestinal tissue was less than sixteen years, and the age of their muscles was just over fifteen years. Further aspects of brain growth and death are presented in Subsection 4.E, page 119.

Brain Shrinkage

Surprisingly, the human brain begins to die, in a sense, even before it is born. One's brain contains the largest number of brain cells that it will ever have at the fourth month in utero, and though the brain will increase in volume by a factor of three by the time an infant reaches adulthood, brain cells are dying by apoptosis (Subsection 3.A, page 32) in a programmed way at a rate of up to a million per day. As mentioned above, until very recently, it was thought that neurons do not reproduce themselves once we have reached maturity, however, this static picture is changing as stem-cell research proceeds. Also see Section 24.B, page 817, in this regard.

Each neuron in the brain (on average) has about 2,500 synaptic connections at birth, but this number increases to 15,000 by age three years, and then this number is reduced to about a few thousand per neuron in the average adult. As we age, synaptic connections are deleted in a process called synaptic pruning, which eliminates weaker synaptic connections in the brain in favor of stronger ones, using the process of programmed neural apoptosis. In this apoptotic process, the weaker connections are those that are infrequently or never used, whereas the stronger ones are stronger because they are used frequently. Neural circuits that are not used eventually disappear, with their places in the brain replaced by the expansion of other brain functions that are used more often. In this way, the brain is shaped by our practice, our learning, our culture, and our environment. This "use it or lose it" scenario is played out most strongly in the years of early childhood and is reason enough to engage children in some form of *yogasana* practice at an early age.[4]

---

4   More than 2,400 years ago, Greek physician Hippocrates anticipated this plasticity of the brain when he taught, "That which is used is developed; that which is not used wastes away." As applied to

Plasticity

An otherwise popular idea in regard to the brain has been shown to be a myth; i.e., that we use only 10 percent of our brain power, implying that we could be much smarter if we were not so lazy mentally. The brain has a demonstrable plasticity, and because of this, people have come to believe that since brain function can be changed with time, there must be vacant, passive parts of the brain waiting to be called into service as needed. Instead, it is closer to the truth to say that because different parts of the brain **compete** with one another for space, a gain in one arena of brain function reflects a loss in another. The brain's plasticity allows transformations of brain function as the needs of the individual change, but this plasticity does not imply the existence of vacant space waiting to be used.[5]

The importance of the brain's plasticity cannot be exaggerated, for this plasticity allows changes of the connectivity patterns on the basis of experience and learning and so allows each of us to evolve continuously in time, in our own unique ways. In regard to plasticity, it has been observed that the brain can break and then remake a new neural synapse in a matter of minutes, thereby reinventing itself as it goes, depending on the experiences of its owner/caretaker. For example, with three months' practice at juggling, the visual center of the brain associated with this action grows in volume by 34 percent due to the formation of new synapses. However, this volume increase falls to 1.5–2 percent once the jugglers cease practicing for

three months [78]. It has been estimated that our brains form about one million new synaptic connections every second of our lives in response to the everyday events within which we are embedded. The plasticity observed in the brains of professional musicians is especially noteworthy (Subsection 18.A, page 692).

In contrast to the plasticity of the higher-brain functions occurring in the midbrain, in the association areas, and in the thalamus, which allow free will, the lower-brain functions occurring in the human brainstem areas are more or less hardwired and so are resistant to change. However, as discussed in Subsection 1.B, page 12, even the lower-brain functions eventually can be changed or controlled through the practice of the *yogasanas,* especially those in the limbic system. The effects of plasticity of the brain in regard to consolidation and long-term memory are presented in Subsection 4.F, page 130.

Redundancy and Flexibility

On studying the various functions of the major parts of the brain, one is struck by how much overlap of functions there is among the parts. This decentralization or redundancy of brain function undoubtedly results in increased mental flexibility, as it allows many alternate paths to the same end. This, in turn, is significant, for it allows a particular small area of the brain to malfunction or even die without there being a corresponding loss of brain function.

The Limbic System

Location

Between the levels of the primitive vegetative brainstem and the sophisticated cortex lies the level of the limbic system, containing the motor-control centers and the centers of emotion and memory. The limbic system appeared about fifty million years after the vegetative brainstem and is considered to be a phylogenetically primitive cortex of sorts. Since the position of the limbic system lies physically between the unconscious brainstem and the high consciousness of the cor-

---

small children, for example, it appears that if a child is separated from its parents, so that there is little or no bonding, then the neurons reserved for bonding in the right cerebral hemisphere are eliminated, the result being that the child cannot regulate its emotions, is vulnerable to stress, and especially tends toward a violent lifestyle.

5   On the other hand, the largest fraction of the brain's cells are neuroglia (Subsection 3.A, page 37), which function, in most instances, as housekeepers, with little or no direct role in "thinking."

tex, it is no surprise that sensations and actions in the limbic system are but shallowly buried in the subconscious.

It is most difficult to define the anatomic boundaries of the limbic system, because many distant structures are so closely connected neurally to the more obvious limbic centers that it seems logical to include them too. Thus, there is no agreement over just what is to be included in the "limbic system" [107, 199, 360, 427]. Guyton [308] states that the limbic system is generally defined as those brain structures lying above the hypothalamus and below the cortex; however, because the limbic system and the hypothalamus work so closely together, we can just as logically define the limbic system as the entire basal system of the brain including the hypothalamus, which together serve to control one's emotional behaviors and many basic physiological drives.

Taking the components of the limbic system to rest below the corpus callosum of the cerebrum but above the midbrain of the brainstem, the limbic system encircles the brainstem at its upper end, close to the inner border of the cerebrum, and includes the hippocampus, the amygdala, and the mammillary bodies. A simple picture of the area generally held to be within the limbic system is shown in figure 2.B-1.

Component Parts

The limbic system has several components. Our text, however, deals with only that small number of nuclei within the limbic system that are most relevant to performing the *yogasanas*. Lying just below the corpus callosum of the cortex (figures 2.B-1 and 4.B-1) are three internal regions of the limbic system: the basal ganglia, which regulate motor performance (discussed below, page 83); the hippocampus, involved with memory storage; and the amygdala, which coordinates autonomic and endocrine responses with emotional states.

The Hippocampus

Our cognitive memories are strongly influenced by the interaction of the hippocampus with the surrounding cortex, which interaction is critical to consciousness. The hippocampus is especially involved with our memories of personal experiences, from which we form our sense of Self and self-awareness, because it forms, stores, and accesses emotional memories. In contrast, memories of situations not directly related to Self, people, locations, or time reside largely in the cingulate cortex surrounding the hippocampus and are considered in this work as part of the association areas of the cerebral hemispheres (figure 4.B-1). Thus, that part of the right hippocampus responsible for route planning was found to be unusually large among London's taxicab drivers, in proportion to their years of driving experience.

Aspects of environmental context in regard to balancing (Subsection 4.G, page 139) quite possibly relate to the phenomenon of "place cells" in the hippocampus [427a]. When we are in a confined space, we tend to divide the space into smaller spatial elements, and when in a particular element, there is a firing of a particular subset of the pyramidal place cells within the hippocampus. As we walk about, moving from one spatial element to the next, there is a different subset of place cells that fire within the hippocampus. We will always know where we are at any moment by the subset of hippocampal place cells that are firing at that moment. Should we walk into a new situation, a new spatial map develops in about ten to fifteen minutes, and its persistence lasts from hours to months, depending upon how intently we scrutinize our space. In this way, the development of a spatial map in the hippocampus is closely related to memory.

Though our "knowledge of space is central to behavior" [427a], there is no specific sensor for searching the environment to locate the details of a spatial map. Thus, formation of the map is a multisensory affair. At the same time, the brain's capacity for processing the signals of the multisensory net is far smaller than the receptors' ability to measure and report on the environment. For this reason, it is essential that one be highly focused, paying attention to those important features of the environment and filtering out those of lesser importance.[6] The relevance of these ideas to the act of balancing and the importance of environmental context in this regard is pursued further in Subsection V.C, page 891.

Amygdala

Because the amygdala (figure 4.B-1) is closely associated with fear, it is a major factor in aversive learning; i.e., when the learning situation involves negative, unpleasant, or otherwise stressful circumstances. The amygdala is central to emotions and is driven by signals that are either terrifying or are possibly physically damaging. It also is rife with receptors for opioids and anti-anxiety drugs, and so taking such substances can provide a momentary release from our anxieties. Being located within the limbic system, the amygdala is a place of neither words, cognition, nor consciousness.

The amygdala is involved in memories having strong emotional content, such as happiness, sadness, fear, anger, and possibly tenderness and disgust. Our emotions surface when the environment changes in a way that is personally important to us. When a person is emotionally distressed, as when angry, anxious, or depressed, there is an increased blood flow to the amygdala and to the right cerebral cortex; whereas when people are upbeat, enthusiastic, energetic, and happy, the blood flow is strong in the left prefrontal cortex. Similarly, whereas the amygdala is home to arousal and excitement, the orbitofrontal part of the brain modulates aggression. It is notable that the

amygdale is smaller in women than in men, and that the ratio of the volumes of the amygdala and the orbitofrontal cortex is smaller in women than in men, implying a rationale for gender-related differences in aggressive behavior.

Other Limbic Functions

The limbic system contains the visceral and emotional centers of the brain, being involved in behavioral and emotional expression, reproduction and memory, drives and motivations; our senses of pleasure and reward involve stimulation of centers in the limbic system [432]. When we first fall in love, the brain centers for motivation and reward become overactive when we view a picture of the loved one; a similar response occurs when we eat chocolate or when we display obsessive-compulsive behavior. The limbic system is in continuous contact with the upward-moving sensory signals from the reticular formation and affects the skeletal muscles, the visceral smooth muscles, and the endocrine glands.

Memory

The limbic system decides which fragments of our experience are to be stored as memories, and these memories in turn form the basis of our sense of reality. Because the limbic system stresses those memories that involve our perceptions of others in our group, individual perceptions and memories untainted by the influence of others seem not to exist. In this way, we learn from each other and from our teachers and become firmly integrated into our groups [66]. At the same time, we also learn to ignore truths that are otherwise obvious to our senses and instead bow to the popular opinions within our group, as discussed in Box 1.A-1, page 5.

Emotion

Emotions are shaped subcortically; i.e., they begin in the limbic system and then project upward to the cortex to become part of the memories of one's experiences. Thus, emotions such as anger, fear, pleasure, contentment, and sadness and drives such as sexual arousal all have their origins in this little-understood part of the brain.

---

6   Said William James in 1890 (as quoted in [427a]), "Millions of items ... are present to my senses which never properly enter into my experience. Why? Because they have no interest for me. My experience is what I agree to attend to.... Everyone knows what attention is. It is the taking possession by the mind, in clear and vivid form, of one out of what seem several simultaneously possible objects or trains of thought. Focalization, concentration of consciousness, are of its essence. It implies withdrawal from some things in order to deal effectively with others." Said differently, paying deliberate attention to specific aspects of thought is the doorway leading to bringing subconscious mental sensations and processes into the conscious sphere (Subsection 1.B, page 12).

Performing passive versions of the *yogasanas,* such as chair-supported *halasana,* for example, apparently defuses the emotional centers within the limbic system. Thus it is said that it is impossible to remain angry after ten minutes in *halasana* [724]. Though emotions have been long associated with the limbic centers, it is now known [270] that the cortex also contributes to our emotions, moods, and drives. A possible explanation for why passive postures release emotions better than the more vigorous ones is discussed in terms of blood flow through the brain in Subsection 4.E, page 110.

The pleasure center responsible for stimulating the cravings of those suffering from addiction is situated in the nucleus accumbens, lying at the crossroads between the dopamine system (which mediates the pleasurable sensations when ingesting drugs or food) and the limbic system (which involves motivation, emotion, and memory).

The Basal Ganglia

Those parts of the limbic system involved with body posture are found in the basal ganglia (figures 2.B-1 and 4.B-1). One of the many functions of the basal ganglia is to limit muscle tone throughout the body by inhibiting the γ-motor excitation of the muscle spindles in the resting state (Subsection 11.B, page 429).

If the basal ganglia are inoperative for any reason, then the inhibition on muscle tone is lifted, and the body becomes rigid due to global contraction of the flexional muscles, as witnessed by the mask-like face and shuffling gait of those with Parkinson's disease. The rigidity associated with many forms of basal-ganglia disease relate closely to a poor sense of balance, for the rigidity implies that the rapid muscular responses necessary to prevent a fall are not functional.

When performing complex actions requiring the proper muscle selection, sequencing, timing, and activation (e.g., *yogasana*), the basal ganglia are of the greatest importance. Some programs of the basal ganglia are inborn (swallowing), whereas others are learned by practice (the straight-leg lift into *sirsasana,* for example). Three nuclei within the basal ganglia, the globus pallidus, the substan-

tia nigra, and the striate body, each with its own specific function, are particularly relevant to our discussion.

There is an interesting example of the different muscular effects that appear depending upon whether an action is driven consciously by the cortex or subconsciously by the basal ganglia. When we are forced to smile in spite of our natural inclination not to, the forced smile is driven by the cortex and has a totally artificial look [221, 350]. On the other hand, given a good joke, the spontaneous smile is orchestrated by the basal ganglia and has a much more natural appearance; i.e., only genuine smiles involve the activation of the orbicularis oculi muscles that crinkle the skin around the eyes. Should cranial nerve VII, the facial nerve, be injured in some way, then conscious, forced smiling may be impossible; however, in this case, the second path to smiling [671a] via the basal ganglia and the emotions, allows the involuntary smile to appear even though the voluntary smile is forbidden! One can only wonder at how these two centers, the forced pretension of the cortex and the naturalness of the basal ganglia, might compete with one another as we perform the *yogasanas.*[7] See Subsection 4.D (page 102) for mention of how cerebral laterality affects the symmetry of your smile.

The Globus Pallidus

The globus pallidus controls the muscle action when certain body positions are to be held for extended times without moving. Also, whenever there is body movement, certain muscles must be braced to support the movement, and this bracing action also is under the control of the globus pallidus. Both the static and bracing aspects of the globus pallidus are clearly of great import to the performance of the *yogasanas,* where the positions are held for long periods and where we often sup-

---

7   This competition between our natural inner Self and the false and pretentious façade of our public persona may relate to B. K. S. Iyengar's recent comments about the two I's within each of us and how we must work to let the hidden, inner *I* shine brightly in our *yogasana* practice (Appendix VI, page 934).

port the posture with a strong, bracing foundation. This bracing action of the globus pallidus may relate to the macroscopic resistance developed in support of muscle stretching, as discussed in Subsection 11.F, page 468.

As we age, certain holding patterns within the globus pallidus become more comfortable than others, and we tend then to hold these comfortable postures to the exclusion of others. This acts to freeze us in the preferred posture, so that postural change becomes nearly impossible. To an extent, the stiffness of the aged is, in reality, a stiffness of the neurological circuits in the globus pallidus controlling posture rather than a stiffness of the muscles themselves; as such, the stiffness is a disadvantageous form of "muscle memory" (Subsection 4.G, page 140). Similarly, the dancer-turned-*yogasana*-student may find herself in conflict with the instructions of the *yogasana* teacher because she has encoded the "proper" attitude of the body for dance into the globus pallidus, and this must be overcome in order to make room for the ascendancy of the postural attitudes of *yogasana*. However, through the practice of *yogasana*, sooner or later, the globus pallidus can learn how to support a great variety of body postures, and in this way, one keeps viable the options for body posture, regardless of age or circumstance.

The Substantia Nigra

All of the information from which the proprioceptive maps of body position (Section 11.C, page 441) are generated is sent to the substantia nigra, a nucleus that is rich in the neurotransmitter dopamine. Though this mass of proprioceptive information (muscle lengths, rates of change of length, muscle tensions, and joint angles) is handled subconsciously, if the substantia nigra is not working properly, then the fine control of the muscles is lost, movement is jerky, and the limbs tremble.

The Striate Body

A third nucleus within the basal ganglia, the striate body, controls the manner of movement. Though we tend to fall into stereotypical movements, such as how we fold the legs when watching television or how we interlace the fingers for *parvatasana,* the patterns of which are stored in the striate body, a healthy variety of such patterns can be available to us through a varied *yogasana* practice. Strangely, the striate-body brain center is also a factor in obsessive-compulsive behavior and in generating a feeling of disgust.

The Diencephalon

The Hypothalamus

Though the hypothalamus is geographically located within the limbic system, it has been awarded its own specific region, the diencephalon, along with the thalamus. The hypothalamus is functionally a very important component of the autonomic nervous system; the reader is referred to Chapter 5, page 165, for a more detailed discussion of this nucleus than is given here.

The hypothalamus regulates the autonomic, endocrine, and visceral functions. Because the hypothalamus has an intimate relationship with both the autonomic nervous system and with the endocrine system, it is a very prominent but subconscious player in regulating our behavior [427]. The hypothalamus is active earlier in girls and leads to them entering puberty earlier than do boys. The hypothalamus is of special interest to the *yogasana* student, as it is the central organ controlling such reflex actions as holding the breath when straining to achieve a posture or the tendency toward flexing the knee in *trikonasana*; reflex actions such as this can be brought under conscious control through *yogasana* practice. The many functions of the hypothalamus and the connections between it and the higher cerebral centers are discussed in Section 5.B, page 166.

Though the pituitary gland formally is not a part of the brain, it is connected to the brain by a stalk. It often is referred to as "the master gland," because it appears to control the other glands but is itself controlled by hormonal secretions from the hypothalamus into the hypophyseal stalk (figure 5.E-1a).

Returning to the discussion of the student in *virabhadrasana I* first mentioned in Box

2.D-1 (page 27), changes are being wrought in the body at the subconscious level as directed by the hypothalamus when in this *yogasana*. In response to the work of the globus pallidus in maintaining the posture, the hypothalamus commands the heart rate to increase along with the blood pressure, the blood to leave the gut and go to the skeletal muscles instead, the respiration rate to increase along with the diameters of bronchial vessels, etc., all without any conscious direction from the cortex. At the same time, memories of the action are being stored in the substantia nigra of the basal ganglia and the hippocampus of the limbic system. Interactions between the hippocampus and the cortex lead to "learning" of the posture (Section 4.F, page 134).

One assumes that once *virabhadrasana I* has been performed satisfactorily, there is a consequent stimulation of the pleasure center in the hypothalamus that simultaneously activates the muscles of expression (a smile [432]) and reinforces the motivational and physical factors that brought the posture to a satisfying conclusion (Section 5.B, page 169).

Specific cells acting in the hypothalamus initiate sleep. Our wakefulness is controlled by a small cluster of cells called the ventrolateral preoptic area (VLPO, figure 5.B-1), which is located on the undersurface of the brain, behind the eyes. The VLPO has inhibitory links to all other major cell groups involved in promoting wakefulness. Thus, the VLPO is the master switch that turns off all arousal systems in the brain, including parts of the reticular formation [763] (Section 23.D, page 797).

The Thalamus

Consciousness as we know it persists even when most of the forebrain has been excised; the essential brain area for consciousness is the thalamus, sitting just above the brainstem (figure 4.B-1) and acting as a switching station for neural impulses moving between higher and lower brain centers [672]. One can lose the sensory cortex with little or no effect on the sensations of pain or temperature, since it is the thalamus that plays the

major role in discrimination of these senses. All of the sensory signals except those from the eyes, ears, taste, and the somatic senses pass through thalamic nuclei.

The Cerebral Hemispheres

The Cortical Lobes

At the highest of the four levels of the brain, one has the cerebral hemispheres, consisting of all structures lying above the thalamus; i.e., the cerebral cortices and the association areas that lie just below them (figure 4.B-1). The most obvious physical characteristic of the human cerebral hemisphere is the deeply folded nature of the cortex and the constancy of the topography formed by its fissures (sulci) and mounds (gyri). Each hemisphere of the cortex can be conveniently divided both by its various sulci and by its functionally into four lobes: the frontal, parietal, temporal, and occipital. Such an approach not only divides the cortex geometrically but also serves to delineate the areas specific to certain brain functions. Thus, the occipital lobe is concerned mainly with vision, the temporal lobe mainly with sound and speech, the parietal lobe with movement, touch, and recognition, and the frontal lobe with thinking and planning. These lobes of the cerebral hemispheres are congruent with the corresponding bones of the neurocranium (figure 9.A-1); i.e., the sutures of the neurocranium closely follow the sulci defining the cerebral lobes.

Each of the four lobes in one hemisphere of the brain is separated from the corresponding lobes in the other hemisphere by the front-to-back longitudinal fissure. The central fissure, also called the central sulcus (figure 2.B-2), is a deep trench in the cortex of each of the cerebral hemispheres, runs perpendicular to the longitudinal fissure, and serves to separate the frontal lobes from the parietal lobes; similarly, the parietal-occipital sulci separate the parietal lobes from the occipital lobes. The various cortical lobes have association areas that are responsible for different types of consciousness. For example, the associa-

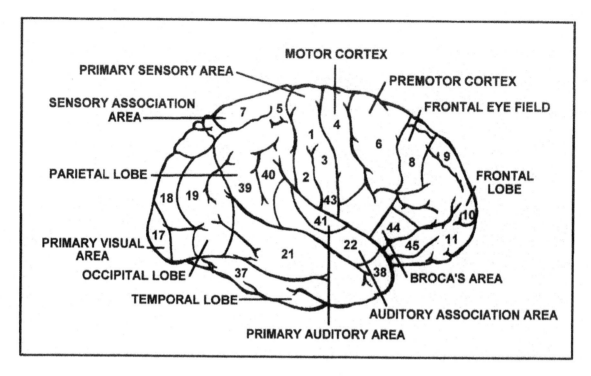

Figure 4.C-1. Brodmann's areas by the numbers and identified by name for the left cerebral hemisphere as seen from the side.

tion cortex in the temporal lobe is the seat of consciousness for sight and hearing.

Brodmann's Areas

More than 200 different areas of the cortex have been assigned specific functions, which makes for a very complex map of the brain; however, Brodmann has offered a simplified and reasonable division of the cortical surface into fifty-two overlapping areas according to function (figure 4.C-1). For example, the visual cortex is found in Brodmann's areas 17, 18, and 19, whereas areas 4, 6, and 8 correspond to the motor cortex and areas 41 and 42 are the auditory cortex. As is appropriate for the extreme importance of the visual sense, the primary visual cortex contains twice as many neurons as any other Brodmann's area. Note that Broca's area, Brodmann's number 44, is found in the left frontal lobe in most people, but not in the right, and that Wernicke's area also is found in the left temporal lobe; the two are involved with language and are connected by a dedicated neural bundle though they are separated by 8 centimeters (3 inches). As this connection does not

form until age one, there is no speech before this age is reached. Wernicke's area is involved with understanding speech and sign language; in the latter case, the signals are first received by the visual cortex and then sent to Wernicke's area for processing.

In order to pick up a yoga strap from the floor, three successive cortical brain processes must be activated. First, the object to be picked up must be identified in some way; this is accomplished in Brodmann's areas 5 and 7 (figure 4.C-1) in the posterior parietal lobe. Next, a muscular plan of action must be formulated in Brodmann's area 6, the premotor area of the frontal cortex. Finally, the planned movement is executed using the primary motor cortex, Brodmann's area 4.

Though many brain functions, such as those involved in picking up a strap from the floor, can be pinpointed as occurring in highly specific areas of the cortex, there also can be a delocalization of strongly related brain function over several seemingly unconnected areas. Thus, for example, the brain centers related to hearing words, seeing words, speaking words, and generating words are seen in figure 4.C-2c to be located in very different neighborhoods of the cortex [360]. As shown by Geschwind [270], when speaking a written word, the signal begins in the primary visual area (17), moves to the angular gyrus (area 19),[8] then to Broca's area 44, and finally to the motor cortex (area 4, figure 4.C-2a). On the other hand, when one speaks a heard word, the cortical signal begins in the primary auditory area (41), moves to Wernicke's area (22), thence to Broca's area (44), and finally on to the motor cortex (area 4, figure 4.C-2b) [308]. Damage to area 44 leads to motor aphasia and an inability to speak, except to swear, and in the same vein, people with aphasia of Broca's area 44 (figure 4.C-1) have great difficulty speaking but can sing with ease and elegance [270].

Wernicke's area, being a combination of Brodmann's areas 22, 39, and 40 in the left cerebral hemisphere, is of special interest, as all of the sensory signals in the brain (including those proprioceptive signals so useful in *yogasana* practice) eventually end up in this area for interpretation. As discussed below, there are alternatives to Brodmann's scheme for dividing the brain, some going back millennia.

---

8   Interestingly, electrical stimulation of the angular gyrus in the right hemisphere (area 19) leads to the sensation of an "out-of-body experience," in which subjects sense that they have left the body and are floating, looking down at the inert body left behind. As this area of the brain is close to the vestibular area of the cortex dealing with balance and touch, it is thought that excitation within the angular gyrus interferes with the vestibular functions nearby, and the result is an out-of-body experience.

Some workers propose that the near-death experience arises due to brain hypoxia. When in crisis and experiencing extreme levels of either oxygen or carbon dioxide, the vagus nerve is stimulated, and this leads to REM intrusion into the awake state (Subsection 23.D, page 800), as occurs in narcolepsy. In times of such possibly fatal stress, the higher brain centers could suffer hypoxia and pass out (sleep paralysis), whereas the brainstem remains active, leading to the experience of near-death. Others implicate a flood of endorphins in the amygdala (which lights up during REM sleep), leading to euphoria and detachment.

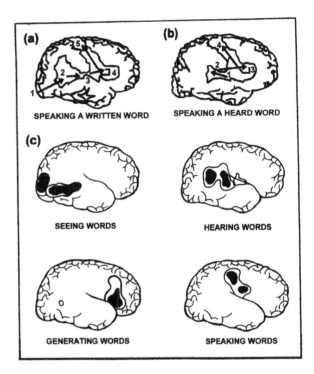

Figure 4.C-2. (a) The four-step neural pathway originating in the left frontal lobe when speaking a written word and (b) the three-step neural pathway originating in the left parietal lobe when speaking a heard word. (c) The PET scans of the cerebral blood flow through the left hemisphere of the cortex highlight the functional areas involved in performing various language-related tasks. These scans clearly illustrate how language ability is localized in different areas of the brain depending upon function; i.e., seeing words (occipital lobe), hearing words (temporal lobe), generating words (frontal lobe), and speaking words (parietal lobe).

Patanjali Division

The three levels of the tripartite brain (brainstem, limbic system, and cerebral hemispheres), first put forward by Dr. Paul McLean in 1972, are not as separate as was first proposed. It is now known that considerable communication takes place among all three levels, and so it has become more difficult than ever to assign a particular function to a particular area of the brain. The various substructures within the three major levels of the brain are discussed more completely below, with the understanding that structures at all levels more or less share in the brain's functioning. As Llinas [24] has responded to the question "Where in the brain is the seat of consciousness?" saying "Where in the bicycle is the seat of bicycleness?" so too is it clear that one cannot be too specific about location and function in regard to the functional subunits of the brain.

It is interesting to note that more than 2,000 years prior to our own time, Patanjali already had described the brain as consisting of four main geographic and functional components: (1) the front brain, devoted to analytical thinking; (2) the back brain, devoted to reasoning; (3) the bottom brain, the seat of pleasure and bliss; and (4) the top brain, the seat of creativity and individuality [391] (figure 4.C-3a).

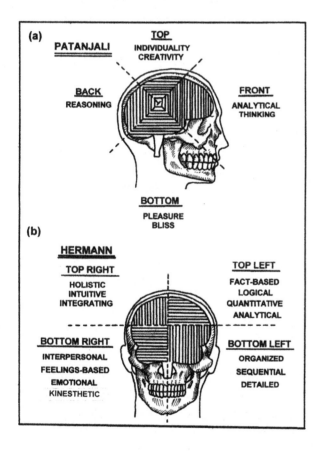

Figure 4.C-3. (a) Patanjali's division of the brain into four quadrants [391] and the characteristics of each, to be compared with (b) Hermann's [365] division into four quadrants and the characteristics of each.

On the other hand, Hermann [365] offers a more modern dissection of the functional characteristics of the brain, again into four components (figure 4.C-3b): (a) The upper-left quadrant is logical, analytical, fact-based, and quantitative; (b) the upper-right quadrant is holistic, intuitive, integrating, and synthesizing; (c) the lower-left quadrant is organized and sequential and deals with planning and details; and (d) the lower-right quadrant is interpersonal, feeling-based, kinesthetic, and emotional. The focus of the bottom-right quadrant on kinesthetic phenomena is in agreement with the eyes turning to that direction when recalling kinesthetic experiences (figure 17.D-2).

Though Hermann's division of brain topography and function is based upon a multitude of sophisticated neurological experiments, the near-agreement with Patanjali's ideas is satisfying. Patanjali's four-part division of the brain can be brought into agreement with Hermann's modern division into four topographical areas if Patanjali's terms "front," "back," "top," and "bottom" are replaced by the modern divisions "top/left," "bottom/left," "top/right," and "bottom/right," respectively. Needless to say, the Hermann dissection correctly recognizes the left-right and top-bottom asymmetries of the brain, whereas the yogic scientists of Patanjali's time only recognized the second of these, having replaced the left-right division with a front-back division.

As seen from the Hermann perspective, it would appear sensible to guide students in *savasana* to relax the brain both from front to back **and** from left to right in order to encourage a relaxed state.

Frontal Lobes

The frontal lobes, the largest of the four types, are located forward of the central sulci and are the locales for absorbing new information and on this basis, planning new strategies; they allow the neural flexibility lacking in the hardwired brains of lesser creatures. The frontal lobes also deal with social behavior and higher mental activities such as analysis, planning, and decision making, whereas speech, sign-language production, and articulation (Broca's area 44) are localized in the left frontal lobe. Frontal-lobe functions include reining in impulses, regulating aggression, mental flexibility, abstract thinking, and the mental capacity to simultaneously hold related pieces of information; the frontal lobes also may be the sites for forming moral judgments. It appears that "general intelligence" resides in the lateral flanks of the frontal lobes in both hemispheres, and it has been proposed that the amount of information that can be stored in short-term memory relates to such general intelligence (Subsection 4.F, page 126).

Size

Note the increasing prominence of the frontal lobe (figure 4.C-4) on going from striped bass to human being. In the great apes, from man to orangutan, the frontal lobes are approximately 36 percent of the total brain volume; whereas in the lower apes, it is less than 30 percent. Among humans, women have about 20 percent more frontal-lobe neurons than do men.

It is presently thought that the cortical lobes of notable thinkers such as Albert Einstein can show deviations in size from the norm. Thus, Einstein's brain showed large, unusually shaped inferior parietal lobes, just those areas in which one performs spatial reasoning and harbors intuitions about numbers. Similarly, violent sociopaths have retarded development of the prefrontal cortex and so have lowered abilities in both decision making and inhibiting impulsive behavior [666], and it has been found that the prefrontal cortices of pathological liars have higher levels of white matter, which speeds neural signaling, and lower levels of gray matter, which may regulate remorse.

Just forward of the central fissure in the frontal lobes are the premotor and motor areas; all of the skeletal muscles of the body can be activated by neural signals originating in these areas. However, due to a decussation of the neural paths in either the spinal cord or the brainstem, activation of the motor centers in one frontal lobe leads to contraction of muscles on the opposite (contralateral) side of the body.

Our abilities to perform the *yogasanas* with the maximum awareness and finesse will relate directly to the sizes of the sensory and motor areas in the cortices devoted to the relevant sensors and muscles. Indeed, when in an environment rich in the variety of its experiences, the cortical layers have been found to thicken noticeably. As these cortical areas will increase in size with increased *yogasana* practice, *yogasanas* should be counted among those experiences that enrich the cortex and thereby make it thicker. Though the cortex in general thins with increasing old age, the prefrontal cortices of experienced meditators actually increase in thickness as they age!

Adolescent Growth

During childhood, the cortices of children first thicken and then thin again in the teen years, as shown by functional-MRI studies. In those children with superior intelligence, the thickening occurs several years later (at age eleven years) than in children of normal intelligence (at age six years), but in all cases, the thickening was then followed by thinning. This thinning involves neural pruning, also called apoptosis (Subsection 3.A, page 32), in which unneeded neural paths are excised. This cortical transformation is strongest in the prefrontal cortex, the site of executive functions such as decision making, developing and executing detailed plans, higher-level cognition, and inhibiting irrelevant or ill-advised actions.

Motor Homunculus

A map representing the motor neurons that activate the muscles on the contralateral side of the body is found just forward of the central sulcus in each of the frontal lobes (figure 4.C-5) and is most interesting. In this map of the motor centers, those body parts having the greatest spatial resolution in regard to finesse and control of motion have the largest areas in the frontal lobes. From such a map of the positions and sizes of the motor-cortex areas dedicated to each of the body's parts, one can draw a human-like gremlin (the homunculus), in which the body parts have sizes that reflect their areas in the motor cortex within the frontal lobes. Thus, one sees in such a

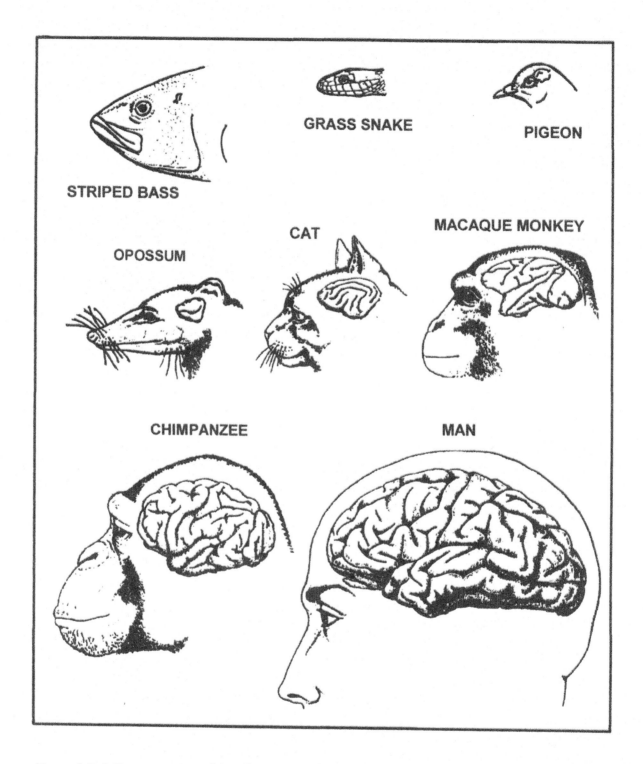

Figure 4.C-4. Demonstration of the relative sizes of the brains of water animals (striped bass), land animals that crawl (grass snake), and animals that fly (pigeon), each having a brain size and location as indicated. The cerebral cortices for the striped bass and the grass snake are too small to appear in the drawing. Brains also are shown for quadrupeds that walk (opossum, cat), for the bipeds (chimpanzee and macaque), and for man [422]. Note the evolutionary development of the forebrain and the increasingly convoluted nature of the cerebral cortices in these higher animals. Humans have the largest cortex in the animal kingdom relative to their body size.

homunculus (figure 4.C-5) that the mouth, hand, and fingers occupy disproportionately large areas in the motor cortex, whereas the back of the thorax occupies a disproportionately small area in the motor cortex. That the mouth, hands, and fingers of humans require disproportionately large shares of the cortical area in the homunculus representation, reflects our high levels of manual dexterity and language skills. On the other hand, the muscles of the back body are given relatively little space in the cortex, since they are used largely for maintaining posture and so operate at a low level of muscular finesse.

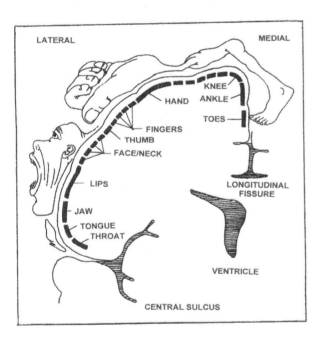

Figure 4.C-5. A map of the motor cortex (Brodmann's area 4), showing quantitatively how it is divided with respect to innervation of the appropriate muscles in the body (see also figure 4.C-6). Shown is a cross section of the motor cortex taken parallel to the central sulcus (figure 2.B-2) within the right cerebral hemisphere, with the size of the cortical arc reflecting the relative size of the cortex devoted to that particular body part. The homunculus drawn above the relevant cortical arcs expresses the relative importance of the various body parts to motor excitation originating within the frontal lobes of the cerebral cortex.

These distorted homunculi within the motor centers are discussed further in Subsection 11.A, page 372. It is most relevant that the specialized practice of a body part, such as the muscles depressing the scapulae in virtually all of the *yogasana* postures, will result in the expansion of the area dedicated to these muscles in the motor homunculus of the practicing student. It would be very interesting to see how much the homunculus of the veteran *yogasana* practitioner differs from that of the average non-practitioner. This difference is said to be substantial when comparing the cortical homunculi of the musician and the non-musician (Subsection 18.A, page 691).

The Prefrontal Cortex

The association area of the prefrontal cortex is found just forward of the premotor area of the frontal lobe (figure 4.B-1) and is the locus of activity for problem solving, planning, short-term memory, and general intelligence, i.e., "brain power," as well as high-level thinking, creativity, and emotion [600]. Many of our sensations are fed into the prefrontal cortex for evaluation, and the signal is then forwarded to the basal ganglia, which in turn send the signal back to the premotor and motor cortices in the rear of the frontal lobes in order to initiate movement, if that is called for [25]. Short-term memory is controlled by the prefrontal cortex and serves to coordinate long-term memories with sights, sounds, feelings, etc.

The prefrontal cortex is very important to our social behavior. Thus, people afflicted with antisocial personality behavior (showing impulsive aggression, for example) have a noticeable deficit of gray matter in the prefrontal areas and reduced neural activity in those areas, especially in areas known to involve inhibition of actions. The prefrontal cortex is larger and matures earlier in women.

Premotor Cortex

Whenever there is a conscious decision to contract a particular muscle, there is an activation of the relevant neurons in the premotor cortex (Brodmann's area 6, figure 4.C-1); following this, the relevant neurons in the motor cortex (Brodmann's area 4, figure 4.C-1) are excited, and the muscle contraction then begins. The motivation for such a muscular act originates in the part of the prefrontal cortex just forward of the eye sockets. Excitation of the premotor cortex is also involved in the phenomenon of so-called mirror neurons (Subsection 4.C, page 94, and Subsection 4.G, page 142).

Strangely, the conscious decision to activate a particular muscle at a particular time is preceded by a subconscious mental event that serves to either negate or reinforce the conscious decision. This subconscious neural event is initiated about 400 milliseconds **before** the action and would seem to make all conscious actions really subconscious! One might assume that the initiating event is a rapid reflexive action that may or may not lead to the conscious action, just as with reflex in many other body systems. See Subsection 4.C, page 96, for more on this aspect of consciousness.

Parietal Lobes

Just posterior to the central sulci and lying between the frontal and occipital lobes are the parietal lobes, into which all conscious sensory inputs (such as those of touch, pressure, and pain) are deposited, again in contralateral ways. The parietal lobes are the sites for mathematical calculation, body awareness, and, most importantly, the ability to integrate experiences. See Appendix VI, page 938, for the possible role of the parietal lobes in regard to Iyengar's statement, "You can see the external world with the eyes, the internal world with the ears." The parietal lobes also are called upon when one estimates the size, shape, and texture of an object, and they also deal with symbolic aspects of language, such as the deciphering of a string of letters into a word. The parietal lobes have different physical structures in the two hemispheres.

Sensory Homunculus

Just as the homunculus within the motor cortex in the frontal lobe reflects the relative resolution of muscle actions in the various body parts, the homunculus of the sensory cortex within the parietal lobe (but just behind the central sulcus) reflects the relative resolution of the tactile sensors in the same body parts. The sensory homunculus in humans has been mapped in detail and is found to be laid out in an orderly array (figure 4.C-6), again with the area dedicated to a particular sensory location being in proportion not to the true area of that location in the body, but rather being proportional to the sensory resolution required of that area, i.e., proportional to the density of tactile sensors in the patch of skin overlying the particular organ or limb. Thus, sensations from the tongue, lips, and hands have a disproportionately large space in the human sensory cortex, due to the high density of tactile sensors in these places, whereas those for the back of the body and trunk are disproportionately small, just as was seen in the motor-cortex homunculus (figure 4.C-5). What the relative sensory importance of the organs of communication and the organs of posture have come to be in the average, non-yogic human body is clear from such cortical maps. Interestingly, the kidney, heart, and spleen do not have cortical sensory representations, but sensory (pain) signals from them are instead referred to the corresponding skin dermatomes (Section 13.D, page 530).

In the homunculus representation, the hands, fingers, and mouth require disproportionately large shares of the cortical area, reflecting our needs for high levels of sensory information regarding manual dexterity and language skills. Intriguing sensory homunculi also have been determined for various other animals; for example, the rabbit, in which the sensory homunculus has a huge face and snout but very small feet, and the cat, the sensory homunculus of which has a large face and snout but, compared to the rabbit, much larger paws. The monkey's homunculus seems most in proportion to its physical form, while that for man shows huge tongue, lips, big toe, hand, and thumb but very small feet and back body [427]. One sees that the disproportions of the sensory homunculi reflect the neural adaptations made by each of these mammalian species in order to secure its niche and guarantee its survival.

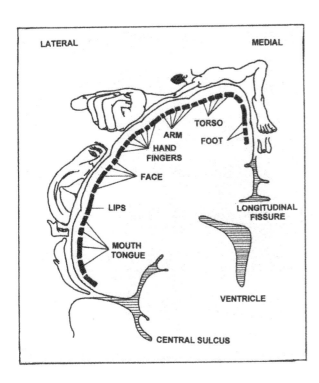

Figure 4.C-6. A map of the sensory cortex (Brodmann's area 1, right hemisphere), showing semi-quantitatively how it is divided with respect to the densities of tactile sensors (superficial and deep-pressure) from different areas of the body and terminating within the parietal lobes of the cerebral cortex. The homunculus drawn above the relevant cortical arcs expresses the relative spatial resolutions and tactile-sensor densities in the skin covering the various body parts.

Temporal Lobes

The temporal lobes are located below the lateral fissure, below the frontal and parietal lobes, and at the temples just above each ear. They receive the auditory signals from the ears, albeit in a largely contralateral way. The temporal lobes are involved in aspects of language communication (Wernicke's area in the left hemisphere in most people and Brodmann's area 22 in figure 4.C-1), in arranging for the storage of learned material in short-term memory in the hippocampus, and in interpreting olfactory signals. When sensations of sight and hearing reach the association areas of the temporal lobes, they are then sensed consciously.

Tactile information is processed in the temporal lobes, possibly relating to B. K. S. Iyengar's comment about the ears and feelings (Subsection VI.B, page 938).

Occipital Lobes

The occipital lobes are positioned at the rear of the brain and are concerned exclusively with processing the visual signals from the eyes in sighted individuals. In a beautiful demonstration of the plasticity of the neural wiring in the brain, the visual areas of the occipital lobes in the blind are used instead to handle either the auditory signals from the ears or the tactile signals from the fingertips. Damage to the occipital lobes usually results in blindness, for the signals sent from the retina are not processed into meaningful images in this case. (However, also see Subsection 17.B, page 669, for an alternate, reflexive route to vision.)

Effects of Alcohol

As alcohol is readily transported from the stomach and into the brain and has significant negative effects on the various lobes of the brain, its use and abuse is clearly at odds with the goals of *yogasana* practice. It is first of all a sedative/hypnotic, leading to sleep apnea and hypoxia. It is also a stimulant, leading to violence and abusive behavior. At low concentrations, alcohol is a vasodilator, but it becomes vasoconstrictive at higher levels, with symptoms including increased blood pressure, worsening migraine, and higher susceptibility to frostbite. With alcohol intake, the frontal lobe suffers losses of reason, caution, inhibition, and intelligence; the parietal lobe loses fine motor skills; the temporal lobe exhibits slurred speech and impaired hearing; the occipital lobe suffers blurred vision and poor distance sense; the cerebellum exhibits lack of muscle coordination and balance; and the brainstem loses vital functions [190]. In persons addicted to alcohol, the limbic system has an abnormally strong response to drinking, especially the nucleus accumbens, the rewards center, which shows a strong gratification response. See Subsection 3.D, page 59, for more on the effects of alcohol on the brain.

Eighty percent of ingested alcohol is metabolized by the liver via the enzyme alcohol dehydrogenase; however, because women have significantly less of this enzyme than do men and because they cannot increase the level of this enzyme by increased drinking (unlike men), their cortical lobes are more at risk for the consequences of alcohol abuse than are those of men.

The Cortex: Seat of Conscious Sensation, Thought, and Action

The cerebral cortex is a thin layer of tissue, heavily folded and creased, covering each of the cerebral hemispheres with a very high density of neurons. Also known as the neocortex, the cerebral cortex is the newest and largest of the brain's additions. The cortical network consists of three main types of neural wiring: (i) those cortical areas reserved for sensory and motor functions, for which there is little or no conscious sensation involved; (ii) the associative areas of the cortex, in which one cortical area is connected to one or more of the other cortical areas, this being the arena of conscious action; and (iii) the projection neurons, which connect the cortex to lower brain centers, such as the thalamus. It is in the association areas of the cortex (ii) that we find the conscious perception of one's own body, the planning of our movements, planning and making decisions, spatial perception, orientation, and imagination, all of which are of great relevance to *yogasana* practice [722].

The all-inclusive term "the cortex" will be used without further delineation in regard to points (i), (ii), and (iii) above, unless specifically noted to the contrary. With that said, it can be stated that, as the conscious reception site for all of the sensory-signal changes in the body, the cortex is the seat of consciousness; it is in control of many of the motor and sensory activities and of all voluntary and many involuntary motions, and it is the site for mental activities such as memory, learning, reasoning, and language.

Topography

On the evolutionary time scale, the cortex is a relatively recent refinement of brain structure, and it is the crowning achievement of the evolutionary process. The evolutionary development of the cerebral cortex is clear in figure 4.C-4, showing that both the relative size and the convoluted nature of the cortex increase as one ascends the evolutionary ladder, reaching the apex in man. It is the cortex that has changed the most as the brain evolved. Many of its unique properties can be traced to its many folds, the true surface area of the cortex being significantly larger than what it appears to be when nestled within the skull. In the human, the surface area of the cortex is 2,500 square centimeters, whereas in the cat it is 83 square centimeters, and it is only 6 square centimeters in the rat; animals larger than humans (elephants, bottlenose dolphins, whales) have correspondingly larger cortical areas than do humans. Note that though the cortices covering the two cerebral hemispheres appear to be identical, they can differ greatly in their functions, as discussed in Subsection 4.D, page 98).

Much of the brain's work is carried out in the thin layer of the cortex, with the underlying cells serving as point-to-point connections within the brain or as housekeeper cells (neuroglia) with custodial duties. The number of "housekeeping" glial cells in the human brain is twice as large as the number of neurons and can be ten times as large in specific areas. However, recent experimental work suggests that in addition to housekeeping, glial cells also are able to communicate among themselves, influence the formation and strength of synaptic connections, and possibly promote neuropathic pain as well as mirror-image pain (see page 520). Though filled with neural tissue, there are no pain receptors in the cortex [199, 528, 801].

Six distinct neural layers have been identified within the 2–4 millimeter thickness of the cortex, with each layer being responsible for different functions in different parts of the cortex. Being of a gray hue, the outer layer of the cortex is the "gray matter" of which we speak when referring to intellectual powers. Because the gray matter of the cortex controls the motor nerves, stroke damage within the gray matter of the brain can paralyze any muscle in the body that otherwise could be moved voluntarily. Lying within the cerebral hemispheres but below the gray matter of the cortex are thick webs of myelinated white matter, the association areas. The significant differences within the gray and white matter of female and male brains are displayed in Subsection 4.E, page 121.

Cortical Folding

In the course of human fetal development, the cortex starts smooth, but by the sixth month in utero, it starts to fold, in accord with the concept of "ontogeny recapitulates phylogeny," as presented in Box 8.A-1. As the brain evolved, the size of the cerebrum increased, as did the extent of convolution of the cerebral tissue, as is evident in figure 4.C-4. At present, there are about three billion neurons in each hemisphere of the human cortex. If the cortex were to be laid flat, it would be about the size of a large pizza, and so it must be very crumpled in order to fit within the skull. This brain folding (convolution) follows the biological principle that allows a person who is only 150 centimeters (five feet) tall to have an intestine that is 900 centimeters (thirty feet) long [343].

The cortex is especially folded and fissured in those animals that have high intelligence and great needs for brain power. In human beings, these folds and fissures are constants of the cortex's topography and so serve to divide it into identifiable lobes (figure 2.B-2). With a maximum thickness of only 4 millimeters (0.16 inches), the cortex and its associated white matter nonetheless are the largest single structure in the brain, accounting for approximately half its volume. This seems at first sight contradictory for an object so thin, but the cortex is so folded and convoluted that only 25 percent of the brain's cortical area is visible on its surface; the remaining 75 percent of the cortex's area is hidden in the sulci (grooves) of the folded sheet [360].

Many believe that the cortex folds so as to minimize the lengths of neural wiring between its many parts and that the folding is a consequence of the brain's tendency to follow this minimizing principle. Thus, strongly interacting areas are pulled more closely together by folding appropriately, and weakly interacting ones become more separated. Recent studies show that the frontal and parietal lobes of females are more strongly folded than those of males, possibly relating to the higher verbal fluency of women compared to men.

Cortical Functions

Consider now the functions of the cortex in the context of practicing *virabhadrasana I* (Box 2.D-1, page 28), for example. A typical sensory signal moving through the various control centers of the brain, going as high as the motor and sensory cortices and then returning back to the effector organ, as would be appropriate for the performance of *virabhadrasana I*, is shown schematically in figure 4.C-7. In this, the sensory signal from some outlying body part enters the spinal cord and then bifurcates, with part of the signal ascending as high as the cortex and the other part exiting the spinal cord as a reflexive signal to the muscles (figure 4.C-7**a**). The descending signals from the motor cortex and the cerebellum then interact in the brainstem before entering the descending tracts of the spinal cord (figure 4.C-7**b**). The final signal activates muscles with a strength that reflects the sum of the influences of many centers in the brain operating at very different levels of consciousness, with the α-motor signal that exits the spinal cord in figure 4.C-7**a** being subconscious and reflexive and that exiting the spinal cord in figure 4.C-7**b** being under conscious control. Note the left-right decussation in both ascending and descending paths.

Cortical Inhibition

Signals also originate at the cortex and travel downward to lower centers in order to inhibit certain sensations by controlling the sensitivity of the relevant synapses. Thus, in *virabhadrasana I*, one can focus on the balancing sensations in the ankle of the front leg to the exclusion of the stretching sensations in the quadriceps of the rear leg, etc. In

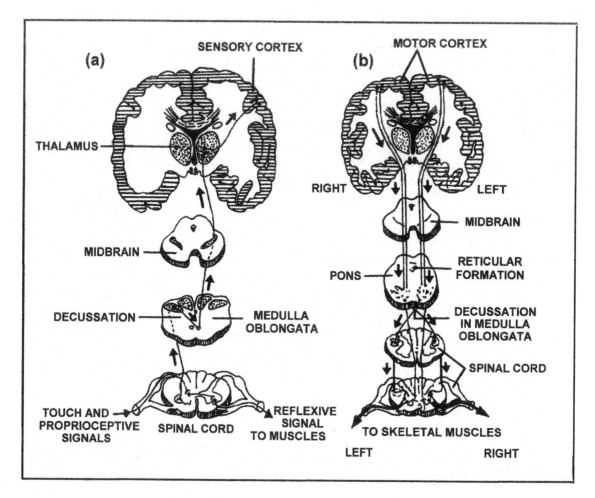

Figure 4.C-7. (a) The path of a tactile sensory signal, one part of which enters the spinal cord, decusses in the medulla oblongata and then moves upward to the sensory cortex via the thalamus. This part of the signal then moves to the motor cortex, where it will begin its downward descent. A second part of the initial sensory signal stays within the spinal cord and reflexively activates skeletal muscles without having ascended even to the brainstem. (b) Having reached the sensory cortex, ascending signals then cross to the motor cortices of both hemispheres and pass sequentially downward to the limbic system, brainstem, and spinal cord, where they exit appropriately to activate the skeletal muscles.

fact, a large fraction of the cortex's function is inhibitory, especially of the right hemisphere by the left. In some cases, one is born with the inhibitions only partially functioning, and this unleashes the amazing performance of the autistic individual demonstrating the savant syndrome; in this case, there is an under-development of the frontotemporal lobe of the left cerebral hemisphere, and this allows the right hemisphere to function at an incredibly high level without inhibition from the left (see Subsection 4.D, page 99, and Subsection 3.C, page 51, for further discussions of cerebral inhibition).

Free Will versus Free Won't

Detailed analysis of a specific excitation of the motor cortex and the resultant muscle contraction [516a] shows that there is a wave of excitation (the readiness potential) within the area of the motor cortex that appears about 300 to 400 milliseconds **before** there is any conscious sense that the decision has been made to contract the muscle! The immediate implication of this undisputed fact would appear to be that there is no such thing as free will, for muscular actions apparently are begun before we can think them through consciously and then initiate them. However, further study shows that within the 300-millisecond window, a decision is made within a subconscious center as to whether the impending action is to be inhibited or not. In this way, it is seen that what we have called "free will" more properly should be called "free won't," as it involves a choice as to whether to inhibit the impending action or not. Though this work by Lisbet [516a] is technically elegant, it is clear from ordinary experience that we routinely act in a subconscious mode; when playing tennis, for example, we act to return the ball in a certain manner far more rapidly than would be the case if conscious thought alone were driving the action. That is, if we had to think out the response to a volley and then react, the ball long ago would have bounced past us before we responded! We almost always make a preliminary reflexive evaluation of our conscious action before we initiate the action.

Note that a voluntary wrist action has been measured to have a latency delay of 200 to 250 milliseconds, whereas the same muscle action, when activated in the reflex mode, has a latency of only 30 to 35 milliseconds. This difference reflects the additional time required to evaluate a conscious muscle action as compared to the same action that bypasses the cognitive apparatus, as when reflexive. When balancing in various *yogasanas*, this difference between conscious and subconscious response times becomes a decisive factor (Subsection V.B, page 883).

Spindle Cells and Social Emotions

The spindle cells are extraordinarily long, spindle-shaped cells found in small clusters in only two places in the brain: in the anterior cingulate cortex and in the orbitofrontal cortex (behind the orbits of the eyes). Those primates closest to humans on the evolutionary tree also have spindle cells in very small numbers, whereas the more distant primates and all of the other mammals (except for certain whales) are lacking entirely in these special cells. The two centers in which spindle cells are found are known to moderate complex social emotions. It appears that, as with many systems of the body, we have brain centers, which operate in a delib-

erate way, controlling our emotions in regard to issues such as fairness, punishment, and moral judgments, and we have the spindle cells, which control real-time instantaneous behaviors in complex social situations. That is to say, regarding social interactions, we have both a slow, thoughtful thinking mode and a more rapid reflexive response (our "gut feeling"), the latter of which is located among the spindle cells. The spindle cells carry receptors for the neurotransmitters serotonin, dopamine, and vasopressin, all of which are important in the neurochemistry of emotion [659], and also have direct connections to the autonomic nervous system.

Below the Cortex

The areas of the brain above the thalamus but below the cortex in figure 4.B-1, the cingulate cortex and the association areas, play central roles in the development of consciousness. These subcortical regions have very strong neural connections to both the hippocampus (the organizer of cognitive memory) and to the amygdala (the organizer and center of emotional memory) within the limbic system. The association region is especially rich in connections between its own neurons (80 percent) rather than with neurons in other regions (20 percent); i.e., it communicates much more with itself than with other parts of the cerebral cortex. Association neurons are found only in the brain and spinal cord.

Association and Commissural Fibers

Though any two Brodmann's areas inscribed upon the cortex may appear to be isolated from one another, they are not isolated in any sense whatsoever. Association fibers connect one cortical area with another in the same hemisphere, and commissural fibers connect a cortical area in one hemisphere with a cortical area in the other hemisphere. The association areas are especially important in that they are the primary sites for converting our sensations into consciousness. This is apparent in the results of recent experiments by Tononi et al. [82, 543], who first stimulated the prefrontal cortices of awake subjects using transcranial magnetic stimulation (Subsection 4.D, page 105) and found that in the few seconds following the initial stimulation, the localized excitation spread to four other brain regions via the association fibers. In contrast, when the same stimulation was applied to the subjects while asleep, there was an initial localized excitation but no spreading to the adjacent areas. Apparently, consciousness arises when the initial neural signal migrates from one brain area to several of the others in a sequential fashion along the association fibers.

Chief among the commissural connections is the corpus callosum (figure 4.B-1), a large bundle of interhemispheric, myelinated fibers containing about 300 million distinct fibers. This bundle allows the rapid interhemispheric transfer of information and learning about motor actions and sensations involving all parts of the body, with the exception of the hands and the feet, strangely; presumably, these communicate using a different path, such as the posterior or anterior commissures. Those parts of the corpus callosum involved with learning language develop at a very high rate during adolescence, but this growth slows thereafter. This may explain why learning a new language is so much more difficult after the age of twelve years.

The Cingulate Cortex

As the cingulate cortex sits between the limbic system and the cortex (figure 4.B-1), it adds an emotional coloring to the conscious sensations of the cortex, as when experiencing pain. During hypnosis to reduce pain, the blood flow to the cingulate cortex is greatly increased, whereas that to the cortex is lessened. See also Subsection 13.C, page 515, for more on the roles of the cingulate cortex in pain, and in recognizing and correcting mistakes.

Projection Fibers

Finally, there are projection fibers in the brain that connect the cortical areas with subcortical areas. For example, the projection fibers carry the heavy neural traffic between the cortex and the thalamus. These fibers should be of great interest to the *yogasana* student, as they are the link

between the consciousness of the cortex and the subconsciousness of the lower-brain centers and they offer the possibility for the conscious direction of subconscious functions! See Section 1.B, page 12, for more on this aspect of the interaction of *yogasana* with brain function. The thalamo-cortical neural pathways are discussed further in Subsection 4.H, page 153. As most parts of the body have sensory afferents that project onto the cortex, the cortex is not devoted to a single mode of sense but integrates all major sensory signals, including those for motor, proprioceptive, auditory, and visual sensations, as well as speech and interpretation.

Because each functional area of the cortex is connected by both afferent and efferent neurons to the thalamus, the cortex can be thought of as an outgrowth of the thalamus [308]. However, as there is no body map in the thalamus, pain signals can be sensed in this center, but there is no conscious sense of how intense the pain is or where the pain originated. These aspects of intensity and location are apparent only when the pain signal has traveled beyond the thalamus to the cingulate cortex.

Section 4.D: Cerebral Hemispheric Laterality

Lateral Asymmetry of the Brain

Though the two cerebral hemispheres of the brain may appear at first to be identical in structure and function, there is now abundant evidence that this is not the case. It was first noticed in 1968 that the planum temporale in the left hemisphere is, on average, significantly larger than that in the right hemisphere [269]. Moreover, at birth, the size of the Wernicke's area and adjacent angular-gyrus areas (see below) in the temporal lobes are substantially larger in the left hemispheres of 90 to 95 percent of all babies; these babies grow up to be overwhelmingly right-handed.

Even in adults, there are about 200 million more neurons in the left hemisphere than in the

Table 4.D-1: Functions of the Cerebral Hemispheres [427, 432]

Right Hemisphere	Left Hemisphere
Feminine (nurture, intuitive, read faces, raise children)	Masculine (hunt, track, chase prey)
Parallel processing (simultaneity)	Linear processing (logical, sequential)
Humorous	Analytical
Yin	Yang
Moon	Sun
Shakti	Shiva
East	West
Parasympathetic nervous system	Sympathetic nervous system
Alpha-wave EEG	Beta-wave EEG
Spatial reasoning	Language functions (vocabulary, speech, alphabet)
Nonlinguistic (rhythm, accent, melody, prosody)	Musical lyrics
Perception of emotions (tone of voice, attitudes)	Manual control; motor dominance, gestures
Recognition of the faces of friends or celebrities	Recognition of one's own face
Holistic	
Proprioception; interoception	
Kinesthesia (muscle memory)	
Imaginative/creative	

right. Anatomic studies and experiments in brain function agree unanimously that the two cerebral hemispheres of the brain show many functional differences that reflect the brain's lack of left-right symmetry; the two hemispheres operate independently and in very different arenas, though remaining in close contact.[9] It is supposed that this

lateralization of brain function results in increased efficiency; however, there is no experimental proof of this. See table 4.D-1 for a detailed listing of the differing functions of the right and left cerebral hemispheres.

In the simplest terms, the left hemisphere of

---

9   Severing the corpus callosum, which otherwise allows the two cerebral hemispheres to communicate with one another, reveals that the two hemispheres have very different functions. The left hemisphere is logical, analytical, quantitative, rational, linear, and verbal. On the other hand, the right hemisphere is conceptual, holistic, imaginative, and nonverbal.

However, in a more complete picture of the brain, the left-right split also must incorporate an upper-lower split; that is, a cerebral/limbic distinction must be made as well. In fact, parts of the lower limbic system (hippocampus, thalamus, and amygdala) are also bilateral, being connected left-right via the hippocampal commissure. Thus, the better model divides the brain into four mutually interactive quadrants [365], as discussed in Subsection 4.C, page 87.

the brain is essentially objective and analytical, dealing best with subjects such as math, the spoken and written word, critical thought, and analytical reasoning of the sort found in the physical sciences. By contrast, the right hemisphere is essentially subjective and intuitive, being most active when dealing with creativity in music and the arts, imagination and insight, and the three-dimensional aspects of objects. In contrast to the situation in the left hemisphere, several areas of the right hemisphere can work simultaneously in a parallel manner [635], as is best for integrating visual, kinesthetic, proprioceptive, and interoceptive information about body posture, body motion, etc. The right cerebral hemisphere also is the seat of the emotions, personality, and non-literal language; damage to the right frontal lobes (especially the medial ventral prefrontal cortex on the right) leads to a loss of the sense of humor [417]. Though the motor functions and interpretive functions are more strongly developed in the left cerebral hemisphere, the sensory signals relevant to these functions are received equally from both sides of the body.

Note, however, that the assignment of the right cerebral hemisphere to emotional matters is a rather crude approximation, because emotional communication involves many different brain regions and channels of communication.

It is interesting to note that the characteristics assigned to the functions of the right and left hemispheres in table 4.D-1 closely match those assigned intuitively in the introduction (table 1.A-2) to World View I and World View II, with the former corresponding to the dominant functions of the right hemisphere and the latter to the dominant functions of the left hemisphere. We see as well that the dominance of the right hemisphere corresponds to parasympathetic excitation of the autonomic nervous system, whereas that of the left hemisphere corresponds to dominance of the sympathetic nervous system (Section 5.C, page 170). Thus, the scientific evidence for different functions of the two cerebral hemispheres supports the more intuitive idea of the dual consciousness within each of us [635].

Handedness

The bilateral asymmetry of the cerebral hemispheres also correlates with the dominance of one hand over the other, because it is the left hemisphere that specializes in manual skills in right-handed people. Topologically, the brain does show an obvious left-right asymmetry in right-handed people; whereas in left-handed people, the asymmetry is much less pronounced [270]. This higher asymmetry may be why right-handed people are much more strongly committed to their right hands than are left-handed people committed to their left hands (see also Section III. C, page 848). In those who are right-handed, the left cerebral hemisphere dominates; in the left-handed, the right hemisphere or neither dominates. Dominance, however, can be specific for particular manual functions, so that for certain manual tasks, it can be the right hemisphere that is dominant in the right-handed rather than the left. Because being right-handed implies a stronger commitment to the dominant hand than does being left-handed, and because the stronger the dominant hand is, the stronger is that side of the body, the differences felt between asymmetric *yogasanas* done on the left and right sides generally will be larger for right-handed practitioners than for the left-handed.

The picture of the effects of hemispherical laterality on handedness recently has been reoriented by the consideration of the corpus callosum connecting the two hemispheres. It appears that the expression of handedness, as assigned to one or the other of the two hemispheres, is strongly modulated by the thickness of the corpus callosum connecting the two, with a thin corpus correlating with a strong handedness preference and a large diameter of the corpus correlating with a much weaker preference in that regard [902].

A person's general preference for one hand over the other extends to the other body parts as well: nine out of ten people are right-handed, eight out of ten are right-footed, seven out of ten are right-eyed, and six out of ten are right-eared [159]. Judging from studies of ancient artwork, the 90-percent proportion of the right-handed in

Table 4.D-2: Left- and Right-Handedness (%) versus the Dominant Hemisphere for Speech [427]

	Dominant Hemisphere for Speech		
	Right	Left	Both
Right-handed	4	96	0
Left-handed	15	70	15

the human population has been constant at least for the past fifty centuries. It is the essential differences between the functions of the left and right cerebral hemispheres, as expressed in table 4.D-1, that underlie all of these left-right outward asymmetries of the body.

Recent studies show that at the age of ten weeks, the fetus in the womb begins to suck either its right or left thumb, and that this act determines the handedness of the child at age ten years. After only ten weeks in utero, there are no connections from the brain to the limbs, and so one sees that handedness develops long before the brain has any control over limb movement; i.e., the causative determinant for handedness in the fetus cannot have any direct relationship to cerebral-hemispheric lateralization [820].

As table 4.D-2 shows, there is a strong but imperfect correlation between handedness and the dominant hemisphere for speech. Because 90 percent of the population is right-handed, it is no surprise that 96 percent of the population is left-hemisphere dominant for speech, as this hemisphere is dominant for motor control. Left-handed people also are largely left-hemisphere dominant in regard speech, whereas some 15 percent of the left-handed have no hemispheric dominance in this regard, and 15 percent exhibit reversed dominance. Individuals with reversed dominance for speech show no cortical dysfunction but simply illustrate the range of normal variation in brain organization. Though language skills appear to be largely localized in the left hemisphere, if this hemisphere is damaged in an infant under two years old, the language skills develop instead in the right hemisphere, without any apparent problems. However, if the damage

occurs at an age beyond ten years, it cannot be compensated for at all [204].

Language

Because language can be used in so many different ways, it is no surprise that damage to a cerebral area dedicated to a particular language skill can leave other language-skill areas untouched. For example, see figure 4.C-2c, where different aspects of speech are shown to be located in very different areas of the cortex. It is also found that the hearing of speech is best in the left hemisphere, whereas the hearing of music is largely confined to the right hemisphere. The integration of certain sounds other than speaking—sounds such as coughing, crying, and the chanting of Om and of melodies—are handled best by the right hemisphere, the meditative, imaginative, and creative side. In regard to music appreciation, the hippocampus of the left hemisphere appears to prefer dissonance, in contrast to the hippocampus of the right hemisphere, which prefers the harmonies of the barbershop quartet [30].

Both vision and hearing are asymmetrical, in the sense that learning or performing nonverbal tasks is better learned through the left eye, as expected for right-hemisphere dominance (table 4.D-1); whereas verbal material is better handled through the right ear, as expected for left-hemisphere dominance [427]. See Box 17.D-1, page 677, in order to determine the symmetry of your visual dominance.

When adults speak and babies babble, they both tend to open the right side of the mouth more than the left, because the muscles of the right side of the face are controlled by the left cerebral hemisphere, which is dominant when language is used, meaningfully or not. On the other hand, when smiling, the left side of the mouth opens wider, since it is the right cerebral hemisphere and its emotional content that are controlling the smile musculature. The right cerebral hemisphere also perceives touch and visual relations better than the left hemisphere and is more accurate in both proprioception and interoception.

Moods and Emotions

Mood is lateral. Drugging (inhibiting) the left hemisphere with a barbiturate leads to temporary depression, whereas drugging the right hemisphere leads to temporary elation [427]. From this, we see that performing an energy-elevating *yogasana* such as *chaturanga dandasana* has its effect essentially as a left-brain stimulant (i.e., it is stimulating to the sympathetic nervous system), whereas performing a passive, cooling posture such as *savasana* is a right-brain stimulant, specifically activating the parasympathetic system (Chapter 5, page 181).

Inasmuch as the turning of the eyes to the right or to the left correlates with accessing either the left or right cerebral hemispheres (respectively) and their attendant moods, one might logically expect that when doing *trikonasana* to the right and looking up toward the left hand, we are accessing the right hemisphere and so visually promoting a relaxed feeling; whereas when we do *trikonasana* to the left and look up toward the right, we are engaging the left hemisphere and so visually promoting an up-lifting energy.

When one is asked an emotional question about oneself, the eyes look to the left consistently, suggesting that the right hemisphere plays a special role in emotions [204], and showing how strongly a purely cerebral process can be coupled to motion of the eyes. Eye movement to the right during thought correlates with left-hemispheric activity, whereas that to the left signals right-hemispheric activity [513, 721]. When thinking logically about a problem, the eyes tend to shift to the right, as if manipulating information in the left hemisphere; when thinking analogically, the shift of the eyes is to the left, as if working in the right hemisphere [721]. Note, however, that

because the optic nerve does not travel through the spinal cord, it cannot decussate in the normal neural sense, so as to send its input only to the opposite cerebral hemisphere. A possible mechanism for this visual crossover far above the brainstem is given in Subsection 17.D, page 676.

When we are happy, the left prefrontal cortex is electrically active, whereas when we are in a negative mood, it is the right prefrontal cortex that is the more active site. Thus, in cases of depression, it has been found that the intensity of the alpha EEG waves (Subsection 4.H, page 154) that signal a lack of outer awareness and alertness are very strong in the left prefrontal cortex as compared with that in the right prefrontal cortex. On the other hand, when one is depressed, beta-wave activity is high in the right hemisphere. Procedures or postures such as *urdhva dhanurasana* that energize the left frontal lobe of the cortex, switching its activity from alpha to beta waves through stimulation of the sympathetic nervous system, can be curative for depression [705].

Note too that when movie films are viewed through either one eye or the other, the view through the left eye is perceived as more catastrophic and emotional than when the same movie is viewed through the right eye. This is in line with the thought that the view of the left eye is processed in the visual center of the right hemisphere, where depressive visions reign. In binocular vision, the depressing vision of the right hemisphere is dominated by the joyous vision of the left hemisphere [204], except perhaps in depressed individuals (Section 22.A, page 756). Perhaps a depressed *yogasana* student should wear an eye patch over the left eye while practicing, in order to accentuate right-eye vision.

Results recently have been reported [362] in regard to experiments that clearly show that instead of the strong hemispheric lateralization of alphabetic letter memory (left hemisphere) and of letter location (right hemisphere) in college students, these occur in **both** hemispheres simultaneously in people sixty-two to seventy-three years old. Moreover, in certain other mental tasks, seniors who were able to use both hemispheres simultaneously could respond faster than younger

---

Box 4.D-1: Cerebral Laterality in Other Animals

In several animals in which the brain is divided into hemispheres, the separate and independent functions of the two hemispheres have been demonstrated [427]. For example, in some birds, the hemispheric laterality allows them to put one half of their brain to sleep and to close the opposite eye, while the contralateral hemisphere and contralateral eye remain alert for predators! [614]. For ducks and penguins sleeping in groups, those on the outer edges of the group keep the outside eye open for predators while the others sleep with both eyes closed [700].

In dolphins and seals, one half of the brain sleeps while the other half stays awake so as to control breathing and other basic functions. Keeping one hemisphere awake while the other sleeps allows the aquatic mammals to surface, to keep one flipper paddling, and to breathe, all the while keeping one eye open during this sleep phase as a security measure. In this half-asleep/half-awake state, it is not known to what extent the brain is capable of processing information. Clearly, the two cerebral hemispheres in humans have very different functions than those in other animals.

In regard to the unihemispheric sleep in animals mentioned above, EEG alpha waves are observed in only one hemisphere during such sleep. In keeping with the neural decussation of the optic signal, the hemisphere opposite the open eye stays alert. In addition to birds and aquatic mammals, reptiles also show unihemispheric sleep. Thus, lizards sleep with one eye open, apparently on the watch for predators. In the invertebrate octopus, there is an easily demonstrable eye preference as well, but it is thought to be related to the fact that the octopus prefers to dwell in small cavities, from which it can look out with only one eye.

Cats and dogs show a strong paw preference, but it is approximately 50 percent right and 50 percent left across each of the populations, unlike that in humans, where the proportions of handedness are 90 percent right and 10 percent left [159]. In the horse, the dog, and the chimpanzee, the preferences for handedness in each of these animals are opposite in the male and female.

---

students, who were limited to using just one side of the cerebrum at a time. It appears that older people adapt their neutral circuitry to accommodate the mental deterioration of aging. See Box 4.D-1 above for a discussion of the evidence for cerebral laterality in animals other than humans.

Beliefs

It has been proposed by Ramachandran that the left cerebral hemisphere is strongly tied to the old ways of doing things and so seeks consistency, resisting new approaches or new ideas, i.e., it holds strongly to World View II (Subsection 1.A, page 3). In contrast, the right cerebral hemisphere operates in a questioning way and so is naturally skeptical of the older ways of thinking; i.e., it holds strongly to World View I (Subsection 1.A, page 3). In a healthy brain, the two ways of thinking are in constant opposition, which works to keep us balanced mentally; however, if the right hemisphere is damaged, then the left hemisphere is unopposed, and the result is delusion: an unshakeable belief held in spite of clear evidence to the contrary [598]. As examples, he mentions patients who are completely emaciated by their anorexia, yet who see themselves as fat when they look in the mirror; he also mentions those with a sense of grandiosity felt when in the manic phase of bipolar disorder. This brings us full circle to the Tomato Effect discussed in Box 1.A-1, page

5, wherein obvious truths are denied regardless of how clearly correct they are to others.

If this hemispheric imbalance were mild but grew progressively more important as we aged, then it could possibly explain the increasing difficulty people have in accepting new ideas as they grow older (Subsection 4.E, page 119).

Cerebral Hemispheric Interactions

Though the two cerebral hemispheres have distinctly different functions, it is not to say that they do not interact, for they do, in two significant ways. In many situations, the distinct functions of the cerebral hemispheres are masked by the significant neural connections between the hemispheres provided by the corpus callosum, which tends to distribute information and function more evenly between the two hemispheres. In those cases where the corpus callosum has been severed to reduce the intensity of epileptic seizures, the inherent differences between the hemispheres become far more obvious. The corpus callosum connects areas of the cortex that are activated by sensors on the midline of the body (the trunk, back, and face), but it does not connect to the extremities (feet or hands). Moreover, the corpus callosum is the vehicle by which the left hemisphere inhibits the right hemisphere, as in the case of the mentally-impaired savant (Subsection 4.D, page 105). Interestingly, an MRI study of the brain of a savant with a phenomenal memory showed no signs of the corpus callosum or the commissures, suggesting that the release of interhemispheric inhibition by destruction of the corpus callosum and the commissures [869] has resulted in an incredible memory in a person who otherwise is mentally lacking in many other ways.

In addition to the corpus callosum, there is a second, smaller neural bundle that joins the two cerebral hemispheres: the anterior commissure. The two connectors differ, in that the corpus callosum deals with sensations at the higher cerebral levels, and the anterior commissure works instead at the level of the emotional responses within the limbic regions of the two cerebral hemispheres.

Though the basic characteristics of the two cerebral hemispheres can be neatly set out, in fact almost all tasks rely on both hemispheres and their interactions. Thus, to play the piano well, one must have not only the left-brain technical skills by which the keys and pedals are manipulated in the proper order but also the feeling and nuance for the fine shading that can come in a personal, intuitive way only from the right hemisphere. With the two hemispheres working together, the result can be beautiful music.

Yogasana

Yogasana practice can be very much like music. In the beginning, we work in a left-brain, robotic way, following the detailed instructions of the teacher or the book, without any sense of our own uniqueness. This is not bad, but as we mature in the practice, we should allow room for right-brain input into the process, so that as we experiment and inquire as to what *yogasana* practice is about, each of us will come by our own path to that most exciting discovery: who we really are and what we can become if we choose! As in all things done well, we need both the analytical and objective functions of the left brain and the intuitive and subjective creativity of the right brain in appropriate proportions when performing the *yogasanas*.

Pert [654] mentions something that may be of use to *yogasana* students. She finds that she is able to get information flowing readily between the left and right hemispheres by walking with the arms swinging oppositely to the legs; i.e., when the left leg is forward, the right arm should have swung forward with it, and similarly with the right leg and the left arm. This simultaneous and deliberate action of the limbs on opposite sides of the body breaks up old patterns of thought and worry and opens the mind and body to new thoughts and points of view. If true universally, this could be a most useful aid in teaching *yogasanas* to older students (Subsection 4.G, page 149), who otherwise might have developed a resistance to new ideas.

In addition to the instantaneous communication between the cerebral hemispheres via the corpus callosum, there is a second, longer-lasting mode of interaction. In this second mode, the inherent character of one of the hemispheres dominates that of the other for a period of a few hours, and then the dominance is reversed (Subsection 4.D, page 105).

The shapes of the brains of right-handed and left-handed people are quite different. In particular, for right-handers, the left cerebral hemisphere is larger than that of the right side, especially in the Broca's and Wernicke's areas (figure 4.C-2) dedicated to the use of language. In contrast to right-handers, left-handers have noticeably more symmetric brains than do right-handers. This correlates with the fact that right-handers are much more strongly committed to their handedness than are left-handers. It is for this reason that right-handers have a more difficult time placing the right arm behind the back when in *gomukhasana* than the left, whereas for left-handers, there is little or no difference as to which arm is placed behind the back. It seems likely to the author that *yogasana* students who are right-handed will experience asymmetric postures such as *trikonasana* as feeling much more different when performed on the two sides than will the left-handed students.

Transcranial Magnetic Stimulation

In the past, the specific functions of various brain centers were determined through the deliberate or accidental destruction of such a center and the operational deficit then assessed; often it was the reverse, with an operational deficit being assessed, and then the damaged site that correlates with the deficit determined years later by autopsy. Such studies are no longer necessary, for nondestructive methods are now available that quickly and painlessly reveal the correlation between function and site. Among the newest of these is transcranial magnetic stimulation, in which a specific area of the brain can be temporarily disabled (or stimulated) by applying an external pulsed magnetic field of appropriate intensity to that spot on the brain.

When one hemisphere of the brain has been momentarily disabled, as when using an external magnetic field, it is observed that mental function in the opposite hemisphere rises above that observed when the two hemispheres are in their normal states. It appears that the two cerebral hemispheres compete with one another and that when one side is inhibited, the other is then free to perform at higher than normal levels [369]. Apparently something of this sort occurs in certain autistic individuals in whom the left hemisphere is largely nonfunctioning; i.e., not strong enough to inhibit the right hemisphere, thereby allowing the right hemisphere to appear amazingly adept at functions that are nonsymbolic, artistic, visual, and motor. These include exceptional talents in the areas of music (especially the piano), art, mathematics, and spatial skills. On the other hand, these same individuals are deficient in left-brain functions such as logical and symbolic reasoning and language and speech skills. Such savants are most often male, and the condition is thought to relate to the effects of excess testosterone on left-hemisphere development, especially of the left frontotemporal lobe while in utero (see Subsection 6.B, page 221) [868].

Oscillating Dominance of Cerebral Hemispheric Laterality

In addition to the hemispheric lateralities detailed above that are constant in time (handedness, vision, emotions, etc.), there are others that just as clearly oscillate in time between dominance of the right and left hemispheres, with periods of a few hours. Such oscillating processes in the body are termed "ultradian rhythms" (Subsection 23.B, page 772). Chief among the ultradian rhythms is the periodic shifting of the flow of the breath between the left and right nostrils, which occurs every few hours. As might be expected, nasal laterality relates closely to hemispheric laterality, with due regard for decussation. The phenomenon of nasal laterality is discussed in detail in Section 15.E, page 627.

Bilateral Cerebral Asymmetry and Unilateral Breathing

It is no surprise that breathing through one or the other of the two nostrils can have significant effects on cerebral hemispheric dominance. Thus, breathing only through the right nostril increases heart rate, systolic blood pressure, and consumption of oxygen, as appropriate for stimulation of the sympathetic nervous system residing in the left hemisphere [775, 852, 855]. Spatial task performance is enhanced during left-nostril breathing, whereas verbal task performance is enhanced during right-nostril breathing [412]. Left-nostril breathing promotes a higher electrical resistance on the surfaces of the palms, indicating less sweating due to increased parasympathetic excitation [852, 855]. Comparison of the entries in table 4.D-1 with those in table 15.E-1 suggests that hemispheric and nasal lateralities are closely related and that by breathing only through a particular nostril, one can dictate which cerebral hemisphere is to be dominant at that moment. It also has been shown [620] that breathing through one nostril while the second is held closed, called forced unilateral breathing, increases spatial memory but does so equally on the two sides of the cerebrum. Note, however, that one cannot change the dominance of one's handedness by unilateral breathing, as it is only certain of the autonomic functions (Chapter 5, page 192) that can be changed in this way. This is discussed more fully in Section 15.E, page 634.

Using Cerebral Hemispheric Laterality in *Yogasana* Practice

Note first two things: (a) the effects of cerebral and nasal laterality are very subtle and can easily be missed unless one is very inwardly directed, and (b) the nasal laterality on one side can be promoted either by pressing the armpit on the opposite side or by using forced unilateral breathing (Subsection 15.E, page 635).

How can we use the effects of hemispheric laterality in our *yogasana* practice? First, following *Swara* yoga [410], it is known that nasal laterality can be obtained easily by lying on one side of the body or the other (Subsection 15.E, page 634). Given this, it seems reasonable to spend the first ten minutes of *savasana* lying first on the left side to warm the body (right nostril open, left hemi-

sphere stimulated along with the sympathetic nervous system), and then lying on the right to relax the body (left nostril open, right hemisphere stimulated along with the parasympathetic nervous system), provided there is sufficient time to switch nasal laterality, and provided the left-right dominance in the student is strong.

The crutch-in-the-armpit reflexive closing of the nostril on that side (Subsection 15.E, page 634) would seem to be active in any posture in which one has the *ardha baddha padma* grip; i.e., right hand holding the right foot from behind so as to put pressure on the right armpit. This should open the left nostril and promote relaxation, whereas the opposite grip will open the right nostril and promote a lifting of energy, all other things being equal. Similar effects are to be expected in *pasasana, parivrtta parsvakonasana, gomukhasana,* and perhaps *maricyasana III,* but only after being in the position for at least two to five minutes.

Though deliberate shifting of nasal lateralization is expected to be especially effective in *yoga-dandasana,* in other laterally asymmetric *yogasanas* such as *trikonasana,* where there is no direct pressure on the axillae, the lateralization effect will be energizing or calming, depending upon which nostril happens to be open at that moment, all other things being equal. In any event, the rather subtle shift in the relative activity levels of sympathetic and parasympathetic autonomic systems in the course of a *yogasana* practice may or may not be apparent to the student, depending upon their sensitivity to subtle changes in physiological, mental, and emotional states.

Lateral Transfer of Yogasana Posture

B. K. S. Iyengar often states that the learning of the posture on the right side can help to teach the left side (Appendix VI, page 945); perhaps the lateral *yogasanas* such as *trikonasana* are more easily learned on first going to the right, and then this learning is transferred via the corpus callosum and anterior commissure to the other hemisphere to help teach the posture to the left side. There are two interesting new reports in the literature regarding asymmetric neural activity, which eventually may prove to be of some relevance to the question of "one side learning from the other." As there are no known **direct** anatomic connections between those neurons that innervate muscles on the right side of the body and those that innervate muscles on the left side, it is odd to read [628] that there often is clear distal nerve damage and pain at the contralateral site when there is a unilateral nerve injury initiated on only one side of the body. Damage at the contralateral site appears within a week after the initial unilateral injury. A second study [627] reports that in the case of unilateral facial shingles (herpes zoster), there is not only a large decrease in the density of sensory neurites in the affected area but a corresponding loss of neurites on the contralateral side, though the pain is localized on just one side. In each of these two studies, there is the suggestion of neural communication between the left and right sides of the body; perhaps one or both of these studies showing that injury to nerves on one side can injure those on the other will prove to be in line with the yogic concept of the nerves on one side communicating with those on the other.

To the extent that *yogasana* practice involves a reconnection of the mind to the body and may work in part like the placebo response in medicine (Subsection 5.F, page 196), it may be relevant to note that the placebo effect is strongest in those with a right-hemisphere dominance; i.e., those who hold World View I (Subsection 1.A, page 3). The same subclass of people is the most easily hypnotized [721]. As certain aspects of hemispheric dominance oscillate, *yogasana* learning may be better at some times (when right-hemispheric dominant) than at others (when left-hemispheric dominant).

Brain/Body Laterality

It is known that in the general population, there is greater strength, coordination, and balance on the side of the body corresponding to the dominant hand [7]. Hand grip is stronger, bone density is higher, and the muscles are larger on the dominant side. One of the tasks, then, in *yogasana* practice is to work to bring the right and left sides of the body more into balance in regard to the above factors. To the extent that the lateralities of the brain and the body are related, practicing the *yogasanas* to achieve a more nearly equal balance on the two sides of the body also may work to achieve a similar balance on the two sides of the brain.

When the body and brain are strongly lateralized, then such simple actions as interlacing the fingers but changing which index finger is uppermost when entering *parvatasana* can have startling effects on the brain, as the "wrong" hemisphere becomes involved in the mechanics of the process. In this regard, the goal in *yogasana* practice should not be to force the "wrong" side of the brain to do work it is not meant to do, but rather to speed the transfer of neural activities between the two hemispheres via the corpus callosum and anterior commissure; some phenomena in the body are meant to show oscillating laterality on the time scale of hours, and some are not.

The yogic and medical approaches to this subject seem not to be aware of one another, especially in that the yogic approach dwells upon the oscillating character of hemispheric dominance and the medical approach dwells on the static aspects of dominance; only rarely does one mention the other. The subject of overall body symmetry is discussed in Appendix III, page 843.

Section 4.E: Aspects of Brain Structure and Function

Cerebrospinal Fluid

Function and Composition

The central nervous system, composed of the brain, the brainstem, and the spinal cord, is surrounded by several continuous layers of tissue that surround it as if it were in a sack. The innermost layer of that sack is called the pia mater, while the outermost layer is the dura mater. These two layers are separated by the arachnoid mater, and a thin void, the subarachnoid space. The outermost layer of this waterproof sack, also called the dural membrane, is a tough layer of randomly oriented fibers of great strength that cover the central nervous system and the arterioles and venules within, down to the level of the spinal-nerve roots. A clear, colorless cerebrospinal fluid (CSF) generated and stored in the four ventricles of the brain (figure 4.C-5, for example) fills the subarachnoid space, the spinal canal, and a small channel running down the gray matter of the spinal cord [878] (see also Section 17.B, page 665).

The composition of CSF is somewhat like that of blood but lacking the red and white corpuscles and virtually all proteinaceous material. In this, it resembles more closely the aqueous humor of the eyeball (Subsection 17.A, page 661), reinforcing the concept of the eye tissue being derived directly from the brain. However, CSF does differ quantitatively from filtered blood and aqueous humor in the concentrations of certain simple ions [187].

Pressure

Because the choroid plexus that lines the ventricles of the brain produces a steady stream of CSF, and because the brain and spinal canal are otherwise a closed system, there must be a mechanism for the reabsorption of the CSF, lest the internal pressure of CSF builds to dangerous levels. This reabsorption of the CSF is accomplished by structures in the arachnoid layer called villi, which absorb CSF and empty their burden into the nearby venous blood supply. CSF pressure in the spinal canal is regulated by the rate of absorption of the CSF by the arachnoid villi, the rate of CSF production being constant at approximately 500 milliliters per day. Though the volume of the cranium and spinal canal taken together amounts to about 1,650 milliliters, it requires only approximately 125 milliliters of CSF to fill the subarachnoid and spinal space, and this amount is reabsorbed in about four to six hours. If the CSF volume is low by only 15 milliliters, then when in inverted *yogasanas*, the forces on the brain tissues change significantly, and severe headache follows immediately.

The pressure of the CSF within the spinal canal is readily measured by lumbar puncture; hydrostatic pressures of only 5 to 15 millimeters Hg are reported when at rest [360, 427]. The pressure of the CSF in the brain cannot be allowed to rise above the pressure within the arteries (around 120 millimeters Hg), lest the arteries collapse and the flow of blood to the brain be diminished. For this reason, there are pressure receptors in the brain that act to promote a higher arterial pressure should the CSF pressure rise too high [308]. Increases of CSF pressure may be due to brain tumors, meningitis, or malformations in the circulatory system of the brain.

Shock Absorption

The CSF serves to cushion the brain and spinal cord from mechanical shocks. Note too that because the CSF has a density 4 percent greater than that of the brain, the brain floats in the CSF. Due to this flotation effect, the average brain of 1,400 grams (3.1 pounds) in air has a weight of only 50 grams (0.11 pound) when floating in the CSF [427]. Due to the flotation of the brain in CSF, if a particular point on the skull is pressed (as in *sirsasana*), the pressure on the CSF is transmitted equally to all parts of the brain, not just to that part closest to the point being pressed.

The difference in density between the CSF and the brain has several ramifications. First, due to its lower density, the brain in any static position will assume the uppermost attitude. When in *tadasana*, the brain will rest closer to the top of the skull; when in *sirsasana*, the brain will rest farthest from the top of the skull, and it will tend to float so as to be closer to the forehead in *savasana* but further from the forehead when in *chaturanga dandasana*.

Because the brain has a lower density than the surrounding CSF, a sharp blow to the forehead sends the CSF forward and the brain backward, so that the primary effect of such a blow to the forehead will be an impact injury to the occipital lobes in the posterior brain. For this reason, brain damage to boxers often is not in the frontal regions where they are struck but in the occipital regions instead. However, if the impact is strong enough, a rebound of the brain can follow, resulting in a collision of its frontal lobes with the anterior skull [8]. If you were to fall backward from *parivrtta trikonasana* and strike the back of your head on the floor, any injury to the brain would first appear in the frontal lobes and only incidentally in the occipital lobes.

Hydrostatic Pressure

Yet another important function of the CSF concerns the inward pressure exerted by the CSF on the brain of a *yogasana* student in an inverted posture. Because the fluid at the top of a column of fluid rests upon the fluid at the bottom of the column, a pressure at the bottom of the column arises due to the weight of fluid above; this is known as hydrostatic pressure. When inverted, the hydrostatic pressure of the blood within the blood vessel in the brain is added to that of the blood pressure coming from the heart action, the combination of these two yielding a high pressure that might lead to an aneurysm. However, when inverted, the CSF in the brain, being outside the highly pressurized blood vessel, exerts an **inward** hydrostatic pressure on the vessel and so partially compensates the excess blood pressure in the brain. The very important function of CSF in countering the hydrostatic pressure of the blood in the brain's vascular system when inverted is discussed further in Section 14.F, page 584.

The Blood-CSF Barrier

In addition to mechanically cushioning the brain and spinal cord, the CSF also is active in transferring brain metabolites into and out of the deeper recesses of the central nervous system, nourishing the cells in the 2–4 millimeters-thick (0.1–0.2 inches) outer layer of the brain's surface (Subsection 4.C, page 95), and otherwise maintaining a constant environment for the various brain cells. Noxious substances are kept out of the CSF thanks to the blood-CSF barrier, a system much like the blood-brain barrier (Section 14.B, page 560). These barriers keep neuroactive substances such as norepinephrine or acetylcholine from crossing from external sources into the brain, where they would have devastating effects [308]. On the other hand, brain centers are able

to release pain-relieving endorphins into the CSF, following which they are carried to all parts of the central nervous system.

Yogasana and CSF Pulsations

The dural membrane enclosing the brain presses against the sagittal suture, the front-to-back line in the skull where the left and right parietal bones meet (figure 9.A-1). Should the production of CSF proceed too far, then pressurization of the dural membrane would press to open the saggital suture wider. However, the suture contains pressure sensors; when overpressurized by the CSF, the sensors report the condition to the hypothalamus, which then slows the production of CSF and accelerates its reabsorption. Once the reabsorption that lowers the pressure at the suture proceeds too far, the sensors report the low-pressure condition, and the reabsorption of CSF stops and production begins again; this is shown schematically in figure 23.B-1.

As a result of the processes described above, the pressure of CSF in the central nervous system oscillates at a frequency of about ten cycles per minute, and so too does the opening of the sagittal suture! The monitoring of this CSF pulse is a prime concern of craniosacral therapy [871], the first step of which is to manipulate the bones of the skull so as to release any jamming at the sutures. Adjustment of the craniosacral pulse is then possible in the hands of a trained worker, so as to restore good health. This pulse rate of about 0.17 hertz is known as the Mayer wave and appears in many places in the body (Subsection 14.A, page 550). In contrast to this, work on cadavers of the elderly shows these cranial sutures to be cemented closed by solid bone. This appears to be another case of flexibility lost through disuse [275, 871].

The general level of muscle tension can manifest itself as a resistance of the sagittal sutures to open and close in response to CSF pulsation [871]. However, the fact that the sutures of the skull contain blood vessels, innervated pressure receptors, collagen, and elastic fibers suggests that the sutures were meant to be opened, rather than cemented shut. One easily can imagine that the practice of *sirsasana I* and its variations could be a very effective means of keeping the sutures of the skull open, supple, and free of calcification while reducing muscle tension as well.

The position of many in the medical establishment is to vigorously deny the existence of the CSF pulse and the movement of the cranial plates about the sutures. For example, consider the assertion by a Western medical doctor that "cranial therapy [is] a quack method of 'manipulating' the bones of the skull. As anyone who has studied anatomy ought to know, the bones of the skull are fused together and cannot be manipulated" [206]. This is perhaps another example of the Tomato Effect (Box 1.A-1, page 5), still in operation to this day. If the sutures are indeed closed, one wonders "Why is the area in question rife with elastic tissue and pressure and stretch receptors?" Most recently, the amplitude of the parietal-suture motion induced by CSF pulsation has been measured experimentally to be about 250 μ (0.01 inches) [111], a distance so small as to be easily missed by the untrained eye or insensitive hand.

Also within the realm of reason is the idea that the significant rise and fall of CSF pressure might involve a corresponding rise and fall of the CSF level in the subarachnoid space. As subconscious signals regarding the status of the CSF are sent to the nerve centers in the hypothalamus [721], it is imaginable that one could sense the level of CSF in the subarachnoid space by sensing the level of tension in the dural membrane or at the sagittal suture resulting from the pressurization. Perhaps this is the mechanism whereby B. K. S. Iyengar is able to convert normally subconscious signals sent to the hypothalamus into consciousness, thereby sensing the level of CSF in the spinal canal in various *yogasanas*.

CSF Flow

Experiments show that the CSF is in motion within its space, especially so when the body is in motion, so as to produce different pressures in different parts of the system [187]. Much as energy can be felt to follow a circular path, moving up the front of the chest and down the back in the *yogasanas*, the CSF is known to flow up the ante-

rior side of the spinal cord and down the posterior side [431]. Through this action, the brain and spinal cord are bathed in a constantly refreshed pool of CSF, which aids the blood in the maintenance of the brain cells. The health benefits of *yogasanas* in regard to keeping the CSF in circulation must be appreciable, especially in *sirsasana I*. However, should this circulation be blocked in some way, then intracranial pools of stagnant CSF are pressurized by the incoming fluid from the ventricles, and should the pressure regulation system malfunction at this point, the result is a high-pressure hydrocephalic condition known as "water on the brain." Dangerously high pressures of CSF can extrude the brain through the foramen magnum, the opening in the base of the skull.

Blood Flow through the Brain

Constancy

Physically, the brain is only 2 percent of an adult's body weight, yet this organ receives 15 percent of the cardiac output and accounts for 20 percent of the body's demand for oxygen [427]. The adult brain requires approximately 0.75 liters (almost a quart) of freshly oxygenated blood every minute in order to function properly, with a four-fold larger flow of blood through the gray matter of the brain as compared to that through the white matter. Cessation of this flow of fresh blood to the brain for only five seconds induces a change in mental state, cessation for ten seconds leads to unconsciousness, cessation for five minutes leads to irreversible damage, and cessation for ten minutes leads to the permanent loss of most, if not all, mental powers [199]. It is thought that blood flow to the brain could be interrupted for thirty minutes without damage were it not for the clots formed in the stagnant blood, which then damage the brain once blood flow is resumed [308]. By comparison, blood flow to the spinal cord can be interrupted for up to thirty minutes without permanent damage. It seems likely that the brain's sensitivity to blood flow lies behind the altered mental states so readily achieved in meditative postures such as *virasana* and *padmasana*

(Box 10.B-1, page 352), as these possibly would involve a shift of blood flow to the brain due to the reduced circulation of the blood in the legs.

The brain's demands on the body are simple but non-negotiable: it must be supplied with oxygen and glucose, delivered by a circulatory system that can be depended upon indefinitely and without qualification. Blood carrying oxygen and glucose to the brain from the heart moves through two main channels, the internal carotid arteries and the vertebral arteries (figure 4.E-1). The carotid arteries are found on either side of the neck, whereas the vertebral arteries pass through the transverse foramina of the C1 to C6 vertebrae on each side, bypassing C7. The vertebral and carotid arteries supply the Circle of Willis, a circular structure within the brain from which many smaller arteries branch in order to serve both exterior and interior structures [199]. About 75 percent of the arterial blood flow to the brain is via the internal carotid arteries and 25 percent is via the vertebral arteries. Metabolic waste products are carried out of the brain by a complex venous system converging upon the jugular veins. The cortex within the brain is served by three arteries: the posterior, middle, and anterior arteries (figure 4.E-1).

Redistributing the Flow

Blood flow to the brain at age sixty-five years may be as small as one-third that at age twenty-five years [250]. One would guess that this long-term diminution of the blood flow to the brain might be slowed by yogic inversions; however, there is no proof that I can find that supports the popular view that standing on one's head increases the short-term flow of blood to the brain or promotes mental clarity. In fact, given the very tight control of the homeostatic conditions in the brain, it would be surprising if inversion were effective in changing the homeostatic blood flow rate. This is supported by the data in table 14.A-2 showing that the blood flow through the heart may be increased sixfold by heavy exercise, yet the blood flow through the brain (0.75 liters per minute) remains constant! On the other hand, when in the REM phase of sleep, blood flow

through the brainstem and cerebellum are said to increase by 47 percent and by 41 percent in the cerebral hemispheres, respectively [30]. Perhaps the oft-stated clearing of the mind that follows from inversion is a consequence of a significant **redistribution** of blood flow, wherein the total blood flow through the brain is held constant but increases in certain local areas at the expense of the blood flow in other areas [112a]. Indeed, experiments show that blood flow is constant, irrespective of the level of mental work being performed, and it has been suggested that the redistribution takes place through an appropriate shift of certain arterial and venous diameters [112a]. Thus, for example, if the blood flow to the emotional center, the amygdala, increases due to an emotional response to a specific situation, there will be a corresponding decrease of blood flow to the more rational area of the brain, the frontal lobe. As a consequence of this shift of blood flow from the rational center to the emotional center of the brain, we then have a more difficult time maintaining rational control of the situation. On the other hand, a good *yogasana* practice is not only a benefit for the body but should redirect blood away from the amygdala, so as to give the emotional part of the brain a rest. This may be relevant to the release of emotional tension attendant to doing *halasana* [724] and other passive *yogasanas* as restorative postures.

It is known that heavy exercise enhances the growth of the capillary system serving the newly used muscle in order to deliver fresh blood (Subsection 11.A, page 375); it seems possible that because such physical exercise implies increased work for the motor cortex, which drives the muscles, the motor cortex, in such a situation, also might experience an enhancement of its vascular system [793]. This may relate in turn to the positive effects exercise has on the cognitive performance of older people. Brain-imaging techniques have shown that blood flow through the brain can be noticeably altered within seconds in response to neural activities. For example, making a fist of the right hand results in an immediate increase in the flow of blood in the left motor cortex, while reading causes an imme-

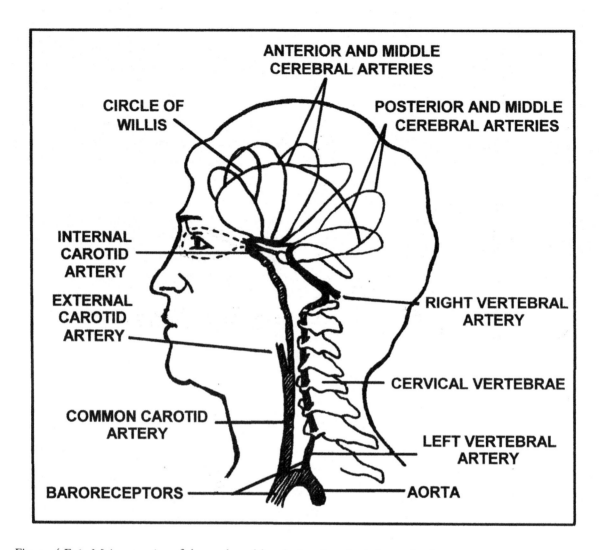

Figure 4.E-1. Major arteries of the neck and head, showing the left vertebral artery within the foramina on the left sides of the cervical vertebrae and the external and internal carotid arteries. The blood flow through the internal carotid and vertebral arteries is roughly in the ratio 3:1. The internal carotid arterial branches about the eye socket are shown schematically by dashed lines.

diate flow of blood to the occipital cortex and to the language areas of the left temporal cortex (Wernicke's area, figure 4.C-2a).

Effects of Exercise

Recent research on the effects of exercise on brain function in the aged reports that aerobic exercise (walking three times a week) has a strongly positive effect on increasing blood flow to those parts of the frontal cortex that are known to be used for allocating attention, and decreasing blood flow to those regions involved in situations of indecision. A comparative study in which the aerobic work was replaced by "stretching and toning exercises," presumably of the *yogasana* sort but so mild as not to cause heavy breathing, showed no noticeable changes in the same brain centers [80]. Presumably, *yogasana* practice by seniors done with enough challenge so as to result in aerobic breathing for about thirty to forty-five minutes three times a week would result in the same improvement in attentiveness and decision making as was found in the aerobic walking study.

Brain Fuel

Unlike other organs, which burn fuels such as fats and proteins, the brain functions only by combining glucose with oxygen. Thus, fats and fatty acids in muscles can be oxidized in the absence of oxygen by an anaerobic process (Subsection 11.A, page 393), but this is not so in the brain, where the blood-brain barrier blocks the transport of fats and fatty acids from the blood into the brain.[10] The brain's insistent demand for the oxidation of glucose by oxygen can be met only by an adequate rate of flow of glucose-laden blood. In fact, when deprived of sustenance, the body can continue to live for weeks or even months by metabolizing fats and proteins, whereas the brain immediately runs into serious trouble when the supply of glucose or oxygen is blocked for ten minutes.

Due to the impermeability of the blood-brain barrier to many of the mobile cells of the immune system, the brain has an immune system that is separate from that of the rest of the body; see Subsection 14.B, page 558, and Subsection 16.D, page 646.

Heat Dissipation

As can be seen in table 14.A-2, the brain burns glucose with oxygen at a great rate (estimated at generating a heat load of 10 watts when fully functional), and so the brain runs hot; when the air temperature is 21.1° C (70.0° F) the temperature is only 21.0° C (69.8° F) at one's foot, but it is 33.3° C (91.4° F) at one's head. At the same time, the brain is very sensitive to overheating, with damage being evident at just 33.8° C (92.8° F) and brain death occurring at temperatures above 41.1° C (106° F). In order to avoid overheating, there must be a very efficient transfer of heat from the neurons to the circulation system within the brain; it is thought that this transfer of heat from neural tissues to blood vessels is aided by the large area of the convoluted cortex.

The heat transfer from the neural elements to the brain's blood presents the problem of how to cool the blood. The high flow rate of the blood through the brain helps in keeping the interior of the brain cool, for the heat load otherwise is quite high (see table 14.A-2 in regard to oxygen demands by various parts of the body during exercise). This heat load generated by the brain and transferred to the vascular system is handled in part by large-area structures within the nose (nasal conchae, Subsection 15.A, page 600), which efficiently transfer the heat of the blood in the brain to the inspired and expired air passing through the nose.

Baroreceptors

That there is sufficient blood pressure to maintain optimum flow through the brain is monitored by the baroreceptor organs (Section 14.E, page 580), which are located within the carotid arteries close to the brain itself (figure 4.E-1). If the neck is squeezed at the carotid arteries, the baroreceptors in that location mistakenly report a high pressure to the brain, which in turn adjusts the heart's action and the associated vascular plumbing so that less blood flows to the brain. As a consequence, the brain is starved for blood in the extreme situation, and the person faints, thereby assuming a horizontal position that once more promotes the flow of blood through the brain. In less severe situations, as when in *sarvangasana,* the increased pressure in the carotid arteries results in reduced heart action and a lowered blood pressure, all other aspects of the posture remaining calm. When practiced in this way, *sarvangasana* is a strongly relaxing posture.

In *yogasana* practice, the momentary throttling of the blood supply to the brain by virtue of the neck posture can have both negative and positive consequences. For example, in the head-forward (flexion) position, as in *karnapidasana,* etc., the mild throttling of the blood flow through the carotid arteries generally slows the heart as the baroreceptors within the arteries report a high pressure to the hypothalamus. This slowing of the heartbeat is welcome, as it promotes relaxation (Section 14.F, page 585). On the other hand, when the head is held in extension, as when thrown backward in *ustrasana,* the throttling of blood flow through the vertebral arteries within

_____

10   Given this, how strange it is to read that brain tissue is 60 percent fatty substances!

the cervical vertebrae can lead to nausea and dizziness, especially if the scapulae are not pulled away from the base of the skull so as to relieve the congestion at the back of the neck (Appendix II, page 838).

Headaches

Sources of Pain

Though the brain is a complex web of neurons and records the sensations of pain from all of the other parts of the body, it can feel no pain generated within itself, because it has no sensors for touch, local pressure, or pain among its neurons. However, pain in the immediate area surrounding the brain often is interpreted as brain pain (headache). That is to say, headache often involves distress in areas surrounding the brain, resulting from dilation or distension of the blood vessels in the scalp or the meninges (the three-fold protective covering of the brain); from spasms of the muscles of the scalp, neck, shoulders, jaw, or face; or from compression of the nerves. There also appear to be pain receptors within the arteries serving the brain, which become painful during vasoconstriction.

Head pain originating outside the brain involves the stimulation of free nerve endings in the area of the head, the transmission of the pain signal downward into the spinal cord, and then its return up the spinal cord, brainstem, and thalamus to finally register in the cingulate cortex [326]. Headache is thus the pain referred from superficial structures of the head to deeper structures (Section 13.D, page 532).

The sensation of headache also can result when arteries or veins in the brain are pulled, displaced, dilated, or disturbed, or when the trigeminal (cranial nerve V), vagus (cranial nerve X), or glossopharyngeal (cranial nerve IX) (Subsection 2.C, page 24) is pulled, compressed, or inflamed [621]. Headaches that involve the state of mechanical tension in the blood vessels are called vascular headaches, whereas those involving muscle tension are called muscle-contraction headaches [200]. Among these two, the more common head-

ache is of the muscle-contraction variety [313]. It is also felt that disruptions to the regular day-to-day pattern of biorhythms (Subsection 23.B, page 771) can precipitate headaches. Fortunately for the headache sufferer, the frequency and intensity of headaches decrease as one ages.

Muscle-Contraction Headache

As the muscle-contraction headache is often brought on by muscle tension in the neck, shoulder, and cranial areas, the symptomatic posture is one in which the head and shoulders are carried well forward, with the chest collapsed and the thoracic curve exaggerated. As a result of poor cervical posture, nerve compression between the occiput and the atlas also can contribute to headache [494]. It comes as no surprise that excessive contractions of the muscles of the neck also can pull on the base of the skull in a way that leads to headache. In particular, the bilateral cervical muscles rectus capitis posterior minor connect the dura mater surrounding the central nervous system to the occiput of the skull. Placing the head and neck in extreme extension by contraction of the capitis muscles interferes with the recirculation pattern of the cerebrospinal fluid within the central nervous system (Subsection 4.E, page 110), and the result is headache. Thus, Gudmestad [303] finds that some students, while in *urdhva dhanurasana*, place the neck into extension (occiput toward the shoulder blades) to such an extent that headache results. Temporomandibular joint (TMJ) dysfunction and dental problems also can cause headaches.

Contraction headaches usually are daytime events and last about thirty minutes; pain is nagging but mild, and the tension patterns in the dura mater that lead to such headaches are largely due to muscular stress. Because headaches of the contraction type are promoted by muscle tension in the upper body, a regular practice of *yogasana* that works to reduce muscular tension in the upper body also works to erase what otherwise would be triggers for this headache type.

Depression and Anxiety Headaches

One of the more frequent types of persistent headache is closely associated with ongoing depression and anxiety [326]. As discussed in Subsection 22.A, page 756, depression is due largely to a lack of several neurotransmitters in the brain (mainly epinephrine and possibly serotonin), and this chemical imbalance can lead to sleep disturbances, etc. (table 22.A-1). When in the throes of depression, the sufferer easily falls asleep, but the depression headache typically begins at 4:00 to 5:00 AM, arousing the sufferer, who then cannot go back to sleep. In contrast, anxiety sufferers have headaches at bedtime and have trouble falling asleep. Note that the early-hour time of 4:00 to 5:00 AM corresponds to the time at which the autonomic nervous system switches from parasympathetic to sympathetic dominance, and the early-evening hours are when the autonomic nervous system switches from sympathetic to parasympathetic balance (Subsection 23.B, page 774).

The diffuse pain of the depression headache is due to muscular contraction of the band of muscles surrounding the head like a hatband and most often affects the frontal and occipital lobes. This headache type is treated medically with analgesics, antidepressants, and muscle relaxants, all of which prompt the sympathetic nervous system to raise the levels of catecholamines in the brain and/or modify the serotonin levels [565].[11] The increase of the catecholamines also can be achieved by performing a vigorous set of *yogasanas* that emphasize motion of the cervical vertebrae (*halasana, dwi pada viparita dandasana, ustrasana,* etc.), followed by an extended relaxation.

---

11   The standard medical therapy for depression involves taking drugs (Prozac, Zoloft, etc.) aimed at retarding the destruction or reuptake of serotonin in certain of the brain's synapses, thereby giving a boost to the effectiveness of the serotonin. However, several workers in this field point out that the effectiveness of such serotonin re-uptake inhibitors is only slightly higher than that of placebos, and thus their effectiveness in reducing depression is due largely to psychological rather than to physiological factors.

Vascular Headache

The nerves surrounding the large blood vessels of the head are exquisitely sensitive to vascular pressure and readily give rise to vascular pain as the blood vessels expand. In vascular headaches, the precipitating cause is an overexpansion of the blood vessels of the brain itself, or of the vessels of the scalp and meninges, due to vasodilation brought on by the release of neurotransmitters such as serotonin and norepinephrine. One can imagine that in the fixed volume of the skull, dilation of the arteries in the brain leads to an increased internal pressure that expresses itself as a headache and which is released when treated in a way that lowers the vascular pressure within the skull.

Cluster headaches (in which the pain localizes around one eye) and some migraine cases fall into the vascular headache category. Often, mild vascular headaches (but not migraines) are associated with excessive sympathetic tone in the body and can be eased by the passive performance of a few *yogasanas* in which the forehead is supported on a hard surface; e.g., *adho mukha svanasana* with the forehead on a block or *adho mukha virasana* with the forehead on the floor. These postures, in which the forehead and/or the orbits of the eyes receive external mechanical pressure, stimulate the ocular-vagal heart-slowing reflex (Subsection 11.D, page 457) and so lower the blood pressure; the acupressure points bladder 2 just above the eyebrows are used for headache relief in that type of therapy. Among people having chronic headache, 65 percent felt that the source of their headache was stress (on the job and otherwise), and for such people, a general stress-relieving *yogasana* practice should be beneficial.

Iyengar [398] recommends a *yogasana* routine as therapy for headache that consists of fourteen postures; in almost every one, the head is supported on either the front surface or the back. Presumably, those postures that cradle the skull from behind (*supta virasana, setu bandha* in *sarvangasana,* etc.) work to release muscle tension in the area of the skull, neck, and shoulders, while those which support from the front (the supported forward bends) invoke the ocular-vagal heart-slowing reflex (Subsection 11.D, page 457) in order to reduce blood pressure in the brain. Drug therapy of the vascular headache is centered on regaining a measure of vasoconstriction by using alpha agonists, beta blockers, ergotamine, and caffeine, all of which act to constrict the smooth muscle of the blood vessels.

As suggested above, certain vascular headaches, if not too intense, can be relieved by drinking a cup of regular caffeinated coffee but are intensified by drinking a decaffeinated brew. The quickest and longest-lasting relief from a vascular-tension headache is obtained by taking ibuprofen and caffeinated coffee simultaneously [917]. However, the more effective a cup of coffee is in alleviating headache symptoms, the stronger is the rebound headache when coffee is withheld [704]. As alcohol is a strong vasodilator, overindulgence leads to arterial vasodilation in and about the brain and the hangover headache that follows heavy drinking. The pain of a vascular headache also will be exacerbated by the vasodilation that follows low atmospheric pressure.

Sinus Headache

Another type of headache related to over-pressurization of the vascular system is found in sinus headaches, where the fluid pressure and/or pressure gradients stretch the nerves in the sinuses; this can involve excess cerebrospinal fluid (CSF). Also, if the body is dehydrated, then the CSF chemical/osmotic balance is upset, and headache can result. Headache related to sinus congestion can be either exacerbated or relieved by inverted *yogasanas;* you must try them for a minute or two and see if the symptoms intensify or fade away.

Migraine

It appears that the migraine headache begins with a hypersensitivity of the visual area of the occipital lobe of the cortex, which, when stimulated, leads to vasodilation, production of the prostaglandins, and pain. Most often, migraines strike in the hours between 6:00 AM and noon; i.e., at a time when the sympathetic nervous system is in ascendance. Easing the distress of migraine headaches through *yogasana* involves passive positions, well supported, with eyes bandaged, minimal movement, and minimal external input of sensations, all aimed at minimal activation of the reticular formation and the sympathetic nervous system [693].

Yogasana

Yogasanas that work to release tension in the neck, shoulder, and chest areas can be effective therapy for headaches. So, for example, *setu bandha sarvangasana, viparita karani, savasana,* and the arm positions for *gomukhasana* and *garudasana* are effective in reducing the effects of muscle-contraction headaches [494, 773], as they release muscle tension in these critical areas. To the extent that prolotherapy (Subsection 7.E, page 251) strengthens ligaments that have been pulled into stressed positions by faulty postures, it too can be used successfully to treat muscle-contraction headaches [2]. There is anecdotal evidence that the protracted practice of *sarvangasana, sirsasana,* and *savasana* is effective in reducing or eliminating attacks of migraine [112a].

Brain Injury

The brain can be injured in several ways. Rapid head movement followed by rapid deceleration (as when in auto accident) can lead to a shearing force in the brain due to a torque on the upper reticular formation, leading to loss of consciousness. It is easy to imagine that such an injury also might result from trying to turn the head suddenly while in *halasana* or *sarvangasana.* Because the brain shrinks as we age but the skull maintains its size, the veins from the brain can be easily overstretched by rapid head movements, and this can lead to a slow but serious leakage of venous blood into the subarachnoid or subdural spaces.

If, instead, a student falls and suffers a blow to the point of the chin, the force of the blow may be transmitted through the jaw directly to the brainstem, where it passes through the foramen magnum. The shock of such a blow can interrupt the continuity of the reticular formation and so lead to a loss of consciousness. Injuries incurred by a blow to the head also can sever or strain other neural fibers; the longer the path of the neurons, the greater the chance of injury, especially as between the afferent and efferent neural centers in the brain. In the event that some neurons die as a result of a blow to the head, recovery is still possible, thanks to the plasticity of the brain, which allows the establishment of alternate neural paths.

Blunt-Force Trauma

In blunt-force trauma to the head, the rapidly moving head is forced onto a hard surface, and the brain is forced into contact with the skull at the point of contact of the skull with the surface and also at the pole point diametrically opposite, where it is forced away from the point of contact. Injuries from this sort of trauma can be healed using antioxidant therapy and free-radical scavengers [799].

Blunt-force neural trauma is distinctly different from the vascular injuries to the brain that can originate in the cervical spine, for example, when the head is turned while in *sarvangasana* (see, for example, Subsection II.B, page 835). In this latter case, injury can result from two scenarios. First, when the cervical vertebrae are both loaded and twisted, the flow of oxygen to the brain via the vertebral arteries is insufficient for the complete oxidation of the glucose used as fuel, and harmful waste products accumulate (Subsection 11.A, page 376). This can lead to neural injury and neural death. Second, there may be direct injury of the spinal cord in the cervical section of the spinal canal on twisting. Either of these situations can be more serious than falling and striking the head on the floor.

Stroke

When blood flow within the brain is totally disrupted locally, brain function in that locality is nil and the person is said to have had a stroke. Later resumption of blood flow through the

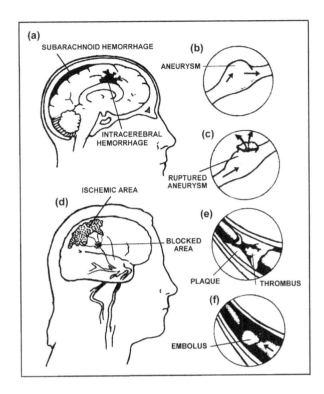

Figure 4.E-2. (a) Sites of either subarachnoid or intracerebral hemorrhages, (b) the weak site of a possible aneurysm in the vascular plumbing, and (c) the aneurysm ruptures. (d) Arterial blockage leading to ischemia due to either (e) the buildup of plaque to form a thrombus or (f) the detachment of the thrombus to form a mobile embolus.

stroke region can cause further injury. A stroke occurs when blood flow is interrupted by either a vascular hemorrhage, called a hemorrhagic stroke (figure 4.E-2), in which a vessel in the brain ruptures, or by blockage to the flow (an ischemic stroke).

Twenty percent of strokes are hemorrhagic and eighty percent are ischemic in nature [203]. The effect of a stroke varies depending upon which part of the brain suffers the stroke, and because of the brain's bilaterality, the effect often is limited to one side of the body. More than half of all ischemic strokes and a third of all brain hemorrhages occur between the hours of 6:00 AM and noon, in line with the blood pressure surge at this time (tables 23.B-1 and 23.B-2).

Note that a small stroke in the left cerebral

hemisphere will likely interfere with the motor co-ordination of the dominant right hand and cause damage to the language centers in the left hemisphere as well; thus a small, left hemisphere stroke will be much more evident than a small stroke in the right cerebral hemisphere, where the effect is more likely to be something like an increase in absentmindedness. In fact, an extensive study has shown that left-hemisphere stroke is 13 percent **more** common than right-hemisphere stroke.

Should there be either a stroke in the brain or a heart attack due to restriction of the blood flow in the heart, the neurons in the affected areas continue to die for days after the blood flow has been restored. This self-induced dying is known as apoptosis (Subsection 3.A, page 32) and is due in these cases to a malfunction within the mitochondria [249].

Hemorrhagic Stroke

As shown in figure 4.E-2, there are two possible types of brain hemorrhage, the first involving the pooling of blood in the subarachnoid space, and the second involving the pooling of blood in a ventricle of the brain. In either case, the hemorrhage is a consequence of the rupture of a blood vessel. Hemorrhagic strokes involve dying red blood cells that injure and kill neurons due to free radicals formed from the iron in the released hemoglobin; this leads to blood-filled swellings known as hematoma. A hematoma pressing on the brain can force it through the foramen magnum, and at the very least, cause an ischemic blockage due to the high pressure. As discussed in Subsection 24.A, page 812, formation of a hematoma between the dura mater and the arachnoid layer is seen in the brains of older citizens who fall or otherwise shear neural tissues, and is due to the strain placed on the cranial veins as the brain ages.

Ischemic Stroke

Ischemic strokes are caused by atherosclerosis and the formation of blood clots (thrombi). If the vascular wall bulges to form an aneurysm, then the turbulent swirl of blood around the obstruction and the quiescent blood within it can lead to

the formation of a blood clot that in turn can embolize (figures 4.E-2d, 4.E-2e, and 4.E-2f). Once the embolized clot lodges in the brain, it impedes blood flow to the downstream areas, resulting in ischemic symptoms; i.e., inflammation and neural death.

Clot formation also can occur in the heart, and the clots then are carried to the brain; however, small clots that form in the heart are often cleared in the vascular web of the lungs before they can get to the brain. Clot formation is also encouraged by holding *yogasana* postures that locally can slow the flow of blood for long periods of time; e.g., in the lower legs when performing *padmasana* for an hour or more. See Subsection II.B, page 838, for more on this topic.

Prevention and Healing

Should part of the cortex suffer a stroke and so erase sensation or motor control over a part of the body, then nearby areas will eventually move into the vacated cortical space, unless a heroic effort is made to hold onto it. Actually, following a stroke, the dead part of the cortex is surrounded by an area that is not dead but is in shock. Through vigorous physical therapy involving the lost function, the shocked part of the cortex can be brought back to functionality, often in the mode of the lost brain cells [816].

Keeping in mind how the affected area in a stroke may recover its functionality if it is exercised with great intensity, it seems possible that our brains are constantly suffering microstrokes and that our *yogasana* practice keeps the affected areas and their surroundings functional and in doing so, heals the brain without any outward signs of disability. In a way parallel to bone remodeling (or Iyengar's general idea in regard to injury and healing; see Section 16.E, page 650), this "brain remodeling" would take advantage of the plasticity of the brain, just as plasticity is involved with bone remodeling and muscle remodeling. Following an injury to the brain, an induced plasticity works toward maximizing the functionality of the brain in spite of the injury; i.e., a work-around can be initiated. This scenario is much like that proposed by R. Mehta [557a] for the mechanism behind yoga therapy in general (Subsection 14.C, page 573).

Small daily doses of aspirin are effective in preventing stroke in women, but not in men. On the other hand, men benefit from similar doses in regard to heart attack, whereas women receive no protection in this regard. This latter fact is related to the very different symptoms experienced by men and women at the onset of a heart attack (Subsection 14.A, page 556).

The interesting phenomenon of preconditioning (Subsection 16.F, page 655) operates in regard to stroke, for the outcome following a major stroke is significantly more positive if the brain has been preconditioned for this injury by having survived a number of smaller strokes. If there has been no preconditioning, then the consequences following the major stroke event are more serious.

Maturation, Aging, and Gender Effects on the Brain

Brain Growth and Death

Regardless of one's age, every individual is a work in progress, as both our genes and the environment continue to be important to our development throughout our lives. During prenatal development, the brain produces an average of 250,000 new brain cells each minute, and at some points in the development, the rate of neurogenesis may reach 50,000 neurons per second! By the twentieth week of fetal life (the second trimester), more than 200 billion neurons have been set in place, after which a cutting back occurs. At week 26, the number of neurons is reduced by 50 percent, and the number of neurons in the brain then remains at 100 billion until full term; the number of synapses (Section 3.C, page 48) is far larger than the number of neurons.

The amazing power of the human brain comes not only from the huge number of neurons but also from the immense number of connections (Section 3.C, page 48) possible in such a collection of neurons. At age eight months, the infant brain has 1,000 trillion synapses, but

the brain has only half that by age ten years. Even more amazing is the fact that the brain of a three-year-old child has more synapses and a higher density of neurons than does the brain of an adult and consumes 225 percent more energy daily than does the adult brain! Everything that the child learns is transformed immediately into a new pattern of connectivity, and the more we learn, the more we are capable of learning the same sort of material.

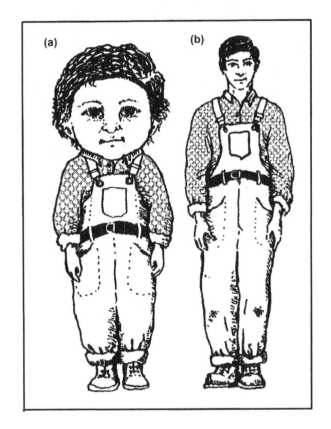

Figure 4.E-3. Comparison of the relative sizes of body parts in a five-month-old infant drawn to the same height as a grown adult male [876], both in *tadasana*. Each of the figures is drawn with the proportions appropriate to its age.

Beginning at the fetal stage, an invasive innervation of the muscle fibers takes place, with each motor neuron connected to several muscle fibers; however, with time and use of the muscles, the innervation resolves, so that each muscle fiber has only one neuron to stimulate it. Similarly, in the autonomic ganglia, neurons at first have many presynaptic connections, but this later resolves to one per ganglion [427].

The general picture, then, is that one is born with a brain that has the potential to develop in many different directions, but once the pattern has been set, excess baggage is shed. This means that anatomically, the brain of a newborn infant is very much oversized as compared to that of an adult, as can be seen in figure 4.E-3, in which a five-month-old infant has been drawn to the scale of an adult male. In a newborn, the area of the head is 19 percent of the body's surface area, whereas in the adult, it is only 7 percent of the surface area, and so the head is disproportionately larger in the infant by almost a factor of three.

In African societies where there is little or no use of calendars, it is decided that a child is ready for school (age five to seven years) when his body proportions are such that he can reach his hand across the top of his head and hold the opposite ear. Clearly, the infant in the figure has several years to go, whereas the adult is more than ready for school.

In the infant brain, there is considerable rewiring in the first two years, with less obvious changes for a few years after that. During these early years, there is considerable reorganization as neural paths are developed, unneeded neurons are shed, and frequently used circuits are strengthened. Myelination in the brain continues up to ages seven to ten years, and at this age, the corpus callosum (Subsection 4.C, page 97) is fully active in connecting the verbal capacities of one hemisphere with the nonverbal capacities of the other hemisphere. Once beyond this point, the learning of language becomes much more difficult.

Adolescence

It has only recently been appreciated that significant changes in brain makeup and function can continue into the teenage years [551]. Between the ages of ten and twelve years, a considerable increase in the sizes of the parietal and frontal lobes occurs by virtue of an explosion of brain-cell numbers and the numbers of their syn-

apses. These are the lobes that are responsible for such functions as planning, social judgment, and self-control. There then follows a shrinking of these lobes up to the mid-twenties, by which time the brain circuitry has again pared away unneeded neurons (by excitotoxicity and/or by apoptosis; Subsection 3.A, page 32) and has completed its myelination of those neurons that remain. This then is its final configuration. It is assumed that this remodeling of the brain during adolescence is responsible for the moody and impulsive actions (and depression) of children during these years [290]. Though wholesale paring away of unused neurons in our early years slows or stops altogether in adulthood, this is not to say that rewiring of existing neurons does not occur, for we maintain the ability to learn and remember throughout life.

Aging

The effects of aging on the mature brain are played out in three arenas: the chemical, the physical, and the mental (see also Chapter 24, page 805). Chemically, the neurotransmitter dopamine in the brain is very important for movement control, and consequently, loss of dopamine on aging can lead to Parkinson's-like motor problems; in the aging brain, dopamine levels drop by 40 percent. Because dopamine is a critical neurotransmitter in the sense of pleasure, loss of pleasure due to loss of dopamine is another problem to be faced by the aged. On the other hand, the level of monoamine oxidase in the brain, a neurotransmitter which helps manage depression, increases with age, though depression nonetheless can be a serious problem in the elderly.

Physically, seventy-year-olds (on average) have 11 percent smaller brains than forty-year-olds, with the weight of brain tissue decreasing as the ventricular volumes increase. This shrinkage appears to be due to an irreversible loss of neurons. The number of neurons in the locus ceruleus, sensitive to norepinephrine, decrease by 35 percent in the elderly. The largest changes are in the most important of the brain's regions, i.e., in the cortex. Here, the number of cells decreases by 40 percent by age seventy-five years, as compared with a twenty-year-old. Within the cortex, the largest drop is in the temporal lobe, one of the sites for storage of memories and where the sulci widen with age.

There is still discussion of what exactly is going on in the aging brain, for it is argued by some that the shrinkage of the brain is not a decrease of numbers but only of size and form of the neurons. Thus, Restak and Mahoney [702] argue that the loss is of neurons not involved in thinking and that the mature brain is organized differently, has different strengths, and can remodel itself. In the past twenty years, it has been realized that the populations studied in earlier brain research involved significant numbers of people with various illnesses that can affect brain function [327]. For example, chronic stress can damage the hippocampus, and chronically high blood pressure can lead to cognitive decline. On the other hand, in a population of healthy but elderly subjects, there was no neural loss of any sort apparent, and evidence is becoming stronger that neurogenesis in the brain occurs not only into adulthood but in the hippocampus, even for several days after one dies! In any event, it is agreed that on aging, there is a general shrinkage of the dendritic trees connecting a particular neuron to its neighbors and a lowered response to neurotransmitters [266], both of which will impact one's ability to progress in *yogasana* practice.

Despite the obvious outward physical changes in the brain as it ages, its functioning remains relatively unchanged. Thus, the EEG activity (Section 4.H, page 149) of the brain begins to decrease only at age eighty years and beyond. As one ages, the verbal IQ stays intact, as does the knowledge (semantic) memory in the cerebral cortex, whereas the episodic memory (Subsection 4.F, page 132) in the hippocampus fades.

It is readily apparent that with age, the brain's speed slows down more than anything else. With age, memory recall slows, as do the reaction times for all sorts of mental tests. Still, the aged can often do the job; it is just that they need more time to focus their mental resources on the problem at hand. One theory of brain aging posits that the effects are due to stress [702] and the excess corti-

sol (Subsection 5.C, page 176) that it can generate [44], and that yogic relaxation techniques can retard brain aging by lowering cortisol levels in the brain. See Subsection 4.G, page 149, for more on teaching *yogasanas* to older students.

Tart [848] points out that as adults, we have become enculturated to see things in a culturally approved way, and in response, to act on them in a culturally approved way.[12] For this reason, older students are more rigid psychologically and so are less able to see things differently from what they have been brought up to see. This may appear as a problem when older students try to learn the new ways of thinking inherent in *yogasana* practice, especially when trying to shift from convergent to divergent thinking (Subsection 4.E, page 124).

Neural Transmission

Whereas aging seems not to affect the numbers of neurons in the brains of healthy subjects, there is a measurable decrease of the levels of several key neurotransmitters and a decreased affinity at the receptor sites involved in memory and learning. With age, plaques also can form within the axons of the neurons, interfering with axonal transport and the transmission of the action potential, eventually leading to Alzheimer's disease.

Gender Differences in Anatomy and Physiology

First, let it be said that there is no known brain function that is found in all members of one sex and not at all in members of the opposite sex; i.e., the gender differences in regard to the brain

---

12   This is related, perhaps, to the experiments that show how culturally different people (Americans and Chinese) focus on different aspects when viewing a common visual scene (Subsection 17.B, page 668). With this idea in mind, Sapolsky and Cape [740] have interviewed many young and middle-aged people and found that the barrier to new ideas occurs at age thirty-five years in regard to new music, at age thirty-nine years for new food, and at age twenty-three years for body decorations such as piercings or tattoos. One concludes that our taste for adventure is one of the first casualties of aging.

are quantitative rather than qualitative, and none are 100 percent gender-specific. Nonetheless, significant anatomic differences (on average) in the brains of men and women can be cited.

In regard to the role of gender in neural anatomy, men's brains on average are somewhat larger than those of women (by approximately 10 percent), reflecting their larger body weight;[13] however, women's brains are cortically more folded, with a larger surface area than men's brains, especially in the frontal and parietal lobes [80a]. Still, the female cortex has 12 percent more neurons in the temporal lobe of the cortex, an area important to language. On the other hand, the male brain is proportionally larger in the frontal cortex, the amygdala, and the hypothalamus. The rate of blood flow through the brains of women is 15 percent larger than it is in men.

Two areas within the hypothalamus are unarguably different in the brains of men and women. The preoptic area (figure 5.B-1) controls sexual behavior in both men and women but is much larger and contains about twice as many cells in men; however, the specific consequences of this are not clear. The suprachiasmatic nucleus of the hypothalamus is spherical in men but much elongated in women. As discussed in Subsection 23.B, page 787, this nucleus is involved with setting the circadian clock in daily body rhythms and reproductive cycles.

Within the brain, gray matter consists of the cell bodies of those neurons that process neural information, whereas the white matter consists of those neurons that transmit but do not process neural signals. The absolute amount of gray matter is the same in the brains of the two genders; however, this amounts to 55.4 percent of the total brain mass in women but only 50.8 percent in men. All of the gray matter we will ever have is present at birth, and it is the gray matter that is pruned in the infant. On average, the corpus callosum (composed of white matter) of the female brain is larger than that of the male, and it is more connected, more integrative, and more organized in the female. With age, the mass of gray matter of the brain decreases at a faster rate; this begins earlier in men than in women.

As girls age from six to seventeen years, there is a 17 percent increase in white matter and a 4.7 percent decrease in gray matter, and the corpus callosum increases in mass by 27.4 percent; for boys in the same age range, there is a 45 percent increase in white matter, a 19 percent decrease in gray matter, and a 58.5 percent increase in the mass of the corpus callosum.

Gender Differences in Cognition

Just as the apparent left-right symmetry of the brain is illusory (Subsections 4.D, page 98, and III.B, page 847), so too is the apparent congruency of the brain functions of men and women. Evidence is accumulating to show that identical brain functions in men and women can occur in very dissimilar areas of their brains. Thus, for example, men use the left hippocampus to find their way out of a virtual maze, whereas women accomplish the same task using the right frontal cortex [591]. Also, it is now known that both of the frontal lobes are used much more by women in the comprehension of language than by men, and that their frontal lobes contain about 20 percent more neurons than those of men. The differences in the brains of men and women are expressed in regions specific for language, memory, emotion, and vision.

In regard to the two cerebral hemispheres, men's brains tend to have a dominant side when hearing words; under the same conditions, women tend to use the two hemispheres more equally. The difference is thought to be related to the higher levels of testosterone in the male brain during development. Clearly, the divisions of labor in the male and female brains are not congruent [590].

On average, the brains of men contain a larger proportion of white matter as compared to women, and this correlates with the superior ability of men, on average, at spatial problem solving. This appears to be related to cognitive functions and long-distance connections (the association fibers). When solving problems, women

---

13 Brain weight is directly proportional to the 2/3 power of the body weight, which is larger on average in men.

are found to use a much larger number of distinct brain areas than do men; i.e., women use more of a consultative scheme in problem solving than do men. However, men and women often use totally different approaches to problem solving.

Gender Differences in Emotion

The brains of men produce serotonin at a rate 50 percent faster than do those of women. This may correlate with the fact that a low level of serotonin can be a significant factor in depression and that women suffer much more often than do men from this condition. Gender differences in brain function are so prominent that it is thought that medical treatments for conditions such as schizophrenia, depression, etc., may well become gender-specific in the future [100]. Should this prove to be the case, then the stage also will be set for gender-specific yoga therapy.

Functional MRI studies of the activation of brain centers in men and women when shown various cartoons revealed that for women, humor was best appreciated when it was rooted in language, lighting up the left prefrontal cortex more intensely as compared with the responses in men.

Amygdala

Gender differences in the brain's emotional sphere are even larger than in the cognitive sphere. Women not only read the emotions in a face more quickly than do men, but they also do so with less effort. The tendency toward aggression begins in the amygdala but is inhibited or modulated by actions in the orbitofrontal cortex; this important action of the orbitofrontal cortex is stronger in women (on average) than in men. Moreover, the decisions that women make based on "gut feelings" actually originate in the amygdala, and because women are more adept verbally, they can more easily establish emotional access to others. In scenes in which a "bad person" receives an electric shock, women react with feelings of empathy, whereas men instead have feelings of retribution.

In general, the orbitofrontal cortex (the seat of higher cognitive functions) and the amygdala

and hippocampus of the limbic system are proportionally larger than other parts of the brains in women than they are in men. The ratio of the volumes of the orbitalfrontal cortex to the amygdala in women is significantly larger than in men, and these ratios are rather different in men and women who are schizophrenic. Women also have a higher density of neurons in two layers of the cortex as compared with the same layers in men.

Though emotionally arousing situations are stored in the amygdalas of both men and women, men store these memories in the right amygdala, and women store the same memories in the left amygdala. Note that unlike the connections to the cerebral hemispheres, those to the hemispheres of the amygdala do not decussate. The right amygdala is concerned with the more global view of the remembered event and the left amygdala with its finer details. These emotional responses within the amygdala occur in only 300 milliseconds and so are too rapid to be part of the conscious picture in real time.

Hormones

Certain regions of the brain show large numbers of receptors for sex hormones, suggesting that brain differences in men and women can be driven by hormonal balances in utero. Indeed, those areas that are functionally most different in men and women show the largest numbers of sex-hormone receptors. Many of the anatomic, physiological, and psychological differences between men and women have been traced back to the levels of testosterone in utero during fetal development.

Creativity

It is implicit that in trying to keep one's *yogasana* practice fresh and interesting from one day to the next, a creative approach in the broadest sense is necessary. Consequently, it is not out of line to dwell for a moment on those aspects of the thinking process that encourage creativity [466]. In adults, it is generally held that centers within the frontal and temporal lobes of the left cerebral hemisphere exert a strong inhibition upon speech, social behavior, and memory, and that when these centers are diseased, these inhibitions are lifted. When so lifted, the negation of these contralateral inhibitions can result in the blossoming of a person's creativity!

This is not to say that one must be brain-damaged to be creative, for there are a number of rational approaches to altering one's modes of thinking that result in increasing one's originality. In this, high intelligence is not a prerequisite, and there are ways of thinking that can appreciably enhance our creativity as we search for solutions to life's problems. In the broadest sense, there are two distinct ways of approaching the solution to a problem: by thinking either in a convergent manner or in a divergent manner.

Convergent Thinking

When thinking in the convergent mode, we try to find the one best solution to a problem, usually using logic and reason to finally arrive at a suitable but orthodox solution. For example, a student complains that something (anything!) in the forward leg hurts while in *trikonasana,* and so we reply with the standard advice: "Lift the knee-cap and, pressing the big-toe mound of the foot more into the floor, roll the front thigh back." Though this may in fact be effective in easing the discomfort, it is formulaic thinking and so does not allow the possibility of finding an answer that is more original and perhaps even more effective. Convergent thinking in *yogasana* practice is just a form of "one size fits all" thinking, as described in Subsection 1.B, page 8, and as described there, its narrow view of the solution can easily lead to an inaccurate diagnosis of the problem, and at the very least, to a solution that is far from optimal. Thinking in the convergent mode is bereft of any abstract connections to other facts other than those as stated in the problem being solved and is largely a left-brain, World View-II activity (table 1.A-2). The map of convergent neural connections shown in figure 3.C-2b can be taken to represent the convergent path to reaching a solution to a problem.

Divergent Thinking

In contrast to the sterile rationality of convergent thinking, divergent thinking is wildly imaginative and opens one up to manifold possible solutions. Of course, this can lead to so many possible solutions that one is paralyzed by the number of choices, but, on the other hand, it also can be the gateway to new ideas, new perspectives, and undreamed-of connections to other phenomena. Perhaps the discomfort mentioned above while in *trikonasana* is a result of over-rotation of the thorax, or improper angular placement of the foot on the ground, or too-wide separation of the feet; perhaps a correction of one of these elements of the posture would serve the student better than the standard explanation for leg pain. It is easier to think in a convergent way but more profitable in the end to think in a divergent way, especially in a field such as *yogasana* practice, where there is such a long tradition of how to do things. Just as convergent thinking is a left-hemisphere activity, divergent thinking (figure 3.C-2a) is a right-hemisphere activity (table 1.A-2).

All of us have a right cerebral hemisphere, but not all of us are creative in our thinking about our practice of *yogasana*. It appears that we are very creative in our younger years, but that as we mature to the point where a serious *yogasana* practice is possible, our abilities in regard to curiosity, experimentation, playfulness, risk taking, mental flexibility (Subsection 11.E, page 466), metaphorical thinking, and aesthetic appreciation become more and more inhibited. Moreover, it is the unimaginative left cerebral hemisphere that blocks the creativity of the right cerebral hemisphere! As divergent modes of thinking are repressed, the relevant neural connections in the right cerebral hemisphere wither and become harder to activate. Note too, that purely divergent thinking leads to too many choices and difficulty in settling on a final solution to one's problem. Because of this, the best approach seems to be to apply the right cerebral hemisphere to bring all of the reasonable solutions into consciousness and then use the left cerebral hemisphere to decide which of these imaginative solutions have the possibility of opening new doors to understanding. This two-phase approach to creativity has been described as inspiration originating in the subconscious, accompanied by a relaxed conscious level, followed by a developmental stage that is strongly conscious. Creativity will involve the entire brain if each side is given an opportunity to function in totally imaginative ways; cleavage of the corpus callosum, which normally connects the two cerebral hemispheres, can lead to incredible feats of rote memory, but extinguishes creativity.

In addition to this left-right interaction, creative thinking also involves a significant front-to-back component, i.e., transfer of stimulation from the frontal lobes to the temporal lobes.

Students of Guruji are specifically advised by him to bring the following four points to their practice in order to stimulate their creativity:

1. **Wonderment**. Try to retain a spirit of discovery—a childlike curiosity about the world—and question understandings that others consider obvious.
2. **Motivation**. As soon as a spark of interest arises in something, follow it.
3. **Intellectual Courage**. Strive to think outside accepted principles and habitual perspectives, such as "We've always done it that way."
4. **Relaxation**. Take the time to daydream and ponder, because that is often when the best ideas arise. Look for ways to relax and consciously put them into practice.

To this list, one can add the following adjuncts to creativity: wide range of interests, ability to handle conflicting ideas, patience, openness to divergent thinking, low levels of norepinephrine in the brain, positive mood, manic depression, bright-light therapy (SAD therapy; Subsection 17.E, page 685), and transcranial magnetic stimulation (Subsection 4.D, page 105).

Section 4.F: Memory

The capacity to learn is one of the fundamental activities of man's higher mental functions. Each of us is the individual that he or she is by virtue of what he or she has learned and what he or she remembers of that; our experiences shape us, often in important ways of which we are not even conscious. In regard to the experiences that shape our view of the world, when one sees order and purpose in an activity such as *yogasana* practice, one comes to expect and respect that order and purpose; order is essential for a person to function physically, and purpose is essential for a person to function spiritually [578].

Our personalities are shaped by the knowledge of the world that we have acquired through our senses, our storage of that information in the brain as a memory, and the retrieval of that memory. Thus, memory and learning are two sides of the same coin: you cannot learn what you do not store in your memory (conscious or subconscious), and you cannot remember what you have not learned (consciously or subconsciously). It is also relevant to *yogasana* practice that you cannot remember or learn what you do not observe (see Subsection 4.G, page 135), unless you do not observe it repeatedly!

Note that although memory and learning are closely related, they do differ in at least one significant respect: if we reserve the word "memory" for some neural pattern that can be recalled in the conscious sphere, then there are still many neural patterns that are embedded deeply in our subconscious centers in the limbic system, the brainstem, and the spinal cord. These buried patterns are learned, but they generally cannot be remembered using the conscious parts of our brains. (However, see Subsection 1.B, page 12.)

Each of us has a unique pattern of synaptic connections in the brain, and the expression of these neural patterns is the unique character that each of us has come to be. Certain of these patterns are inborn and hardwired, but others are changeable and allow us to learn (the ability to modify our behavior on the basis of our experience) and to remember (the ability to store and retrieve this modification over time) [426]. We are who we are largely on the basis of what we have learned and what we remember; i.e., on the basis of the patterns of synaptic connection that we have formed and maintained in the brain. Through *yogasana* practice, we will learn and remember important information about ourselves, thus transforming the brain's wiring and so transforming our entire being in the process.

Memory and Time

Memory has three stages, in each of which time is an important factor (figure 4.F-1). First, sensory information is fed into the immediate memory; if it is deemed relevant, it is passed on to short-term memory. A second filtering process in short-term memory then occurs, and if the information passes the second test for novelty and

relevance, it is then consolidated into long-term memory, where it is available for recall long after the event. Information in either the long-term or the short-term memory banks can be searched for, read, and retrieved; this is what we remember of the stored experience days later. Loss of memory is due either to erasure of the memory or poor performance of the search-and-retrieve function. The physiological and structural characteristics of the immediate, short-term, and long-term modes of storage are discussed further in the subsections that follow.

Immediate Memory

Sensory information is first fed into the immediate memory, a site having a huge capacity but a retention time of about two seconds or less. With such a short retention time, it is useful only for sensing rapid changes in sensory input. Far less than 1 percent of the items in the immediate memory are selected for transfer to short-term

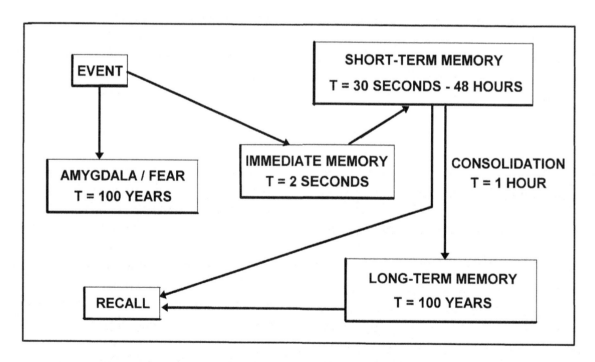

Figure 4.F-1. Information in the immediate memory lasts only for a few seconds, following which, it may be transferred to short-term memory. The details of an event are stored for about twenty-four hours in short-term memory and are available for recall during that time. After twenty-four hours, the details are consolidated in long-term memory (largely during sleep), where they are available for recall at times as long as several decades later.

memory. It is not at all clear where in the brain the immediate memory is located.

Short-Term Memory

Following a brief sojourn in immediate memory, meaningful sensations are transferred to short-term memory. Data in short-term memory is held only for a few seconds before it starts to lose detail, and it fades after a short time unless the sensation is repeated and repeated, as when one rehearses an action. It is said that we must repeat an action ten times in order to "learn" it, and we must perform it every day for ninety days before it becomes a "habit." If it is so rehearsed or is otherwise just very memorable, it can survive in short-term memory for up to twenty-four hours, just long enough to be transferred to long-term memory [342].

Physiology

Physiologically, "to place an item into short-term memory in a meaningful way" implies that it is practiced so that its neural pathway is reinforced. This means the synapses involved in this short-term neural circuit are more conducting of the neural excitation current, because there is a stronger than normal release of neurotransmitter, a heightened sensitivity to the neurotransmitter, or a slower degradation of the neurotransmitter in the synaptic cleft (Section 3.D, page 54). In some way, the learned action in short-term memory is translated into enhanced neural transmission along a specific path. However, the enhancement is fleeting, and if it is not transferred into long-term memory within a few days, the memory will be lost forever. It is proposed that reverberatory neural circuits (Section 3.C, page 50) are the active components of short-term memory that keep the memory bright. In general, short-term memory is based upon instantaneous but transitory chemical and electrical changes but does not involve a long-term modification of neural proteins or the formation of new synapses.

Capacity and Permanence

Short-term memory can hold approximately seven distinct items simultaneously—certainly fewer than a dozen items—and depending upon the definition of the term "item," some say only three or four items will fit in short-term memory at any one time. Given that short-term memory is so limited in capacity, one sees immediately that when teaching the intricacies of a particular *yogasana* to beginners, if one gives more than a few details to the students at one time, their short-term memories will become overloaded and they will abandon the earlier instructions in order to make room for the more recent ones. This is not so much a problem for more experienced students, who have laid down permanent memories of the instructions through earlier practices.

What we call short-term memory also is known in the trade as "working memory" and is widely thought to relate to general intelligence, in that general intelligence increases as the number of items that one can hold simultaneously in working memory increases. Special training can increase this number, and with it, one's level of general intelligence is strengthened.

Consolidation and Long-Term Memory

Information in short-term memory that has not already been erased is transferred to long-term memory in a process called consolidation. If an activity is practiced so that the memory of it is stored first in short-term memory and then consolidated into long-term memory, it becomes a permanent part of the cortical brain's mode of action. Norepinephrine and dopamine in the brain act as neuromodulators to cement our experiences in long-term memory and to hold them there for a lifetime.

When we are first born, we have very little cortical development and very little memory of events. The formation of long-term memories begins at about age four, and because most of the growth of the cortex is completed by age eight, it is at this time that most long-term memories begin to be stored for the future. These memories appear first in the hippocampus and then are transferred, over a matter of time from days to years, to the temporal lobes of the cortex [552]. It has been estimated that only 1 percent of all of the information that makes its way into our consciousness is committed to long-term memory and that much of that is soon forgotten anyway [863]. Given these odds, it is clear that one cannot be a mild-mannered *yogasana* teacher and still make a lasting impression on the quality of one's students' practice. (B. K. S. Iyengar states, "To make the pupil *sattvic*, the teacher must be *rajasic*.") On the other hand, it has not yet been shown that the capacity for long-term memories is anything less than infinite.

The long-term consolidation of memories is complete in about one hour but is well on its way only ten or fifteen minutes after the memorable event occurs, provided there is no interruption or mental fatigue [308]. This fits nicely with the use of *savasana* for fifteen minutes or so at the end of *yogasana* practice. Most recent research suggests that sleep is an essential ingredient of memory consolidation, with sleep restoring many memories for recall the next day, even if they were forgotten during the day on which they were experienced. If you have been awake for twenty-one hours without a rest, your mental powers are essentially at the level they would be at if you were legally drunk.

Protein Synthesis

Though all electrical aspects of brain activity can be shut down by deep anesthesia, by cooling, by coma, by electroconvulsive shock, or by lack of oxygen, upon recovery, all of the memories in long-term storage are present and available for recall, unlike those stored in short-term memory. This strongly suggests that unlike the situation with short-term memory, long-term memory involves permanent changes in the brain's morphology, chemistry, and/or connectivity. Noting that the ingestion of chemicals that inhibit protein synthesis have a detrimental effect on long-term memory and that the brain otherwise is rich in protein, it was hypothesized and then proven that the deposition of long-term memories in the

brain involves the site-specific generation of proteins within specific synapses of the brain. Drugs that inhibit protein production have no effect on short-term memory but inhibit long-term memory if given just after learning; clearly, long-term memory is dependent on protein synthesis, but short-term memory has no such dependence.

Biochemically, the deposition of a memory in the short-term bank involves the strengthening of existing synapses, whereas the deposition of a memory in the long-term bank requires that the experience being remembered either is very novel or has been repeated a number of times. In either of these cases, the relevant synapses are first primed for reconstruction, then genes within the cell nucleus manufacture the new neural proteins, and these are broadcast so that they can reinforce the synaptic strength at any and all synapses in the area that have been primed earlier [242a, 427a]. As shown in figure 4.F-2, "strengthening of the synapse" due to sensitization (figure 4.F-2c), as compared to that prior to the long-term stimulus (figure 4.F-2a), arises through the increase of presynaptic terminals by more than 100 percent, by the increase of the fraction of active terminals by 50 percent, and by the growth of new postsynaptic terminals on the target neuron.

The protein synthesis necessary for facilitation of the synaptic strength clearly is used for the construction of more efficient and larger numbers of presynaptic and postsynaptic terminals and their contents. A very similar process is at work in the infant brain, wherein those synapses that have been useful are strengthened with neural protein in a way analogous to the situation in regard to long-term memories, but those that are otherwise of little use are pruned by apoptosis.

The long-term stimulus that drives the construction or destruction of additional synaptic terminals is quite simple: it is the repeated activation of the relevant neural circuit, as when performing *yogasana* practice! Furthermore, these synaptic changes are basic not only to the facilitation of the movements, but to the cementing of the memory of how to do them.

Unambiguous experiments have shown that, even in cells that last a lifetime, there is a constant

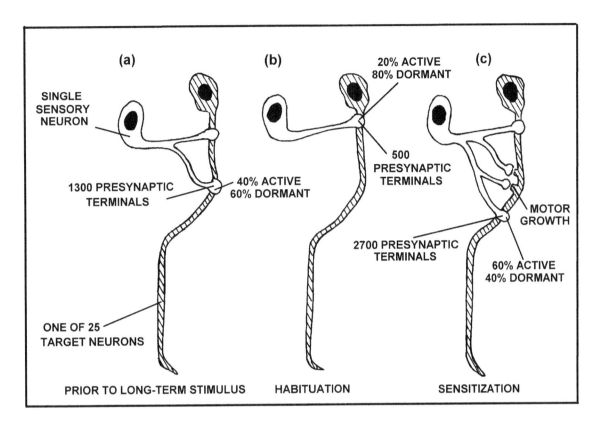

Figure 4.F-2. (a) The short-term presynaptic connections between a single sensory neuron and one of twenty-five target neurons in the brain prior to any long-term stimulus. (b) The quantitative transformation of the same presynaptic connections after long-term habituation. (c) The quantitative transformation of the terminals shown in (a) following long-term sensitization. See also the discussion in this subsection.

but lifelong replacement of almost all the material in the cell. Thus, in the human being, though a brain cell may exist for ninety years, half of its protein is regenerated anew every eighty days. The reproduction of the protein in this process is so exact that memories persist clearly for decades, even though the proteins that are responsible for them have been reproduced many, many times over [876]. The old idea that the neurons of the brain must not reproduce themselves, for if they did, memories could not be sustained for long periods, is now held to be fallacious. It is known that glucose, epinephrine, and caffeine help to increase the strength of memory and in the performance of mental tasks.

Branching

It has been shown repeatedly that when a task is practiced, the branching patterns of neurons involved in the long-term storage of the experience are changed in number and in type. When a synapse is used a few times, it tends to develop more axonal terminals, more dendrites, and more vesicles holding the appropriate neurotransmitters. As the neural event is repeated over and over, the synapses become sensitized, and swellings of the relevant synapses rapidly form as the numbers of vesicles and receptors in each synapse increase. After only a few hours' time, these inflamed synapses begin to deposit fresh protein in order to build new and thicker connections, thereby cementing the memory of the practice in the brain.

It also appears that the various motor circuits compete with one another for space within the brain, so that a task that is practiced tends to occupy more area within the brain (thus allowing for a fine-tuning of the actions in the task), at the expense of those that are not practiced. In this regard, it is interesting to look at the effects of long-term stimulation of an afferent-efferent synapse, as shown in figure 4.F-2. As seen there, when the long-term stimulus is somewhat annoying but not noxious, as with the startle response, for example, the synapse tends to change as shown in figures 4.F-2a and 4.F-2b; i.e., the strength of the synaptic connection decreases. This situation is termed habituation. If, on the other hand, the stimulus is truly noxious and warrants avoidance, then the synaptic connection becomes sensitized and takes the strengthened form shown in figure 4.F-2c. In both cases, one has "learned" by a physical adaptation of the neural circuitry. Changes such as these are discussed from the point of view of chronic pain in Subsection 13.C, page 520.

Recall

The availability of memories for recall from long-term storage is dependent upon many factors, such as level of stress, the environment at the time of learning, the level of mental concentration, repetition, and how important the information is to the learner. In regard to memory, mental exercise limbers the brain and allows easy recall, just as *yogasana* practice limbers the body and allows easy action. Though recall from short-term memory is essentially instantaneous, recall from long-term memory may require several minutes as the contents are scanned. The filing system in long-term memory places similar items (how to perform the various *yogasanas,* for example) in closely associated positions in the brain.

When we attempt to recall items from memory that we have seen earlier, such as faces, colors, or scenes, and then hold these memories in our imaginations, the same places in the visual cortex are stimulated as when the objects were first seen; however, the signals are weaker in imagination than when witnessing them firsthand. Thus, creating mental images is much like seeing, only less powerful [597]. If functioning of the visual cortex is blocked by transcranial magnetic stimulation (Subsection 4.D, page 105), then the ability to imagine past scenes is blocked as well.

Our long-term memories of emotionally laden moments are stronger than when there is less emotional content. Moreover, as actors know all too well, the actor's recall of the lines when acting out an emotional event is stronger still if it is accompanied at the time by relevant body movements.

Editing and Revision

Note, however, that recent experiments [552] strongly suggest that even the memories in long-term storage can be erased or edited for content rather easily. Each time a memory is recalled from long-term storage, it then must be reconsolidated; during this act of reconsolidation, it can be edited to suit a person's fancy, and the newer version then is returned to long-term memory, replacing the earlier version. Thus, if we tell a story of a past event and embellish it with the telling, the new edition of what really happened will become the new memory and over time will replace the older version in long-term memory. As applied to *yogasana* practice, when we learn a new aspect of the practice, it naturally and smoothly replaces the older ideas stored in our long-term memory, and so we advance in our practice. However, this shifting of points of view apparently does not occur as easily or as often in the aged (Subsection 4.G, page 149).

Forgetting

Forgetting the more ordinary types of events in our lives occurs in two phases. First, there is a rapid forgetting during the first hour after learning, and then there is a second, much slower forgetting during the next month. We interpret this as forgetting in the short-term and the long-term memories, respectively. However, if the shock of the event is "unforgettable," there will be no forgetting at all. If some action that was first learned and then put into memory is forgotten, it can be relearned more easily the second time than when first learned.

Interestingly, when one purposely tries to forget a memory, as when trying to forget the lessons of a previous *yogasana* teaching in favor of a new one, the blood flow to the prefrontal cortex shows a particularly intense flow, whereas that to the hippocampus is particularly slight, implying a backward flow of neural action from the cortex to the hippocampus; stabilization of long-term memory requires activation of both the cortex and the hippocampus to approximately equal degrees. The act of forgetting an already implanted memory may involve a weakening of the synaptic connections due to habituation, as in figure 4.F-2b, or due to outright severing of synaptic connections, as occurs during apoptosis.

Plasticity

Consolidation of a lesson into long-term memory involves plastic changes in the brain, by which is meant a detectable alteration of the synaptic circuitry in the central nervous system. By virtue of the different learning experiences we all have had, each of us has a unique synaptic brain structure, and each of us is therefore a unique person.

The plastic changes in the brain that occur once something is learned and stored are deposited simultaneously in several different parts of the brain and may involve not only neurons but glia and vascular cells as well. Furthermore, whereas some lessons are stored in the higher brain centers, others may be stored as low as the spinal cord (see the discussion on central-pattern generators in Subsection 4.A, page 71) and may be active even in a brain-dead person. That experience can change the brain's morphology reflects its plasticity. As with the bones (Subsection 7.C, page 237), the brain is undergoing constant modification in response to the environment, to stimuli, and to learning, and it is able to change its architecture in response to these pressures. To learn something, anything, is to permanently change the circuitry within the brain; conversely, without the brain's plasticity, nothing can be learned.

Once having learned something, we are often tested on that material. Interestingly, it has been found that students solve problems fastest when lying down as compared to when they are sitting or standing. The difference is attributed to the sympathetic excitation (Subsection 5.C, page 170) unavoidably present when sitting or standing and its burden of epinephrine, which is known to re-duce the ability to reason and to pay attention to details. Perhaps this too is an advantage of doing *savasana* following *yogasana* practice.

Conscious and Subconscious Memories

Reflexive Memory

In the broadest sense, there are two basic types of memory and learning [427], both of which involve long-term memory. In the first type, called reflexive or procedural memory, the learning accumulates slowly by repetition over many practice sessions, and the memory of the lesson learned has an automatic quality to it, in that it is not dependent on awareness, consciousness, or cognitive properties. Involving perceptual and motor skills, reflexive memory and learning lead to improved performance in many tasks, yet the train of actions necessary for successfully performing a task cannot be articulated. For example, with practice, one can learn how to jump into *adho mukha vrksasana* with straight legs, and though the sequences of muscle actions are stored in memory in the basal ganglia and cerebellum, one is unable to describe verbally what is going on, except at the simplest level. Even certain verbal skills can become reflexive if repeated enough, as when speaking with a regional accent. Much of our practice of the *yogasanas* is reflexive learning, and lessons learned reflexively, such as riding a bicycle or keeping the legs straight in *trikonasana,* are only rarely forgotten.

Declarative Memory

The second basic type of memory and learning is declarative, this being the type in which one makes a conscious effort to recall learning effects and experiences that can be described verbally. This type of learning/memory depends upon cognitive processes such as evaluation, comparison, and inference. Declarative memory is being accessed when the teacher recites to the class the list of points to be attended to when performing a *yogasana.*

Reflexive and declarative memories involve different neural circuits. Thus, the amygdala, the basal ganglia, and the cerebellum are active in reflexive memory, whereas declarative memory involves the temporal lobe and the diencephalon. As such, one may assign reflexive memory largely to the subconscious realm and declarative memory somewhat more to the conscious realm. It is thought by some that the various modes of learning and remembering involve different areas of the brain; nonetheless, many learning experiences have both reflexive and declarative elements operating simultaneously, though not necessarily in equal proportions, and these seem to be mapped onto many, if not all, areas of the brain. Memory is distributed rather than localized.

Episodic Memory

The acquisition of facts about ourselves and about other people, places, events, etc., is called episodic memory and takes place in the hippocampus [180], a part of the limbic system that is the among the most structured and regular within the brain. Because the hippocampus encodes information and experiences regarding self-awareness, which are then stored in long-term memories elsewhere in the cortex (possibly during sleep), it is a center of great importance to the *yogasana* practitioner. Because one of the effects of recurrent depression is a shrinking of the hippocampus, it also may have a negative effect on the ability to learn and remember *yogasana* principles; antidepressants may work to reverse this shrinkage [333]. Given enough practice, memories can be moved between reflexive and declarative forms of storage, in accord with the subconscious-conscious mixing described in Subsection 1.B, pages 12 and 15.

Emotional Memory

As discussed in Subsection 4.C, page 80, the limbic system, which operates on the subconscious level, is involved deeply in the emotions; it is no surprise, then, that memories having a strong emotional content are stored subconsciously in the limbic system. For example, the memory of the shock and fear attendant to coming face to face with a rattlesnake in the woods is stored both in the conscious regions of the prefrontal cortex

and in the subconscious region of the amygdala [418]; the thalamus and hypothalamus also are involved in registering fear. On next meeting a snake in the woods, the subconscious memory of it in the amygdala will prompt an immediate reflexive freezing of the posture and the all-out activation of the fight-or-flight response (Subsection 5.C, page 173) in the body. At a longer time thereafter, the conscious mind will also be alerted to the danger, but at a time so removed from the event as to be almost useless. It is the cingulate cortex that is intermediate between the cortex and the limbic systems and which controls the emotional content of the conscious sensations. The more one tries to control the emotions attached to what is being witnessed, the less accurate is the memory of the event.

The lack of simultaneity of subconscious and conscious memories of the same event parallels that of the reflexive and conscious responses to being stuck with a pin, for example, where the reflexive neural action occurs first at the level of the spinal cord, leading to the appropriate muscles being activated subconsciously, and only later does the conscious mind recognize the situation. It is also similar to the two types of smiling, one consciously involving the cortex and one subconsciously involving the limbic system. Subconscious reflex actions followed by conscious actions are also known to occur within the visual system (Subsection 17.B, page 669) and the balancing system within the inner ears (Section 18.B, page 699).

Fear

We are capable of learning fear in a strictly verbal way. Thus, being told that backbends are part of the *yogasana* practice program can generate a fear response in the amygdala, though no physical stress has been applied. Moreover, because there are far fewer neural connections that run from the cortex to the amygdala than run from the amygdala to the cortex, rational thought has only a very small effect in controlling the emotion of fear. Part of our heritage is that we, as humans, are extremely effective at fashioning fearful memories from dangerous situations, but we likely have many more fears than we need.

Recent experiments strongly suggest that when we experience an emotional event and it is stored in the emotional memory for later recall, in fact there is an immediate time period, just previous to the event, during which the memory has been cleansed of the elements leading up to the event. This is a stronger effect in women than in men [75]. It is reminiscent of the amnesia induced in the normal memory by head trauma. Emotion-induced memory effects involve the activity of adrenergic stress hormones functioning as neuromodulators on the amygdala. Furthermore, it appears that recall from the subconscious memory may be more accurate than that from the conscious memory [658].

When events are experienced that recall the initial trauma, the amygdala stress response is activated, but the prefrontal cortex often is able to extinguish the stress after it happens a number of times and one comes to recognize that the threat is not real. If the prefrontal cortex is unable to control the amygdala, then the result is post-traumatic stress disorder (PTSD).

The Sense of Self

Recent experiments using magnetic-resonance imaging [930] show that each of us has a much stronger memory for questions about ourselves than for others, no matter how close they may be to us, and that different brain regions are activated when we think about ourselves and when we think about others. For example, when we think about ourselves, there is stimulation of the medial prefrontal cortex, this being located in the cleft between the cerebral hemispheres, just behind the eyes; whereas this region is not stimulated when thinking about others. Experiments such as these show that there are distinct differences in brain function when thinking about ourselves and when thinking about others; the Self is not just a more familiar object to the brain but is, in fact, a unique object.

Memory and Sleep

Recent research [657] shows that certain phases of the sleep cycle are intimately involved with the consolidation phase of learning; especially relevant is the REM (rapid eye movement) phase (Subsection 23.D, page 800), a phase that we go through perhaps a half-dozen times in a night's sleep. This research shows that slow-wave stage-2 sleep and REM sleep both participate in the memory consolidation process, especially so when the material to be remembered is reflexive or procedural; i.e., how to do something such as a *yogasana,* rather than a more abstract storage of fact (the square root of 2 is 1.414) [536, 831]. The retention of emotional memories also is supported by REM sleep. Simple skills that are just a refinement of skills learned earlier require stage-2 sleep within twenty-four hours if they are to be retained, whereas when learning totally new skills, there must be a REM-sleep phase within twenty-four hours if the practiced technique is to be retained. It is hypothesized that as learning proceeds, not only are specific synapses strengthened, but inappropriate synapses formed previously are pruned from the neural net. See Subsection 4.G, page 137, for further discussion of this topic.

The memory trace held in long-term memory remains fragile and transitory when sleep does not intervene. During sleep, there is an active exchange of information back and forth between the hippocampus and the cortex (this also occurs during the day), finally leading to permanent changes of protein structure in the cortex during the hippocampus-to-cortex transfer. The transfer of information between the cortex and the hippocampus occurs during the REM phase of sleep, whereas the transfer in the opposite direction occurs during the stage-2 phase of the sleep cycle. The devastating loss of memory in Alzheimer's patients is associated with lesions that act to cut off the hippocampus from all other brain centers.

Though a sleep session that immediately follows a reflexive lesson, such as a *yogasana* practice, increases the amount of time spent in REM sleep, drugs that are known to decrease the length of REM sleep nonetheless have no effect on reflexive learning [536]. Apparently, REM sleep has functions that go beyond the consolidation of memories [831], and Siegel [789] has raised many questions in regard to the hypothesis associating REM sleep with learning and memory.

In contrast to reflexive learning, declarative learning seems not to involve consolidation of information during REM sleep, for REM-sleep deprivation has no effect on retention of declarative information [536, 831]. Thus, sitting and listening to your teacher describe aspects of *yogasana* practice can be a true learning experience; however, it will not require a REM period for consolidation, whereas what you learn from your own *yogasana* practice will require such a REM period. The role of rest and relaxation in the consolidation of what has been learned in the previous twenty-four hours is discussed further in Subsection 4.G, page 139.

Recycling

The repeated cycling of information back and forth between the hippocampus and the cortex (perhaps this is another form of a reverberating neural circuit) not only transfers information into long-term memory but also allows the brain to explore meaning and to integrate the new information with earlier memories, often in creative ways. Learning and remembering the instructions and techniques of *yogasana* practice thus are seen to be a twenty-four-hour per day job, significant portions of which are completed while we sleep! It is interesting to speculate as to what meaning this has, if any, for the apparent REM-like action of the eyes while relaxing in *savasana;* perhaps this signals the start of the hippocampal-cortical transfer of the information learned during the *yogasana* practice.

Hormones

Hormones also play a role in memory and learning. The hypothalamus activates the pituitary to release vasopressin, a hormone that not only regulates kidney action and water balance but also is a vasoconstrictor for regulating blood flow (Subsection 6.B, page 215). In the brain, vasopressin enhances memory and learning, perhaps working as a neuromodulator. The levels of vasopressin in the cerebrospinal fluid show a circadian rhythm (Section 23.B, page 774), no doubt correlating with the circadian rhythms of memory and learning abilities that rise and fall during the day [721].

If one experiences a frightening situation calling for the activation of the sympathetic branch of the autonomic nervous system (Section 5.C, page 173), the release of vasopressin into the bloodstream will assure that the memory of the event will be retained, so that one will act to avoid it in the future [716]; thanks to vasopressin, lessons learned in pain or fear are not forgotten. The release of ACTH into the bloodstream during periods of crisis also works to retain the memory of the crisis, and so helps to avoid it in the future. Oxytocin, another pituitary hormone, works to produce short-term amnesia, among other things. Its concentration in the body is greatest for women in labor and can act to make them forget the pain of childbirth. However, oxytocin also is a potent hormone involved in bonding between mother and child, and woman and lover, and so is responsible for many pleasurably unforgettable moments as well. The positive role of oxytocin in bonding is supported by the release of dopamine, the neurotransmitter involved in stimulating the brain's pleasure centers.

Stress Effects

Mild to moderate stressors activate the amygdala, leading to the stimulation of both the adrenal medulla and the adrenal cortex; this dual stimulation results in a rapid increase of the concentration of the catecholamines (epinephrine and norepinephrine) in the bloodstream and a slow increase in released corticosteroids (largely cortisol). Through these two actions of the sympathetic nervous system, one component of which reacts quickly and the other of which reacts on a much longer time scale, the hippocampus is activated, and the memory of the event is more easily consolidated. In this way, moderate stress is known to enhance the strength of the associated memories, making one feel alert and focused. If, however, the stress is intense or frequent, the positive effects of the cortisol become largely negative, especially in regard to the declarative memory, and especially so if there exists a neural projection from the amygdala to the hippocampus (figure 4.B-1). Excess cortisol has the effect of withering the dendritic trees so necessary for communication within the hippocampus [738]; it also acts on the locus ceruleus, stimulating it to release norepinephrine, which stimulates the amygdala in turn, thus boosting the intensity of the fight-or-flight effect. For these reasons, the production of excess cortisol in general is to be avoided in our *yogasana* practice.

Section 4.G: Teaching, Observing, Remembering, and Learning in *Yogasana* Practice

Learning and Observation

Motivation

Because you need to know something in order to learn something, all learning occurs by comparison of the old with the new. Thus, re-learning something that already has been studied is always faster than it was the first time the material was approached. It is also clear that there is a motivational aspect to successful learning (figure 2.B-1) and that the motivation will be minimal if the material to be learned is meaningless. In line with this, it follows that certain aspects of *yogasana* practice will be more meaningful (i.e., more easily learned) if the neurological, physiological, and anatomic reasons for doing them as we do are more clearly understood by teachers (and their students), rather than just being handed down ex cathedra[14] (Subsection 4.G, page 146).

The impact that a motivated *yogasana* practice can have on manual dexterity (and hence on anxiety), as compared with an unmotivated practice, is evident in the work of Manjunath and Telles [533]. These workers measured the results of a test of manual dexterity in two groups, one of which consisted of students who volunteered to practice yoga and a second group consisting of workers who underwent the same month-long training, but not by choice. At the end of the training period, substantially higher scores were recorded by the volunteer group, presumably because their motivation to practice yoga was more effective in reducing test-taking anxiety than was the case in the unmotivated group.

As mentioned above, the undertaking of *a yogasana* practice is predicated upon the notion that one is motivated to do so. In the very beginning, explanations of anatomy and physiology are moot, and a more emotional approach instead may be used to stimulate and motivate. Motivation to undertake such a strenuous course is unnatural in those who tend to be more or less lazy, thereby conserving energy whenever possible. Such students may be attracted to a vigorous activity only if they see that the rewards are larger than the price to be paid, and such reward/punishment decisions are made largely in the emotional realm, rather than in the rational realm. Thus statements such as "Yoga is good for your health" or "Isn't it interesting that your blood pressure drops in this posture?" are rational but may not be very persuasive to a beginner, whereas the emotional arguments that "Yoga can make you more attractive to the opposite sex" or "This posture can ease your sciatic pain" can capture the attention of beginners and lead them to want to give it a try [176].

Even when motivated to practice, it seems to be our nature that when left alone, we choose to practice those postures that are least appropriate to our condition [610]. Thus, one must be aware that some but not all students with low muscle tone, when left to themselves, will prefer to prac-

14   It was my seeking to answer the question of how to increase the strength of the motivational factor in learning and teaching *yogasana* to beginners that was my original motivation for writing this handbook. At the time, I did not understand how much it would motivate and energize my own practice as well!

tice relaxation rather than muscle-toning postures, and that some but not all depressed students will prefer to practice forward bends rather than backbends, even though their normal posture is rife with forward flexion. Similarly, overconfident people with a prevailing spinal extension in their posture will gravitate toward backbends and shy away from forward bends, if given the choice. In situations such as these, the *yogasana* teacher must emphasize those postures that will bring the student more into balance.

Extensive studies have been reported on the characteristics of the grandmaster in chess [720a] and how these characteristics are present as well in the "grandmasters" of other fields such as classical music, painting, sports, and mathematics. It is reported that such very-top-of-the-field performers are more often made rather than born, requiring a minimum of ten years of complete dedication to study of their field, during which they accumulate a vast memory of their experiences through effortful study. They can call on this vast storehouse of structured knowledge whenever they need to, and most relevant to yoga is the fact that their study is based upon years of continually tackling challenges that lie just beyond their competence, in contrast to those who become very good at their field because they are willing to put in the hours of practice but who do little or nothing to challenge themselves to go beyond their perceived limits. This last point, regarding the necessity of going beyond, is abundantly clear in the philosophy of B. K. S. Iyengar, who says, "When you feel you have attained the maximum stretch, go beyond it. Break the barrier to go further. Today's maximum should become tomorrow's minimum." Furthermore, it is said that such practitioners become "grandmasters" of their fields more by their motivation to succeed that by their innate natural ability.

Visual Observation

Note that even though we scan a scene with our eyes wide open, with all aspects of the scene in view, our attention may be focused on a much smaller part of the scene, as if the scene were being viewed through a soda straw. A student may be watching you demonstrate a particular posture in full view; nonetheless, their attention may be fully on the strange way your ankle is turned on the floor. This is undoubtedly related to the saccadic motions of the eyes (Subsection 17.B, page 667), which focus the eye's attention on a few relevant (or irrelevant) details of the scene and ignore all others.

When we learn visually from our teachers or teach visually to our students, there is an implied conscious observation of the relevant point, and if this point is not observed by the student, then it is moot in regard to conscious learning. Factors that influence the observability of what is being demonstrated depend first on our limited capacity to observe; it is said that humans can observe only one object at a time. For example, if shown a picture containing many faces, you will not know immediately if yours is among them unless you make a one-by-one facial scan of the assemblage. Second, when asked to compare two related scenes, the differences between them will be missed unless the difference was previously pointed out as being an object of attention, or if it changes the meaning of the scene. (See also the argument involving the competition for attention in the visual cortex in Subsection 17.B, page 671.) In summary, our visual perception is highly selective and preprogrammed to perceive certain specific facets of the scene while subconsciously filtering out what has not been preprogrammed as important [848].[15]

It is clear from the above that we often must draw specific attention to the point we wish to make when teaching a *yogasana,* otherwise the point will not necessarily register with the student. We cannot rely on the students being so

---

15   Tart [848] describes the situation wherein most Westerners show special acuity for horizontal and vertical lines but less so for slanted lines, whereas Cree Indians who grow up in teepees built of slanted lines have equal acuity for horizontal, vertical, and skewed lines! Enculturation affects perception, beginning with consciousness even in infancy, and then extending beyond that. See also Subsection 17.B, page 668, for how different the observations of a common scene can be when viewed by Americans and by Chinese.

aware that they will learn without their attention being directed to specific aspects of the posture, and we cannot rely on the possibility that the learning and remembering will be subconscious. However, see the discussion on neural priming in Subsection 4.G, page 144.

Recall of a learned experience is also known to be strongly dependent on the congruency of environmental factors when learning and recalling; this is discussed further in Subsection 4.G, page 139.

Taking Notes versus "Sleeping On It"

Recent experiments on decision making also may be of relevance to *yogasana* students. When making important decisions on complex matters, one should not try to gather all of the facts and then think logically about the benefits of different courses of action, because the conscious brain does not have the capacity to think about such a large amount of material. Instead, it is better to consciously absorb all of the information as it is presented, and then sleep on it, allowing the subconscious to work over the data and come to some decision.[16] It appears that, done in this way, the decisions are often better than trying to work in the totally conscious mode.

This subconscious approach to learning *yogasana* techniques is most relevant to learning in beginners who want to turn to teaching. The more enthused of these students will attempt to capture more of the lore of teaching by taking copious notes in class. In many Iyengar yoga classes, this exuberance is discouraged by the teacher, and the students are told to pay attention in class and let the information percolate in the subconscious instead. Support for this point of view has been presented in work recently published [83], where it was shown that when the number of choices is small, conscious consideration of the relative merits leads to a small advantage in making an intelligent choice; whereas when the amount of in-

formation is very large, then the conscious mind cannot cope, and it is more profitable to simply pay attention from moment to moment and then let the subconscious mind digest it during sleep.

Note as well that when a person is sleep-deprived, excess cortisol is generated, and this in turn retards neurogenesis in the hippocampus, thereby impairing certain types of learning and memory.

Learning and Neuroplasticity

Plasticity

Up to this point, the brain has been pictured as hardwired, with every particular region of the brain dedicated to a specific role (see, for example, the implicit assignment of specific brain areas in the motor and sensory cortices to specific body parts, as shown by the homunculi in figures 4.C-5 and 4.C-6, respectively). Until recently, it was believed that once the brain matured, new synapses and new neurons could not be formed and that the extant neurons were frozen in their shapes, sizes, and connections. However, were this true, then learning new material would be impossible, because learning implies a **change** in the neural structure of the brain, and change is inconsistent with the brain being hardwired. In fact, the brain must be mutable if learning is to be accomplished. This mutability can be termed "neuroplasticity." Being neuroplastic, the brain can be remodeled by internal or external pressures, just as the muscles (Subsection 11.A, page 398) and bones (Subsection 7.C, page 237) respond to stress.

Thus, for example, a portion of the brain that has been silenced by a stroke can be recreated in another portion of the brain and the original function thereby regained through the intense practice of mental and physical exercises [377]. Plasticity is also found outside the motor and sensory cortices, for the brains of people cured of obsessive/compulsive disorder through behavioral training have demonstrably different structures following the training. The plasticity of the human brain is higher for children than for adults, and the

---

16   This sounds very much like being faced with a decision to be made and "praying on it," so that the subconscious can come to the best decision, largely free of the control of the conscious mind.

limit to which the brain can be remodeled is not known.

Experiments in humans have since shown that when a cortical area of the brain is disconnected from the relevant organ, not only can adjacent neural areas take over the unused cortical area, but the takeover may involve areas that are far removed from one another. Thus, in musicians playing a stringed instrument, the fingering hand in one hemisphere has a larger area in the motor cortex than the bowing hand in the other hemisphere, and the most-used fingers have the largest areas (see Subsection 18.A, page 692).

In the blind who read by Braille, the visual cortex (Brodmann's area 17, figure 4.C-1) becomes active when the fingers are passed over the Braille characters; and when a person loses a limb, the sensory cortex serving that limb may develop to serve the face instead. These changes could not occur were it not for the plasticity of the brain.

To the extent that *yogasana* practice is about transformation of the body, mind, and spirit, it is implicit that the brain's plasticity will play a huge role. Without this plasticity, there will be no learning, no satisfaction, little or no motivation to practice, no emotional release, no muscular stimulation or relaxation, no stress reduction, etc. Without this plasticity, one would not be able to turn a feeling of dread toward a particular *yogasana* (*eka pada adho mukha svanasana,* in my case) into a deeply satisfying feeling through constant practice.

Synaptic Strength

As discussed in Subsection 4.F, page 128, the learning of a particular skill involves selecting, from among a large collection of neurons (all having synapses already in place), a much smaller subset of neurons in which the strengths of the synaptic connections (called facilitation) are altered in ways specific to the skill being learned. Moreover, the persistence of such synaptic facilitation within the central nervous system is the basis not only for learning but also for memory, both long-term and short-term. Kandel [427a] points out that the results of learning will be the strengthening of certain synapses and the weakening of others, and that the changes of synaptic

strength are widely distributed throughout the affected neural network, rather than being localized at one or a few synapses. When increasing the synaptic strength in either short-term or long-term memories, a transport of material from within the cell body to the axonal tips is involved; this is accomplished by the microtubular axonal transport system (Subsection 3.A, page 35).

Though the same synapses are involved in both long-term and short-term memories, they differ in a quantitative sense. Not only do the changes attending storage in long-term memory last longer than those in short-term memory, but there are more synapses of higher activity if the stimulus results in a strengthening of the synapses (sensitization), and there are fewer synapses and they are weaker if the stimulus results in a weakening of the synapses (habituation). For example, consider the situation shown in figure 4.F-2a. In the brain, a single sensory neuron typically has about 1,300 presynaptic terminals contacting about twenty-five different target neurons (muscle cells, interneurons, etc.). Of these terminals, only 40 percent are loaded with neurotransmitters, the rest being dormant. "Neural habituation" is learning to recognize that a repeated stimulus is nonthreatening and, though it may be obnoxious, that it can be safely ignored. As an example, our awareness of the heartbeat is minimal due to habituation, and so we avoid an unnecessarily exaggerated defensive response. In the case of the sensory neuron synapsed to a motor neuron, as in figure 4.F-2a, habituation leads to a weakened synaptic potential in the motor neuron. Quantitatively, this means that the number of presynaptic terminals drops to 850, and the number of active terminals drops from 500 to only 100. Thus it is seen that the number and strength of the synapses changes in accord with habituation to the stimulus.

Sensitization is the response opposite to that of habituation; i.e., if one is once put on strong alert by a frightening stimulus, then almost any other stimulus results in an increased response by reflex. When sensitizing the synapse between a sensory and a motor neuron, one generates a stronger synaptic potential in the motor neuron. At the synaptic level, following long-term sensitization (figure

4.F-2c), the number of presynaptic terminals increases from 1,300 to 2,700, and the proportion of such terminals that are active is now 60 percent. Simultaneous with the large-scale changes in the sensory neuron, the postsynaptic neuron also grows new dendrites to interact with the new presynaptic terminals. Again, there have been highly visible changes in the synaptic region, due to the nature of the stimulus. Should this sensitizing stimulus fade, the number of presynaptic terminals eventually would drop back to about 1,500.

The Genes Speak

Whatever you have learned from studying this chapter is the result of physical alterations within your brain, through a rearrangement of the strengths of certain synapses as they are used in short-term memory and the permanent changes in the their physical structures as they are then consolidated in long-term memory. In the case of long-term consolidation, the manufacture of the new proteins of the sort that are used in synaptic facilitation involves the turning on of a particular gene in the cell's nucleus and turning off another in the nucleus. Thus, the learning we undergo when either practicing the *yogasanas* or reading about *yogasana* practice comes about as a direct consequence of the stimulation of certain genes directing protein synthesis within the nuclei of our brain cells!

Meditation

Meditation is known to slow the rate of the cortical thinning involved in the degeneration of the white matter of the brain on aging. In general, those parts of the brain that are often used show a thickness larger than normal. Though plastic changes in brain structure can be driven by our physical experiences, it is also true that mental exercises involving thoughts of the physical action can lead to the same plastic changes. (See Subsection 4.G, page 140, for more on this subject.)

Rest and Recall

When studying for an examination, it is known that students do better if they study less and then get a fair night's sleep, rather than study for an extended period right up to the time of the exam. When we rest for a short period before the exam, there is time for the studied information to be strengthened in short-term memory and thus be readily available during the exam. On the other hand, if one were to study up to the time of the exam, there would be no time for the learned information to settle into short-term storage, where it might then be available to one during the test. Indeed, psychological studies show quite clearly that the memory of what has been studied is clearest after a quiet period following a study session, and that **any** activity in this final period before the exam lowers one's score [227].

From the discussion given above, it is seen that one of the physiological benefits of doing *savasana* at the end of *yogasana* practice is that it offers the calm conditions necessary for implanting the learned neural pattern into short-term memory. Though not proven, it seems reasonable to think that such short-term consolidation occurs most readily when the mind has shifted from beta-state arousal to alpha-state calm (Section 4.H, page 152). On the other hand, information is best remembered if it is perceived at a time of high mental arousal and is best recalled later if one again is in a state of high mental arousal [30].

Ideally, one sleeps before the exam, so that the consolidating benefits of REM sleep to long-term memory will be in place when one will need them most (Subsection 4.G, page 139). Indeed, in regard to "learning" the motor skills inherent to the *yogasanas,* it has been reported [316] that learning takes place most efficiently following an adequate sleep on the day of the practice, thus allowing for proper and complete consolidation of the learned material in long-term memory. As Shakespeare said, one should experience the "sleep that knits up the ravel'd sleeve of care."

Learning and Environmental Context

Yet another aspect of learning involves what we might call "the environmental context factor." It has been shown repeatedly that when students study for an examination in the cafeteria, for example, they will do better on the test for that material when tested in the cafeteria than when tested in the gymnasium. A similar association has been made between learning specific material in the presence of an odor (say, chocolate) and then taking an examination on that material in the presence of that odor or in its absence. Apparently the learned material is associated in the brain with the environmental cues (the cafeteria or the smell of chocolate) prevailing at the time it was learned and is most readily recalled from memory when the environment at the time of testing is congruent with that at the time of learning. This association between environment and recall holds whether the lesson learned was a success or a failure, for in the latter case, the association of the environment with failure was found to persist in spite of further attempts to succeed in that environment. Finally, if the lesson was learned while under the influence of a certain drug, then the lesson will be best remembered while under the influence of that drug!

The environmental factor is most obvious in the *yogasanas* when practicing the balancing postures, for both the balancing and the environment involve strong visual inputs. When these *yogasanas* are learned in a particular setting, and the eyes are used to establish visual anchors for balancing (Subsection 17.B, page 666, and Subsection V.C, page 888), there is a strong mental association of the learning environment, as sensed visually, with the technical details of the *yogasana*. In that case, it is often found that the balancing is easiest when done while looking at the same environment that was present when the *yogasana* was learned and that trying to perform the balance in another room (or in the same room, but facing another view) can be more difficult. Needless to say, the *yogasanas* ideally should be practiced with the eyes not holding onto external objects, so that the *yogasanas* can be performed equally well in all environments and with relaxed eyes.[17]

Muscle Memory, Real and Imagined

The more often a movement is made (this is called practice), the more accurate and discriminating it becomes (this is called learning), which is why we must practice our *yogasanas* with all of our senses wide open if we hope to learn more about ourselves. It also must be remembered that though the muscles move the body, these movements in turn rely on the nerves for their initiation; if the nervous system is hibernating, then the muscles will not move, regardless of how large and glorious they might be. On the other hand, the task at hand may involve an intricate pattern of neural activation, unseen but nonetheless necessary for the act. Because the pattern of neural impulses may not develop for a long time, the practice of an activity may do very little for apparent muscle strength but much for the development of the necessary neural control.

The efficiency of the process that changes neurological activity into movement can be slow to respond to training; which is to say, neural efficiency improves relatively slowly as the neural patterns are refined. B. K. S. Iyengar, well into his eighties [395], relates how his aging has lessened his strength, but by constant practice, he continues to increase his neural efficiency and mental strength and so maintains his level of performance.

Once the neural pattern for a particular action is set in place, then the act may be performed

---

17   That environmental context could be a factor in *yogasana* practice can be rationalized in part by noting that within the hippocampus, there is a set of neurons called the "place cells" that are involved with recognizing local environments (Subsection 4.C, page 81). When facing one wall and learning *vrksasana*, certain of the place cells will be excited as appropriate to the view at that moment, whereas when turned to face the window in the same posture, a different subset of the place cells will be activated. This difference, in which place cells are excited depending upon the scene one views, would seem to give the performance advantage to that view and place-cell excitation that was present when the posture was first learned. The nature of the possible connection between place-sensitive neural excitations and the effects they may have on *yogasana* performance presently is vague to nonexistent; however, I feel that it eventually will prove to be of significant value to *yogasana* practitioners.

easily and repeatedly without a deliberate effort at recall. This refinement of the neural circuitry by practice, and its storage and recall from the appropriate places in the nervous system, is called muscle memory. Gorman [288] describes muscle memory in the following way:

> The organization of a fully developed innervation pattern requires afferent impulses from proprioceptors and touch receptors, in particular, by body parts participating in the movement; i.e., the entire sensory impulse flow released when the movement is performed in its proper context. With repetition, the outflow to muscles facilitating movement becomes better balanced, as do inhibitory impulses to muscles antagonistic to the movement. Gradually, movements become more and more fluid as the interplay between agonists and antagonists facilitating and inhibiting movements and those stabilizing the joints are perfected and become economical.

The muscle-memory point of view stresses the importance of neural aspects in what otherwise appears to be a purely muscular display; the increase of muscle efficiency and apparent strength with practice often is actually due to a refinement of the neural apparatus driving the muscles.

This priming of the muscular system through exercise of one's muscle memory, either through slow, almost passive movement or through the use of the imagination, is the pivotal idea behind the Feldenkrais [29] and the ideokinesis [719] approaches to bodywork. At first, the cerebellum is very important from the neural point of view when learning a muscular sequence, but later, it only plays an initiating role, as other centers then take control.

There is a general inhibition of the α-motor nerve impulses from the brain (Subsection 11.A, page 377), but with exercise, more motor units can be activated on demand, and there is a better integration of the work patterns of the motor units. For women and adolescents, it has been ob-served that their apparent strength does increase with physical training but without any noticeable increase in the size of their muscles. It is thought that the effect involves the development of a more complete and efficient use of the nerves driving the muscles rather than an accumulation of more muscle fiber; i.e., it is a case of the strengthening of muscle memory. One also can think of muscle memory as a long-term warm-up benefit, comparable to those listed by Peterson [655] for short-term exercise (Subsection 11.E, page 467); however, the gains of muscular exercise are lost through lack of activity about as fast as they were gained, whereas muscle memory is active far beyond the time when it was discontinued, as when one is able to ride a bicycle or type long after one has ceased their practice.

Unfortunately, the constant mental replaying of an unfortunate stressful event also primes the neural circuitry so as to more readily play out the eventual physiological response; e.g., elevated blood pressure (Subsection 14.D, page 576).

Strength versus Finesse

In the untrained *yogasana* student, one can make progress in increasing the apparent strengths of the muscles in a short time, due to the effects of muscle memory and neural repatterning. Even the strength gained from the repeated practice of weightlifting has a strong component of muscle memory [726], but in this case, it involves the ability to recruit more motor units to the lifting rather than to a refinement of a complex neural pattern. In either case, with continued exercise, there is not only a repatterning of the neural proteins, but also an enhanced accumulation of contractile proteins entering existing muscle fibers, the end result being what might rightly be called "an increase in muscle strength" (Subsection 11.A, page 399), but which is due to increases of **both** muscle girth and neural efficiency. Though there is always a decrease in strength when one detrains, thanks to the muscle memory, one still will be significantly stronger than when one first began training [90].

Memory and Imagination

A second aspect of the muscle-memory phenomenon of importance is that the practice of the actions through the use of the imagination also may strengthen the neural circuits, so that the muscle action in real time is smoother and stronger. It has been shown in several non-yogic studies that the neuromuscular skills of the sort that we work to perfect in *yogasana* practice are in fact enhanced by passive visualization of the activity prior to practice [602], and that the visualization practice in fact exercises the motor neurons involved in the actual practice. This enhancement is possible if one considers that one might visualize actions so that when the real act is performed, the neural currents are stronger than they would be otherwise.[18] Indeed, in an experiment in which half of a group of students did nothing, whereas the other half meditated on contracting the biceps, the first group showed no increase in strength after a few weeks, but the second showed an increase of 13 percent in biceps strength, which was maintained for months after the training was ended [138]. In this case, the increase in strength must be due to neural repatterning, as no muscular biceps work was practiced.

Passive neural patterning is an interesting idea that is well worth exploring as an adjunct to *yogasana* practice. Presumably, exercising the thought processes involved in the activity without actually activating the requisite muscles can be of value, thanks to the strengthening effect it may have on the neural patterning that eventually will drive the muscles.[19]

It is becoming more and more recognized that optimizing athletic performance not only involves muscle strength but also involves a certain amount of psychological/neurological conditioning and warm-up. To take advantage of this, for example, just prior to attempting a balancing *yogasana* that is difficult for you, meditate sequentially on the actions you will take leading to the successful outcome of that attempt. The effect of such warm-up imagery is to program the neurological system so as to perform optimally the first time it is called upon.

In a similar vein, it also has been shown that practicing an exercise on only one side actually works to improve the performance on the second side, through a transfer of the neuromuscular pattern refined on the first side.[20] This may relate eventually to the observations of a symmetric pain developing in some people when only one side of the body has been injured (Subsection 13.C, page 520). Perhaps something like this is at work when *yogasana* students are asked to be still and just watch the teacher perform the *yogasana*. In observing in this way, the students' neurological systems are primed to do the work asked of them through the use of the "mirror neurons" phenomenon (see below). Neurological practice through imagery can be used to advantage in reinforcing the neurological patterns necessary for particular muscular actions, as with Iyengar's idea in regard

18   Studies have shown that the recall of odors, taste, and auditory and visual sensations occur in the brain in locations very close to those originally activated by the initial perceptions. The more detail there is in the imagery, the closer is the correspondence of the brain areas involved in the imagery with those involved in the original perception. Presumably, then, the same close association exists between the neural patterns activated in performing a *yogasana* and those activated when imagining the performance of the same *yogasana*.

19   Mary Dalziel tells me of a woman who was severely injured in an auto accident and who came to yoga for recovery. Her teacher had her lie in the corner of the yoga room, listening to the class and just visualizing herself performing the postures. She worked in this way for three months before trying to perform in real time and space. She is now a yoga teacher.

20   Perhaps one can imagine that when one side of the body is active in performing a *yogasana*, the second side is "watching" and is able to refine its neural pattern by using its "imagination"; i.e., the second side also goes through the appropriate neural sequences, but without excitation of the corresponding muscles!

to a *yogasana* done to one side, which then teaches the second side.

Interestingly, imagining the normal functioning of an arm otherwise paralyzed by a cerebral stroke has been shown to be highly effective in restoring action [641a].

Learning and Mirror Neurons

At the neurological level, astounding new discoveries shed significant light on the learning process as it might be applied to *yogasana* practice. Experiments recently have shown that when we perform a meaningful action, such as bending at the hip and coming into *trikonasana*, the relevant muscular actions that are driven by the motor cortex are preceded by neural firings of complementary neurons (called mirror neurons) in a warm-up area, the premotor cortex in the frontal lobes (figure 4.C-1). Most interestingly, if, instead of doing *trikonasana*, we stand and watch intently as our teacher demonstrates the posture, our premotor cortices nonetheless display the characteristic neural firing pattern present when performing the posture! In essence, by first observing the posture being done by the teacher, we prime our neural systems for performing the posture on our own.[21] It also has been shown that the appropriate section of the premotor cortex is energized when verbs are read that refer to motor actions, such as "dance," or "kick," or "lift your chest" [79]. The tendency to imitate is less when watching a videotape [411] or when watching a robot perform the action [846] than when seeing it done live. Functional MRI studies show that though the viewing may be binocular, the involved premotor areas can be strongly localized in one or the other cerebral hemisphere; for example, the mirroring of another's emotional state (empathy), when viewed by both eyes, is observed

to occur in the viewer's right cerebral hemisphere, as appropriate for emotions [509] (table 4.D-1).

The mirror-neuron effect on learning has a strong resonance with Iyengar's prescription for teaching the *yogasanas* by first having the students witness the silent performance of the *yogasana* by the teacher. We see now that such an approach relies on the subconscious interactions of the mirror neurons of the teacher and those of the students to prime the neural systems of the latter for the appropriate actions. This approach not only helps us understand at a deeper level how we learn from our teachers, but also why we come to resemble them to such a high degree in doing the postures. The infectious nature of yawning also may involve mirror neurons, as might subconsciously walking in step with a partner and other entrainment phenomena.

Mirror neurons not only play a very important role in reading the physical intentions of others but also in empathy, imitation learning, deciphering facial cues, language development, social skills, and cultural rules. These neurons are active when we complete a sentence begun by someone else; even if the last part of the action spectrum is truncated, the observer will sense a complete set, thus operating on a sense of inferred action [870a]. In this way, mirror-neuron learning can be thought of as a form of mind reading!

So far, in humans, the mirror-neuron effect has been observed in which hand, arm, foot, and mouth movements are mirrored, and in touching, provided the movements are meaningful and goal-related rather than random. The mirror neurons found in the ventral premotor cortex specifically involve hand and mouth movements and are not involved with the execution of contractions of individual muscle groups. These motor neurons appear to form a cortical system that matches observation and execution of motor actions. Thus, every time we observe someone performing an action, the motor circuits activated in the performer are also activated in us. Observation of grasping in humans using PET scans showed activation in Brodmann's areas 21, 40, and 45; these areas are traditionally associated with language (figure 4.C-2).

---

21 The mirror-neuron phenomenon was first observed in macaque monkeys, and so mirror neurons also have been called "monkey see, monkey do" neurons. In humans, women have a larger number of mirror neurons than do men.

A possible goal in *yogasana* teaching could be to teach by imitation, for when new motor skills are to be learned, one often spends the first training session trying to reproduce the actions of an observed instructor. In this situation, a muscular plan of action is formulated in the observer, but carrying it out is inhibited, except in those with prefrontal lesions, who lack the necessary inhibition. These people will copy in detail what is shown to them, rather than observing without moving [261]. The known response of the mirror neurons to hand actions may be of relevance to hand *mudras* in yoga practice (Subsection 10.A, page 339) and to the use of finger pressure to dictate how the shoulder blades press onto the rib cage (Subsection 10.A, page 331). It will be very interesting to see how far the mirror-neuron concept can take one in regard to learning and teaching the *yogasanas*.

A phenomenon rather close to that of mirror neurons also occurs in the emotional sphere. Thus, if you imitate the facial expression of someone telling you an emotional tale while it is being told, then you will be more empathetic with that person and their emotion. Your conscious imitation of their subconsciously-derived facial expressions allows you to share their emotional state more easily.

Autism

Experiments suggest that a malfunctioning of the mirror neurons is behind the difficulty autistic children often have in imitating other people's actions and in reading their intentions and feelings. In this case, there is an overreliance on interpretation by the parietal lobes and neglect of the prefrontal lobes; this combination leads to diminished social interactions [82a, 691a]. It is felt that the observed dysfunction of the mirror-neuron system in the mildly autistic, as revealed by blood-flow studies within the brain, is a serious factor in their difficulty in learning social skills, as learning by watching is nonfunctional. Deficits in the mirror-neuron systems of autistic children also have been shown to severely limit their abilities to empathize with the emotional states of others [294, 691a]. Similarly, antisocial individuals

also show very little activity in the mirror-neuron region of the brain.

It has also been observed that in nonautistic subjects, either the movement of their hands or the observation of others moving their hands results in a quenching of the mu waves in the EEG (Subsection 4.H, page 152); whereas in autistic subjects, moving of the hands quenched the mu-wave intensity, but observing others perform this action did not. Thus, it was concluded that the autistic suffer from some sort of mirror-neuron impairment and that this is closely related to mu-wave stimulation or lack thereof [691a]. Postmortem study of the brains of adult autistic males showed that their brains are significantly deficient in neurons in the amygdala, a region that is very important in memory and emotion.

Priming

Priming is another relevant aspect of subconscious processing of information. In this phenomenon, a fragment of visual information is glimpsed so quickly that it registers only in the subconscious. Later on, when the same information is presented at a slower rate, so that it registers in the conscious sphere, it is found to be more strongly remembered because of the previous subconscious priming of the learning process. The subconscious processing of subliminally perceived information allows for the same information to be recognized and processed at a faster rate in the conscious sphere when it is seen a second time. This process possibly could be relevant to the efficacy of using subliminal effects in teaching *yogasana*.

Sports Philosophy and *Yogasana* Practice

The very interesting book by Murphy and White [601] mentions two aspects of sports involving mental imagery that should be applicable to *yogasana* practice. Distance runners, football players, golfers, and other athletes report that on occasion, they have caught glimpses of their viscera, tendons, muscles, or blood vessels and even sensed cellular structures. The mechanism whereby such views can be sensed most likely involves the interoceptive sensors, as discussed in Subsections 11.C, page 444, and 19.C, page 716. Athletes in many sports employ interoceptive visualization of the inner body in regard to healing and recuperation following a hard practice, and they report that such a coupling of mental and physical work seems to speed recovery. This is perhaps not too distant from visualizing the relaxation of the muscles in *savasana* following a *yogasana* practice and Cousins' visualization of the T cells of the immune system multiplying and fighting cancer cells [170]. It seems to me that such mental pictures of one's internal architecture would be of immense value to *yogasana* students, especially in regard to a second phenomenon, discussed below.

Bodybuilders of the class of Arnold Schwarzenegger report that they are able to visualize the muscle shape they desire in a particular muscle and that this shape then materializes about ten times faster with the visualization (and work) than with work without visualization! One can only wonder at the possible gains to be won by an imaginative but active *yogasana* practice during which the shapes of the postures are the focus of attention.

It is most interesting to read [602] about how aspects of Western sport can become pathways to exalted states of mind and heightened abilities to move the body. These aspects of self-transformation through sport are listed below, because I feel they are equally applicable to transformation through *yogasana* practice and so are well worth consideration by *yogasana* students and teachers.

- » Regular practice of particular physical movements with the intent to improve them
- » Sustained and unbroken attention/concentration; freedom from distraction while practicing
- » Imagery rehearsal
- » Abandoning cognitive, volitional, emotional, and sensorimotor patterns that can limit performance
- » Practiced detachment from results
- » Long-term commitment

- » Boundedness of sport and sacredness of sport venues
- » New integration of mind and body

Practice of the above eight aspects of sport brings sportsmen to a state beyond their normal functioning, a state of extraordinary clarity and focus often called "the zone" (Section 5.C, page 172). Application of the same principles to *yogasana* practice, I suspect, can bring one a step closer to *samadhi*.

Attentiveness and Mental Concentration

Your level of attentiveness (the second point above) is dependent upon the level of arousal. This level, in turn, is controlled by the levels of norepinephrine and dopamine in the brain, with the former leading to a state of outward-looking vigilance (sympathetic dominance, beta-wave EEG), whereas the former promotes a state of persistent goal-oriented behavior (parasympathetic dominance, alpha-wave EEG). Anything that raises the dopamine level increases concentration. In general, concentration is best achieved by sleeping well, eating foods with high levels of slow-release sugars, and taking lots of exercise. This fits nicely with the ideal yogic lifestyle. Furthermore, it helps if the subject on which one is concentrating is something that you find interesting—another plus for *yogasana* practice.

External factors that work against concentration are interruptions such as telephone calls and working too close to a refrigerator filled with tempting treats. As background noise also works against concentrating, soft but innocuous music can be of some help in drowning out otherwise bothersome noise. Neurofeedback, which involves making brain activity visible (biofeedback) and then mentally shifting the balance of activities, has been shown to be effective in improving the memories of medical students and improving the techniques of musicians and dancers, and it is being tested on opera singers and surgeons [210]. Perhaps *yogasana* practitioners will be next.

Interestingly, we crack under pressure when we are too deliberately focused on what we are doing muscularly and so block the automatic or reflexive processes that otherwise would occur. To perform without cracking or choking, we must act with less self-consciousness [293] and less attention to proceduralized routines, and we must minimize anxieties about our performance [48]. B. K. S. Iyengar speaks of this in Subsection VI.A, page 934, where he points out that we must allow our intuitive Self to guide us in performing the *yogasanas* rather than the deliberate, conscious Self [4a].

Over-Motivation

It is possible to be overly motivated in one's *yogasana* practice; i.e., to become so addicted to the practice that one abuses it, perhaps in an effort to avoid depression. In this regard, the neurological response to exercise is the release of dopamine, the "feel good" neurotransmitter. Possibly, certain students receive an extra lift from the dopamine release and are addicted to this feeling. In this way, they become compulsive practitioners.

Learning and Teaching *Yogasana*

At the neurological level, the repeated excitation of a pathway in the central nervous system (also called "practice") results gradually in an increased ease of transmission of that particular neural impulse to muscles through that pathway, due both to the decrease in synaptic resistance and to the increase of the synaptic potential. This strengthening of the pathway is the basis for the formation of habits and memory and for learning, all the while explaining the efficacy of practice [181]. Specific pathways for learning and performing are shown in figure 11.A-7**b** and discussed in Section 11.C, page 441.

In regard to the more specific subject of learning and *yogasana,* it is interesting to note that yoga practice has been shown to impact positively on what are seemingly unrelated frontal-lobe mental functions, such as planning and execution of motor tasks, visual and spatial memory, attention, and concentration [533a].

Motivation

Learning can take place by mere repetition, but it is faster still and more enjoyable when there is a motivation to learn (Subsection 4.G, page 136). An event (lesson) must be meaningful for successful learning to take place. The application of this idea to teaching the *yogasanas* is obvious and straightforward. There is a good reason behind the way we do each of the *yogasanas,* and there are many good reasons for making *yogasana* work a lifelong activity. The teacher, at every opportunity, should stress why we are doing this work and the physiological and psychological benefits that come from doing it in our particular way. By doing so, the skeptical student will be won over, and the converted student will find even more reason for dedicated work. Brief comments in this regard show the student immediately that the *yogasanas* go far beyond geometry and exercise and will speed their realization of the benefits (see Subsection 5.F, page 193).

It recently has been found that damage to certain brain centers results in patients having a lack of motivation to act and a loss of the ability to act unless provoked from outside themselves. The critical center for motivation to act lies within the basal ganglia, with the frontal lobe also contributing to the lack of action if it is brought into the picture by the basal ganglia; i.e., one cannot decide to act if the frontal lobe is inactivated by the basal ganglia. On the other hand, if directions are given verbally to such a person, the directions travel directly from Wernicke's area to the frontal lobes without input from the basal ganglia and hence are acted upon in the normal way. The sort of motivation needed to advance to the level of a "grandmaster" in *yogasana* is discussed in Subsection 4.G, page 136.

Reward and Punishment

People tend to repeat behaviors that are rewarded. In the context of *yogasana* teaching, attention or praise from the teacher can act as positive reinforcement and so can help students learn more quickly and completely. Though it is also a truism of psychology that we will retain forever those lessons we learn while in a state of fear or panic, this is not a good basis on which to build one's teaching technique. In a similar vein, it has been shown that lessons are best remembered when the lesson contains a surprise of some sort, the relevant area of the brain being the frontal cortex (Section 4.F, page 125).[22]

It is no surprise that most of us learn best by watching with our eyes; almost 90 percent of our information from outside the body reaches us through the eyes. As a teacher of the *yogasanas,* you should encourage your students to watch you closely as you demonstrate the posture of the moment. In showing the students a new posture, ask them specifically not to try to do it with you as you demonstrate it for the first time, so that their awareness is totally on what you are doing and not divided between what you do and what they feel at the moment; see Subsection 4.G, page 142, for an interesting aspect of visual learning in this way. Perhaps it is also relevant that certain brain regions are activated when students consciously choose to learn by seeing and that these centers are muted when we choose to learn instead by hearing.

Not only will the students learn the proper way to perform the *yogasana* by watching you as the teacher,[23] but they will subconsciously begin to look more and more like you. Though it may seem to be a compliment to the teacher, it is a truism that students will follow their teacher to such an extent that they will come to resemble the teacher in their performance of the *yogasanas* (Subsection 4.G, page 142). This means that any weakness of the teacher is transferred to the students, to their detriment. It is for this reason (and others as well) that students should be encouraged to work with other teachers who teach the same or related forms of *yogasana*. It often happens that another teacher, by chance, will be able to say something in a different way that just makes everything clear to a student who otherwise was not able to get the message. Another teacher may introduce postures to your students that you ignore because you do not do them well, because you dislike them for personal reasons, or because you are too injured to demonstrate them.

For those students who learn better through the auditory channel than through the visual channel, ask the class to watch closely and listen carefully as you demonstrate and explain the intricacies of the new posture. When teaching, allow some silent space for reflection and digestion of the previously given information—we all can catch the seven-digit phone number when given the first time if the giver will only stop talking briefly after giving it [878]!

As *yogasana* practice in a group setting is undeniably a social situation, it is understandable that there are many opportunities for conversation among the students. However, the impulse to chatter can interfere with the subtleties of the practice and so must be postponed. The power of silence has been expressed by other practitioners or teachers [30] in sayings such as:

Better an inch of practice than a foot of preaching.

Ancient Zen saying

Use words to explain thoughts but silence once thoughts have been absorbed...those qualified to seek the truth will grasp the fish and discard the fishing net.

Tao-sheng, China, 360–434

---

22   Perhaps this relates to the apparent success of the Iyengar approach, in which students who do not learn are swatted on the dead part of their anatomy in order to raise their awareness in that place. Indeed, it has been found that a process called "superlearning" occurs with regard to new material when this material is presented in a surprising way. Note also Iyengar's statement that in order to make the student *sattvic,* the teacher must be *rajasic!*

23   Note, however, that what students can focus on visually is limited due to the nature of saccadic motion of the eyes (Subsection 17.B, page 667), unless they are pointedly directed to the aspects of the posture that you want to imprint on their consciousness (Subsection 4.G, page 136). This verbal instruction can precede the demonstration of the posture first done in silence. See also Subsection 4.G, page 145.

Do not require a description of the countries toward which you sail. The description does not describe them to you and tomorrow you arrive there and know them by inhabiting them.

Ralph Waldo Emerson, 1926

These dicta in regard to the power of silence refer not only to the student attempting to learn, but also to the teacher attempting to teach.

Body Image

For those students who learn most easily using the visual channel, their internal body image is essentially that of their external visual image. They will be enchanted by their image in the mirror, the more so if they can see their image in profile or from the back. Such students are rarely at rest in front of the mirror, for they are constantly making adjustments so as to "look better" [764]. On the other hand, those who learn more easily through the auditory channel are more often aware of internal sensations and imbalances and compare their postures to mental pictures constructed from auditory cues. This parallels the dreams in sighted-but-deaf and hearing-but-blind individuals, with the former dreaming in visual pictures, whereas the dreams of the latter are auditory rather than visual.

Intention and Action

When the brain initiates a command to activate a particular muscle in the performance of a particular *yogasana,* the signal is split into two and follows two distinct paths. One of these paths leads to the motor cortex (that part of the brain that activates a particular muscle contraction), and the other leads to the cerebellum (that part of the brain that records the movement and evaluates its appropriateness). It appears that the cerebellum understands which proprioceptive signals are to be expected in regard to body geometry, muscle tension, etc. if the posture is being done correctly, and then compares that with the reality of the posture at that moment. That is, the brain is wired to activate muscles and at the same time to compare this muscle activation with our intentions, in order to

see that our actions and intentions are congruent. If we are sufficiently aware, differences between our intentions and our actions will result in corrective actions [930]. I postulate that the initial template for our intentions, against which our actions are to be gauged, is planted within the cerebellum when we first see our teacher demonstrate the posture (Subsection 4.G, page 135).

Forming Habits

It must be understood that memory and learning do not necessarily function only in the conscious sphere. Thus, through practice, we learn and never forget how to ride a bicycle, how to type a letter, or how to walk. In these cases, the neural circuits for such "automatic" muscle actions can reside in the spine and lower centers of the brain rather than in the more conscious centers, and once they are activated by higher centers in the brain (consciously or subconsciously), they operate without further control from the higher centers until turned off by them. Such motor-memory effects are examples of the mixing of conscious and subconscious actions depicted schematically in figure 1.B-1. As *yogasana* students become more practiced in the postures, they will find that certain aspects of the postures become more subconsciously attended to, so that the conscious awareness can be turned to more subtle aspects. It is also possible that with practice, certain aspects of the postures become more subconsciously attended to, but the conscious awareness is not turned to more subtle aspects; in this case, one is working out of habit (*yogasana* as physical maintenance) rather than as an adventure (*yogasana* as a journey into the unknown), Subsection 11.C, page 441.

As we work with a new *yogasana* and become more adept at its performance, it may seem that we are "expanding our consciousness" through practice; however, as one becomes more practiced, this "new" neural pattern associated with the *yogasana* will become more and more a subconscious one (Subsection 1.B, page 12). Thus the "expansion" is temporary if the action is practiced often, without the addition of new elements of awareness.

The task faced by a teacher in one *yogasana* style having to teach a student with experience in a second style is formidable, because the student must learn to inhibit what was learned previously and replace that with new information on the relevant style. This is very much like what is faced by a person with competence in one language who is trying to learn a second language. The ability to inhibit one brain function while learning a second alternative function is carried out by the prefrontal cortex acting in concert with other areas, largely the hippocampus. See also this page, below, where failure to inhibit irrelevant thoughts is discussed as a factor in teaching *yogasanas* to senior citizens, and Subsection V.H, page 930, where the negative impact of irrelevant thoughts on balance is discussed.

Sleep

During sleep, your brain processes the recent memories of what you have just learned in your *yogasana* practice (Subsection 4.F, page 133). While asleep, the circuits activated during practice will be reactivated, in essence putting the brain through mental rehearsals of the previous physical actions and then shuttling the rehearsed neural patterns into long-term memory. In this process, totally new and creative patterns may appear as well. Even a short *savasana* can help in the various neural processes that otherwise take place during sleep.

Aging

One truly significant difference induced by aging is that the aged in general have a problem with accepting new information, unless it is a simple extension of what they already know to be true. As we age, we are less able or willing to try out new ideas and find them acceptable; which is to say, we become mentally inflexible and are discomfited by new thoughts or new ways of doing things (Subsection 4.E, page 121). As teachers of aging students, we must be aware of this possible stumbling block to learning and find ways to make the new material seem not so new that learning it is resisted. See Subsection 4.E, page 123, for a possible way to overcome

this situation. Further, since the aging brain finds it harder to stick to a single line of thought and so requires more frequent rest breaks, teaching *yogasana* to seniors should be broken into smaller steps, punctuated by more frequent rest periods [702].

Time of Day

Another factor that must be kept in mind when working with senior citizens is that most elder students are "morning people," who are best able to arouse and apply themselves to *yogasana* work in the early hours of the day and who are correspondingly least able to do this type of work in the evening hours. This steady decline throughout the day in the ability of seniors to perform physically applies as well to the memory. By contrast, young adults are more able, physically and mentally, in the evening hours and least able in the early morning! It is thought that in seniors, there is a declining ability to keep the mind focused on the work at hand as the day unwinds, for the inhibition of irrelevant thoughts is strongest for them in the morning and weakest in the evening.

Section 4.H: Brain Waves and the Electroencephalogram (EEG)

Characteristics of the EEG

When the cortex is functioning properly, there is a simultaneous electrical activity of large populations of neurons acting more or less in synchronicity. Such large-scale electrical activity actually can be observed as variations in electrical potential (voltage) on areas of the scalp overlying the active area of the cortex. The pattern of such voltage changes over short time periods (minutes) is called the electroencephalogram (EEG). The cerebral currents associated with the cerebral voltages also have magnetic fields associated with

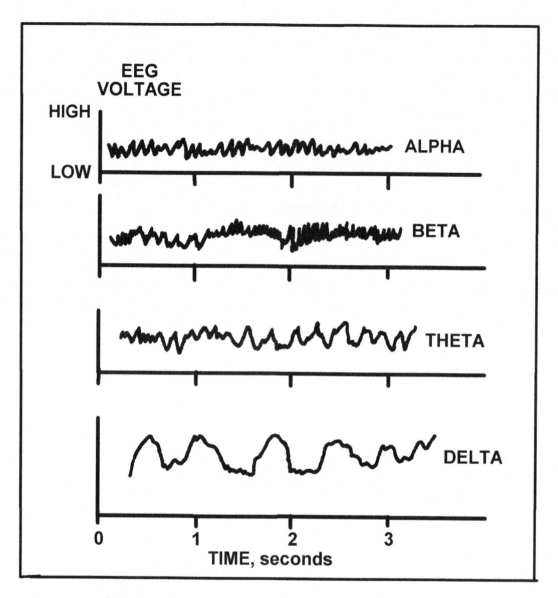

Figure 4.H-1. Four of the five recognized brain-wave patterns, showing a preponderance of either alpha, beta, theta, or delta waveforms.

them, and these too can be measured externally, as a magnetoencephalogram (MEG) [637]. The frequencies of the component waves in the EEG or MEG are indicative of the mental state of the subject at that moment. Similar but not as detailed information can be obtained by measuring electrical activity in the gut rather than in the scalp; for example, when telling a lie, there is a very intense (high voltage) electrogastrogram, whereas this is much subdued when telling the truth.

The origin of the EEG signals involves the postsynaptic potentials in the pyramidal cells of the cortex and ionic conduction in the extracellular fluid [427]. As the pyramidal cells of the cortex are all oriented in parallel fashion, their synaptic voltages can be summed over a large area to produce a significant net voltage, in contrast to other active cortical cells, which are not as well oriented and so have voltage contributions that algebraically sum to a near-zero value on the scalp.

The pacemaker for the EEG signals resides in the thalamus. When Ca^{2+} ions first enter channels in the thalamic cells, the brain-wave oscillations begin and last for between one and a half and twenty-five seconds, followed by a second period

Table 4.H-1: Characteristics of EEG Brain Waves [22, 427, 432, 860]

Name	Frequency, Hertz	Amplitude	Synchronicity	Mental State
Alpha	8–13	High	Synchronized	Relaxed wakefulness; tranquility; nonarousal; meditative
Beta	15–40	Low	Desynchronized	Mental activity of normal wakefulness; aroused, metabolically active; strong mental engagement
Gamma	40–90		Synchronized	Sensory integration; memory consolidation; meditation
Theta	4–7	Very high	Desynchronized	Dreaming state; reverie and creativity while awake
Delta	1.5–4	High	Desynchronized	Stage of dreamless sleep

of approximately five to twenty-five seconds, during which the oscillations continue in a free-running mode. It is thought that while in this second mode, the brain-wave pattern can be entrained and driven by an external electromagnetic field, so as to have the frequency and phase of the external field [637]; i.e., in this way, external physical fields can influence inner mental states! See also Subsection 4.H, page 149, for additional information on the external generation, reception, and control of EEG waves and their effects on the human body.

Typical EEG patterns (figure 4.H-1) are complex and cannot be easily interpreted. In fact, each observed pattern is a combination of other, more basic patterns that are not necessarily obvious in the raw data but which can be teased out of it using the mathematical technique called Fourier analysis (Subsection 14.A, page 549). At any moment, five major distinct mental states can be identified in the EEG, present simultaneously but in varying proportions depending upon the situation [366], with each characterized by a particular brain-wave frequency and shape. Furthermore, the characteristic EEG wave patterns may be more or less localized in specific areas of the brain.

The characteristics of the five basic EEG brain-wave patterns corresponding to the five different wave frequencies are as shown in table 4.H-1 and described below. The spatial patterns of the various basic frequencies may be global or very local with respect to various areas of the scalp. The brain waves described in table 4.H-1 are also prominent in various phases of sleep (Subsection 23.D, page 795). Such electrical data potentially could be of great use to those studying the relationships between the *yogasanas* and their physiological correlates, because shifts between different EEG levels largely involve changes of levels of excitation in the reticular formation (Subsection 4.B, page 74) within the brainstem and also reflect the relative levels of autonomic dominance. That is to say, the EEG directly indicates the level of mental arousal and awareness, whereas a flatline EEG is taken as a sign of brain death. Unfortunately, there is very little data available concerning the EEGs of students while performing the *yogasanas*, though Galle [260a] does mention that yoga adepts can readily shift their brain-wave patterns among alpha, beta, and theta waves using EEG feedback.

Alpha Waves

In the alpha-wave EEG pattern, there is a voltage fluctuation with a frequency of 8–13 hertz, the waves are synchronized across the scalp, and the waves are prominent when one is relaxed, with the eyes closed but the mind awake. In this state of nonarousal, one is resting and meditative. In general, the alpha state is attainable only when the eyes are closed, as any visual, auditory, or tactile stimulation will desynchronize the EEG waveform and raise its frequency into the range of the beta-wave or possibly the gamma-wave state [371, 427, 432]. However, for those who are adept at meditation and yogic discipline [860], there is a more conscious control of the brain-wave EEG state, and the above statement does not necessarily hold true (Section 4.B, page 76). Because the tranquility of the alpha state also is disturbed by muscle potentials [371], students in deeply relaxing postures such as *savasana* should avoid any muscle excitation (shifting of the weight, scratching, coughing, opening of the eyes, motions of the eyes, swallowing, etc.) other than that required for breathing and circulation of the blood. When in the alpha-wave state, the heart rate and blood pressure decrease, and respiration has a decreased rate and becomes more even, while gastrointestinal activity increases. As shown in table 5.A-2, all of these responses are characteristic of stimulation by the parasympathetic nervous system.

Cole [141] discusses how stimulation of the baroreceptors in the carotid sinus and the aortic arch (Section 14.E, page 582), as when doing wall *padasana,* leads to synchronous alpha waves in the EEG; contrarily, when one goes from the supine position toward standing, the lessening of the baroreceptor signal promotes a shift of the EEG waveform from alpha relaxation to beta alertness. Among yoga instructors at their practice, it was found that as the level of cortisol fell, the intensity of the alpha waves in their EEGs increased [425]. On the other hand, for depressed students, a rise of the cortisol level (up to a certain level) in the morning and the movement of the brain waves toward beta frequency are considered to be hopeful signs.

As already demonstrated with meditators, it may be assumed that a strong *yogasana* practice with many moments of deep alpha-wave activity can make *yogasana* students mentally stable and unflappable, in spite of whatever might be going on around them. Considering the ease with which babies are rocked to sleep, it is no surprise that an alpha-wave EEG is promoted by mild, low-frequency stimulation of the skin, as by rocking, which also may be a stimulus to the perineural nervous system (Section 2.C, page 26).

Mu Waves

A variant of the alpha wave is the so-called mu wave, consisting of short bursts of synchronous, wicket-shaped waves of 9–11 hertz frequency originating in the cortex. Simply opening the eyes does not diminish the intensity of mu waves, in contrast to the case for alpha waves. However, mu waves are repressed by movements of the hands or arms, by thinking of moving the arms or legs, and by seeing someone move their arms or legs. The inhibition of mu waves appears to be intimately related to the function of the mirror neurons (Subsection 4.G, page 140). The quenching of mu waves undoubtedly occurs when we perform or think of performing the *yogasanas* or watch someone else perform them. However, it is difficult to see what function this serves.

Beta Waves

Once the eyes are opened in the alpha state or one is engaged in intense mental activity or social interactions, the desynchronized beta waves of 15–40 hertz appear, characterizing a state of mental arousal [371]. Beta waves are characteristic of metabolic activity, mental arousal, a strongly engaged mind, and sympathetic dominance of the autonomic nervous system [143]. Beta waves are observed at the high-frequency end of the beta EEG spectrum during a grand-mal seizure, when suffering confusion, and when under the effects of light-ether anesthesia. Beta waves are observed at the low-frequency end of the beta EEG spectrum when paying attention or when frightened, as when in the fight-or-flight mode (Chapter 5, page 173). *Yogasana* teachers, while teaching, are in a beta state of high arousal; their students in *savasana* are in an alpha state of deep relaxation. When going to sleep, the EEG states move successively from low beta to alpha to theta and finally to delta, running a course of monotonically decreasing EEG frequencies. Cole [142] has observed that placing a student in supported *setu bandha sarvangasana* leads to an immediate shift of EEG from beta to theta type, implying a shift from an aroused state to either a deeply relaxed state or to sleep itself.

In those students who are new to *yogasana* practice, the brain-wave patterns for almost all postures will be dominated by beta waves, reflecting the intensity of effort required in their performance. After much practice, the goal shifts toward being as relaxed in all of the other postures as one is in *savasana;* i.e., it shifts toward the alpha state.

During moderate aerobic exercise, the EEG pattern is reported to shift from beta waves to alpha waves, indicating a shift toward a more meditative state [618], and the alpha state persists beyond the cessation of the exercise. As the *yogasana* student becomes more adept at meditation, there is a shift of the EEG brain-wave pattern from that of beta-wave alertness to alpha-wave inner awareness and then to theta and delta states of inward quietude and harmony [860].

Theta Waves

The theta-wave state has a frequency of 4–7 hertz and is prominent when daydreaming; it is induced by repetitive, nonthinking actions such as freeway driving. This is the state of creative ideas (and freeway accidents). In the theta state, manual tasks become highly automatic and the brain disengages and follows another path without guilt or censorship. It is a very positive state, and time spent with theta waves is time of significant creative mental activity. Theta waves are localized to the temporal lobes and are observed in infants, deteriorated epileptics, and as the slow component of petit-mal epilepsy (the fast component of which is a high-frequency beta wave).

A recent study has shown that the brain areas excited during daydreaming in young, healthy adults are also those that eventually fill with the amyloid beta plaque in those who will contract Alzheimer's disease.

Delta Waves

The delta-wave state is characterized by an EEG wave of 1.5–4 hertz frequency, which never goes to zero frequency, as this would correspond to being brain dead. The delta-state EEG is observed when in a stupor, when under surgical anesthesia, and when asleep. As the delta-state frequency shifts upward toward theta, we pass into a phase of REM sleep (Subsection 23.D, page 800). The delta and theta waves are desynchronized, have relatively low frequencies (table 4.H-1), and appear in the deeper stages of dreamless sleep and meditation, respectively.

Gamma Waves

An EEG state of high frequency has recently been reported; the gamma state is strongly synchronized with a characteristic frequency of 40–90 hertz and appears for brief periods while one is integrating visual or other sensory sensations [22, 125] or is meditating [205]. The gamma waves in the EEGs of meditators were more intense, longer lasting, and more widely synchronized the longer the meditators had practiced their art. The breadth of the gamma-wave synchronicity increases as the degree of mental concentration increases, whereas in a condition such as schizophrenia, there is a preponderance of discordant mental activity and a corresponding lack of gamma synchronicity. Such studies show that meditation is not a relaxation, but a deep, serene inward attentiveness, and that trained musicians also experience a similar calm but strong inner awareness as their gamma-wave function intensifies and spreads as they play. It would be fascinating to see just how prominent gamma waves become in the EEG spectra of trained *yogasana* practitioners when in challenging balancing postures (Appendix V, page 930).

Sleep

Interestingly, several of the electrical activities signaled by the EEG waveforms described in figure 4.H-1 and table 4.H-1 are seen as well in various stages of sleep (Subsection 23.D, page 794). It is also reported that the nature of the EEG wave pattern can be changed at will [204]. This ability is related to that which allows the yogi to defeat the lie detector (Box 5.E-1, page 192).

Brain-Wave Frequencies and Mental Functioning

A very new and exciting idea has recently appeared involving EEG waves and a wide variety of serious neurological and psychological disorders [24, 125]. As discussed briefly in Section 4.C, (page 97), there is a constant transfer of information between the conscious levels of the cortex and various lower-level nuclei in the brain. In particular, there are direct neural connections between the thalamus and the cortex, along which the thalamus offers information to the cortical centers, which decide which elements of the information are truly useful and important and then return this information to the thalamus. The thalamus next edits the information received from the cortex and transmits the abbreviated information a second time to the cortex, thereby reinforcing the important aspects of the original message. All of this happens in the space of a few seconds and involves considerable high-frequency gamma excitation in the EEGs of both the thalamus and the cortex. There are known to be separate and dedicated thalamo-cortical neural pathways for visual information, for auditory information, for touch, etc., all operating in the waking state at the gamma-EEG frequency of 40 hertz. In this process, the thalamus acts as a high-level filter (much like the reticular formation at a lower level), screening out useless sensory signals that otherwise might overload the capacity of the frontal cortex for decision making.

When we fall asleep, the thalamus blocks almost all of the information flow to the cortex, as the frequency of the thalamic signal drops into the range of the theta EEG waves (4–7 hertz), and the neural circuits are barely kept simmering. There are no alpha waves in the sleeping state.

Psychological Problems

What is new and exciting here is that in subjects having any one of several psychological conditions, it has been found that in the waking state, information over one of the ascending thalamo-cortical loops remains at the sleeping theta level, whereas the cortical return signal is at the appropriate gamma frequency and increased in intensity. This sort of dysrhythmia (see Section 22.A, page 761) between the thalamus and the cortex has been found in subjects displaying symptoms as widely disparate as depression, schizophrenia, tinnitus, obsessive-compulsive disorder, Parkinson's, migraine, and epilepsy [73, 705]. In all such conditions, it appears that specific parts of the thalamus have "fallen asleep" in the waking state, leading to a communications mismatch between the thalamus and the cortex for specific sensory modes.

In a variation on the above theme, in psychotic subjects, there is a rapid shifting of the EEG patterns between alpha and beta states [860]. In the epileptic state, all electrical brain activity has been synchronized and entrained, whereas in the normal state, different brain areas have different tasks, EEG frequencies, phases, etc. After an epileptic attack, the neurons resume their normal electrical patterns, and the areas function independently once again [840]. The gamma-wave frequency is very strong in the EEGs of meditators but is weak to nonexistent in those suffering from schizophrenia [81a]. As the gamma-wave intensity and synchronicity increase with meditative training, it is possible that such training (with or without a soft *yogasana* practice) could be of help to students suffering from schizophrenia.

Assuming that the above descriptions hold up to further scrutiny, it has been proposed that the cures for these conditions rest in either pharmacology or electrode implants to reset the thalamic frequencies in rhythm with those of the cortex, much as a cardiac pacemaker guides the heart. As it is already known that the more relaxing *yogasana* postures, such as *savasana, setu bandha sarvangasana,* and *viparita karani,* are effective in switching the brain's EEG level from beta toward theta [142], it may be that through the more arousing *yogasanas* performed in an inversion and backbend practice, the "sleeping" EEG of the thalamus can be raised from theta to gamma frequency. This possibly is a factor in how arousing *yogasanas* such as *urdhva dhanurasana* work to overcome depression (Section 22.A, page 761).

The transfer of information back and forth between higher and lower brain centers in the waking state also brings to mind the shuttling of information at gamma-wave frequencies between the cortex and the hippocampus during sleep, leading to consolidation of the information in long-term memory (Subsection 4.F, page 127).

Schumann Resonances, Brain Waves, and the Atmosphere

Several decades ago (1952), W. O. Schumann, an atmospheric physicist, deduced theoretically that the electromagnetic disturbances caused by lightning strikes around the globe should be trapped between the earth and its ionosphere in a standing-wave pattern, and that given the diameter of the earth and the height of the ionosphere, the pattern would have an oscillating frequency of 7–8 hertz. Ten years later [637], such "Schumann resonances" of lightning-driven electromagnetic waves were observed in the 7–10 hertz range, but subject to slight shifts of frequency and intensity, due to perturbations such as sunspot activity, lunar position, atmospheric conditions, location, time of day, celestial conditions, etc.

The relevance of Schumann resonances to the study of yoga is not immediately apparent until one realizes that such waves have a frequency very close to that of the electromagnetic alpha brainwave state (8–13 hertz; table 4.H-1) and so might actually entrain the brain waves of humans during those times that their brain waves are "free running." This means that one's brain would tend to move to the alpha state when in the vicinity of high-intensity Schumann waves!

Schumann waves are easily generated in the laboratory and are found to have astounding effects on the subjects. Thus, for example, reaction times are readily shown to be altered by the application of external electromagnetic Schumann-like fields of approximately 10 hertz, whereas at 3 hertz, the effects are headaches, sweating, and tightness of the chest. It is thought that it is the magnetic component of the electromagnetic Schumann wave that is effective in coupling with the brain through the agency of the magnetic center in the brain, the pineal gland. Mechanical stimulation of the brain, using a helmet and motor arrangement run at 10 hertz, also has a strongly sedating effect, as does a long ride over a rough road, during which there is much shaking [13].

Healing

Moreover, when energized by Schumann waves at the alpha frequency, the body appears to be capable of healing at an accelerated rate. When a person's EEG is in the alpha-wave state, it has been shown repeatedly that the hands broadcast intense amounts of what are essentially magnetic Schumann waves at the alpha frequency and that these can be received by another person, either nearby or in contact. It appears that this transfer of biomagnetic energy at the alpha frequency lies behind the miraculous cures achieved by the "laying on of hands" by body workers, etc. It would appear to tie in as well with the concept of sacred sites of high energy, for it has been observed that such sites carry anomalously intense Schumann resonances. Though all of this sounds like science fiction, there is considerable good science behind it, and it could be of great consequence to understanding the subtleties of *yogasana* practice, healing, and teaching.

The Autonomic Nervous System

5

Section 5.A: Introduction to the Autonomic Nervous System

Origin

Through evolution over time, various older brain functions are superseded by newer, more useful ones. Though eclipsed by these new brain functions, the ancestral brains have remained in the newer animals to perform their functions in less obvious ways. In insects and reptiles, there has never been anything more than this ancestral brain and its associated nervous system; in humans today, the reptilian brain has survived intact as a part of the autonomic nervous system. In addition to this, humans also have the somewhat newer brain of the limbic system and the most modern addition, the cortex, the function of which is largely inhibitory with respect to the other two [574] (Chapter 4, page 95).

Subconscious Action

When the autonomic nervous system was first uncovered, it was so named because it was believed that its actions were totally automatic and independent of any outside control, in contrast to the central nervous system (figure 2.A-1). In the first approximation, the autonomic nervous system in humans does work without any conscious control, is inaccessible to conscious inspection, and operates independently of the central nervous system. Working independently

of the central nervous system, it is able to sense the status of the internal body apparatus and then signal adjustments to be made, so as to keep the body's parameters coordinated and within certain preset bounds. This process, called homeostasis (see below), involves a large number of visceral reflexes. The autonomic nervous system controls the smooth muscles found in the skin, within the blood vessel walls, in the iris of the eye, in the stomach, in the cardiac muscle of the heart, and in the glands of the body. This system functions twenty-four hours per day, every day, largely sight unseen.

The huge number of autonomic functions that are being monitored continuously (for deviations from their homeostatic values) suggests why this function is normally assigned to the subconscious. If all of this information were to appear in the conscious realm, the knowing and thinking mind would be so swamped with information regarding homeostasis as to be rendered nonfunctional for making other conscious decisions.

Conscious Action

Though activation of much of the autonomic nervous system originates at the lower centers in the spine, brainstem, and hypothalamus, some autonomic functions also can be influenced indirectly by higher brain centers in the cerebral cortex. In agreement with the findings of the yoga masters of past millennia, medical doctors today acknowledge that the supposed independence of the autonomic nervous system is unrealistic, for there is likely a strong mixing of the subconscious autonomic and conscious central

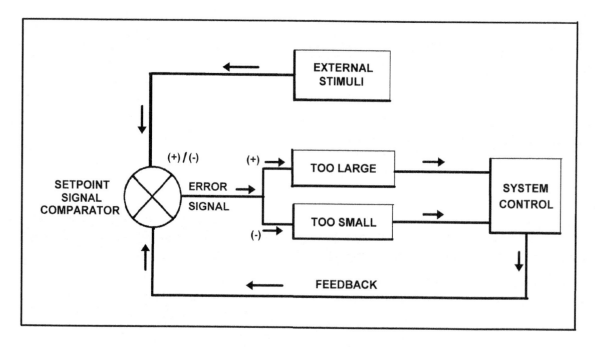

Figure 5.A-1. A typical feedback circuit for the autonomic nervous system. In this, an external stimulus acts to change a physiological parameter of the system, as revealed by comparison of the altered parameter with its set-point value. This comparison generates an error signal, which drives the system controller, which in turn alters the system physiology toward the set-point value via feedback, thereby reducing the error signal to zero. In this way, the set-point value is maintained subconsciously, in spite of external forces to the contrary.

nervous system functions, as in figures 1.B-1 and 1.B-2. This deliberate, conscious access to autonomic functions can be one of the great practical benefits of *yogasana* practice, especially when the practice is performed with autonomic control in mind.

Homeostatic Control and Feedback

Though the human body can survive under a wide range of conditions, there is a single set of narrowly defined conditions under which it operates best. Should any of the body's parameters fall outside the optimum range, due to either external or internal forces, then the body reacts automatically to regain the optimum value, in a general process called "homeostatic control" [427, 574]. For example, the various systems of the body automatically adjust so as to keep the body's core temperature optimal (37.0° C, 98.6° F) regardless of the external weather or internal chemistry. The core temperature of the body is

monitored by a sensor in the aortic arch, at a point between the aorta and the brain. In this case, autonomic adjustments may include shivering, sweating, readjustment of vascular diameters to shift blood flow, etc., each of which works to drive the core temperature in one direction or the other. Though normal core temperature is 37.0° C (98.6° F), during vigorous exercise this may rise momentarily to 40.0° C (104.0° F). However, the body will react to this as best it can to return the core temperature to the homeostatic value, 37.0° C (98.6° F).

Other body systems under homeostatic control are the kidneys, which regulate the salt content of the body fluids; the cardiovascular system, which concerns itself with the heart rate, blood pressure, and vascular diameters; the respiratory system, which is involved with breathing rate and oxygen and carbon dioxide levels in the blood; and the appetites for water and food.

The Feedback Mechanism

Control of autonomic functions is by the mechanism called feedback, as illustrated in figure 5.A-1. For a particular body function, there is an optimum set-point value for this function. A detector for the level of the function in question detects any deviation from the set-point value and so produces an error signal, either positive or negative, depending on the sense of the deviation. This error signal is then fed back to the controlling center, thereby either raising or lowering the level of the function until the value of the function is brought back into agreement with the set point. For example, sensors in the brain monitor the concentrations of oxygen and carbon dioxide in the blood. If these concentrations are not within the set-point ranges for optimum brain health, the sensors report error signals, and the respiratory centers then alter the rates and amplitudes of the breath and the heartbeat until the gas concentrations are within the prescribed limits and homeostasis is achieved. The set points for various functions can be reset, as by pyrogens, for example, which induce and maintain fevers when the body is fighting an infection, or by a constant stress over a long period, which acts to raise the set point referring to blood pressure, for example.

A related set-point mechanism for automatic regulation involves the internal body clock, which dictates physiological changes on the basis of the transitions between light and darkness, as observed visually at sunrise and sunset (figure 23.B-1). In this more realistic scenario, rather than having a set-point value, the system moves between an upper and a lower set point, and though the system control is homeostatic, the monitored function is always oscillating between the higher and lower limits. In a broader sense, homeostasis consists of a regular oscillation of the level of a controlled function between the high and low set points, and though it may momentarily be at just the prescribed set-point value, more generally it is kept within a narrow but nonzero range of set-point values.

Resetting Limits

Elasticity is built into the feedback loops of the body, so that every time a limit is exceeded, there is a tendency toward readjustment of the set-point range in the direction of the error. If there is a chronic tendency to stray in a specific direction from a set point (i.e., if a chronic stress is present in the body), there will follow a long-term resetting of the set point to an accommodating value. This shift of the set point to an extreme value can be unhealthy, for the extreme value will lead to a homeostatic adjustment only when the function being monitored takes an even more extreme value. This is why we need periods of rest and relaxation, for these activities break the tendency of set points to be constantly nudged to new, unhealthy values.

Fortunately, through *yogasana* practice, one can deliberately shift the homeostatic set points of autonomic functions, so that the body maintains homeostasis about a new mean value of the functional variable that is healthier. This is a mechanistic description of the effect illustrated in figure 1.B-1 of the mixing between conscious and subconscious actions through *yogasana* practice.

Lest the reader get the idea that the homeostatic set-point range is truly static, it must be pointed out that under certain conditions, the set-point ranges may be instantly adjusted to accommodate instantly changing external situations (Subsection 5.A, page 158).

Interoception

As discussed in Section 11.C, page 441, there is a detailed picture of the body's posture and motion that is assembled in the mind from moment to moment and is accessible to the subconscious mind in the *yogasana* beginner, and to the conscious mind as well in more adept practitioners. This sense of the body's external form is called proprioception. A more internalized form of proprioception involving the sense of the physiological states of the **internal** body organs, glands, chemistry, etc. is known as interoception [173] and is discussed further in Subsection 11.C, page 444. Using the autonomic nervous system, interoception is the physiological signal that alerts the body to homeostatic imbalance, though its signals may be sensed as high as the cortex. Interoception involves the experiential sense of one's body image, the changes in the physiological parameters that define homeostasis, and the feelings of energy flow in the body, energy intensity, or diffuseness. Interoceptive signals are deposited in the cerebral hemispheres, with some (those from the sympathetic afferents) going to lower cortical centers in the right hemisphere, and those from others (the parasympathetic afferents) going to lower cortical centers in the left hemisphere.

The Anatomic Center

The main center for autonomic control of body functions is the hypothalamus, in the diencephalon at the base of the brain (figure 4.B-1). Additionally, input from the hypothalamus impacts on higher brain centers; for example, information on drives (sex, hunger, thirst) and emotions and control of these drives and emotions travels from the limbic system to the hypothalamus, where it is modified and then returned to the limbic system. Ascending sensory input to the hypothalamus regarding the status of the internal organs is via the reticular formation (Subsection 4.B, page 74) and then output again via the autonomic nervous system.

Signals from the hypothalamus also stimulate the pituitary gland to secrete hormones to regulate water, salt, and the metabolic and other hormonal parameters of the body. It is seen from this that though the hypothalamus is the primary autonomic control center, weighing input from both above and below and then directing the autonomic nervous system on this basis, other centers, such as the medulla oblongata in the brainstem (Subsection 4.B, page 72), also are important in regard to autonomic control.

Hypothalamic Nuclei

Most of the centers involved in maintaining the status quo (i.e., homeostasis) are located in the hypothalamus (figure 4.B-1), the center for autonomic action. Nuclei in the hypothalamus receive afferent signals in regard to the status of the body's systems, and then, via hormonal secretions, neural efferents to target organs, and consciously directed motivational systems, the internal climate of the body is changed so as to bring it back to optimum functioning. Higher centers in the brain help direct the hypothalamus in its work, interfacing with it through the limbic system.

As with the central nervous system, the autonomic nervous system uses the frequency of the efferent signal as the measure of the intensity of the effect it is employed to induce. However, in the autonomic system, the frequency range of the effector signals is only 1–20 hertz, to be compared with a range of 50–200 hertz in the more modern central nervous system [308]. The frequency difference reflects the fact that the older autonomic system uses neurons of much slower conduction velocity than does the newer central nervous system (table 3.B-3). The anatomy and function of the hypothalamus are described in detail in Section 5.B, page 165.

Autonomic Branches

Sympathetic

The autonomic nervous system consists of three main branches, the sympathetic, the parasympathetic, and the enteric (figure 2.A-1), the characteristics of which are compared among themselves and with the central nervous system in table 5.A-1. The sympathetic nervous system is responsible for the "fight or flight" response [54]. In this reflexive response, the body and mind shift away from the normal homeostatic condition to one that optimizes the body and mind to either fight to defend itself or to flee from some threat. All of the sympathetic reflexes originate with the fight-or-flight response and so can be understood initially in terms of offering better chances for survival when threatened. From the evolutionary point of view, the sympathetic nervous system is the oldest part of our modern nervous system, older than either the central nervous system or the parasympathetic nervous system.

In case of imminent danger, the sympathetic nervous system quickly prepares us to either defend ourselves against the threat or to run from it. To this end, norepinephrine is released into the neural synapses, making them conductive for a brief moment. Following this, epinephrine and norepinephrine are released from the medulla of the adrenal glands for circulation in the vascular system for several minutes, in support of the initial reaction. When in this state, heart and respiration rates increase so as to furnish oxygen to the muscles, mental alertness increases, and the pupils of the eyes dilate, as do the bronchioles of the lungs. And this is only the abbreviated list! In our present-day life, some of these responses are no longer logical or necessary, but they are present, nonetheless, as the "normal" responses to the stresses of modern-day living.

Whereas most *yogasana* teachers are more or less familiar with the fight or flight reflex, the general attitude among them is that it is only a factor in times of great danger and so is rarely active; however, it is closer to the truth that it is activated when there is **any** arousal of the senses, as when walking across the room or when performing most *yogasanas;* it is at its weakest only when in *savasana* or at certain moments during sleep [275].

Arousal in the sympathetic nervous system is largely an all-or-nothing affair, in that when the system is activated, virtually all of the responses under its control are activated simultaneously, all with one goal: to protect the body from an outside threat. If the threat is in the form of an emotional stress rather than physical, the sympathetic response nonetheless is the same: all systems go, albeit the response can be graded as to the degree of threat. It appears that there is some selective excitation possible in the sympathetic nervous system, but not much. The sympathetic nervous system is discussed in more detail in Section 5.C, page 170.

Parasympathetic

The global arousal of the body's defenses by the sympathetic nervous system is moderated by the responses of the body to the parasympathetic nervous system (Section 5.D, page 178).

This system restores calm to the body's internal workings, slowing the heart and lowering the blood pressure, among other things. In general, the two subsystems of the autonomic nervous system are working simultaneously in a cooperative way, balanced as is appropriate to the situation at hand. Though not all of the body's organs are innervated by both the sympathetic and parasympathetic branches, where there is dual innervation, the relative amounts of sympathetic and parasympathetic excitation can be altered so that the net effect is the dominance of the sympathetic nervous system, at one end of the spectrum, to sympathetic/parasympathetic parity at the other end. These contrary functions of the sympathetic and parasympathetic branches of the autonomic nervous system are discussed in detail below, together with the evidence that in humans, the autonomic control of these internal functions can be brought under conscious control, especially through the practice of the *yogasanas* and also through acupuncture [567a]. The characteristics of the autonomic, enteric, and central nervous systems are compared in table 5.A-1 [863], and the parasympathetic system is discussed in detail in Section 5.D, page 178.

Enteric

The enteric nervous system controls the involuntary actions of the digestive system and is often classified as part of the parasympathetic nervous system; however, it has been shown to be able to operate efficiently without any connection to the central nervous system or to the vagus nerve of the parasympathetic nervous system. The enteric system has more neurons in it than does the spinal cord and uses serotonin as a neurotransmitter (Subsection 3.D, page 55), a compound that is active in the brain but is not found in either the sympathetic or parasympathetic autonomic branches. Thus, the enteric system would seem to be worthy of recognition as an independent third branch of the autonomic nervous system [268], though its actions appear to be largely parasympathetic and localized in the gastrointestinal tract.

Table 5.A-1: Comparison of the Somatic and Autonomic Nervous Systems [268]

Nervous System	Final Neurotransmitter	Target Organs
Somatic	Acetylcholine	Skeletal muscles
Sympathetic	Norepinephrine	Glands, blood vessels, heart, smooth muscles
Parasympathetic	Acetylcholine	Glands, blood vessels, heart, smooth muscles
Cardiac	Acetylcholine or norepinephrine	Heart
Enteric	Serotonin	Gastrointestinal organs

Table 5.A-2: Influences of the Sympathetic and Parasympathetic Nervous Systems on Body Functions[a]

Site/Function	Sym	Parasym	Source/Target[b]	References
Heart rate	+	–	T1–T4	[143, 273, 360, 431, 432]
Atrial contraction force	+	–		[432]
Ventricular contraction force	+	0		[275]
Artery diameter (alpha)	–	0	T1–T4	[432]
Artery diameter (beta)	+	0	T1–T4	[432]
Vascular resistance	+	–		[143]
Stroke volume	+	–		[360]
Blood				
Clotting	+	0		[273, 626, 851]
Blood pressure	+	–	T1–T4	[143, 273, 360, 626]
O$_2$ concentration	+			[626]
Red cell count	+			[582]
Core temperature	–	+		
Intestinal circulation	–	+		[878]
Brain				
Brain waves, left hemisphere (beta)	+	–		[143]
Brain waves, right hemisphere (alpha)	–	+		[143]
Reticular formation	+	–		[143]
Posterior hypothalamus	+	–		[143]
Anterior hypothalamus	–	+		[143]
Preoptic hypothalamus	–	+		[143]
Basal forebrain	–	+		[143]
Solitary tract	–	+		[143]

Site/Function	Sym	Parasym	Source/Target[b]	References
Alertness	+	−		[626]
EEG				
High-frequency beta	+	−		[143]
Low-frequency alpha	−	+		[143]
Habituation	−	+		[143]
Synchronicity	−	+		[143]
Sleep stages 1–4	−	+		[860]
REM sleep	+			[427]
Eyes				
Pupil diameter	+	−	C N III	[273, 360, 431, 582]
Lens curvature	−			
Ciliary tone	−	+	C N III	[360, 431, 432]
Blink rate	+			[267]
Lachrymal output	+			[431]
Eyelid elevation	+	−		[143]
Intraocular pressure	+	−		
Sphincter pupillae tone	0	+		
Dilator sphincter tone	+	−		
Gastrointestinal tract				
Peristalsis	−	+		[360]
Spasticity	+	−		[851]
Lumen sphincter tone	+	−		[432]
Gallbladder tone	−	+		[432]
Bile duct tone	−	+		[432]
Secretions	−	+		[273, 360]
Nutrient absorption	−	+		[878]
Anal sphincter tone	+	−		[878]
Metabolism				
Glucose	+	0	Liver	[273, 432, 582]
Fat	+			[273, 626]
Basal	+	−		[143, 432]
Glycogen synthesis	+	0	Liver	[432]
Skeletal Muscles				
Tone	+	−		[143, 273, 626]
O_2 consumption	+			
Vasoconstriction, alpha arteries	+	0		[360, 431, 432]
Vasodilation, beta arteries	+	0		[432]
Lactic acid production	+	−		[143]

Site/Function	Sym	Parasym	Source/Target[b]	References
Smooth Muscles				
Vasoconstriction	+			[268, 431, 432]
Lungs/respiration				
Rate	+	−		[143, 273, 431]
Glandular secretions	+			[360]
Bronchiole diameter	+	−		[431, 432]
Nasal erection	+	0		[36, 687]
Nasal laterality, R open/L closed	+	−		[143, 687]
Nasal laterality, L open/R closed	−	+		[143, 687]
Glandular secretions				
Nasal mucus	−	+		[431, 582]
Salivation	+	++	C N VII	[427, 431, 582]
Lachrymal	0	+		
Gastric	−	+		[273, 626]
Adrenal	++	0	T10–T12	[626]
Pineal	+			[360]
Immunity	+/−	+		[143]
Chemical release				
Insulin	−	+	Pancreas	[580, 626, 778]
Thyroxine	+			[626]
Epinephrine	+	0	Adrenal medulla	[143, 360, 626]
Norepinephrine	+	0	Adrenal medulla	[143, 360, 626]
Cortisol	+	−	Adrenal cortex	[143]
Glucose	+	−	Liver	[427, 432]
ACTH	+		Pituitary	
Aldosterone	+			
CRF	+			
Lactic acid	+	0		[143]
Glycogen	0	+		[432]
Beta endorphin	+	0		[432]
Thyroid hormone	+	−		[143]
Oxytocin	+			[360]
Vasopressin	+			[360, 427]
Fatty acids	+	0	Adrenal cortex	[273, 360, 432]
Glucagon	+		Liver	[626]
Skin				
Finger temperature	−	+		[431, 432]
Sweating	++	0	T1–L3	[273, 360, 431, 432, 582]
Piloerection	+	0	T1–L3	[432]

Site/Function	Sym	Parasym	Source/Target[b]	References
Vasoconstriction	+	0	T1–L3	[273, 360, 431, 582]
Shivering	–			[626]
Kidney, bladder, genitalia				
Urinary output	–	0		[432]
Urinary sphincter release	0	+		[582, 878]
Detrussor tone	0	+		[432]
Anal sphincter	0	+		[582]
Trigone tone	+	0		[432]
Penile/clitoral erection	0	+		[431, 432, 878]
Ejaculation	+	0		[360, 432, 878]

a Lists the effects of activation of either the sympathetic (Sym) or parasympathetic (Parasym) nervous system on the site, function, process, or event as either enhancing/increasing (+), no effect (0), or inhibiting/decreasing (-).

b Lists the neural paths used in the activation and the target organ, if there is one.

Subsystem Comparisons

Aspects of the somatic and the various branches of the autonomic nervous system are compared in table 5.A-1. The effects of autonomic action on the functions of the body are manifold, and many, if not all, of these are within the reach of the *yogasana* practitioner. The results of an extended search of the medical literature in regard to the effects of sympathetic and parasympathetic excitations on various organs and bodily processes are presented in table 5.A-2. For each of the functions listed in the table, there are one or more sensors reporting the status of the function on a continuous basis; i.e., all of these functions are being controlled homeostatically. Notice that there are a few functions that are stimulated by the sympathetic branch of the autonomic system but for which there is no compensating parasympathetic balancing. For a more detailed account of the interaction between mind and body vis-à-vis the autonomic nervous system, see Section 5.F, page 193.

Classical Interpretation

The roles of the sympathetic and parasympathetic nervous systems have been interpreted by Iyengar [391] using the classical Indian concepts of the *nadis* (Section 5.G, page 201) with the sympathetic nervous system corresponding to the *ida nadi* and the parasympathetic to the *pingala nadi*, respectively. When, through *yogasana* practice, the energies of these two *nadis* become "fused," they generate energy that is available to all parts of the body through the *sushumna nadi*, the central nervous system.

Section 5.B: The Hypothalamus

Location and Properties

The hypothalamus is the head ganglion of the autonomic system. As such, it is responsible for an amazingly large number of regulatory functions, all aimed at homeostasis and carried out largely in the subconscious, so that we are hardly aware of their occurrence until something goes wrong. A list of the hypothalamic responsibilities would include regulation of the body's core temperature, water balance, energy resources, feeding behavior, and rates of heart action and breathing. This is accomplished using both neural and hormonal signaling. Speaking

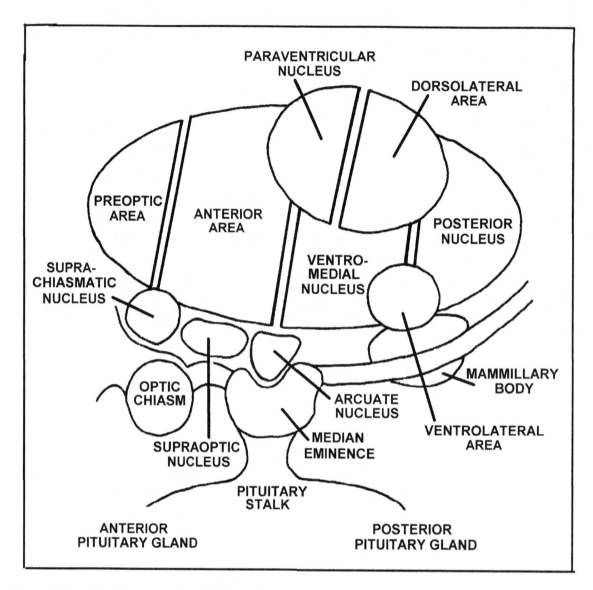

Figure 5.B-1. Component nuclei of the hypothalamus within the brain and their relation to the pituitary gland, as seen from the left side; the entire organ weighs only 4 grams. See table 5.B-1 for descriptions of several of these nuclei.

geographically, the anterior part of the hypothalamus is reserved for the control of the parasympathetic system, whereas the posterior part is reserved for control of the sympathetic system [625]. As mentioned in Chapter 4, the hypothalamus may be considered not only as a part of the diencephalon, but also as a part of the brain's limbic system, and as such, it would be the most important origin for efferent motor pathways within that system.

Anatomy

The hypothalamus is a rather poorly defined organ lying at the base of the forebrain (figure 4.B-1). Rossi [721] states, "One seeks in vain for clarity regarding the basic anatomy and functions of the hypothalamus." It is composed of a poorly organized mass of subregions; its nuclei (figure 5.B-1 and table 5.B-1), all of which communicate with one another, are used for regulation of the autonomic, neuropeptide, endocrine, and immune systems, all of which again communicate

Table 5.B-1: Functions of Nuclei within the Hypothalamus [360, 432, 721]

Center	Function
Lateral hypothalamus	Triggers increased heart rate and blood pressure, peripheral vasoconstriction, skeletal muscle vasodilation, general sympathetic activity
Posterior nucleus	Sympathetic autonomic excitation, cutaneous vasoconstriction, piloerection, promotes release of epinephrine and thyroxine, increase of metabolic rate, generates and conserves body heat
Dorsolateral area	Adjusts salt concentrations in body fluids
Anterior area	Parasympathetic autonomic excitation, activates heat-loss centers, reduces heart rate and blood pressure, increases gastrointestinal secretions, initiates sweating, inhibits thyroid
Preoptic area	Controls sexual and maternal behavior, causes body to cool, affects sleep/wake cycle
Supraoptic nucleus	Secretes hormones
Paraventricular nucleus	Controls water, salt, and thirst, secretes hormones, promotes eating of carbohydrates
Suprachiasmatic nucleus	Drives circadian rhythms, vision
Median eminence	Excretes hormones to pituitary
Solitary tract nucleus	Receives interoceptive information from viscera

with one another. Note too that certain vegetative and endocrine functions are governed by subcortical structures connected to but outside the hypothalamus.

With neural connections to centers both higher and lower than itself, a chain of command can be drawn up for the hypothalamus: it is controlled by the amygdala and the thalamus, which in turn are controlled by the cortex, and the hypothalamus is in direct control of the autonomic nervous system and the pituitary gland.

Importance

Its small size (occupying less than 1 percent of the brain's volume and weighing only a few grams) belies the importance of the hypothalamus to the body's well being, for on a volume-to-volume basis, no other part of the brain receives as much blood as is pumped through the hypothalamus. Furthermore, Swanson [843] states, "It may very

well be that gram for gram the hypothalamus is the most important piece of tissue in any organism." In lower creatures such as insects and reptiles, the hypothalamus is the highest brain center in the nervous system. In a more modern vein, it is said by present-day neuroscientist E. L. Rossi [721], "The hypothalamus is thus the major output pathway of the limbic system. It integrates the sensory-perceptual, emotional and cognitive functions of the mind with the biology of the body." Is not this statement just that of the yogi defining yoga as the union of body, mind and spirit?

Emotion and Behavior

In addition to its effects on the purely physical parameters of the body, the hypothalamus also affects the emotional climate, for it is intimately connected to the amygdala (emotions) and the hippocampus (memory and learning) within the limbic system. In turn, the hypothalamus is influ-

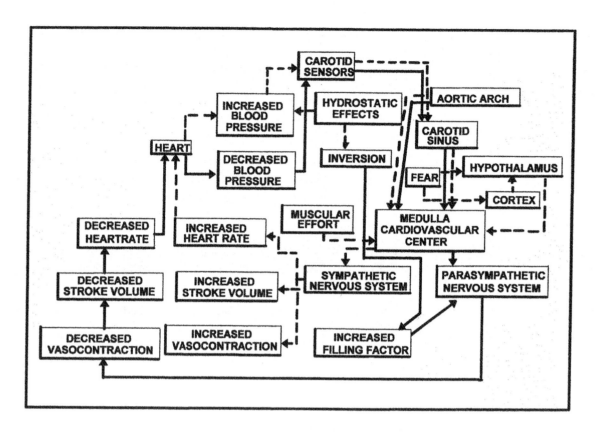

Figure 5.B-2. The multiple effects of inversion on various autonomic functions. The dashed lines indicate the paths of sympathetic excitation, and the full lines indicate the paths for parasympathetic excitation. See text for explanation.

enced by direct connection to the olfactory nerve (cranial nerve I, emotional memory of odors) and to the eyes (where it dilates the pupils and sets the internal clock according to the changes in light intensity as sensed by the eyes upon going from night to day). In humans, the hypothalamus controls the emotions of anger, fear, pleasure, contentment and placidity, the sex drive, etc., but with an overlying inhibitory control by the forebrain, so as to make the expression of the emotions socially acceptable and appropriate. It also integrates emotional and visceral responses to emotional stress.

Through its hormonal connection to the brain's pituitary gland and its hormones, the hypothalamus is indirectly responsible for autonomic functions such as blood pressure, heart rate, breathing rate, metabolism, and muscle tone.

There also are connections between the hypothalamus and the limbic system (which deals with emotions) and through the limbic system, with the prefrontal cortex (which deals with thoughts and decision making).

Neurologically, sympathetic excitation is associated with increased beta-wave activity in the EEG of the left cerebral hemisphere, and parasympathetic activity is associated with increased alpha-wave activity in the EEG of the right cerebral hemisphere (Section 4.H, page 152). The many aspects of such cerebral laterality, as well as mood, the breath, and autonomic dominance are discussed in Section 4.D, page 98, and Section 15.E, page 629. It is through this web of interconnections between cerebral hemispheres, EEG activity, the emotions, and homeostasis that bodily reactions, thoughts, emotions, and behaviors all come together in the autonomic system to influence one another in nonlinear ways. For example, given the map in figure 5.B-2, one can trace the connection between fears hidden within the limbic system, the flexional reflex, and the sympathetic response of the autonomic nervous system, all of which can be activated when faced with performing *sirsasana I* (Section 11.D, page 450).

Reward and Punishment

Sensations and feelings of reward are promoted in the lateral and ventromedial nucleus of the hypothalamus (figure 5.B-1). Apparently either punishment/rage or reward are sensed, depending upon the intensity of the stimulating signal received in the ventromedial centers; the sense of punishment and fear can be so strong that it can overcome any sense of pleasure and reward. All of our actions (yogic or otherwise) ultimately have consequences in the reward and punishment centers of the hypothalamus. If the behaviors are rewarding, they will be repeated, but if they are punishing, they will be abandoned; and in either case, they will leave more or less of a memory trace in the cortex, the more so if the behavior has been repeated. Thus, behaviors that are only mildly rewarding or punishing are not remembered or learned (Subsection 4.G, page 146), as we become habituated to them, whereas the stronger responses to the behavior, positive or negative, are reinforced and so are well learned. It is thought that the hippocampus plays a large role in the consolidation of such pleasure/pain signals in long-term memory (Section 4.F, page 127).

Biorhythm

As discussed in Subsection 23.B, page 774, hormonal levels in the body rise and fall in patterns that are keyed to the light/dark cycles of sunrise and sunset. This timing is accomplished by neurological signals from the eyes that go directly to the suprachiasmatic nucleus in the hypothalamus (figure 5.B-1), which then is able to turn hormone levels on and off at the proper times by reference to the phase of the day/night sun cycle. The pineal gland (Subsection 6.B, page 215) and its hormone melatonin also are involved in this timing scheme. In a well-regulated body, the hormonal levels as controlled by the hypothalamus are optimum for *yogasana* practice between the hours of 6:00 to 8:00 AM (Subsection 23.B, page 779).

Connectivity and Function

As there are ascending and descending neural fibers both entering and leaving the hypothalamus, it is one of the central information hubs within the brain. Being the major output pathway of the limbic system, the hypothalamus integrates the sensory-perceptual, emotional, and cognitive signals of the mind with the biology of the body [721].[1] But not all of the hypothalamic nuclei are connected to the autonomic nervous system, for some are involved only with the endocrine, neuropeptide, somatic, or immune systems in nonautonomic ways.

Centers within the hypothalamus regulate the feeding reflex (generating hunger and satiety sensations to promote and inhibit eating), adjust the levels of sugar in the blood and stored in tissues (mobilizing the release of sugar into the blood from storage sites and vice versa), control the water balance in the body via control of the release of hormones from the kidneys (creating a thirst sensation when the body is deficient in water, and increasing urination when there is a surplus), raise and lower the blood pressure, and initiate shivering in order to raise the body's muscle tone and thereby generate heat, or initiate sweating in order to cool the body.

Hypothalamic centers can decrease the heart rate, inhibit thyroid function, maintain the health of the sex organs, promote the secondary sexual characteristics, promote breast feeding and uterine contractions, and regulate the menstrual cycle. The hypothalamus regulates metabolism via the thyroid gland, the sensations of hunger and satiety, and the general level of digestive action at any one time. And all of this is controlled by an organ the size of a pea!

---

1   Note how closely this matches the aim of yoga, phrased as the union of the body, the mind, and the emotions/spirit! As we shall see, the hypothalamic control of the autonomic system is indeed a very important factor in understanding how *yogasana* affects the body, mind, and emotions and vice versa.

Modes of Action

Interestingly, the information flowing into and out of the hypothalamus is of two sorts: neural impulses flowing through the body's network of nerves, and chemical hormones circulating through the body's fluids. It follows from this that there are four possible modes of hypothalamic action: neural input/neural output, neural input/hormonal output, hormonal input/neural output, and hormonal input/hormonal output. All four of these modes are used by the hypothalamus.

Pituitary Hormones

Hormonally, the pituitary gland is thought to be the master gland controlling the levels of hormones in the body and thereby controlling the body's growth, reproductive capabilities, metabolism, and response to trauma and stress. However, even the pituitary is under the control of the hypothalamus. Thus, the hypothalamus releases hormones directly and specifically to the pituitary gland to either stimulate or inhibit its secondary release of hormones into the bloodstream. In particular, the hypothalamus dictates the pituitary's control over growth hormone, follicular stimulating hormone (FSH), luteinizing hormone (LH), adrenocorticotropic hormone (ACTH), thyroid stimulating hormone (TSH), prolactin, antidiuretic hormone (ADH, vasopressin), and oxytocin (Chapter 6, page 213).

In its only inhibitory action, the hypothalamus inhibits the pituitary from releasing prolactin, a hormone that otherwise stimulates the flow of breast milk in women [621] and relaxation following orgasm in men.

Section 5.C: The Sympathetic Nervous System

It is understandable that the hypothalamus is more concerned with excitations in the sympathetic nervous system than with excitations in the parasympathetic, because sympathetic excitations are immediate and can save one's life in an emergency, whereas parasympathetic excitations only save one's life in the long run. And though the sympathetic alarm response does have its place in emergency situations, it also can lead to problems if it is continued for an unnecessarily long time. Though one can exist without activation of the sympathetic nervous system, without it, one cannot do strenuous work, cannot defend oneself, and cannot survive in a harsh environment.

Innervation

Efferents

The efferent fibers of the sympathetic branch of the autonomic nervous system originate in the gray matter of the spinal cord at levels between T1 and L2. Exiting through the ventral horns of the cord (figure 4.A-2), they immediately synapse in chain structures that parallel the spinal column, forming the paravertebral ganglia of the sympathetic trunk (figure 5.C-1a). Fibers from the spinal column enter the paravertebral trunk and may continue through without synapse; may enter at one level and then leave at another; or may enter, synapse, and leave at the same level. It is characteristic of the sympathetic nervous system that there is a synapse close to the vertebrae, followed by a long postganglionic axon to the effector organ and a second synapse to the organ. In contrast, each neural component of the parasympathetic nervous system has but a single synapse between the vertebral column and the effector organ, with the synapse much closer to the organ than to the vertebrae (figure 5.C-1b). As the efferent sympathetic fibers travel from the paravertebral ganglia to the effector organs, they branch in a divergent way (figure 3.C-2a) as many as twenty times, so that many sites can be activated in cascade fashion by one initiating efferent neural impulse (figure 5.C-1a). Though most organs have both sympathetic and parasympathetic innervation, only the former is found in the sweat glands, in the piloerector muscles surrounding each hair, and in the walls of blood vessels.

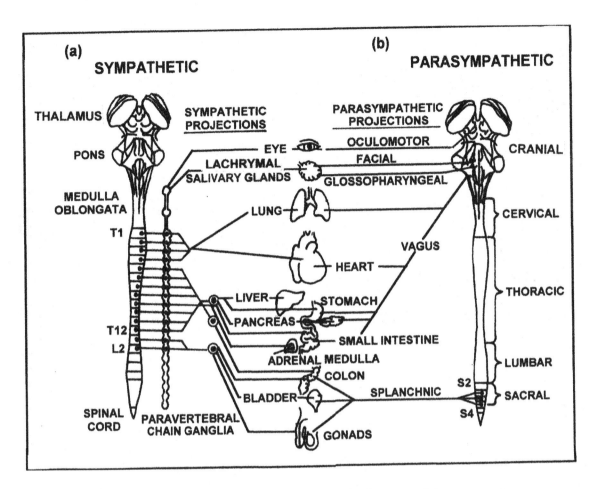

Figure 5.C-1. The sympathetic (a) and parasympathetic (b) divisions of the autonomic nervous system. Note that several organs are innervated by both systems and that the two subsystems use very different points of entry and exit on the spinal cord. Only a small number of the organs and muscles innervated by the autonomic nervous system are shown.

Note that the efferent sympathetic fibers that exit the spinal cord at a specific vertebra do not necessarily follow the same track as the α-motor neurons of the central nervous system exiting at that vertebra. Thus, the sympathetic fibers exiting at T1 go to the head, those from T2 go to the neck, T3–T6 go into the thorax, T7–T11 go to the abdomen, and T12–L2 go to the legs. Compare these with the α-motor neuron destinations shown in table 13.D-1.

Afferents

The various effector organs and sites also send afferent nerves to the spinal cord and thence to the hypothalamus, as input to hypothalamic nuclei in the decision-making process that leads eventually to the excitation or inhibition of the organ's function. There are few ganglia that are not bundled with the other spinal nerves; namely, the afferent nerves from the pupil of the eye, the salivary glands, and the blood vessels of the head, heart, and bronchi (figure 5.C-1).

Modulation

The nerves of the sympathetic nervous system are disynaptic; they synapse once at the paravertebral chain ganglia and a second time at ganglia close to the effector organs (figures 5.C-1 and 5.C-2). By contrast, nerves in the α-motor system are monosynaptic, with axons that travel long distances from the spinal cord to finally synapse at the relevant muscles. In the autonomic system, the intermediate synapse allows for a modulating influence, due to the dendrites from

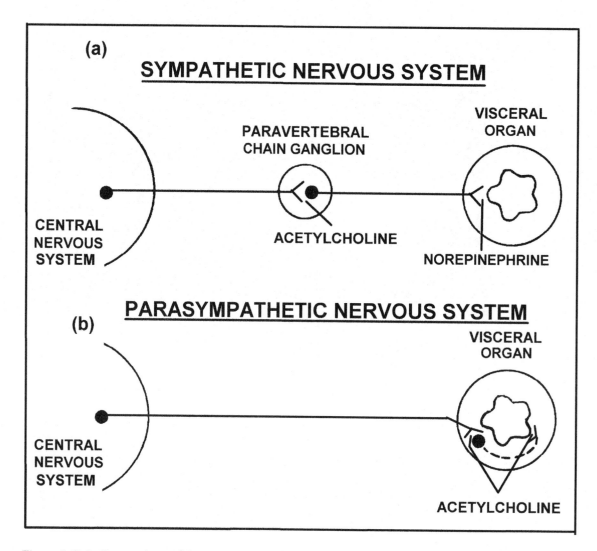

Figure 5.C-2. Comparison of the innervation existing between the central nervous system and the visceral organs in the sympathetic and parasympathetic branches of the autonomic nervous system. Note the different neurotransmitters used in the two branches and the relative positions of the synapses.

other neurons in the ganglia, which contribute to the eventual neural signal. Thus, the additional synapse allows for subtle fine-tuning of the transmitted signal strength [268]. It follows that the control of the body attained through the autonomic system may be of a finer sort than that possible through direct somatic control from the cortex. If so, then one possibly has an explanation for the quality of the performance when an athlete is in "the zone," an unusual mental state in which the consciousness has shifted from the norm and is working in a rather independent way, as appropriate for the autonomic nervous system [601].

The release of norepinephrine in the course of sympathetic excitation leads to a short-term mental jumpiness that works against sustained attention to a task and to details that may be involved in the task. On the other hand, a sharply focused attention is the base of the mental pyramid, so that if this can be achieved, then all of the higher mental functions above the level of attention are boosted. This brings us back to the goal of *yogasana* practice as expounded by Patanjali (Subsection 4.B, page 76); i.e., to work so as to quiet the fluctuations of the mind and achieve a state of sharply focused attention.

On the other hand, there is divergent branching of the axonal terminals of the efferents in the sympathetic and parasympathetic systems, which results in a rather indiscriminate spraying of the neurotransmitters over a broad area of the innervated organ. Thus, autonomic innervation of an organ can result in a global muscular excitation; for example, in the urinary bladder, on command from the autonomic nervous system, all of the muscle fibers encircling the bladder are energized simultaneously, and the bladder empties.

Neurotransmitters

All synapses in the sympathetic paravertebral chain ganglion use acetylcholine as the neurotransmitter. A second set of synapses is found in the sympathetic system, close to the target organs, but the neurotransmitters used here are the catecholamines, except for the sweat glands and in the vascular systems of the muscles, where acetylcholine again is the neurotransmitter (figure 5.C-2).

Alpha and Beta Receptors

The effector organs activated by the autonomic nervous system have two types of receptors, termed alpha and beta. In general, the activation of an alpha receptor involves an increased permeability of the postsynaptic membrane to Na^+ ions and is therefore excitatory. In contrast, activation of a beta receptor involves an increased permeability of the same membrane to the outward flow of K^+ ions and the inward flow of Cl^- ions and is generally inhibitory. Alpha receptors are activated by the neurotransmitters norepinephrine and epinephrine (Subsection 3.D, page 55), whereas beta receptors are activated by epinephrine; though epinephrine activates both alpha and beta receptors, the beta receptors are more strongly activated by epinephrine than are the alpha receptors. The types of receptors involved in various activities of the autonomic nervous system are presented in table 5.A-2.

Excitation of the beta receptors by epinephrine leads to relaxation of the bronchial airways, increased muscle strength, a dry mouth, and increased heart rate and blood pressure. Excitation of the alpha receptors by norepinephrine leads to vasoconstriction, pupillary dilation, and contrac-

tion of the vascular systems within the skin and muscles.

The Effects of Sympathetic Excitation

Immediate Effects

A creature drops out of the trees just in front of you and snarls. The fight or flight sympathetic response is activated, but you must make a decision: will you fight or will you take flight? In order to make a rational decision, you must weigh the options: relative speeds, relative sizes, relative number of threats, relative lethality, etc. In the time that it takes to evaluate the options and make a decision, you will have been attacked and eaten! The fight or flight response is of no protective value unless you can make a life-saving decision in less than a second; i.e., unless you can act subconsciously, intuitively, and reflexively rather than consciously and deliberately.

Just as with the muscles (Chapter 11, page 446), vision (Chapter 17, page 669), and hearing (Chapter 18, page 691), we have both a slow, rational, conscious neural mode and a second neural mode that is fast, reflexive, and subconscious [277]. Making decisions with the subconscious mode lies beyond chance, for it can be influenced by the intelligence of the deliberate mode by conscious/subconscious mixing (Subsection 1.B, page 12), yet remain very fast.

If the sympathetic nervous system is to be of some use in a fight or flight situation, it must be able to respond very quickly to a threat. Indeed, the heart rate can be doubled by the sympathetic system in just three to five seconds and the arterial pressure can be doubled in ten to fifteen seconds. On the other hand, the arterial pressure can be lowered so rapidly by vasodilation that a faint is induced in four to five seconds. Sweating is induced in a matter of seconds, as is bladder voiding. Such rapid changes of physiological variables when driven by emotional shifts (as when one tells a lie) form the basis for the operation of most lie detectors (Box 5.E-1, page 192) [308].

One can abstract table 5.A-2 to list nine principal and immediate effects on the body and mind once the fight or flight response has been triggered [626]. Others, no less important, work on a longer time scale:

1. Sugar and fat enter the blood stream, as fuel for the muscles and brain

2. Respiration rate increases, to raise the level of oxygen in the blood

3. Heart rate and blood pressure increase, to speed the delivery of oxygen and fuel to the cells

4. Blood-clotting mechanisms are activated, in anticipation of injury

5. Muscle tone increases, in anticipation of muscular effort; sweating increases

6. The pituitary increases hormonal output; epinephrine and glucagon production also increase

7. Digestive processes (peristalsis, etc.) are put on hold as blood is diverted from the gastrointestinal tract to the muscles and brain

8. The pupils of the eyes dilate

9. Attention and alertness on a short time scale increase, as beta waves become prominent in the EEG of the left cerebral hemisphere.

Blood Flow

The sympathetic nervous system readily initiates the flow of epinephrine and norepinephrine from the adrenal medulla into the bloodstream, and these hormones can strongly affect blood flow. Once the hypothalamus is signaled by the cortex to do so, its release of the hormones into the bloodstream is rapid (on the scale of seconds) and affects target organs throughout the entire body. As can be seen from table 5.A-2, excitations in the sympathetic nervous system favor blood flow to skeletal muscles, to the heart, and to the brain, all in expectation of an attack of some sort. At the same time, the epinephrine released from the adrenal glands by the sympathetic excitation directs blood out of the digestive system and into muscles by inhibiting peristalsis in the gut (Subsection 19.A-1, page 711). Rossi [721] states that the practice of focused attention, imagery,

biofeedback, and therapeutic hypnosis (and presumably *yogasana* practice) all involve redirection of blood flow. Arguing that this type of practice is a common factor in the resolution of most, if not all, body/mind problems, he lists sixteen healing processes that are dramatically aided by redirection of the blood flow, all via the effects of the mind on the autonomic nervous system. (See Subsection 5.F, page 193 for a complete list of these healing processes.)[2]

The autonomic nervous system affects blood flow by dilating some vascular components and constricting others, using neurotransmitters in the sympathetic nervous branch. The most significant parasympathetic input to this is via the vagus nerve (cranial nerve X) to the heart, which works to decrease the heart rate and contractility (table 5.A-2). Because the postganglionic synapses of the sympathetic nervous system respond strongly to nicotine, cigarette smoke is very effective in activating the sympathetic nervous system.

Emotions

Emotions can work to excite one or the other branch of the autonomic nervous system, and these emotions can be brought to the surface by imitating their attributes using the facial muscles, even though the true emotion is not there [221]. It is interesting that when in different emotional states, the response of the autonomic nervous system is not necessarily consistent. Thus, when either angry or fearful, the heart and perspiration rates increase as appropriate for sympathetic excitation; however, when angry, the blood flow to the hands increases (as if preparing to fight), whereas when fearful, the blood flow increases to the legs instead (as if preparing for flight) [221].

Sudomotor Effects

The expectation that all of the symptoms of sympathetic excitation given above will appear in

---

2   It is left as an exercise for the student to review the *yogasana* therapy postures in any of the many texts available [388, 398, 404] in order to determine which shifts of blood flow might be involved in particular therapies.

concert when any one of them is present is not necessarily realized. Thus, as Telles et al. [856] have shown, meditation on the meaningful word "Om" results in decreases in the heart and respiration rates, as expected for a parasympathetic response; whereas the palmar skin resistance also decreases significantly, as expected for an increase in sympathetic tone. Because meditation on a meaningless word such as "one" decreases the heart and respiration rates but not the skin resistance, it was felt that "Om" has a special cognitive significance involving higher mental centers, implying that the skin response in the latter case was not totally autonomic. Measurement of the electrical resistance of the skin is strongly dependent upon the sweat on the skin ("sudo" means sweat), and sudomotor responses may not necessarily follow those of other sympathetic responses, as their control may lie with higher cortical centers. Thus, activation of the sweat glands in the palms of the hands and the soles of the feet is based on the sympathetic cholinergic activation, whereas most other sympathetic activations are based on norepinephrine as the neurotransmitter (figure 5.C-2a). Because of this, the sweat glands can be activated independently of other sympathetically driven subsystems, such as the heart rate. In line with this, detailed study shows that the autonomic heart rate is closely tied to somatomotor and respiratory systems, whereas palmar conductance is tied to four different psycho-physiological systems (motor, attentional, motivational, and cognitive) and so may not always follow the same patterns, depending upon circumstances [472].

Because there are no muscles in the fingertips, blood circulation ceases in the fingertips when the sympathetic system is activated, just as happens in the gastrointestinal system under the same conditions. This is why the fingers turn cold when under sympathetic control.

There is a wide spectrum of sympathetic intensity possible, with the full-fledged fight or flight reaction being at the very strong end, whereas sunlight entering the eyes at sunrise will induce a weak but noticeable sympathetic response at the opposite pole. A similarly broad

spectrum exists for the parasympathetic system. In the case of the sunlight entering the eyes, one has a weak sympathetic response; which is to say, a weak activation of a weak fight or flight response, even though there is no obvious emergency situation that must be attended to [275]. Its origin must lie very far in our past, when the rising sun might have revealed our hiding place while we rested, or signaled us as to the earliest time to begin the hunt for food.

Note, however, that because the limbs show only sympathetic innervation, only the sympathetic autonomic system will be active in controlling functions such as the diameters of smooth-muscle blood vessels, sweating on the hands and feet, and piloerection (Subsections 20.D, page 725, and 20.E, page 727) [275].

Release of the Catecholamines

The hypothalamus-mediated release of the important hormones epinephrine and norepinephrine upon stimulation of the sympathetic nervous system warrants a more detailed discussion. Once the hypothalamus is aroused by the appropriate signal coming either from below (via the reticular formation) or above (via the limbic and cortical systems), among other things, there is a direct neural signal to the adrenal medullas, glands that sit on top of each of the kidneys (figure 5.E-1). Actually, within each adrenal cap, there are two glands, the adrenal medulla and the adrenal cortex, having different structures, embryonic origins, and hormonal secretions. On command from the hypothalamus, the adrenal medulla releases a mixture of epinephrine (80 percent) and norepinephrine (20 percent) into the bloodstream. This mixture of the adrenal hormones is often called the catecholamines. A measurable amount of analgesic endorphin is also released from the adrenal medulla at this time. As epinephrine preferentially binds to the beta receptors in cell walls, and norepinephrine preferentially binds to the alpha receptors in cell walls, and the materials circulate freely throughout the body, several immediate effects are triggered once these materials are released (table 5.C-1).

Table 5.C-1: Effects of Releasing Epinephrine and Norepinephrine into the Bloodstream

Effects of Epinephrine	Effects of Norepinephrine
Vasoconstriction in the skin, kidney, gastrointestinal tract, and spleen	Vasoconstriction in the skin, kidney, gastrointestinal tract, and spleen
Vasodilation in muscles	Decreased digestive action
Bronchiole dilation	Hair erection
Glycogenolysis	Glycogenolysis
Increased heart activity	Increased heart activity
Blood pressure rises	Blood pressure rises
Increased blood clotting	
Dilation of pupils	

As summarized in table 5.C-1, the catecholamines constrict the blood vessels in the skin and the viscera (mostly due to norepinephrine binding to alpha-cell receptors), thus leaving more blood for the muscles, the blood vessels of which are covered with beta receptors and so are dilated by the epinephrine.[3] The epinephrine (common in bronchial inhalers) acts to open the bronchioles, thereby making it easier for oxygen to come into the lungs and carbon dioxide to leave. At the same time, the heart rate and cardiac contractility are increased, the arterioles in the heart expand with more blood, and the systolic blood pressure rises. The blood will now clot more readily (in case there is any spilled), and the pupils of the eyes dilate, so as to offer the widest field of view. Under the influence of the catecholamines, glycogenolysis turns glycogen in the liver into glucose for the brain, while lipolysis turns fatty acids into glucose, again for use by the brain in its time of emergency. At the same time, the brain is aroused

and is unusually alert. Note, however, that these hormonal effects are rather slow to act, as they depend upon the circulation of the blood for their distribution (see Section 5.E, page 183).

Activation of the sympathetic nervous system tends to turn all functions on (or off) in one concerted action, because the circulating catecholamines released into the bloodstream by the adrenals energize the synapses of all components of the sympathetic nervous system (except the sudomotor system). Whereas acetylcholine is cleared in just a few seconds from the synapses, once triggered, it may take twenty minutes or so for the epinephrine and norepinephrine to be cleared from the bloodstream and the synapses. Clearly, in this single process, activation of the sympathetic nervous system prepares the body for a physical and mental challenge of the sort we may face in our daily *yogasana* practice! But there is much more going on (see below).

Cortisol

Even when the body is resting and there is no mental or physical stress on it, the hypothalamus slowly releases a hormone called corticotropin releasing factor (CRF) into a duct leading to the pituitary. The action of CRF in the pituitary is to release a second hormone, ACTH (adrenocortico-

---

3   By having two types of cell-wall receptors (alpha and beta), the body manages to constrict some blood vessels while simultaneously dilating others, using the same epinephrine-norepinephrine mixture. The shift among those vessels that are dilated and those that are constricted acts to shift blood flow throughout the body as well as to change temperatures locally.

tropic hormone) into the bloodstream, and once ACTH reaches the adrenal cortex, three other corticosteroids are released. The most important of these is cortisol (hydrocortisone), which is a potent stress reliever on a short time scale when working along with the catecholamines, as when doing *yogasanas*.

ACTH acting on the adrenal cortex also produces aldosterone, which works within the kidney to maintain the proper concentrations of K^+ and Na^+ in the body fluids and also regulates the sex hormones released by the ovaries, which hormones in women are important sources of estrogen but are much less important in men, for whom the sex hormones come instead from the testes.

In the short term, cortisol in the blood relieves stress, and its level is very sensitive to one's psychological state. In addition to being necessary for repeated muscle contraction, cortisol redirects glucose to the brain, breaks down protein into constituent amino acids for bodily repair, and raises blood pressure if stress happens to lower it (falling blood pressure is the instantaneous response to stress).

Were the hypothalamus to overproduce CRF, then high cortisol levels could result. When at too-high concentrations, cortisol acts to turn off the release of CRF from the hypothalamus and of ACTH from the pituitary, so that the body systems can be brought back into balance through negative feedback.[4] As the unstressed release of CRF from the hypothalamus is regulated by the circadian clock (Chapter 23, page 787), there is a diurnal variation in the body's cortisol level, being maximal in the early morning and minimal twelve hours later [565]. The traditional time for *yogasana* practice (4:00 to 7:00 AM) corresponds with the peak levels of cortisol in the body; i.e., these are times of high energy and alertness.

In times of momentary high stress, the hypothalamus floods the body with CRF, leading to very high cortisol levels. Such high levels of cortisol in the body are appropriate for real health emergencies such as freezing cold, hemorrhage, broken bones, and wounds. If the *yogasana* practice is so intense as to reach this level of cortisol in the body, you have gone from the response-to-challenge mode to the response-to-threat mode (Section 5.F, page 193), and you should moderate your practice.

If the body is subject to chronic stress, then the cortisol levels will tend to remain high in spite of the negative-feedback effect of cortisol on CRF and ACTH production. In this case, the cortisol set-point is reset upward, so that one now has a chronic elevation of the cortisol level; in this case, one can expect ulcers, lymphatic atrophy, protein imbalance, hypertension, and vascular disorders, along with the consequences of a depressed immune system [266].

Yogasana

In an interesting preliminary study [88], a one-hour *yogasana* practice with both experienced and inexperienced students showed significant lowering of plasma cortisol at the end of the hour (11:00 AM to noon) in both groups, suggesting that the practice worked to reduce stress in these students. However, the study seems to have neglected the fact that cortisol is released in spurts and so is subject to rapid fluctuations (figure 6.A-3). A similar study among students suffering depression reports that cortisol in the saliva showed a noticeable rise following Iyengar yoga classes [903].

The hippocampus, an organ responsible for transferring short-term memory to long-term storage, is studded with cortisol receptors, suggesting a role for cortisol in memory [266]. Indeed, it is now known that whenever we experience an especially important event in our life, there is an accompanying brief but intense release of cortisol, which works to implant the event in the memory bank of the hippocampus. On the other hand, when the release of cortisol is chronic, then the memories of special events in our lives become generalized and are not remembered specifically.

---

4   However, the situation is a little more complicated, as leukocytes within the immune system also are now known to release CRF in addition to that coming from the hypothalamus.

Whatever the positive effects of exercise on supporting the powers of the brain, it is largest in the hippocampus, the organ involved in memory and learning. Correspondingly, the chronic elevation of cortisol levels works on the hippocampus to undo the good effects of exercise. Perhaps it is the wonder of *yogasana* done in moderation that it offers the benefits of exercise but at the same time relaxes the body and mind so that excessive levels of cortisol are not generated.

Renin

In addition to the catecholamines, the adrenal glands are able to excrete renin through the stimulation of the adrenal glands by the sympathetic nervous system, as when performing *yogasanas* or otherwise being under stress. Renin is an enzyme that acts on the angiotensins, eventually leading to the production of aldosterone, a hormone having an effect on the water retention abilities of the kidneys and affecting the salt and water balance in the body. This is discussed further in Chapter 6, page 220.

Section 5.D: The Parasympathetic Nervous System

The anatomy of the parasympathetic branch of the autonomic nervous system is shown in figure 5.C-1**b**. If the sympathetic nervous system can be thought of in terms of fight or flight, then the appropriate phrases for the parasympathetic nervous system are "rest and digest" [191] or the "relaxation response." Benson describes the relaxation response in prayer, meditation, and yoga as being due to "an integrated hypothalamic response resulting in generalized **decreased** sympathetic nervous system activity" [54]. Hypothalamic real estate is divided neatly into regions that contain centers critical to sympathetic functions and those critical to parasympathetic functions. Thus, the sympathetic division is found in the posterior and

lateral parts of the hypothalamus, whereas parasympathetic actions are controlled from the anterior and medial portions of the hypothalamus.

The parasympathetic nervous system plays a more passive role in the body than does the sympathetic, for its main job is to moderate sympathetic responses and to bring the body back to homeostasis once the sympathetic stimulation of an emergency has passed. Actually, the two competing nervous systems are always "on" to some extent, with the relative proportions of each ready to change at a moment's notice, to accommodate whatever the situation. One sees in figure 5.C-1 that several organs are innervated by both the sympathetic and parasympathetic autonomic branches. The parasympathetic branch of the autonomic nervous system has efferents issuing from the four cranial nerves III, VII, IX, and X and from vertebrae S2–S4.

Note that with respect to several organ systems under the competitive control of both the sympathetic and parasympathetic nervous systems, the sympathetic is dominant in the sense that it can function without compensation by the parasympathetic, whereas the effect of the parasympathetic can be no stronger than to just cancel the prevailing sympathetic tone. For example, the muscles controlling the pupils of the eye generally have a purely sympathetic muscle tone that enlarges the pupils to about twice the diameter they would have if there were no such tone present. In this case, the effect of parasympathetic excitation then would be to reduce the pupil diameters, but not beyond their untoned values [308]. As table 5.A-2 shows, there are many sympathetic processes for which there are no balancing parasympathetic processes.

Though the actions of the parasympathetic system are strongly localized in the visceral organs, they would appear not to encroach on the functions of the enteric system, which system is independent of the autonomic system. In the parasympathetic arena, the actions are largely subconscious; however, signals regarding hunger, nausea, and the need for elimination can rise to the conscious domain. When the parasympathetic relaxation response is active, then the general physiologic and behavioral short-term changes are as follows [626]:

1. Decreases in heart rate, blood pressure, and sweat production
2. Pupils of the eyes contract; many tears and much saliva
3. Increased peristalsis and digestive enzyme production
4. Body's sphincters open; relative lack of control over defecation, urination, and ejaculation
5. EEG brain waves in the right cerebral hemisphere shift toward the alpha state
6. Skeletal muscle tone decreases
7. Insulin production increases (but exercise is good for diabetics!)
8. Sense of inactivity, relaxation, drowsiness; lowered level of arousal

As there are no visceral organs in the arms or legs, there are no parasympathetic fibers to these limbs, nor is such parasympathetic innervation found for the sweat glands, the piloerector hair muscles, or within the walls of the blood vessels.

It is not unusual to find that as a *yogasana* class draws to an end and the students lie down for *savasana*, a student may break into muffled sobs and copious tears, for when the muscle tension is relaxed through the *yogasanas,* previously buried emotional upheavals that lead to muscle tension can be brought to the surface and released. These tears and saliva are promoted by the parasympathetic response accompanying relaxation (point 2 above); the generally positive effect of parasympathetic relaxation on external secretions (Chapter 20, page 721) is obvious as well in *sarvangasana* and *savasana,* as a tendency to salivate excessively.

In the parasympathetic system, the proportion of afferent nerve fibers is unusually large, being as much as 85 to 90 percent in the vagus nerve, the main nerve of the parasympathetic system stretching from the neck to the genitals. These afferent nerves may be either myelinated or not and can carry information on pain, distress, or discomfort in the visceral organs. As discussed

in Section 13.D, page 532, the visceral pain may be referred to the skin overlying another area of the body; e.g., the pain of a urinary infection may appear on the skin at the backs of the upper thighs (figure 13.D-3). As parasympathetic innervation does not extend to the sweat glands or the muscles that make hairs stand on end (piloerection), there is only more or less sympathetic excitation in these cases (see table 5.A-2).

Innervation

The nerve fibers forming the parasympathetic nervous system originate in the brainstem (figure 4.B-2) and then exit both from the brainstem (bypassing the upper vertebrae), so as to form part or all of four cranial nerves and also exit between S2 and S4 in the lumbar spine (figure 5.C-1**b**). Unlike the case with the ganglia in the sympathetic system, all of the ganglia in the parasympathetic system have synapses based on acetylcholine as neurotransmitter (figure 5.C-2**a**) rather than norepinephrine, and so they are not activated when the blood is rich in this latter hormone. Some neurons of both the sympathetic and parasympathetic nervous systems rely upon nitric oxide as neurotransmitter—the nerves controlling penile erection, peristalsis, and vasodilation, for example [450].

The nerve structure of the parasympathetic system is different too from that of the sympathetic, in that there is only one ganglion between the brainstem and the effector organ, and that single ganglion is quite close to the target organ (figure 5.C-2**b**). Unlike the situation with the sympathetic nervous system, which is distributed globally over the body, the parasympathetic nervous system is distributed primarily in the head and in the viscera of the thorax, abdomen, and pelvis. The various neuronal components of the parasympathetic nervous system and their effector organs and sites are listed in table 5.D-1. In contrast to the all-on/all-off aspect of the sympathetic nervous system, the parasympathetic nervous system is wired so that those parts of the system can be activated that are needed at the moment, while the other parts remain dormant.

Table 5.D-1: Parasympathetic Nerves and their Effector Sites and Organs

Nerve-Fiber Bundle	Organ or Site
Cranial Nerve III	Ciliary muscle of the eye
	Sphincter pupillae of the eye
	Extraocular recti muscles of the eye
Cranial Nerve VII	Lachrymal gland
	Nasal and oral secretions
Cranial Nerve IX	Nasal and oral secretions
Cranial Nerve X (Vagus)	Heart
	Bronchioles of the lungs
	Stomach
	Liver, gallbladder, and pancreas
	Intestine and colon
S2, S3, S4	Descending and sigmoid colon
	Rectum and bladder
	Genitals

The Vagus Nerves

Eighty percent of all of the parasympathetic nerve fibers in the body are found in cranial nerve X, called the vagus nerve. Actually, there are two vagus nerves, the left and the right. Both go to the throat area, the lungs, heart, and upper stomach; however, the left one stops at the upper stomach, whereas the right vagus nerve continues into the abdominal cavity and connects with digestive and reproductive organs all the way down to the perineum [626]. The word "vagus" is related to the word "vagabond," as the nerve seems to wander a great distance in the body [107].

The vagus nerves pass through the chest cavity, and the motions of the chest while breathing seem to stimulate this nerve, with a subsequent effect on the heart rate. Thus, it is known that on inhalation, there is a sympathetic excitation of the heart, and the heart rate increases; whereas on exhalation, the sympathetic excitation wanes as the parasympathetic response via the vagus nerves is activated, and the heart rate decreases [626]. This alternating effect of the two phases of the breathing cycle on the heart rate is known as "respiratory sinus arrhythmia" and is discussed further in Subsections 14.A, page 549, and 15.C, page 619.

Respiratory sinus arrhythmia illustrates the principle of reciprocal innervation of an organ. Both sympathetic and parasympathetic nerves innervate the heart, the first to raise the heart rate and the second to depress it. At rest, both are active, and the resting heart rate is a reflection of this balance. In times of stress, the parasympathetic signal decreases in favor of the sympathetic signal, and the heart rate increases. Once the stress has passed, the parasympathetic system is activated, and the heart rate then descends to normal, but not below it, unless one is meditating or in *savasana*. The relative strengths of these two branches of the autonomic nervous system shift as the need arises, provided one is in good health.

Because the vagus nerve also passes through the center of the neck, it is possible that it is influenced as well by the pressure in the neck in *sarvangasana* [448], especially if the posture is done without blankets under the shoulders. Inasmuch as *sarvangasana* is considered to be a relaxing posture, we may take it to mean that the pressure on the vagus nerve in the region of the neck serves to stimulate a parasympathetic response. However, it is more likely that the vagus nerve plays an indirect role in the changes in respiration and blood circulation that occur whenever one is inverted in any *yogasana*. In brief, when certain pressure receptors in the neck and chest (Subsection 14.E, page 580) sense that the blood pressure is rising, they signal the hypothalamus as to the situation, and the response via the vagus nerve is to slow the heart rate and dilate the blood vessels accordingly. This is explained in more detail in Section 14.F, page 586.

The vagus nerve similarly is prominent in the stimulation of peristalsis and gastric secretion in the gut; however, it should be noted that peristalsis takes place even after the vagus nerve is severed (Subsection 19.A, page 711); in this case, the enteric branch of the autonomic nervous system drives the peristaltic action in the absence of the parasympathetic branch. It is somewhat surprising, but it appears that the vagus nerve is also active in controlling the release of certain cytokines within the immune systems of the abdominal organs.

Syncope

In some situations, the vagal-nerve stimulation may slow the heart rate and dilate the arterioles so that the blood pressure in the vicinity of the brain falls so far that the person faints; this is called "vasovagal syncope." This syncope may also occur when the carotid arteries are compressed, as when in *halasana* or *sarvangasana*; in this case, the effect is called "cardiac sinus syncope." In a similar way, "orthostatic syncope" involves fainting following the drop of blood pressure to the brain on quickly standing up from lying, sitting or positions such as *savasana, dandasana,* or *uttanasana* [330]. The various syncopes would most likely present themselves in *yogasana* students who ordinarily have low blood pressures, especially in students who also tend to close their eyes in the postures.

Ocular-Vagal Reflex

As discussed more fully in Subsection 11.D, page 457, the vagus nerve plays a second but no less important role in regulating heart action in certain *yogasanas*. Thanks to the ocular-vagal heart-slowing reflex, pressure applied to various points around the orbits of the eyes (as when one performs *adho mukha svanasana* with the forehead resting upon a block) leads to a rapid activation of the vagus nerve and slowing of the heart rate. This shift toward cardiac relaxation through parasympathetic excitation is most evident when infants (and adults) rub their eyes with the fists in preparation for sleep. The close association of the rectus muscles that move the eyes and the vagus nerves that lead to a more parasympathetic, passive attitude is used by the police in the control of violent individuals and by martial artists, massage therapists, and hypnotists.

The Effects of Parasympathetic Excitation

Interestingly, all of the sympathetic reactions are bound together, so that if one of them is excited, all of them are excited; whereas the parasympathetic reactions are not necessarily bound to one another in this way. Consequently, if one particular body function can be turned from sympathetic control to parasympathetic balance, it then can have the effect of turning off all or most sympathetic functions! That is to say, if we are sympathetically energized and then consciously work with the breath so that the respiration rate becomes parasympathetically significant, most other sympathetic functions will assume their subservient roles as well, and one has relaxed globally.

An important difference between sympathetic and parasympathetic dominance resides in the idea that anything that promotes parasympathetic dominance will act to steady the cardiac rhythm, whereas sympathetic dominance often leads to cardiac arrhythmia, leading sooner or later to death. This benefit of parasympathetic activity is so noteworthy that in a recent editorial in the English medical journal *The Lancet,* it was suggested that increasing parasympathetic activity should be a therapeutic target when treating cardiovascular disease. This is a clear area in which a *yogasana* practice performed so as to stimulate the parasympathetic response could make an important contribution to cardiac health [837]. Note, however, that though long-term cardiac stability is good, cardiac stability in the very short term (from one breath to the next) indicates a lack of autonomic flexibility and is a signal of impending ill health (Subsection 14.A, page 549).

Emotions

Our emotions are tied strongly to the momentary dominance of one or the other of the two autonomic branches. For example, recent experiments on the sites of specific brain functions [705] show that the right prefrontal cortex is the site for negative, fearful thoughts, whereas the left prefrontal cortex is the site for positive thoughts. In depression, the EEG of the left prefrontal cortex is overly intense in the relaxing alpha-wave rhythm characteristic of parasympathetic dominance, whereas the right prefrontal cortex is deficient in this brainwave. In a sense, in depression, the left prefrontal hemisphere has gone to sleep, and the therapy for depression then is a *yogasana* routine that stimulates the sympathetic nervous system, leading to an alert state of mind (Subsection 22.A, page 761).

Autonomic Inflexibility

It was mentioned in Section 5.B, page 167, that the emotions within the hypothalamus are held in check by the prefrontal cortex. However, in those for whom the prefrontal cortex is underdeveloped, there is a strong parasympathetic dominance across the entire body and mind, and the emotional control takes an odd turn. In such people, sympathetic arousal is difficult, and the people are remorseless and lack any feelings of guilt. Lacking inhibitions, they thrive on violence [592], i.e., they lack stimulation of the sympathetic nervous system and so are unable to show any sympathy for the plight of others. Alternatively, one might describe this condition as an inflexibility of the autonomic system, being frozen in the parasympathetic mode. In this regard, see also Subsection 5.E, page 186.

Laughter

When we laugh, the following physiological changes are found to take place: endorphins are released by the pituitary gland in order to dull

pain, the levels of cortisol and of epinephrine in the body are dramatically reduced, the levels of immune cells in the blood (killer T cells, for example) and of antibodies in the blood and saliva increase, and the need to urinate becomes stronger (Box 14.F-3, page 594). These changes can be safely attributed to parasympathetic excitation as stimulated by laughter.

Section 5.E: Autonomic Balance: Stress and *Yogasana*

Stress

Stress is the reaction to any action or situation (called the stressor) that tends to unbalance a person either physiologically or psychologically, the effect being beneficial or harmful or both in varying amounts. The thought that a particular stressor is either "good" or "bad" is not a useful one, because a stressor may be good for one person and bad for another and in fact may have both good and bad aspects at the same time. In general, we may take a stressor to be equivalent to excitation within the sympathetic nervous system. However, not everyone reacts to stress in the same way. In fact, some respond to stress by withdrawal; i.e., they roll over and play dead rather than fight or flee. When stressed, such people display decreased physiological function, loss of muscle tone, mental lassitude, inactivity, and eventually, depression. The totality of these responses implicates a parasympathetic response (the possum response) to stress rather than a sympathetic one [626].

It must be understood that stress is not necessarily a bad thing, for as Selye has said, "Stress... gives an excellent chance to develop potential talents, no matter where they may be slumbering in the mind or body. In fact, it is only in the heat of stress that individuality can be perfectly molded" [772].

Continuing in this vein, Councilman says, "We are what we are because of the stresses placed upon us and the adaptations we have made to these stresses, both physically and otherwise. The state of our bodies, our minds, and our personalities is the result of this adaptation [169]." All stresses leave us somewhat changed, sometimes for the better and sometimes for the worse.

Neural and Hormonal Paths

When reacting to a stressor, the body follows a hard-wired program, the fight or flight response, which follows two courses simultaneously, one of them hormonal and one of them neural (figure 5.E-1). In either case, the action begins in the hypothalamus [618] (Sections 5.A, page 160, and 5.B, page 165).

One sees from figure 5.E-1**b** that the simulation of both the hormonal and neural paths begins with excitations driven by the solitary tract nucleus within the hypothalamus (table 5.B-1), this nucleus being activated in turn by signals from visceral afferents and from nuclei within the limbic system. In this scheme, neural excitations need go no higher than the limbic system in the subconscious realm.

In the case of the hormonal response to the stressor, the hypothalamus releases the hormone CRF directly into the pituitary gland, which in turn releases the hormone ACTH into the bloodstream. On reaching the adrenal glands, the ACTH promotes the release of epinephrine and norepinephrine from the adrenal medulla into the bloodstream. Once released, these hormones trigger many other physiological effects, all of which (see table 5.A-2 for a complete list) are in aid of protecting the body in the face of an emergency, be it real or imagined.

The second route to sympathetic arousal, the neural route, is energized simultaneously with the hormonal route. Here, the hypothalamus energizes the spinal cord, which leads immediately to the release of cortisol from the adrenal cortex, leading in turn to increased muscle tone, heart and respiration rates, blood pressure, and perspiration; whereas digestive processes and saliva secretion stop. The neural route is activated more quickly than the hormonal route but has a much shorter lifetime. The competing paths of hormonal and neural excitation of the adrenal glands by the hy-

pothalamus is also discussed in Subsection 5.F, page 193.

Physiological Consequences

Once a stressor triggers the release of hormones into the bloodstream from the adrenal medulla, the epinephrine and norepinephrine act on the short term to increase heart rate, blood pressure, muscle tone, core body temperature, and the consumption of oxygen. Additionally, these hormones stimulate the liver to increase glucose and fatty acid levels in the blood, to divert blood from the digestive tract to the muscles, and to increase perspiration.

The long-term physiological effects of stress are manifold and include the following:

- » Some forms of baldness have been related to high levels of stress
- » Mouth ulcers, oral fungus growth, and trench mouth are stress-related
- » Mental or emotional stress can worsen symptoms of asthma
- » Angina and heart arrhythmia can correlate with stress
- » Gastritis, irritable colon, etc., are related to stress
- » Menstrual disorders and impotence are related to stress
- » Irritable bladder
- » Muscle twitches and tics are more noticeable when under stress
- » Outbreaks of many types on the skin are due to excessive stress

Most importantly, activation of the sympathetic nervous system by intense stress can have an adverse effect on the immune system, leading to increased susceptibility to colds and minor infections. Indeed, with moderate exercise, the spleen is activated to release more red blood cells, while blood-clotting ability and white blood-cell production also increase.

Emotional Consequences

We are subconsciously aware at all times of events that may serve as triggers for an emotion-

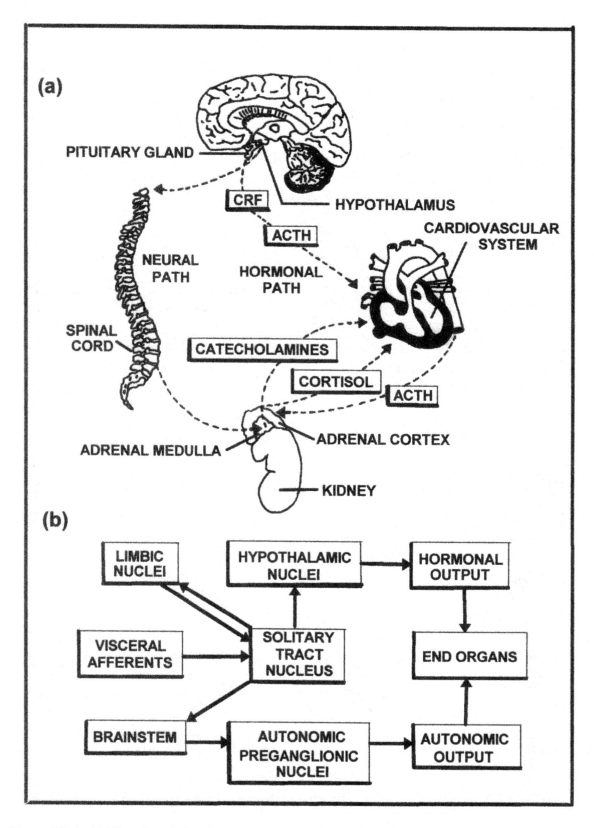

Figure 5.E-1. (a) The adrenal gland's response to a signal originating at the hypothalamus can be both hormonal (using the endocrine pathway) and neural (using the autonomic nervous system). In the former case, the end result is the release of cortisol from the adrenal cortex, and in the latter case, it is the release of the catecholamines from the adrenal medulla. (b) The various nuclei involved in the activation of the adrenal glands by both the hormonal and neural routes.

Table 5.E-1: Comparison of the Effects of Chronic and Acute Stressors [739]

Body System	Chronic Stress	Acute Stress
Brain	Impaired memory, increased risk of depression, lowered level of cognition	Increased alertness and lowered perception of pain
Immune system	Lowered immune response	Arms itself in expectation of injury
Circulatory	Elevated blood pressure and increased risk of cardiovascular disease	Increased heart rate and general vasodilation to bring more oxygen to muscles
Gastrointestinal	GI disorders	Digestion temporarily ceases
Adrenal glands	High hormone levels slow recovery from acute stress	Releases hormones that mobilize energy supplies
Gonads	Increased risk of infertility and miscarriage	Reproduction temporarily suppressed

al response. If such a threatening situation does occur, then the body can react within milliseconds in order to defend itself. In effect, this is a subconscious reflexive response to an external threat. Just as is the case with muscular reflexes (Section 11.D, page 446), it is the case with the emotions that with practice, one can make the emotional response more cerebral, more deliberate, more controlled, and less subconscious; however, this will take more time to activate than does the purely reflexive response. Thus it is an aim of Buddhist practice [221] to avoid the reflexive-autonomic emotional response and lift it into the conscious realm for cool-headed consideration, as in figure 1.B-1.

Psychologically, one has an increased level of anxiety and a sense of foreboding when in the stressed state, and stress may work in the brain to promote depression through the agency of cytokines (see Subsection 16.B, page 644).

Chronic versus Acute Stressors

Schatz [751] has earlier pointed out how the global stress response can develop as a wide variety of body-function changes interact among themselves and with brain functions to place all of the body's systems on attack alert. It is exci-

tation of the sympathetic nervous system due to stress that sets these changes in motion.

When functioning properly, the vital functions within the human body are in homeostatic balance. Within this context, a stressor is anything that threatens to interfere with the homeostatic processes. Moreover, the consequences of stressor interference with homeostasis can be very different depending upon whether they are chronic or acute. These differences are presented in table 5.E-1.

It occasionally happens that there is a perception within a person that particular events of his or her life are so upsetting that the sympathetic nervous system remains activated even though the events are long past and no longer life-threatening. If this stimulation is ongoing and not resolved, then the physiological and psychological (psychosomatic) consequences of such chronic stress may include hypertension, cardiac arrhythmia, indigestion, headache, backache, poor sleep, anxiety, depression, autoimmune disease, low resistance to cancer, and memory and cognitive deficits in old age [139].

Chronic stress leaves tissues damaged; for example, males who subject themselves to ongoing physical strain produce fewer sperm, and their testosterone levels fall; women who chronically stress their bodies produce fewer ova, while their menstrual cycles become more irregular. Constant stress on the energy systems of the body raises the risk for and severity of type 2 diabetes.

Mechanism of Response

Ideally, the release of the glucocorticoids from the adrenals represses the release of CRF and ACTH from the brainstem, but this is not always the case. Thus, the stress response can be unnecessarily intense and long-lasting if the glucocorticoids do not perform their roles. If the hypothalamus is overactive, then the excess CRF decreases the growth-hormone supply, impedes digestion, and promotes problems of depression due to a chronic excess of cortisol [226].

If the source of stress is visual, auditory, or involves certain thoughts, there is a chain reaction that again begins in the hypothalamus and involves the amygdala, the pituitary, and the adrenal glands by both the hormonal and the neural pathways (Subsection 5.E, page 183). The locus ceruleus within the limbic system steers emotional stressors such as fear from the amygdala to the solitary tract nucleus within the hypothalamus, which then stimulates the vagus nerve at the same time that the adrenal hormones are released.

Excess Stress

Though stress can be useful as a tool for learning or performance at a certain level, it can be overdone. When we overwork, the physiological effect is illness, whereas the psychological effects are boredom and a sense of anticlimax. In competitive sports and the performing arts, the boredom of training is relieved by the excitement and release to be found in competition and performance; however, in *yogasana* training we have no such avenues. It is then the responsibility of the teacher to be aware of incipient boredom and to make every effort to keep *yogasana* practice fresh and interesting, both for herself and her students.

Autonomic Plasticity

When the autonomic nervous system is working properly in a healthy body, it has a responsiveness that allows one to move easily between sympathetic dominance and parasympathetic balance in either direction. In contrast, in the unhealthy body, the dominant neural mode is set either too high (sympathetic) or too low (parasympathetic), and the body is unable to easily switch from one dominance to the other. Thus, we see in figure 5.E-2 the healthy responsiveness of a balanced person, as measured by fingertip temperature and muscle tension as he or she goes through cycles of stress and relaxation. As shown there, the flexibility of response is significantly different for the balanced person as compared with responses for subjects who are chronically excited in either the sympathetic or parasympathetic modes, regardless of the stress.

People who are either depressed or have high anxiety are relatively insensitive to external stressors and so remain either strongly parasympathetic or strongly sympathetic, respectively, as seen in figure 5.E-2. In contrast, healthier people are able to cycle easily between the two neural states; i.e., they are balanced, because their neural systems are more flexible. Similarly, when we practice our *yogasanas,* with accompanying sympathetic excitation, and then finish with a deep relaxation such as *savasana* and its accompanying parasympathetic excitation, we are exercising the autonomic neural system in a way that encourages sympathetic/parasympathetic neural flexibility and its accompanying good health.

Other health-related aspects of the responsiveness of the autonomic nervous system to changing dominance involve respiratory sinus arrhythmia (Subsection 14.A, page 549, and Section 15.C, page 619) and the alternation of nasal laterality in breathing (Section 15.E, page 627).

General Adaptation Syndrome

Activation of the fight or flight response is useful in some situations, no doubt. However, Selye [772] has shown that the fight or flight response can be a first step in a four-stage process, the end

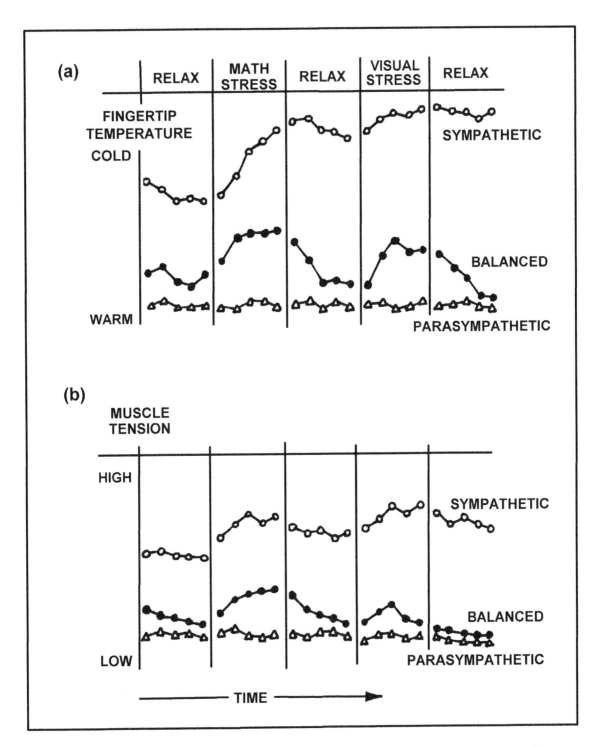

Figure 5.E-2. Responsiveness of three subjects having different autonomic types (sympathetic dominant, parasympathetic dominant, and balanced) to repeated stress and relaxation cycles as measured by (**a**) finger temperature and by (**b**) muscle tension [626].

result of which can be a tragedy. Selye defines the four stages of response to stress in what he calls the general adaptation syndrome (GAS):

Stage 1: The alarm reaction, in which all aspects of sympathetic activation are turned on (table 5.A-2) in response to a stressor. These are the short-term adaptations our bodies make in doing the challenging work of the *yogasanas.*

Stage 2: A resistance stage in which the body appears to resist the changes wrought by stage 1 by attempting to reverse its symptoms and so regain homeostasis. For students of *yogasana,* this takes place during our relaxation (*savasana,* etc.).

Stage 3: If the stress of the stage 1 fight or flight situation is continual and ongoing, then efforts to achieve homeostasis act to deplete the body's reserves and so lead to a state of exhaustion. As one has a depleted ability to adapt to the initial stressor, the body systems begin to break down in the long term. It is the chronic stress reached in stage 3 that can eventually prove to be a serious health threat. Should our levels of stress be sufficiently high and sufficiently long so as to enter Selye's stage 3, there will follow three general, nonspecific physiological long-term responses to the stress: (a) enlargement of the adrenomedullar glands with increased output of cortisol, leading to anxiety and hypertension; (b) shrinking of the lymphatic tissue, with a decrease of lymphocytes in the blood and a consequent decrease in the strength of the immune system; and (c) ulceration of the stomach lining, especially in the upper part of the duodenum, due to minor ruptures of small blood vessels.

Stage 4: If sympathetic arousal continues beyond stage 3, the organism will die from the stressor.

All of the above assumes that there is no conscious control of the stress or of the reaction to the stress. However, as stated above, a person's response to a particular stressor and recovery from that stressor are unique to that person, and so one cannot assign a particular quality to a stressor or a strategy of recovery and expect it to apply to everyone [336]. The response to stress can vary from individual to individual; in some, but not all, the response of the immune system is negative,

reducing the resistance to both viral and bacterial attack. Those who respond to stress with extreme increases in heart rate and blood pressure are significantly more likely to have frequent minor illnesses, as compared with those whose response is more moderate.

The effects of stress are cumulative, and if we spend a certain amount of our adaptability on dealing with external stressors such as those that accompany bad living, anger, or worry, less will be available for handling the demands of *yogasana* practice.

Rephrasing the GAS

The causes and consequences of the general adaptation syndrome can be restated in terms of sympathetic-parasympathetic balance within the autonomic nervous system, as shown in figure 5.E-3. In this scheme, GAS stage 1 is represented by "Alarm Response" and by "Fight or Flight" response, GAS stage 2 by "Adaptation, Activation, and Harmonization," stage 3 by "Fatigue and Atrophication," and stage 4 by "Pathology." Note that in the GAS scheme, there is no room for beneficial responses to minimal stress, as occurs in the phenomena of hormesis or preconditioning (Section 16.F, page 653).

Yogasana

In the 1950s, Wenger and Bagchi traveled to India to study, in a most scientific way, the claims that Indian mystics and yogis were able to voluntarily control aspects of the autonomic nervous system [891]. Their confirmation of these claims has opened somewhat the door of respectability to yoga in the West.

It is at this point—where a discussion of the autonomic system, stress, relaxation, and *yogasana* intersects a discussion of the control of subconscious centers by conscious ones—that the heart of this handbook is revealed. In virtually all of the *yogasana* work that a beginning student may be taught by her teacher, performing the postures has a direct and understandable impact on the autonomic system. If one has an understanding of the physiology of the body at the level of the

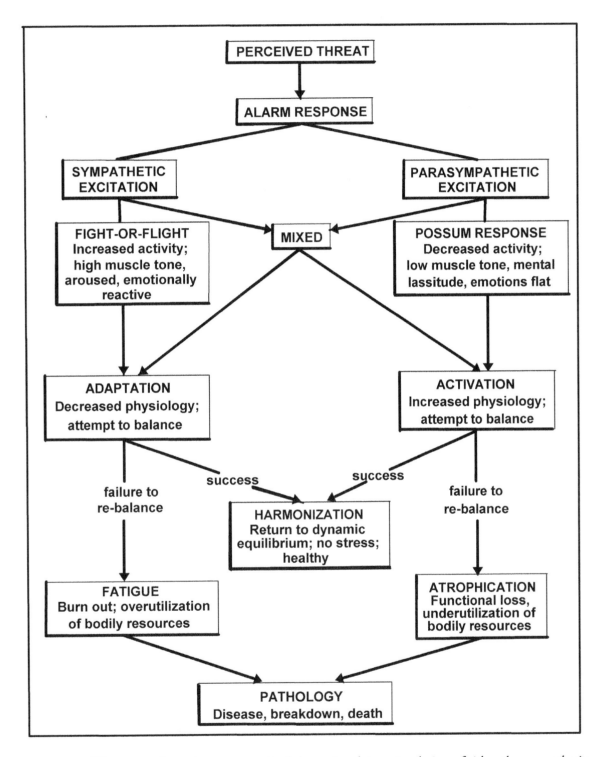

Figure 5.E-3. The stages of reaction to a perceived threat, involving stimulation of either the sympathetic or parasympathetic nervous systems and leading eventually to pathology if balance is not achieved.

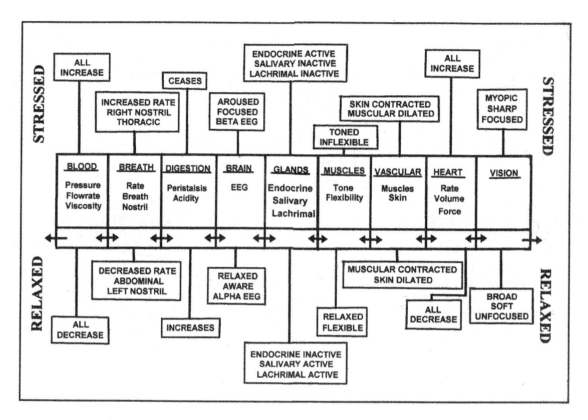

Figure 5.E-4. Because the subsystems of the body/brain are strongly interconnected (center panel), a change in one of them toward either a more stressed state (upper panels) or a more relaxed state (lower panels) will drive the others in the same direction. Thus, through *yogasana* practice, the shift toward the relaxed state (or the stressed state) of one subsystem will pull all of the others more or less in the same direction.

autonomic nervous system and an understanding of the *yogasana* postures in terms of their alignment, their effects on the energy of the body, and their effects on changes in blood flow, then one can work the postures so as to deliberately produce changes in the autonomic balance. For example, because the body is generally cold in the winter and warm in the summer, the *yogasana* program should be arranged to excite the sympathetic nervous system in order to warm the body in the winter months and to excite the parasympathetic nervous system in order to cool the body in the summer months. To these ends, the winter program should focus on the standing postures, backbends, spinal twists, and the more challenging inverted postures; whereas in the summer, it is time for supported postures, forward bends, and cooling inversions, such as *halasana* and *sarvangasana* [851].

Referring to figure 1.B-2, we realize now that the psychological space labeled "unconscious" in the beginning student contains all of the autonomic adjustments of the body and mind, and that through the conscious practice of the *yogasanas,* certain subconscious physical, mental, and emotional factors can be lifted into the conscious sphere. At the same time, certain of the deliberate, conscious actions of the *yogasanas,* after much practice, will become intuitive and automatic.

As can be seen in figure 5.E-4, the concerted actions of many interacting body-mind functions can conspire to make one stressed, or the conspiracy can be reversed, leaving one calm and relaxed. The parasympathetic activation that is necessary for this reversal can be attained through *yogasana* practice, most especially through the control of the breath and the tension in the muscles.

It is interesting to consider what the autonomic balance might be like for a beginning student performing *sarvangasana,* for example. To make the example more concrete, consider the student's blood pressure in *sarvangasana* as representing the level of autonomic balance, with high pressure signaling sympathetic excitation and low pressure signaling a parasympathetic counterbalance. The plot in figure 5.E-5 shows how one might expect the pressure to change year after year, as the student becomes more experienced. At first, the newness of the inverted position adds an element of fear to the posture, and the pressure is higher than when standing (time 0 to time A). However, with several years' practice (time A to time B), the essential relaxing quality of the posture exerts itself and the pressure drops. With more practice following this, one enters a period starting at time B in the figure, in which the conscious control over the autonomic nervous system gradually becomes so complete that as one moves from time B to time C, one can make the pressure either go up or go down depending on one's will to have it rise or fall!

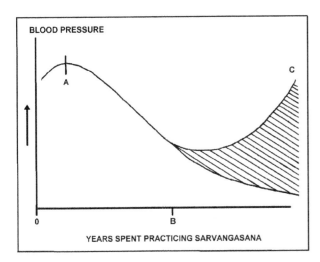

Figure 5.E-5. With only a few years of practice, *sarvangasana* may raise the blood pressure (time 0 to time A), but with further practice (time A to time B), it becomes relaxing, and the blood pressure falls. As one continues to practice and gains control over the autonomic system (point B to point C), one can then consciously control the change of blood pressure in *sarvangasana,* making it either rise or fall (shaded area).

In general, the beginner's practice of the *yogasanas* results in a stimulation of the sympathetic nervous system, with the challenge or threat of the *yogasanas* leading to all of the classic fight or flight responses on a rather short time scale. However, once we deliberately choose to go from the active *yogasanas* to *savasana,* the parasympathetic nervous system then exerts its effect and brings the body back to a balanced physiological and psychological state, though not as rapidly as did the sympathetic system to create that imbalanced state. Obviously, the body's need is for a quick response to danger, but there is no rush to restore calm in the aroused body.

As *yogasana* practice can have a direct effect on the body's balance between sympathetic and parasympathetic dominance, those students who suffer from an autonomic imbalance can profit from a *yogasana* program that stresses whichever branch is deficient. That is to say, a depressed student will profit from a practice that is rich in sympathetic-stimulating backbends (Subsection 22.A, page 761), whereas students who bring anxiety to class will profit from parasympathetic-stimulating supported relaxation (Subsection 22.C, page 766), and students who are autonomically well-balanced profit from a program that is first sympathetically active and then parasympathetically active (Subsection 5.E, page 182).

Often, the body seems constantly stressed, implying rigidity in the autonomic balance in favor of sympathetic excitation. Through practice of *yogasana* with awareness, we can learn to relax through excitation of the parasympathetic system. In this, we develop an autonomic/neural flexibility, in addition to physiological/somatic and psychological/mental flexibilities. As described in Box 5.E-1, page 192, for example, occasions may arise when the well-developed autonomic flexibility can be of great value to the *yogasana* practitioner.

Box 5.E-1: *Yogasana* Practitioners Can Beat the Lie Detector

The lie detector (polygraph) works on the assumption that when one answers a question truthfully, there is little or no change in the level of sympathetic excitation in the body, but that when one knowingly lies in answer to a question, there is an unavoidable rise in the level of anxiety and a corresponding shift toward sympathetic excitation that easily can be measured as changes in palmar conductance, blood pressure, respiration rate, muscle tension, etc. The technique is generally successful in identifying those who lie but who cannot consciously control the balance in their autonomic nervous systems [45].

On the other hand, it seems quite reasonable that a *yogasana* student adept at sympathetic-parasympathetic shifting could easily manipulate his or her nervous system so as to foil the machine; see Section 4.H, page 149. Such a student could raise the baseline readings during innocuous questions by right-nostril breathing, tightening the quadriceps, biting the tongue, making a fist, compressing the chest, crossing the legs and squeezing, contracting the anal sphincter, etc., all of which will lead to intense sympathetic signals. Alternatively, the usual effects of a lie could be hidden and go undetected by the parasympathetic release of autonomic tensions by left-nostril breathing, silently repeating a mantra, etc., all the while telling a huge lie. However, only healthy liars may have the autonomic flexibility and control needed to fool the lie detector!

Read Box 14.A-2, page 546, in regard to Swami Rama and his exquisite control of the autonomic system, and then imagine the futility of giving him a lie-detector test! See also Box 20.A-1, page 722, for information on the use of the autonomic response as a lie detector in ancient times.

Most recently, investigators have found that when there is an excitation in the sympathetic nervous system, as when telling a lie, there is a rush of warm blood to the areas surrounding the eyes, and this readily can be sensed using a thermal-imaging camera. Note, however, that as shown in figure 14.A-5a, swamis have control of differential blood flow and so can move warm blood in and out of specific areas of the body at will.

Conscious Switching of Autonomic States Using the Laterality of Breath, Body, and Mind

Because the autonomic nervous system has its own twenty-four-hour internal clock, it will switch back and forth between sympathetic and parasympathetic dominance every four to six hours without outside prompting (Subsection 15.E, page 630). In addition to this automatic shift, one also can shift the state of autonomic balance at any time, using certain asymmetric aspects of the body and the breath. First, one can shift the balance between sympathetic and parasympathetic states by constricting the flow of blood through one or the other of the armpits (Subsection 15.E, page 634); and second, one can shift by manually constricting the flow of air through one or the other of the nostrils (Subsection 15.E, page 635). This laterality of autonomic excitation is odd, because the outer body appears to be so left-to-right symmetric. However, the inner body is very asymmetric, and so the oddness lies in why the exterior body appears so symmetric. There may be an evolutionary factor at work here, since it is known that in almost all animals that select a mate, the left-right symmetry is a key visual indicator of the mate's good health and strength and so offers the promise of strong, healthy children (Appendix III, page 843).

Section 5.F: The Reciprocal Effects of Emotions, Attitudes, and Stress on One Another

Psychology Influences Physiology

Threat versus Challenge

In regard the question of the impact of one's attitude on stress, experiments show a great biochemical difference in the response when the stressor is seen as a challenge versus the response when the stressor is seen as a threat [721]. When the source of the stress is seen as a threat, both catecholamines and cortisol are released from the adrenal glands, whereas when the stress is viewed as a challenge, catecholamines are released from the adrenal medulla, but there is no increase in cortisol! As one works on *yogasanas,* it is clear that one always wants to regard the work as a challenge and not as a threat as long as one is not depressed; one now sees that the distinction between threat and challenge has a biochemical basis. That is to say, one wants a neural excitation of the sympathetic nervous system from the hypothalamus to the adrenal medulla, in order to release the catecholamines, but one does not want the hypothalamic release of CRF, which leads to ACTH and cortisol via the hormonal route (figure 5.E-1). Note that this is accomplished by a shift in attitude; we must convert the negative stress of threat into the positive coping experience of challenge. This is one of the basic principles of psychobiological therapy: "reframe threat into challenge." Looked at in another way, one wants to avoid the sympathetic autonomic reflex that is the concomitant to dealing with a "threat" and instead use the responses dictated by the higher mental centers that are implicit in considering how to deal in a conscious, rational way with a "challenge." Also see Subsection 5.E, page 183.

Of course, the mind can be engaged in several ways to sway the autonomic balance. Thus, just thinking of a scary event in one's past will initiate a fear response, and fight or flight symptoms will follow from that; whereas thinking of a calm and happy situation will slow the breath and relax the autonomic tension.

Lethal Threats

Though Gazzaniga [266] says that "from a host of other studies we know that it is virtually impossible to teach the autonomic nervous system anything," Rossi points out that in fact the limbic-hypothalamus system is the connection between the mind and the body and so can be a very active teacher in using the mind to modulate the functions of the autonomic nervous system [721]. The strong influence that the psyche can play on the operation and direction of action of the autonomic nervous system is clear in several phenomena. Besides the positive example of Iyengar yoga, two negative examples will suffice to illustrate this point.

In voodoo death, a person of unchallenged authority decrees another person will die at a prescribed time, and the prediction comes true to the minute. The cause of death is psychological stress, in which there are rapid shifts between sympathetic and parasympathetic activities [104, 721]; collapse of the immune and endocrine systems also are involved in this assault. On a longer time scale, there is the related phenomenon of the "defeat reaction" [360]. This is a pathophysiological syndrome brought on by repeated or prolonged psychic stress, which induces a complicated pattern of fluctuating sympathetic and parasympathetic responses which eventually harm the blood vessels and decrease the level of sex hormones; while levels of ACTH and glucocorticoids rise, the immune system is depressed, and infection or tumors follow.

Voodoo death, and possibly the defeat reaction, are examples of the "nocebo effect" (Subsection 5.F, page 201). The opposite effect (the "placebo effect," below, page 196, and Subsection 13.C, page 528) also is well known. Further examples of the effects of mental attitude on the strength of the immune system, the ability to fend off disease, or the ability to recover from an illness are presented in Chapter 16, page 641, and in Subsection 5.F, page 193, while examples of the same approach in regard to hypertension are given in Subsection 14.D, page 575.

Gender Differences

Note that an external stressor does not necessarily create the autonomic response; it is the individual who does that, and so, depending upon the individual's psychological makeup, the response can vary from person to person [618], being autonomic and reflexive in some and involving higher centers only in others. In this regard, it is interesting to note that the catecholamine level in men rises most sharply when triggered by competition and intellectual challenges, whereas for women, the most rapid rise is found during stressful personal situations. Men's catecholamine and blood-pressure levels also fall drastically when they leave the workplace, whereas women's levels for these two markers for stress stay elevated when returning home to face family responsibilities. For men, the rise in blood pressure is most rapid when angry, whereas it is most rapid for women when anxious. Still, women appear to be less vulnerable to stress, because they are more likely to contemplate, discuss, and then act on stressful problems using higher mental and emotional centers than are men.

The Breath

One way to control the autonomic nervous system is through willpower [687]. By being single-minded and focused, one can direct the autonomic nervous system; however, the lungs and diaphragm are easier to control for most of us than is the will. Considering the ease with which the breathing pattern can be changed by a simple emotional event, it is obvious that the autonomic nervous system controls the respiration process, influencing the respiration rate and the opening and closing of the airways. However, through *pranayama*, one can consciously control the breath, and in so doing, one gains conscious access to the functions of the autonomic nervous system. Control of the breath through *pranayama* becomes the doorway to conscious control over

many, if not all, of the processes of the autonomic nervous system [692].

Of course, consciously choosing to perform the proper *yogasana* will lead to predictable excitation of one or the other of the two autonomic branches. If one chooses, for example, to perform *yoganidra*, one can expect a general parasympathetic response from the body, for this process takes one from wakefulness toward a state of sleep (table 5.A-2) [388]. On going from a normal resting state to *yoganidra*, the blood flow in the brain shifts from the frontal lobes and the brainstem to cortical areas in the posterior brain [585]. If, on the other hand, one chooses to do *urdhva dhanurasana*, the body will shift toward sympathetic excitation, with all of its attendant characteristics (Box 11.D-1, page 453).

Psychologists have shown that there is a connection between personality type and breathing type. But according to yoga experience, the interaction between breath and the mind is mutual, so that each can be influenced by the other. Thus, one concludes that by changing the breathing pattern, one can change not only the mind, but the personality [687].

Blood Flow

Rossi [721] lists the well-documented healing effects of increased blood circulation that are facilitated by modulation of the physiology by one's psychology:

» Warming and cooling of different body parts to lessen the pain of headache
» Controlling blushing and blanching of the skin
» Stimulating the enlargement and apparent growth of women's breasts
» Stimulation of sexual excitation and penile erection
» The amelioration of bruises
» Controlling the loss of blood during surgery
» Minimizing and healing burns
» Producing localized skin inflammations
» Curing warts
» Producing and curing forms of dermatitis

» Ameliorating congenital ichthyosis (dry, scaly skin)

» Aiding blood coagulation in hemophiliacs

» Ameliorating the fight or flight alarm response

» Ameliorating hypertension and cardiac problems

» Ameliorating Raynaud's disease (a vascular spasm of the superficial vessels)

» Enhancing the immune response

References to the original literature are given in Rossi's work [721].

Inasmuch as the blood's circulation can be stimulated and directed through the proper use of *yogasana* and the mind, one presumably can influence some or possibly all of the items in Rossi's list above through such practice.

As pointed out by Telles and Desiraju [851a], meditation can have strong effects on one's physiology (blood pressure, heart rate, respiration rate, etc.), but the specific effects will depend strongly on what form of meditation one practices. The same can be said in regard to the physiological and psychological effects of different forms of *yogasana* practice.

Physiology Influences Psychology

There is abundant evidence (as stated above) that our psychology or frame of mind can have a direct and immediate effect on our state of the body or physiology. Similarly, one can influence the state of the mind by changing the state of the body in some way. The truth of this is clear to anyone who has practiced *yogasana* while alert to the psychological changes that attend such practice. Thus, within the *yogasana* practice, one has both energizing, arousing postures and those that are sedating and relaxing. With a proper choice and sequence of *yogasana*, one can play the body like a violin, exploring all of the notes possible in the course of several hours. As therapy for mental conditions, *yogasana* routines have been put forth for the treatment of depression and anxiety (Chapter 22, page 753).

Yogasana practice rivets our attention on the present moment, as it energizes the body and then leads to overall body relaxation; it is preferable to working out on a stationary exercise machine, for example, which is mentally defocusing and so allows one to become tense as one thinks obsessively about one's problems.

Facial Expression Influences Mood

Ekman [221] describes the strong influence on physiology that is exerted by one's facial expression. If one artificially forms a face appropriate to moods such as fear, anger, or sadness, the body responds to these shows of mood with physiological changes that characterize the body and mind when in the throes of the truly felt moods. By mimicking the emotions with the features of the face, one activates the various autonomic responses, such as increased heart rate, change of skin temperature, and sudomotor changes, that otherwise would accompany the true mood or emotion. Viewers of artificial facial expressions also undergo parallel changes in their physiological states, through the activation of their mirror neurons (Subsection 4.G, page 142); however, autistic children are largely lacking in this activation of the mirror neurons and so do not respond to such changes of facial expressions [82a]. It is theorized that the tensing of the facial muscles affects blood flow to the brain and so changes the states of mental activation affecting mood.

Psychoanatomy

Given the close connections between the body and the mind, it is no surprise that close connections exist between specific body areas and specific emotions, attitudes, and psychology. This is the field of psychoanatomy, with close relations to the ancient study of the *chakras* and their attributes (Section 5.G, page 201). A brief listing of these psychoanatomical body/mind connections is given below [265, 764].

» **Feet:** connect us to the ground and give us a sense of security.

» **Legs:** mobilizers that stabilize us and keep us in touch with reality. The thighs are synonymous with independence, and strong legs imply that one has strong determination and may be excessively controlling.

» **Pelvis:** the center of power, energy, and sexuality. Relates to our sexual image and our relations to others.

» **Abdomen:** the emotional center, expressing vulnerability and helplessness. The emotional responses are blunted by the overdevelopment of the abdomen.

» **Lower Back:** the control center. When tight, behavior is compulsive, and when loose, behavior is impulsive.

» **Chest:** an amplifier and a form of muscular armoring, shielding one from emotional experiences of Self, such as a sense of inferiority or behavior that is assertive or aggressive.

» **Shoulders:** are protective, with rounding indicating fear.

» **Arms and Hands:** are clutching, reflecting our inability to hold on or to control.

» **Upper Back and Armpits:** an area of conflicted emotions (anger, rage, hatred, resentment, etc.) being held in check.

» **Neck:** the mediator between the thought center and the feeling center. When the neck is very strong, there is a repression of the emotions.

» **Head:** the locale for obsessive worry and Self analysis, leading to bodily tension.

Given the above connections between body and mind, it is easy to see how the practice of the *yogasanas,* through stretching and releasing and through strengthening of specific areas of the body, can influence the emotions and attitudes. For psychoanatomical reasons, we are often reluctant to occupy the full space open to us; i.e., we often have less than the full potential of open chest, full height, etc.

The Placebo Effect

Efficacy

Because positive attitudes are known to effect cures in very ill patients, the "placebo effect," in which medically inert pills cure real illnesses, is not unexpected. The U.S. Food and Drug Administration (FDA) reports, "People are often helped, not by the food or drug being tested but by a profound belief it will help" [618]. In essence, this is the placebo effect. In fact, many in the medical field hold that our belief in our own health is the most important predictor of health outcomes [525], though strong religious beliefs also can be a factor. As Murphy states, the psychological and somatic changes that can be induced by placebos attest to our capacity for self-transformation [602].

Statistics

It is most noteworthy that in a huge number of totally unrelated placebo studies, the success rate using nonspecific placebos is very often found to be approximately 35 percent, indicating a common remedial factor in the use of placebos, regardless of the affliction. The reliance of the Western medical community on ascribing significant medical results as "due only to the placebo effect" in fact attests to the undeniable connection between mind and body, an idea quite prominent in Eastern thinking.

An average of 35 percent of the members of any large group will respond favorably to the administration of a "drug" when the drug in fact is nothing but water or sugar [266, 618]. Though the percentage of placebo effectiveness rises to 50 percent when the problem being treated is headache, it is seen to be exceptional even at 35 percent, considering that strong morphine is successful in only 75 percent of the cases for which it is prescribed [562]. As applied to somatic (muscle) pain, the taking of a placebo does reduce muscle pain to an extent beyond the 35-percent statistical expectation [266]. The greater the implicit or explicit suggestion that pain will be relieved, the more effective is the placebo;

Box 5.F-1: Examples of Material and Psychological Placebo Effects

Material

» Patients who were on blood-pressure medication were not told for three weeks that they would be given a placebo instead. In spite of this, their blood pressure returned to normal.

» Patients who received pretend knee surgery, but were not actually operated on, uniformly reported pain relief and said they would recommend the operation to their friends.

» Patients in pain are relieved by the injection of morphine; however, when further injections are given with saline solution instead, pain relief is still experienced. Placebo saline solutions are also effective in reducing the tremors and stiffness of Parkinson's disease. If naloxone, known to cancel the effects of morphine, is added to the saline solution, the analgesic effects of the saline are cancelled [93]!

» Placebos do 75–100 percent as well as SSRIs such as Prozac in relieving symptoms of depression.

» Saline injection was an effective anesthetic for 30–40 percent of the people it was given to who were undergoing wisdom-tooth extraction.

» Doctors today are relying on the placebo effect when they prescribe antibiotics for viral infections and recommend drinking milk for gastric ulcers.

Psychological

» Thousands of elderly Chinese Americans in California who were born in years with poor astrological qualities died sooner from cancer than did a similar group born under "good" astrological signs. Caucasians born in the same years showed no such tendency to die sooner when born in "poor" years as compared with "good" years.

» Chinese and Japanese Americans have a rate of dying on the fourth day of any month of a heart attack or heart disease that is 7 percent higher than the rates on other days of that month [919]. In the Chinese and Japanese languages, the sound of the number "four" is close to that of the sound of the word for "death" and is not spoken in polite company. In Japanese, the number four is pronounced as "yon" rather than as "shi," the latter being the root of the verb "to die." On the other hand, Chinese Americans and Japanese Americans die with lower frequencies on the days just preceding important symbolic events such as holidays.

» Acupuncture seems effective in relieving headache, no matter where or how the needles are manipulated; most surprisingly, placebo treatment is also effective in replacing the missing dopamine in the basal ganglia of Parkinson's patients [598].

» Exercise is good for the body if and when one is motivated to work so as to achieve its benefits, but what if one does the work but has only an incidental interest or knowledge about its physical benefits? To explore this, eighty-four female hotel workers were divided into two groups and each was told about how to do their cleaning. However, only one of the groups was told incidentally that the work, which was physically taxing, would be good exercise for them. Given this brief explanation of their work, and the exercise involved in doing it, after one month, the exercise-informed group of women experienced greater degrees of weight loss, drops in blood pressure and body-fat percentage, and several other health improvements than did the group that was not informed in regard to the benefits of the exercise component of their work. The observed difference in increased health between the two groups demonstrates the psychological placebo effect that benign verbal instruction can exert through physical work.

These examples show that people's expectation that they will get well, that cultural beliefs, and that the doctor's enthusiasm for the treatment are all contributing factors to the placebo effect.

however, it is less effective each time it is used thereafter [562].

Pain

When we experience a "real" pain, there is an increased blood flow through an area within the frontal lobe of the brain known as the anterior cingulate, and when treated with a pain analgesic, the blood flow and the pain are correspondingly reduced. If, instead, one is given an inert placebo that is presented as an analgesic, the pain is relieved, and the blood flow through the anterior cingulate falls. Thus, through a purely mental action (the suggestion that "this will help you"), both the sensation of pain and the cortical evidence of pain signals, as shown by cingulate blood flow, are reduced.

It is thought that a specific mental state is promoted by being sold on a placebo pain-killer, and that this state releases endorphins, the body's own opioids. The endorphins in turn activate cells in the midbrain to block pain sensations, while suppressing the immune system [266] (Subsection 13.C, page 515). The strength of binding of opioids that have been released through the action of a placebo and bind to pain receptors varies linearly with the sense of pain relief.

Placebo effectiveness also has been related to the stress that many patients feel is released once they are in the hands of a warm, caring, and authoritative figure [847]; this is most true for patients suffering from asthma, hypertension, depression, and anxiety. Placebos are highly effective not only in the treatment of pain and depression, but also for some heart ailments and gastric ulcers and other stomach complaints, achieving success rates of more than 60 percent. In some cases, the placebo success rate is even higher than that of the best drugs for the condition!

The phenomena of placebo action can be divided into those that encompass the use of a material substance and those that bypass the material and work directly on the psyche of the patient. These are listed as "material" and "psychological" in the examples given in Box 5.F-1, above. Other examples related more or less to the placebo effect appear in Box 13.C-1, page 529.

It has been shown that the placebo effect can be effective in combating hypertension, stress, cardiac pain, low blood-cell counts, headaches, and pupillary dilation, all with the help of the placebo-induced activation of the autonomic nervous system. The placebo effect has been especially successful in treating depression and anxiety [562], with success rates that rival those of the best and most modern drug therapies [847] (Chapter 22, page 753). As is the case with genuine drug treatment, the use of placebos can have toxic side effects (see subtopic "Nocebos" below) and can have totally negative effects if that is the goal of the medical officers in charge [602]. It also appears that each time a placebo cure is disparaged by the medical community as just a "frivolous psychosomatic effect," the measurable effectiveness of the cure decreases. On the other hand, the placebo effect is still strong and active in subjects who have been told beforehand that they are just being treated with placebos! This latter effect is reminiscent of the Tomato Effect, in which one holds strongly to an idea that is demonstrably in conflict with reality (Box 1.A-1, page 5, and Subsection 4.D, page 103).

The efficacy of the placebo effect on the physical plane is shown by a study in which warts were eliminated by painting them with an innocuous but brightly colored dye and telling the patients that the warts would disappear when the color of the dye wore off. Similarly, dilation of the bronchial airways results in many people when they are told that the inhaled substance is a powerful bronchodilator, though in fact it is a placebo [847].

The role of placebos in medicine revolves about the distinction between illness and disease: illness is what the patient feels, whereas disease is what the doctor finds. Placebos are effective in first softening the effects of illness by reducing the patient's distress; with this reduced level of distress, the body then has a better chance to heal itself of the disease [557a] (Chapter 13, page 528).

It has been determined that, with regard to the placebo effect, injections are more effective than pills, with capsules in between; among pills, small, yellow ones are best for depression, whereas large, blue ones work best for sedation (see Subsection 13.C, page 528). As might be expected, the more bitter is the pill being swallowed, the stronger the placebo effect [635]. In the same vein, though large placebo pills usually are more effective than small pills, placebo injections are yet more effective, and placebo surgery is the most effective course of treatment [847].

Rossi [721] proposes that about half of all the cures effected by Western medicine are due to the placebo effect and involve the limbic-hypothalamic bridge between mind and body. Indeed,

Western medicine, in its earlier days, operated totally on the placebo effect, and with strongly positive results, as both the physician and the patient were convinced of the efficacy of the treatments! Though a certain amount of credit must also be given to the natural course of illness, which causes it to wax and then wane, the placebo effect nonetheless is a real and useful tool, with results that often go well beyond the natural cure rates.

Mechanisms

The magic of modern imaging techniques recently has been applied to the mechanism of pain reduction when using placebos, and it is now clear that the placebo-induced release of endorphins is a key factor, with the release being both larger and wider-ranging than is the case for untreated pain. When the placebo effect is set in motion by suggesting that the subject can expect pain relief, the anterior cingulate (sensitive to intensity of the pain), the prefrontal cortex (site of decision making and interpretation), the insular cortex, and the nucleus accumbens (sensitive to the importance of the pain) all become bathed in endorphins [930]. Moreover, the pain relief was largest in those who expected to receive the largest benefit from the "treatment" and was lowest in the skeptical. Placebo treatments of those who do not know that they are being treated are completely ineffective, but they are maximally effective in those who have had previous successful outcomes when taking medicines [598].

The placebo effect is more effective with those who have right-cerebral hemisphere dominance, as is hypnotizability.[5] To the extent that

---

5   In fact, the autonomic nervous system is regarded as a major factor in the physiological effects of hypnosis [721]. This must have some meaning for *yogasana* practice. Notice that a therapeutic hypnotist uses phrases such as "getting more and more comfortable and your eyes close," which would be perfectly appropriate for a *yogasana* teacher to tell the class when entering *savasana*. This suggestion initiates a shift from sympathetic to parasympathetic dominance, because the arousal of the reticular formation is lower and proprioceptive and kinesthetic signals are sparse, while closing the eyes stimulates alpha and finally theta

our *yogasana* student-teacher relationship also involves a strong element of suggestibility, this will probably be true for yoga students as well. In this regard, it is known medically that a treatment can have an active healing effect just by the nature of the personal interaction between the doctor and the patient. It appears that the doctor-patient relationship may stimulate the innate self-healing powers within all of us [64], independent of the efficacy of the technological treatment. Inasmuch as the laying on of hands is one of the most basic actions offering human comfort and the annual physical checkup is one of the tried-and-true bonding rituals between doctor and patient, it is no surprise that the bond between *yogasana* teacher and student also can be a curative one. As *yogasana* teachers, we in the United States are not allowed to function as doctors; however, it is within the law to state that certain postures are known to stimulate certain organs, for example, and to expect that though we do not prescribe them for our students, they nonetheless will take

---

brain waves (Section 4.H, page 149). The signals from awareness of feeling and imagistic experience shift one from external (proprioceptive) to internal (interoceptive) awareness, and the activity of the cerebral hemispheres (Section 4.D, page 105) shifts from the left to the right, all of this through the agency of the vascular system. Presumably, the hemispheric shift is accompanied by a corresponding shift in nasal dominance (Section 15.E, page 629).

In hypnosis, as in *savasana,* once the eyes are closed, there is generally considerable motion of the eyeballs and eyelids, suggesting a search of the inner landscape. Rossi [721] lists many such signs of "inner work" as they appear in a hypnotized subject; the list is not too different from what is observed in *yogasana* students when in *savasana.* Slede and Pomerantz [799] and Galle [260a] speak in detail of the similarities of yoga and hypnosis, especially in the arena of pain management. Deeply hypnotized subjects are known to have a very high tolerance for pain if this is suggested to them by others [562].

To the extent that there is a placebo component to *yogasana* teaching, note that the effect is directly psychological rather than material: there is no pill involved, just the direct engagement of the student's psyche by the teacher.

to heart what we say and possibly heal themselves on the basis of the teacher-student (authority-patient) relationship.

The social conditions under which the placebo effect is most efficacious have been listed by Murphy [602], and very little effort was required on my part to rephrase them for application by the teacher to the *yogasana* student:

» Enlarging *yogasana* classes can improve the response to placebo-like suggestions, probably due to the increased power of suggestion fostered by the increased number of participants. This also relates to the well-known benefits that individuals receive from belonging to a cohesive, supportive group.

» The power of a *yogasana* teacher's placebo suggestions will depend upon the teacher's interest in the ailing student, positive expectations that the *yogasanas* will work to relieve the problem, concern about the student's recovery, and the student's interest in the science of *yogasana.* The teacher's comment in regard to the level of pain a student may experience in a particular *yogasana* will act as a placebo and so may have a strong influence on the level of discomfort the student perceives.

» Teacher comments that promote positive images, positive emotions, and behaviors that promote healing all will aid in the transformation to health.

» A placebo's power is increased when the modality of delivery has a good reputation.

Expectant faith, as expressed by the teacher in regard to performing the *yogasanas,* is a powerful stimulant to both healing and performance (Subsection 4.G, page 146). Brooks [93] states, "The relationship between expectation and therapeutic outcome is a wonderful model to understand mind-body interactions." Because the success of the placebo effect for pain reduction is tied to the expectation of a reward, in Alzheimer's patients in whom the prefrontal brain region (the locus for expectation and reward) does not function, no placebo effects for pain reduction are present. Many other examples of the intimate connection between the mental centers and the autonomic nervous system quickly come to mind: thinking of delicious food promotes salivation via the parasympathetic system, embarrassment leads to blushing due to activation of the vascular system, sudden psychic stress leads to a change in the heart rate due to sympathetic excitation, etc. Though the repeated activation of some of the innocuous sympathetic reflex actions can lead to pathological changes in the visceral organs [360] (e.g., peptic ulcers, asthma, hypertension, and coronary problems), the real importance of the placebo effect is in its demonstration that each of us has a self-healing mechanism already in place, if only we can find a way to trigger it into action.

Nocebos

To the extent that the placebo effect is the positive response to a psychological suggestion by someone in authority, one might expect that negative suggestions by someone with a malicious intent might provoke negative responses [41]. Such responses are known as "nocebos," from the Latin word meaning "I will harm." A well-known nocebo is the voodoo curse in which a victim is told that he will die on a certain day at a certain time, and the curse often comes true (Subsection 5.F, page 193.) As *yogasana* teachers, we must choose our words carefully so that we encourage the concept of "think well, be well" and avoid comments that could lead to a "think sick, be sick" point of view in our students.

Section 5.G: *Nadis, Chakras, and Prana*

Historical Perspective

Long before the art of dissection was practiced, the ancient yogis were able to deduce certain subtle aspects of human anatomy and physiology,

through close observation of their own bodies [47, 222, 263, 392, 687, 689, 741]. These yogis of old divided the body and mind into five layers or sheaths, going from the external to the internal aspects. The two external sheaths, called the *annamaya kosha* and the *pranamaya kosha,* are interpreted by B. K. S. Iyengar as corresponding to the Western concepts of the anatomy and the physiology of the body, respectively [401].

The ancient yogis estimated that within the body, there were up to 350,000 channels called *nadis,* the *nadis* being pathways of sensation along which the life force *(prana)* travels. Of the 72,000 *nadis* that radiate from the navel, the three most important are the *ida,* the *pingala,* and the *sushumna* [410]. When the *prana* can move freely through the *nadis* with little or no resistance, then mental and physical health are optimal. For our purposes, the first of the three most important *nadis* is the *sushumna* (figure 5.G-1a), located within the *merudanda,* a column extending from the occiput (at the base of the skull) to the coccyx. The *sushumna* bifurcates at the throat, with branches that ascend both anteriorly and posteriorly, to rejoin at the *brahmarandra,* a cavity within the skull.

The two other major *nadis,* ida and *pingala,* lie essentially parallel to the *merudanda,* but with each weaving back and forth so as to cross each other and the *merudanda* between five and eight times. The *ida* originates at the right side of the coccyx, terminates at the left nostril, and is said to carry the cooling moon energy; whereas *pingala* originates at the left side of the coccyx, terminates at the right nostril, and carries the warming sun energy. Those points along the *merudanda* where the *ida, pingala,* and *sushumna nadis* intersect (figure 5.G-1a) are called *chakras.* The *chakras* are also referred to as wheels, for they are the points from which many other *nadis* radiate.

The seven generally recognized *chakras* and their associated properties are listed in table 5.G-1. When a *chakra* is open to the flow of *prana,* the characteristics of the *chakra* become manifest in the individual. For example, those people for whom the heart *chakra (anahata)* is optimally open are healthy, compassionate, and

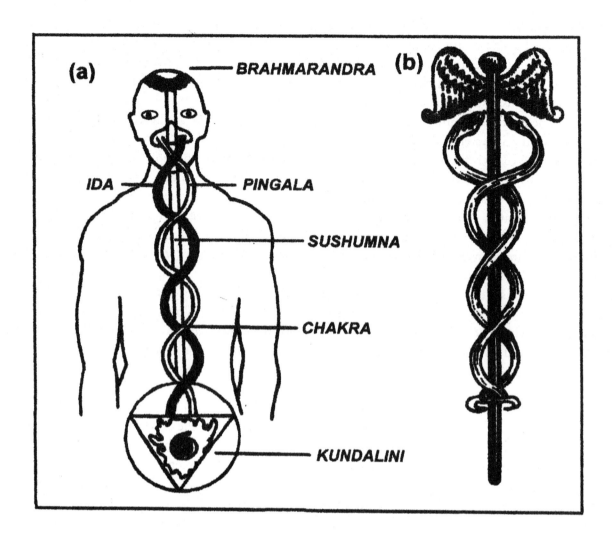

Figure 5.G-1. (a) The vertical *sushumna* and the oscillating *ida* and *pingala nadis* ascend the spine. The *chakras* are those points at which the *sushumna, ida,* and *pingala nadis* cross. *Kundalini,* resting at the bottom of the *sushumna,* ascends the *chakras,* finally reaching *brahmarandra,* the crown *chakra* at the top of the skull. (b) The ancient caduceus, the wand of the god Hermes or Mercury and presently the symbol of the U.S. Army Medical Corps and the medical symbol of the Western world, has a close relation to the symbol (a) of the Ayurvedic physicians of the Eastern world.

psychologically stable and centered. The heart *chakra* is associated with the color green and the air element. In contrast, for someone whose highest open *chakra* is the belly *chakra (swadisthana),* their personality is friendly and creative, with strong emotional feelings. The color of this *chakra* is orange, and the element is water. It must be said that many other interpretations of the *chakras* are available other than those given in table 5.G-1.

The importance of the *chakras* is understood to be that when they all are open, as through op-

timum physiological and psychological health, then *prana* can flow unimpeded through *ida* and *pingala* to reach the nostrils. Given this state, a super energy called *kundalini* can flow up the *sushumna* to the crown *chakra,* resulting in a state of bliss. This sounds at first remarkably like the discussion of nasal laterality (Section 15.E, page 627), but one must remember that with respect to *nadis, chakras,* and *prana,* one is dealing with structures or substances that do not necessarily exist on the physical plane.

It is the goal of the aspiring student to suc-

Table 5.G-1: Characteristics of the Seven Chakras [687, 689, 824]

Chakra Name	Position on Spine	Terminal Plexus	Organ/ Gland Innervated	Autonomic Association	Color/ Element	Effect on Opening
Crown *Sahasrara*	Crown of head		Cerebral cortex	-	Violet/ Electric	Universal love, power, influence, transcend-ence
Third Eye *Ajna*	C1	Nasociliary	Pituitary, pineal, brain, ears	-	Indigo/ Electric	Intuitive, charismatic, knowing, detached
Throat *Vishuddha*	C3	Pharyngeal	Thyroid, parathyroid, throat, eyes	Parasympa-thetic cranial	Blue/Ether	Commu-nication, creativity, contented-ness, nerves centered
Heart *Anahata*	T1	Cardiac	Heart, thymus, lungs, lymph glands	Parasympa-thetic vagus nerves	Green/Air	Healing, compassion, centered
Solar Plexus *Manipura*	T8	Celiac	Adrenals, diaphragm, skin	Adrenals T10-T12 sympathetic, vagus nerve	Yellow/Fire	Outgoing, elevation, vitality, psychic awareness
Belly *Svadhisthana*	L1	Hypogastric	Pancreas, ovaries, intestines	Sympathetic from lumbar	Orange/ Water	Feelings, friendliness, intuitive
Root *Muladhara*	S4	Sacral	Testes	L1-L3 sympathetic; S2-S4 para-sympathetic	Red/ Earth	Healthy, sexual power, passion, confidence

cessively reopen the higher *chakras*. To the extent that yoga can influence this flow of nervous ener-gy, *yogasana* and *pranayama* are of use in opening the higher *chakras*. Needless to say, this is but a very brief abstract of a subject that has been stud-ied for thousands of years. For deeper discussions, see for example [222] and/or [851].

Possible Relations of *Chakras* to Anatomic Features

In trying to set this interesting but inferred to-pography of *nadis*, *chakras*, and *prana* into corre-spondence with modern anatomic understanding, *ida* and *pingala* may be taken to refer to the para-sympathetic and sympathetic nervous systems, respectively, and the *chakras* to the known nerve plexuses radiating from the spine. Iyengar [391] further identifies the efferent nerves as the *karma nadi* (nerves of action) and the afferent nerves as the *jnana nadi* (nerves of knowledge) and states, "Perfect understanding between nerves of action and nerves of knowledge, working together in concord, is yoga." The *prana* currents within the *ida* and *pingala nadis* can be brought to a healthful balance by performing either the appropriate choice of *yogasanas* or by practicing *nadi shodana* (Section 15.F, page 637) [34]. With reference to the Chinese system of acupuncture, the yogic concepts of *prana, nadi, ida,* and *pingala* correspond to qi, meridians, yin, and yang, respectively.

For the sake of simplicity, one might associate the *nadis* with nerves,[6] the *chakras* with nerve plexuses, and *prana* with nerve impulses. Telang [851] points out that *prana* is not oxygen but is a spiritual material that is carried by oxygen. With this in mind, note that as discussed in Box 3.B-1, page 43, what moves from one end of an excited nerve to the other is not a material substance but is explained by Western scientists as a voltage difference, which is physically effective and can be sensed using real-world instruments but is so insubstantial that it cannot be analyzed, weighed, or captured in a bottle. Can this be the Western analog of *prana*?

Pushing the analogy further, the *merudanda* is the spinal cord, the *brahmarandra* is a ventricular

---

6   As explained to me by Gilmore [275], it was Swami Kuvalayananda who first sought the connection between Western medicine and Eastern yoga in the 1920s and who, at that time, first published drawings of the nerves and called them *nadis*. However, Gilmore stresses that the nerves and the *nadis* are concepts on very different planes and should not be compared with one another, no matter how tempting it is to do so. On the other hand, Iyengar [394] assigns some *nadis* to the physical body (arteries, capillaries, bronchioles, etc.), carrying physical substances (air, blood, etc.), and others that are to be found in the spiritual body transporting energies, etc., as with the nervous system. Yet other *nadis* are assigned as existing on and within more subtle levels not yet recognized by Western scientists.

space in the brain, and *ida* and *pingala* are the two branches of the autonomic nervous system, the sympathetic and parasympathetic. Indeed, as listed in table 5.G-1, the seven *chakras* can be put into one-to-one correspondence with known anatomic neural plexuses having origins at known levels along the spine (and above it) and both sympathetic and parasympathetic innervation (figure 5.G-2). Each of these plexuses (*chakras*) is known to innervate one or more glands or visceral organs, just as explained by the ancient yogis. Thus for example, *anahata,* the heart *chakra* of the ancients, can be thought to originate in the vicinity of T1 and to sympathetically innervate the heart, lungs, thymus gland, and the lymph glands. Parasympathetic innervation of the same area involves branches of the vagus nerve originating at cranial nerve X (Subsection 5.D, page 180). On the other hand, the belly *chakra* anatomically has sympathetic innervation at the L1 level and corresponds to the hypogastric plexus encompassing the pancreas, the intestines, and the ovaries of women. The eight hierarchical *chakras* of the Ayurvedic system correspond closely to the eight hierarchical levels of *Ashtanga* yoga.

The possible scientific significance of the colors assigned to the various *chakras* in table 5.G-1 is discussed further in Subsection 17.E, page 681.

The sympathetic and parasympathetic nervous systems affect every tissue and practically every cell in the body, irrespective of function. By controlling the balance between sympathetic and parasympathetic actions through *yogasana* practice, we can control physiology at the cellular level [751]. It is tempting to equate the three *gunas* (*rajasic, tamasic,* and *sattvic,* as used broadly in describing the *yogasanas* [388]) with the dominance of the sympathetic nervous system, the dominance of the parasympathetic nervous system, and a balanced state between the two extremes, respectively. In turn, neural flexibility within the autonomic nervous system, so necessary for good health, has its analog in the classical picture wherein blockage of the *pranic* flow through either the *ida nadi* or *pingala nadi* stymies the eventual raising of the kundalini energy in the *merudanda* (figure 5.G-2).

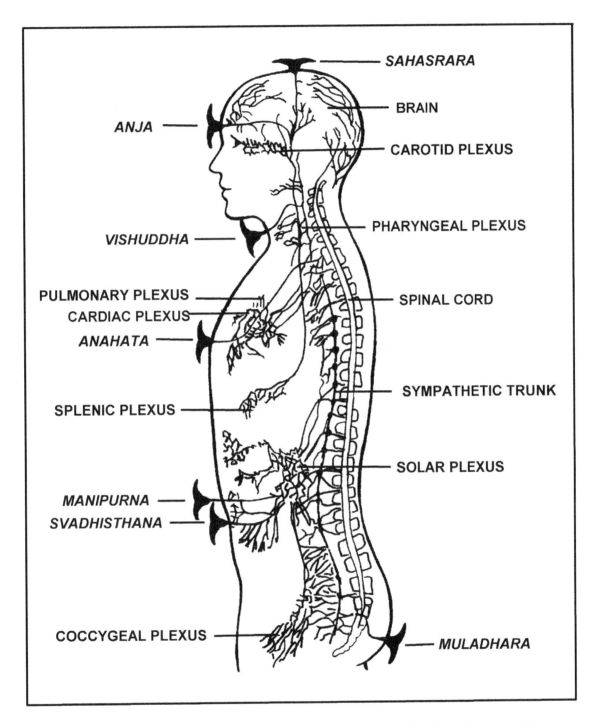

Figure 5.G-2. Correspondence of the major *chakras* residing at the sites of the lotus flowers and the various nerve plexuses in the body.

The Endocrine Glands and Hormones

6

Section 6.A: General Features of Endocrine Glands and Their Hormones

As primitive organisms became larger and more complex, cell functions became more specialized and spatially separated from one another. In order to coordinate the functions of such specialized but widely separated groups of cells, two paths of communication evolved, both using chemical messengers: the neural pathway and the hormonal pathway. In the neural pathway, both electrical impulses and chemical means are invoked to alter the activities of muscles and glands; in the hormonal pathway, chemicals are released into the blood to alter cell metabolism.

Two Types of Glands

In addition to the neural mechanism discussed in Chapter 3, page 29, cells separated by large distances in the body can communicate with one another without synapses, using glands and their hormonal secretions. In this case, the communication is not cell-to-cell specific and rapid; instead, it is more like organ-to-organ and is relatively slow, as compared with the neural route. Rather than using neurotransmitters released into the synapse between each pair of communicating cells and chemical-specific receptors as the signal-carrying means, the glands release substances into the body fluids more or less indiscriminately, often sensed by molecule-specific receptors. There are two general types of glandular structure.

Exocrine Glands

In an exocrine gland, there is a well-defined duct that leads the secretion from some reservoir to its target cells (Chapter 20, page 721). In contrast to the situation in the endocrine glands, the exocrine glands release their active substances onto either a free surface of the body, such as the skin, or into ducts that deliver the hormone into the lumens of the body [863]. Only the secretions of the endocrine glands are called hormones.

As examples, the exocrine sweat glands and sebaceous glands deliver their messengers to the skin surface through distinct ducts, as do the exocrine tear ducts, which carry tears to the surface of the eye; similarly, the bile within the gallbladder is delivered to the small intestine through such a duct. In the case of the gallbladder, stimulation of the parasympathetic vagus nerve to the liver simultaneously releases the sphincter to the gallbladder and contracts the muscles of the gallbladder walls, so that the bile stored in the bladder is expelled into the small intestine [107]. These, however, are not endocrine glands, and their outputs are not hormones.

Endocrine Glands

In the endocrine glands of the human body, there is no duct evident, and the hormones are simply released into the extracellular fluid surrounding the local capillaries, and these then absorb the hormone and distribute it widely through the circulatory system. In one sense,

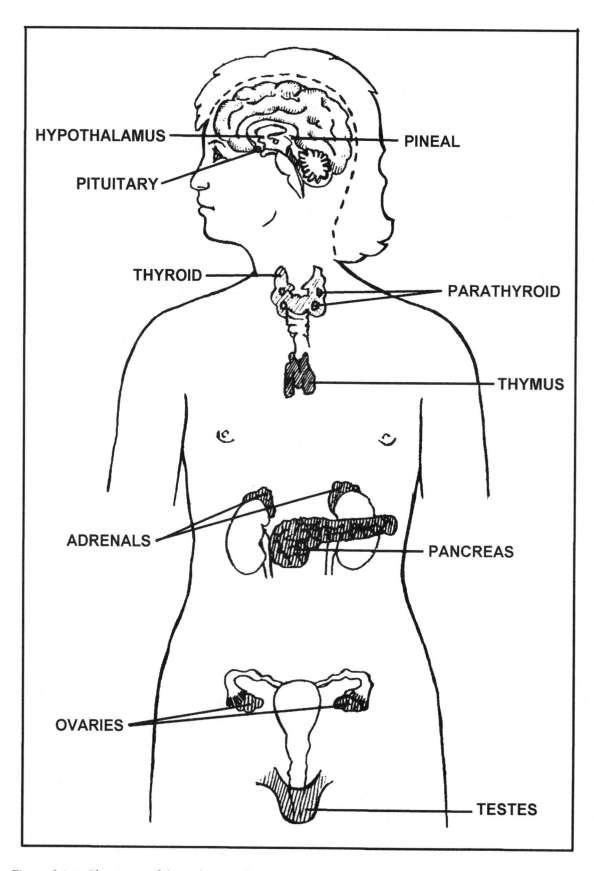

Figure 6.A-1. Placement of the endocrine glands in the body.

the hormonal release mechanism of endocrine glands closely resembles that of the neural release of neurotransmitters (figure 3.C-1), for in both cases, the active substance is stored in vesicles, and when needed, the vesicles migrate to the outer surface of the gland or axon, fuse with the membrane, and then open to release their contents into the neighboring area, to eventually find a receptor site [107]. The positions of these endocrine glands in the body are shown in figure 6.A-1.

Even within the class of endocrine glands, there is a subclass of glands within organs that largely serve just that organ hormonally. This is so for the hypothalamus, the liver, the thymus, the heart, the kidney, the stomach, and the duodenum [432]. Almost all glands are controlled by subcortical brain structures such as the hypothalamus and pituitary.

The Hormones

Hormones are chemical messengers connecting glands in one part of the body with receptive cells in far distant places within the body. In this communication mode, the hormone is released into the bloodstream by the relevant endocrine gland and is carried to the receptor site by the circulation of the blood. Receptor sites might be other endocrine glands, which are stimulated to release other hormones in turn; or they might be organs within the body. Once the hormone is bound to the receptor site, physiological changes are initiated, as the hormone is a modulator of the cell's potential function. Though the same molecule can serve in the human body as both a messenger in the hormonal system and a neurotransmitter in the neural system, the functions triggered by the molecule in the two systems will not be the same [806]. The ultimate purpose of the hormones is to regulate the body's chemistry (i.e., the cell's physiology), so as to keep it in homeostatic balance (Subsection 5.A, page 158).

Neural/Hormonal Interactions

It was long held that the neural and the hormonal systems of the body were rigidly separate,

but with more studies, this is seen to be less and less the case. Thus, for example, stimulation of the adrenal glands by the hypothalamus is now known to occur both neurally on a short time scale and hormonally on a long time scale (Section 5.E, page 183, and figure 5.E-1). The modes of action in conventional neural conduction and in hormonal signaling involving the hypothalamus are compared in figure 6.A-2. Moreover, the hormone insulin, known to originate in the pancreas, is now known also to be produced by some cells in the brain, implying a neural modality as well.

As compared with the direct link between the originating cell and the target cell in the neural network, the action in the hormonal system is more indirect, for in the latter, the general action is a release of the messenger molecules into the bloodstream for distribution throughout the body. Reflecting the different modes of deployment, the neural effects are apparent in times of a few milliseconds; whereas for hormonal deployment, hours may pass before the effect is apparent. Though hormonal stimulation is a much slower process than neural stimulation, it can last for a much longer time; however, both modes operate on the basis of transmitter molecules binding sooner or later to receptor sites on adjacent or distant cells and thereby activating the cells to a specific function.

Hormonal Signaling Mechanism

Initial stimulation of an endocrine gland begins with afferent neural signals that originate in the visceral organs and go first to the nuclei of the solitary tract, which in turn either stimulate the hypothalamus to release hormones that release other hormones or stimulate the brainstem nuclei, ending in an autonomic neural output that stimulates an end organ (figure 5.E-1**b**). When these two modes (neural and endocrine) function simultaneously, the result is a neuroendocrine function.

Activation of the afferent visceral nerves promotes sympathetic responses, most likely via endocrine stimulation within the hypothalamus. As many *yogasanas* could easily stimulate the afferent

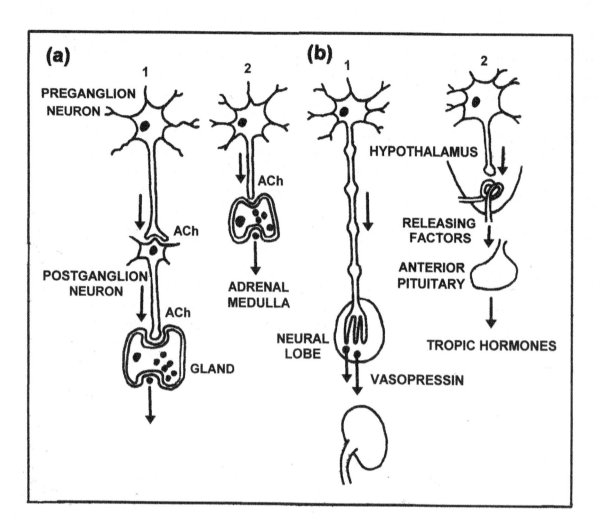

Figure 6.A-2. (a) In the conventional autonomic system, acetylcholine (ACh) serves as the neurotransmitter, inducing the release of hormones as in (1) and (2). (b) The two modes of neuroendocrine release in the hypothalamus: (1) the direct release of hormone from the neural lobe of a neural cell; and (2) the hypothalamus stimulates the hormonal release into the anterior pituitary, which then releases the specific hormone into the general circulation.

visceral nerves, they easily could result in endocrine shifts [155].

Yogasana

From the yogic point of view, the glands and their excretions are held to be of the highest importance, and though there is little or no scientific evidence to support the idea, it is generally held that a stimulating hormonal effect of a *yogasana* posture is gained through increased release of the hormone due to compression of the appropriate gland. In particular, this is discussed in regard to the release of the catecholamines from the adrenal glands by backbending in Box 11.D-1, page 453.

However, there is no medical evidence to support the common yogic point of view that applying external pressure to an endocrine gland will stimulate it to release its hormonal load, unless the pressure is so extreme that the glandular cells are ruptured. In this regard, the endocrine glands differ from the exocrine glands (see below). It is more likely that if there is a positive effect of a specific posture on a hormone-releasing gland, it is due to increased vascular circulation in the area of the gland [914].

Table 6.A-1: Times of Maximum and Minimum Concentrations of Hormones in Blood Plasma [584]

Hormone	Time for Maximum	Time for Minimum
Cortisol	4:00 AM	10:00 PM
Growth hormone	10:00 PM	All day
Aldosterone	4:00 AM	All day
Prolactin	4:00 AM	All day
Testosterone	2:00 AM	6:00 PM
Luteinizing hormone, male	No peak	No peak
Follicle stimulating hormone, male	No peak	No peak
Thyrotropin	10:00 PM	All day

Hormone Types

Steroidal Hormones

Chemically, there are two general types of hormones, the peptides and the steroids. The peptides are composed of long chains of amino acids, as is the case with insulin and gastrin, for example. The steroidal hormones have chemical structures that are based upon that of cholesterol and include the important molecules cortisol, corticosterone, aldosterone, progesterone, testosterone, and estrogen. As discussed in Subsection 4.G, page 135, hormones not only influence cell metabolism but also can play active roles in memory and learning.

Peptide Hormones

The peptide hormones are hydrophilic and so have very little affinity for the lipid membrane surrounding a cell, other than for the proteinaceous transmembrane receptors embedded within the membranes (figure 3.A-2). In contrast, the steroidal hormones are hydrophobic and so are able to freely diffuse through the fatty-lipid membranes surrounding cells, finding receptors within. The steroidal hormones are transported in the blood as protein complexes [450].

Rhythmic Release of Hormones

The release of the endocrine hormones in the body follows the twenty-four-hour circadian clock (Section 23.B, page 774), but with a one- to two-hour ultradian rhythm superposed. Thus, at the time in the twenty-four-hour cycle of a hormone's maximum release, there will be a release of several spurts of hormone, with a delay of one to two hours between spurts (figure 6.A-3). Rapid fall of the hormone levels is a consequence of the rapid clearing of hormones from the receptor sites through metabolic processes. The times of maximum and minimum release of various hormones are listed in table 6.A-1, and the periodic release of specific hormones is discussed in more detail in Section 6.B, page 213.

The basic ninety-minute rest-and-activity rhythm that characterizes the release of hormones in the human body is also found operating in regard to our awareness and cognitive skills and was first observed in a soil amoeba and later shown to be active in yeast cells and other such cell lines. The ninety-minute rhythm appears to be a largely genetically controlled process and a near-universal attribute of life.

Slow Release

Remembering that a hormone is released into the bloodstream and can affect an organ in the body only after it has been circulated through the

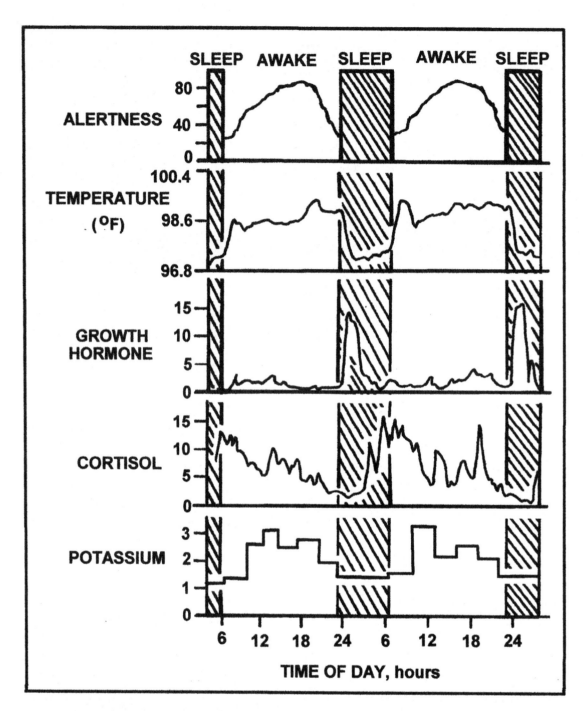

Figure 6.A-3. Comparison of the release of spurts of growth hormone and cortisol with several nonhormonal parameters of body function over a two-day period.

bloodstream to reach that organ, one then sees that the slow release of the hormone in small spurts allows for the hormone's effect to be realized and measured by the body before another may be launched. This prevents overdosing, provided the relevant subsystems are working properly. If a *yogasana* position were to stimulate a hormone release (as has been postulated for *urdhva dhanurasana* and the catecholamines; Box 11.D-1, page 453) by mechanically squeezing the gland, then the effect would not appear any sooner than thirty to sixty seconds thereafter, this being the time for a round-trip circulation of the blood through the body.

The hormones CRF and ACTH involved along the hypothalamus-pituitary axis (Section 5.B, page 165) also have plasma concentrations that are tied to the circadian clock. Though the corticosteroids in humans peak just as the day begins and then fall to a minimum in the evening, it is just the reverse in nocturnal animals.

Hormonal Control

Three homeostatic mechanisms limit the concentrations of hormones in circulation:

1. In this scenario, a hormone is set free in the blood and promotes the release of a second hormone, which then inhibits the further release of the first. For example, FSH (see below) promotes the release of estrogen from the ovarian follicle, and the resultant high level of estrogen then inhibits the production of more FSH.
2. There also may be antagonistic pairs of hormones at work; for example, insulin causes blood sugar to drop, and the hormone glucagon causes it to rise. Thus, insulin and glucagon form an antagonistic hormonal pair working together to maintain a near-constant level of glucose in the body fluids.
3. A substance may be set free by the action of a hormone, and the substance is then an inhibitor of the hormone's release, as with Ca^{2+} and the parathyroid hormone (PTH), Subsection 7.B, page 235.

Section 6.B: Specific Glands and Their Hormones

The Hypothalamus

Located just above the pineal and the pituitary glands (figure 5.E-1a), the hypothalamus integrates neurological information from other neural centers and chemical information from the bloodstream into a coherent course of action for the other glands. It acts as the primary coordination center between the nervous and the endocrine systems. Through the release of its hormones into the pituitary stalk (figure 5.B-1), the hypothalamus regulates not only the hormone production of the pituitary but of the adrenal glands as well. The functioning of this gland is described in detail in Section 5.B, page 165, and its key role in several body processes is shown in figures 5.E-1a and 6.B-1. All three hormones involved in the interactions along the hypothalamus-pituitary-adrenal cortex (HPA) axis shown in figure 5.E-1a follow circadian rhythms dictated by the suprachiasmatic nucleus, which in turn is keyed to the light-dark cycle of the sun, as sensed by the eyes (Subsection 23.B, page 787).

Many hypothalamic hormones are first released into the duct going directly to the anterior and posterior lobes of the pituitary (a gland within the brain but not a part of the brain), which then releases hormones into general circulation. These pituitary hormones eventually find their target organs in the ovaries, testes, thyroid, bones, skin, kidneys, and breasts. The intended action at the target organ then releases yet another hormone, which acts in an inhibitory way with the hypothalamus so as to regulate its actions through feedback [431], as discussed for homeostatic mechanism 2 in Subsection 6.A, page 210. Along with several other hormones, the hypothalamus releases the following directly to the pituitary gland: (a) gonadotropin releasing hormone (GnRH), which promotes the subsequent release from the pituitary of luteinizing hormone (LH) and follicle stimulating hormone (FSH); (b) corticotropin releasing factor (CRF), which promotes the release of ACTH corticotropin from the anterior pituitary, eventually to influence the adrenal cortex; (c) thyrotropin releasing hormone (TRH), which releases thyroid stimulating hormone (TSH) from the pituitary [432, 806]; (d) growth-hormone releasing hormone (GHRH), acting to promote the release of growth hormone;[1] and (e) somatostatin

---

1   Careful X-ray measurements on the lengths of the long bones in teenagers actually show the incremental lengthening of these bones with spurts of GHRH

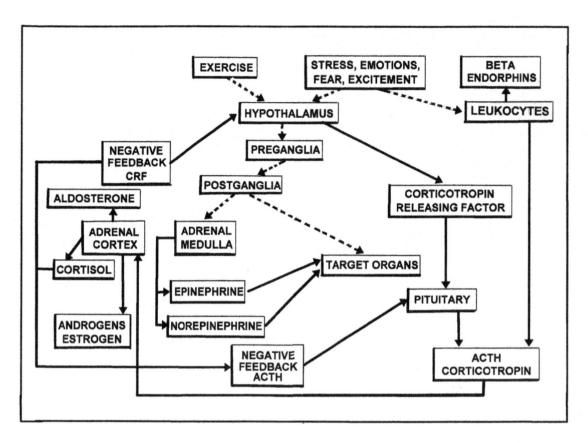

Figure 6.B-1. A flow chart showing the neural (dashed arrows) and hormonal (full-line arrows) consequences of stress and exercise on the body and the interactions between neural and hormonal processes.

and dopamine, the principal hormonal functions of which in the hypothalamus are to inhibit the release of prolactin from the anterior pituitary. All of the above hypothalamic hormones are released in ninety-minute spurts, and in fact, they have no physiological effect if administered externally at a constant rate. Two other hormones, vasopressin and oxytocin, when stimulated by the hypothalamus, are released from the posterior pituitary into the general circulation.

The Pituitary Gland

This endocrine gland is widely known as the master gland; however, it is activated by hormonal

secretions from the hypothalamus just above it in the midbrain. Though situated between the left and right temporal lobes of the brain, the pituitary gland is not a part of the neurological apparatus, nor does it function as part of the brain. Hormonal action of the pituitary gland is readily divided into that governed largely by its anterior portion and that governed by its posterior portion. Secretions from the anterior pituitary include growth hormone, ACTH, prolactin, and thyroid-stimulating hormone (TSH), whereas secretions from the posterior pituitary include oxytocin and vasopressin (also known as antidiuretic hormone or ADH).

The sex hormones that are active at the onset of puberty and throughout the adult reproductive period also originate with signals at the hypothalamus and pituitary gland [432, 806, 858]. On command from the hypothalamus, the pituitary releases follicle stimulating hormone (FSH) to stimulate the growth of follicles in the ovaries,

---

growth hormone largely during the sleeping hours (figure 6.A-3). It is well known among professional cyclists that short naps of one to two hours are especially restorative, as they promote the release of spurts of growth hormone.

luteinizing hormone (LH) to convert a follicle in the ovary to a corpus luteum, and corticotropin (ACTH) to the adrenal cortex in order to promote the release of cortisol.

Vasopressin and Oxytocin

The pituitary is also the source of vasopressin, a very powerful hormone that not only acts on the kidneys to retain water, but constricts the vascular system to raise the blood pressure (especially at times of heavy blood loss) and works on the liver to break down glycogen, a polymeric form of glucose. Vasopressin is released by cells in the posterior pituitary and serves as a messenger in both neural and hormonal circuits. As a neurotransmitter, vasopressin is found in the synapses of the brain and is assumed to play some role in memory [174, 806].

Oxytocin is both a hormone and a neurotransmitter. Massive amounts of oxytocin are released from the uterus during copulation and during orgasm. Moreover, the release of oxytocin is responsible for the contractions of the uterus during labor and for lactation thereafter. Because oxytocin tends to produce amnesia, many mothers are said to have little or no memory of having given birth to a child [721].

At lower concentrations, oxytocin promotes and regulates social memory and social relations and is an integral part of the memory process when sexual or maternal bonds are being formed [137]. It also induces relaxation and lowers anxiety; thus, for example, warm hugs, for women, promote higher levels of oxytocin in the blood and lower blood pressures. Inhalation of an oxytocin spray reduces the level of cortisol in the blood.

Oxytocin is released by men as well as by women; however, in a woman, the effects of oxytocin are enhanced by her female hormones, whereas in a man, the effects are blocked by his male hormones. Among men, the inhalation of oxytocin spray promotes an atmosphere of mutual trust in financial transactions and political situations, as it blunts the activity of the amygdala, the center of the brain that signals fear in social situations [9a]. Many women who have lifelong troubles with close relationships have low levels of oxytocin, as do many autistic individuals.

Surges in oxytocin levels attendant to social or sexual relations are accompanied by stimulation of the nucleus accumbens lying just beneath the frontal cortex. This in turn releases dopamine into the reward circuits of the brain (Subsection 3.D, page 56) and thereby stamps the event into our memories.

The Pineal Gland

Photosensitivity

Located deep in the brain, the pineal gland is at about the level of the eyes. In the dark, the pineal gland secretes the hormone melatonin, a natural antidepressant and a factor in setting the biological clock (Subsection 23.B, page 788). The production and release of melatonin by the pineal gland promotes sleep and is blocked by irradiation of the eyes with light of wavelengths of 420–460 nanometers (figure 17.B-2), close to the peak of sensitivity of the blue-sensitive cones in the retina. During adolescence, melatonin concentrations peak later in the day than they do in either children or adults, resulting in the need for late nights and long morning lie-ins. The inhibition of melatonin production by exposure of the eyes to light also induces puberty whereas melatonin release otherwise inhibits the onset of puberty.

The pineal gland is not only photosensitive, but also psychosensitive, for it also releases melatonin during meditation (and presumably during yogic relaxation). Evidence suggests that melatonin is an active agent in fighting prostate and breast cancers [139]; the incidence of breast cancer is 50 percent higher in women who work the night shift and so have a reduced melatonin production.

The Thyroid Gland

The thyroid gland is located at the base of the throat, and its hormones are regulators of human growth, levels of activity, and metabolism. The thyroid synthesizes and excretes triiodothyronine

(T3), thyroxine (T4), and calcitonin. T3 and T4 increase the metabolic rate; i.e., they increase the rate of oxygen consumption and increase the rate and strength of the heartbeat. The T3 and T4 thyroid hormones generate heat in the body through the regulation of the body's rate of metabolism and promotion of protein synthesis. In addition to increasing heart action, these hormones also act to increase the brain's excitability [71, 432]. Circulation in the vicinity of the thyroid would be promoted by inverted *yogasanas* such as *sarvangasana* and *halasana*, which force the chin into the chest just over the thyroid gland. Excessive T3 and T4 production leads to the thyroid condition known as Graves' disease [450].[2]

The hormone calcitonin is also released by the thyroid when the level of Ca^{2+} in the blood rises too high. Calcitonin serves to lower the level of Ca^{2+} in the blood by encouraging the osteoblasts to incorporate Ca^{2+} in bone formation and simultaneously discouraging the release of Ca^{2+} from the bones by the osteoclasts [71, 432] (Subsection 7.B, page 233).

The Parathyroid Gland

Parathyroid hormone (PTH) regulates the Ca^{2+} and PO_4^{3-} levels in the blood (Subsection 7.B, page 235) and activates the synthesis of vita-

---

2   If, in fact, simple mechanical pressure is sufficient to stimulate a gland to excrete its hormone, then students with excessive T3 and T4 production should avoid postures such as *halasana*, *sarvangasana*, and *setu bandha*, as these postures place the neck into flexion and so press the chin strongly into the sternum. Strangely, postures such as *urdhva dhanurasana*, *ustrasana*, and *viparita dandasana*, in which the neck is in extension, also are said to be stimulating to the thyroid even though there is no pressure of the chin on the sternum [398]. Accepting this argues for a mechanism of thyroid stimulation in which the simple pressing of the gland by either flexion or extension of the neck exerts its effect by stimulation of the circulation in the area and not by a pressure-stimulated release of the hormone. See Box 11.D-1, page 453, for related arguments as to why hormones are not necessarily secreted by mechanical pressure.

min D. In order to increase the level of Ca^{2+} in the body fluids, parathyroid hormone stimulates the osteoclasts to dissolve bone, thus setting free the Ca^{2+} ions in the bone. When the proper level of Ca^{2+} in the body fluids is reached, the parathyroid ceases to release its hormone. On the other hand, an overactive parathyroid leads to brittle bones [450].

Calcitonin promotes storage of Ca^{2+} in the bones. Parathyroid hormone from the parathyroid acts to inhibit the action of calcitonin, as PTH promotes transfer of Ca^{2+} from bones to blood; in this way, calcitonin and PTH form an antagonistic hormone pair, working in accord with mechanism 1 in Subsection 6.A, page 210.

The Thymus Gland

Being located just behind the heart, the thymus gland is a component of the heart *chakra* (*anahata*). Its only function appears to be an association with the immune system in the subadult, for whom lymphocytes that pass through the thymus gland are transformed into T cells, while thymosin hormones can be released by the gland, which then stimulate T cells in their protective functions. Moreover, the thymus appears to program the T cells of the body so as not to attack other cells of the body, and it is possibly a depot for the storage of the T cells of the immune system [432] (Chapter 16, page 643).

Degeneration

Though the thymus is formally a part of the lymphatic system, its activity and size wane considerably after puberty, becoming a small knot of yellow, fibrous tissue in the adult. Some hold that the general failure of the immune system with age correlates with the degeneration of the thymus gland. *Yogasana* exercises designed to stimulate the adult immune system by virtue of increased vascular circulation to the thymus would seem to have minimal value in view of this early degeneration [431], unless it helps to unleash a hidden supply of T cells from the atrophied gland or promotes the release of hormones which in turn stimulate the T cells. It would be very useful to see a scientific study aimed at determining any changes in either T cell numbers or their effectiveness following the practice of supposed thymus-stimulating postures such as *halasana* or *sarvangasana*.

The Adrenocortical Glands

A cluster of glands that play highly significant roles in the body's response to stresses of various kinds sits atop the kidneys. This glandular complex, among the most highly vascularized organs of the body, is divided into a central part (the adrenal medulla) and a wrapping about the medulla (the adrenal cortex). Though side by side, the adrenomedullar and adrenocortical glands differ in their structures, embryonic origin, the hormones they release, and the hormones to which they respond [432, 806, 858]. The adrenal cortex is the origin of the hormones known as the corticosteroids and the mineralocorticoids, whereas the adrenal medulla is the origin of the hormones known as the catecholamines (Subsection 3.D, page 54). As discussed in Subsection 5.F, page 193, if the driving force for adrenal action is an immediate threat to one's safety, it is the adrenal cortex that is activated; whereas if the driving force is a challenge to be met by conscious action, then the adrenal medulla is activated instead. Moreover, the excitation in the first case is hormonal, whereas in the second case, it is neural (figure 5.E-1**a**).

Hormones

The adrenal cortex is divisible into three zones. Once prompted to do so by the hypothalamus, ACTH (adrenocorticotrophic hormone) from the anterior pituitary gland (Section 5.C, page 170) activates cells within the adrenal cortex to release hormones (largely testosterone or estrogen) in very small amounts, glucocorticoids (largely cortisol, also known as hydrocortisone), and mineralocorticoids (largely aldosterone) into the bloodstream for transport to all of the cells of the body.

The middle zone of the adrenal cortex is responsible for the release of cortisol, a hormone that is very important in resisting stress when in low concentration and that increases the glucose supply for the brain and heart in times of stress. As the glucocorticoids have a potent effect against inflammation and depress the immune response, these hormones are used to fight the inflammation of autoimmune problems associated with rheumatoid arthritis and asthma (Subsection 16.D, page 648).

The outer zone of the cortex releases the hormone aldosterone, which acts within the kidney to regulate the concentration of Na^+ and K^+ ions in the body fluids, increasing the former and reducing the latter. It is released only in cases of dire emergency involving loss of blood or blood pressure. Because aldosterone promotes reabsorption of Na^+ in the kidney and so promotes water retention, it is also known as antidiuretic hormone (ADH). Aldosterone also acts on the sweat glands to slow the loss of Na^+ and is released from the adrenal glands by the actions of ACTH and angiotensin II. As seen in table 6.A-1, other than for emergencies, the peak release of aldosterone is almost coincident with the time of general early-morning (4:00 AM) arousal of the entire body.

Cortisol

The effects of cortisol begin at the moment of birth. When the baby is ready to be born, its adrenal cortex releases cortisol into the common bloodstream of mother and baby. With increased cortisol in the blood, the mother's progesterone level falls, while estrogen remains high. Uterine contractions then begin, and a baby is delivered who is alert, charged with life, and ready to meet life's challenges [878]. The circadian release of cortisol does not develop in children until the age of two to three years.

Under heavy exercise, the hypothalamus triggers a cascade of hormonal events that end with the release of cortisol from the adrenal cortex (figure 6.B-1). The best-known action of cortisol is to increase the levels of glucose in the blood and at the same time inhibit the uptake of glucose by the muscles, in order to insure adequate fuel supplies for the brain and heart under conditions of stress. For a given level of stress, the largest stress-stimulated release of cortisol occurs at times of lowest ambient cortisol level (10:00 PM, table 6.A-

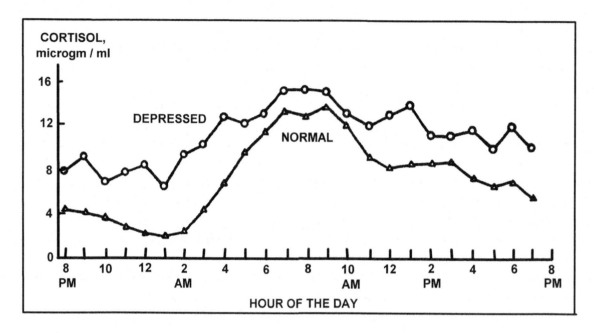

Figure 6.B-2. The course of the cortisol levels measured hourly throughout the day in normal and depressed subjects. Note the relatively elevated levels in the morning and evening hours and the erratic variations in the depressed subjects as compared with the norm. The apparent differences in the cortisol-release curves versus time (figure 6.A-3) reflect the temporal resolution (continuous versus hourly monitoring) used in gathering the data in the two cases.

1); the release is lowest when the level of ambient cortisol is highest (4:00 AM). Accordingly, one would guess that the amount of cortisol generated by *yogasana* practice would be largest for a morning practice and least for an evening practice.

Ideally, too high a level of cortisol turns off the initiating event in the hypothalamus, the release of ACTH; however this is not the case for those under chronic stress. When our stress is chronic, so too is the elevation of the cortisol level in the blood. In this case, the middle zone of the adrenal cortex becomes hypertrophied, and one faces increased risk of stomach ulcers, loss of immunity due to shrinkage of the lymph glands, hypertension and other vascular disorders, excess sugar in the blood, heart disease, upper respiratory infection, and the accumulation of abdominal fat. The significant differences in the cortisol levels throughout the twenty-four-hour day in normal and chronically depressed subjects is clear in figure 6.B-2.

Brainard et al. [88] have measured the amounts of cortisol in the blood of three groups of subjects: a group of beginning *yogasana* students, a group of experienced *yogasana* students, and a control group. The first two groups were to perform their *yogasana* practice, while the control group was to sit and read. Cortisol measurements were made before and after a one-hour *yogasana* practice, and it was found that the control group showed a slight cortisol drop between 11:00 AM and noon (see figure 6.B-2 as well), as is normal for the circadian rhythm. On the other hand, the beginners showed a much more substantial decrease in cortisol, and the more experienced students showed an even larger decrease. The authors concluded tentatively that *yogasana* practice could be an antidote to the many stressful scenarios that otherwise raise the levels of this stress hormone. In a somewhat related study on the effects of Iyengar *yogasana* practice on the mood of depressed, cortisol-deficient subjects [903], it was found that there was a rise in the cortisol levels following a morning practice. It is not clear what the relation is between the more complete data of figure 6.B-2, comparing the levels between depressed and the norm (both without exercise), and the truncated studies of Woolery et al. [903] and of Brainard et al. [88], comparing the level before and after *yogasana* practice. However, it must be pointed out that if the rapidly changing levels of cortisol release shown in figure 6.A-3 are reliable, it means that one must measure cortisol at time intervals much shorter than one hour and be assured that the sharp peaks come at the same times in different subjects, if one wants to accurately assess the relative effects of *yogasana* practice on levels of plasma cortisol.

Cortisol Surge

The adrenal hormone cortisol is of great interest to the teacher of *yogasana*. The circadian rhythm describing the early-morning release of cortisol is very strongly tied to the rising and setting of the sun, even in blind people, and is very resistant to perturbation from the outside. The surge of cortisol concentration with the rising sun has many ramifications for our health as the day unfolds. First, cortisol in the blood acts to keep the muscles surrounding the airways relaxed, so that one can breathe easily. With little or no cortisol in the blood in the evening hours, one is then prone to an asthma attack in the hours before sunrise. Similarly, cortisol is an anti-inflammatory, and since it is low in the hours before sunrise, one often wakes up with sniffling and a stuffy, runny nose. These symptoms of cold and flu disappear as the cortisol surge asserts itself. The early-morning cortisol surge is also key in making the late-morning hours pain-free for those with osteoarthritis. As the cortisol level rises abruptly in the morning, so too does the glucose level.

Cortisol and Stress

It is ironic that whereas the levels of almost all other significant hormones in the body decrease as we age, that of the stress hormone cortisol shows little or no drop-off with age. Moreover, when older people are subjected to stress, they generate even more cortisol than when they were younger, but are less able to recover from the stress and its associated hormone! As we age, we become even more proficient at becoming stressed and less able to let go of its consequences, unless we are engaged in physical activities specifically aimed at relaxation, such as *yogasana* practice; as might be expected, laughter and smiling reduce cortisol levels.

The Adrenomedullar Glands

Sympathetic Neural Excitation

In contrast to the situation with the adrenal cortex, which is activated hormonally, the adrenal medulla only can be activated neurally. Under stress, the medulla is signaled by the sympathetic nervous system (Section 5.E, page 182) to release the catecholamines epinephrine and norepinephrine (earlier known as adrenaline and noradrenaline, respectively) into the bloodstream, typically in the proportions 80 percent epinephrine to 20 percent norepinephrine [432]. In this excitation, the released catecholamines lead to an increased rate and strength of the heartbeat and to a heightened blood pressure. Further, blood is shunted from the skin and viscera to the muscles, coronary arteries, the liver, and the brain; blood sugar and metabolic rate rises, and there is an increase in the release of ACTH from the pituitary. Sympathetic excitation also leads to dilation of the bronchi of the lungs and pupils of the eyes, stands body hair on end (piloerection), and decreases the clotting time of the blood (Section 5.C, page 173) [450].

Epinephrine

Epinephrine is released from the adrenal medulla into the bloodstream when triggered to do so by the neurally driven opening of K^+ channels; the triggering level is highly variable between species and between individuals within a species. It is hypothesized [762] that among thrill seekers, for whom ordinary life is too boring without the excitement of risking life and limb, the trigger level is set extraordinarily high, so that one must be close to death in order to feel the epinephrine rush. Though epinephrine cannot pass from the bloodstream into the brain, its presence in the blood leads to the release of dopamine in the brain—always a pleasurable sensation. The epinephrine rush can be triggered by physical, emotional, or intellectual means.

Epinephrine is targeted toward tissues carrying beta receptors, whereas norepinephrine targets tissues with alpha receptors. Thus, epinephrine acts on the beta receptors of the heart, causing an increased pumping rate and a more forceful contraction, and on the beta receptors of the smooth muscles of the bronchioles to relax and so dilate them (see also Subsection 5.C, page 173). Epinephrine also promotes the breakdown of glycogen and the conversion of fat to glucose for use as fuel.

The generally inhibiting actions of epinephrine on the beta receptors of the body can be blocked by compounds fittingly called beta blockers. Working throughout the body, beta blockers have the following effects: inhibition of vasodilation in the brain, reduction of fluid pressure within the eye, constriction of bronchial airways, slowing of the rate and force of the heartbeat, lowering of the blood pressure, reduction of the activity of the thyroid, and reduction of muscle tremor due to anxiety. Beta blockers are often prescribed for hypertension.

Norepinephrine

The alpha receptors of the visceral blood vessels are stimulated by norepinephrine to contract the vessels, thereby rerouting blood from viscera to the large muscles and raising the blood pressure; this effect is stronger yet in the presence of cortisol. The alpha receptors in the heart react to norepinephrine, stimulating contraction and working to increase the strength of contraction of the muscles in the arms and legs [806, 858]. In keeping with the fight or flight syndrome, the sympathetic release of catecholamines raises the levels of alertness and excitability in the brain. The catecholamines are the short-term response to stress.

Yogasana

The synapse between the sympathetic preganglionic fiber and the adrenal gland itself is cholinergic; were the synapse adrenergic, the initial release of the catecholamines would stimulate the further release of yet more catecholamines in a cascading fashion. Once the stimulation of the sympathetic nervous system and the release of

catecholamines ceases, about twenty minutes are then required for these hormones to clear the system [878]. This fact suggests that twenty minutes is a reasonable time for performing *savasana* and that ambient catecholamine levels can decrease dramatically in less than half an hour.

Note that contrary to the pronouncements of many *yogasana* teachers, the only proven route to catecholamine release from the adrenal glands is by neural excitation. A simple squeezing of the kidneys, as when in *urdhva dhanurasana*, will not release these hormones (as discussed more fully in Box 11.D-1, page 453) unless there is a psychological fear factor associated with the action. Similarly, it is often argued that the compressive action of *halasana* or *sarvangasana* on the thymus gland (figure 6.A-1) is stimulating to the gland; however, I can find no experimental evidence for this. It is more likely that compression of the glands in *yogasana* work, if beneficial at all, is due to increased circulation in the area of the gland, but not to enhanced glandular output.

Renin

Yet another hormone excreted by the kidneys, when prodded to do so by the sympathetic nervous system, is renin. As described in Subsection 5.C, page 178, renin acts indirectly to produce angiotensin II, which causes blood vessels to constrict and also promotes aldosterone release in order to increase the blood volume, all of which act to raise the blood pressure [107, 140, 584, 858].

The Pancreas and Gastrointestinal Glands

Insulin

The pancreas is a gland that is 99 percent exocrine and 1 percent endocrine, the former providing digestive enzymes to the duodenum and the latter releasing hormones that control the level of glucose in the blood. The glucose level in the blood must be kept relatively constant, as either too much or too little will inhibit its uptake by the body's cells. Were this to happen in the brain, for example, the result would be confusion, convulsions, and coma. If the glucose level in the blood is too low, then the alpha cells[3] of the pancreas release glucagon, a hormone that converts stored glycogen in the liver into glucose [858]. On the other hand, if the glucose level is too high, the pancreatic beta cells then release insulin, which promotes the uptake of glucose by the cells and the conversion of glucose into glycogen and its storage in the liver. Insulin is very important, because it allows the glucose, amino acids, and fatty acids in the blood to cross a cell's lipid membrane and so become fuel within the cell. If, for some reason, there is too little insulin or it is unable to enter the cell, the result is one form or another of diabetes. Thus, the hormonal outputs of the alpha and beta cells of the pancreas work to stabilize the level of glucose in the blood.

Insulin is packaged within the pancreatic beta cells in vesicles that migrate to the cell membrane, fuse with it, and thus release their hormonal burden to the extracellular fluid outside. Release of insulin can be triggered either neurologically or hormonally [858]; however, more than half of the insulin released by the pancreas is scavenged by the liver before it can be of any use to distant cells.

Autonomic Control

The pancreas is innervated by both the sympathetic and parasympathetic nervous systems, with the former inhibiting the release of insulin and the latter promoting its release. On this basis, one would guess that *yogasanas* leading to parasympathetic strengthening might be curative in those cases where there is an insufficiency of insulin. Though there are several reports of the efficacy of *yogasana* practice in regard to diabetes, there is as yet no firm evidence that *yogasanas* can affect insulin production [244, 580], other than the recent work of Manjunatha et al. [535],

which has demonstrated the increased response of the beta cells to blood glucose attendant to the long-term practice of the *yogasanas*. In regard to athletic performance, an overdose of insulin loads the muscles with glycogen and prevents the breakdown of any muscle mass that has been spawned by taking steroids.

Digestive Hormones

Several small glands are scattered about in the stomach, small intestine, and liver, releasing hormones to the digestive system. All gastric hormones are peptides, many of which are also found in the brain. These hormones are dispersed not only throughout the body, but also locally in a paracrine fashion. Gastrin is found in the stomach and duodenum, where it stimulates the release of hydrochloric acid and pepsin. The hormone secretin is secreted in the duodenum, where it encourages the pancreas to secrete the ion HCO_3^- in an exocrine way for acid neutralization. Somatostatin acts in the stomach to inhibit the action of gastrin, acts in the duodenum to inhibit the action of secretin, and is secreted by the hypothalamus [450]; the presence of enkephalins in the intestines controls peristalsis [59].

The Gonads

The glands in question here are the ovaries in women and the testes in men, in both cases being responsible for the growth and development of the reproductive organs and for sexual behavior. The ovaries release the female steroids estrogen, progesterone, and relaxin, whereas the testes release the male steroidal androgens, including testosterone.

Testosterone

In the male, the secretion of testosterone by the testes increases strongly at puberty. As a result, the facial and other hair thickens, the voice becomes deeper, and long bones begin their rapid growth. At this time, the body loses fat and becomes stronger and more muscular, and the generation of sperm is begun [858]. It appears that the level of testosterone in the male body during

---

3   The alpha and beta cells of the pancreas are not to be confused with the alpha and beta cells of the heart and the vascular system, nor with the response of the latter to the catecholamines, as discussed in Subsection 6.B, page 213.

development is just as important a determinant for behavior as is the level in adulthood. Androgen production remains relatively constant in the male into the seventh or eighth decade, especially as compared with the swings of the sex-hormone levels in mature women; i.e., testosterone levels in males fall by only 50 percent on going from age forty years to age seventy years. As the gonadal hormone levels shift in older men and women, they tend to move toward one another, so that in old age, men and women become more alike, from the hormonal point of view.

Normal concentrations of testosterone act to sharpen one's focus and concentration on a particular subject but lessen one's ability to do several things at once; for example, to press out through the big toe, straighten the leg, lift the inner thigh, lift the ribs, pull the shoulder blades down, and lift the chest. Testosterone levels are low in vegetarians, and it is believed that *yogasana* practice also works to lower testosterone levels. Men who proclaim themselves to be madly in love have lower than normal testosterone levels, whereas women who are madly in love have higher than normal testosterone levels. Both sexes, when madly in love, have considerably elevated levels of the stress hormone cortisol.

Because the brain has a huge number of testosterone receptors and shows high levels of testosterone conversion products, it is of interest to ask in what way testosterone functions in the brain. It appears that stressful situations rapidly decrease the level of testosterone in the brain, leading to "irritable male syndrome," a condition that is often attributed instead to changes in cortisol concentrations, resulting in depression; however, testosterone appears to be a strong factor in this as well [623]. On the other hand, ingestion of alcohol leads to an immediate upward spike in the concentration of brain testosterone. High levels of testosterone depress the immune system.

Excess testosterone in utero, either from the mother or the embryo, is known to temporarily inhibit left-cerebral hemisphere development, so that an overly developed right hemisphere and correspondingly underdeveloped left hemisphere can result. As an adult, such asymmetric cerebral development can lead to autism, homosexuality, left-handedness, dyslexia, the ring finger of the right hand being significantly longer than the index finger of that hand, and enhanced musical ability [108a, 593]. Extreme differences in index-finger and ring-finger lengths correlate with physical aggressiveness in men.[4]

Estrogen and Progesterone

Men and women produce both estrogen and testosterone, but in differing amounts. In men, estrogen has a key function in the regulation of sperm production, and estrogen-like compounds in the environment are a real threat to men's fertility. The testosterone normally produced in a woman's body by the adrenal cortex is only 6–8 percent of that normally found in men, but women appear to be much more sensitive to low concentrations of the hormone than are men. The sex hormones also exert actions on nonsexual structures, such as the muscles and skin [858].

In maturing young women, estrogen and progesterone from the ovaries spur the development of breasts, the uterus, the fallopian tubes, and the vagina; at the same time, they slow the growth of

---

4   While in utero, the fetus is exposed to both testosterone and to estrogen, with the first of these hormones promoting the growth of the fourth digit (4d, the ring finger) and the second of these promoting the growth of the second digit (2d, the index finger). The ratio of the lengths of these two digits on the right hand (the 2d:4d ratio) is indicative of the relative masculinization or feminization of a person due to the relative proportions of these two hormones while in utero. Women most often have a 2d:4d ratio of 1.0, whereas for men, it can be as low as 0.96. Among adults of both sexes, high ratios of 2d:4d correlate with a high incidence of neuroticism, whereas low ratios signal a higher than average aerobic efficiency. Gay men tend toward having a high 2d:4d ratio, and lesbian women generally tend toward having a low ratio. Among all men, those with the lowest ratios have the largest number of sexual encounters and the most children; among all women, those with the highest ratios are the most fertile. Women with high ratios seem to be more susceptible to breast and cervical cancers, and men with lower ratios tend to be more susceptible to heart attack [210a].

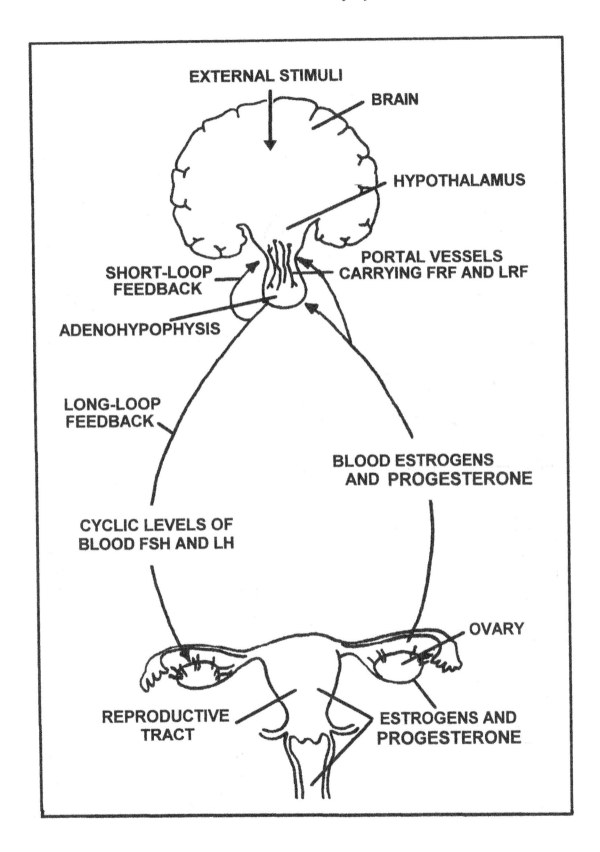

Figure 6.B-3. Hormonal paths by which the brain and the female reproductive tract influence one another. The abbreviations are as follows: FSH is follicle stimulating hormone; LH is luteinizing hormone; FRF is follicle stimulating hormone-releasing factor; and LRF is luteinizing hormone releasing factor.

the long bones, regulate the muscle tone in the urinary tract, control bone density, and regulate fluid retention [71]. The ovaries also produce inhibin, a hormone that acts on the pituitary and hypothalamus to restrict the production of gonadotropin releasing factor and of follicle stimulating hormone. The hormonal paths by which the brain and the female reproductive apparatus influence one another are shown in figure 6.B-3.

Progesterone is secreted by the corpus luteum and the placenta and is responsible for preparing and sustaining the female body for pregnancy. The corpus luteum excretes progesterone after ovulation in order to prepare the endometrium for pregnancy, but if there is no pregnancy, then secretion wanes, and menstruation begins. If a pregnancy is begun, then the placenta takes over and supplies progesterone. The drug RU-486 blocks progesterone receptor sites and so blocks pregnancy [450].

The "estrogens" are really a family of closely related hormones. Before menopause, the key actor is estradiol, a hormone that helps the reproductive system to mature. At menopause, there is a shift of relative importance, with estrone then becoming important; it is the loss of estradiol that brings about hot flashes, etc. The testosterone level in women also falls at menopause, but the sex drive can remain high as long as the ovaries remain intact (see also Section 21.C, page 748).

Excess Hormones

In regard to an excess of the gonadal hormones, if estrogen is present in too large amounts in the womb during a pregnancy, the cerebral asymmetry is opposite to that which occurs if excess testosterone is present, and this can result in a child having an index finger much longer than the ring finger, a feminine personality, and a higher than normal tendency toward breast cancer.

It is strange but interesting that when a gonad is removed in either a male or a female, the intraocular pressure in the opposite eye is significantly lowered [678]. If both gonads are removed, then the intraocular pressure drops in both eyes. This is an example of "pure nervous feedback" from an endocrine organ. Intraocular pressure also can be lowered by meditation and yogic relaxation.

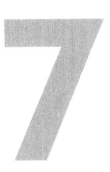

The Bones and Joints

7

Section 7.A: Bone Structure and Development

Importance of Bone

Most people equate "bones" with "skeleton" and so come to think of bones as hard, inert, dead objects—Mother Nature's rigid reinforcing rods. Though Rolf [714] states, "The function of bone, any bone, is to serve as a sophisticated, curved thrusting bar, holding softer myofacial tissue apart," the importance of bone goes far beyond being an inert structural element [582].

True, bone is the mechanically rigid scaffolding holding the body upright against the forces of gravity and other accelerations, and it also acts as the lever arm for muscle action; however, the bones of human beings are themselves very much alive. Compared to flesh, it is easy to think of bone as rigid, but in fact, it too is elastic and can be bent and stretched. In response to internal and external stimuli, bone can be removed and replaced in the processes of growth and repair (Section 7.C, page 235), and as with many other body tissues, bone also is served by a vascular system and nerves; the periosteum surrounding the bone has channels for the transport of blood, lymph, and neural signals into and out of the more solid parts of every bone [450]. Bones also are able to synthesize proteins that are protective against pathogenic organisms that may find their way to the bone surface.

Bone is found only in vertebrate animals; teeth are a form of bone [6].

In addition to bracing the soft tissues of the body, bones such as the ribs and those of the skull also offer protection to more vulnerable internal organs, such as the viscera and the brain. As with the skin (Section 13.A, page 501), and in contrast to the nerves and muscles, the bones are able to renew themselves throughout the life of the body.

Bones also play major roles in many important biochemical processes in the body. As will be seen, several important components of the blood are manufactured within the long and short bones of the body, components that are critical for both respiration and immunity. Bones are the source of all blood cells; bone marrow fills all of the empty pores in cancellous bone.

Finally, the bones are the body's storehouse of calcium and phosphorus, elements essential to skeletal stability, to nerve conduction, and hence to muscle action. Ninety-nine percent of the body's store of Ca^{2+} is in the bones. Most relevant to a discussion of the functioning of bones are the joints formed by two bones that come into end-to-end contact, the ligaments that act to join one bone to its neighbor, and the tendons and aponeuroses that connect the muscles to the bones.

Fetal Development

In the mesoderm phase of fetal development (approximately the first two weeks after fertilization), the body tissue is a soft, jelly-like mass of collagen protein containing areas of more rigid cartilage (Section 12.A, page 481). Wherever this cartilage is penetrated by blood vessels, inorganic

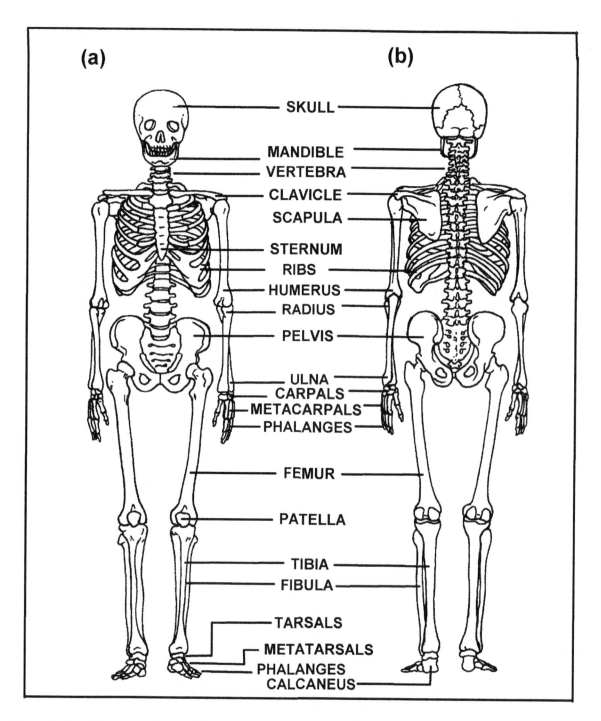

Figure 7.A-1. The major bones of the human body and the cartilage of the rib cage; the scapulae are not visible in the frontal view (**a**) but can be seen in the rear view (**b**).

hydroxyapatite crystals begin to form within the collagen, and ossification (bone formation) takes place, with different long bones forming at different times. Thus, the cartilaginous tissues of the fetus are models for the long bones that are to be formed from them [422, 714, 878]. Because

the cartilaginous tissue is itself laid down in response to mechanical stresses in the fetus [603], this mechanism places the bones just where they can do the most good.

Once an infant is born, the gravitational stress on the infant is ongoing and acts further to convert cartilage into bone. For example, the bones of the pelvis in the newborn are distinct and poorly joined until the infant starts to walk, at which time the gravitational stress on the pelvis initiates the formation and strengthening of the hip sockets by knitting several bones in the area into one. As with the bone remodeling taking place in the pelvis, the shapes of infant and adult vertebrae are significantly different, for those of the infant lack bony processes (figure 8.A-2); however, as the infant sits and then stands, the use of the spinal muscles stresses the spinal cartilage and molds the vertebrae so as to form strong anchors for muscle attachment [714]. The bone remodeling discussed here is also at work in the changes mentioned in Box 8.A-1, page 270.[1]

In contrast to the growth pattern of the long bones, the flat bones of the skull, the mandible, and the collarbone form directly from a tissue called periosteum, without going through the intermediate process of cartilage modeling. Such flat bones are the source of red bone marrow.

Bone Numbers

The bones of the adult human body can be divided into two groups: the eighty bones of the skull, vertebral column, pelvis, and ribs that form the axial skeleton, and the 126 bones of the upper and lower limbs that form the appendicular skeleton. The human skeleton is about 15 percent of the total body weight. The 206 bones of the adult skeleton are derived from the 270 to 300 bones of the infant skeleton by the fusion of many bone pairs. This implies a corresponding decrease in the number of joints in the body and in the body's flexibility on reaching maturity. The major bones of the body are named in figure 7.A-1.

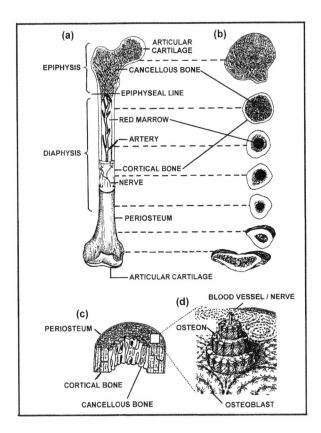

Figure 7.A-2. (a) Structural components of a long but immature bone. (b) Cross sections of the long bone, showing the internal distribution of cortical and cancellous bone and the presence of bone marrow within the bone. (c, d) Microscopic bone structure, showing the osteons (also known as Haversian channels) carrying the blood vessels and nerves within the bone [432].

Long Bones

The major components of the immature long bone, as found in the arms and legs, are shown in figure 7.A-2; such a long bone consists of a long hollow shaft (the diaphysis) constructed of high-density cortical or compact bone and end caps (epiphyses), which are constructed of a rather open network of spongy bone called cancellous or trabecular bone. The flared ends of the long bones offer large surface areas over which to distribute the forces of loading. In the cancellous bone at the ends of long bones and in the vertebrae of the spine, the internal structure of the

---

1   The delayed conversion of cartilage into bone in the infant makes sense if the child's energy is better spent on body growth or brain development rather than on building bones that won't be used for months or years into the future.

spongy cancellous bone at first appears to be randomly aligned; but in fact, the lattice is oriented so as to support external compressive stresses, with struts crossing at right angles for maximum strength (figure 7.A-2**a**). Furthermore, cancellous bone is light in weight and slowly can change the orientation of its struts in order to accommodate new stresses over time, Subsection 7.C, page 235. The diaphysis structure is ideal for resisting bending forces, as the outermost layers of the cortical bone have mutually perpendicular fibril orientations for maximum strength.

Bone Growth

Up to age twenty years, the diaphysis and the epiphyses of a long bone are separated by a cartilaginous region (the growth plate or epiphyseal line; figure 7.A-2**a**), into which they both grow when directed to do so by the growth hormone secreted by the pituitary gland [878] (see Subsection 7.B, page 233). Bone growth is stimulated by the release of spurts of growth hormone at night; amazingly, careful X-ray measurements actually show the hour-by-hour growth of the long bones as the hormone is periodically released in spurts!

When growing, the ends of the bones are coated with fresh cartilage by chondroblast cells, and this is then converted into bone material by the osteoblasts; however, the release of estrogen in both men and women at maturity suppresses the chondroblast action, the active growth areas become calcified, and the long bones then stop their growth [858]. This estrogen-driven union of the epiphyses with the shafts of the long bones causes the skeletons of females to stop growing a few years sooner than those of males, and young women who are deficient in estrogen are often several inches taller than their more normal female friends, in all cases due to the timely or untimely impact of hormonal factors. In contrast, older women who are deficient in estrogen when going through menopause, and older men who are deficient in testosterone, can suffer significant bone loss (see Subsection 7.G, page 254).

Joint Lubrication

Once sexual maturity is reached, the growing face on each end of a long bone fuses under the action of estrogen, and bone growth is terminated. However, this is not to say that mature bone is otherwise inactive, for bone repair and remodeling of extant bone continue into old age. Moreover, even after the cessation of bone growth, a relatively small amount of virgin cartilage remains in the joints of the arms and legs, the front ribs, at the nose and ears, and in the intervertebral discs. The cartilage that remains in the joints serves as a lubricant, insuring frictionless motion around the joints.

Long bones contact one another end to end at their articular surfaces (figure 7.A-2**a**). These surfaces are covered with cartilage and press on one another; however, their relative motion is lubricated not only by the cartilage, but also by the synovial fluid secreted by the lining of the joint's capsule (Subsection 7.D, page 239). In contrast, there is no need for lubrication in the skull and shoulder blades, for they are plate-like bones and derive their strength from a structure in which two layers of stiff cortical bone are sandwiched around a third layer of spongy cancellous bone, much like corrugated cardboard [6]. This offers a high degree of compressive strength against blows from outside the body but does not allow for any significant relative motion of the bone parts.

Bone Marrow

The central channel of long bone is filled with marrow; in adults, this marrow is yellow and fatty and has no recognized function in the body. However, red marrow persists in adults in the cancellous bone of the spine, ribs, and skull. The marrow of the bones of the skull, ribs, and spine produces blood platelets at the rate of ten million per minute, all in aid of fighting invading organisms and repairing any breaks in the vascular plumbing (Subsection 14.B, page 559). Red blood cells also have their origin in the bone marrow. Thus, the red marrow within the bones is seen to be a chemical factory of great importance to our health and well-being. The percentage of cells within various bones producing platelets falls with age, dropping to close to zero for the tibia and femur but remaining relatively high for the vertebrae and sternum. It would be of great interest to know if these percentages were higher in those who practice *yogasana* as compared to the average population.

Periosteum and Endosteum

During the growth phase of a long bone, it is covered on the outside by the periosteum, the outer layer of which is intimately interwoven with the tendons and ligaments bound to the bone; the corresponding covering on the inside of the bone is known as the endosteum and is that part of the bone responsible for radial growth [878]. The bone surface just beneath the periosteum is a thin shell of cortical bone in all bones. In immature bone, solid cortical bone is first deposited in the region of the epiphyseal line (figure 7.A-2**a**) by the osteoblast cells in the endosteum, and on the outer bone surface by osteoblasts in the inner layer of the periosteum. However, osteoclasts in the endosteum then work from the inside out to thin the bone shaft (diaphysis) and to convert cortical to cancellous bone in the epiphyses. The osteoclasts demineralize bone through the action of hydrochloric acid on the inorganic component of the bone (hydroxyapatite). These two bone-cell types, the osteoblasts and the osteoclasts, are active throughout our life, the former depositing bone substance, and the latter destroying it.

The outer covering of bone (periosteum) and the inner lining of bone (endosteum) form a continuous sheath of connective tissue. These inner and outer coverings of the bone are much like the bark of the tree; if the periosteum is breached, the internal bone mass slowly leaks to the outside. Interwoven with this covering is the connective tissue of the ligaments and tendons, the latter of which is contiguous with the connective tissue surrounding the muscles, blood vessels, and organs. The epiphyses are covered with thin layers of hyaline cartilage, which help the bones forming a joint to move easily and with minimum friction; those parts of the bones not in contact with one another are covered instead by periosteum.

Continuity of Connective Tissue

Because almost all muscles are tethered at their ends to different bones, the continuity of the connective tissue extends from one joint to the next, throughout the entire body. In this way, there is formed a continuous head-to-toe web of connective tissue to which bones contribute significantly [632]. The muscle attached to the bone comprising half of a joint has its connective-tissue fibers so tightly interwoven with those of both the periosteum and the endosteum that a contraction of the muscle sufficient to fracture the bone will not pull the muscle's tendon free of the bone. The importance of bones and their connections to other body parts cannot be overestimated. See Rolf [714], Myers [603], and Juhan [422] for further comments on this.

Bone Shapes

The long bones are slightly curved, so that they may serve as shock-absorbing springs, much as the spine is multiply curved (Subsection 8.A, page 268) in order to isolate the brain from the shock of walking, running, etc. The sculpting of a bone into the ideal shape to match its intended function is accomplished using the two complementary cell types, the osteoblasts and the osteoclasts, reacting to the stresses in the bone resulting from its intended use. In contrast to the long bones, the short bones in the body are more often cuboid shaped.

Innervation and Vascularization

As the cartilage of the fetal bones is calcified, narrow passageways are formed within, so that blood vessels and nerves have access to both the outer and the inner regions of the bone. On the microscopic level, the material of the cortical bone is laid down by deposition along the inner surface of the corresponding blood vessel and appears as concentric layers in a cylindrical pattern; each such cylindrical unit is called an osteon (figure 7.A-2**d**). These systems have open central channels, which provide space for connective tissue, afferent and efferent nerve fibers, lymph, and blood vessels and which run not only along the length of the bone, but radially as well, so as to connect the outer periosteum and the inner endosteum. Osteons are not found in the more open structures of cancellous bone [431].

Blood vessels carry raw materials and products to and from the chemical factories active within the bones, whereas the nerves within and upon the bones sense the nature of the mechanical stresses and carry neural signals directing the actions of the bone-building osteoblasts and bone-thinning osteoclasts. Thanks to the stimulation of the pain nerves in the bones, one also can experience bone ache, just as with a headache or a stomach ache. This sensation is especially intense in cases of bone cancer or osteoarthritis. On the other hand, the neurons within the bones also allow the *yogasana* student to sense the extent of the mechanical forces acting on the skeleton while performing the postures. The relevance of *yogasana* practice to maintaining a balance between the opposing actions of the osteoclasts and the osteoblasts is discussed in Subsection 7.B, page 234.

Bone Mechanics

To function in a broad range of situations, bone has to be strong in both compression and tension, and it must combine strength with lightness for reasons of speed and energy. Mother Nature has met these criteria using a composite structure consisting largely of collagen, a flexible organic meshwork (Subsection 12.A, page 483) in which hard microcrystals of the mineral hydroxyapatite are embedded. The synthetic material known as fiberglass is a composite much like Nature's bone, being constructed of inorganic, ceramic hard-glass fibers embedded within a flexible organic-resin matrix [6].

Bone Strength

Mechanically, the collagen component of adult bone offers a material that is strong in tensile stress; it can be stretched reasonably without breaking, but on compression, it buckles easily. On the other hand, because the hydroxyapatite component of bone is a ceramic material that is

strong in compression but weak in tension, the composite matrix of hydroxyapatite crystals suspended within the collagen matrix, as in bone, has the beneficial mechanical properties of each of the component substances. Furthermore, the tensile strength of collagen is doubled by the addition of the mineralization [6]. Compared to cast iron, mature bone is almost as strong, is far more flexible, and is considerably lighter. As all of the forces within a structure must sum to zero when the structure is at mechanical equilibrium, the tensile force of the muscles must be balanced by the compressive resistance of the bones [877]; see Subsection 12.B, page 492. In addition to compressive and tensile stresses, bone is also able to resist shearing and torsional stresses, such as those encountered by the vertebrae when twisting the spine (figures 8.B-4b and 8.B-4c).

Vogel [877] discusses the mechanical properties of materials from two opposing points of view: toughness and stiffness. Toughness refers to the resistance of the material to the propagation of cracks; hard, brittle materials such as glass and pottery are high in stiffness but very low in toughness. In sharp contrast, collagen, the organic component of bone, is very low in stiffness but very high in toughness. Like steel, bone itself is high in toughness, (thanks to its collagen content), and it is also high in stiffness (thanks to its mineral content). The mechanical combination of flexibility and toughness found in bone makes *yogasana* practice possible without too large a risk of injury.

Bone under Stress

For a long bone under compression, the breaking point is about 17 kilograms per square millimeter of cross-sectional area (24,000 pounds per square inch); for the same bone under tension, the breaking point is only about 10 kilograms per square millimeter (14,200 pounds per square inch). Therefore, when a long bone is bent so that the inside of the curved bone is under compression while the outside of the curve is under tension, mechanical failure of the bone occurs on the side under tension; i.e., always on the outer surface of the curved bone. Should a bone be fractured, for obvious reasons, it should be placed under compression (pushing of the two broken bone fragments toward one another) rather than under traction (pulling the broken bones away from one another).

Tubular construction is generally favored for long bones, with the thickness of the bone wall often being 6–20 percent of the bone-shaft radius and the length larger than the width. A bone with a strong, compact shaft offers some resistance to overloading as it bends and twists. However, the apparent strength of long bones is very much dependent upon the tone of the muscles attached to and surrounding the bone in question. Thus, when an inebriated person falls, they are much more likely to break bones than others would, because in the inebriated state, the muscles do not react quickly enough to support the stresses on the bones generated by the fall.

Microstructure

As discussed more fully in Section 7.B, page 233, the collagen in the body takes the form of helical cylinders called fibrils. The relative orientation of the fibrils in the circular layers of the osteons can change in response to local stress. Usually, a layer is composed of, say, right-handed collagen helices, while adjacent layers are built of left-handed helices [6]. Additionally, some bone layers may be rich in collagen in response to the need to support tensile loading, whereas others may be richer in hydroxyapatite in order to supply more compressive resistance locally.

In order for a bone to be strong in all directions, all the fibrils in each layer must lie parallel to one another, and the fibrils in adjacent layers must have directions that are skewed with respect to those of its neighbors. In this way, the bone structure gains strength in the same way that plywood does; i.e., by using a layered structure in which the direction of highest strength varies from one layer to the next due to the orientation of rod-like fibers.

As discussed in Subsection 8.A, page 268, the spine is strengthened by the curvature of its sections (in comparison to a straight rod of the same material) and is also more flexible due to the

alternating curvature. So too does it seem to be with the long bones, for they are all more or less curved, presumably gaining both strength and flexibility thereby.

Applying the above to the *yogasanas,* consider first the practice of *adho mukha vrksasana,* the full-arm balance. Though there is a compressive load on the humeral bones of the upper arms (figure 7.A-1) in this posture as they support the weight of the trunk and legs, these bones do not bow noticeably outward under their load, for the hydroxyapatite within strengthens them so that they can resist compressive forces. Moreover, the practice of this compressive type of posture promotes the formation of a higher proportion of hydroxyapatite within the humeral bones. In contrast, when doing *paschimottanasana* with the arms vigorously extended so as to bring the hands beyond the feet, the tension in the arms is more tensile than compressive, and the effect of the posture on the bones of the arms will be to increase slightly the proportion of collagen in them. Similarly, these bones of the arms are under tensile stress when hanging from the wall ropes and under compressive stress when in *adho mukha svanasana.* All of the stresses on the bones when so loaded in the *yogasanas* will work to raise bone density whether the stresses are tensile or compressive.

When muscular action is constantly drawn upon to hold the bones in place in our everyday posture, the muscles are pulled onto the bones and become more bone-like in their hardness, compaction, and density. Moreover, with the bones and the muscles acting this way, there is no opportunity for openness or fluidity within the body, no flow of the *pranic* energy, no release of the tension, no relaxation, and no meditation. Working as we do in the gravitational field (see Appendix IV, page 851), we must work with the bones in such an intelligent way that the gravitational force is resisted by the bony skeleton, whereas the muscles not only do minimum work in holding the bones in their proper positions [444] but also work to keep the joints from collapsing. These ideas have special relevance when doing the balancing *yogasanas* (Appendix V, page 873).

Bones as Anchors

The desired action of a muscle contraction in *yogasana* practice is to force a movement of a particular bone in a particular direction with respect to the other bones of the body. In order to achieve this desired action, it is necessary that the prime mover muscle have an anchor against which it can work. Most often, it is other bones that serve as the anchors, but only if they are themselves held motionless by yet other muscles (including antagonists) or by the gravitational attraction of a particular body part pressing onto the floor. This is especially true when twisting or lengthening the spine, as discussed below. Other examples of bones serving as anchors are presented in Subsection 11.F, page 469.

The importance of having an anchor against which to rotate is easily demonstrated by sitting with the legs crossed on a yoga mat on a polished floor with the left shoulder close to the wall. If you now turn to face the wall, placing the left hand on the wall and the right hand on the floor, and press the left hand against the wall, your shoulders will turn with respect to your hips, and a deep spinal rotation results. Compare this with the twist obtained by placing an opened blanket instead on the polished floor and sitting with crossed legs on the blanket with the left shoulder close to the wall. Turn to the left to face toward the wall, place the left hand on the wall at shoulder height, and then press the left hand against the wall so as to push the left shoulder further from the wall and so go deeper into the spinal twist. As there is nothing to resist the rotation in this case, pressing the left hand to the wall turns the **entire** body but does not rotate the shoulders with respect to the pelvis. In the first case, one rotates the upper spine with respect to the pelvic anchor formed by the sitting bones on the yoga mat, whereas only a weak twist results in the second example, as there is no resisting pelvic anchor when sitting on a slippery surface.

In a similar way, when sitting sideways on a metal chair seat for *bharadvajasana I* to the left, with the left hand pressing the back of the chair, note that the relative spinal twist of the shoulders with respect to the pelvis is minimal, because the pelvis also tends to rotate in the same direction as the shoulders, as evidenced by the right knee being far forward of the left knee. If, instead, the right femur is pulled into its hip socket so that the knees remain touching, then the pelvic action offers resistance to the rotation of the shoulders by rotating in a disrotatory sense (Subsection 8.B, page 298) with respect to the shoulder girdle. The resistance of the pelvis to rotation of the shoulders leads to a deeper twist. Similarly, placing a belt around the tops of the thighs of a student in *adho mukha svanasana* and pulling the belt up and backward as the student walks the hands forward gives the student an anchor against which to work, so as to lengthen and reduce the curvatures of the spine in this posture. Similar actions against an anchor are resorted to when twisting in *parivrtta parsvakonasana, parivrtta janu sirsasana, maricyasana III, parivrtta trikonasana*, etc.

Spinal rotation when inverted in *sarvangasana* or in *sirsasana* again is possible because the head and shoulders are pinned to the floor, and the feet rotate against this anchor so as to rotate the spine. Indeed, it is risky to allow the neck or shoulders to rotate when the neck bears one's weight, as is the case in these postures.

The use of internal anchors is closely related to the phenomenon of co-contraction (Subsection 11.A, page 422) in which there is a simultaneous contraction of an agonist muscle and its antagonist. Thus, in *tadasana,* there is the simultaneous pressing of the upper thighs backward (figure 9.B-4a) and the pulling of the buttocks toward the heels (figure 9.B-4b); these two actions (simultaneous contraction of both the psoas and the gluteus maximus) working to tip the pelvis in opposite senses also work against one another to lift the pelvis off the femoral heads and the rib cage away from the pelvis (figure 9.B-4c). This subject is also discussed in Subsection 11.F, page 468.

The anchoring of specific parts of the anatomy so that other parts can pull against them while in the *yogasana* postures is also mirrored within each of the muscle sarcomeres, where the myosin myofilaments serve as anchors against which the actin myofilaments work in order to produce motion (Subsection 11.A, page 381).

Bone Density

Bone density is defined as the weight of a bone divided by its volume; the density of cancellous bone is understandably low due to its open, low-mass structure, whereas that of cortical bone is high, for there are no open spaces in it to lower the density. The question of bone density is especially relevant to the condition of osteoporosis faced by the elderly (Section 7.G, page 254) and should not be confused with bone mass, which considers the total weight of bone but not the weight per unit volume. Thus, the bone mass of a large person may be large, while the bone density may be only normal or even subnormal.

When a bone is compressively stressed at a level below that of its breaking point, the general reaction is a thickening and strengthening of the bone to raise its density in the region of maximum stress. This higher bone density is one of the general health benefits of *yogasana* practice vis-à-vis the skeleton (Subsection 7.G, page 256).

Given this, it is understandable that bone mass is lost rapidly when gravitational or muscular stress is removed from the skeleton, as when weightless, resting in bed, or recovering from a spinal cord injury. The loss of bone mass amounts to 1 percent per month of bed rest, but once stress is applied to bone, the piezoelectric effect promotes renewed bone growth (Subsection 7.C, page 237). It is no surprise, then, that the density of the femur bone is largest in weight lifters and decreases in this order: shot and discus throwers, runners and soccer players (who do run considerable distances but who only support their body weight while doing so), cyclists, and is least in swimmers, whose skeletons experience very little gravitational stress due to their neutral buoyancy in water [524]. Because the mineral component of bone has a higher density than does the organic component, a higher percentage of mineralization will translate into a higher bone density, and a lower percentage of mineralization will translate into a lower bone density. However, these changes in the extent of mineralization may have repercussions in regard to the brittleness or toughness of the bone.

The truth of the "use it or lose it" aphorism with respect to bone density is shown clearly by studies of the two arms of tennis players; in these athletes, the bones of the racquet arms have about 20 percent higher bone densities than those of the other arm [69, 618]. The question of the impact of exercise on bone density is addressed further in Section 7.G, page 256.

Section 7.B: Bone Chemistry

Collagen

When fully developed, bone is a chemical mixture of 35 percent organic matter (collagen and cell components) and 65 percent hydroxyapatite [$Ca_{10}(PO_4)_6(OH)_2$ or $3Ca_3(PO_4)_2 \cdot Ca(OH)_2$]. If the inorganic hydroxyapatite component of bone is removed by soaking in acid (try a chicken bone in vinegar, for example), the remaining cartilaginous "bone" is so flexible that it can be tied into a knot! Correspondingly, a bone deprived of its organic content by incineration is easily broken by twisting or bending. Within the spectrum of connective-tissue elements based on collagen (see also Subsection 12.A, page 483), bone is among the hardest of them all, as it contains a very high proportion of mineralization; tooth enamel is the hardest material within the body, as it has the largest ratio of hydroxyapatite to organic matter of any structure in the body.

Chemical Structure

Collagen is a protein composed largely of units of the amino acids glycine and proline, strung together in long chains. In the body, the collagen chains intertwine three at a time to form rod-like fibers known as triple helices. In turn, clusters of the triple helices in which the helix axes are parallel are known as fibrils. In the formation of bone, the hydroxyapatite microcrystals are laid down in the 400-angstrom gap that exists between the end of one fibril and its neighbor. Collagen is also a primary component of various other connective

Box 7.B-1: Detoxification of Bone and Tissue

Lead

Because the chemistries of calcium ions (Ca^{2+}) and lead ions (Pb^{2+}) are very similar, a portion of the Ca^{2+} in hydroxyapatite readily can be replaced by Pb^{2+}, if Pb^{2+} should be ingested. This sequestering of the lead in the bones is fortunate, for Pb^{2+} otherwise interferes with brain function, most especially in young children. However, as the bones demineralize in the osteoporotic process (Section 7.G, page 254) or during bed rest, there is a rapid release of stored Pb^{2+} into the body fluids, which can lead to lead intoxication and neuropathy if the lead is not otherwise chelated [878]. On the other hand, as *yogasana* practice promotes bone mineralization and so works against osteoporosis, it can be prophylactic for lead poisoning from bone demineralization.

Organic Toxins

In a way similar to the situation in the bones, ingested pesticides and other organic toxins are stored in part in body fat and may be released during extreme dieting. The effects of *yogasana* work can be similar to dieting, in that *yogasana* work may promote a short period of detoxification as both the liver and the body fat release their toxic burdens into the circulatory system. The detoxification is evident in beginning students as a momentary nausea following a demanding *yogasana* practice centered on backbending and spinal twists, both of which tend to have a wringing action on the liver. Concomitant with this detoxification in beginners, there is a foul odor released into the air through the skin and breath, such that the studio must be aired out before others can come in to work. This detoxification reaction may be present for a month or two, until the body finally clears itself of its toxic burden.

Toxins also may be trapped within the web of connective tissue, specifically within the ground substance (Section 12.A, page 485) [764], and the *yogasanas* may then act to release them into the lymphatic system for eventual excretion.

---

tissues in the body and is discussed as such in Section 12.A, page 483.

The bones and several of the internal organs of the body function in part as storehouses for chemicals that are either intentionally or unintentionally present in the body. On occasion, these stores may be emptied on a relatively short time scale, with the inadvertent release of high levels of toxins into the bloodstream. See Box 7.B-1 (above), for a discussion of this detoxification process in the beginning *yogasana* student.

Hormonal Control of Ca^{2+} in Body Fluids

In contrast to the bone-building action of the osteoblasts, the osteoclasts within bone function to demineralize bone by locally excreting concentrated hydrochloric acid [878], which acts both to loosen the collagen matrix and to dissolve the hydroxyapatite. This destructive action can be beneficial or harmful, depending upon many factors, but generally serves an important and useful purpose: the bones are the body's storehouse of Ca^{2+}

and, on receiving a hormonal signal, the osteoclasts can be activated to demineralize the bones and so supply Ca^{2+} to the body fluids. Thus, as the fetus develops within a pregnant woman, in order to form its own bones, its drawing of Ca^{2+} from the mother's skeleton is made possible by osteoclastic action in the mother's body. In contrast, the osteoblasts remove Ca^{2+} from the body fluids and sequester it in the hydroxyapatite of the bones. As seen from the chemical formula for hydroxyapatite given above, the removal or deposition of hydroxyapatite is accompanied by the corresponding removal or deposition of phosphorus as PO_4^{3-} ion.

Parathyroid Hormone

Ninety-nine percent of the body's Ca^{2+} is stored within the bones. In order to maintain Ca^{2+} homeostasis in the body fluids, there is an ongoing absorption of Ca^{2+} from the body fluids into the bones and a release of the Ca^{2+} from the bones, each driven by hormonal regulation of the osteoblasts and osteoclasts, respectively [431, 858]. The parathyroid glands (figure 6.A-1) release a simple polypeptide hormone (parathyroid hormone or PTH; Section 6.B, page 216) when the concentration of Ca^{2+} is too low in the blood; PHT simultaneously represses the bone-building of the osteoblasts while activating the Ca^{2+}-releasing actions of the osteoclasts. If the Ca^{2+} concentration were to remain too low in the blood due to inadequate parathyroid secretion, then muscle twitching, stiffness, spasm, and convulsions could follow. On the other hand, if the parathyroid is overactive, too much Ca^{2+} is leached from the bones, and they weaken, as do the muscles. PTH is the engine that drives the bone loss that results in osteoporosis; when a body is sedentary, as when confined to bed, the action of PTH continues, and the bones are thinned.

Calcitonin

A second hormone, calcitonin, originates in the thyroid gland (figure 6.A-1) and acts to counter the effects of excess PTH; i.e., it inhibits osteoclast activity and leads to a stabilization of the concentration of Ca^{2+} in the blood; see also

Section 6.B, page 216. The importance of maintaining the proper levels of Ca^{2+} throughout the body cannot be exaggerated, for not only is Ca^{2+} a major constituent of bone, but it is also an important player in muscle and nerve function; is involved in the release and actions of many hormones, neurotransmitters and enzymes; affects membrane permeability; is active in the acid/base pH buffering of the blood; and is essential for blood clotting [858].

Section 7.C: Bone Repair and Remodeling

Injury and Repair

Microfractures

When, in the normal course of an active life, a bone should suffer a microfracture, the local osteoclasts first clear damaged material from the site by reabsorption (figure 7.C-1a). The bone-building osteoblasts then fill the cavity formed by the osteoclastic action with an organic matrix (hyaline cartilage), which is then mineralized to form new bone (figure 7.C-1e) [524]. This process of absorption and redeposition of bone works not only to repair fractured bone but also to remove bone from areas of little use and then to redeposit it in distant areas needing more mechanical support; the process occurs most often while one sleeps.

The wear and tear of an active lifestyle leads unavoidably to small cracks and tears in our bones, and these microfractures are under constant repair; as mentioned in Subsection 7.A, page 230, bone is not only stiff but is also tough, due to its ability to repair microfractures. However, if there is unreasonably high stress for a long time on a bone without a rest period for repair, a stress fracture may occur in which the insignificant bone crack finally becomes a significant bone fracture.

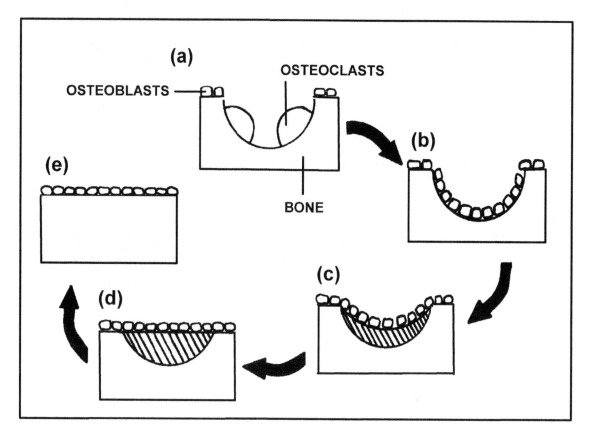

Figure 7.C-1. The bone-remodeling process begins with the site of a microfracture being cleared by osteoclasts (**a**), followed by osteoblastic activity at the site to backfill the cavity with organic material, (**b**) and (**c**), which is then mineralized (**d**) to form new bone (**e**).

Bone Fracture

Once a bone is fractured, primitive bone cells and macrophages gather at the point of fracture in order to span the gap with collagen bridges. At the same time, the osteoclasts and osteoblasts work in the area of the break in order to remodel nearby bone damage. Growth hormones then work to strengthen the new bone growth. The directions of the osteons (figure 7.A-2**d**) in the new bone growth do not necessarily follow those of the surrounding older bone and so can resist fracture along the old fault line. Though formal bone lengthening ceases at about age twenty-five years, the osteoblasts and osteoclasts remain active as the agents for repair and remodeling, albeit at slower rates as we age. The entire skeleton will be remodeled in a period of about ten years on average, meaning that the shape of a bone can be changed significantly in that time if the stress on it is significant and ongoing for ten years or so.

In the young child, the bones have a higher proportion of collagen, giving them more tensile strength in regard to bending or breaking, and also a mechanism for rapid healing, should they break. On the other hand, in the older person, the collagen of the bones is more frayed, and the proportion of collagen is lower than in the bones of the young; i.e., the percentage of brittle hydroxyapatite is higher in the older body, and so its bones are more easily broken by tensile stress. When broken in an older person, such bones are slow to heal, unless the broken ends are pinned together [603].

Atrophy and Inactivity

Bones generally respond to submaximal stress by becoming thicker and stronger, with osteoblasts becoming more active than osteoclasts. However, the balance between these two cell functions is reversed when there is no stress on the bone in question. If a bone is not used as a structural element, demineralization and consequent weakening soon follow. Thus, in both space flight and in horizontal bed rest, osteoblast activity declines and bones atrophy, often along the lines of previous fractures.

Healing

With respect to the repair of broken bones, perhaps the largest benefit of *yogasana* practice is in the increased circulation of body fluids that occurs during the practice. Thus, for example, one would not want to do *vrksasana* on a leg having a broken ankle, but *viparita karani* (and other inversions that can be sustained for minutes on end) would be nonthreatening to the injury yet would encourage healing by promoting the flow of blood through the injured area. Interestingly, bone surgeons can use the phenomenon of negative bone stress (compression) to promote rapid healing of fractures. In this, they hold the two ends of the broken bone immobile and in close proximity, using an external mechanical clamp that allows normal use of the bone while it is under compressive stress.

Low-frequency (20–50 hertz) mechanical stimulation of injured bone also speeds recovery. Cats often purr when injured, and the purr frequency is often in this range; it is postulated that this purring is self-healing. It is also well known that the external application of voltage at the site of a broken bone speeds mending of the fracture [863].

The Remodeling Response to Mechanical Stress

As was pointed out above, there are several ways in which bone is alive. To this list must be added the remarkable property of "remodeling," a process most active before reaching sexual maturity. At any one time, it is estimated that 5 percent of the bone mass of the body is undergoing regular reabsorption and redeposition through remodeling [878]. When remodeling, cancellous bone reforms under pressure, dissolving in one place and growing in another. However, it is also possible that if the stress is constant and excessive, then the bone in the stressed region will atrophy rather than grow [288].

As an example of bone remodeling, suppose a foot injury causes one to walk on the left outer heel (the calcaneus, figure 7.A-1**b**). Under direction of the autonomic system, bone remodeling will commence with reinforcement of the bone strength in that area, by dissolving bone from the left inner heel, where it is no longer needed, and redepositing it on the left outer heel. Assuming that the bone deposition was "normal" before the injury, one sees that after bone remodeling, the bone has been encouraged to take an abnormal shape (strong on the outside, weak on the inside), which, in special situations, may prove to be a problem (say, balancing on that foot and ankle in *virabhadrasana III*).

If the stress on a bone changes slowly in magnitude or direction, the affected bone can change its internal architecture through remodeling, so as to accommodate the shifting stress. In this way, bones can be reshaped, lengthened, and realigned (or misaligned), even though there has been no separation of bone substance as in a fracture.

The remodeling of bone in response to an externally applied stress has its analog in the world of trees, where Japanese horticulturists hang weights on tree limbs in order to coax them into more aesthetic positions. In this process, the wood structure of cellulose and lignin slowly is altered to accommodate the stress, much as in the case of the collagen and hydroxyapatite in bone.

Piezoelectric Signaling

How do the osteoclasts know where to dissolve bone and the osteoblasts know where to lay down a cancellous web of bone so that it is mechanically most supportive? I hypothesize that this is accomplished using the known piezoelectric properties of bone [515]. A large number of biological materials are known to be piezoelectric; when these materials are stressed mechanically, they develop a significant electrical voltage on their surfaces in proportion to the extent of the stress, with the voltage having an electrical sign (+ or -) depending upon whether the stress is tensile (positive) or compressive (negative).[2] Because bone is piezoelectric, applying stress to a bone leads to a particular pattern of induced positive and negative local voltages on its surface, due to the particular local pattern of tension and compression. When the afferent nerve endings within the bone detect these stress-induced voltage changes, the signals are sent to subconscious areas of the brain for processing. Following this, the proper nerves are energized via the autonomic nervous system, activating the osteoclasts to remove bone in areas of lowered stress and the osteoblasts to deposit bone in areas of higher stress, thus remodeling the bone so as to be more supportive of the stress. It is known that the osteoblasts and osteoclasts in the body communicate with and influence one another using two neuroproteins that bind to the receptor sites on the bone-cell surfaces [866].

The thinning of bone by the osteoclastic cells is performed by these cells through the agency of hydrochloric acid, the same substance used in digestion within the stomach (Subsection 19.A, page 707). However, because no hydrochloric acid is released in the vicinity of bone that bears the appropriate piezoelectric charge, bones that are stressed through exercise remain thick (or even becomes thicker); whereas bones that are not stressed, such as those of astronauts in orbit or patients lying in their sickbeds, are weakened by acidic dissolution, exactly as with the chicken bone dissolving in vinegar (Subsection 7.B, page 233).

It should be pointed out that the bone remodeling process involving both osteoblasts and osteoclasts is a distinctly different process from that involving these cells to change the Ca^{2+} levels

in the blood. In the latter situation (Subsection 7.B, page 234), there is hormonal activation or inhibition on a global scale in order to satisfy the body's need for Ca^{2+} homeostasis in the blood; whereas in the case of remodeling, the action is local, probably is driven by neural signals, and is aimed at reconfiguring local bone structure in response to local mechanical stresses.

Chronic Loading

It is obvious from what is said above that if one were to always carry a heavy weight from the left shoulder while walking, there would be a slow but definite asymmetric remodeling response of the bones in the skeleton in support of the asymmetric load. Though not as obvious, it is just as true that the "load" on the skeleton can be a chronic asymmetric tension in the muscles, which results in a chronic pull on the bones to which they are attached, resulting in a slow but definite asymmetric remodeling response of the bones to the perceived loading. In this way, the shapes of bones and the orientations of their structural elements also can be changed by excessive and chronic muscle tension [422].

Effects of Muscle Stress

As a corollary to the above, when the muscular stresses on the bones are released or realigned, as through *yogasana* practice, the internal structures of the relevant bones will change to accommodate the shifting stress. In this way, the proper practice of *yogasana*, with attention to elongation and alignment, will slowly pull the elements of the body into a new and more functional shape with a tendency toward higher symmetry.

The normal pull of the muscles on the bones is sufficient over time to remodel the bones to suit the particular pattern of stress that they apply to the bone. That level of stress can be multiplied and the remodeling speeded if the muscles so involved work in an active and long-lasting way to stress the bones. This occurs for the ankle, for example, when one stands on one foot in *vrksasana* or on two feet on a vibrating platform [683], where one works the muscles around the ankle to maintain balance in both cases.

---

2   In fact, according to Oschman [637], almost all of the tissues of the body are capable of developing electrical charges on their surfaces when stressed mechanically. For piezoelectric materials such as these, the body then has a simple means of determining the patterns of induced mechanical stress if it can read the voltage pattern. This piezoelectric phenomenon is invoked in the discussion of the sensing of stress in the perineural nervous system (Subsection 2.C, page 26).

Yet another factor in bone health is mentioned by Lasater [736]; when the body is under stress, the acidity of the blood increases (pH decreases), and this tends then to slowly destroy bone, much as the osteoclasts use hydrochloric acid to thin bone; however, in this case, performing the relaxing *yogasanas* brings the pH back to the basic side.

Section 7.D: The Joints

The Bones Form the Joints

Tendons connect muscle to bone and serve to convert muscle power into motion of the bone. Adjacent bones that are in contact at their articular surfaces form a joint; the joints between bones are generally of two types [295, 431, 632]. In the first type, there is little or no motion intended (as between the plates of the skull or between the tibia and fibula of the lower leg), and the joint is held together by strong bands of fibrous or cartilaginous tissue, as is also the case in the cartilaginous joint of the pubic symphysis under normal conditions. The second type of joint is the synovial joint. Synovial joints have a rather open structure bone-to-bone compared to the fibrous or cartilaginous joint and are able to move through relatively large ranges of motion.

Synovial Joints

In joints in which movement of the bones is relatively large (as with the knee, hip, and shoulder joints), the ends of the bones not only are covered with smooth cartilaginous coatings, but the joint is further provided with an internal system of lubrication. Such synovial joints are encapsulated by a stout outer covering (the joint capsule) and an inner synovial membrane that lubricates the joint by exuding synovial fluid into the joint capsule (figure 7.D-1a). This fluid reduces the friction between the bones in a joint when moving against one another by keeping the coverings of the ends of the bones soft and

moist; it is also the medium by which nutrients move from surrounding tissue into the cartilage of the joint, which otherwise has no direct access to nutrients, as it is avascular. The synovial fluid also contains phagocytes of the immune system, which remove cellular debris and envelop any invading organisms. The volume of fluid in the synovial capsule (only 3.5 milliliters in the knee joint) is just sufficient to coat the inner aspects of the joint.

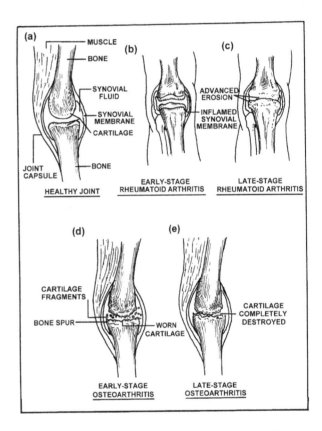

Figure 7.D-1. (a) The internal structure of a normal synovial joint, showing the two bones separated by a cartilage coating and the synovial lining that supplies the joint with lubricating synovial fluid. (b and c) In rheumatoid arthritis, the synovial lining is inflamed and the joint is over-pressured with excess synovial fluid. (d and e) In osteoarthritis, the cartilage has degenerated, and painful spurs may form as the eroded bone in the damaged area attempts to repair itself.

In the healthy hip joint (figure 10.B-1**a**), the lubrication can be so complete that the friction between the ball and socket is less than that between one ice cube sliding on another. When there is no movement in the joint, the synovial fluid becomes as viscous as egg white, eventually allowing the two bones to fuse; however, this viscosity decreases once the joint is used.

Most synovial joints place a concave surface of one bone onto the convex surface of the other, so as to more or less simulate the ball-and-socket arrangement, a configuration of high mechanical stability [878]. For example, this principle is approximated in the knee joint (figure 7.D-1**a**) and, to a much greater extent, in the hip joint, where the ball (the femoral head) is set deeply into the socket, called the acetabulum (figure 10.B-1**a**). In the former, motion is allowed only around one axis, as in a hinge; in the latter it is allowed in two directions, as with a true ball and socket.

There are four factors acting to hold a synovial joint together: (1) ligaments, especially in hinge joints such as those in the knee and elbow; (2) muscles; (3) fascial structures that cover the muscles; and (4) atmospheric pressure. As an example of factor 4, if all of the tissue holding the hip joint together is severed, the femoral head still does not fall out of the acetabulum, thanks to the inward force of the atmospheric pressure (14.7 pounds per square inch) surrounding the joint. Similarly, it is atmospheric pressure that helps to hold the shoulder blade against the rib cage.

Frozen Joints

If there is pain in a synovial joint, then we tend to avoid moving it. However, when a synovial joint is not used, the joint capsule shrinks and stiffens, the viscosity of the lubricating fluid increases, and the range of motion around that joint tends toward zero. The end result of shying away from a painful joint in the long term is a "frozen joint" in which little or no motion is possible [745]. If a joint has been injured and is in pain, it is best to accept this as the body's way of insuring sufficient rest for the injury; but if the joint is allowed to rest so completely that it goes into retirement, then its action may be lost forever.

Interestingly, even in the hip joint, the archetype of the synovial joint, there is a ligament between the center of the femoral head and the back of the acetabulum that helps bind the two together, much as with the fibrous type of joint. Integrity of the hip joint also is maintained by atmospheric pressure against the partial vacuum within the joint. Because there is no equilibration possible between the gas pressures on the outside and inside of a joint capsule, changes in external atmospheric pressure may be felt in sensitive joints as the capsules swell or shrink. There are many pressure and pain sensors in the joint-capsule tissues.

General Bone Movement

By widening the bones at their ends (the epiphyses), bones are better able to resist oblique compressive stresses transferred across synovial joints [878, 884]. Because the forces are spread over a large area at the epiphyses, the ends of long bones can be built lighter; i.e., they can be made of cancellous bone. In this way, larger joints are more easily stabilized and cushioned. As described more fully in Section 11.B, page 428, the joints play a major role in the body's proprioceptive system, for they carry important sensors for determining body position and motion. Further, the joint capsules contain sensors that report on the angle of the joint and the velocity of the bones as the joint angle changes.

Generally, movements in the joints are rotatory motions around the joint centers, which are then transformed into the translations of the distal ends of the bones. When the distal ends of two bones in a joint move toward one another, the joint is moving toward a position of flexion; and when they move away from one another, the joint moves toward a position of extension. This restricted definition does not allow for opening of the joints as occurs in the *yogasanas,* a topic discussed in Subsection 11.A, page 425. Rotatory motion is the primary motion of the joint, whereas the opening of the joint is a secondary and hence more complex action.

When a muscle contracts, both of the bones in the corresponding joint tend to move, but the relative degrees of motion are inversely dependent upon the ratios of the masses being moved. Thus, when a leg is swung forward by contraction of the abdominal muscles, as when lifting the leg in *hasta padangusthasana,* both the leg and the torso move to close the hip joint; however, the mass of the leg is only one-tenth that of the torso, and so it moves ten times as far as the torso moves, all other things being constant. When moving into *ardha navasana* from *dandasana,* the legs would be thought to move through a much larger angle than does the torso, due to the relatively smaller weight of the legs; however, the point of contact with the floor also moves from the ischial tuberosities toward the lumbar spine, thus upsetting the simple picture painted by considering mass alone.

In general, in a joint consisting of two bones spanned by a contracting muscle, one of them is essentially immobile in spite of the pull on it by the muscle, whereas the muscle action forces the second bone of the joint to move relative to the first (Subsection 7.D, page 242). Were this the only way that a muscle could cause movement, then a crab that has molted its exoskeleton could not move until its new exoskeleton has hardened, nor could an elephant move its trunk, for in neither case is there a bony anchor against which the relevant muscles can work. In both these cases, it is known that movement is possible because certain internal structures are pumped full of fluid or air, so that they become so taut momentarily that they become stiff as bone and so can act as anchors against which work can be done by the attached muscles. Very similar situations are found in the Valsalva maneuver in the human body (page 616) and in penile and clitoral erection. These are general examples of the more common macroscopic resistance in support of muscle action, discussed in Subsections 7.A, page 232, 10.A, page 331, and 11.F, page 468.

Stability versus Mobility

There would appear to be a reciprocal relation between the stability and the mobility of a joint. Thus, for example, because the shoulder joint is a much shallower ball-and-socket joint than the corresponding hip joint, the shoulder joint is much more mobile in allowing motion of the attached arm, as compared with the motion allowed by the hip joint to the attached leg (figure 10.A-3). On the other hand, the shoulder is much more unstable with respect to dislocation than is the hip, which is bound by large muscles for stability but which muscles inhibit motion [484]. If the muscles surrounding the hip (the gluteals, the quadriceps, the hamstrings, the psoas, and the abdominals) are strong, then they can assume certain of the functions of the hip or knee joints, should they be injured. Thus, for example, strong quadriceps can function effectively as shock absorbers if the menisci in the knee joints fail in this regard. If there is a hip or knee injury, the first muscles to lose strength are the antigravity muscles, the gluteals and the quadriceps.

Congruence

If the congruency between the ends of the bones forming a joint is high (i.e., there is a good match of shapes as in the elbow, hip, vertebral articulations, etc.), then there is not much stress placed on the lubricating cartilage within the joint. If, however, the congruency is low, then on pressurizing the joint, there will be a strong demand for the cartilage to deform, as in the knee and ankle joints [288].

Flexibility

Flexibility is joint-specific [7]; the range of motion achieved in one joint is no indicator of the range of motion achievable in the other joints. Flexibility in the right hip joint is no indicator of flexibility in the left hip joint, and the flexibility for one shoulder movement is no indicator for flexibility of another movement in the same shoulder. Indeed, for the beginner student, one often sees that a high degree of flexibility in one mode is accompanied by a high degree of inflexibility in the complementary mode. For the *yogasana* beginner, one can in no way assess whole-body flexibility by looking at just one joint in one particular movement; this will be less true as the beginner progresses in the *yogasanas* and the pattern of tensions in the agonist and antagonist muscles become more balanced.

Joint Injury

Complete dislocation of the bones of a joint involves tearing of the tissues in the joint area and is called luxation, whereas partial dislocation is called subluxation. In either case, the joint function is minimal to nonexistent, with significant pain in the area of the joint. Twisting or wrenching a joint is often sufficient to result in a sprain; i.e., damage to the ligamentous attachments surrounding the joint, but without subluxation of the articulating bones. Sprains are often accompanied by swelling and discoloration and most often occur in the ankle and lower back.

With a high concentration of mechanoreceptors in the ankle, an ankle sprain can result in the loss of proprioceptive sensing in the affected ankle, with the size of the proprioceptive loss depending upon the severity of the sprain. Due to the enhanced circulation that it promotes, early (but not too early) practice of *vrksasana* following an ankle sprain not only helps the ankle to heal quickly once it has been rested but also helps in the recovery of the balancing sense at this joint.

Misalignment

The proper alignment of the bones comprising a joint is important in that misalignment can lead to swelling and/or thickening of the surrounding tissue, which in the vicinity of the joints is rich in both nerves and blood vessels. Compression of these tissues can be deleterious, especially in the vertebral joints of the spine [422]. A particularly obvious misalignment of a joint often is seen in women who insist on wearing pointed shoes. In this case, the result is a big toe (the hallux) that is strongly angled inward toward the second toe, while the joint between the big toe and the first metatarsal head moves outward, forming a bunion; technically, the condition is known as hallux valgus. The corresponding condition resulting from the inward turning of the little toe with respect to the fifth metatarsal head is called a bunionette. The misalignment can be reversed by working the feet in

the *yogasanas* so as to broaden across the base of the foot, by wearing non-tapered shoes,[3] and by inserting and leaving spacers between the toes at night, so as to encourage the toes toward alignment [724]. Lacking this, the solution is surgical. Yet another shoe-related joint problem stems from the wearing of high heels by women (see Subsection 7.D, page 250). The consequences of joint misalignment on the neighboring soft tissues are described in Subsection 7.D, page 244.

Definitions of Joint Motions

Joint Opening and Closing

Angular movements of the joints can involve flexion, extension, abduction, and adduction; the muscles responsible for these motions are called flexors, extensors, abductors, and adductors, respectively (figures 11.A-1, 11.A-2, and 11.A-3). In flexion, there is most often a decrease in the angle between the anterior surfaces of the articulating bones of the joint in question; for example, the closing of the anterior angles of the hip joints when forward bending in *prasarita padottanasana*. However, when the angles at the knees or the angles of the toe joints are in flexion, it is the posterior surfaces of the bones that approach one another, rather than the anterior surfaces.

If the posterior surfaces of the bones in a joint approach one another, then one has a case of extension of the joint, again with the exception of the knees and toes. For example, as one drops the head back in *ustrasana*, the cervical vertebrae are put into extension. If a joint has been flexed, then extension returns the joint to its anatomic position, and extension beyond the anatomic position (figure 7.A-1) can result in hyperextension of the joint, as shown in figure 7.D-2 for the neck.

Specific motions around the joints and within their normal ranges of motion are readily classi-

---

3   In more than 80 percent of humans, the tip of the big toe (first metatarsal) is more forward than any other on the foot, whereas pointed shoes are fabricated on the assumption that the tip of the middle toe (third metatarsal) is the most forward.

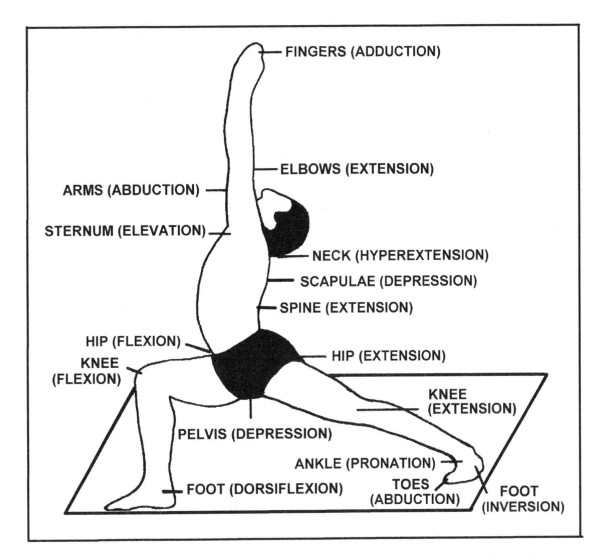

Figure 7.D-2. Joint motions and positions as demonstrated by the student in *virabhadrasana I.*

fied below; however, the motion about a particular joint often is a combination of the motions described here [863]. The classification is with respect to the so-called anatomic position.

Flexion and Extension

If the toes are pulled upward toward the knees, the foot is in dorsiflexion; whereas when pointed toward the floor, as in *setu bandha sarvangasana,* the action is one of plantar flexion. When forward bending, the spine is in flexion, whereas when in any type of backbend, the spine is placed in extension. Extension of the hip joint, which moves the relevant leg either backward or to the side, involves contraction of the gluteus maximus and/or the hamstrings. Flexion of the hip joint,

which moves the relevant leg forward and up, involves contraction of the hip flexors running from the lower back to the front of the thigh.

Abduction and Adduction

Abduction involves a movement of a bone away from the medial line of the body, as when lifting the leg in *vasisthasana I.* Abduction of the fingers and toes involves a spreading of the relevant fingers or toes, as when one sets the hands for *adho mukha svanasana* or sets the foot for balancing in *vrksasana.* Being in essence the opposite of abduction, adduction involves a bringing of the appendages closer to the center line of the body. As one raises the arms sideways in moving from *tadasana* to *udhva hastasana,* the arms first are abducted to reach the horizontal position and then are adducted to reach the vertical position.

Joint Rotation

There are two general types of rotation within a joint. One speaks of rotation when the motion is about a long axis of one of the bones of a joint, as when turning the head around the neck when shaking the head "no." Motion of the anterior aspect of a bone toward the center line of the body is termed medial rotation, as opposed to rotation of the same aspect of the bone away from the center line, termed lateral rotation. If one rolls the front thighs inward in *tadasana,* the rotation is medial.[4]

A second type of rotation, called circumduction, involves the motion of one end of a bone in a circular arc around the unmoving opposite end, as when swinging the straight arm about the humeral head through 360° with the arm sweeping out a cone of circumduction in the air, as in figure 10.A-3a. If the ankle is rolled inward around the long axis of the foot so that the inner ankle drops toward the floor (the tendency of the ankle of the back leg in *virabhadrasana I,* figures 7.D-2 and V.B-1), the position is referred to as pronated; whereas if the weight is on the little-toe side of the foot (*baddha konasana*), the ankle position is referred to as everted. With respect to the hands on arms hanging at the sides, if the forearm is rotated so that the palm is facing forward, the action is termed supination; whereas the pronated position of the hand has the palm facing backward (figure 10.A-4).

Translation

In certain situations, bones move with respect to one another by translation only, without rotation, as when gliding. This is the case as the scapulae are raised and lowered with respect to the rib cage. When the scapulae are lifted or dropped, they are said to have been elevated or depressed, respectively. Examples of almost all of the above motions around the joints are illustrated by referring to the student in *virabhadrasana I* in figure 7.D-2.

Range of Motion

When practicing *yogasana,* it is useful to remember that the range of angular motion at a synovial joint is largest when the joint is most open; i.e., when the ball and socket are most disengaged (but not dislocated!). Thus, in *baddha konasana,* each femur is extended from the groin to the knee, and with the hip joints opened in this way, the anterior thighs are rotated laterally, so as to bring the knees toward the floor. Similarly, in *ustrasana,* while upright, lengthen the spine by lifting the rib cage up and away from the pelvis, and with the vertebrae disengaged in this way, maintain this opening as the spine is bent backward in extension.

Factors Limiting Motion

Motion around a synovial joint is inhibited by several factors: (1) the pressing of one soft body part against another, as when the leg is bent and the calf of the lower leg presses on the hamstrings of the thigh in *vajrasana;* (2) the pressing of one hard body part against another, as when the straightening of the supporting arm in *vasisthasana* is arrested by the contact of the bones of the upper and lower arms at the elbow (see Section 7.F, page 252); (3) tensile stress in the muscles and associated ligaments and tendons of a joint, as experienced by the hamstrings when bringing the angle at the knee to 180° in *uttanasana.*

Ligaments and Tendons

Two adjacent or nearby bones forming a joint are joined by one or more of three different types of collagenous strap. A joint may be spanned by a muscle, with each end of the muscle being tightly interwoven with the periosteum of one of the two

---

4   Note that when the front thighs rotate inward so as to produce a medial rotation, the same action as seen from the back is an **outward** rotation of the thighs and so produces a lateral rotation! Thus, it is meaningless and confusing to instruct students to "roll their thighs medially" or "roll their thighs in" without specifying whether it is the fronts or the backs of the thighs that are to be rolled.

bones. If the collagenous material at the end of a muscle that is bound to the periosteum of the bone is a relatively narrow strap (as with the biceps), it is called a tendon; but if it is a broad band (as with the latissimus dorsi), then the structure is called an aponeurosis. Aponeuroses also may function as bones, being anchors for muscle attachment. A third possibility is that the collagenous band contains no muscle yet spans the two bones in question; in this case, the structure is called a ligament. Ligaments cannot contract but are supplied with many tensile-stress, type-IV sensors (Section 7.E, page 251), the outputs of which are used in the construction of the proprioceptive map in the cerebellum.

Microstructure

Collagen is one of the main constituents not only of bone but of many ligaments, tendons, and cartilage as well. Indeed, as described in Section 7.A, page 225, bone is formed by the incorporation of microcrystals of the mineral hydroxyapatite into a matrix of collagen fibers. Being collagenous materials but totally lacking in mineralization, ligaments and tendons are somewhat elastic, but not overly so: untreated tendon can extend only 8 percent before rupturing; i.e., it can be strained only 8 percent before separating, whereas the comparable figure for rubber is 200–300 percent.[5] See Section 12.A, page 482, for more on the chemistry and structure of connective tissue such as is found in ligaments and tendons.

The semi-rigidity of the ligaments and tendons serves us well, as these elements are used as straps to hold one bone close to another (ligament) or to tie a muscle onto a nearby bone (tendon). As collagenous material can withstand strong tensile forces with minimum strain, it is ideal for this purpose, but of course, it buckles immediately under a compressive force.

If the tensile limit is not exceeded, then

stretching a tendon is quite reversible, returning as heat about 93 percent of the energy invested in stretching it. Energy storage in the stretched tendons of the foot and leg are of significance when we walk or run. Tendons cannot afford to be too flexible, however, because if they were so, then the tendons would stretch on contracting a muscle, but the bones would hardly move at all, just the opposite of our intention when contracting a muscle [877]. The Achilles tendon (also called the calcaneal tendon) anchoring the gastrocnemius muscle onto the posterior calcaneus heel bone is the strongest tendon in the body, being able to resist tearing under a 450-kilogram (1,000-pound) load, yet it is the tendon in the body most often ruptured [863].[6]

It is worth repeating that, although a ligament is unable to contract on its own the way a muscle can, when stretched, a ligament can return to its resting length if the initial stretch was not too extreme; i.e., it did not exceed the elastic limit. If, on the other hand, the strain approaches 8 percent or so, the elastic limit is exceeded, and the ligament will be permanently lengthened or even may be torn apart. Note that though ligaments are protected by embedded type-III sensors against damage by overstretching (Section 7.D, page 249), this protection can be defeated by stretching when one is willful, reckless, and hasty.

The ligaments in the body of an adolescent are unusually flexible, as they must keep up with the rapid growth of the bones in the growing body. This flexibility is aided by the high concentrations of growth hormone so prominent at this time. In the adult body, there is much less growth hormone, and so the body is less flexible; however, the integrity of the joints is higher.

---

5 Actually, the ligamentum nuchae in the neck (figure 8.A-5a) stretches by almost 200 percent when the neck is flexed so as to place the chin on the chest, as in *sarvangasana*, but this is quite atypical of ligaments.

6 This apparent discrepancy can be understood in the following way. Suppose the tendon is actually viscoelastic (i.e., it is able to extend elastically if the stress is applied slowly); however, if the load is applied quickly, it acts like a solid and simply fractures. One assumes then that the 450-kilogram (1,000-pound) load is applied slowly, whereas frequent injuries to this tendon are the result of the too-rapid application of tensile stress.

Torn Ligaments

An injury to a joint, as from a too-sudden contraction, a rapid twisting, or a forceful blow, can partially or totally tear the associated ligament. Such a torn ligament is most common in the knee joint, especially in young adults who are not in good physical condition. If the injury to the ligament is mild (shows tenderness, swelling, and pain when stressed), then the cure would be the application of heat and cold, elevation of the joint, and early use of the joint. On the other hand, for a fully torn ligament, treatment instead involves a forced immobility of the joint, followed eventually by physical therapy.

Bursa and Tendon Sheaths

At several places in the body, the muscles and their attendant tendons are forcefully pressed onto nearby bone when the muscle is contracted. In order to soften the contact of bone on muscle and tendon, the body has incorporated about 150 small sacs, filled with synovial fluid, at these critical points, which serve to lessen the friction of the motion of the soft tissues against the bones. For example, there is such a sac in the pelvic area where the gluteus maximus muscle crosses the greater trochanter of the femur bone. These sacs are called bursae, and when they become inflamed and sensitive, one has bursitis. The discomfort of trochanteric bursitis will be apparent in forward bends such as *prasarita padottanasana* or *parsvottanasana*.

In many tendons, there is a surrounding structure known as the tendon sheath, which is made of tubes of fibrous connective tissue, each having an inner and an outer layer separated by a very thin film of synovial fluid. Acting like bursae, the sheaths allow tendons to move easily over one another; however, excessive exercise of the muscle may lead to swelling of the attendant tendon sheaths, due to the accumulation of synovial fluid. This condition is known as tendinitis [863]. In situations where a tendon is under tensile stress and is pulled around or over another bone, the tendon sheath is compressed. Excess traction of such a tendon compressed on the bone results in inflammation of the tendon at that spot and the formation of adhesions between the tendon and its sheath, so that when stretched, the adhesions are broken, with a consequent sharp pain at the spot. This condition is known as tenosynovitis.

In general, the ligaments and tendons lack distinct vascularization and are nourished by diffusion. In fact, were these tissues vascularized, they would have been converted into bone in the fetus! Because of this lack of vascularization, once broken or ruptured, ligaments and tendons heal only by a long, slow process. Note that since the ligaments are essentially collagenous, they do not have the ability to contract rapidly, as might a muscle. As a consequence, if they are overstretched, as when postures are done by hanging on the joints (as when doing *trikonasana* with the quadriceps limp, for example), they can be fatigued and in pain long after the stretching has ended [483].

Misalignment

The mechanical integrity of a joint will depend upon the proper tensioning of the stabilizing ligaments and tendons, which in turn will depend upon proper alignment of the relevant bones. If one performs *yogasanas* with the bones of the joints out of alignment, over time, a corresponding misalignment and relaxation of the relevant ligaments and a corresponding destabilization of the joint will occur [445]. As often happens with students doing "hang-out" yoga, the ligaments about the joints can learn the wrong lesson and be stretched excessively, leading to serious joint problems down the road. In fact, an entire treatment protocol for joint pain has been developed based on the premise that joint pain is the result of weak, loose ligaments and that tightening of these structures by injection of innocuous substances (sugar, etc.) will reduce the pain [232].

The instability at the joint extends to the muscles too. If the bones of a joint do not bear weight properly, then muscular action will be called upon. Over time, this incorrectly used muscle will become short and hard (like a bone), while its antagonist (Subsection 11.A, page 420) at the same time will become weaker through lack of use. This muscular asymmetry will then work to further destabilize the joint, with the problem eventually spreading to other joints in the body [445]. On the other hand, proper alignment can release the tension at the joint and restore the proper weight-bearing relationship between bone and muscle.

Achilles Tendon

The largest and strongest tendon in the body is the Achilles tendon behind the ankle, this being 15 centimeters (six inches) in length. As with most tendons, there are few nerves in the Achilles tendon, so that total rupture may be painless! Rupture of this tendon is more likely in middle age, when tendons are stiffer and more easily overstretched to the point of damage. Though damage to the Achilles tendon can occur if the stress on the tendon is applied rapidly and is intense, as when the high heel on a woman's shoe breaks off and the heel instantly drops several inches to the floor, this would not seem to be much of a problem when stretching the same ligament slowly, as when the heel of the back leg descends to the floor in *parsvottanasana*. Lacking vascularization, a torn Achilles tendon heals slowly, if at all, and often has to be repaired surgically. Keeping this tendon long and flexible, along with its associated muscle (the gastrocnemius), through practice of *yogasanas* such as *parsvottanasana* will help in avoiding such a tear. Of course, if any posture is done to the extent of having gone from discomfort into pain, one then runs the risk of tearing a tendon rather than lengthening and strengthening it.

One can estimate the relative importance of ligaments and muscle tendons in holding a joint together from a comment made by Juhan [422]. He notes that when a hospital patient is given a general anesthetic that relaxes the muscles, hospital personnel must be very careful in moving the patient, as without the ordinary muscle tone (Subsection 11.B, page 434), the patient's joints can be easily dislocated. Assuming that the non-contractile ligaments are unaffected by the anesthetic, this can be taken to demonstrate that the muscle's tendons play the major role in stabilizing joints with respect to dislocation. The effects of pregnancy on joints and ancillary structures are discussed in Subsection 21.B, page 745.

Joint Noises

When a joint is formed by two bones articulating end to end and is surrounded by synovial fluid within which oxygen, nitrogen, and carbon dioxide gases are dissolved, pulling the joint apart ("cracking" it) produces an audible pop, otherwise called crepitation. X-ray pictures show that when such a joint is cracked, a gas bubble is formed in the joint that increases the volume of the joint by 15–20 percent [7]. Bubble formation is followed by an explosive collapse of the bubble and the generation of sound waves. Once popped, the joint is in the subluxed open position for about twenty minutes as the remainder of the gas bubble redissolves; the joint cannot be cracked again until the gas within this bubble has dissolved. During this time, the joint is unstable and is subject to trauma. Repetitive cracking of a joint may adversely affect the soft tissue around the joint, leading to swelling and loss of strength. If the above mechanism is correct, it would appear that cracking of a joint does not release any tension in the body and otherwise leaves the joint susceptible to damage for a short time after the cracking.

Vertebral joints often crack the first time one goes into *urdhva dhanurasana,* but it is difficult to see how these joints might be pulled apart to form bubbles. Perhaps it is better to view this cracking sound as due to the realignment of overlying muscles and tendons after a night of relaxation. As the joint is pulled open, tendons and ligaments that have relaxed into abnormal positions return to their original aligned positions with a snap of the ligaments and tendons onto the bone. In this case, it is not necessary for the volume of the joint to increase in order to produce a popping sound. This second type of joint cracking, as in the spine, would appear to be the more beneficial one for *yogasana* students, as it is a consequence of the proper realignment of the tendons and ligaments about the joint in question [91]. In contrast, joint cracking in the ankles, knees, elbows, or shoulders is not thought to be a good sign.

If a joint pops or cracks, and there is no associated pain or swelling, then one may assume that there is no problem; however, if the sound appears at the moment of an injury that leads to pain or swelling, then you may have damaged the joint.

Extremes of Joint Position

If the muscles, tendons, and/or ligaments that bind two bones into a joint are not too strong mechanically, one can make the mistake of applying either a momentary or an ongoing stress to the joint (in either the bending or stretching coordinates) that compromises its stability. It is useful to distinguish between an extreme opening of the joint angle (hyperextension) and an extreme end-to-end opening of the joint space (overstretching).

A joint at the extreme end of its range of motion is a joint at risk, especially when practicing *yogasana*, because the joint capsule, tendons, and ligaments surrounding such a joint can be stressed to such an extent that the joint is easily pulled apart (dislocated or luxed) if one is willful. Once dislocated or overstretched, nerves in the area of the joint may be impinged, resulting in radiating pain; and being in an area that is relatively avascular, such joint injuries can be very slow to heal. Dislocation or overstretching may even injure the bones forming the joint.

It is especially important that students of *yogasana* realize that placing a joint in an extreme position is dangerous, as this can injure nearby soft tissue or allow catastrophic collapse of the joint when the student works at maximum intensity. Such collapse is resisted in part by the ligaments and tendons around a joint, which act as collagenous straps to maintain its integrity. Improper practice of the *yogasanas* over a long period of time, with the joint in question being stressed but not reinforced (as with the knee of the forward leg in *trikonasana*, for example, done with the quadriceps relaxed), can overcome this safety factor, with disastrous results, as can lifting the bent leg to place it in *padmasana* (Box 10.B-1, page 352). In this regard, also see, for example, Lasater's work [492] on spinal rotation

(Subsection 8.B, page 298). Of course, there are a variety of mechanoreceptors in and around a joint (Section 11.B, page 440), the functions of which are to monitor and signal unusually high tensile stress or torque in the joint. However, an ambitious student can consciously override these signals.

Hyperextension

Popularly known as "double-jointedness" or hypermobility, hyperextension spans a wide spectrum of angular range of motion [490]. Technically, hyperextension is defined as an angular range of motion for one or many joints that is beyond the ninety-fifth percentile in the general population. Tests for hyperextension involve measuring the bending of the joints, as when bending the fingers and thumb backward toward the elbow, bending the knee of the straight leg backward (as can happen in *trikonasana*), and bending the elbow of the straight arm inward, resulting in an angle between humerus and the lower arm larger than 180 degrees (as can happen for the supporting arm in *vasisthasana*). If there is bone-on-bone contact at the extreme of joint bending, then too vigorous an action may result in bone fracture (Sections 7.F, page 252, and 8.A, page 293).

Hyperextension is seen more often in the young than in the old, in women much more than in men, and in all ethnic groups, but especially in Asians. At its most serious, hyperextension (and easy overstretching) are characteristics of Ehlers-Danlos syndrome, of Marfan syndrome, and of Down syndrome, each of which involves a component of connective-tissue pathology (Subsection 12.A, page 483). At the opposite end of the health spectrum, hyperextension may be only an amusing, innocuous aspect of one's body, brought out for parties, etc.

It also may be that extreme joint positions are due to unusually high levels of the pregnancy hormone relaxin in the body, that the connective tissue is high in elastin (Subsection 12.A, page 484), or that the muscles spanning the joint are simply lacking in tone. There is also a very strong genetic component at work in hyperextension, with the syndrome readily passing from either or both parents to their children.

In order to open a joint and keep it in alignment without hyperextending it, one must simultaneously contract the agonist and antagonist muscles surrounding the joint (Subsections 7.D, page 248, and 11.A, page 422), so as to offer resistance to the hyperextending action and thereby bring stabilization to the joint. If there is no such co-contraction operating, then one is simply "hanging on the joint." When a joint lacks flexibility due to a weakness of its prime mover, use of the joint often results in taking the path of least resistance in changing the joint angle; i.e., a relative flexibility is developed, in which synergist muscles rather than the prime mover are used until they too are injured by their inappropriate overuse.

Joints that are hyperextendable do not hold chiropractic adjustments very well, and because high levels of estrogen promote such laxity, it can become more of a problem during the menstrual period and during pregnancy when estrogen levels are high. One must be especially careful when working the *yogasanas* with students having Down syndrome, for the ligaments globally in such students are highly elastic, and such students all too easily can be placed in positions that further reduce the stability of their joints.

Overstretching

Injury of a joint by tensile overstretching is unusual, for this implies an overstretching of the muscle fiber as well, and it is more likely that the muscle will be injured before the joint. However, it is also possible that both the joint and the muscles spanning it could suffer injury simultaneously.

An unusually supple joint may involve the shallow insertion of one bone into the cavity of another. For example, the shoulder joint is far more mobile than the hip joint because it has a much shallower setting of the humerus into the glenoid fossa than is the case for the femoral head in the acetabulum. Thus, the arm—any arm—may be overstretched with respect to the leg, meaning that it would not be unusual for the gle-

nohumeral joint to dislocate while elongating in *virabhadrasana III*, whereas it would be extremely unusual for the hip joint of the horizontal leg in this posture to dislocate.

Overstretching is especially serious when it occurs in the sacroiliac joints, for these joints have little else to hold them together if the ligaments are overstretched; the end result of overstretching the sacroiliac joint is certain lower-back pain.

Joint Lubrication and Arthritis

Rheumatoid Arthritis

The two general types of joint degeneration, called rheumatoid arthritis and osteoarthritis, are shown graphically in figures 7.D-1b and 7.D-1e, respectively. In rheumatoid arthritis, there is inflammation of the synovial joint capsule, due to an autoimmune reaction in which the white blood cells of the immune system mistakenly recognize the collagen within the joint as a foreign substance and attack it. This reaction leads to overproduction of synovial fluid, a thickening of the synovium tissue, and increased temperature and pain. Enzymes released by inflamed cells then destroy cartilage and bone, leading to the swelling and stretching of the joint and the weakening of the ligaments and tendons in its vicinity. Once the ligaments and tendons have loosened, the alignment at the joint is compromised, the bones fall out of alignment, the normal range of motion is severely curtailed, and the characteristic joint distortions of rheumatoid arthritis become evident.

The effects of rheumatoid arthritis are usually right-left symmetric in the body and are three times more prevalent in women than in men [415]. The lubrication quality of the synovial fluid also declines in rheumatoid arthritis, and with that, so too does its ability to supply nourishment to the joints' cartilage. Drugs that suppress the immune system often reverse the effects of rheumatoid arthritis, supporting the idea that the condition is due to an autoimmune reaction; several experts in the field consider rheumatoid arthritis to be caused by an infectious organism, but this has not been proved [884].

The stress hormone cortisol is virtually absent in the blood in the evening hours, and consequently, the pain and discomfort of rheumatoid arthritis can be maximal upon awakening. However, the early-morning spurt of this hormone (Subsection 6.A, page 211) then works to ease the pain by midmorning; the time between 5:00 and 6:00 PM is the most pain-free and so is the best time for a light *yogasana* practice for those with rheumatoid arthritis. At this time, they will experience increased flexibility and joint motion, as well as an elevation of mood. Though there is evidence that *yogasana* practice can work to increase the strength around joints afflicted with rheumatoid arthritis [357], the inflamed joints must not be worked directly. Because rheumatoid arthritis is neither necessarily progressive nor deforming, earlier reliance on an appropriate *yogasana* practice may be very valuable in this regard.

When the barometer is reading low, as it would be when a storm is approaching, the low pressure experienced by the hermetically sealed joint allows the tissue cells to expand and irritate any inflamed tissue or adhesions in or close to the joint. When coupled with high humidity and atmospheric electrical disturbances (phase 4, meteorologically), this combination can be very painful to those with rheumatoid arthritis; however, there is as yet no convincing explanation as regards the general mechanism.[7] It has been reported that deterioration of the intervertebral discs can lead to accumulation of gas in the intervertebral space and that lower-back pain can appear when the weather becomes humid, the atmospheric pressure drops, and the gas within the intervertebral space therefore expands [434].

Osteoarthritis

In osteoarthritis, there is an erosion of the cartilage and the epiphyseal surfaces (but not the synovial membrane), leading eventually to bone spurs, or projections that are painful when the joint is moved. The erosion is initiated by overloading of the joint, as often happens in obesity or by poor alignment of the joint surfaces, which causes the protective cartilage to wear away. This in turn can lead to thickening of the ends of the bone and a rubbing of bone on bone, with little or no intervening lubrication. Erosion of the epiphyses is promoted by chronic muscle tension, which acts to close the joints, figure 7.D-1e [12].

Osteoarthritis commonly affects the hands, hips, knees, neck, and lower back and usually is worse upon awakening or getting up after a long rest but improves quickly as one begins to move. It is the knee joint that is most commonly affected by osteoarthritis, followed by the hip joint and that between the trapezium of the hand and the metacarpal of the thumb. Osteoarthritis of the knee is experienced by twice as many women as men, whereas osteoarthritis of the hip joint is more common in men than in women. Severe osteoarthritis of the hip is a significant factor in obese women; however, recreational physical activities, such as running or *yogasana* practice, seem not to be factors in this condition.

Experiments show that walking in high-heeled shoes reduces torque at the ankle, as compared with walking barefoot, but increases it at the knee, all the while inducing lower-back pain. It is conjectured that the significantly higher incidence of bilateral osteoarthritis in the knees of women can be traced to their frequent walking in high-heeled shoes [441].

Circadian Rhythm

In contradistinction to the situation with rheumatoid arthritis, the pain and discomfort of osteoarthritis are maximal in the hours between

---

7   Other physical and mental responses to changing weather have been reported [475]. For example, alertness and wakefulness as measured by response times both noticeably decreased in a period of phase-4 weather, possibly involving parasympathetic excitation. Industrial accidents rise noticeably when the temperature goes outside the range 12–24° C (54–75° F), and the effect of cold weather on many people is to increase the blood pressure. It also is known that very small changes in atmospheric pressure of the order of 0.001 atmosphere (less than 1 millimeter Hg) can have demonstrable effects on the abilities of test takers to solve puzzles, etc.

mid-afternoon and mid-evening and are least in the early morning hours.[8] Again, it is the early-morning release of cortisol that is so effective in easing the pain and restoring mobility to those afflicted with osteoarthritis, but apparently the times at which it becomes most effective are different in the two arthritis types. Persons with osteoarthritis should take a light *yogasana* practice in late morning and remember that "motion is lotion."

As shown in tables 23.B-1, 23.B-2, 23.B-3, and 23.B-4, the symptoms of rheumatoid arthritis are most intense at 6:00 to 7:00 AM, whereas those of osteoarthritis are most intense at 6:00 to 7:00 PM. The hour between 6:00 and 7:00 AM is the time during which the autonomic nervous system switches from parasympathetic to sympathetic dominance, whereas the hour between 6:00 and 7:00 PM is the time during which the autonomic nervous system switches from sympathetic to parasympathetic dominance.

The tendency in osteoarthritis to avoid movement in order to avoid pain quickly leads to immobility. For those with osteoarthritis, it is best to do range-of-motion exercises that do not stress the joints. All of these movements should be low impact, smooth, and rhythmic. Clearly, *yogasana* has a great potential use here in maintaining range of motion [239] and in reducing muscle tension at the joints, so that bone-on-bone contact within a joint is minimized.

Loading

Practically everyone who is chronically 9 kilograms (twenty pounds) or more overweight will show signs of osteoarthritis due to the pressure

of the added weight on the joints, which acts to wear away the protective coating on the ends of the bone, especially at the knee [415]. One would guess that *yogasanas* done with special attention to keeping the joints open would work to resist the collapse of the joints and so reduce wear on the protective cartilage. Indeed, a pilot study aimed at assessing the value of Iyengar training for reducing knee pain and disability in obese subjects over fifty years old showed some promise in this regard [459]. It is also possible that *yogasana* done while suspended in water can reduce the pain on overloaded arthritic joints.

Section 7.E: Mechanoreceptors in the Joint Capsules and Ligaments

Alter [7] presents a concise description of the four types of mechanoreceptors that are found in and around the joint capsules (figure 7.D-1a) surrounding each of the synovial joints within the body. The first three types of joint-capsule receptors (types I, II, and III) essentially monitor mechanical stress at the joint, whereas the fourth (type IV) registers pain. Signals from these receptors provide input to the proprioceptive centers in regard to joint position and movement and so aid the construction of the proprioceptive map.

Type I receptors are found in the tissue of the joint capsules, more so in the tissues of the hips and spine than in the more distal joints; they signal joint angle, velocity of joint movement, and changes in joint pressure. As they are highly sensitive, are active for every joint position, whether moving or not, and are slowly adapting, they will be easily activated in every *yogasana* and the signal will be long lasting. They apparently are a variation of the Ruffini corpuscle (Subsection 11.B, page 440), with each consisting of a knot of three capsules interwoven with the connective tissue, muscle, and tendon fibers within the capsule, so that any motion of the joint compresses or stretches at least one component of the sensor.

Type II receptors are found in the deeper tis-

---

8   The pattern of pain and fatigue experienced in fibromyalgia closely resembles that of osteoarthritis; however, in the former, the fatigue elements seem related to poor sleep, with alpha waves in the EEG interrupting the delta waves of deep sleep. Sufferers of fibromyalgia also have a morning cortisol release that is often too little and too early. As is the case with osteoarthritis, *yogasana* practice for fibromyalgia sufferers will be best when done in the late morning to early afternoon.

sue of the joint capsule, and because they respond only when the joint is in motion and are rapidly adapting, they will be most active when moving into and out of the *yogasanas*. Presumably, type II receptors will play a role as proprioceptive elements when balancing.

The type III receptors function much like the Golgi tendon organs, except that they are located in the joint capsule and the ligaments of each joint. Being dynamic sensors, with a high threshold and slow adaptation, the type III sensors work largely at the extremes of joint angle position and may act as inhibitors of joint motion, if such motion is extreme. In this sense, they function much like the muscle spindles and the Golgi tendon organs in protecting the musculoskeletal system from extreme stresses.

When joint motion is extreme, and the surrounding tissue is injured, then high-threshold, slowly adapting pain receptors (type IV) are activated in the articular tissue, and joint pain is sensed. These sensors are present in synovial tissue, menisci, and the ligaments of the joints; however, by a pain-gate mechanism (Subsection 13.C, page 525), their pain signal can be inhibited or diluted by mixing with the signals from type I sensors.

Section 7.F: Bone-on-Bone Contact

The Problem

As you stretch in the *yogasanas*, it occasionally happens that you come to a point in a posture where further depth in the posture seems unattainable, no matter how much you practice it. When you are up against such a dead end, it is possible that the posture is being done in such a way that a bone is being pressed against a second bone (either a partner in a common joint or not) and that progress stops because such bone-on-bone contact is an insurmountable stone wall. For example:

» **(A)** You are working in *trikonasana*-to-the-right, trying to get the hand further down the leg, but with the right and left feet **parallel** to one another and turned forward, as in *tadasana*. In this case, the right hand cannot go further down the right leg, because with the feet in parallel position, the upper rim of the acetabulum on the right presses into the femoral neck on the right as one leans to the right (figure 10.B-2c), and it is impossible to go deeper once this bone-on-bone contact has been made.

» **(B)** You are working in *parivrtta janu sirsasana* over the straight leg and can go no further, because the ribs on the right side are in contact with the right frontal pelvic bone.

» **(C)** You fold the legs into *padmasana* only with difficulty, and then the pain of the pressure of one shin on the other is too much to bear.

» **(D)** You are pushing up into *urdhva dhanurasana*, but the entire spine is in pain, because the spinous processes in the thoracic region press on one another, and the lumbar spine is so strongly compressed that the lumbar vertebrae also press on one another. In spite of the discomfort, no further extension seems possible.

» **(E)** You cannot descend beyond a certain point in *paschimottanasana*, because the ribs have collapsed and adjacent ribs press onto one another. You cannot go any deeper into *ardha baddha padma paschimottanasana*, because of the contact of the ankle of the bent leg with the xiphoid process of the sternum.

In each of the above all-too-possible situations, progress in the posture has come to a halt because one bone has come into contact with another.

In one instance, bone-on-bone contact is avoided due to the odd shape of one of the bones; when the forearm and the hand are in the supinate orientation, the ulna and radius bones are parallel and not in contact. On rotation from the supinate to the pronate position (figure 10.A-4), the radius of the forearm crosses over the ulna, with the positions of the distal bones (at the wrist) being reversed by 180°, i.e., the distal end of the radius moves from the lateral position to the medial position. In this crossing of the bones, direct bone-on-bone contact is avoided by the severe curvature of the radius, which allows it to curve around the ulna without contact in the pronate position.

The Solution

Rather than wait the decades necessary for the bones to change their shapes by remodeling and then progressing from there, it is far better to find new approaches to the *yogasanas* listed above that redirect the action away from bone-on-bone compression and toward muscle and connective-tissue tensile stretching. This rephrasing of the problem is a wise choice, for tensile stretching will sooner or later respond to practice, whereas the response to bone-on-bone compression can take a lifetime. With the idea of overcoming bone-on-bone compression, the following solutions might be of some help:

» **(A)** For *tikonasana,* as shown in figure 10.B-2e, the lateral rotation of the anterior right foot and thigh moves the femoral neck out of the path of the rim of the acetabulum so that the upper body can then descend to the right if the hamstring stretch on that side will allow.[9]

» **(B)** Progress toward going deeper into *parivrtta janu sirsasana* is possible if one will first concentrate on lifting the right ribs even more to the right before descending toward the right foot. With this adjustment, the ribs fall beyond the frontal pelvic bone, thereby transforming bone-on-bone (ribs-on-pelvis) compression into opposite-side muscle stretching.

» **(C)** With practice at loosening the external-rotator muscles in the hips (Box 10.B-1, page 352), the pressure of the top shin on the bottom shin when in *padmasana* will disappear.

» **(D)** As the spinal discomfort of backbending involves considerable intervertebral compression, this can be released by focusing on pulling the back rim of the pelvis toward the knees, pubis pressed forward and frontal pelvic bones pulled toward the front ribs. This action lengthens the spine, as it reduces the spinal compression but transfers the stress of the posture to the quadriceps muscles of the anterior upper legs, which can more easily learn how to deal with the stress than can the bony vertebrae.

» **(E)** The descent in *paschimottanasana* is stalled by rib-on-rib contact as a result of going into the posture by bending at the mid-body upper hinge. The rib-on-rib contact in forward bending is avoided by bending forward from the lower hinge instead (Subsection 9.B, page 321, and

---

9   With the legs separated left to right, if the feet are set so that the left foot is pointing forward but the right leg is turned to the right, then one can fold deeply on the lower hinge of the right hip so as to enter *parsvakonasana*-to-the-right. In this posture, 71 percent of the body weight appears on the right foot and only 28 percent appears on the left foot (figure IV.D-1), which is qualitatively reasonable because the folding movement presses the upper body to the right side. Keeping the legs in the above starting orientation but instead folding in on the lower hinge of the left hip places one in *virabhadrasana II*, in which case the weight distribution on the feet becomes 63 percent

on the right foot and 35 percent on the left foot. The fact that the weight on the left foot in *virabhadrasana II* performed to the right remains less than that on the right foot, even though the weight of the upper body is being pulled to the left in this posture, is due to the limiting effect of bone-on-bone contact in the left hip joint when trying to fold in that direction. However, if one turns both feet fully to the right so as to be in *virabhadrasana I*, the bone-on-bone contact in the left hip joint is relieved (as in *trikonasana,* figure 10.B-2e) and the weight distribution then becomes more even, i.e., 53 percent right foot and 46 percent left foot (figure IV.D-1).

figure 9.B-5). The solution to the problem of bone-on-bone (sternum-on-ankle) contact in *ardha baddha padma paschimottanasana* should now be obvious to the reader.

Section 7.G: Osteoporosis

Definition, Statistics, and Causes

As women reach middle age (at approximately fifty years) and go through menopause, the levels of estrogen and progesterone in their bodies fall precipitously. Because estrogen activates the osteoblasts, inhibits the osteoclasts, and speeds the absorption of Ca^{2+} into the bones, its loss following the onset of menopause often leads to thinning of the bones, a condition called osteoporosis [836]. Osteoporotic bones have a density (Subsection 7.A, page 233) substantially lower than the norm for younger adult bone. In premenopausal women, the bone-destroying actions of the osteoclasts are held in check by circulating estrogen.

Figure 7.C-1 illustrates the manner in which osteoclasts and osteoblasts normally work together to remodel a flaw in bone structure. However, with increasing age and hormonal shifts due to menopause, a state of osteoclastic overactivity and/or osteoblastic underactivity often leads to the formation of deep fissures in the bone and a dangerously low bone density; i.e., osteoporosis. As the demineralization of osteoporosis proceeds more rapidly with cancellous bone than with compact (cortical) bone, a person with osteoporosis has heightened risk of stress fractures of the cancellous bony features, such as the spinal vertebrae, pelvis, and wrist [524, 754, 878]. The differences between normal and osteoporotic thinning of cancellous bone structures and the effects of osteoporosis on the structure of the spine are shown in figure 7.G-1.

It recently has been found that activation of the T cells of the immune system (Subsection

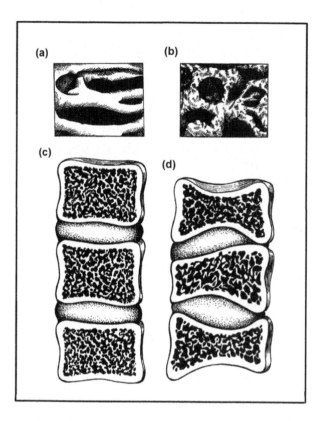

Figure 7.G-1. Comparison of the microscopic structures of normal cancellous bone (**a**) and the same bone afflicted with osteoporosis (**b**). Expanded view of the vertebrae and intervertebral discs in a normal spine (**c**) and the effects of osteoporosis on these spinal structures (**d**).

16.B, page 643) leads to the production of an immunotransmitter that is preferentially stimulating to the osteoclasts of the bone, leading to osteoporosis. As the action of this immunotransmitter is blocked by estrogen, the close relation between osteoporosis and menopause [866] is understandable. In regard to drugs for osteoporosis, the best today are the bis-phosphonates, which bond to bone and induce apoptosis (Subsection 16.F, page 653) in any osteoclasts that may attempt to dissolve the bone.

If only Ca^{2+} is leached from bones, then the result is osteomalacia, a softening of the bones. However, in osteoporosis, there is a loss of Ca^{2+} and a loss of the organic collagen matrix as well, resulting in brittleness and a low density. As the countries with the highest level of dairy consumption in the world also have the highest rates

Table 7.G-1: Risk Factors for Osteoporosis in Women[a] [618]

Well Established	Moderate Evidence	Inconclusive
Age (+)	Alcohol (+)	Moderate exercise (-)
Removal of ovaries (+)	Cigarette smoking (+)	Asian ethnicity (+)
Use of steroids (+)	Low dietary Ca^{2+} (+)	Diabetes (+)
Bed rest (+)	Heavy exercise (-)	Progestin use (-)
Obesity (-)	Short stature, small bones (+)	Fluoridated water (-)
Black ethnicity (-)		Caffeine (+)
Estrogen use (-)		Lean body (+)

a The (+) sign signifies an increased risk, whereas the (-) sign signifies a decreased risk for osteoporosis.

of hip fractures among its older citizens, it is clear that fighting osteoporosis may involve more than just ingesting high-calcium dairy products. Furthermore, high levels of vitamin A in the diet of the elderly raise the risk factor by almost 50 percent for hip fracture from falling.

If bone loss is not stopped, 90 percent of women and 50 percent of men will have osteoporosis by age eighty years [524]. Elderly women subject to osteoporosis will eventually lose 50 percent of the Ca^{2+} in their cancellous bone and 30 percent in their cortical bone. For elderly men, the corresponding figures are only 30 percent and 20 percent, respectively. For women who are five to ten years postmenopausal, the bone loss can amount to 2–3 percent per year. Elderly men also incur a bone thinning with age and increased risk of fracture, but at only half the rate experienced by women [754]. Osteoporosis becomes a heightened risk for men having abnormally low levels of testosterone [754], and injections of this hormone can halt the progress of osteoporosis while increasing the risk of other unfavorable conditions. It is known that for women, about 70 percent of the bone-density change is attributable to genetic factors, but lack of exercise and poor diet also play significant parts.

Symptoms and End Results

There are no obvious symptoms in the early stages of osteoporosis, but with advancing age, osteoporosis becomes more and more of an im-

portant health factor. At age forty years, bones inevitably begin to lose mass, though not as fast as after age fifty years. Nieman [618] presents a table of risk factors for osteoporosis, divided according to the strength of the evidence supporting each claim, as shown in table 7.G-1. Schatz [754] also lists a more complete list of such risk factors but does not comment on how conclusive these various factors might or might not be.

It is very interesting to note from the table that it is well established that though old age, alcohol, and smoking increase the risk for osteoporosis in women, the risk is also increased by bed rest but is decreased by obesity! This is understandable from the point of view that bed rest essentially negates the gravitational pull on the skeleton and so promotes bone weakness, whereas the extra weight carried by obese people stresses the skeleton and so leads to both an increased density of the weight-bearing bones and a higher risk for osteoarthritis. Regarding osteoporosis and loading of the skeleton, it is felt that a situation parallel to that of obesity results from performing the *yogasanas*, with the bones of the skeleton being stressed in a beneficial way so as to provide an antidote to osteoporosis.[10] It is known [836] that

---

10   Note that in the obesity situation, the extra weight that promotes stronger bones also acts to collapse the relevant joints, rubbing bone against bone, thus promoting osteoarthritis as well (Subsection 7.D, page 249); whereas in the practice of *yogasana*, one works to keep the joints open and well lubricated, so

if the bone mass of a young woman is low due to a lack of exercise, she will have a much higher risk of severe osteoporosis in her later years. Thus, the years of *yogasana* work done by a young woman when premenopausal—and an appropriate high-calcium intake at that time—lead to bone density in the bank for her later years.

A second significant effect of aging on the skeletal system involves the reduced rate of the production of the protein collagen in old age. In this case, the proportion of hydroxyapatite in the older bone becomes higher, and the bone is more brittle and more easily broken through falling [863].

Yogasana, Western Exercise, and Osteoporosis

Of course, the strengthening of osteoporotic bone or the maintenance of high bone density will depend in part upon the diet supplying an amount and form of Ca^{2+} adequate for serious bone building. At the same time, fending off osteoporosis will involve applying stress to the bony skeleton, for the body's response to this type of stress is to build bone density. Though walking and running provide weight-bearing exercise for the legs of the aging but active senior, only *yogasana* can do as much not only for the legs, pelvis, and spine but for the arms and upper body as well, through the practice of inversions and hand balances. Schatz [754] gives a detailed *yogasana* program for those having osteoporosis or who are at risk for this condition.

To the increased bone strength created by *yogasana* practice should be added the increases in neuromuscular control and balance (Appendix V, page 865), which make a fall less likely, and the increased muscle strength, which can make the impact of a fall less serious. The importance of avoiding, if possible, such an accident is clear in

---

that the conditions for the formation of osteoarthritis are discouraged. Interestingly, the physical symptoms of weightlessness can be mimicked by prolonged rest with the head inclined downward by six degrees [893].

the statistics [524], which show that for the elderly, the morbidity following a hip fracture is 20 percent! Note too that it has been found recently that in middle-aged and older women, hip fractures are reduced by 30 percent in those women whose diets are rich in vitamin K (the blood-clotting factor), as found in leafy green vegetables. A similar beneficial effect of vitamin K is found for astronauts in space. Interestingly, fluoride ion at a level of one part per million has a strongly positive strengthening effect on teeth, making them resistant to dental caries through the formation of fluorohydroxyapatite. At much higher levels (4–50 milligrams), fluoride ion stimulates osteoblast formation (especially in the spine!) and the renewed formation of strong bone [69, 524]. Thus, fluoride ion at the appropriate low level has become a prime member of the anti-osteoporosis chemical armamentarium.

Loss of Height

It must be noted that whereas hip and wrist fractures often result from falls by the osteoporotic, fractures and collapse of the spinal vertebrae (figures 7.G-1c and 7.G-1d) can occur without falls [69]. Thus, the osteoporotic woman can fracture vertebrae just bending over to pick up the newspaper or even can awaken to find her vertebrae broken during sleep. A multiplicity of such fractures in the vulnerable senior can result in a deep spinal kyphosis (also called dowager's hump, figure 8.A-3) and the loss of several inches of height. The care with which such vulnerable *yogasana* students must be guided by their teachers is obvious. In particular, older students in danger of osteoporotic collapse should perform their standing postures with wall support or even sitting.

When osteoporosis is active, there is a gradual collapse of the spinal column, which is outwardly evident as a loss of height as one ages. However, even without osteoporosis, if the musculature is atrophied, weak, and sagging, then it is not able to support the bones, and there will be a general collapse of the skeleton, even though the bones themselves are not osteoporotic. The implications of a loss of height due to osteoporosis upon mortality by compromised breathing and digestion are discussed in Subsection 24.A, page 811.

Gender Effects

Osteoporosis is less of a problem for older men, because as children, they were, on average, more active physically and so have a larger bone density from the start, and also because the decrease in testosterone levels in men is not as precipitous as the decrease of estrogen levels in women [69]. With almost equal certainty, it can be said that the postmenopausal risk for osteoporosis among women can be avoided by taking an external source of estrogen [69], and it is now known that the hormone-replacement therapy so effective for older women also works for older men.

Western Exercise

Though heavy exercise does increase bone density, young women who are extremely active physically and so have low fat-to-muscle ratios still may suffer from osteoporosis. Under heavy exercise, a young woman can become amenhorreic, because the body acts to prevent an undernourished woman (one with a low fat-to-muscle ratio) from becoming pregnant; in losing her menstrual period, this woman also loses the bone-protective effect of having estrogen released into her system [836, 878].

Note that the bone-building effects of exercise are site specific; i.e., running strengthens the bones of the legs but not of the arms. Note too that the exercise must be weight bearing; i.e., swimmers' bones are not strengthened at all by their exercise, as only their cardiovascular fitness increases [69]. The phenomenon of a 20-percent higher bone density demonstrated in the racquet arm of an active tennis player, as compared with the other arm, is interesting in itself; moreover, it suggests that a well-rounded *yogasana* practice can be a positive factor against osteoporosis in all of the long bones in a woman's body.

Yogasana

The power of *yogasana* to build a stronger and more dense bone mass is evident in the variety of weight-bearing positions it takes. In what other activity is weight placed for a long period of time on the head so as to load the cervical vertebrae? In what other activity is the spine twisted for an extended time while in alignment? *Yogasana* practice is also beneficial because the weight-bearing positions often can be held for relatively long times, rather than just being experienced impulsively, as when one swings at a tennis ball. In contrast, a complete lack of loading (no work done against the force of gravity, as when confined to bed) acts to thin and weaken bone. Arguing in reverse, it seems likely that bone also will demineralize if one does only "hanging" postures while holding weights, which puts bones under tensile stress rather than compressive stress. This will be a small effect unless one hangs often for hours at a time using heavy weights. Large increases in bone density are reported for the leg bones when the subject stands on a vibrating plate, and the bone growth stimulated by the passage of mechanical shock waves through the soft tissue of the body is thought to be related to that stimulated by yogic stretching and the application of external pressure.

It is almost certainly true that larger, stronger muscles do lead to larger, stronger bones, because the pull of such muscles on the bones, when they do work, acts as loading on the bones and so strengthens them. In this regard, *yogasana* is again valuable, for it will strengthen the bones as it strengthens the muscles. On the other hand, while a large frame does signify large bones, it does not necessarily signify a high bone density, which is the more relevant factor for osteoporosis [325].

A recent study [684] has shown that resistance exercise increases the strength of the muscles but has little or no positive effect on bone density. In contrast, those practicing high-impact step aerobics showed significant increases in the bone densities of their heels and lower spines. This correlates nicely with the findings that externally applied shock (as when jumping in *surya namaskar*) is very stimulating to bone growth.

In somewhat related research [335], it has been shown that passively standing upon a plate vibrating at 30 hertz for ten minutes a day for a year increases the bone density in the pelvis and spine by 3 percent, while adjacent muscle mass increases by 4 percent. Apparently, the vibrations act to stimulate the balancing sensors, so that when vibrating, there are constant small-muscle contractions in response to the balance sensors, and these contractions stimulate bone and muscle growth. In this way, it suggests that vigorous exercise is not a necessary ingredient of a program to fight osteoporosis; moreover, the vibrating-plate treatment parallels the yogic advice to bring circulation to a sprained ankle by practicing *vrksa-sana,* again using the small-muscle contractions inherent in maintaining balance (Subsection V.B, page 878.)

In regard to osteoporosis, we conclude that the advantage of *yogasana* practice is the total-body aspect of the practice, but the quickest route to local increases in bone density comes from high-impact approaches. Thinking in this vein, one would guess that one can gain the high-impact advantage of rapid increase of bone density by incorporating a significant amount of jumping in the *yogasana* practice, such as when repeating the *surya namaskar* series.

Section 8.A: The Spinal Column

The spinal column (also known as the vertebral column) has the highest priority for our attention in the *yogasanas*, for it is the principal postural axis of the body's skeleton, and the spinal cord within it is a conduit for many of the brain's lines of communication to and from the muscles, glands, and sensory and visceral organs. The function of the spine is both neurological, in regard to the spinal cord, and mechanical, in regard to the spinal column; and it is important that the *yogasana* teacher understands each of these aspects separately as well as how they might interact. The spinal column additionally serves as the site for the attachment of many major muscles, including the diaphragm; to the extent that the breath is controlled by the emotions, the emotions impact on that part of the spine closest to the diaphragm; i.e., the middle back and vice versa [10]. In the broadest sense possible, the spine and its components are the principal axis of our existence, secondary in importance only to the upper half of the central nervous system, the brain (Chapter 2, page 21, and Chapter 4, page 78).

Mechanically, the spinal column is anchored at its base to the pelvis, which serves as the point of attachment of the legs to the torso. The pelvis is not only a bowl holding the viscera of the abdomen but is also a participant in a major joint (the sacroiliac), allowing flexion (forward bending), extension (backward bend-

ing),[1] lateral bending, and twisting around the spine. At the opposite end, the spinal column supports the skull; more indirectly, the arms, scapulae, and ribs also articulate with the spinal column. While the spinal column proper is discussed in this chapter, the skull and pelvis are discussed in Chapter 9, page 311, the arms and legs in Chapter 10, page 323, and the ribs in Subsection 15.A, page 606.

Though the joints between the spinal column and the skull, pelvis, arms, legs, and ribs are synovial joints allowing wide ranges of motion, the main purpose of the synovial joints within the spine is to bear weight, to lubricate, and to act as shock absorbers [884], often within relatively small ranges of motion.

The spinal column is also important in another way, for as it evolved over the past five million years to allow humans to assume an upright bipedal posture, it altered the lungs and respiration so as to allow speech, and it freed the arms and hands for those manual activities that mark us as human. Moreover, once the hand was free to begin to fully develop its abilities in the biped, the brain was then stimulated to develop in order

---

1   In this work, the term "extension" is taken as the opposite of flexion; with respect to the spinal column, flexion refers to forward bending at the hips, and extension refers only to backward bending and not to lengthening or elongation of the spine. The terms "extension" and "flexion" are also used (somewhat arbitrarily) in describing arm position, with the arms-over-head position as in *urdhva hastasana* being called flexion and the positioning of the arms behind the back as in *purvottanasana* or *sarvangasana* being called extension [305].

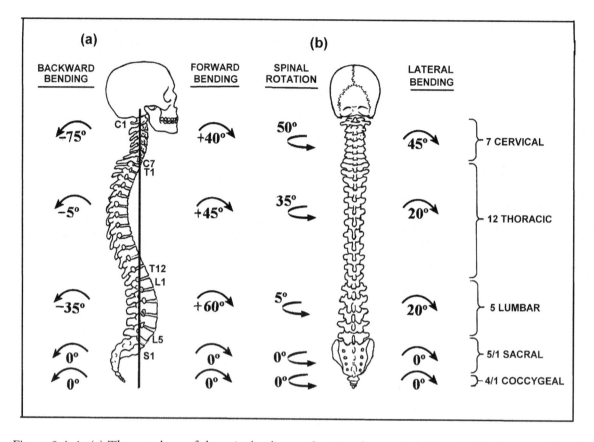

Figure 8.A-1. (**a**) The vertebrae of the spinal column, showing the cervical, thoracic, lumbar, sacral, and coccygeal sections in lateral view. The vertical line is drawn through each of the transitional points in the column where the vertebral type changes. Also shown are the maximal angular extension (on the left-hand side of the figure) and maximal angular flexion (on the right-hand side of the figure) in the five regions of the spine, as measured on a normal population. (**b**) Posterior view of the vertebrae of the spinal column. Also shown are the maximal angles for rotation about the spinal axis (on the left-hand side of the figure) and for lateral bending (on the right-hand side of the figure) in the five regions of the spine [428]. Note that these values were measured on non-yogic subjects and so likely represent bending at the upper hinge (the waist), whereas *yogasana* students are encouraged to bend at the lower hinge (the hips), Subsection 9.B, page 321.

to keep pace with the increasing dexterity of the hand [787]. Moreover, the modern spinal column has interlocking vertebrae, giving it a rigidity lacking, for example, in fish and reptiles where the vertebrae are noninterlocking.

Vertebral Structure and Motion

The Spinal Column

Considered at the simplest level, the spine consists of a bony yet flexible spinal column supporting the weight of the upper body (figures 8.A-1**a** and 8.A-1**b**) and a channel within this bony structure through which the bundle of spinal nerves (the spinal cord, figure 8.A-2**a**) passes. This spinal column is composed of bony vertebral building blocks set one on top of another, but with offsets front and back, which give the spine its characteristic front-to-back alternating curvatures. As with the ends of the long bones, such as the femur of the leg and the radius of the arm, the vertebrae are composed of cancellous (porous) bone (Subsection 7.A, page 225), with internal struts aligned to withstand the gravitational stress in the vertical direction [288]. However, if the spinal column comes under a chronic stress in a direction different from that of gravity, in time,

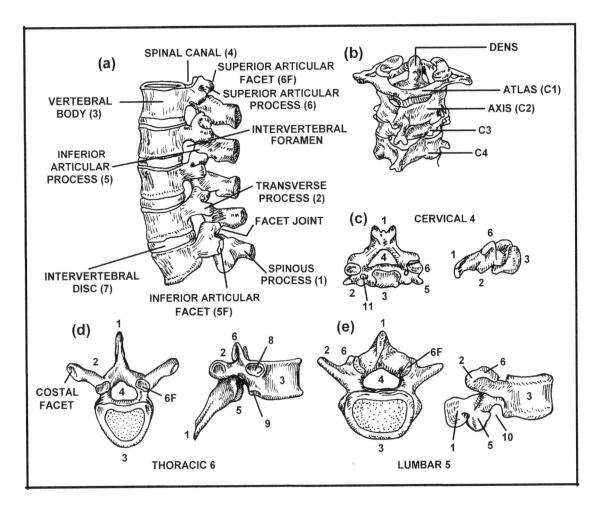

Figure 8.A-2. (a) Stacking of the lumbar vertebrae and the intervertebral discs so as to form facet joints, as seen with the posterior spine to the right. Numbers in parentheses in (a) correspond to those shown in drawings (b), (c), (d), and (e). (b) Superior view of the cervical vertebrae showing the atlas and dens. (c) Superior and lateral views of the architecture of the C4 vertebra. (d) Superior and lateral views of the T6 vertebra. (e) Superior and lateral views of the L5 vertebra. Key to numbered features: (1) spinous process, (2) transverse process, (3) vertebral body, (4) vertebral foramen (spinal canal), (5) inferior articular process, (5F) inferior articular facet, (6) superior articular process, (6F) superior articular facet, (7) vertebral disc, (8) and (9) facets for the formation of synovial joints to the ribs, (10) intervertebral foramen, and (11) transverse foramen for the vertebral artery. Adapted from [613].

it will remodel itself: the shape of the vertebrae will change, as will the direction of the supporting struts within the cancellous bone, so as to optimally support the stress and thus avoid collapse (Subsection 7.C, page 237).

Vertebral Numbering

There are seven vertebrae in the cervical region (labeled C1–C7), twelve in the thoracic region (labeled T1–T12), and five in the lumbar region (labeled L1–L5); whereas in the sacral region of the adult, five vertebrae (S1–S5) are fused into one, forming the sacrum, and four vertebrae are fused into one, forming the coccyx. The rigid bony structure of the spine is softened by the presence of twenty-three deformable intervertebral discs (figure 8.A-2a and Section 8.C, page 303). The numbering of exiting spinal nerves and the corresponding vertebrae can be confusing, because there are eight cervical nerves and only seven cervical vertebrae. The first cervical nerve exits between the occiput and the atlas (C1); i.e., it lies above the cervical vertebra with the corresponding number. The same situation holds for the other C2 to C7 cervical nerves and their corresponding vertebrae (figure 8.A-1a). However, the nerve C8 emerges from between C7 and T1, and all lower nerves are numbered according to the numbering of the vertebrae below them. This numbering system makes internal sense if one considers that the nerve labeled C1 is to be associated with the occiput rather than with the vertebra labeled C1, as in figure 8.A-1a.

The discrete vertebrae in the cervical, thoracic, and lumbar regions have a common architecture yet distinctly different shapes (figures 8.A-2c, 8.A-2d, and 8.A-2e) and ranges of motion, all of which can be rationalized in terms of the details of their functions. Note especially the vertebral facets 8 and 9 in the thoracic region (figure 8.A-2d), which are used to bind the ribs to the spinal column in that region. The ranges of motion of the various spinal sections are discussed in Section 8.B, page 281.

Spinal Functions

In humans, the various spinal sections function in the following ways: the cervical spinal column is highly mobile, assisting the visual apparatus by allowing wide-angle viewing due to the mobility of the head in the up/down and left/right directions; the thoracic spinal column supports the ribs, which protect the heart and lungs; the lumbar vertebrae mechanically support the structures above the pelvis and are shaped so as to allow deep forward bending, as in the quadrupedal stance; the sacral plate connects the spine to the pelvis; and the coccyx is a vestigial tail. Surgical removal of the coccyx has no discernible effect on one's health, though some have suggested that it serves to anchor minor muscles and so may be important to advanced *yogasana* students. Because each spinal section has a unique function and is shaped to optimize the performance of that function, the points of transition where vertebral types change sharply from one to the next (occiput to C1, C7 to T1, T12 to L1, L5 to S1) are especially weak in regard to misalignment (subluxation). Interestingly, each of these weak transi-

tional points lies on a vertical straight line (figure 8.A-1a).

Structural Elements

The Vertebral Body

Within each vertebra there is anteriorly a body of cancellous bone (3), which commonly is held to serve for weight bearing; posteriorly to this, there is an encircling arch of bone, which forms a small section of the vertebral foramen (4); the foramina of adjacent vertebrae are aligned so as to form the spinal canal. The delicate spinal cord is protected within the canal formed by the vertebral bodies and the neural arches of the vertebral blocks (figure 8.A-2a). Neural roots exit and enter the spinal cord through the transverse intervertebral foramina (10).

The Spinous Process

Each of the discrete vertebrae except C1 has a "spinous process" (1) projecting posteriorly (to the left in figure 8.A-1a and to the right in figure 8.A-2a), and it is this aspect of the vertebrae that one feels when palpating the spinal column from behind when in *dandasana* or *ardha uttanasana*, for example. The spinous processes can be very prominent in regard to palpation in the region C7–T1. Between vertebrae, there also are intervertebral foramina (10) for the lateral entry and exit of local nerve branches to and from the spinal cord, as distinct from the vertebral foramen, which runs the length of the spinal column (4). In each of the cervical vertebrae (C1–C7), two foramina in the transverse processes (11) allow the vertebral arteries access to the base of the skull and thence the brain (figure 4.E-1).

Articular Processes and their Facets

In addition to the spinous process, each vertebra also has a pair of transverse processes (2) extending laterally from the vertebral bodies; the upper and lower surfaces of each transverse process have protruding facets, called the superior articular facet and the inferior articular facet, respectively (figure 8.A-2a). These superior and in-

Table 8.A-1: Geometric Parameters and Dimensions of the Spine [428]

Property	Cervical	Thoracic	Lumbar	Sacral	Coccygeal
Number of vertebrae	7	12	5	5/1[a]	4/1[b]
Anterior curvature at given age					
Age					
1 day	Convex	Convex	Convex	Straight	Straight
13 months		Convex	Straight	Straight	Straight
3 years		Convex	Concave[c]	Concave[c]	Convex
10 years	Concave	Convex	Concave	Convex	
Adult	Concave	Convex	Concave	Convex	Convex
Forward displacement from posterior[d]	33	25	50	Slight	Slight
Kg (lb) weight carried in 100-Kg (220 lb) man[e]	9 (20)	17 (37)	47 (81)	-	-
Disc thickness, mm	3	5	9	0	0
Thickness/height[f]	0.4	0.2	0.33	0	0
Position of nucleus pulposus[g]	5.5	5.5	6	-	-
Flexion, degrees	40	45	60	0	0
Flexion per vertebra, degrees	5.7	3.8	12	0	0
Extension, degrees	-75	-5	-35	0	0
Extension per vertebra, degrees	10.7	0.4	7	0	0
Lateral flexion range, degrees	+/- 45	+/-20	+/-20	0	0
Lateral flexion per vertebra, degrees	6.4	1.7	4	0	0
Axial rotation range, degrees	+/-50	+/-35	+/-5	0	0
Axial rotation per vertebra, degrees	7.1	2.9	1	0	0

a Five vertebrae fused into one
b Four vertebrae fused into one
c Very slightly so
d The forward distance of the vertebrae from the back body, as a percentage of the back-to-front distance
e The weight carried by each of the spinal sections in a 100-kilogram (220-pound) man
f Ratio of disc thickness to vertebral height
g Relative to 0.0 representing the front of the vertebral body, and 10.0 representing the back of the vertebral body

ferior articular facets on a particular vertebra form synovial joints (Section 7.D, page 239) with the articular facets on adjacent vertebrae, in order to align and stabilize the spinal column. In particular, the superior articular facets of a given vertebra form facet joints with the inferior articular facets of the vertebra above it, and its inferior articular facets form facet joints with the superior articular facets of the vertebra below it. These facet joints are very stabilizing mechanically for the spinal column, but in turn, they can severely limit the range of motion for *yogasana* students. The transverse processes in the cervical region are also the sites for many bilateral muscle attachments.

The situation in regard to synovial joints in the spine is considerably changed in the thoracic region, for the thoracic vertebrae are joined not only to one another by synovial joints, but also to a set of twelve ribs, again through synovial joints. This is discussed further in Subsection 15.A, page 605.

Intervertebral Discs

Each of the vertebrae is separated from its neighbor by a soft pad of tissue known as the intervertebral disc. This disc serves both as a shock absorber and as a cushion around which adjacent vertebrae enjoy a certain amount of motion, thanks to the increased distance between neighbors.

Mechanical Stability

Though one often works in *yogasana* to make the spine more flexible, the spine's inherent rigidity is actually the key to its mechanical stability; the strong spine is both flexible and mechanically well braced. The spine would have little mechanical stability were it not for the facet joints and the array of muscles and ligaments (Subsection 8.A, page 259) that bind the vertebrae to one another and to the ribs via the transverse and spinous processes [428]. Additionally, the fibrous intervertebral discs (Section 8.C, page 303) act as symphysis joints, holding adjacent vertebrae in their proper positions while allowing limited motion.

The direction and amount of vertebral movement is dictated largely by the interactions among the articular facets of the transverse processes. The interlocking nature of the vertebrae, on the one hand, stabilizes the spine by limiting its possible motion; but on the other hand, the limited nature of its motion can be a frustration to the *yogasana* student, as when backbending or twisting. The various geometric parameters and ranges of motion of the spinal segments in the average population are summarized in table 8.A-1.

Loading

A spinal loading of 600 kilograms (1,300 pounds) is sufficient to crush or fracture the anterior portions of the vertebrae, and at 800 kilogram (1,800 pounds), the entire vertebra is crushed. Unfortunately, at loading far less than this, the osteoporotic vertebrae of the elderly are readily fractured and collapsed. See Section 7.G, page 254, for more discussion of this. Axial loading on the cervical vertebrae, as when in *sirsasana*, is considered in the subsection below.

The Cervical Spinal Section

Vertebral Joints

The uppermost seven vertebrae in the spinal column are called the cervical vertebrae, with the upper two being unique in their deviation from the norm (figure 9.A-2b). The uppermost vertebra, C1, also called the "atlas," forms the joint between the spinal column and the occiput of the skull, with the facets of the atlas mating with the condyles of the occiput. The atlas, the smallest of the moveable vertebrae, is somewhat ring-like, with a large vertebral foramen; because C1 has no vertebral body, there is no vertebral disc between it and the occiput above. C2, the "axis," also is unique in the spinal column, having an upward-pointing spike 1.5 centimeters (0.6 inches) long called the "dens." This spike rests within the foramen of the atlas (figure 9.A-2b), where it functions as a cranial pivot. Because the spinal cord and the dens of C2 both occupy the vertebral foramen of the atlas, the integrity of the dens within the foramen of the atlas is very important, for if the dens were fractured, then the spinal cord within the foramen might be compressed by fragments of the dens, and death could result.

The joint between the skull and C1, the atlanto-occipital joint, is relatively immobile, allowing only slight rotation. In this joint, the condyles of the occiput and the mating surfaces of the atlas form saddle-shaped joints of limited three-dimensional motion. The mating surfaces of the C1 atlas and the C2 axis form the atlanto-axoid joint, and when the head is rotated around the dens, the atlas sinks onto the axis by 2–3 millimeters (one-eighth inch), meaning that the "rotational" motion of the head actually is helical rather than purely rotatory [288]. There are five ligaments connecting the atlas to the axis.

The structural mismatch between the cervical and thoracic vertebrae is filled by the unique structure of C7, with its large spinous process. When C7 is displaced posteriorly and becomes covered with a thick pad of nonfunctional tissue, the stage is set for the development of a dowager's hump (see Subsection 8.A, page 271, [599]). In most spines, the C7 vertebra is at the level of the clavicle bones.

The presence of small muscles connecting the occiput to various prominences of the atlas and axis are very important to the practice of the *yogasanas*, due to their high concentrations of muscle spindles used in proprioceptive sensing of balance (see Subsection 11.B, page 428).

Motion

As can be seen in figure 8.A-1**a**, the spinous processes of the cervical vertebrae are inclined about 45–90° with respect to the line of the spinal column itself, looking much like a set of Venetian blinds; whereas the planes of the articular facets (figure 8.A-2**b**) have angles with respect to the line of the spinal column that are nearly 90°. The articular facet joints allow movement of the cervical vertebrae, but only by sliding one vertebra upward and forward or backward and downward with respect to its neighbors. For example, when the chin is dropped into the *jalandhara-bandha* position, the cervical vertebrae slide upward and forward; when the head is tipped backward (in

extension), as in *ustrasana*, the same vertebrae slide downward and backward. With facet joints such as these, cervical spinal rotation is achieved by the facet joints on one side of the spine going forward and upward while those on the opposite side go backward and downward. It is clear from their architecture that the spinal facet joints work best when the motions are simple linear movements of one transverse process with respect to the next along lines parallel or perpendicular to the spinal axis. Note that the articular processes, though made of bone, nonetheless have a certain flexibility that allows one facet to be pressed against the adjacent one, with a consequent bending of the bone. Working the facet joints in this manner, however, is risking the chance of a broken vertebra and so should be avoided. Moreover, 360° neck rolls are to be discouraged, as this is a motion appropriate to a ball-and-socket joint such as the glenoid fossa of the shoulder (figure 10.A-1), and this is certainly not the case in the cervical spine [495].

One can divide the cervical spine into two parts. The upper cervical spine consists of the occiput, the atlas (C1), and the axis (C2); the lower cervical spine consists of vertebrae C3 to C7. These two sections have somewhat opposite curvature and can be moved independently of one another. When rotating the head by 90° around the spinal axis, the upper section is responsible for 20–30° and the lower for 60–70° of the full rotation.

Loading

The weight of the head is supported by the facet joints between the occiput and C1 and between C1 and C2, whereas the dens acts as a central pivot, keeping the vertebral array in alignment [288]. The uppermost two cervical vertebrae carry the weight of the skull (about 9 kilograms, or twenty pounds) with ease; however, when inverted in *sirsasana*, the weight can be considerably over 45 kilograms (100 pounds), as all of the body weight, save that of the skull and arms, is now supported by these vertebrae. Even when much of the body weight is born instead by the action of the arms on the floor, *sirsasana I* can still be a challenge to the cervical vertebrae. In any event, in such an inversion, the body weight is first distributed onto the two atlanto-occipital joints (left and right), thence to the two atlanto-axoid joints (left and right), and from there, it is redistributed onto the three pillars of C3 and the lower vertebrae; i.e., onto the vertebral bodies and the articular facet joints. In general, most of the body weight is born by the vertebral bodies and their associated vertebral discs when in *sirsasana I*. In this case, the thoracic and lumbar facet joints are kept open and mobile, as might be needed for performing *sirsasana* variations; however, also see Appendix IV, page 862.

Nepalese porters are reported to carry even heavier loads on their heads than do African women. These men carried loads from 93 to 183 percent of their body weights on footpaths up to 2,800 meters (8,400 feet) high; women's loads under these conditions average 66 percent of body weight. The porters carry these large loads for many hours by walking slowly and resting often [568]. By comparison, beginning *yogasana* students with no understanding of how to work the arms to reduce weight on the head and neck place about 50 percent of their full body weight on the head in *sirsasana I*; intermediate-level students commit only 35 percent or less of their total weight to the head in this posture (Subsection IV.D, page 858).

As a consequence of excessive muscle tone in the upper trapezius, levator scapulae, and rhomboid-minor muscles of many of those without *yogasana* training, the scapulae and shoulders can be pulled up around the ears. Because these muscles have their origins on the cervical vertebrae, excessive tightness results in a compressive load on these vertebrae, with negative consequences for the intervertebral discs and joints [410a].

Injury

Because the articular facets in the cervical spine are essentially horizontal (figure 8.A-2b) and the spinous processes do not strongly overlap, when in a "whiplash" situation (as when seated in a stopped auto and then struck from behind), the adjacent cervical vertebrae can eas-ily be subluxed in the front-to-back direction without breaking. As discussed in Subsection 11.D, page 458, the injuries suffered in a whiplash situation relate strongly to the consequences of the startle reflex.

The atlas and axis are the two vertebrae in the spinal column most vulnerable to subluxation, because they are the only two vertebrae which do not have strongly interlocking bony facets. Death from whiplash often is due to the dens of the axis being driven into the medulla oblongata of the spinal cord at the level of the atlas (figure 8.A-2b). The C1 and C2 vertebrae also are very susceptible to subluxation if the head is tilted to the side with weight on the head, as might occur when in *sirsasana* with the head placed off center on the floor, or if the head is turned while in *sarvangasana*.

The Thoracic Spinal Section

Vertebral Joints

The shapes of the thoracic vertebrae are unique due to their attachments to the ribs (Subsection 15.A, page 606). In this spinal section, the body of a thoracic vertebra carries both a superior and an inferior costal facet (figure 8.A-2d) in addition to the normal articular facets found in vertebrae of the cervical (figure 8.A-2c) and lumbar sections (figure 8.A-2e). In turn, the posterior ends of each rib bear two facets, one of which is joined to the superior costal facet of a thoracic vertebra and the other of which is joined to the inferior costal facet of the higher neighboring vertebra (figures 15.A-3c and 15.A-3d). Thus, each rib in the group T1 to T12 is bound posteriorly between two neighboring vertebrae by synovial joints, but only ribs T1 to T10 are bound anteriorly to the sternum. In 8 percent of adults, there is a thirteenth rib (issuing from either C7 or L1) and the superior and inferior angles of the scapulae in most spines are at the levels of the T2 and T7 vertebrae, respectively. Viewed from the front, the sternal notch of the rib cage is at the level of T2 and the xiphoid process is at the level of T10.

Motion

The ribs not only are attached to the posterior surfaces of the thoracic vertebrae in a way that binds each vertebra to its neighbors (figure 8.A-2**d**), but the articular facet joints also bind each thoracic vertebra to its nearest neighbors. Moreover, the anterior end of each of the ribs is bound firmly to the cartilage of the sternum. Consequently, motions of the thoracic vertebrae are severely limited by their connections to the rib cage. A second important factor arises in regard to the thoracic vertebrae if forward, backward, or lateral bending is allowed to occur at the upper hinge (figure 9.B-5**a**). In this case, the chest tends to collapse in the direction of the bending, and the ribs then collide with one another on the side to which one is bending. This rib-on-rib contact is avoided if the chest is kept lifted and the spine kept as left-to-right symmetric as possible, even though the posture might be inherently asymmetric. This is discussed further in Section 7.F, page 252, and Subsection 9.B, page 321.

Looking at the spinous processes in figure 8.A-1**a**, it is seen that in the cervical and lumbar regions the spinous processes are more or less perpendicular to the line of their vertebral bodies, whereas in the thoracic region, they are more strongly angled down and more closely approach one another. Thus, the clamping effects on the rib cage of the thoracic vertebrae, which contribute so significantly to the rigidity of the thoracic spine, are enhanced by the bone-on-bone contact among the spinous processes when backbending (unless the vertebrae can be pulled further apart so as to avoid bone-on-bone contact). Indeed, only 2.9° of backbending (table 8.A-1) can be generated by each of the twelve thoracic vertebrae, due to the bone-on-bone contacts between adjacent spinous processes.

Loading

Thanks to the presence in the thorax of the lungs and the diaphragm, it is readily possible to strengthen the spine in the thoracic region whenever the spine is loaded externally. Known as the Valsalva maneuver, it involves taking a deep breath, closing the glottis, and tightening the abdominal muscles, all simultaneously. When in the Valsalva mode, the thorax is inflated, so that large weights can be lifted with the arms, all the while sparing the thoracic vertebrae from compressional loading. Needless to say, the Valsalva maneuver is inappropriate for *yogasana* practice and should be avoided when possible. See Subsection 15.C, page 616, for more on how inappropriate this common maneuver is to *yogasana* practice.

Injury

The effects of whiplash on the thoracic and lumbar vertebrae differ from those on the cervical vertebrae. During whiplash, the thoracic and lumbar vertebrae may well be pressed forward (dislocated or subluxed); however, because the spinous processes point downward and adjacent processes strongly overlap one another (figure 8.A-1**a**), the tendencies toward subluxation, luxation, and injury to the spinal cord in the thoracic region are diminished.

The Lumbar Spinal Section

Vertebral Joints

The lumbar vertebrae are three-dimensional and massive compared with those in the higher spinal sections (figure 8.A-1), as would be expected for those at the base of the spinal column. In most spines, the L4 vertebra is at the level of the line connecting the iliac crests.

Motion

Note that the planes of the articular facets face differently in the different spinal regions. For example, for the lumbar vertebrae, the planes of the facets are essentially vertical, allowing easy forward and backward bending (+60° and -35°, table 8.A-1) in this section; whereas spinal rotation drives one lumbar facet into that of its neighbor and so is much more difficult in this region (only 1° per vertebra, table 8.A-1).

Injury

Because the L5–S1 intervertebral disc is very thick and wedge-shaped, with the thicker edge being anterior, there is a resulting concave curvature to the lumbar spine as viewed posteriorly. Moreover, because of the curvature of the lower spinal column, the intervertebral surface between L5 and S1 is inclined by only 30° from vertical (figure 8.A-1a), so that L5 tends to slide forward and downward with little resistance. Consequently, the L5-S1 joint is relatively very weak in regard to subluxation, the L5 spinous process not withstanding. The resistance of L5 to sliding is offered by bone-on-bone contact in the vertebral arch, but if this arch fractures, then one develops spondylothesis and spasms of the erector spinae muscles [288]. Discussion of lower-back pain is deferred to Subsection 8.C, page 307.

The Sacral and Coccygeal Spinal Sections

Vertebral Joints

The five individual sacral vertebrae are connected by cartilage in childhood and are transformed into a single bone (the sacrum) in the adult spinal column. The coccyx has three to five (usually four) fused, rudimentary vertebrae, with the joint between the coccyx and the sacrum being of the fibrocartilage type, thus allowing front-back movement during defecation or labor. The sacrum also is held to the coccyx by many ligaments. In the male, the sacral-coccygeal joint ossifies at an early age, but in females, it remains open and moveable until much later, to allow for pregnancy and delivery. This gender difference in the ossification of the sacral-coccygeal joint may be a factor in determining the relative ease of backbending in the two genders. Four distinct muscles connect to the coccyx, including the gluteus maximus; these are largely vestigial from our tailed relatives [288] but nonetheless would seem to allow deliberate motion of this part of the spinal column.

As they develop in utero, all vertebrates have the ability to form a vertebral tail. However, only in humans is this development brought to a halt and then reversed. In this case, the tail is evident in the five-week-old fetus, but this appendage is then destroyed by apoptosis and the remaining tissue fused to become the coccyx; nonetheless, approximately a hundred cases have been reported in the medical literature of human infants born with functional tails (vertebra, muscles, ligaments, etc.) which were then removed after birth. See also Box 8.A-1, page 270, regarding the amphibian phase of human evolutionary development.

Injury

The sacrum is bound to the pelvis by the sacroiliac joint, a structure that is rather easily injured by overly vigorous action in the spinal twists. This is discussed further in Subsection 8.B, page 298.

Normal Curvature

Though the spinal column ideally is as straight as a yardstick when viewed either anteriorly or posteriorly, it shows an alternating curvature in the front-to-back direction when viewed from the side (figure 8.A-1a). When viewed posteriorly, the cervical and lumbar regions are curved concavely, whereas the thoracic and sacral regions, when viewed posteriorly, are curved convexly (figure 8.A-1a and table 8.A-1).[2]

If, in the standing adult, one imagines cross sections taken through the neck, chest, and abdomen, one will see quantitatively where the ver-

---

2   Descriptions of spinal curvature as "convex" or "concave" are arbitrary, depending upon the viewer's points of view of the spine and the meanings of these words. Throughout this handbook, the spine will be viewed from the posterior position, and when curved toward the observer, the curvature is termed "convex," and when curved away from the viewer, the curvature is termed "concave." When standing erect in *tadasana* and viewed from behind, the cervical, thoracic, lumbar, and sacral regions are observed/defined as having concave, convex, concave, and convex curvatures, respectively. Others have used definitions that are opposite to those used here.

tebral bodies are placed along a horizontal line going from the very back of the body to the front of the body at that elevation; these values appear as "Forward displacement from posterior, %" in table 8.A-1. In the region of the cervical spine, the vertebral bodies are seen on average to be about 33 percent forward from the back of the neck toward the front of the throat, resulting in the concave curvature of the cervical section. This position places the cervical bodies almost under the center of gravity of the head (the sella turcica, figure 9.A-2a). In the thorax, the spine is pressed back so that its vertebral bodies on average are only 25 percent of the way forward along the back-to-chest line. This posterior displacement accommodates the heart and lungs within the chest cavity and leads to convex curvature when viewed posteriorly.

The spine is again pressed forward in the lumbar region, being situated 50 percent along the back-to-front line on average, again the placement being such as to position the vertebral bodies just under the torso's center of gravity and resulting in significant concavity when viewed posteriorly.

The alternating curvatures of the spinal column are a mechanical simulation of a flexible spring and in fact work to dissipate the vertical forces inherent in standing, walking, running, jumping, carrying, etc. These changing curvatures of the spinal column (table 8.A-1 and figure 8.A-1a) reflect not only the historic development of the individual but the historic development of the individual's species, as discussed in Box 8.A-1, below.

Alternating Curvature

As the infant matures, the spinal curves develop in a way such that the spinal column becomes more like a spring, in large part isolating the brain from the mechanical stresses inherent in walking [10]. As pointed out by Kapandji [428], the alternating curvatures of the adult spine actually strengthen it mechanically by approximately a factor of ten, compared to a straight rod of the same material and dimensions. Were the spine a straight metal rod, its shock-absorbing capacity would be nil; whereas when the rod is curved

in imitation of a spring, the same metal "spine" can then be an excellent shock absorber, thanks to the flexibility implicit in its curves and its ability to convert the energy of flexion into heat [884]. Were the spine to grow into a rigid, straight rod,[3] then walking would be difficult, for the jolt of every footstep would be transmitted directly to the brain. The various alternating curvatures in the adult spine can be brought into correspondence with the five lowest *chakras* as indicated in table 5.G-1 [10].

This springiness of the spine due to its unique series of curves is mirrored in the feet, where the arches of the feet act as springs to absorb the shock to the spine and higher structures when walking or running (see Section 10.B, page 359). Additionally, each pair of adjacent vertebrae in the spinal column is separated by a resilient pad of soft tissue, the intervertebral disc, which also can function as a shock absorber between the feet and the skull, as long as it is kept well nourished and healthy (Subsection 8.A, page 264, and Section 8.C, page 303).

Though the curvatures of the spine are clearly advantageous from the aspects of mechanical strength, stability, mobility, and shock absorption, there is also a price to be paid. In allowing motion of the spine in many directions, motions also may occur in directions that result in misalignment of the component vertebrae (subluxation) and the woes of "back trouble" (Subsection 8.C, page 307), especially at those points of transition between vertebral types and opposing curvatures (figure 8.A-1a).

Abnormal Curvature

Lordosis

The most obvious deviations of the spine from the norm involve either the exaggeration or

---

3   In certain cases of severe spinal misalignment, rigid metal rods actually are inserted in the spinal column to brace and straighten it. This artificial rigidity must result in reduced shock absorption, among other things.

Box 8.A-1: Ontogeny Recapitulates Phylogeny

It is a long-considered principle of evolutionary development that "ontogeny recapitulates phylogeny," meaning that as a fetus and an infant mature, they tend to go through developmental stages that mimic stages in the evolution of its phylum and species. These stages have their analogs in the *yogasana* lexicon.

In utero, the fetus has frog-like gills, a tail, and webbed hands and feet, as appropriate to an amphibian (*mandukasana*); see Subsection 8.A, page 268, for a discussion of humans born with such amphibian appendages. The sacral and coccygeal regions of the spinal column are essentially straight at this early time. However, in the newborn infant, the curvature in the cervical, thoracic, and lumbar regions of the spine has become posteriorly convex (table 8.A-1): the curvature is that of the fetal position (*garbhasana*), appropriate to fitting the fetus into the small space of the womb [433, 469].

The first notable accomplishment of the infant is the lifting of its head, which strengthens the muscles of the neck and reverses the cervical curve from posteriorly convex to posteriorly concave. With the head and the upper part of its body lifted in this early stage, the infant's posture is now reptilian, resembling *bhujangasana*. This change of cervical curvature is effected in spite of the off-center nature of the head as it is mounted on the atlas; i.e., the center of gravity (Section V.C, page 887) of the head lies forward of the atlas, resulting in the head dropping forward unless the muscles at the back of the neck are sufficiently toned so as to pull the head into the erect position, thereby generating a cervical concavity (figure V.C-1).

Sitting as in *muktasana* then follows, representing a simian phase in which the lumbar region is strengthened and the lumbar curvature reverses to concave [288]. Later, the infant develops the ability to rise onto all fours. With this, the lumbar concavity develops further, and the stance is quadrupedal (*adho mukha svanasana*). Finally, the infant rises to stand in *tadasana* and moves on two feet, as befits a bipedal species. Once the spinal curves have begun to develop, and the infant stands and begins to walk, then the hands can be used for more important tasks than just support [68]. All of the *yogasana* practices of the infant are punctuated with deep, intensely restorative sessions of *savasana*.

When standing erect in *tadasana*, the line connecting the centers of gravity of the body and of the earth (Section III.B, page 845) runs from the base of the ankle through the external opening in the ear and passes through each of the spinal transitions: the atlanto-occipital joint, C7–T1, T12–L1 and L5–S1 (figure 8.A-1**a**), as well as the hip joint, the knee, and the ankle [288] (figure 9.B-4**c**). The front-to-back curvature of the spine is such that the center of gravity of the upper body is centered front to back over the hip joints. As a person ages normally, the cervical and lumbar curves tend to reverse, going from posteriorly concave to posteriorly convex, moving one back toward the fetal posture.

the reversal of the cervical, lumbar, and thoracic curves (figure 4.A-1a) or the deviation of the spine from strict left-right symmetry (figure 4.A-1b). As for the lumbar curvature, when standing with the heels, buttocks, shoulder blades, and back of the head to the wall, the lumbar vertebrae, when in proper curvature, should be no further from the wall than the thickness of the metacarpal heads where they join the palm of the hand (about 2 centimeters, or one inch). A similar criterion for ideal lumbar curvature holds when lying face up on the floor.

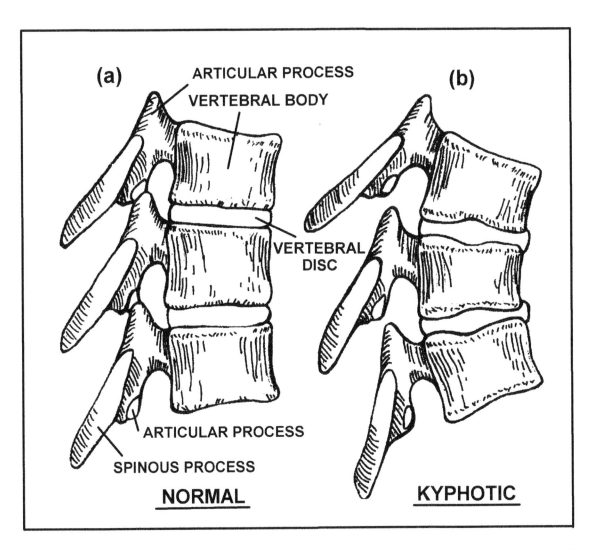

Figure 8.A-3. (a) Normal curvature in the thoracic spine, as seen with the posterior to the left. (b) The thoracic kyphosis that results from a wedging of the vertebrae and/or the discs (being thicker on the posterior left-hand edges), leading to a dowager's hump.

Extreme concave curvature of the lumbar spine is called lordosis or, more commonly, "swayback" and involves rotations of the articular facet joints in the lumbar region around the left-to-right horizontal line, even in the relaxed position. Though one may suspect lordosis in a student with overly large buttocks, the bony part of the back body still may have just the normal curvature. Students who have noticeable lordosis in their normal posture often suffer from lower-back pain; they can relieve the compression of their lumbar spine when standing by pulling their navel backward onto the spine, especially in the *yogasanas*. The same recipe holds for adjusting

lordosis when it accompanies a *yogasana* posture in a student who otherwise does not display this lumbar condition. Thus, for example, when the arms come over the head in *urdhva hastasana*, the lumbar often goes lordotic; again, the adjustment is to pull the navel toward the spine as the lowest back ribs and the back rim of the pelvis move away from one another.

Kyphosis

Spinal concavity in the cervical and lumbar regions is promoted by intervertebral discs that are thicker anteriorly and thinner posteriorly in these regions. For example, the posterior axis of the sacrum is set at 30° to vertical, and as a consequence of this, the joint between the lowest lumbar vertebra (L5) and the sacrum is padded with a disc that is strongly wedge-shaped, creating a strongly concave curvature in the lumbar area. In contrast, if the vertebrae or the discs themselves in the thoracic region are wedged oppositely to those in the cervical and lumbar regions, a kyphotic posterior convexity known as "dowager's hump" results (figure 8.A-3b). Medically, the kyphotic condition is defined as having an angle between the upper thoracic spine and the center line of the spine that is equal to or larger than 40°. The "normal" spinal column shown in figure 8.A-1a shows a value of 20° for the angle in question.

Kyphosis is most often a problem in the elderly suffering from osteoporosis (Subsection 7.G, page 254). In this case, the anterior edges of the thoracic vertebrae collapse, so as to produce excessively wedged vertebrae and accentuated convex curvature. Vertebral fractures are also a significant contributing cause of kyphosis.

Schatz [757] outlines the postural consequences of having a kyphotic back. In this condition, the neck is thrust forward while the chest collapses, leaving little room for the lungs, which instead push downward on the diaphragm and the abdominal organs, forcing the latter to push the abdominal muscles forward, impeding circulation and leading to constipation. Spinal rotation is hindered in an upper back in this collapsed state. Furthermore, when the head is chronically carried in the forward position, there is a possible interference with the blood flow to the thymus gland and to the brain via the vertebral arteries, and possibly a compromised immune system [482].

Though the kyphosis resulting from a wedging of the thoracic vertebrae is largely irreversible, there is also a reversible kyphosis that results from muscle imbalance. For example, young women who are overly self-conscious may try to hide their breasts by assuming a rounded upper back and a collapsed chest. In such a case, yogic opening of the chest and strengthening of the muscles of the upper back, as with *ustrasana* and *urdhva*

dhanurasana, can reverse the kyphotic curvature of the spinal column.

Cervical Curvature

Standing erect, the proper cervical curvature is attained when the line between the tip of the chin and the forehead is vertical, or when in *savasana*, this line is horizontal. However, in various other postures, the neck is properly placed in extreme curvature, as when flexed in *halasana* or *sarvangasana*, or as when extended in *salabhasana*, *vrschikasana*, etc.

Scoliosis

In students with scoliosis sufficiently severe to require treatment (90 percent are female and 10 percent are male), sections of the thoracic and/or lumbar spines are offset from the medial plane to the right, to the left, or both. In 90 percent of teenagers with a scoliotic displacement of only the thoracic spine, the sense of displacement is to the right, as if the spine is being pulled away from the heart; and in 80 percent of those with only a lumbar displacement, it is to the left, as if it is being pulled away from the liver. Curves also appear in which both the thoracic and the lumbar curvatures are to the right; less often, the thoracic curve is to the right and the lumbar to the left [570, 571, 572, 572a]. Adolescent scoliosis involves wedge-shaped vertebrae, with the thicker parts of the vertebrae oriented to the side toward which the spine is bent [275], just as lordosis and kyphosis involve orientation of the thicker portions of the vertebral wedges either forward or backward, respectively.

As an added complication, the left-right displacement of scoliosis is often accompanied by a front-to-back asymmetry, in which the ribs on one side protrude forward and the ribs on the other side protrude backward; i.e., in which a section of the spine is both laterally displaced and rotated about the central axis. For example, in a right-thoracic scoliosis in which the thoracic vertebrae are displaced to the right, the ribs on the right side will be more widely separated and rotated forward, whereas the ribs on the left side will be pressed toward one another and rotated backward. This is in accord with the generality expressed in Box 8.B-1, page 299, which relates lateral bending and spinal rotation.

External signs of scoliosis may include a high shoulder, a prominent shoulder blade, a prominent breast, a high iliac crest, a prominent buttock, and poor overall posture. Should the scoliosis be severe, the curvature may press on the spinal cord, with resultant neurological complications. Though various postural imbalances involving the shoulders, pelvis, head, etc. may be associated with these spinal distortions, it is not clear to the novice observer what is "cause" and what is "effect." The spinal asymmetry of scoliosis is most easily seen by the *yogasana* teacher from behind, while the student is bending forward, as in *adho mukha svanasana*.

Sixty-five to 80 percent of scoliosis cases are deemed to be idiopathic; i.e., "of unknown cause." Western medical scientists agree with *yogasana* practitioners that the year-to-year rate of scoliotic deviation, if it is not too large, can be resisted by postural manipulation. However, they find that corrective bracing to simply reduce the rate of enlargement of the scoliotic angle requires twenty-three hours a day of realigning force applied for a year or more, whereas we as *yogasana* teachers generally subject our clients daily to only one to two hours of corrective stress. Consequently, the yogic approach may be effective in preventing an increase in the problem, but only very slowly, over the course of many years. In accord with this, Kiley [442] mentions that a breath-centered yogic practice may be able to affect the body so as to slow the progression of the deformity but not reverse it.

Note too that the scoliotic torsion of the spine may have its origin in asymmetric muscular imbalances in far distant sites; e.g., in the shoulders and legs. Moreover, a small study has suggested that scoliosis in some adolescents may be a consequence of a vestibular dysfunction (Section 18.B, page 701) that hampers the person's ability to orient symmetrically in the earth's gravitational field [676], resulting in a spine that is pulled asymmetrically out of alignment in an effort to negate a perceived postural imbalance. A similar scoliosis

would follow if the muscle-spindle signals of the left and right capitis muscles at the back of the neck, normally used to keep the head in an upright position (Subsection V.C, page 887), were neurologically imbalanced, thereby inducing a local twisting of the spinal column in response to a falsely perceived imbalance of the head position.

Yogasana

Because the range-of-motion data in table 8.A-1 was assembled from a population of "normal" individuals, *yogasana* students, with their mastery of the spine, may far exceed the values given there (see below), whereas students with spinal problems such as scoliosis may not be able to achieve "the norm" without significant effort, if at all.

For students with lordosis, kyphosis, or scoliosis, *yogasana* practice can be difficult, for each implies that in the displaced region, the adjacent vertebral facets or the ribs are already in close contact and so will resist further motion. This is especially true in backward-bending *yogasanas* and in *yogasanas* involving spinal twisting. Indeed, as Schatz has pointed out [756], in a student with an abnormal spinal displacement, rotation can be painful in the region of the displacement; in a more normal region of the spine, the student may over-rotate in an effort to compensate, and so be injured. In either case, one should encourage a more normal alignment and spinal lengthening (Section 8.A, page 272), if possible, before trying to rotate fully. Realignment of the scoliotic spine is much simpler in those rare cases where there is only left-right displacement without rotation. Because the act of breathing requires an extra effort when the spine is strongly scoliotic or kyphotic, allowance must be made for *yogasana* students who are burdened with such abnormal curvatures.

When the scoliosis is slight, it is said that its curvature and the discomfort associated with it can be minimized by twisting into the concavity of the displacement; i.e., twisting oppositely to the twist inherent in the scoliosis [577]. Note also that in scoliosis, there often is a partial collapse of the lung on one side of the chest, which spinal twisting and *pranayama* can help to open again. Miller gives advice on how to alter the *yogasanas* to accommodate any of four different scoliosis types [572a].

Spinal Elongation and *Yogasana*

Lumbar curvature is a balance between the muscle tone of the abdominal muscles encouraging lumbar convexity on the one hand, and the tone of the paravertebral erector spinae (figure 10.A-2**b**) and psoas muscles (figure 9.B-2**b**), each encouraging lumbar concavity. Electromyographic studies reveal that when standing in a relaxed position, the spinal curvature is controlled almost totally by the paravertebral muscles; however, when in *tadasana*, not only the abdominal muscles come into play, but the gluteus maximus and hamstrings also activate, as well as the paravertebral muscles. As lengthening of the spine is one of the postural goals in *tadasana*, it is advantageous in this posture to reduce any and all excess curvature and muscle tone in all of the spinal sections. Thus, in *tadasana*, the muscles in the posterior neck relax, so as to reduce cervical curvature, thereby increasing the cervical length; the sternum is lifted away from the pelvis (which also may reduce cramping of the heart and lungs that otherwise follows from exaggerated thoracic curvature); psoas tension is reduced, so as to reduce excess lumbar curvature; and at the same time, the tone in the abdominals, gluteus, and hamstrings increases, so as to aid flattening and elongation of the lumbar spine. The total effect of these actions in *tadasana* is maximal elongation of the spine while preserving the spirit of the natural spinal curves.

Questions of hydration aside, the spine, when in its normal curvature, is only 95 percent as long as the fully elongated spine. Virtually all of the 5-percent deficit in the spinal length can be recovered by conscious yogic elongation.

Note that at the extreme ends of the spinal column, the curvature of the spine will be strongly dictated by the tilt of the head and pelvis. Thus, when sitting in a slumped position in *dandasana*, the spine can be lengthened, in part, by a rotation of the pelvis around the hip joints, which lifts the back rim of the pelvis upward while reversing the lumbar curvature from convex to concave. Pelvic tilt in general is dictated by the combined actions of the hip rotators, adductors, abductors, flexors, and extensors of the legs and pelvis. While in *dandasana*, extreme concave curvature of the cervical spine can be reduced by rotating the head more toward a flexional posture.

When standing on one leg, as in *vrksasana*, the lumbar naturally falls to the unsupported side, the thorax shifts to the supported side, and the cervical spine then moves again to the unsupported side. Again, in the interest of increasing spinal length, these lateral curves induced by the posture's asymmetric geometry may be minimized by pulling the independent body parts onto the common center line. Lying on one side of the body (*anantasana*, for example) again results in a lateral alteration of spinal curvatures and so does not relax all of the muscles the way that *savasana* can. It also can interfere with breathing. However, even in *savasana*, those with high psoas tension will demonstrate too large a lumbar curvature; in this case, the students will have to flex their knees and put their feet on the floor in order to release lumbar compression and so feel relaxed.

In several situations (*paripurna navasana*, for example), it can be a problem for students to control the convex lumbar spine so as to move it more toward concavity. In this case, spinal length can be increased by releasing most of the tension in the abdominal muscles by holding the legs up with the hands or a belt, anchoring the thighs by pressing them away from the rib cage, and activating the psoas, so as to move the lumbar toward concavity.

Spinal Muscles, Tendons, and Ligaments

Muscles

There are three major groups of muscles in the back body, all of which attach to the spinal column [447]. The first group (figure 8.A-4**a**) has fibers that run almost perpendicular to the spine (latissimus, trapezius, rhomboids, etc.) and

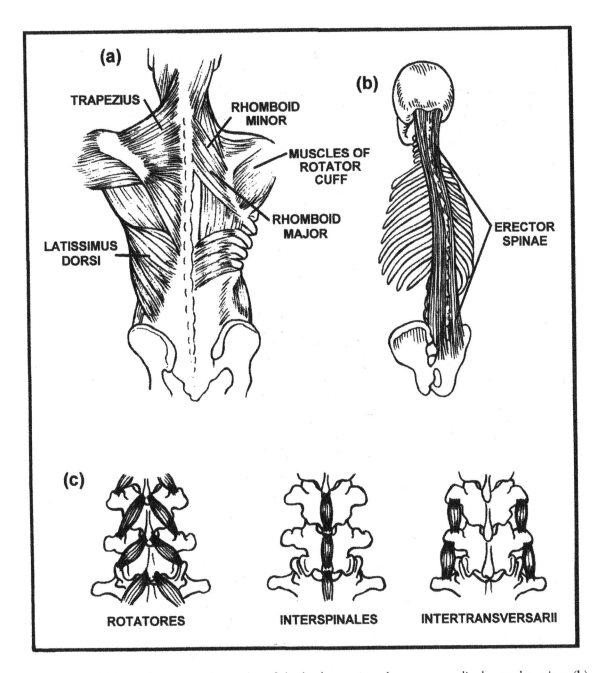

Figure 8.A-4. (a) Posterior views of muscles of the back running almost perpendicular to the spine. (b) Muscles of the back running parallel to the spine along its length. (c) Posterior views of muscles connecting transverse and spinous processes of neighboring vertebrae. Not shown are the multifidus muscles, which run obliquely from the transverse processes of each vertebra to one, two, three, or four of the spinous processes above it.

work to connect the actions of the arms to the spine. The three members of the second muscle group (figure 8.A-4b), the erector spinae (paraspinal) muscles are superficial and run parallel to the spine over its entire length, lying within the channels between the spinous process and

the transverse processes. Contraction or lengthening of these muscles induces backward or forward bending, respectively. Muscles of the third group (figure 8.A-4c) are deep and connect the transverse and spinous processes of each vertebra with those of its neighbors in either an up-and-down or in crossing patterns, so that contraction of these muscles can act either to rotate the spine about its axis or to pull the adjacent vertebrae closer to one another in either extension, flexion, or lateral bending. See Kilmurray's comments in regard to keeping the muscles in the third group relaxed during spinal twisting (Subsection 8.B, page 294).

The muscles connecting one vertebra to the next (figure 8.A-4c) are largely postural. Of these, there are two types, i.e., those that, when acting unilaterally, flex the spine laterally and pull more or less of the spine into extension, and those that, when acting unilaterally, rotate the spine and pull it more or less into extension. In the first group, we have the intertransversarii muscles, found only in the cervical and lumbar regions, where they connect adjacent transverse processes; and the interspinalis muscles, again found only in the cervical and lumbar regions, where they connect adjacent spinous processes; the later are situated on the spinal axis and so do not appear as bilateral pairs. In the second group of intervertebral muscles, we have the multifidus and the rotatores muscles, the unilateral actions of which induce a rotation of the spine abut the column axis.

The bilateral contraction of the paraspinal erector spinae muscles also leads to spinal extension. This latter contraction is resisted by stretching of the rectus abdominis muscles of the abdomen, and vice versa, for flexion. That is to say, backbending is front-body stretching and forward bending is back-body stretching. For lateral flexion to one side, resistance comes from the erector spinae and quadratus lumborum muscles on the opposite side [288]. Muscles in the erector spinae group have origins and insertions placed variously on the iliac crests, on the spinous and transverse processes, and on the posterior aspects of the ribs.

Recent experimental work [921] has shown that the transversus abdominis of the abdomen and the deep-layered multifidus muscles of the spinal column work together to support and protect the lumbar spine. However, if one is confined to bed rest or sits for hours in a slumped or collapsed posture (body bent at the upper hinge;

see Subsection 9.B, page 319), these muscles become inactive and cease to support their load, and lower-back weakness and pain result.

The trapezius muscles at the back of the neck have their origins at the occiput and insertions on the shoulder blades (scapulae), figures 8.A-4a and 11.A-2. Bodily tension accumulates readily in the trapezius, as witnessed by those people who chronically carry their shoulders close to their ears. Students for whom the upper trapezius muscles are chronically short will be at a disadvantage in their *yogasana* work, for they will not be able to lower the scapulae into a position where the scapulae can press the rib cage in order to lift and open it (Subsection 10.A, page 328). They also will not be able to relieve the congestion around the neck when the spine is in extension or flexion if they cannot relax the trapezius muscles.

The sternocleidomastoid muscles in the neck (figure 11.A-1) are oriented diagonally, going from the clavicles to the posterior base of the skull on both sides of the neck, and serve as both neck flexors (when contracted bilaterally) and neck rotators (when contracted unilaterally). When one inhales deeply, the sternocleidomastoid and scalenus muscles of the neck are reflexively contracted along with the external intercostals, and this combined action lifts the rib cage upward, away from the pelvis.

The capitis muscles at the posterior of the neck have origins on the occiput and insertions at C1 and C2 (figure V.C-1); they serve to turn the head about the neck and to place the neck in extension. One of these, the posterior rectus capitis, is especially interesting in that it has an extremely high density of muscle spindles, table 11.B-1, and is of great importance because the differences in muscle-spindle tensions on the left and right sides of the cervical vertebrae directly indicate a postural imbalance of the head on the neck.

Order of Recruitment

When bending forward, as in *uttanasana*, the erector spinae are the first muscles to react to slow the descent of the upper body, working in the eccentric isotonic mode, followed by the gluteus, and finally the hamstrings and soleus muscles.

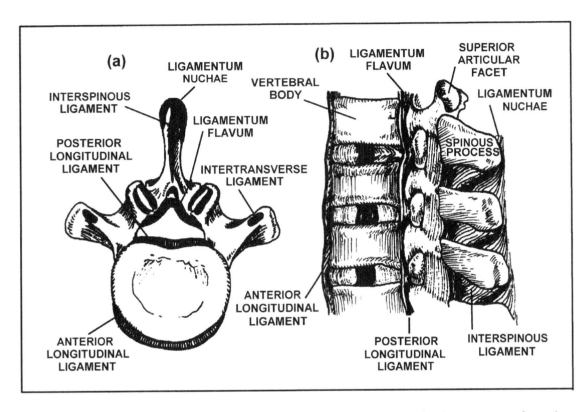

Figure 8.A-5. (a) Disposition of the larger ligaments supporting the spinal column, as seen from the top of the spine and (b) as seen from the left side, with the body facing to the left. In the cervical spine, the ligamentum nuchae also is known as the supraspinous ligament.

On recovery from *uttanasana* to reach *tadasana,* the order of muscle recruitment is the reverse of that listed above, beginning with the soleus and ending with the erector spinae muscles. Provided that the flexion is performed at the lower hinge, so that the ribs do not collide with one another or with the pelvis (Section 8.B, page 283), the limit to flexion in *uttanasana* is dictated by tension in the hamstrings.

Ligaments and Tendons

See Subsection 7.D, page 244, for an extended discussion of the general nature of ligaments and tendons. The ligamentum nuchae is a very thick ligament, enveloping all of the spinous processes from C2 to C7 on the posterior side (C1 has only a stub of a spinous process); below C7, it becomes continuous with the supraspinous ligament, again binding together the spinous processes (figures 8.A-5a and 8.A-5b). It stabilizes the neck and is stretched in *sarvangasana* [478] and even more so in *halasana* and *karnapidasana,* especially if there is no solid support under the neck and shoulders in these postures. The anterior longitudinal ligament runs the length of the spinal column on the forward side and acts to limit the amount of extension possible in backbending postures [101]. The anterior and posterior longitudinal ligaments run the full length of the spine, with the former running on the anterior outer side of the neural arch (the ligamentum flavum is parallel to it but on the inside of the arch) and the latter lying on the anterior inner surface of the spinal canal. The anterior longitudinal ligament limits spinal extension, as in *ustrasana,* and the posterior longitudinal ligament limits spinal flexion, as with the neck when in *sarvangasana.*

The fibroelastic ligamentum flavum connects the vertebral bodies of adjacent vertebrae to one another in a long vertical run along the posterior edges of the spinal canal (figure 8.A-5) and in doing so, helps keep the body erect. It is very thick and very strong but will allow deep flexion if this is done slowly, as we know from our forward-bend practice. That the ligamentum flavum is a highly elastic structure is evident from its name: *flavum* is Latin for "yellow," and yellow connective tissue has a high content of elastin, a highly elastic tissue component (Subsection 12.A, page 484).

The spinal ligaments resist axial rotation and will make the spine shorten in twists if one does not make an effort to keep the spine long. In spinal rotation, the action generally is inhibited in part by those layers of the annulus fibrosus within the intervertebral disc that have the "wrong" orientation for increased twisting (see below, page 294); whereas in the lumbar spine, the degree of rotation is very low, due to the vertically oriented articular facets pressing on one another [288].

It is reported that when the spine is fully flexed, the erector spinae are relaxed and myographically quiet. It is believed that this flexed position is maintained by tension in the ligaments of the spine and by passive resistance to further deformation by the intervertebral discs. In regard to *yogasana* practice, one can interpret this finding as pointing out that when in *paschimottanasana*, there is little or no contraction of the erector spinae muscles; however, the strain felt parallel to the spine is due to overstretching of the ligaments paralleling the spinal column (ligamentum flavum and the posterior longitudinal ligament) and/or to discomfort in the intervertebral discs. However, it must be pointed out that such spinal tension is the result of bending forward at the upper hinge and is much less a factor when bending more properly at the lower hinge (Subsection 9.B, page 321).

The posterior lower back is home to a broad, flat ligament called the thoracolumbar neurosis, figure 10.A-2**b**, covering the posterior thorax from the sacrum up and out to the iliac crests and reaching as high as the lower thoracic vertebrae. It serves as an anchor for muscles such as the latissimus dorsi, and members of the erector spinae group.

Damaged ligaments can allow motions that lead to pain. However, prolotherapy shots can tighten ligaments and increase strength while allowing one to remain pain-free. Much like the situation involving the hyperflexible student, those with loose spinal ligaments can go into spinal postures that are injurious and painful; whereas with the inflexible student, the range of motion is small but always within the safe, pain-free region [725].

Restricted Flow in Spinal Blood Vessels

The Vertebral Arteries

Approximately one-third of the blood going to the brain is carried there by the vertebral arteries passing through the vertebral foramina in the transverse processes of the cervical vertebrae (figure 4.E-1), with the other two-thirds traveling via the internal carotid arteries. Almost any off-axis head movement imaginable has the potential for interfering with the vertebral blood supply to the brain, with resultant dizziness, nausea, or fainting, depending on just how large an oxygen debt is generated in the brain by the movement. Occlusion of the vertebral arteries is especially likely when the neck is in extension with the trapezius muscles pulling the scapulae toward the ears, as often is the case with beginners in *ustrasana*, for example. In the elderly, however, occlusion can occur by just rotating the head while standing erect [57, 889] (Subsection II.B, page 838). The symptoms of occlusion can be eased in a posture such as *ustrasana* by not tipping the head backward and/or by pulling the scapulae away from the cervical vertebrae. Any student experiencing neurological symptoms in any posture where the head is tipped backward in extension should immediately change position. As discussed in Subsections 4.E, page 116, and II.B, page 838, far more serious consequences also are possible, involving the formation of thrombi in occluded vertebral arteries and their transport as emboli to regions of the brain where they induce cerebral strokes.

The Carotid Arteries

In contrast to the occlusion experienced by the vertebral arteries when the cervical spine is in extension, the internal carotid arteries become partially blocked when the cervical spine is in flexion (Subsection 8.A, page 278). In this latter case, the pressure in the carotid arteries is raised locally, and the baroreceptors within the arteries (figure 4.E-1) respond by calling for a lowered blood pressure and heart rate. Carotid flow also can be retarded by applying pressure to the orbits of the eyes. Known as the ocular-vagal heart-slowing reflex, it is discussed further in Subsections 11.D, page 457, and 14.D, page 579. These two effects reinforce one another when one is in the passive forward bends with the head and neck in the *jalandhara bandha* position and the orbits of the eyes rest upon a solid surface, such as a block or bolster.

Cautionary tales regarding serious neck injuries while in *sirsasana*, *halasana*, or *sarvangasana* appear in the medical literature [247, 483] and are discussed further in Section II.B, page 835.

Keeping the Spine Healthy into Old Age

It is often said, "A healthy spine characterizes youthfulness of body and mind, and a rigid spine, old age and senility" [744]. Apparently, if you are looking forward to old age and senility, then you are advised to move minimally and to allow gravity to dictate your posture. On the other hand, old age and senility can be forestalled by resisting gravity, using motions that move the spine maximally but with intelligence; i.e., by *yogasana* practice. This truism comes about in part because as we age, there is a natural shutting down of the vascular system that otherwise nourishes the spinal components. As we age, the nutritional servicing of the spine is less and less by direct delivery of blood via the vascular system and more and more by the indirect and inefficient diffusion of metabolites to and from outlying areas. This diffusion can be speeded up considerably by moving the spine as in *yogasana* practice.

As vascularization retreats in the spinal region with increasing age, the intervertebral discs begin to change. Normally, the nucleus pulposus (Section 8.C, page 303) within a vertebral disc has a tough fibrous covering (the annulus fibrosus); however, the nucleus itself is soft and jelly-like, allowing the structure to function as a shock absorber and also allowing smooth motion between adjacent vertebrae. Over the years, the soft inner part of the disc turns into tough, calcified cartilage, this transformation being complete in some people by the age of sixty years [52]. Once calcified, the spine becomes shorter, more rigid, and more brittle. The effects of aging on the range of motion of the lumbar spine in nonyogic subjects (presumably bending at the upper hinge) are shown in tables 8.A-2 and 8.A-3, where it is seen that the ranges of motion for extension and lateral bending are maximal in the age range two to thirteen years and fall to values significantly less than half the maximal range by sixty-five to seventy-seven years [428].

On average, one loses almost two-thirds of one's lumbar range of motion on going from the youngest age group (two to thirteen years) to the oldest (sixty-five to seventy-seven years), with the largest part of the decrease coming between the age groups two to thirteen years and thirty-five to forty-nine years. Fortunately, *yogasana* students are not "average" and so can expect to do much better than average in this regard. Note too that the values in these tables are those for nonyogic students bending at the upper hinge, whereas *yogasana* students will exceed these values as they learn how to bend at the lower hinge (Subsection 9.B, page 319).

It is satisfying to see the large margins by which serious *yogasana* students can exceed the "maxima" of the anatomists (figure 8.B-5, for example). The difference is due in part to the increased flexibility of the *yogasana* student, but also in part due to the ability of the student to intelligently work other parts of the body in concert with the stretch or bend coordinates in order to achieve extraordinary lengthening or bending, all the while avoiding spinal collapse and bone-on-bone contact.

Because the spine is deeply involved when

Table 8.A-2: Average Range of Motion for Extension in the Lumbar Vertebrae with Increasing Age [428]

Vertebra	Age 2–13	Age 35–49	Age 50–64	Age 65–77
L1	6°	4°	2°	
L2	10°	8°	5°	5°
L3	13°	9°	8°	3°
L4	17°	12°	8°	7°
L5	24°	8°	8°	7°
L1–L5 Total	64°	43°	33°	24°

Table 8.A-3: Average Range of Motion for Lateral Bending in the Lumbar Vertebrae with Increasing Age [428]

Vertebra	Age 2–13	Age 35–49	Age 50–64	Age 65–77
L1	12°	5°	6°	4°
L2	12°	8°	7°	7°
L3	16°	8°	8°	6°
L4	15°	8°	7°	5°
L5	7°	2°	1°	0°
L1–L5 Total	62°	31°	29°	22°

forward bending, backward bending, and in twisting postures, performance of these *yogasanas* improves the circulation of nutrients into and removal of wastes from the spinal region and thereby forestalls premature calcification of the spine. The same *yogasanas* that massage the intervertebral discs also massage the internal organs. A healthy spine not only stays supple but remains elongated, so that the vertebrae do not collapse upon one another; i.e., one's height is maintained on aging. However, maintaining a healthy spine involves both proper exercise and rest [10].

Those *yogasanas* that involve flexion and extension of the spine necessarily involve not only the spine proper, but most, if not all, of the other muscles, organs, and glands within the thorax. Interestingly, the forward bends (flexion) and the backward bends (extension) in many ways have much in common: both involve compression and stimulation of the internal organs, both increase spinal suppleness and spinal length, and both stimulate and release the tension in the associated nerves [747]. The two forms of spinal bending differ, however, in their effects on the articular facet joints, opening the joints in flexion and closing them in extension, and on the intervertebral muscles and ligaments, where the anterior ones are stretched in extension (figure 8.A-6c) and the posterior ones are stretched in flexion (figure 8.A-6f). Moreover, the two forms of spinal bending can differ in their impact on the autonomic nervous system, with supported forward bends in general resulting in parasympathetic relaxation and unsupported backbends resulting in sympathetic excitation (Section 5.E, page 182). However, supported backbends can promote a parasympathetic response, just as with supported forward bends, and unsupported forward bends can promote sympathetic excitation, just as with unsupported backbends. The differences in response of the autonomic nervous system in regard to whether the postures are supported or not is simply a reflection of the amount of muscular effort invested in their performance: i.e., low effort

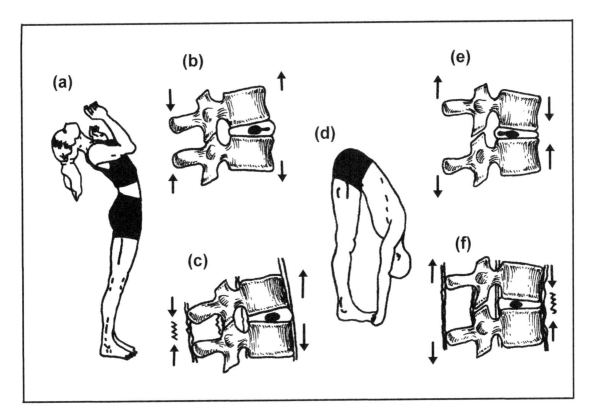

Figure 8.A-6. (**a**) Extension of the spine, resulting in the pressing of the nucleus pulposus in the anterior direction (**b**) and (**c**) with the concomitant stretching of the anterior longitudinal ligament and the relaxation of the posterior longitudinal ligament, the ligamentum flavum, and muscles on the posterior side of the spine. (**d**) Flexion of the spine, resulting in the pressing of the nucleus pulposus in the posterior direction (**e**) and (**f**) with the concomitant stretching of the posterior longitudinal ligament and muscles on the posterior side of the spine and the relaxation of those on the anterior side of the spine [101]. Notice that extension presses the nucleus pulposus away from the spinal cord within the spinal canal and that flexion presses it toward the spinal cord within the spinal canal. More will be made of this difference in Subsection 8.C, page 307.

for supported postures and high effort for unsupported postures.

Section 8.B: Ranges of Motion of the Spinal Column

We now turn to the ranges of motion of the spine when engaged in various *yogasana* postures. As such, it must be remembered that in every case, the action of the spinal column will be just one component of the posture and that the spinal actions in any posture will be more or less coupled to those of the pelvis, arms, legs,

etc. For example, the extent of lumbar curvature in *urdhva dhanurasana* will depend not only on the motions of the spinal sections but also on the tilting of the pelvis, as dictated by actions of the psoas, the quadriceps, and the hamstring muscles of the legs. Nonetheless, we limit our discussion in this chapter to the generalities of spinal motion when involved in forward, backward, lateral, and rotational motions of the spine, regardless of the particular posture.

The configuration of the spinal column while in the various postural types are shown in figure 8.B-1, beginning with the spine when in *tadasana* (figure 8.B-1a). As with the data in table 8.A-1, the spinal postures in figure 8.B-1 are representa-

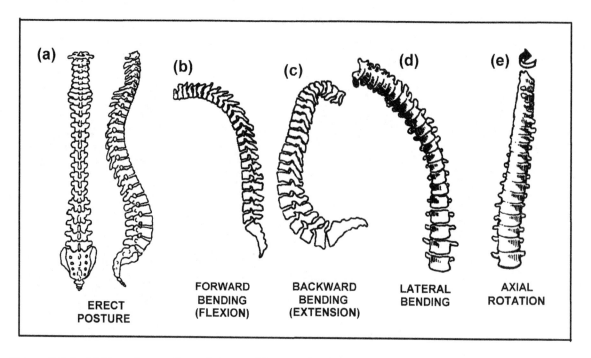

Figure 8.B-1. (a) Posterior and lateral views of the spinal column in *tadasana*. (b) Lateral view of the spine in forward bending, anterior spine facing left. (c) Lateral view of the spine in backward bending, anterior spine facing left. (d) Lateral spinal bending to the left, as seen from the rear. (e) Axial rotation of the spine, as seen from the rear. The bending postures show the spinal architecture when bending at the upper hinge, whereas *yogasana* students will bend at the lower hinge instead.

tive of an average population of nonyogic adults, and so the extent of bending and twisting can be quite different for experienced *yogasana* students, who will have larger ranges of motion and also will be trained to bend from the lower hinge rather than from the upper hinge (Subsection 9.B, page 319), as is most likely in the data that led to these drawings.

Note how very different the spinal shapes are for forward bending and for backward bending (figure 8.B-1). In forward bending, the lumbar spine is shown as somewhat convex, as would be the case when bending forward from the upper hinge (figure 9.B-5a), and the cervical spine is severely flexional and convex, with the chest collapsed; the spine in figure 8.B-1b would be a fair representation of the spine in *ardha uttanasana* done with bending at the upper hinge. In contrast, *ardha uttanasana* done with bending at the lower hinge (figure 9.B-5b) maintains the proper concavity in both the cervical and lumbar regions, leaving the spinal posture more like that of figure

8.B-1a. Indeed, almost all of the *yogasanas* ideally are performed with the spine aligned as closely as possible with that of *tadasana*, the standard of postural excellence for beginners (Subsection 9.B, page 320).

When backbending, were the proper concavity in both the lumbar and cervical regions attained, the thoracic region still would be relatively straight, due to the bracing by the rib cage. Due to this bracing by the rib cage and to the strong interference of the thoracic spinous processes, the spinal concavity demanded by backbending is clearly inhibited in the thoracic region, thereby over-bending the lumbar and cervical regions. Our ongoing work in backbending is then to bend less in the cervical and lumbar regions and more in the thoracic, so that the spine is more evenly curved end to end.

Though the interference of the spinous processes in backward bending is not a factor when forward bending, there is still a strong rib-on-rib interference in this case, unless one can manage flexion at the hip joints rather than in the thoracic spine. It is because it can be so difficult to place the thoracic section in extension that the thoracic posture of beginners is severely flexional in forward bends, whereas it is only weakly or not at all extensional in backbends. Ironically, it is just these thoracic difficulties of forward and backward bending that we work so hard to overcome in our *yogasana* work!

Similarly, the spinal curvature shown for lateral bending in figure 8.B-1**d** is totally a consequence of bending at the upper hinge, as proper lateral bending from the lower hinge keeps the lengths of the two sides of the spinal column more closely the same. Imagine what *trikonasana* would look like were the student's spine bent as in figure 8.B-1**d**!

Rationalizing Ranges of Motion

Motions of and within the spinal column are limited by tension in the ligaments and tendons binding one vertebra to the next and by bone-on-bone (vertebra-on-vertebra and rib-on-rib contact, Section 7.F, page 252) [288]. Furthermore, motion in the spine can be inhibited by contraction of certain muscles; e.g., contraction of the abdominal flexors can inhibit backward bending, and contraction of the hamstrings can inhibit forward bending. Nonetheless, one can qualitatively rationalize the range-of-motion data in figure 8.A-1 and table 8.A-1 from a consideration of nearest-neighbor intervertebral bone-on-bone congestion.[4] Thus, the range of backbending will be limited by the collision of the adjacent spinous processes, and, as shown in figure 8.A-1**a**, this will be less of a problem in the cervical and lumbar regions (10.7° and 7.0° extension per vertebrae, respectively), where the spinous processes are well

separated, as compared to the situation in the thoracic region, where the spinous processes are much closer (only 2.4° extension per vertebrae). When forward bending, one sees that there are relatively few or no bone-on-bone factors operating, and so the various spinal regions contribute about equally; however, on a per-vertebra basis, one sees that the bending in the thoracic region (3.75° flexion per vertebra) is smaller than that in the cervical (5.71° flexion per vertebra) and lumbar regions (12.0° flexion per vertebra), reflecting the effects of the spinal bracing of the thoracic region by the rib cage and the resistance of rib-on-rib contact in this region (see below).

When lateral bending, interference between adjacent transverse processes comes into play, and it is clear from the shapes of the vertebrae (figure 8.A-1**b**) that this is least important in the cervical region and that the lateral bending in the thoracic region (only 1.67° per vertebra) is again impeded by rib-on-rib congestion. The situation is different in the case of spinal twisting, because here, the limiting factor is the spatial orientation of the articular facets, and this is not apparent from the figure. However, the articular facets are more vertical in the lumbar region and more horizontal in the thoracic and cervical regions, and so rotation about a vertical axis is easiest in the two latter regions (4.2° and 5.0° per vertebra, respectively) and most difficult in the lumbar region (1° per vertebra). The sacral and coccygeal regions contribute negligibly to the overall range of spinal motions.

Overcoming Bone-on-Bone Congestion

The problem of overcoming bone-on-bone contact in the *yogasanas* is discussed from a general point of view in Subsection 7.F, page 252, and is reintroduced here in regard to the specifics of intervertebral contact. Once the student is in the region of bone-on-bone contact, going deeper into the posture is largely impossible until she learns a new approach to the posture in which compressive stress is removed from the bones and is replaced by tensile stress on the muscles and connective tissue. This is especially relevant to the spine, where bone-on-bone interactions are a

---

4   In our discussion of bone-on-bone contact within the spine, we are referring here to the contact of adjacent vertebrae at points that are not otherwise parts of a common joint. Thus, the contact between adjacent spinal processes is relevant to our bone-on-bone discussion, but that between adjacent superior and inferior articular processes involved in a common joint is not.

natural aspect of the spine's mechanical integrity. As described above, this type of congestion can be dealt with by transferring spinal motions from the vertebrae to the hip joints (Subsection 9.B, page 314); a second approach to understanding the problem is considered below, phrased in terms of intrinsic dimensions within the spine.

Ratio of Disc Thickness to Vertebral Height

The ranges of motion of the various spinal sections can be rationalized in part by consideration of the ratio of disc thickness to vertebral height in each of the sections. This approach is related to the qualitative discussion given above in regard to how closely the adjacent vertebral parts approach one another. It is no surprise that the lower vertebrae bear more weight, and the cushions between them are thicker. The ratio of the disc thickness to the height of the adjacent vertebra (table 8.A-1) is an interesting quantity, in that large ratios imply a large intervertebral separation and therefore a high mobility around that joint by avoiding bone-on-bone contact. In general, the thicker the disc and the thinner the vertebrae, the larger is the ratio of disc thickness to vertebral height, and one expects the larger will be the range of motion at that joint [101]. From this, one sees that on the basis of the disc-thickness/vertebral-height ratio, flexion and extension motions of the cervical vertebrae will have the largest ranges of motion (thickness/height ratio = 0.4), whereas those in the thorax (ratio = 0.25) are predicted to have even smaller ranges of motion than those in the lumbar region (ratio = 0.33), possibly due to rib-on-rib contact in the thoracic region. That is to say, due to the unavoidable rib-on-rib contact and because adjacent thoracic ribs are joined to one another by the costovertebral joints (figure 15.A-3d), there is no reason for the thoracic joints to show large disc-to-height ratios.

In evaluating the disc-thickness/vertebral-height ratio as a measure of spinal mobility, it is more meaningful to normalize the sectional ranges of motion by calculating the range of motion per vertebra, as in table 8.A-1 and as shown in figure 8.B-2. The figure shows that, considered on the per-vertebra basis, flexion, extension, and lateral bending of the three spinal sections

behave in the same way: the thoracic section is significantly stiffer in these three coordinates than are the other two. The ratio of disc thickness to vertebral height is also plotted there, and it follows the trends for flexion, extension, and lateral bending very nicely. The qualitative agreement of the disc-thickness-to-vertebral-height ratio curve with the observed per-vertebra range of motion averages reported by Kapandji (high, low, high in the cervical, thoracic, and lumbar regions, respectively) supports our basic premise: it is the intervertebral bone-on-bone contact of vertebrae otherwise not in contact in *tadasana* that limits the ranges of spinal motion in bent and twisted postures. However, there is one anomaly: rotation in the lumbar region is far smaller than otherwise expected, leading to a pattern of high, low, then lower on going from the cervical to thoracic and from thoracic to lumbar sections (figure 8.B-2). Remember that because the articular facets are oriented essentially in the vertical plane in the lumbar region, rotation in the lumbar region about a vertical axis will be inhibited regardless of the appropriate disc-thickness-to-vertebral-height ratio, even in *tadasana*. Thus the apparent disagreement between the observed ranges of motion and the ratio of disc thickness to vertebral height when considering spinal rotation in the lumbar region can be rationalized after the fact.

The specific effects of the intervertebral discs on the ranges of motion of the spinal segments are discussed in Subsection 8.C, page 303.

Aspects of Spinal Elongation and Compression

Hydration and Dehydration

Were the spinal column simply a stack of bones, questions regarding spinal elongation and compression would be moot. In fact, the separation of each vertebra from its adjacent vertebrae by soft, water-filled pouches called intervertebral discs (figures 8.A-2a and 8.B-3a) allows for a much more interesting situation. When a vertebral disc is hydrated, it expands, and thus so does the length of the spine. When so expanded, the

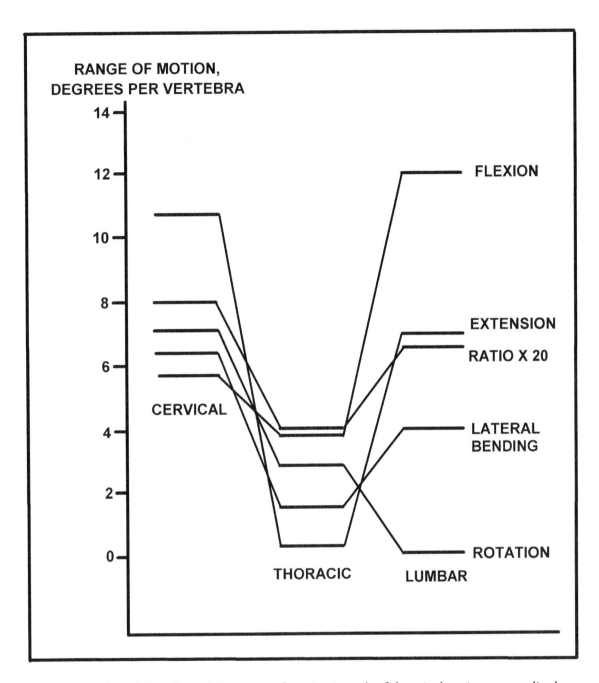

Figure 8.B-2. Display of the values of the ranges of motion in each of the spinal sections, normalized to a per-vertebra basis (table 8.A-1) and comparison with Kapandji's value of the ratio of disc thickness to vertebral height (X 20) in each of these three sections.

ratio of disc height to vertebral body height also increases, and this implies an increased range of mobility in the joint (Section 8.B, page 284).[5]

twists, it is likely that significant dehydration probably does not happen within the short time we normally spend in the spinal twists. Indeed, hydration of a dehydrated disc requires several hours, and so should dehydration of a hydrated disc. Though it is easiest to speak in terms of water movement, in fact the intervertebral joints are surrounded by synovial fluid, and the "hydration and dehydration" of the discs may involve more than just the movement of water.

5   This implies that if the disc is dehydrated on twisting, as is the case when wringing out a wet cloth, the rotational mobility of the spinal joint that it spans would decrease. As this is not our experience in spinal

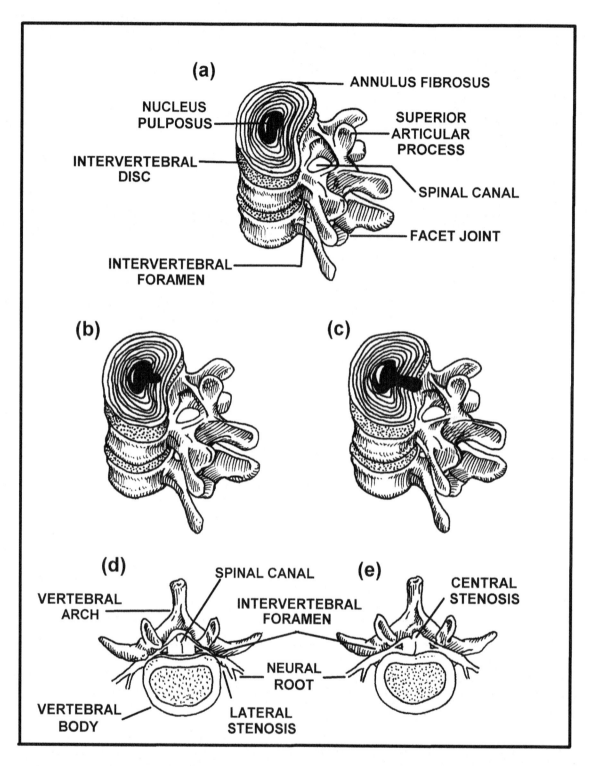

Figure 8.B-3. (**a**) Superior view of a lumbar vertebra, supporting an intervertebral disc and its nucleus pulposus on its upper surface. (**b**) A bulging but not herniated disc pressing posteriorly through the annulus fibrosus toward the spinal canal. (**c**) A herniated disc exudes its nucleus through the torn annulus fibrosus so as to impinge upon the nerve bundle within the spinal canal. (**d**) Stenosis of the nerve roots due to narrowing of the lateral spinal foramina exiting the canal. (**e**) Stenosis of the spinal cord due to narrowing of the spinal canal itself.

Furthermore, the mobility of the vertebrae and the changing curvatures of the various spinal sections upon hydration also open the door to changes of the overall spinal length and the levels of tension and compression in the spine.

For maximum all-around efficiency, the spine must be both rigid and elastic. This mechanical rigidity of the spine is due to the outward (expansive) pressure of the hydrated intervertebral discs (20 percent of the spine's length is due to the thickness of the hydrated intervertebral discs) and the inward (compressive) pressure of the intervertebral ligaments and muscles and the balance between these two opposing forces. This rigidity is also supported by the clamping of the thoracic vertebrae by the rib cage and by the fitting together of the hills and valleys of each vertebra onto the corresponding valleys and hills of its neighbor through the agency of the facet joints.

Each of the plateau surfaces of the intervertebral discs is lined with a thin layer of cartilage, which in turn is perforated by microscopic pores congruent with channels in the cancellous bone of the adjacent vertebrae. With axial compression of the spine, in a matter of a few hours, the pressure drives water from the nucleus pulposus of the intervertebral disc into the pores of the vertebral body and surrounding tissue. As a result of the water loss, the disc thins, and in consequence of this, the overall length decreases. In *yogasana* practice, we work muscularly to increase the disc thickness, not by pumping them up with water, but by pulling adjacent vertebrae away from one another, thereby lessening the local spinal curvatures and increasing the spinal length.[6] In this

process of lengthening, however, the gravitational load on the discs does decrease, and so the lengthening of the spine will indirectly promote the hydration of the discs.

Due to the dehydration of the discs resulting from the external pressure generated by gravity on the vertical spine, the overall height of a person can decrease by as much as 2.5 centimeters (one inch) after a day of standing or sitting. In the lumbar region, where the external pressure (weight) is highest, the disc volume decreases by about 20 percent after a day of standing and sitting [7]. Correspondingly, astronauts measure 5–10 centimeters (two to four inches) taller on return to earth from gravity-free space. The effect of gravity on the length of the spine was first raised when it was noted that the vertical spine of a man on horseback shortened after a day's ride, but the hoof-to-shoulder height of his horse did not.

When lying down at night, the gravitational loading on the discs is relieved (but not the smaller effects of intervertebral resting-muscle tone), and the discs rehydrate so as to assume their larger thickness by morning. When we awaken in the morning, the discs are fully hydrated, the vertebrae are pushed apart by the increased thickness of the discs, and the spine has its maximal length. On the other hand, Carol Wipf points out that this overnight pressurization of the intervertebral discs can be very painful on awakening for a student having a disc herniation of the sort shown in figure 8.B-3c.

Numerous experiments have shown that the simple act of drinking water results in an increased sympathetic muscle tone lasting for an hour thereafter [767]. Consequently, it is not recommended that one drink water during *yogasana*

---

6   This prompts three general statements in regard to spinal motions in the *yogasanas*. (1) If possible, move each spinal segment so as to lessen its curvature and so increase its length. The curvature is least when each end of the segment is pulled away from its opposite end. Carol Wipf points out that this "rule" would not apply to back-bending postures, though one would do well to lengthen each spinal section in these postures, even though the curvature might be increased through this. (2) A modest increase of the vertebral separation in the spine can have the effect of making spinal movement easier and/or less painful, especially when move-

ment is otherwise impeded by bone-on-bone contact. (3) Thoracic deep breathing (inhalation to contract the scalene muscles while pulling the abdomen onto the spine; see Section 15.C, page 615) lifts the ribs away from the pelvis and so lengthens the spine while separating the ribs. It is also necessary to acknowledge that a set of such simplistic mechanistic rules such as given here will be severely limited in regard to explaining movement in the living spine [442a].

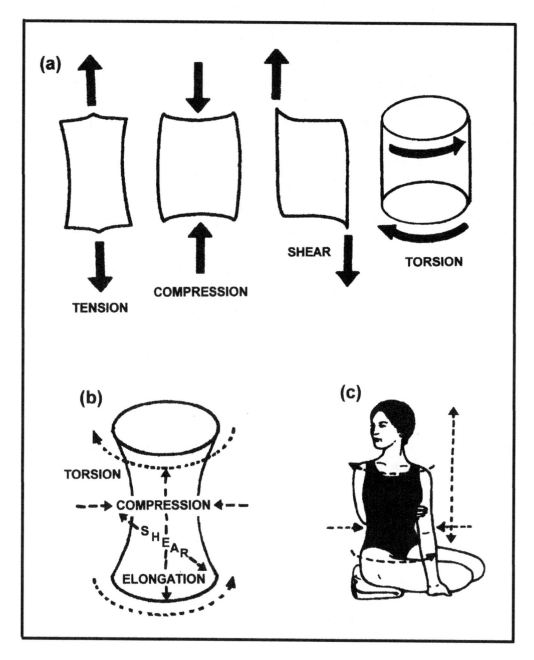

Figure 8.B-4. (a) A two-dimensional sheet of any material can be stressed in one of four ways: tension, when the ends are pulled away from one another; compression, when the ends are pushed toward one another; shear, when opposite corners are pulled away from or pushed toward one another; and torsion, when the two ends of a solid body are twisted oppositely. (b) In a flexible three-dimensional object, torsion compresses it perpendicular to the torsional axis and elongates it along the torsional axis at the same time [876]. (c) The elements of disrotatory spinal torsion applied to the upper body when in *bharadvajasana I*.

practice unless one is dehydrated or has a good reason for stimulating the sympathetic nervous system.

Disc Response to Loading

During and after rest, the vertebral discs rehydrate and attain the preloaded state; in this con-

Table 8.B-1: Lumbar-Disc Pressures in Various Postures [27]

Posture	Pressure (millimeters Hg)
Lying down on back	25
Lying down on side	75
Standing	100
Standing, *ardha uttanasana*	150
Standing, *ardha uttanasana*, weight in hands	220
Seated, 90° chair back	140
Seated, 90° chair back, slumped forward	18
Seated, 90° chair back, slumped forward and weights in hands	275

dition, the spinal column is longer than was the case before resting. When the spine is elongated, as when hanging vertically on the ropes, the internal disc pressure decreases and the annuli fibrosus of the discs become taller and narrower, whereas the nucleus pulposus becomes more spherical. In contrast, when the spine is axially compressed as when in *sirsasana I*, the discs flatten and become wider, and the internal pressure on the nucleus becomes higher, thereby increasing the tension on the innermost annular layers. An asymmetric annular force to one side of the disc moves the nucleus to the opposite side, pulling fibers apart on that side, and in the process, generating a restoring force (figures 8.A-6b, 8.A-6c, 8.A-6e, and 8.A-6f).

In axial rotation of the spine, the obliquely oriented fibers of the annulus that run counter to the direction of the torque are stretched, whereas those running in the same direction are relaxed. Thus, some of the layers of the annulus are under tension, and others are more relaxed, depending upon the relative sense of the twist and the angular orientation of the fibers within a particular layer. The effect of the twist is to compress the nucleus (figure 8.B-4) [288], because the tension of twisting is greatest on the innermost fibers, and this acts to compress the discs. The structure of the disc annulus is such that whatever compressive force is applied to a disc, there is an increase of the internal pressure on the disc, and the stretched annulus then acts to oppose the force and restore balance [288].

Loading and Disc Pressure

The variation of the internal lumbar-disc pressure has been measured in various postures, as per table 8.B-1. As expected, lying down on one's back (*savasana*) generates only a very small pressure within the disc (25 millimeters Hg). Possibly due to lateral bending of the spine, this pressure rises to 75 millimeters when on the side (as when preparing for *anantasana*) but is only slightly larger than this when standing (100 millimeters). When standing, there are many structures in the thorax that help support the body weight and so reduce the pressure on the discs. However, when sitting, these supporting structures are no longer at work, and thus when so relaxed, the disc pressure rises to 140 millimeters Hg; some argue that the disc pressure on going from standing to sitting increases by as much as a factor of ten. It would be very interesting to see if the well-trained *yogasana* student could not reduce the disc pressure when sitting by pressing the thighs into the chair seat and lifting the rib cage, as in *dandasana*.

Spinal Length

The gravitational loading of the spine in the normal standing posture will act not only to flatten the discs, but due to the inherent curvatures of the thoracic and lumbar spines, these curvatures may increase through the course of a day and so contribute substantially, or even overwhelmingly, to the apparent loss of height (and possibly range of motion) by nightfall; indeed, it is estimated that the effect of gravity on spinal curvature is responsible for about 80 percent of the daily spinal shrinkage on standing. In contrast, the yogic goal of working to elongate the spine by reducing the local curvatures of the spine, thereby lengthening it, is seen to be equivalent to achieving the low-curvature posture of the horizontal resting position (*savasana*). It also follows from this that any action or motion that acts to reduce the curvature in any part of the spine will act to increase the distance between adjacent vertebrae and therefore increase the potential range of motion within that section.[7]

It is safe to assume that with higher lumbar disc pressure as one changes posture, the more compact the spine becomes and vice versa. Viewed this way, it is seen from the data in table 8.B-1 that the spine is longer when standing than when sitting, and that it is longer when lying on the back than when lying on the side.

Time of Day

When hydrated, the various muscles and ligaments that bind each vertebra to its neighbors are pulled taut, and consequently, the spine would seem to be at its least flexible in the morning, when hydration is maximal. Conversely, spinal flexibility would seem to be maximal at the end of the day, when the discs are dehydrated, the ligaments and muscles become slack, and the spine assumes a collapsed condition. This supposition would be true for some spinal motions and false for others, because the tautness of the spinal muscles and ligaments are not the only factors determining spinal flexibility. Thus, when the discs expand and tighten the spinal musculature, they also lift the bony transverse processes of each vertebra off of and away from that below it (figure 8.A-2**a**) in the cervical and thoracic regions; i.e., the facet joints open, and this works to increase spinal flexibility for backbending, as stated in Subsection 8.B, page 281. It would appear that the pressing of the transverse processes against one another or the spinous processes is the more important of the two factors, for it is always better to lengthen the spine before twisting or backbending, even if it tightens the spinal musculature. On the other hand, reversing the above argument leads one to expect that because forward bending does not strongly involve the vertebra-on-vertebra interference between the articular processes, it might be easier late in the day, when the spinal muscles and ligaments have relaxed due to the gravitational collapse of the intervertebral discs.[8]

When preparing for either twisting or backbending, the yogic prescription is to lift the cervical end of the spine away from the sacral end while

---

7   My coworkers tell me that the goal in *yogasana* practice is to elongate the spine and yet maintain the *tadasana* curvatures. I may be wrong on this, but I feel that simultaneous elongation while maintaining constant curvature is not possible, and that when we elongate the spine by lifting the rib cage away from the pelvis, for example, there is a corresponding flattening of the curvatures of the spine, especially in the thoracic region. I picture the spine, when horizontal, as a hanging clothesline; we can pull one end away from the other, but only if the line between the ends reduces its curvature. I do not propose that the goal in *yogasana* practice is to flatten the spine, but I do feel that where lengthening of the spine is appropriate, this can be accomplished by **somewhat** flattening its curves while keeping the effort to do so within reason. (Also see the folllowing footnote.) In a similar way, I also argue that when the arm and the leg are straightened or elongated, it again involves reducing the curvatures at the knee or elbow joint, respectively.

---

8   We have a situation here where lengthening the spine by increasing the distance between vertebrae, so as to avoid intervertebral contact, makes the spine more flexible but also tightens the spinal musculature, making it less flexible! On the other hand, if we keep the spine short, so as to keep its musculature soft and flexible, motion is then inhibited by intervertebral bone-on-bone contact. One can imagine that the bone-on-bone aspect is ultimately to be avoided, as there is no way to gain more range of motion when in this situation, whereas if the bone-on-bone contact is avoided by elongation, then one can work in the usual *yogasana* way to increase the range of motion in the spinal-stretch coordinates. That is to say, it is more practical to work to overcome tight musculature in the elongated spine than to work to overcome intervertebral interference in the short spine. Also see footnote 7, this page, regarding this concept.

"grounding" the sacrum. This lengthening moves each vertebra away from its neighbors, opens the distance between contacting facets, and allows a larger range of motion. This lengthening of the lumbar spine in preparation for backbending can lessen the discomfort often felt in that region due to lumbar compression of the facet joints and of the spinous processes. Though easy to say, lengthening of the spine can take years of work.

Because the height of children falls between 9:00 AM and 3:00 PM by about 1 centimeter (0.4 inches), comparative studies of children's height must be done at the same time of day for every measurement [879].

Aspects of Spinal Flexion

As the various spinal sections are activated in the *yogasana* postures, it appears that not all of the vertebrae contribute equally to the action. For example, when flexing the neck in *sarvangasana*, the joint between C4 and C5 is involved primarily, whereas in neck extension, as when in *salabhasana*, it is the joint between C5 and C6 that is paramount [482]. Because the normal flexion angle at the neck is only 40–50° [428, 493], attempts to perform *sarvangasana* or *halasana* with the lines of cervical and thoracic vertebrae perpendicular to one another will induce considerable kyphotic bending around the higher thoracic vertebrae and the consequent collapse of the upper chest in these *yogasanas*. As the atlanto-occipital joint is inherently stiff, flexion at this joint is accompanied by flexion at the atlanto-axoid joint.

In order to avoid rounding of the chest when in *sarvangasana* or *halasana*, it is much better to place blankets under the shoulders and upper arms, as in figure 14.F-2d; with this, the chin can drop back away from the chest, so that the thoracic vertebrae can remain in vertical alignment while there is a strong vertical lift of the viscera off the diaphragm, lungs, and heart [493]. From the point of view of neck flexion, *halasana* will be even more challenging than is *sarvangasana* for the beginner, due to the intense paravertebral stretch of the ligaments in the former. In spinal flexion, inverted or not, the anterior spinal ligament is relaxed, but posteriorly, the longitudinal ligamentum flavum, ligamentum nuchae, and the interspinosus ligaments (figure 8.A-5) are all tensioned and limit movement. Also in tension are the antagonist extensor muscles of the back and the quadratus lumborum muscles connecting the lower-back ribs to the upper-back rim of the pelvis. The change of vertebral type on going from T12 to L1 very strongly limits the motion about this joint, except for flexion [288].

Unlike the situation in extension, flexion is not limited by vertebral-vertebral interaction, but rather by the tension in the posterior spinal ligaments (figure 8.A-5) and by the tendency of adjacent ribs to collapse onto one another, especially if the flexion takes place at the upper hinge. Thus, when bending forward (*paschimottanasana*, etc.), flexion is limited, especially by rib-on-rib contact, if the rectus abdominis muscles (Subsection 15.A, page 608) are contracted. However, if the rectus muscles are relaxed, so that the ribs can be lifted up and forward by contraction of the external intercostal muscles, then the ribs both elevate and separate, and one can achieve a tighter forward-bending angle at the lower-hinge hip joints, as with the model in figure 8.B-5b who readily bends the average line of the thorax through 174° with respect to the line of the standing leg in *ruchikasana* [913]. In this case, it is tension in the spinal ligaments, in the quadratus lumborum and in the hamstrings that limit the range of flexion.

Kapandji reports 115° as the maximum angle for the simultaneous flexion of the thoracic and lumbar spines (table 8.A-1) by rounding each of them maximally. Compare this now with the yogic postures shown in figure 8.B-5. As a comparative standard, first consider *tadasana* and measure the angle between the femur of the leg and the average line of the thoracic vertebrae (figure 8.B-5a). As these lines are parallel, the angle in question is 180°. For the model in *ruchikasana* (figure 8.B-5b), the thoracic-lumbar line displays an angle of 150° with respect to the femur of the standing leg and is very close to 180° to the femur in the leg in *eka pada sirsasana* [913]!

With the spine placed in extension, the circus

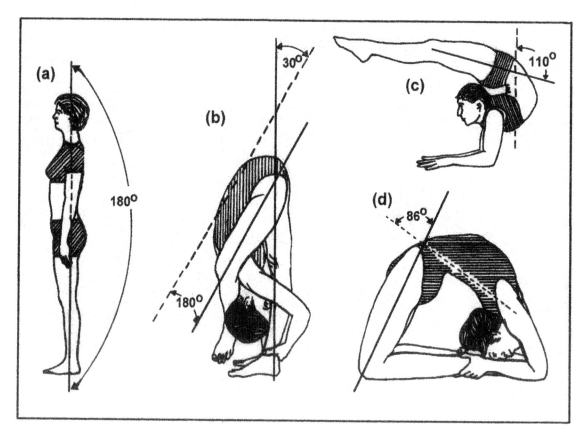

Figure 8.B-5. Angles formed by the femur bones (full lines) and the lumbar spine (dashed lines) in *tadasana* (a), for each of the legs in *ruchikasana* (b), and in *kapotasana* (d). The model in (b) and (d) is Patricia Walden. (c) *Pincha mayurasana* as performed in the circus contortionist style, showing an angle of 110° between lumbar and femur.

performer in *pincha mayurasana* can generate an angle of 110° between the lumbar spine and the femur (figure 8.B-5c); whereas in *kapotasana* performed by an expert in the Iyengar yoga approach (figure 8.B-5d), the corresponding angle is only 86°; however, the spinal collapse so obvious in the former has been avoided in the latter.

When beginners bend forward, they often cannot reach their hands to their feet without putting their lumbar spines so far into flexion that the curvature reverts to convex. This flexion results from bending around the L1 to L5 lumbar vertebral joints (the upper hinge; see Subsection 9.B, page 319) rather than bending about the hip joints (the lower hinge). Kapandji places the maximal flexional curvature of the lumbar spine at 60° (table 8.A-1); i.e., severely convex. However, *yogasana* students must be encouraged to have a minimally convex curvature in this spinal section rather than the maximum when bending forward. If the students will hold belts placed around their feet, then they can still work with the spine having the normal curvatures; in the Iyengar approach, it is better to use a belt and maintain lumbar extension/concavity as best as one can, than to hold the toes with the hands and thereby make the lumbar spine strongly convex.

Aspects of Spinal Extension

The compressive load on the facet joints of the lumbar vertebrae can be relieved by spinal flexion, whereas extension magnifies the forces that shear the joints (figure 8.B-4a) and jam the spinous processes onto one another. This latter can be avoided in backbends by working to keep the lumbar spine elongated, as occurs when tipping the back rim of the pelvis toward the knees (figure 9.B-4**b**). Backbending (extension) in the thoracic region especially is limited by the bone-on-bone pressure of adjacent spinous processes on one another [101, 884].

In extension, the articular processes of the upper and lower vertebrae are more tightly interlocked as the spinous processes contact one another. Extension is limited, not only by this bone-on-bone contact between adjacent vertebrae, but also by tension in the anterior ligaments (figure 8.A-5). Nonetheless, extension still can be high in the angular sense in the lumbar and cervical regions.

Cervical extension is limited by the contact of the posterior arch of the atlas with the occiput above and the axis below. When in cervical extension, as in *ustrasana*, the arch of the atlas may be caught between that of the axis and the occiput and can be crushed if the extension is too forceful; this especially would be the case in extreme postures such as *salabhasana* or *sayanasana*. Tipping the head back tends to clamp down on the vertebral arteries delivering blood to the brain (Subsection 8.A, page 278) as the cervical vertebra slide down on one another in collapse [483]. The joints other than the atlanto-occipital and that between C1 and C2 are the potential sites for herniated-disc problems in the neck (Section 8.C, page 307) and for the birth of an embolus.

As seen from table 8.A-1, in the average neophyte student attempting *urdhva dhanurasana*, there will be only 60° (25° thoracic plus 35° lumbar) of angular extension available in the thoracic and lumbar regions in order to complete the full backbend. However, if the spine can be deliberately lengthened in the *yogasanas*, the disc-to-bone thickness ratio increases, and one's spinal mobility increases along with it. Thus, *urdhva dhanurasana* becomes possible for the beginner who will work to lengthen the spine.

Inasmuch as the spinous and transverse processes are posterior to the vertebral bodies, backbending acts to close the intervertebral joints, forcing bone onto bone at the facets and at the spinous processes. This can be accommodated in part by the flexing of the bony processes. However, rotation around the spine when the posterior spinal column is strongly compressed, as with spinal rotation while in *urdhva dhanurasana*, focuses the pressure unevenly on the transverse processes and so puts them at risk for fracture. Consequently this combination of rotation and backbending (as when in *mandalasana*) is a risky venture for beginning students who are unable either to lift their body weight off of their heads or to keep the inherent twist in this maneuver from going into their cervical vertebrae.

Yogasana versus Contortion

In terms of yogic backbending, the total angle of extension is not as important as the evenness of the distribution of this angle among all of the vertebrae. Thus, it is better and safer to have an angle of spinal extension of only 60°, with this extension distributed approximately evenly among twenty or so vertebral joints, as compared with a deeper spinal extension of, say, 120°, where the largest part of this bend occurs among a much smaller number of relatively weaker vertebral joints, as in figure 8.B-1**c**. This is but one of many aspects of spinal extension that differentiate *yogasana* practice from contortionism; compare the postures in figures 8.B-5**c** and 8.B-5**d**, the first of which is performed by a contortionist and the second of which is performed by an Iyengar-trained yogini. In the former, the thoracic spine is not activated at all, whereas virtually all of the extension would appear to be 90° bends at both the T12–L1 and the L5–S1 points of spinal weakness. In contrast, the yoga student in figure 8.B-5**d** shows considerable elevation of the rib cage and much more equal contributions to the extension by the three spinal sections. Compare also the inversions illustrated in figure V.G-1, performed with yogic alignment (figure V.G-1**a**) versus those done using circus contortion (figures V.G-1**b**, V.G-1**c**, and V.G-1**d**).

In certain postures, one of the legs performs a forward bend while the second leg is in a backward bend; e.g., as in *eka pada setu bandha sarvangasana*. Postures of this sort can be difficult, because the pelvis is structurally unitary and so resists having its two ends being rotated in opposite senses; i.e., in a disrotatory way.

Aspects of Lateral Bending

In lateral flexion, the limit is set by the stretching of the antagonist muscles and their ligaments on the contralateral side. Flexion accompanied by lumbar rotation is relatively slight, because lumbar rotation is difficult in any case; but lateral flexion is large in the lumbar region, for the same reason that lumbar twisting is small in this region (vertical facet joints). Lateral flexion at the upper hinge (Subsection 9.B, page 319) is strongly inhibited by the iliolumbar ligaments binding L4 and L5 to the ilium (figure 9.B-1a), and lateral movement in the thorax is limited by collision of the articular facets on the side to which one bends, as well as by rib-on-rib interaction in the thoracic region. Thus, these factors allow only 40° of thoracic-lumbar lateral bending relative to the line of the sacrum. Lateral movement at the upper hinge also decreases respiratory amplitude, which in turn hinders spinal elongation. If, however, one bends at the lower hinge instead (figure 9.B-5b), the ribs stay separated on the lower side, and interference among the articular facets is no longer a problem. When bending laterally to the side, the abdominal obliques and the quadratus lumborum muscles on that side can be an aid in this movement, if they are used intelligently.

The combination of lateral bending and spinal rotation involves both the intervertebral disc and the vertebral body. These discs are wedge-shaped, being thicker in the front, as one might guess from the curvature in the lumbar and cervical regions. As one bends laterally, the thinner parts of the wedges move toward the site of compression, and because the discs are bonded to the vertebrae, the spine in that spinal section also tends to rotate. This is the case for lumbar and especially cervical vertebrae. Also, the intertransversarii ligaments connect adjacent vertebrae (figure 8.A-4c), and when bending laterally, these are stretched on one side and loosened on the other; any spinal rotation that then occurs will act to tighten the loose side and loosen the tight side. Parallel with the sharply decreasing extensional angles with increasing age (table 8.A-2), the same decrease is seen for the lumbar vertebrae when bending laterally (table 8.A-3). Values

in these tables are not to be interpreted as those appropriate to *yogasana* bending, as the values listed here most likely are for upper-hinge bending, and *yogasana* students will bend laterally at the lower hinge (Subsection 9.B, page 319).

Aspects of Spinal Rotation

Spinal rotation (twisting of the spine) is an important aspect of *yogasana* practice, because circulation of blood is negligible within the intervertebral discs in the adult spine, and nutrition and clearing of metabolic wastes from these organs is only by diffusion. This slow process can be aided by a squeezing of the discs, as when in spinal rotation, and then releasing the rotation, so that fresh fluid can move into the discs. It is supposed that this squeezing and releasing action, even in the short term, protects the flexible discs from ossification.

Note that when it is said that rotation in the cervical spine is 50°, this means on average, each vertebra rotates by about 7° beyond that of the one below it. That is, with respect to T1, C7 rotates by 7°; C6 rotates by 7° with respect to C7, but by 14° with respect to T1; and C1 rotates by 7° with respect to C2, but by 50° with respect to T1. Thus, the total amount of twisting at each vertebra within a spinal section increases with respect to the lowest vertebra on going from the next lowest vertebra to the highest.

Of course, when the elements of the spine are wrung out by twisting, so too are the internal organs; however, the effects of twisting and shearing on the viscera will be weak below the diaphragm, where the twisting is minimal (only 5° possible in the lumbar region: 1° per vertebra), only somewhat stronger in the thoracic region (35° possible in the thoracic region: 2.9° per vertebra), and strongest on organs within the neck (50° possible in the cervical region: 7.1° per vertebra). (See table 8.A-1.) Within each region, it will be weakest at the lowest vertebra and strongest at the highest.

Muscles Involved

In order to twist about the spine when standing erect, one must use muscles that are oriented diagonally across the body, as opposed to those running either horizontally or vertically. Furthermore, in order to rotate the thorax around the spine, the rotator muscles either must be large or there must be many of them. When the spine is twisted in the lumbar and thoracic regions, the abdominal obliques, the rotatores, and the muscles of the scapulae on one side of the body contract, and the sacroiliac ligaments on that side relax, whereas the same muscles and ligaments on the opposite side of the body are stretched.

The Cervical Region

The spine in the cervical region is not coupled to the actions of the abdominal obliques, but it is twisted by the action of the sternocleidomastoid muscles (figure 11.A-1) in the neck, these also being inclined left to right and front to back. Twisting to face to the side implies contraction of the sternocleidomastoid muscles on that side of the body while stretching the antagonist sternocleidomastoid muscles on the opposite side.

Large rotation about the cervical vertebrae will be strongly hindered by any actions in the upper body that lift the scapulae toward the ears. Thus, in order to get the full range of motion in cervical rotation, as when doing *trikonasana* with the head turned to look at the up-stretched hand, one must depress the scapulae by relaxing the upper trapezius and contracting the lower trapezius (figure 10.A-2b). In contrast, spinal twisting while in *sarvangasana*, *halasana*, *sirsasana*, or their variations should not involve any twisting about the cervical vertebrae; i.e., for safety reasons, we do not twist about the cervical vertebrae while this part of the spinal column is under load.

The Thoracic Region

In the cervical and lumbar regions, we speak of "spinal rotation" with the unspoken understanding that in these two regions, there is also the collateral twisting and shearing of all of the organs, muscles, ligaments, etc. within the neck and the lower abdomen, respectively; the rotation in each of these regions is around the spinal column as axis. However, the unspoken understanding of the phrases "spinal rotation" or

"spinal twisting," when applied to the thoracic region, cries out for a more explicit discussion, for in this region, the thoracic cylinder has a posterior aspect (the spinal column), an anterior aspect (the sternal axis), and an intermediate aspect (the central vertical axis of the rib cage), and one must consider how these three axes are affected during "spinal rotation."

As mentioned above, the situation in the thoracic region vis-à-vis spinal twisting is rather different from those in the cervical and lumbar regions. Through costovertebral facets, vertebrae T1–T12 are jointed to twelve pairs of ribs at the costovertebral hinge joints. Furthermore, the uppermost ten of these ribs wrap around the organs of the upper thorax and join again anteriorly onto the sternum. This structure, together with the diaphragm, is discussed in regard to respiration in Section 15.C, page 613. Spinal twisting is difficult in the thoracic region, because ten of the twelve ribs are attached to the vertebrae posteriorly and to the sternum anteriorly, so that when one rotates about the spinal column, there also is a forced but strongly limited rotation of the ribs about the sternum (figure 8.B-6).

Twisting the Rib Cage

It is interesting to consider the purely mechanical consequences of twisting the spine. As shown in figure 8.B-4**b**, when the opposite ends of a cylinder are rotated with respect to one another and about the central axis, the curved surface of the cylinder experiences both tension and a shearing force, and the body of the cylinder experiences a radial compression as well. It is this compressive component that squeezes the water out of a wrung-out washcloth while the fibers of the cloth clearly are under tension.

Applied to spinal twisting, the compressive force will narrow the thorax,[9] will tend to dehy-

---

9   The shape produced by the shearing of the two ends of a cylinder is a hyperboloid of rotation figure 8.B-4**b**), a shape that is curved in two dimensions and which is used in the building of industrial cooling towers because of its mechanical strength and stability in regard to outside forces. Due to the wringing

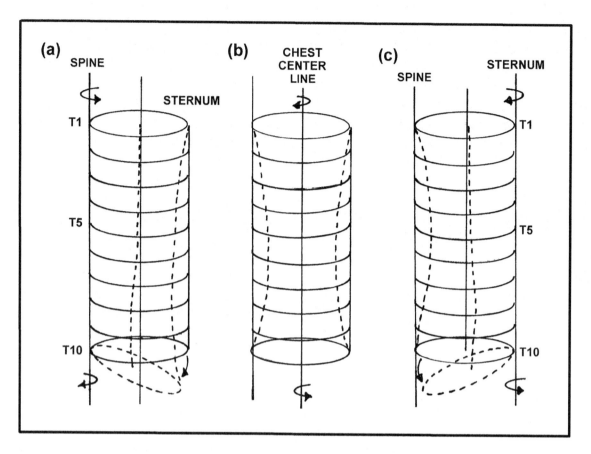

Figure 8.B-6. (a) Distortions of the sternum and the center line of the thorax as the base of the thoracic cylinder is disrotated about the spinal column; (b) distortions of the spinal column and the sternum as the thoracic cylinder is disrotated about the center line of the thorax; (c) distortions of the spinal column and the center line of the thorax as the thoracic cylinder is disrotated about the sternum, as viewed obliquely.

drate the spinal discs (as disc volume and spinal length decrease on twisting), and also will shear the skin of the torso. It is for this reason that students with herniated disc problems are able to twist without pain only if they consciously lift and lengthen the spine before turning. Lifting the abdomen inward and upward while doing the twist helps compress the waist, and this will allow a larger angular rotation to be achieved. On releasing from the twist, the discs and organs will then rehydrate with fresh, healthful fluid.

_____

action inherent in the spinal twist, the chest will also become compressed, thereby making it difficult to breathe deeply. This throttling of the breath is also due to the elongation of the external intercostals when in a spinal twist, for in this condition, the intercostals are weak muscularly due to poor myofilament overlap (Subsection 11.A, page 384).

The mechanics of twisting the thoracic cylinder are much more complicated and asymmetric, as shown in figure 8.B-6. I look at it this way. In the cervical and lumbar regions, it is fair to picture spinal rotation as turning about the vertebral axes in those areas; however, this does not make sense for the thoracic area. In this area, I picture the uppermost thoracic vertebrae rotating strongly along with the cervical vertebrae, whereas the lower thoracic vertebrae are more or less anchored along with the lumbar vertebrae. Even if the spinal rotation begins with the spinal column as rotational axis, very quickly, the centers of the top and bottom surfaces of the thoracic cylinder no longer lie over one another, and both the central axis of the chest and the axis of the sternum become twisted and pulled off center (figure 8.B-6a).

When the thorax is twisted, each of the possibilities shown in figure 8.B-6 should be considered as participating; however, the mechanism shown in figure 8.B-6**b** can be dismissed, as it demands that axial rotation about the weak centerline is able to distort both the spine and sternum. Of the two remaining, (a) requires that the spine stays straight while the sternum is distorted and pulled toward the spine, whereas in (c), the sternum remains straight and the spine is pulled in toward the sternum. Clearly, it is (a) that is closest to our experience, and just a clearly, twisting about the thoracic spine is unavoidably accompanied by a twisting of the sternum (figure 8.B-6**a**). As one approaches the age of forty, the sternum normally begins to stiffen and ossify, and this will impede spinal twisting in this section; but again, it seems reasonable that a twisting practice started before ossification establishes itself will help forestall this eventuality [395].

Among the intervertebral joints in the thoracic spine, that between T11 and T12 is especially mobile in regard to flexion, extension, lateral bending, and spinal rotation. This is so because the lowest two ribs attached posteriorly to these vertebrae are "floating" anteriorly and so are not bound to the sternum as tightly (figure 15.B-1**a**). The intervertebral joint at T11–T12 is the one that is most likely to be stressed when the spine is excessively rotated [101]. The sacrum and coccyx have no mobility to speak of, save for that at the L5–S1 joint and that between the sacrum and the coccyx in women but not necessarily operational in men.

Because there are no large muscles in the thorax that run front to back and left to right with which one could develop a rotational torque in that part of the spine, thoracic twisting is limited. Moreover, rotation about the spinal column in the thorax implies an unavoidable rotation of the horizontal plane at the top of the thorax, so that it is no longer centered over the horizontal plane of the bottom of the thorax (figure 8.B-6**a**). Said differently, when twisting, the two ends of the thoracic cylinder are rotated oppositely about an axis on the vertical surface of the cylinder, and this acts to shear the cylinder and strongly distort the sternum. Inasmuch as the sternum may well

be ossified in the older adult, this too will hamper spinal twisting in the thoracic region. These two factors (clamping by the rib cage and the resistance of the sternum to distortion) will tend to limit severely the amount of twist that can be generated in the thoracic region (only 1.8° per vertebra; see table 8.A-1). Spinal rotation is easiest in the young, for whom the cartilage in the rib cage is flexible, but this advantage is not granted the older student.

The ultimate rotation of the axis of the shoulders, with respect to the axis of the pelvis, can be increased significantly if the rib cage and the skin over it as a whole are wrapped with a long but narrow band of yoga mat and the thorax is rotated by pulling on the mat when in a twisted posture such as *parivrtta trikonasana* [255] (Box 13.A-1, page 504).

The Lumbar Region

When rotating the spine, rotation is very minimal (approximately 1° per vertebra) in the lumbar region, due to the angle at which the articular facets meet. It is generally true that rotation about the vertical spine is easy around vertebrae in which the articular facets are horizontal, and so the rotational motion is a horizontal gliding motion of one vertebra with respect to its neighbors; it is difficult when these facets are oriented vertically, as they are in the lumbar region. The wedge shape of L5 accommodates the transition to S1, which is nearly horizontal on its upper surface.

Prime among the large muscles serving rotation in the lumbar region are the internal and external obliques of the abdominal area (Subsection 15.A, page 608). As shown in figure 10.A-2**a**, the obliques are bilateral, with the internal oblique on the left originating on the left side of the pelvis and crossing the abdomen so as to terminate on the lower (floating) ribs on the right side, and with the internal oblique on the right crisscrossing it to terminate on the lower (floating) ribs on the left. The left external oblique parallels the right internal oblique, and the right external oblique parallels the left internal oblique. With the internal and external obliques working together in contraction, considerable torque can be generated so as to twist the lumbar spine and the T11–T12 vertebrae carrying the floating ribs strongly to the right or to the left. Note, however, that the lumbar vertebrae will rotate only 5° in total. The joint capsules between adjacent vertebrae and between vertebrae and ribs will resist this twisting motion, as will the presence of the iliolumbar ligaments anchoring the L4 and L5 vertebrae to the upper rims of the pelvis.

Beating the Averages

It is interesting to compare the range-of-motion values reported by Kapandji (figure 8.A-1 and table 8.A-1) as measured on an "average" population with those attained by accomplished students of *yogasana*. Thus, Kapandji lists the maximal rotation about the cervical vertebrae at +/- 50°, whereas students of *yogasana* routinely rotate through +/- 90° at the cervical vertebrae when doing *virabhadrasana II*. According to Kapandji, maximum rotation about the thoracic and lower sections of the spine combined amount to 40°, whereas *yogasana* students rotate by 90° in *maricyasana III*. Although *yogasana* students readily can eclipse these "maximum" ranges of spinal rotation when doing spinal twists such as *maricyasana III*, even in these students, it nonetheless appears that the cervical vertebrae rotate about ten times farther than the lumbar. With fourteen cervical vertebrae, the owl can turn its head more than twice as far angularly (270°) as can *yogasana* students with only seven such vertebrae [878]. Kilmurray [447] presents a second point of view on spinal rotation. He considers the second and fourth *chakras* (the *swadisthana* belly and *anahata* heart centers; see table 5.G-1) to be muscular centers that are to be used to drive the rotation, whereas the spine itself acts passively to receive the torsion. In this way, the spine is twisted, but it does not twist itself (presumably using the intervertebral rotatores muscles shown in figure 8.A-4c), as it remains relaxed and is acted upon by larger muscles in the upper and lower spine.

Preferred Sense of Rotation

While still in the womb, infants show an obvious preference for turning the head to one side over the other. In a related vein, twice as many people tilt their heads to the right when they kiss as do those who tilt their heads to the left. In right-handed people, twisting the front body to the left is the easier direction in general, with the right arm wrapping around the front of the body in this twist as the left arm goes behind the back [7]. Perhaps this tendency may result in different sensations being felt when we turn the head to the left or to the right in *yogasanas* such as *maricyasana III* or *bharadvajasana*. This twisting preference may reflect the dominant right-handedness among 90 percent of people.

Rotation and Lateral Bending

When the spine is twisted, there is a tendency for the spine to bend laterally as well; for a twist that will face in a given direction, the direction of the lateral bend is in the same direction and largely in the lumbar spine [447]. Furthermore, not only does twisting promote lateral bending, but lateral bending promotes twisting. The consequences of this coupling of bending and rotation in two *yogasanas* and in scoliosis are presented in Box 8.B-1, next page.

Conrotatory and Disrotatory Actions

In the Spine

As the spinal column is twisted, there is an unavoidable twisting of the sacral plate in the sacroiliac joint (figure 8.B-7), which tends to misalign it (or align it, if misaligned); this twisting is accompanied by a loosening of the ligaments of the sacroiliac upon which the joint is dependent for stability [492]. Intense twisting action can painfully misalign this important joint.

When we perform spinal twists, such as *bharadvajasana I*, the pelvis often rotates along with the rotation of the rib cage. For the sake of concreteness, imagine the rotation of the anterior spine to be toward the right, in which case, the left knee will be thrust forward, as the anterior pelvis rotates to the right as well. To accommodate this unwelcome rotation of the pelvis, one often resets the left femur into the hip joint so that a

Box 8.B-1: Spinal Rotation Can Be Induced by Lateral Bending and Vice Versa

There is a psychological component to everything, including the tendency to bend forward in *trikonasana:* the area in front psychologically represents the known and familiar, whereas the area behind is dark, unknown, and frightening. The beginning student in *trikonasana* must be brave enough to pull the upper body backward, going from the region of safe-and-sure into the unknown, so that the torso is above the triangle of the legs, thus bringing the entire back body into two-dimensional alignment (Box III.B-1, page 846).

A second factor in regard to the tendency to bend forward in *trikonasana* is not psychological in nature, but nonetheless works to align the ribs in this posture. The concave lumbar curve results in part because the discs in the lumbar region are wedge-shaped, with the thinner aspect of the wedges pointing to the rear [52, 884]. As one bends laterally, the bending is assisted by a rotation of the lumbar wedges so as to place the thinner parts of the wedges to that side on which the intervertebral discs are more compressed; i.e., the side toward which one bends.[1] Correspondingly, the thicker parts of the wedges move toward the opposite side, where the vertebral discs are more expanded. The tendency of the thick and thin parts of the discs to change positions when bending laterally results in a rotation of the lumbar vertebrae, which pulls the ribs forward on the side toward which one is bending. Application of the same argument to the thoracic spine, where the thin part of the vertebral wedges point forward (rather than backward, as with the lumbar wedges), leads to the conclusion that the thoracic spine will tend to rotate oppositely to that induced in the lumbar spine.

This coupling of the lateral bending with twisting is especially synergistic in *trikonasana* and in *parivrtta janu sirsasana*, where the lateral motion in the lumbar spine tends to turn the rib cage to face forward or upward, as these *yogasanas* require. On the other hand, in *parivrtta trikonasana*, the rotation induced by the lateral bending is in the direction opposite to that demanded by the pose, and so one must overcome this tendency with awareness and practice. The bending-rotation connection described above can be countered by unilateral contraction of the psoas muscle (Section 9.B, page 317); if the right-hand psoas is contracted, this acts to pull the torso to the right and rotate it to face left, as when doing *parivrtta janu sirsasana*. This bending and twisting action of the contracted psoas is a result of its diagonal orientations in both the left-to-right and front-to-back directions.

The simultaneous occurrence of lateral flexing and rotation of the spinal vertebrae often is apparent in the spines of those with scoliosis (see Subsection 8.A, page 272), where lateral curvature is always accompanied by spinal rotation. In this case, the spine is pushed largely to one side and forward when in the neutral position (*tadasana*), with other spinal segments also displaced oppositely in compensation for the primary displacement. The condition of scoliosis is outwardly much like that experienced by beginners in

---

1   Actually, this will be more the case when bending laterally at the upper hinge, whereas bending at the lower hinge does not accent any wedginess in the lumbar discs. Thus, this discussion is more appropriate to *trikonasana* performed by beginning students bending at the upper hinge.

trikonasana, except that the rotation and lateral flexion is very difficult to reverse, and the misalignment may have a long-term effect on the internal organs.

Just as is the case in the lower spine, rotation of the head about the cervical vertebrae is accompanied by a lateral flexion of the same vertebrae. Pure rotation is allowed at the C7–T1 joint due to the horizontal facets at that place, but at the level of C2 and C3, the proportions of rotation and flexion are about equal [288].

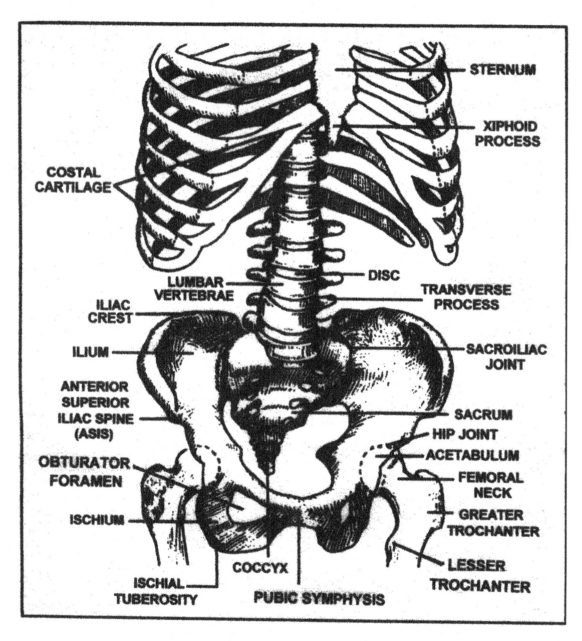

Figure 8.B-7. The bones of the pelvis, attached to the sacral spine above and to the femoral heads below, as seen from the front [428].

counter-rotation of the pelvis occurs with respect to that of the rib cage; i.e., a disrotatory action is set in motion. In this way, the intensity of the twist is amplified by oppositely twisting the two ends of the spine, as in figure 8.B-8**a**. However, in doing this counter-rotation, one must keep in mind the huge torque that this produces within the sacroiliac joint and that the opposite relative rotation—conrotatory action (figure 8.A-8**c**) rather than disrotatory—may be better suited to students with lower-back weakness and/or pain.

For safety's sake, in sitting or standing twists where one could forcefully counter-rotate the pelvis with respect to the rib cage (a disrotatory action), the two ends of the spine instead may be mildly rotated in the same direction (a conrotatory action), as, for example, when doing *maricyasana III*. This action will keep the lumbar vertebrae, the sacrum, and the ilium bones in *tadasana*-like alignment and so will not unduly torque the sacroiliac joint [447, 492]. On the other hand, in twists where the body is lying on the floor so that there is no pressing of the sacrum into the sacroiliac joint (*jatara parivartanasana*, for example) or is inverted (*parsva sirsasana*, for example), the disrotatory twist is more acceptable but still should not be overdone. For those who wish to rotate the spine with neither conrotatory nor disrotatory motion of the pelvis, the pelvis can be locked into the neural position by twisting with the legs immobilized, as when sitting in *vajrasana* or *baddha konasana*.

An element of disrotatory action of the pelvis can be found in *hanumanasana*, for the forward leg has the hamstrings in high tension, whereas the leg in back has the quadriceps in high tension. As a consequence of the connection of these muscles to the pelvis, the two sides of the pelvis, left and right, are being rotated oppositely in this posture. As a result of this disrotatory action in the pelvis, the upper body tends to rotate to face away from the forward leg in *hanumanasana* when there is tension in the each of the relevant quadriceps and hamstring muscles.

In *hasta padangusthasana*, the lifted leg rotates the pelvis on its side in a particular sense and, due to the rigidity of the pelvis, the standing leg tends to rotate in the same sense, i.e., they ro-

tate together in a conrotatory way about the axis between the hip joints. That is to say, the thigh of the standing leg tends to rise so as to be parallel to that of the raised leg. This action not only tends to bend the standing leg, which is rapidly tiring (as when in *utkatasana*), but also encourages congestion between the raised thigh and the lower abdomen. What is called for here is an opposing conrotatory action of the thighs about the line of the hip joints. On both legs, press the thighs away from the frontal pelvic bones, bending only at the lower hinge, and bring the back rim of the pelvis forward and down. On both legs, press the front thighs to the back thighs. This conrotatory action of the two thighs will work to make the thigh of the standing leg vertical and that of the lifted leg horizontal (assuming that it has been lifted too high), all the while relieving congestion in the area between the thighs and the lower abdomen.

In the Limbs

As discussed at length in Chapter 10 (page 331) and in Subsection 11.F (page 468), motions of the pelvis and rib cage are aided by disrotatory actions within the legs and arms, respectively. Thus, in *adho mukha svanasana*, a disrotatory arm action, in which the backs of the hands are rotated medially while the anterior aspects of the upper arms are rotated laterally (figures 8.A-8**b** and 8.A-8**d**), is key to pressing the scapulae onto the rib cage; see Subsection 10.A, page 328, for more on this. This disrotatory action of the arm also is appropriate to the arm action in *trikonasana* to the right, where the lower part of the right arm is rotated medially and the upper arm is rotated laterally, as seen from the front; the right shoulder is pressed more forward so as to be positioned just below the left shoulder, if the right arm is worked in a disrotatory way.

The disrotatory action of the arm described for *trikonasana* is quite parallel to that initiated in the leg, where the anterior femur of the leg is rotated laterally while the lower leg is rotated medially in order to press the groin on that side forward (Subsection 10.A, page 337).

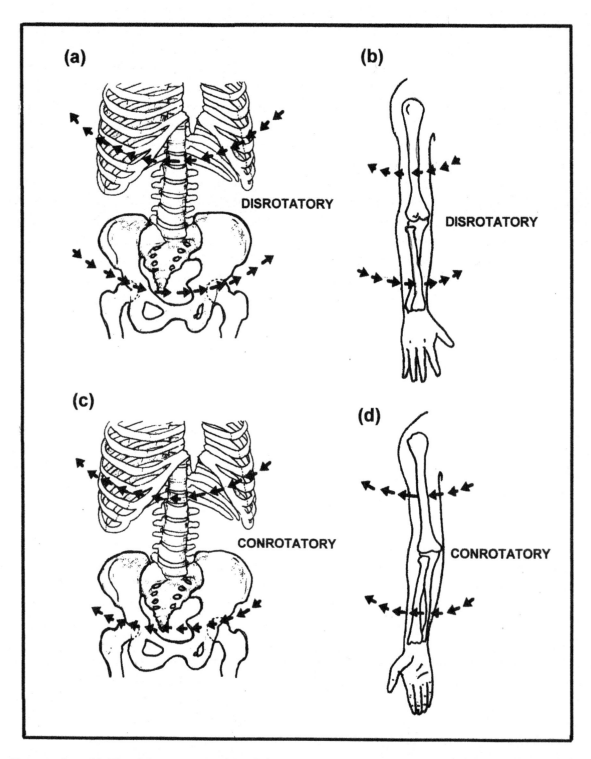

Figure 8.B-8. (a) The disrotatory rotation of the spine torquing the sacrum within the sacroiliac joint, as might occur in *bharadvajasana I*; (b) disrotatory action in the right arm, with the upper arm and the lower arm rotated oppositely, as for *adho mukha svanasana*; (c) the conrotatory rotation of the spine with reduced torque in the sacroiliac joint; and (d) conrotatory rotation of the right arm—in this case, in the lateral sense in regard to the biceps.

In the Neck

The conrotatory and disrotatory aspects of twisting are relevant not only to the relative motions of pelvis and rib cage, but also to the relative motion of the rib cage and the head. Moreover, it is not always true that the conrotatory action is the one that is kinder to the body. Thus, if the anterior rib cage is twisted to the right, the head may be twisted to the right (conrotatory) or to the left (disrotatory) in beginner's *trikonasana*. Turning the head to look down at the forward foot involves a disrotatory turn of the head with respect to the rotation of the rib cage, whereas in the more advanced form of the posture, the face turns toward the upwardly extended arm, and the head rotation is conrotatory with respect to the rotation of the chest.

Walking and Running

It is now felt by researchers in the field that spinal rotation is an integral part of walking and running, with the pelvis and shoulder girdle performing a disrotatory twisting action centered about T7. In this, the lumbar curve is twisted first in one sense and then the other with each step, so as to place each foot alternately ahead of the other. In this act, the lumbar spine is twisted so as to place the center of gravity of the body over the leg that is on the ground at that moment, and in compensation, the thorax above T7 rotates in a disrotatory sense. This twisting is aided by the curvature of the lumbar spine and by swinging of the arms.

Section 8.C: The Intervertebral Discs

Several factors combine to determine the overall mobility of the cervical, thoracic, and lumbar sections of the spine. Thus, in the cervical region, the orientation of the facet joints and short transverse and spinous processes all combine to infer a large range of motion to the cervical spine. In contrast, motion in the thorax is highly restricted by the overlapping of the spinous processes, the

binding effects of the ribs, possible rib-on-rib contact, and possible torsion of the sternum. In the lumbar region, the facet orientation strongly restricts spinal rotation but allows large movements in directions perpendicular to the spinal axis. Additionally, the mobility in the various spinal regions is affected strongly by the physical state of the soft, springy discs positioned between the vertebrae; these discs are designed to act as shock absorbers and as integral parts of the synovial joints between vertebrae, as discussed below.

Structure and Shapes

A semirigid element called the intervertebral disc (figure 8.B-1**a**) is positioned between each adjacent pair of vertebrae in the spine, except between the occiput and C1 and between C1 and C2. This disc, composed of a central ball-shaped portion (the nucleus pulposus) surrounded by the stout but flexible annulus fibrosus, sits between the relatively flat surfaces of adjacent vertebral bodies (figure 8.A-2**a**). Thanks to the elastic nature of the intervertebral disc, all motions of adjacent vertebrae are more or less allowed, with the nucleus pulposus being the center about which the motion occurs [288].

The nucleus pulposus, a jelly-like hydrophilic (water-loving) material consisting of up to 88 percent water, is surrounded by the seven sheaths of the annulus fibrosus (figure 8.B-3**a**). The latter sheaths are made of fibrocartilage, with their fibers set at different angles in each of the inner layers. The fibers in the outermost annulus are oriented vertically, unlike the inner ones, which are alternately tilted at +/-65° to vertical. This anti-parallel arrangement of fibers in the successive layers of the annulus strengthens it, just as it does within the different layers of bone (Section 7.A, page 225). That the annular sheaths have superior strength with respect to shear (thanks to the fibers' mixed orientations) is advantageous, for the annulus serves as a casing to keep the nucleus pulposus intact while under pressure; i.e., its job is to resist herniation of the disc.

In the adult spine, no blood vessels serve the discs, the vascular system having disappeared by age twenty years. Instead, the discs are nourished by the diffusion of nutrients and wastes into and out of neighboring tissues [478, 756]. Weight bearing on the spine wrings fluid from the discs, whereas rest restores the discs by bathing them in fresh fluid. Note that this fluid is not cerebrospinal fluid, which is contained within the vertebral canal (Subsection 4.E, page 107), whereas the vertebral discs lie outside of the vertebral canal but are within the synovial capsules and so are bathed in synovial fluid instead. If the discs are not wrung out and then restored by fresh fluid, they become thin, brittle, and easily damaged [756].

Characteristics and Functions

Height and Load

In humans, the intervertebral discs account for approximately 20 percent of the length of the spine and so are a significant structural element in addition to serving as shock absorbers [582]; however, the discs lose their elasticity and height as we age. Being somewhat flexible, the intervertebral discs are also important components of the intervertebral joints and the resultant spinal flexibility. The semirigid nucleus pulposus acts like a swivel ball between the two near-planar surfaces of the relevant vertebral bodies. As a swivel, it allows relative tilt, rotation, and shearing motion of the two vertebral plates. Though these reorientations may be of small magnitude at one joint, the combined effect along the length of the spine can be substantial (table 8.A-1).

The facet joints of the spinal column not only distribute the compressive load on the spine among all of the component joints but also protect the nucleus pulposus from injury during extreme motions. If the nucleus pulposus degenerates or becomes dehydrated and so reduces its thickness, the facet joint closes and so bears more of the weight compressing the spine. When the discs are healthy, 16 percent of the compressive load of the body weight is carried on the facet joints of the lumbar spine but this fraction increases to 70 percent when the discs in the lumbar spine lose their thickness, and thereby allow the

facet joints to close [884]. The increased bone-to-bone contacts experienced when the discs collapse can be very painful and strongly limit the range of spinal motions, as one might guess from their smaller ratios of disc thickness to vertebral heights (Subsection 8.B, page 284).

Under axial (head-to-toe) compression, the nucleus pulposus bears 75 percent of that part of the load borne by the discs, the annulus 25 percent. When the top of the spine is externally loaded with 40 kilograms (ninety pounds), there is an axial compression of 1 millimeter (0.04 inches) per disc, while each disc correspondingly expands radially by 0.5 millimeters (0.02 inches). In a healthy disc, the thickness will decrease by about 1.4 millimeters (0.06 inches) for a 100-kilogram (220-pound) load; whereas in a diseased disc the loss of disc height is closer to 2.0 millimeters (0.08 inches), and recovery will be incomplete on releasing the load. If the spine is lengthened, the gravitational loading on the discs is decreased, and their nuclei are expanded to a more spherical shape.

Diseased or not, as the axially loaded disc broadens as when in *tadasana*, it presses radially (left to right) on the annulus, thereby transforming a vertical stress into a horizontal stress. Both the vertebrae and the discs that separate them can be damaged by aging or by overloading. Thus, the compressive strength of the lumbar vertebrae in those aged sixty to seventy is only half that in those aged twenty to thirty, and lumbar herniation is encouraged in the latter when stoop-lifting with the legs straight or when returning to *tadasana* from *uttanasana* with the legs straight and the back rounded.

Loading on the intervertebral discs also may be asymmetric front to back. Thus, for example, the forward slump so common when sitting will act to compress the anterior portions of the intervertebral discs (and to relieve the pressure of one vertebra pressing posteriorly on its neighbor); whereas backbending will act to compress the posterior portions of the same discs [487] (figures 8.A-6b and -6e). Indeed, the discs are said to be wedge-shaped front to back in the cervical and lumbar regions, with the thick edges of the wedges forward, even when the spine is held vertically. This wedging leads to the concave spinal curvature observed in these two regions. Though heavy loading may be sufficient to force one vertebra onto the one below it, even the bony vertebrae themselves have nonzero elasticity and can deform in response to modest loading [483].

Shock Absorption

The vertebral disc acts as a shock absorber, damping impulsive shocks and spreading its load over a larger area by spreading laterally on compression. It has a broad range of responsiveness, being equally effective in damping the shock of an instantaneous footstep and the daily long-term downward stress of gravity when standing or sitting. Ideally, the disc itself is very springy, as one would expect for a shock-absorbing structure; however, this useful property tends to degrade with age.

Spinal Misalignment

When the vertebrae are out of alignment (subluxed), a heightened risk of pressure applied to the spinal cord in the vicinity of the displacement results. Not surprisingly, there is a clear correlation between the location of the misalignment along the spinal column, the area of the body affected by the misalignment, and the effects that can appear in that area. Tables 8.C-1, 8.C-2, and 8.C-3 list these correlations for misalignment of the cervical, thoracic, and lumbar vertebrae, respectively [647]. Misalignment of the cervical vertebrae (Subsection 8.A, page 264) also can adversely affect the blood flow through the vertebral arteries to the brain, with consequent neurological problems in that organ (see Subsection 8.A, page 278).

When the intervertebral discs have degenerated but not herniated, the vertebrae may come to rub on one another, leading to the growth of painful bone spurs and even the fusion of adjacent vertebrae. This occurs most often in the cervical region [478]. *Yogasana* postures that challenge the strength or flexibility of the spine must be approached gingerly with students who experience problems of this sort.

Disc Deformation

The intervertebral disc is firmly bound to the upper and lower surfaces of the vertebral bodies confining it. This means that when the spine is twisted, the upper and lower ends of the disc are twisted in a disrotatory way, so that the disc tends to be wrung out (dehydrated) and shrinks at the waist (figure 8.B-4c). This also is supported by the twisting of the joint capsule. On returning to the untwisted state, the disc imbibes fresh fluid from within the synovial capsule surrounding the joint and from water stored within the pores of the cancellous vertebral bone. This most likely is the scenario if the twist is held for a matter of hours, but it also may be a factor when held for only a matter of minutes.

Intervertebral discs show viscoelastic behavior, much like that shown by the muscles (Subsection 11.E, page 462). That is to say, when a disc is loaded and then released quickly, it first compresses and then expands elastically, so that there is no net change in its thickness. However, if the loading is heavy and long lasting, then the disc behaves viscoelastically (Subsection 11.E, page 462), losing water during the compression and then regaining its full thickness only after a long-term rest, if at all.

Actually, even in near-zero gravity, as when one is prone, there is a strong outward pressure on the annulus due to water in the discs, and this acts to pre-stress (preload) them in anticipation of the compressive gravitational loading from the outside as one goes from prone to a more erect posture. Because the preloading is most marked in the morning, this is the time when the discs are at their thickest, the spine is at its longest, the facet joints are most open, and the tension on the intervertebral musculature is maximal. (As discussed in Subsection 23.C, page 791, there are other physiological markers that suggest that *yogasanas* are best done in the early morning).

With increasing age, the discs are less able to achieve the preloaded state during rest, and thus they do not inflate well; the result is loss of height, loss of spinal flexibility, and changing spinal curvature in the aged (see also Section

Table 8.C-1: Effects of Cervical Misalignment [647]

Vertebra Misaligned	Area	Effect
C1	Blood supply to the head, pituitary gland, scalp, bones of the face, brain, inner and middle ear, sympathetic nervous system	Headaches, nervousness, insomnia, head colds, high blood pressure, migraine headaches, nervous breakdown, amnesia, chronic tiredness, dizziness
C2	Eyes, optic nerves, auditory nerves, sinuses, mastoid bones, tongue, forehead	Sinus trouble, allergies, crossed eyes, deafness, eye troubles, earache, fainting, blindness
C3	Cheeks, outer ear, face bones, teeth, trigeminal nerve	Neuralgia, neuritis, acne, pimples, eczema
C4	Nose, lips, mouth, Eustachian tube	Hay fever, catarrh, hearing loss, adenoids
C5	Vocal cords, neck glands, pharynx	Laryngitis, hoarseness, sore throat
C6	Neck muscles, shoulder, tonsils	Stiff neck, upper-arm pain, tonsillitis, whooping cough, croup
C7	Thyroid, shoulder bursae, elbow bursae	Bursitis, colds

Table 8.C-2: Effects of Thoracic Misalignment [647]

Vertebra Misaligned	Area	Effect
T1	Forearms, hands, wrists, fingers, esophagus, trachea	Pain in lower arms and hands, asthma, cough, difficult breathing, shortness of breath
T2	Heart, heart covering, coronary arteries	Heart conditions, chest conditions
T3	Lungs, bronchial tubes, pleura, chest, breasts	Bronchitis, pleurisy, pneumonia, congestion, influenza
T4	Gallbladder, common duct	Gallbladder conditions, jaundice, shingles
T5	Liver, solar plexus, blood	Liver conditions, fevers, low blood pressure, anemia, poor circulation, arthritis
T6	Stomach	Stomach troubles, nervous stomach, indigestion, heartburn, dyspepsia
T7	Pancreas, duodenum	Ulcers, gastritis
T8	Spleen	Lowered immunological resistance
T9	Adrenal and supra-adrenal glands	Allergies, hives
T10	Kidneys	Kidney trouble, hardening of the arteries, chronic tiredness, nephritis, pyelitis
T11	Kidneys, ureters	Acne, pimples, eczema, boils
T12	Small intestines, lymph	Rheumatism, gas pains, sterility

Table 8.C-3: Effects of Lumbar, Sacral, and Coccygeal Misalignment [647]

Vertebra Misaligned	Area	Effect
L1	Colon, inguinal rings	Constipation, colitis, dysentery, diarrhea, hernias
L2	Appendix, abdomen, upper leg	Cramps, difficulty breathing, acidosis, varicose veins
L3	Sex organs, uterus, bladder, knee	Bladder trouble, menstrual troubles, bed wetting, knee pains
L4	Prostate gland, muscles of lower back, sciatic nerve	Sciatica, lumbago, difficult, painful or too frequent urination, backaches
L5	Lower legs, ankles, feet	Poor circulation in legs, swollen ankles, weak ankles and arches, cold feet, weak legs, leg cramps
S1–S5	Hip bones, buttocks	Sacroiliac problems, spinal curvatures
Coccyx	Rectum, anus	Hemorrhoids, pruritis, pain on sitting

24.A, page 807); this normal degeneration is accelerated by osteoporosis. Even in a young person, under conditions of constant loading, the discs tend toward collapse, simulating old age. In view of the above, practicing *yogasana* is seen as practicing preventive medicine, thanks to the emphasis placed by the *yogasanas* on the lengthening of the spine, the release of chronic pressure on the vertebral discs, and the stimulation of fluid circulation in their vicinity.

Herniation, Nerve Impingement, and Lower-Back Pain

Disc Herniation

Surgical treatment of lower-back pain is the most common neurosurgical procedure performed in the United States, with 300,000 such operations taking place each year. These procedures follow from fifteen million physician visits per year, with a total annual cost to society for such treatments of fifty billion dollars. A certain part of this lower-back pain can be traced to disc herniation and consequent nerve impingement, or to damage of the spinal muscles.

As the axial compression on the discs increases from the cervical to the lumbar vertebrae (table 8.A-1), the discs at the base of the spine may rupture on loading, especially in the elderly. In this case, the annulus bulges or tears to release the nucleus pulposus into the intervertebral space, and a herniated disc is born (figure 8.B-3c). Note that if the herniation is posterior, as in figure 8.B-3c, the nucleus pulposus will press on elements of the spinal cord, whereas if the herniation is forward, there is no direct compression of the spinal cord.

There are many points of view as to the seriousness of the herniation of an intervertebral disc (also called disc prolapse). As there are no nerves serving the discs, there is no direct pain signal to be felt when a disc is injured. However, because of the injury, the load bearing may shift away from the injured site, thereby impinging upon a nearby site instead, and this site may then respond to the impingement with pain, tingling, or numbness.

A herniated disc can be the cause of lower-back pain (lumbago) or buttock and leg pain (sciatica). These are often precipitated by a flexion injury, and as the stress of flexion is greatest in the lumbar region (table 8.A-1), herniation of the discs is most often seen at L4–L5 and L5–S1; cervical herniation is most often seen at C5–C6 and C6–C7 [360], and thoracic herniation occurs most often at T12 [433]. It is said that the disc between L5 and S1 is more or less degenerated in most people by the age of twenty years [553]. It appears that disc problems are often found in or adjacent to the transitional regions of spinal vertebral types, such as at C7–T1, T12–L1, and L5–S1. Research has recently has shown that there is an inheritable gene variation involving the structure of intervertebral cartilage that encourages lumbar-disc herniation.

Sciatica

Nearly 90 percent of sciatica problems originate either with the rupture of an intervertebral disc and the pressing of the disc contents onto the sciatic nerve (figure 8.B-3c) or with osteoarthritis of the lumbo-sacral vertebrae [565]. Pain from nerve impingement also may occur when the diameter of the vertebral canal shrinks, as with spinal stenosis (figures 8.B-3d and 8.B-3e) [588]. Moreover, in certain positions requiring pelvic flexion (*supta padangusthasana*, for example), the herniated disc may trap the rootlet to the sciatic nerve, so that it does not move through the intervertebral foramen, and so becomes painful as the leg is stretched. Nerve impingement on the components of the sciatic nerve due to a herniated disc can result in pain on the front, side, or rear of the affected leg (corresponding to impingement on neural roots at L4, L5, or S1, respectively) or to numbness at the inner knee, the side of the calf, or on the back of the calf, depending again on whether it is the disc between L4 and L5 or L5 and S1 that is involved [323].

It is something of an open question as to whether students with lower-back pain should bend forward or backward for relief. A recent study [671] showed statistically that better results were obtained with mild backbending; however, a significant number of subjects did better with mild forward bending. The backbending result is understandable in terms of a disc that is herniated backward but is pushed forward, away from

the spinal cord, by increasing the lordosis (figure 8.A-6b); this in turn lessens the pain and shortens the time to regain the pain-free range of motion of the spine.[10] For most disc-herniation problems, forward bends are not recommended, but supported backbends, done with much less than maximum angular extension, are often effective at reducing discomfort [464].

Because the vertebral discs are bonded tightly to the vertebrae, the discs themselves are torqued when the spine is twisted, as in *maricyasana III*, for example [447]. This torquing of the intervertebral discs results in an additional compressive radial force when one rotates about the spine; however, this compression can be avoided if spinal elongation is performed as a prelude to the twists. In any case, during spinal rotation, some of the sheaths in the annulus are stretched, while others are relaxed, depending on the clockwise or counterclockwise sense of the twist and on the fiber orientations within each of the sheaths. Extreme twisting, as in *ardha matsyendrasana I*, can also lead to tears in the annular sheaths, thus weakening them and setting the stage for herniation; this is less likely if such twists are performed in a conrotatory rather than in a disrotatory manner (page 298).

Impingement and Referred Pain

Though the pain of a herniated disc often follows from the disc contents being forced backward into the spinal canal and impinging on the spinal nerves, impingement also can be on the nerves serving the pelvis [323], with referred pain then sensed as coming from the groin, rectum, bladder, etc. (Subsection 13.D, page 532). When this is the case, the pain should be relieved by mild backbends, such as *setu bandha sarvangasana*, which force the expelled nucleus forward again [577, 671]. However, such *yogasanas* must be done with deliberate spinal lengthening to be effective pain relievers [110].

---

10   In fact, Iyengar specifically mentions in his book Light on Yoga [388] that he recommends regular practice of *salabhasana* without recourse to surgical intervention for lower-back pain.

Pain Symptoms

Note too that pain is a very subjective sensation, with strong modulation of its intensity made possible by psychological factors (Section 13.C, page 528). Many experiments show that our response to pain is a learned behavior and that through the connection of the spine to the diaphragm and the breathing process, the spine is very strongly involved with problems of a psychological origin [10].

That lower-back pain is a complex phenomenon is shown by the fact that there is a frequent lack of correlation between pain and herniation. Many people have herniated discs but report no symptoms, and many others have undergone surgical repair of their herniation without any diminution of the pain, suggesting that mechanisms other than that shown in figure 8.B-3c may be at work. The picture of lower-back pain is further complicated by the fact that pressure on the sciatic nerve may originate not with a herniated disc or a subluxation of the vertebrae, but rather with the pressure of the piriformis muscle within the buttocks on the sciatic nerve bundle as it traverses the buttocks region [745]. As discussed further in Section 9.B, page 314, this particular scenario is readily treated by the practice of the appropriate *yogasanas*. At the cervical end of the spine, "pinched nerves" may result from the pressure of the trapezius muscles on nerve roots at a distance from the spinal column, rather than from the pressure of a herniated cervical disc. In this case, there often is a lack of sensation in the arm or hand. At the lumbar end of the spine, one often sees a stenosis of the vertebrae, so that nerves are pinched either within the vertebral canal or as they pass through the intervertebral foramen (figures 8.B-3d and 8.B-3e).

It has been observed that the pressure of a herniated disc on a sensory nerve in the spinal cord sometimes increases the frequency of its action potential and sometimes decreases this frequency, yet both create the sensation of lower-back pain. Further, even removal of the offending disc may not remove the pain if there are other psychological factors at work [266, 745].

Yet another possible mechanism for lower-back pain is advanced by Faber and Walker [232], who claim that the spinal ligaments (figure 8.A-5) normally hold the discs in their centered positions between the vertebrae. If the intraspinal ligaments (figure 8.A-4c) become overstretched, their grip on the relevant vertebra is loosened, and the disc is then free to move backward and press on the vulnerable nerves. In this case, one needs joint-proliferant therapy (prolotherapy) to rebuild ligaments and so strengthen the spine. Sarno [745] also argues that sciatic pain is the result of a high resting muscle tone (Subsection 11.B, page 434) due to psychological tension, and that resolution of the psychological problem will resolve the pain problem.

Though there is a high degree of bacterial infection in herniated discs [105], it is not clear if it is incidental to the herniation or is causative. Lower-back pain also may be the result of the imperfect fitting of the sacral plate into the sacroiliac joint, the plate being either poorly centered left to right or falling forward. Carbonnel [105] claims that most vertebral herniations are self-healing if they are given six weeks of rest. It also is possible that when the annulus tears, there follows a reaction generating swelling of the torn tissue, and that this swollen tissue then impinges on the sciatic nerve, rather than material from the nucleus pulposus.

Circadian Effects

Often, lower-back pain is worse in the evening and mildest when first awakening. In this case, the pain is circadian (Subsection 23.B, page 774) and is due to the gradual compression of the spinal vertebrae over the course of the day and the decompression upon lying down at night. It is the lower back that suffers most when loaded like this, since it carries most of the weight when erect, but carries no weight when lying down or in a quadrupedal stance. Just as with the other joints in the body, the vertebral joints also may suffer from osteoarthritis (Subsection 7.D, page 250), which arises from a wearing away of the cushioning cartilage between adjacent vertebrae. For those whose lower-back pain is most intense on awakening, the situation may be that the hydration of the intervertebral discs and/or shrinkage of the spinal ligaments during the night increases the intervertebral pressure, and this in turn presses more strongly on the herniated nucleus pulposus, pressing it against the spinal cord.

Spinal Arthritis

A second type of spinal arthritis, known as ankylosing spondylitis, is found overwhelmingly in males and resembles rheumatoid arthritis in that it has similar symptoms. It too is thought to be caused by an autoimmune attack by the body on itself. In this case, the ligaments and tendons binding the vertebrae to one another are damaged and swell, leading eventually to the fusion of adjacent vertebrae. The pain here too is circadian; however, it is worse in the morning hours between 6:00 and 9:00 and least between noon and 3:00 PM, much like rheumatoid arthritis, but in contrast to spinal osteoarthritis. Symptoms are more serious in the winter months and least so during the summer (table 23.E-1).

Pain Treatment

Regarding lower-back pain, there are many possible treatments available. In a recent study, 492 patients complaining of lower-back pain were questioned as to the methods of treatment they had tried and the efficacy of each. The study found that among those who tried treatment by yoga instructors, 96 percent of the cases had moderate to long-term relief from symptoms, compared to 65 percent who reported the same level of relief when they were treated by physical therapists, 28 percent who were treated by chiropractors, 10 percent who were treated by massage therapists, and only 4 percent who were treated by neurologists [455]. Qualitatively similar results also have been reported by Williams et al. [897, 897a], in regard to Iyengar *yogasana* therapy. The clear superiority of yoga and physical therapy in regard to lower-back pain is likely due to their emphasis on exercises that strengthen the muscles of the back and the supporting muscles of the abdomen; the more fit you are in terms of yogic conditioning, the less likely you are to suffer from lower-back pain.

It recently has been shown that enduring years of lower-back pain works to shrink two key areas in the brain, the thalamus and the prefrontal cortex, which are known to be involved in the perception of pain (Chapter 4, page 85). This pain-induced shrinkage is about ten times larger than that which occurs naturally through aging.

Axial Appendages to the Spine

Section 9.A: The Skull

Structure

The skull and pelvis ideally are centered on the axis of the spinal column and so are known as axial appendages of the spine. As shown in figure 9.A-1, the skull can be considered as both a neurocranium (consisting of all structural elements above the plane connecting the occiput and the upper palate) and a visceral cranium (consisting of all structural elements, such as the jaw, eye sockets, and nasal socket, etc., below that plane). The skull is composed of many more bones than one might guess at first; i.e., eight in the neurocranium and fourteen in the visceral cranium. Surprisingly, seven bones in the fetus must come together in the adult to form the eye socket [632], just as collections of individual bones fuse in the adult to form the hip sockets, wrist bones, etc.[1]

Each of the six lobes of the brain (figure 2.B-2) is protected by a bony plate of the skull which is named for the cranial lobe below it: i.e., occipital, parietal, temporal, and frontal, figure 9.A-1. Linked by appropriate fibrous sutures acting much like joints, these plates bring elasticity to the skull, making it a shock absorber, much like the arches of the feet (figure 10.B-8) and the vertebral discs of the spine (figure 8.A-2a). Flexibility of the sutures of the skull is discussed in Subsection 4.E, page 107.

Many of the muscles in the head, upon and within the skull, are energized by the cranial nerves (Section 2.C, page 24), often as parts of the autonomic nervous system (Section 5.A, page 157).

The Mandible

The lower jaw (the mandible) is held to the skull by synovial-temporomandibular joints of the ball-and-socket type (figure 9.A-1), the joint

---

[1] It is odd that as one progresses along the evolutionary path from the lower animals to humans, the numbers of bones in the skull decrease. For example, fish and reptiles have approximately one hundred and seventy bones in the skull, primitive mammals have approximately forty, and humans have only twenty-two bones. Similarly, humans have only four muscles with which to move the ears, whereas the horse has thirteen! This can be rationalized in the following way: humans depend upon the movement of the muscles of the face in order to register emotion, but the muscles activating the ears are not among these. In contrast,

the horse expresses emotion almost totally through movement of its ears, and so it has a large number of such muscles. Think of it as finesse of muscle motion requiring a large number of motor units in the case of the horse, but many fewer in the case of humans (Sections 4.C, page 91, and 11.A, page 369). Though humans have only four muscles dedicated to moving the ears, they have twenty-nine more facial-muscle pairs for expressing emotions, and this is more than any other animal [61a]! A human smile requires the subconscious activation of eight muscles, whereas a frown requires the activation of up to twenty muscles. The brain centers involved in the reading of human facial expressions are discussed further in Section 5.F, page 195.

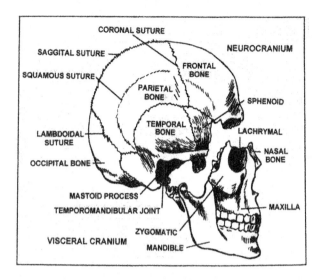

Figure 9.A-1. The various bones of the neurocranium (above) and the visceral cranium (below), shown with exaggerated separation, but not meant to imply a joint. The neurocranium is comprised of the skull and the sutures that define the various cranial lobes. The cranial topography follows the sulci and gyri of the cortex (figure 2.B-2), except that the frontal and occipital bones of the skull are not separated left-to-right in distinction to the corresponding left and right frontal and occipital lobes of the cerebrum.

coming just below the ear on each side of the skull. This joint is closed by contraction of the masseter muscles, which have their origin on the neurocranium and their insertion on the mandible. The temporomandibular joint is the most frequently used joint in the body, estimated to open and close 2,000–3,000 times a day. As such an extensively used joint has a very poor congruence between the condyle of the mandible and the fossa of the skull into which it fits, a donut-shaped meniscus forms between condyle and fossa to reduce the rubbing between the bony parts involved in this joint.

Because gravity encourages the jaw to hang down, contraction of the masseter muscles is necessary to keep the lips pursed and the mouth closed. Excessive tension in the masseters of the jaw and tension in the pelvic floor often are the result of clutching the floor with the toes when

in the standing postures.[2] Long-term spasms of the masseter muscles, known as temporomandibular joint (TMJ) syndrome, are painful, with symptoms that may extend as far as the neck and shoulders.

There are a large number of lymph nodes lying in the area surrounding the ears, just external to the sternocleidomastoid muscles, just below the mandible, and above the clavicles. The various endocrine glands within the head and neck are discussed in Section 6.A, and the excretory glands in Chapter 20, page 721.

The Sinuses

Several cavities called sinuses exist within the skull. These sinuses are lined with mucus membranes, the secretions of which normally drain into the nasal cavities. However, if a sinus cavity is swollen due to infection or to an allergic reaction, it may fill but be unable to release the pressure by draining, thus setting the stage for sinusitis and a sinus headache, (Subsection 4.E, page 116). Such drainage can be initiated by relaxing *yogasana* inversions, such as *sarvangasana*, and by the humming sound produced when one chants "*Om*" in a seated position [44a]. Actually, while in *sarvangasana*, the compression in the neck strongly inhibits drainage from the sinuses, however, once out of the posture, drainage can be rapid and complete. The structures of the nose and throat are discussed more fully in Section 15.A, page 600, and Subsection 19.A, page 705.

Maintaining a Level Head

Note that the center of gravity of the head in *tadasana* is forward of the atlas, (figure 9.A-2a), so that if the muscles of the neck are passive and soft, the head will naturally fall forward when standing. However, were this to happen, the stretch

_____

2   This unexpected connection between the action of the toes and the jaw follows from consideration of Myers's anatomy train called the "deep front line," this being a muscular train running from the flexors of the toes in the soles of the foot, through the inner aspects of the legs, and up the anterior spine, terminating at the temporomandibular joint [442, 603].

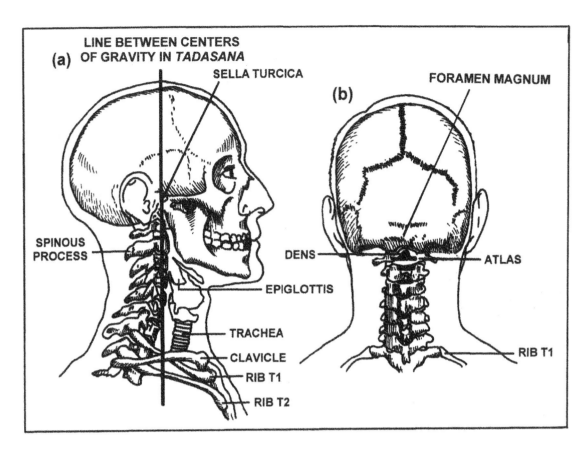

Figure 9.A-2. (a) Relative positions of the center of gravity of the head (the sella turcica) and the support of the head on the vertebral fulcrum, C1, in *tadasana*. The vertical line joins the centers of gravity of head and Earth. (b) Detail of the atlanto-occipital joint as seen from the back of the head and neck.

reflex (Section 11.B, page 429) activates the extensor muscles at the back of the neck (the posterior rectus capitis muscles), so as to return the head to an erect position. The muscle spindles in these muscles are just one set of several sensors that work to sense head imbalance (Section V.C, page 886); however, they are not to be used muscularly for correcting front-to-back balancing or falling in *sirsasana*, as this is the job of the arms and shoulders.

It appears that whenever we are concentrating mentally, there is a strong tendency to keep the head immobile, holding it rigidly, as if we are afraid to allow the retinal streaming (Subsection V.C, page 889) to interfere with the internal image of our thoughts. If this rigidity develops while we are concentrating on performing a standing *yogasana*, it can travel through the torso into the legs and so impede the necessary actions in those distant regions. On the other hand, this type of mental concentration and body immobility is advantageous for the beginning student when learning how to balance (Subsection V.B, page 884).

The Tongue

The tongue within the mouth is controlled by two sets of muscles: a) an external group of three glossus muscles that move the tongue while chewing or swallowing, and b) a set of muscles internal to the tongue that control its shape. As it is an organ of constant volume, these muscles change its shape by increasing certain dimensions while decreasing others.

The Neck

Muscles in the neck are key elements in regard to placement of the cervical vertebrae and the orientation of the head in space; this is discussed in Subsection V.C, page 887. The hyoid bone is located within the neck, just above the larynx, and functions largely to anchor the muscles of the tongue. It is also anchored to muscles that connect the skull to the lower jaw, to the sternum, and to the clavicles. If the muscles surrounding the hyoid are contracted along with the masseters, then the action is a tipping of the head forward, i.e., flexion. On swallowing, the hyoid is elevated.

Relaxing the Face

It will be difficult to relax fully in *savasana* unless the muscles of the face, neck, and scalp release. We briefly consider a few specific areas to be relaxed when in *savasana*. When fully relaxed, the student will feel the jaw's relaxation as the masseter muscles release just below the ears where the jaw is hinged. At the same time, one has a sense that the molars of the jaw are dropping away from those of the upper palate. In addition to the jaw, relaxation in *savasana* also will involve allowing the hyoid bone in the throat and the clavicles to drop toward the back of the neck.

Because we work so often in our *yogasana* practice to lift the upper part of the body up and away from the lower part of the body, there is a subconscious action in aid of the lifting in which we press the tongue against the upper palate of the mouth, as when in *parvatasana,* for example. Of course, this is a wasted effort with no real effect on the lifting and should be avoided. When the tongue is relaxed, it is short but broad and the tip rests against the inside of the front lower teeth, i.e., it does *savasana* on the floor of the mouth.

Any constriction of the airways and/or tension at the back of the throat must be released in order to relax. There should be minimum resistance to airflow through the nose, though the flow does not have to be in any way left-right symmetric (Subsection 15.E, page 627). When in a particularly relaxing *yogasana* position, the mouth can be allowed to open somewhat in order to relax the masseters, but the breath should nonetheless continue to move through the nasal passages on both inhalation and exhalation. Allow the breath to breathe itself in *savasana*.

Relaxing the eyes is especially necessary and interesting. Sympathetic tone in the external muscles of the eye acts to pull the eyeball forward and turn it in toward the nose through the pulley action of the tendon of the superior oblique muscle at the trochlea, (figure 17.A-1a). When sympathetic excitation of the superior oblique turns parasympathetic, the rectus lengthens, and the eyeball falls back into the eye socket and turns more toward the outer corners of the eyes (Subsection 17.A, page 657).

As discussed in Box 18.A-1, page 694, the relaxation of the small muscles of the middle ear can be readily demonstrated by using a radio; when these muscles relax, the perceived volume of a sound will rise significantly, and the student in that state becomes vulnerable to being shocked by the unexpected loudness of a soft sound.

On the face and neck, the wrinkle lines are perpendicular to the directions of the underlying muscles, so that the horizontal furrows caused by stress in the muscles of the forehead reflect high muscle tone in the frontal belly of the epicranius muscles, which run vertically. These muscles are best relaxed by vertical stroking rather than horizontal stroking. Muscles of the scalp also should be released when relaxing the upper body.

Section 9.B: The Pelvis

Structure

As the pelvis must not only support the weight of the body but also allow motion in all directions, its job is a difficult one. As shown in figure 8.B-7, the adult pelvis consists of two bony parts and five moveable joints. The bones of the pelvis are the two symmetric ilium bones, which are joined to one another to form a fibrous joint anteriorly at the pubic symphysis, to the spinal column through the left and right sides of the sacral plate at the base of the spine, and to each of the legs via the hip joints. The bony plate of the coccyx is joined to the base of the sacral plate.

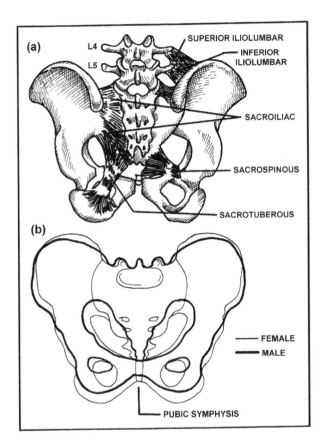

Figure 9.B-1. (a) The various ligaments of the pelvis, binding the sacrum to the ilium, as seen in a posterior view [428]. Not all of the ligaments on the left and right sides of the pelvis are shown, in order to simplify the picture. (b) Anterior view of the pelvis comparing the typical shapes in adult males (heavy line) and adult females (light line).

Gender Differences

Being essentially a bowl (the word "pelvis" stems from the Latin word for basin), the pelvis has a floor that is a web of muscles designed to control various functions; in an upright creature such as man, the pelvis is shaped to carry the organs of digestion, elimination, and reproduction. However, the pelvis in the adult male and female is noticeably different [863]. In males, the pelvis is somewhat lighter, with thinner bones, whereas in the female, it stands taller, is deeper, and has a rounder pelvic outlet to accommodate childbirth (figure 9.B-1b). The joints of the pelvis are not only important in the birthing process, but they

also are important in transmitting the forces of the leg bones to the upper body. Other differences worth noting are that in the female pelvis, there are only two segments of the sacrum bound by ligaments to the ilium bones, whereas for men, the number of ligaments is three, and the sacrum is wider and shorter in women [492]. Moreover, the ischial tuberosities are turned outward in females and inward in males, and the acetabulum in females is relatively small compared to that in males [863].

In adult women, during the latter part of the menstrual cycle, during menopause, and during pregnancy, the pubic symphysis and the sacroiliac joints are relatively destabilized by hormones and so assume larger than normal ranges of motion. Women in general are more flexible in the pelvic area, whether pregnant or not [7]; however, childbirth can misalign their sacroiliac joints [492].

Sacroiliac Joint

Just opposite the joint forming the pubic symphysis (figure 8.B-7), the ilium bones form a wedge-shaped opening in the posterior of the pelvis; the sacral plate, being a wedge-shaped fusion of five spinal vertebrae, just fits into this space, forming a sacroiliac joint at each side. The sacroiliac joints are angled at +/-20° from the vertical and are largely synovial joints supported by ligaments, in contrast to the pubic symphysis, which is a fibrous joint.

In infants, the mating surfaces of the sacroiliac joint are smooth and allow considerable motion; however, as we age, the surfaces become remodeled so as to have many interlocking hills and valleys, which strongly restrict the joint's motion. In old age, the sacroiliac joint actually may become fused and totally immobile. The sacroiliac joint acts as a shock absorber between foot and brain, and then should this joint degenerate, the shock-absorbing task would fall more heavily on the intervertebral joints, overloading them and encouraging their premature degeneration in turn.

The sacrum itself is curved convexly, as viewed from the back, just opposite to the curvature of the lumbar spine. Though the sacroiliac joint is spanned by ligaments, (figure 9.B-1a), there are only two muscles that span the joint: the piriformis (figure 9.B-2c) and the gluteus maximus [295]. Just below the sacrum lies the coccyx, another plate of fused vertebrae; however, it is joined only to the sacrum and not to the pelvis proper [428]. In ancestral animals, the coccyx was responsible for wagging the tail, using the muscle joining it to the ischium. The joint between the coccyx and the sacrum can undergo flexion and extension only, and then only during defecation or childbirth [428].

The pelvis is supported from below by the femur bones of the upper legs, the connection being made at the acetabulum of the hip joint (figure 8.B-7). In the newborn, the ilium and the ischium, are separate bones that later fuse to form the acetabulum, once the legs begin to bear weight [582]; whereas the vertebrae of the sacrum maintain their individuality up to about age twenty-five years, at which time they too fuse into a single plate [492].

Sacroiliac Stability

As the sacrum fits nicely into the crevice provided by the ilium bones and is held in place by relatively few ligaments, (figure 9.B-1a), it is more tightly held when the load on it from above is increased. This means that the sacroiliac joint is most stable when one is standing or sitting and is much less so when lying down. For students who are weak in the sacroiliac joint, when twisting in a seated position, as in *maricyasana III*, the pelvis should be rotated in the same direction as the rib cage (a conrotatory motion; see, figure 8.B-8c) in order to minimize twisting within the sacroiliac joint. Lying twists in which the sacroiliac joint is not loaded are not recommended for a student having a weak, highly mobile sacroiliac joint, as evidenced by either previous experiences or frequent general discomfort in that area.

Sitting

We sit most comfortably when the femur bones make an angle of 125–135° with the vertical. Thus, in *yogasana*, we often sit cross-legged (*muktasana*) on blankets, so that the knees of the

bent legs are **below** the hip sockets, especially so in meditative seated postures. In these positions, the femurs fall away from the hip sockets, and the hip joints are thereby opened without effort [497]. The posture is completed by rotating the pelvis so as to lift and press the top of the sacrum forward, making the lumbar decidedly more lordotic, but not excessively so.

The ischial tuberosity is the bony prominence in each of the buttocks that bears the weight of the body when seated. Just how one sits on the ischial tuberosities is of great importance to the student of *yogasana*, for if one sits on the forward edge in *dandasana*, for example, then the pelvis is tipped so that the lumbar spine is pressed forward somewhat and the proper spinal alignment results, whereas if one sits on the back edge, it is very difficult to pull the lumbar spine into alignment, especially so in related seated postures, such as *krounchasana* or *paripurna navasana*, in which one or both legs are lifted. In contrast to this, one does sit on the back edge of the ischial tuberosity when in *ardha navasana*. The hamstrings, adductor magnus, and sacrotuberous ligaments all are attached to the ischial tuberosities.

There are bursae just beneath the hamstring tendons attaching to the pelvis; inflammation of these bursae leads to ischial bursitis, which makes sitting very painful, but which is relieved by performing crossed-leg, sitting variations of *maricyasana III*.

Muscles of the Lumbar Area

Three important bilateral muscles in the lumbar area are the iliacus, the psoas, and the piriformis. As can be seen in figure 9.B-2a, the iliacus has its origin on the internal surface of the ilium at the back of the pelvis, and has its insertion on the inner upper surface of the lesser trochanter. Depending upon which end of the iliacus is fixed, contraction leads either to flexion of the hip or to the rolling of the iliac crests in the forward-downward direction.

The psoas shares the tendon attachment of the iliacus to the lesser trochanter of the femur; however, its origin is on the anterior aspects of the L1–L5 vertebrae (figure 9.B-2b). It differs in

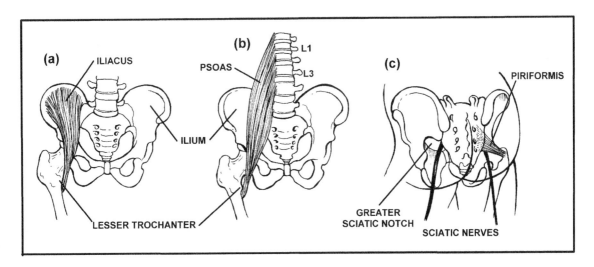

Figure 9.B-2. The origins and insertions of (**a**) the iliacus muscle, as seen anteriorly; (**b**) the psoas muscle, as seen anteriorly; and (**c**) the piriformis muscle, as seen obliquely from the posterior.

its action from that of the iliacus in that with the femur fixed, its action is to pull the lumbar vertebrae into lordosis.

The piriformis muscle operates diagonally in the pelvis, originating on the anterior surface of the sacrum and passing over the sacroiliac joints and the greater sciatic notch, to insert on the greater trochanter of the femur (figure 9.B-2c). Tightness of this muscle impacts negatively on the sciatic nerve passing through the greater sciatic notch, and can readily lead to the pain of sciatica.

The Pubic Symphysis

The pubic symphysis is a joint within the pelvic girdle, lying opposite the sacroiliac and consisting of the two pubic tubercles of the ilium bones separated by a thick, fibrocartilaginous pad; it is relatively immobile, and this rigidity helps to stabilize the sacroiliac joint in turn. However, it occasionally happens that in the course of childbirth, the pubic symphysis separates, allowing the sacrum to move forward. In general, motion around the sacroiliac joints and the pubic symphysis is minimal at best, provided the symphysis joint retains its integrity.

Front-to-back motion in the pelvis is coupled with side-to-side motion, so that when the top of the sacral plate moves backward (as in *bakasana,*

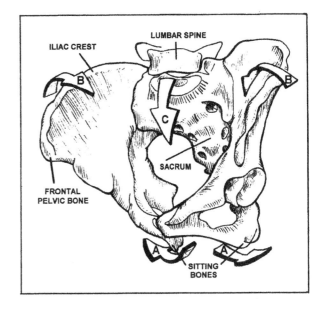

Figure 9.B-3. Anterior view of the pelvis, showing how an inward (medial) rotation of the off-axis anterior femurs (see figure 10.B-1b) increases the separation between the sitting bones (**A**), leading to a decreased separation of the iliac crests (**B**) and a forward thrust of the top of the sacrum (**C**), as when performing *adho mukha svanasana* [428]. These motions of the pelvis are discussed further in Subsection 10.B, page 341.

for example), the two frontal pelvic rims move toward one another, whereas the two ischial tuberosities (the sitting bones) move laterally away from one another (figure 9.B-3). Because these actions are reciprocal, if one rolls the anterior upper thighs outward, as when doing *uttana padasana* [388] with ankles crossed and the outer edges of the feet pressing against one another (Subsection 10.A, page 337), the sitting bones move toward one another, and the top of the sacrum is pulled up toward the navel as the lumbar spine becomes lordotic.

Given that the heads of the femur bones are firmly set into the hip joints, (figure 8.B-7), and that several strong muscles in the pelvic area are attached to the femurs at several points, (figure 9.B-2), it is clear that motion of the pelvis is strongly dependent on leg action (Subsection 10.B, page 341). Thus, lateral opening and closing of the pelvis is dictated by rotation of the legs, and forward-backward tipping of the pelvis is controlled by pressing the thighs backward or forward, respectively. Similarly, with the femur fixed, the muscles of the lumbar area are able to directly move the pelvis and the lumbar spine. Among the more difficult *yogasanas* to perform are those that have one leg positioned so as to encourage the pelvis to tip in one direction, and the other leg positioned so as to encourage it to tip in the opposite direction, e.g., *eka pada urdhva dhanurasana* or *hanumanasana*, in each of which, one leg is encouraged to perform a backbend and the other is encouraged to perform a forward bend.

The Pelvic Seesaw

One can think of the lower spine and the upper legs as forming a seesaw, with the pelvis as the fulcrum around which the others turn. When standing, for example, if the upper thighs are pressed backward, the lumbar is pushed forward, and the spine becomes lordotic (figure 9.B-4a), whereas if the lumbar spine is pressed backward and flattened, then the pelvis rotates, and the upper thighs are pushed forward (figure 9.B-4b). As applied to *tadasana*, the posture requires that there be a co-contraction, so that the posterior rim of the pelvis is raised by contraction of the psoas

and the quadratus lumborum and, **at the same time**, the ischial tuberosities are pulled downward toward the heels by contraction of the gluteus maximus, while the abdomen is pulled up and back onto the spine (figure 9.B-4c). Viewed from the perspective of the internal anchor (Subsection 11.F, page 468), the contraction of the gluteus serves as an anchor against which the contraction of the psoas and quadratus lumborum work (and vice versa!) in order to change the pelvic orientation in *tadasana*.

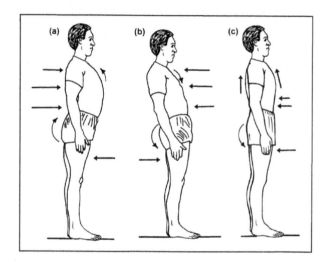

Figure 9.B-4. (a) When the front thighs are pressed backward (and rolled inward) by psoas and quadratus lumborum contraction in *tadasana*, the back rim of the pelvis is lifted upward, and the lumbar spine is pressed forward as it becomes lordotic. (b) If, instead, the thighs are pressed forward in *tadasana* by contraction of the gluteus maximus, the centers of the buttocks descend and the lumbar region is flattened as it is pressed backward. (c) Proper alignment of the pelvis and spine in *tadasana* requires the simultaneous application of the actions of both (a) and (b), i.e., co-contraction of the psoas, quadratus lumborum, and the gluteus muscles, with stabilization of the legs by co-contraction of the quadriceps and hamstrings.

The action shown in figure 9.B-4c, which acts to lengthen and flatten the lumbar curve, is appropriate to all back-bending postures, (Section 7.F, page 252, and Subsection 8.B, page 292).

If, instead, the student comes to *supta baddha konasana* with the anterior thighs rolled laterally, the psoas is stretched and tends to lift the lumbar spine off the floor, so that descending the knees laterally lifts the lumbar spine and vice versa. This seesaw action is unavoidable for the beginner unless a deliberate effort is made to pull the navel down onto the spine by gluteal contraction. Correspondingly, when in *urdhva dhanurasana,* the elevation of the navel toward the ceiling is enhanced by lateral rotation of the front thighs, dropping them toward the floor. However, this seesaw action must be resisted by rolling the feet medially instead and contracting the hamstrings so as to reduce the lumbar curvature by pulling the ischial tuberosities toward the knees.

The pelvic seesaw can be activated in *supta padangusthasana* in the following way. Lie on a sticky mat so that when the legs are straightened along the floor, the feet press against the wall, wedging the body between the wall and the shoulders on the mat. Lift one leg into the vertical position, and with that, the back of the knee and the buttock crease on the other leg will tend to lift from the floor in sympathy with the tensile stress on the hamstrings of the vertical leg. At this point, if the foot against the wall tries to slide up the wall while pinned to the wall, the tendency in the pelvis will be to seesaw or rotate so that the buttock crease and the upper thigh of the horizontal leg are pressed toward the floor. This action brings all parts of the horizontal leg closer to the floor.

Upper and Lower Hinges

Because the pelvis has joints both to the bone above it (the sacrum) and to bones below it (the femurs), it can be bent at either or both of these places; i.e., at the lumbar spine and/or at the hip joints, respectively (figure 9.B-5). Calling these two places for possible mid-body motion "the upper hinge" and "the lower hinge," respectively, the tendency in beginners is to bend forward, sideways, or backward more at the upper hinge; what has to be learned in *yogasana* practice is how to bend more at the lower hinge and less at the

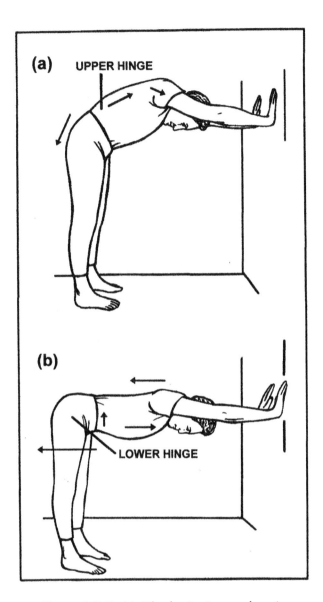

Figure 9.B-5. (a) The beginning student in *ardha uttanasana* bends the torso at the upper hinge and so rounds the back body, as the relationship between pelvis and lumbar spine is altered while collapsing the chest. (b) The more experienced student in *ardha uttanasana* instead bends at the lower hinge, keeping the back relatively straight and the chest open and lifted, as in *tadasana,* the standard posture.

upper. That is to say, the upper hinge is to be kept open, with the spine straight, whereas the lower hinge is closed at the hip joint(s), bending either forward, sideways, or backward as the posture demands. It is an open question as to whether the lower hinge should be involved or not in spinal twisting (Subsection 8.B, page 294). The answer depends upon the integrity of the ligaments binding the sacroiliac joint (figure 9.B-1a) in the student.

Speaking in a muscular sense, forward bending at the upper hinge (as in Figure 9.B-5a) is the result of contraction of the rectus abdominis muscles in the front body; contraction of these muscles pulls the lowest ribs toward the iliac crests of the pelvis and so makes the front body short and changes the lumbar curvature to convex. All postures in which the rectus abdominis is contracted more or less will result in a lower-body posture more or less like that shown in figure 9.B-5a. In contrast, if the rectus is kept long and relaxed, then flexion at the hip joints follows from contraction of the psoas muscles instead, these being joined to the lower vertebrae of the lumbar spine at one end, and to the lesser trochanters at the other (Subsection 9.B, page 317).[3] When the psoas is contracted, it pulls the lumbar spine forward and down toward the thighs, so as to accentuate the concave lumbar curvature. At the same time, the psoas action rotates the front thighs medially, the end result being a posture as in figure 9.B-5b. These actions of the psoas are assisted by co-contraction with the iliacus muscles. If the psoas is contracted on only one side, then the result is a lower-hinge lateral bend.

The beginner's tendency when backbending is to overly arch the lumbar spine, so as to send the lumbar spine into extreme lordosis while pressing the navel toward the ceiling. This is an upper-hinge action, whereas the preferred lower-hinge action is to keep the lumbar spine long by pulling the centers of the buttocks toward the knees via the gluteus maximus. In this way, one bends (in extension) around the hip joints (figure 9.B-4b), so that it is the pubic symphysis

rather than the navel that is pressed up toward the ceiling.

Note that the rotation of figure 9.B-5b around an axis perpendicular to the page results in figures showing the proper lower-hinge bending action for postures such as *navasana, adho mukha svanasana, dandasana* in *adho mukha vrksasana* (half handstand), *dandasana,* and *urdhva prasarita padasana;* bending at the lower hinge in all of these postures is the yogic ideal. The point of view that bending at the lower hinge is preferable to bending at the upper hinge in the *yogasanas* is pointed out specifically in the excellent review of lower-back therapy by Williams et al. [897, 897a].

Tadasana, the Standard Posture

An alternate way to think about bending at the lower hinge is to consider the situation first in *tadasana,* (figure 9.B-4c), which will be taken as the standard for alignment. In this case of the standard, the chest is lifted forward and upward; the spine has its normal alternating curvatures; the navel is pulled up against the lumbar spine; the psoas, gluteus maximus, quadriceps, and hamstrings are co-contracted; and the anterior thighs roll medially and are pressed back. This action results in a spine in which the length is maximal, the curvature is minimal, the horizontal axis of the pelvis and the axis of the spine are mutually perpendicular, the axes of the shoulders and the pelvis are parallel, and the distance between the lowest ribs and the iliac crests on the two sides are equal and maximal. In all other *yogasana* postures, one strives to maintain as many symmetry elements of the standard posture as is possible given whatever asymmetry is inherent in the posture (Section III.B, page 847). Thus, virtually all of these elements are preserved in *ardha uttanasana* as performed in figure 9.B-5b, when bending at the lower hinge; whereas fewer of these elements are preserved when bending at the upper hinge, as in figure 9.B-5a. The use of *tadasana* as a standard for *yogasana* alignment and muscle action is discussed further in Section III.B, page 845.

---

3   If the legs are anchored, then during the contraction of the psoas, the end of the psoas connected to the trochanter becomes the muscle's origin and the end connected to the lumbar becomes the insertion. If, instead, the lumbar spine is anchored, then the designations of the psoas's origin and insertion given above are reversed.

Consequences of Bending at the Two Hinges

Several negative consequences of bending at the upper hinge readily come to mind. First, when working with the lumbar spine in the configuration of figure 9.B-5a, the erector spinae (figure 8.A-4b) may be overstretched, so that there is a low overlap of the myofibrils in their sarcomeres (figures 11.A-10 and 11.A-11). When in this weakened condition and trying to lift the upper body as when recovering from *uttanasana,* for example, the weak erector spinae can be more easily injured. Similarly, even if the erector spinae are not damaged when in the posture shown in figure 9.B-5a, the possibility nonetheless exists that bending only at the upper hinge while loaded can result in herniation of a lumbar disc in the direction of the spinal cord, as shown in figure 8.A-6e. Finally, if one bends at the upper hinge in the forward bends, the rectus abdominis muscles are unnecessarily contracted and the erector spinae are fully stretched, whereas if the forward bend is performed with the lower hinge, the stress is relieved in the lumbar spine and abdomen but instead is transferred to the hamstrings, which are better able to handle the stretch than are the erector spinae.

If one is bending at the upper hinge while backbending, the result is a severe compression of the lumbar vertebrae, which often is suffi-ciently painful to keep the student from going any deeper in the posture. On the other hand, if the backbending is performed at the lower hinge, there is still stress in the posture, but rather than being a painful compression of the lumbar vertebrae, it becomes a strong stretch of the quadriceps muscles, a problem that readily can be solved by practice of the appropriate quadriceps stretches (Section 7.F, page 252).

Lateral bending also can be performed at either the upper or the lower hinges. When bending to the side in *parivrtta janu sirsasana,* for example, if the bending is performed at the upper hinge, the consequence is that the ribs on that side move toward the iliac crest on that side, and the extent of bending is terminated when the lowest ribs and the iliac crest collide. If, instead, the bending is performed at the lower hinge, so that the distance from the lowest ribs to the respective iliac crest on that side is kept constant, then the ribs on the bending side move up and over the iliac crest and come to rest on the thigh, forward of the iliac crest (Section 7.F, page 252). Bending at the lower hinge also avoids any rib-on-rib contact that otherwise impedes bending at the upper hinge.

None of the problems noted here for upper-hinge forward, backward, or lateral bending arise when the bending is performed at the lower hinge so as to preserve the largest number of the symmetry elements of *tadasana.*

The Spinal Appendages 10

Chapter 9 presented the skeletal structures of the spine and the axial attachments thereto, the skull and the pelvis. This chapter briefly outlines the anatomies and mechanics of the spinal appendages, i.e., the arms and legs. The rib cage is considered in Subsection 15.A, page 606.

Section 10.A: The Arms, Shoulders, and Scapulae

Structure of the Shoulder, Chest, and Back

Skeletal Anatomy

The shoulder is the most flexible and most mobile of the joints in the body, and as a corollary to this, it is also the least stable. Because the shoulder and arm are adapted for manipulation rather than locomotion (in contrast to the situation in the leg), and because the arms generally are not weight bearing, they are not attached as directly to the spinal column as are the legs. Specifically, the shoulder girdle is formed from three bones—the scapula, the clavicle, and the humerus—and their associated muscles, tendons, and ligaments (figure 10.A-1). The head of the humerus, the bone of the upper arm, inserts into the cavity formed by the clavicle and the acromion portion of the scapula. Taken together, these bones form the glenoid fossa, otherwise known as the socket of the shoulder joint. When the glenoid fossa is taken together with the humerus of the upper arm, the primary joint of the shoulder, the glenohumeral joint is formed. Because the ends of the bones within this joint so poorly conform to one another in their shapes, all of its motions except that of axial rotation involve combinations of rocking and gliding of the various bones, just as within the knee joint.

The three bones of the glenohumeral joint (the humerus, the scapula, and the clavicle) are lashed together by an array of muscles and ligaments to give strength and a wide range of motion to the shoulder. However, the shallow depth of the glenoid fossa not only confers high mobility but also low stability in regard to dislocation. In contrast, the hip joint is the most stable joint in the body with respect to dislocation; however, in compensation, the arm and shoulder are capable of motions that are totally impossible for the leg and hip.

Due to the large number of components in the shoulder girdle, by which the spine, neck, shoulder, and arm are interconnected, the shoulder is a very complex and easily injured part of the body. As is the case with the knee, the shoulder joint is further destabilized if stretching extends to the inelastic ligaments binding it together. In order to accommodate the large range of motion in the shoulder, the ligaments about this joint are unusually loose, so that the bones within can be separated by 2–3 centimeters (one inch) when relaxed. The individual bones and their contributions to forming the glenoid fossa are described below.

The Clavicle

The clavicle, or collarbone, is connected at its medial end to the manubrium of the sternum;

323

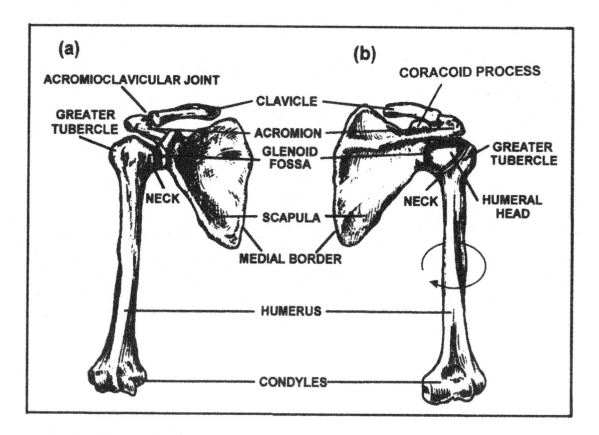

Figure 10.A-1. The clavicle, acromion, and the coracoid process of the scapula are bound together so as to form a shallow cavity (the glenoid fossa), into which the head of the humerus can fit, forming the glenohumeral shoulder joint. The anterior (**a**) and posterior views (**b**) of the right shoulder are shown. Note in drawing (**b**) how the scapula can be pressed forward onto the rib cage by the lateral rotation (arrow) of the humerus.

its lateral end is involved in forming the shoulder joint (figures 10.A-1 and 15.A-3c). The clavicle ("little key," as it keys the shoulder blade to the sternum) is *S* curved in two directions and is the first to begin ossification in the fetus. Moreover, it also is the last bone in the body to be completely ossified, and is the bone most often broken. The lateral end of the clavicle is joined to the scapula at the scapular acromion, and this joint allows further movement of the shoulder complex, once the joint at the sternum has moved maximally through its range of motion. This connection of the clavicle to the glenohumeral joint is the only one connecting the arms directly to the central axis of the body.

In the glenohumeral skeletal complex, the clavicle rotates around the sternum, the scapula rotates around the clavicle, and the humerus rotates around the scapula, thus forming three joints, all interactive and mutually dependent. Movement of the clavicle will always move the scapula, and movement of the scapula will often result in movement of the humerus, and vice versa.

The sternoclavicular joint between the sternum and the clavicle (figure 15.A-3c) is a saddle joint and so allows motion of the clavicle at the shoulder end of 3 centimeters (one inch) in the downward, forward, and backward directions and of up to 10 centimeters (four inches) in the upward direction; rotation around the clavicle axis is possible as well, as when one lifts the rib cage through the use of the scapulae (Subsection 10.A, page 328). The sternoclavicular joint has a meniscal padding for reasons of lubrication and cushioning. The plane of the scapula and the line of the clavicle on the same side form an angle of 60°.

The Scapulae

Each of the scapulae lies close to the rib cage, but rather than articulating with it, each floats on the back ribs of the thoracic spine (figures 7.A-1**b** and 15.A-3**d**), suspended in a web of muscles, tendons, and ligaments; sixteen different muscles are attached to each of the scapulae. The rib cage and the scapulae are separated by several layers of fatty tissue known as glide planes, which serve to lubricate the motion of the scapulae upon the posterior surfaces of the ribs. Interestingly, the strongest force holding the scapulae onto the rib cage is said to be atmospheric pressure, the same force holding the femoral head within the acetabulum of the hip joint (but apparently insignificant in holding the humeral head in the glenoid fossa).

The most important of the connections in the shoulder is the joint between the humeral head and the upper, outer edge of the scapula (figure 10.A-1) [429, 788, 834]; the particular part of the scapula involved in this joint is called the acromion process. The joint between the humerus and the scapula leads to the well-known relationships between arm and shoulder blade actions, so important in the *yogasanas*. (See Subsection 10.A, page 328.)

Using various muscles bound at one end to the scapula and at the other end to either the rib cage or the humerus, the scapula can be elevated (+6 centimeters or 2.4 inches, raised), depressed (-6 centimeters or -2.4 inches, lowered), pulled toward (7.5 centimeters or 3 inches, adduction), or away from the spine (7.5 centimeters or 3 inches, abduction), and the lower tip of the scapula (the inferior angle) can be rotated from medial to lateral through a 60° range [101, 288].[1] The upper

---

1   As is the case with the measurements of range of motion of the spinal column (Subsection 8.B, page 281), those reported in the anatomic literature for the scapulae apply to an average body and are most likely exceeded by far by practicing students of *yogasana*. On the other hand, note that because the scapulae are firmly bound to the humeral heads, the ranges of translational motion given above for the scapulae are more appropriately assigned as those for the shoulder joints rather than for the shoulder blades. That is to

parts of the trapezius muscles (figure 11.A-2) often are chronically tense, resulting in the scapulae and shoulders being lifted upward, toward the ears. This tendency should be countered in all of the *yogasanas* by depressing the scapulae, using the lower portions of the trapezius muscles.

The Humerus

Because the head of the humerus has a surface area approximately three times larger than that of the glenoid fossa, into which it is to be fit (figure 10.A-1**a**), the joint is a shallow one, with a wide range of motion in several directions. As is the case with the other long bones, the epiphyses of the humerus are large and expanded in order to decrease the compressive stress at the ends of the bones, as when supporting weight in *adho mukha vrksasana, purvottanasana,* etc. In spite of the shallow nature of the shoulder joint, there is a point in the circumduction of the arm where the rim of the glenoid cavity interferes with the humeral neck so that the humerus has to be rotated about its long axis in order to relieve the bone-on-bone contact (Section 7.F, page 252), just as with the femoral head in the acetabulum of the pelvis (figure10.B-2**e**).

The Rotator Cuff

The shoulder joint is held together by the deep muscles that surround it, rather than by the shape of the bones involved or their ligaments. The four major muscles that hold the humeral head in the shoulder socket are known collectively as the rotator cuff. This muscular cuff connecting the scapula to the humerus consists of (1) the supraspinatus, (2) the infraspinatus, (3) the teres minor, and (4) the subscapularis muscles (figure 10.A-2**b**), surrounding the joint almost completely; the first three of these are bound to the greater tubercle of the humerus. The muscles of the rotator cuff function essentially as postural muscles of the shoulder, for they are on constant

---

say, when the scapula moves x centimeters in a certain direction, the humeral head also must move x centimeters in that direction, as the two are bound to one another.

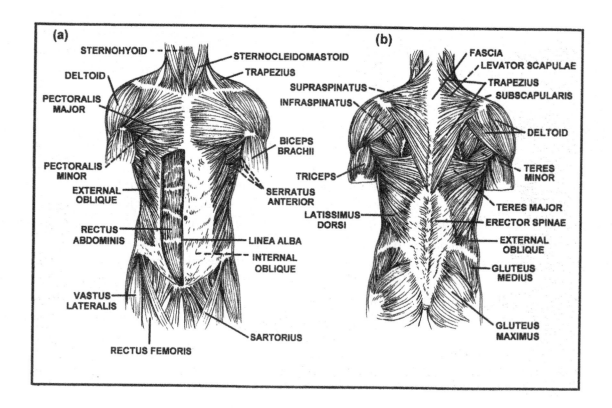

Figure 10.A-2. Details of the muscles of the upper body, (a) with those muscles of the front body tagged with full lines being superficial and those tagged with dashed lines being deeper lying; and (b) the muscles of the back body, with those tagged with full lines being superficial and those tagged with dashed lines being deeper lying.

duty, charged with the job of holding the humeral head in a balanced position within the glenoid socket. The infraspinatus and the teres minor muscles also are responsible for lateral rotation of the upper arms, whereas contraction of subscapularis leads to medial rotation of the upper arm. As the subscapularis muscle passes beneath the joint between the acromion and the clavicle, it is supplied with a bursa separating the bones from this muscle.

If the arms are lifted to the sides, lateral opening of the shoulder joint is most easily accomplished by extending the ring fingers of each hand away from one another [276]. Note that in any position of the arm and shoulder, proper action depends not only on the muscles positioning the limb but also on the antagonist muscles, which stabilize the joint and so make the muscle action precise and steady. For example, the agonist/antagonist pair biceps/triceps works in tandem to precisely to set the angle at the elbow and maintain that angle when one moves from straight-arm to bent-arm *chaturanga dandasana*. In the case of the scapulae, it is the anterior serratus and the rhomboid major muscles that serve as agonist/antagonist partners in stabilizing the position of the scapulae. It is interesting to note the similarity of the muscles of the rotator cuff for rotating and pointing the arm (figure 10.A-2b) and the external muscles of the eye for rotating and pointing the eyeball (figure 17.A-1b) [603].

Other Muscles about the Joint

Nine muscles cross the shoulder joint, seven with origins on the scapula and two with origins on the axial skeleton; all nine have insertions on the humerus. On the upper front body, the pectoralis minor lies deep below the pectoralis major, with its origin on the ribs and its insertion on the coracoid processes of the scapulae (figure 10.A-

2a). When the ribs are held stationary, the pectoralis minor pulls the scapulae down and forward and helps elevate the middle ribs during heavy breathing.

The serratus anterior muscles originate on the T1–T9 ribs, with insertion along the entire medial border of the scapulae; when the ribs are fixed, contraction of the serratus anterior will pull the scapulae to the medial side, whereas if the scapulae are fixed, the contraction works to lift the rib cage during inhalation. Co-contraction of the serratus anterior and the trapezius muscles stabilizes the scapulae. The serratus anterior raises the arm and participates in horizontal arm movements, while the infraspinatus muscle of the back body holds the head of the humerus in place and laterally rotates the upper arm. Contraction of the posterior deltoid muscle pulls the humerus posteriorly and also rotates it laterally, whereas contraction of the latissimus dorsi rotates the humerus medially.

The diamond-shaped trapezius muscle (figure 10.A-2b) has origins stretching from the occiput of the skull down to T12 on the vertebrae, and insertions on the clavicle, acromion, and scapula; excitation and relaxation of the various components of the trapezius dictate the level at which the scapulae rest on the rib cage.

Joint Injuries

The bursa between the rotator cuff tendons and the acromial process can become inflamed (bursitis), and the tendons also can tear; these are typical rotator cuff injuries. When there are rotator cuff problems, it is recommended that one should apply heat before stretching [329]. The glenohumeral joint is protected from impact by the bulk of the deltoid muscle (figure 10.A-2), which otherwise lifts the arm laterally and rotates the humerus either medially or laterally.

Looking down the humeral head into the glenoid fossa, the rotator cuff muscles are centered at 11:00 (supraspinatus), 3:00 (subscapularis), 7:00 (teres minor), and 9:00 (infraspinatus), leaving a noticeable weakness at 5:00. Consequently, subluxation of the glenohumeral joint most often involves the forward-medial motion of the humeral

head, as when the arms are in *gomukhasana* or *garudasana*. By contrast, subluxation of the hip joint is quite rare.

Upper-Arm Rotation

When the anterior thighs roll medially (inward), the action of the femoral neck is to press the pelvis back (as in *adho mukha svanasana*); whereas when the anterior thighs roll laterally (outward), the pelvis is pressed forward (as with the front leg of *trikonasana* or both legs in beginner's *urdhva dhanurasana*). One should also consider the psoas, contraction of which tends to pull the lumbar vertebrae into a more lordotic condition when the anterior thigh is rotated outward (figure 9.B-2b). It is clear from this that leg action controls the orientation of the pelvis. In a way similar to the situation in the leg and hip joint, the scapular/arm action through the glenoid fossa influences the orientation of the rib cage.

The analogy between femur-hip action in the pelvis and the humerus-glenoid fossa action of the shoulder can be expanded. When the arm first hangs down and then is raised backward approximately to shoulder height in the parasagittal plane (parallel to the medial plane) of the body,[2] motion beyond about 90° is impeded by the collision of the exposed humeral head and/or the greater tubercle with the acromion of the glenoid cavity, into which the humeral head fits (figure 10.A-1b). Further lifting of the arm is then accomplished by rotating the biceps of the upper arm laterally, so that the exposed humeral head and/or the greater tubercle is turned back and can fit under the acromion (figure 10.A-3a). If the fingers are interlaced at the small of the back and the arms then lifted toward horizontal, the interlace does not allow the humeral rotation, and it is very difficult to get the wrists up to or beyond the level of the shoulders. It is this bone-on-bone contact at 90° that is responsible for the noncircularity of the bases of the circumduction cones shown in the figure, for

---

2   This action is most easily seen in figure 10.A-1b by visualizing the lifting of the humeral condyles, keeping the humeral head in the plane of the figure, but raising the humeral shaft perpendicular to the plane.

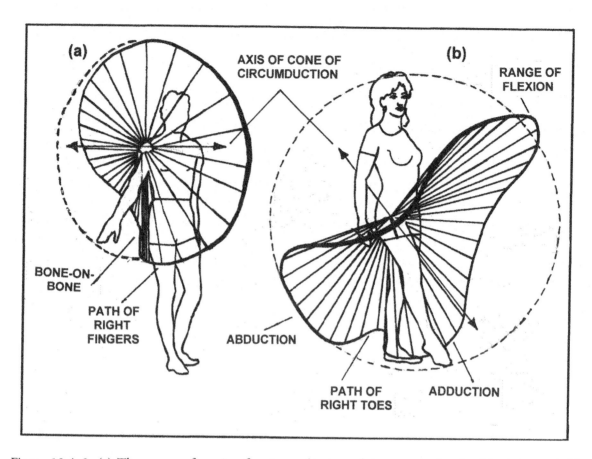

Figure 10.A-3. (a) The ranges of motion for circumduction of the arm at the shoulder joint and (b) ranges of motion for circumduction of the leg at the hip joint. In each figure, the closed loop around the limb being circumduced represents the path in space of the distal end of the limb during circumduction. Drawing adapted from [288]. Dashed lines are ball-and-socket paths.

the cones of circumduction have simple circular cross sections when the joint is simply a ball and socket without any bone-on-bone interference. This bone-on-bone situation in the shoulder joint parallels the necessary lateral rotation of the femur of the forward leg in *trikonasana* so as to avoid a similar collision of the femoral neck with the acetabulum of the hip joint (figure 10.A-3**b** and Subsection 10.B, page 339).

If the arm were a simple pole attached to the body at the shoulder, rotation of the arm would be a constant action along its entire length. In fact, the three-bone compound structure of the arm (figure 10.A-4) is such that it allows either the upper or the lower arm to be rotated either laterally or medially while the opposite end remains stationary, and it is even possible to rotate the two ends oppositely (figure 8.B-8**b**). This

disrotatory action is highly relevant to using the arms to lift and open the chest (see the following subsections).

Using the Arms to Lift and Open the Chest

Femoral and Humeral Necks

Because there is very little congruency between the head of the humerus and the glenoid cavity, the glenohumeral joint itself is only loosely packed, weak but mobile. Notice that the head of the humerus (figure 10.A-1**b**) lies on the medial side of the long axis of the humeral bone shaft, much like the head of the femur bone is offset in the leg (figure 10.B-1**a**). In the femur, the angle between the bone shaft and the neck

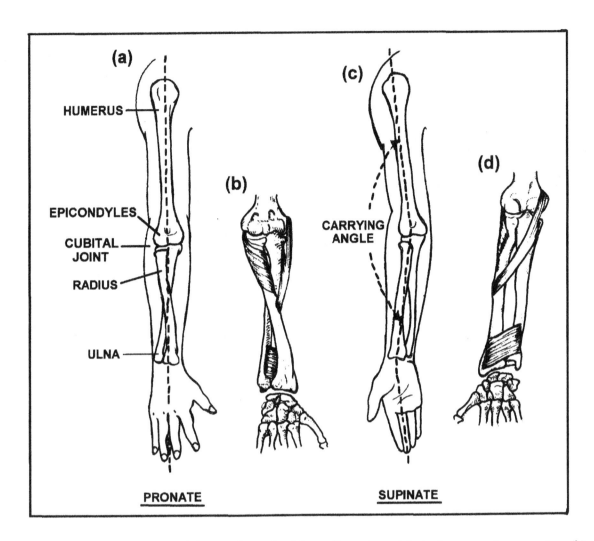

Figure 10.A-4. (**a**) The bones of the arm from shoulder to fingertips, with the lower arm in pronation; (**b**) details of the internal structure of the lower arm with hand in pronation; muscles shown are those active in crossing the radius over the ulna. (**c**) The bones of the arm from shoulder to fingertips, with the lower arm in supination; (**d**) details of the internal structure of the lower arm with hand in supination. Drawing adapted from [613].

at the proximal end of the bone is 125°, and in the humerus, it is 135°. Much like the situation in the femur, when the humerus is rotated about its long axis with the wrist fixed, the off-center head can press the components of its appendicular joint either forward or backward, depending upon the direction of rotation. Moreover, because the ball and socket of the glenohumeral joint are so poorly matched, less than half of the surface area of the humeral head sits within the glenoid fossa, leaving approximately 60 percent of the head exposed; the mismatch of surfaces within the glenohumeral joint is eased by the presence

of a thick fibrocartilaginous ring (the glenoid labrum) resting between the humeral head and the glenoid fossa.

As the humeral neck (also called the anatomical neck; figure 10.A-1) is much shorter than the femoral neck (figure 10.B-1a), it would appear that it cannot exert as much torsional force on the scapula as can the femur on the pelvis; however, note that the humerus has a much larger range of three-dimensional motion in compensation for its shorter neck.

Magnifying Humeral Rotation

Allow the arm to hang straight down, with the biceps facing forward. If the rotation of the humerus turns the biceps to face laterally, then this lateral rotation of the humeral neck also acts to press the scapulae weakly onto the back ribs from behind (figure 10.A-1b) due to the rotation of the anatomical neck of the humerus. This effect of humeral rotation on the scapulae tends to lift the rib cage upward and forward while also spreading the clavicles. Because this open chest position is appropriate for almost all *yogasanas* (Subsection 10.A, page 328), this tendency toward lifting and opening the chest induced by lateral biceps/humeral rotation is an important element of almost all *yogasanas*. On the other hand, because there are relatively few sensors in the back body (figure 13.B-2), it will be difficult for the beginning student to make conscious contact with the back body and thereby activate the muscles necessary for lifting and opening the chest.

The effect of the humeral rotation, however, lacks just one other thing in order to accentuate the pressure on scapulae. To experience that one missing aspect, sit in a chair in front of a table, with your arms hanging down. Note how easy it is to rotate and lift the humerus laterally with little or no effect on the scapulae. Next, set the palms of your hands on the edge of the table, with the thumb braced beneath the front edge of the table, and depress the scapulae. On rotating the humerus laterally while the thumbs resist this action, the depressed scapulae are now pressed maximally into the rib cage! The bracing action of the hands and thumbs in this little exercise arises due to the disrotatory action within the arms, with the lower ends rotated medially and the upper ends rotated laterally. That is to say, the upper and lower parts of the arm, when either straight or bent, when rotated in a **disrotatory** way, with the upper arm rotated laterally and the lower arm rotated medially (as in figure 8.A-7b), and with the hand immobilized and the scapula depressed, impacts the scapulae strongly so as to lift and open the chest. This is an example of the muscle action described in Subsection 11.F, page 468, and discussed in more detail below.

The lateral rotation of the upper arm, when magnified by the disrotatory action of the lower arm, is the appropriate arm, shoulder, and chest action for virtually every *yogasana* that we practice. In order to get the upper-arm rotation to maximally press the scapulae onto the rib cage, it is necessary to press the rotated hand onto a stable surface, such as the floor *(adho mukha svanasana)* or the ankle *(trikonasana)*. This arm-shoulder action with depressed scapulae is quite similar to the rotational action of the femur of the right leg, for example, in order to bring the right groin forward when in *trikonasana* to the right. Just how this disrotatory action of the arms, whether straight or bent, becomes an important factor in performing several key *yogasanas* is discussed in the following subsection, page 331.

Bone-on-Bone Contact in the Shoulder Joint

Keeping the picture of the shoulder joint in mind (figure 10.A-1a), stand in *tadasana* and then lift the arm from vertical to horizontal (keeping it always in the parasagittal plane), and then from the horizontal to the over-head vertical position, again in the parasagittal plane. The circular pattern of arm motion is interrupted at this point as there little or no motion possible allowing one to go from over-head vertical to horizontal-but-behind-the-back. As can readily be seen from figure 10.A-1a, moving the arm yet more backward from the over-head vertical position is blocked by the collision of the humerus with the anterior portion of the acromion of the scapula. Similarly, raising the arm from the vertical position in *tadasana* to horizontal but to the rear is readily accomplished, but no further motion is possible as humeral motion in the parasagittal plane is now blocked by the contact of the humerus with the posterior side of the acromion. It is because of the contact of the acromion with the humerus that the arc of circumduction of the arm shown in figure 10.A-3a is not a simple, symmetric cone. In the hip joint, figure 10.B-1a, a similar bone-on-bone contact between femur and acetabulum occurs, leading again to a complicated shape of the cone of circumduction.

If the bone-on-bone (humerus-on-acromion)

contact is forced as when hanging in the ropes with the arms behind the chest (rope 1), the action of the humerus bones on the acromions of the scapulae is to press them in a way that tends to close the joints between the acromions and the clavicles, while stretching the pectorals and the deltoids. In contrast, when this contact is forced from the front as when in *urdhva dhanurasana*, the bone-on-bone action is to press the anterior acromions away from the clavicles (figure 10.A-1a), thereby opening the joints between them.

Opposable-Thumb Yoga

Note that the chest-opening action is a response to the action of the scapulae as driven by the arms, so that the rib cage receives the action of the arms in an indirect way. In this action, the lower margins of the scapulae (i.e., the inferior angles) press forward more strongly than do the upper margins. When the hand is on the floor and the medially rotated hand action is weak, a cavity forms under the bases of the index and middle fingers, which we may call the "indicial elevation." Experience shows that in order to get maximum pressure of the scapulae on the rib cage, with the hands in pronation and the thumbs strongly in extension (i.e., thumbs on the floor and perpendicular to the second metacarpal by contraction of extensor pollicis longus), one must roll the second and third metacarpals medially and then anchor this firmly while rolling the upper arm laterally. That is, when weight is on the palms of the hands, the indicial elevation must be flattened totally by pressing the heads of the second and third metacarpals of the hand to the floor with the thumbs in extension if a strong effect is to be felt in the scapulae. Details of how to accomplish this flattening of the indicial elevation so as to oppose the humeral rotation are discussed in the context of specific *yogasana* postures below.

Yogasana Examples

This action of the upper arms through the scapulae to help lift and open the chest in the *yogasanas* generally is understood by *yogasana* prac-

titioners, especially when the hands are on the floor and so necessarily offer a certain resistance to the upper-arm action. However, the deliberate contribution of the thumb and index finger actions toward resisting the humeral rotation is less well known. Though the disrotatory action of the arms does have a strongly positive effect on lifting and opening the chest in the *yogasanas* (as discussed below), the maximum effect is achieved by the application of pressure on the thumbs that goes beyond the prescription of simply rotating the humerus.

Thumb-on-Thumb Action

There are a number of examples in which pressure of the tips of the thumbs on one another or on the floor, or the compression of the fleshy mound at the base of the thumb (the thenar eminence), results in additional pressure of the scapula on the rib cage on that side, provided the forearm is pronated and the humerus is rotated laterally. For example, lift the arms in *parvatasana* or *virabhadrasana I*, fingers interlaced, the palms inverted so as to face upward, and the biceps turned laterally; at the same time, lower the scapulae. Then press the tips of the thumbs onto one another as the upper arms are rotated laterally, and feel the stronger bite of the scapulae onto the rib cage as they press the sternum forward and upward. The thumb-on-thumb effect is weak to nonexistent if the scapulae are allowed to rise (upper trapezius contracted) as the arms are extended upward.

When the arms are gently folded behind the back as when entering *paschima namaskarasana*, the upper arms are rotated medially and, in compensation for this, the shoulders press forward and the supraspinatus muscle is lengthened. In order to relieve the flexion imposed by this posture, one must rotate the forearms so as to bring the thumbs onto one another while the biceps are laterally rotated. Once adjusted in this way, the depressed scapulae are pressed onto the rib cage, opening and lifting it. More chest opening also is obtained in the strongly active version of *namaskarasana* (*namaste*) if the lateral edges of the thumbs are pressed against one another as they rest upon the sternum, again with the upper arms rotating in opposition to that of the hands and thumbs.

With the fingers interlocked behind the head in *sirsasana I*, so that the thumbs can not rotate laterally, work the upper arms against this internal anchor by rotating them laterally, and feel the scapulae bite into the rib cage.[3]

Thumb Tips on the Floor

Get stronger chest-opening action in *prasarita padottanasana* by setting the fingertips on the floor under the shoulders, fingernails forward, and while laterally rotating the humerus, oppose this action by pressing the tips of the thumbs into the floor while the scapulae are depressed. A disrotatory action of the upper arms and thumbs in *dandasana* similar to that in *prasarita padottanasana* again is advantageous in regard to lifting and opening the chest. The disrotatory thumb/upperarm action with the thumb on the floor when in *ardha chandrasana* is effective in turning the chest to face more forward in this posture.

Thumb on Bone

In *trikonasana,* place the hand at the ankle so that the thumb can press against the inside of the ankle bone (the medial malleolus, figure 10.B-1a); this unilateral but disrotatory action presses

---

3   In this work, we stress the thumb action that opposes the lateral rotation of the humerus. It has been pointed out by many that one of the most important differences between humans and the other primates is our having evolved the opposable thumb (specifically, contraction of the muscle opponens pollicis that brings the distal tips of the first and fifth phalanges together) which has allowed us extraordinary manual dexterity overall. As Kapandji [429] states that the hands would be essentially useless were we to lose our thumbs, the opposable thumb is said to be the one single quantum leap that has allowed humans to surpass their primate ancestors [101]. In the evolutionary context, the opposition of the thumb that is celebrated is that between tip of the thumb and the other finger tips, as when grasping a small object. *Yogasana* thumb-on-thumb practice now gives the world yet another reason for celebrating the opposable thumb, in this case, the movement being palmar extension, the movement antagonistic to that of the opposable thumb!

the scapula on the side of the forward leg so that the torso is rotated toward the proper position. This action may be what lies behind Iyengar's comment in regard to the use of the thumbs in *trikonasana* (Section VI.A, page 934).

The benefit of thumb action in *paschimottanasana* is especially clear. With the hands holding the feet with the fingers wrapped around the lateral edges of the feet, press the thumbs into the first metatarsal heads. This action serves two important purposes in this posture: the thumb action not only helps the depressed scapulae lift and open the chest but also supports the strongfoot position, which helps straighten the legs and spread the toes (Subsection 10.B, page 362).

In contradistinction to these, when in *sarvangasana*, the hands are necessarily turned into the supinate orientation, and there is no opposable thumb action possible; however, none is required, as the hands in *sarvangasana* can play the role of the scapulae in lifting and opening the rib cage, provided they can be placed on the back of the rib cage close enough to the shoulders!

Palms on the Floor

Pressure of the thumbs on the floor in *adho mukha svanasana* not only works to straighten the arms, but also works to open and lift the chest. The effects of thumb action on the scapulae while in *adho mukha svanasana* is apparent if one places two blocks at the wall and sets the edges of the index fingers and the thumbs along the block's edges, fingers pointed to the wall and thumbs pointed toward one another. This is the *yogasana* equivalent of the seated-at-the-table exercise described in the previous subsection, page 330. The arm action for *adho mukha svanasana* then is thumbs both into the forward edges of the blocks and into the floor, while the biceps rotate laterally. This combination of actions will strongly press the depressed scapulae into the rib cage. In order to take full advantage of the thumbs in opening the chest in *adho mukha svanasana* performed without the blocks, it is best to turn the lower arms medially, point the thumbs at one another, pin the thumbs to the floor, and then rotate the upper arms laterally; i.e., the upper and lower arms again in a disrotatory state.[4] Done in this way, the upper-arm action will tend to rotate the hands laterally; however, the thumbs pressing the floor will resist this motion as the angle between thumb and index finger opens somewhat.

Because the yogic thumb action found in *adho mukha svanasana* is yet more apparent in *adho mukha virasana,* start in this posture, hands on the floor but rotated medially. Maintaining this medial action of the lower arms, with the thumbs colinear and pressed to the floor, rotate the upper arms opposite to that of the lower arms (that is, rotate the upper arms laterally), and feel the strong action of the depressed scapulae on the rib cage. From this point, with the arms fully engaged in *adho mukha virasana,* go onto the toes and straighten the legs to attain *adho mukha svanasana,* but do not let the scapulae come up around the ears.[5]

The effect of opposable thumb action on the scapulae in *adho mukha svanasana* is strongest when (with lateral rotation of the upper arms) the wrists are rotated medially so that the thumbs point at one another (or even somewhat toward the feet); the effect is somewhat weaker when the fingers are straight ahead but the thumbs are pointing toward one another, and it is least when the lower arms are fully rotated laterally, with the thumbs more or less parallel. That is to say, the chest-opening effect in all postures is strongest when the lower and upper arms work in disrotatory opposition (figure 8.B-8**b**), with the thumb pressing an immovable object (floor, bone, or opposite hand), so that the lower arm is pronated

and is held in opposition to the lateral disrotatory action of the anterior upper arm. Not only is the action described here a step more complex than the usual statement given to beginners in *adho mukha svanasana* to "press the thumbs and bases of the index fingers to the floor," but at the same time, it is a perfect example of one muscle working against the macroscopic internal resistance of another to achieve more opening of the body, as discussed in Subsection 11.F, page 468. The same effect is observed in *sirsasana II* as is seen in *paschimottanasana* if the thumbs are pressed into the floor appropriately, so as to oppose the humeral action.

The effect of the thumbs on the rib cage also is found in *paryankasana* and *matsyasana* when performed with the palms of the hands placed on the floor just under the lower back, and it is found in *urdhva dhanurasana,* where it is easiest to feel the effect when the head is resting on the floor. The beneficial opposable thumb action on the scapulae and rib cage also is apparent in *bhujangasana* and *urdhva mukha svanasana.* Though it at first appears easier to do *purvottanasana* with the fingertips facing backward, this fully rotates the wrists laterally, placing the hands in a supinate position, and so offers only weak opposition to rotating the upper arms laterally, as with *sarvangasana* above. If, instead, the fingertips in *purvottanasana* are placed facing **forward** on the floor (the classical position for this posture [388, plate 171]), then the wrists have been rotated medially, the hands are now pronate, and the lateral rotation of the upper arms results in a strong upward action of the scapulae on the rib cage. Further discussion of the use of the opposable thumbs appears in Section 11.F, page 470.

Thumbs in the Air

The prescriptions given above are appropriate to beginners in *yogasana* practice; however, there is a way of doing the thumb action without contact with a stable anchor, and this may be of use to the more sophisticated practitioner. For this, sit in *dandasana* with the arms extended forward, parallel to the floor, and depress the scapulae. As the humerus is rotated laterally, press the palms

---

4   Alternatively, one can set the hands at the wall with the edges of the thumbs and the index fingers touching the wall and then press both to the wall while disrotating the upper arms and depressing the scapulae in *adho mukha svanasana.* When in the position with the hands blocked, if the heels can be blocked as well, then the effects on the scapulae are further magnified.

5   Ellen Kiley [442] points out that if the humerus is rotated appropriately by *yogasana* students but the scapulae are not first depressed, then the result is the development of a chronic tension in the rhomboid muscles of the back.

forward, especially the base of the index finger and the full length of the thumbs; the opposition of the humeral actions and those of the hands will increase the action of the scapulae on the rib cage. Note how closely this arm action resembles that of the lower leg when making the "strong yoga foot" (Subsection 10.B, page 362).

A Possible Mechanism

The following muscles are used in activating the scapular action discussed here. At the glenoid fossa, contraction of the infraspinatus and the teres minor initiates lateral rotation of the humerus, whereas contraction of the subscapularis of the upper back, the latissimus dorsi of the side body, and the pectoralis major muscles all aid in the medial rotation of the arm. The subscapularis is especially relevant as it lies between the scapulae and the posterior ribs (origin on the anterior surface of the scapula and insertion on the deltoid tuberosity of the humerus), and its contraction pulls the scapula forward onto the posterior ribs provided the humeral head is immobilized. In this scenario, the medial rotation of the hand/wrist as assisted by the contraction of the latissimus dorsi and other rotator cuff muscles serves to immobilize the humerus, thereby forming an anchor against which the contraction of the subscapularis muscle promotes the forward motion of the scapula. I propose that the lateral humeral rotation attendant to the infraspinatus and teres minor contractions overcome the medial humeral rotation of subscapularis but not the forward pressure of the scapula on the posterior ribs. In this case, the positions of subscapularis muscle origin and insertion have been reversed through the stabilization of the humerus to rotation. This action, in turn, works in conjunction with the direct scapular pressure resulting from the lateral rotation of the offset humeral head in the glenoid fossa.

Note, however, that if the arm is simply hanging loose at the side when the muscles of the rotator cuff contract, then the hand and wrist wave like a flag on a pole during a windy day while the scapula remains nearly motionless. Thus, it is the bracing of the hand in medial rotation (thumb to the floor) that immobilizes the humerus so that

the action of the rotator-cuff muscles in lateral rotation and the contraction of the subscapularis together turn the humeral head and pull the scapula forward onto the back of the rib cage. This action is strong, but is less so when the hands are free to rotate laterally and so no longer serve as humeral anchors. A similar scenario can be envisaged for the foot and leg in regard to adjusting the pelvis (Section 10.A, page 337).

Looking a little deeper into how an action in the hand/wrist might affect the attitude of the rib cage, consider that in the forearm, contraction of pronator teres (originating on the epimedial condyle of the humerus and inserting on the lateral surface of the radius) is aided by contraction of pronator quadratus (connecting the distal ends of the radius and the ulna), both forcing the lower arm to rotate medially. In the hand itself, the action that collapses the anatomical snuffbox and presses the thumbs, the thenar eminence, and the head of the second metacarpal onto the floor involves contraction of the flexor pollicis brevis and opponens pollicis muscles. Possible muscular connections of this sort are shown in figure 11.A-20.

A somewhat different approach to understanding how the hand and lower arm might work together to lift and open the chest is possible. Return first to the discussion of Subsection 7.D, page 240, and Appendix IV, page 856, where it is shown that when there is a change of the angle between the two bones of a joint, each of the two bones moves, but in inverse proportion to the masses attached to each of the bones. For the arm loosely hanging at the side, activation of the rotator cuff muscles so as to alternately rotate the arm first medially and then laterally around the humeral shaft, readily turns the arm, while the side body and shoulder are unmoved. This follows because the lower arm is of very low mass compared to the shoulder and rib cage. If, on the other hand, the lower arm can be braced by placing the hand on the floor (or on the edge of the table, etc.), then the effective mass of the lower arm can be huge, and it will be the shoulder and rib cage instead that are moved when the appropriate rotator cuff muscles are contracted. I feel that this is at the heart of the opposable-thumb action in lifting and opening the chest.

This medial twist of the radius tends to rotate the biceps medially, but when the medial thumb action is resisted by the floor (or by another bone in the body) on which the thumb is placed, then the lateral rotation of the humeral head is such that the scapula is pressed forward with maximal pressure, with the result that the rib cage is lifted and opened, provided that the scapula has been lowered. One sees from this that the admonition of all *yogasana* teachers to beginners in *adho mukha svanasana* to press the inner aspects of the hands (and indeed the inner aspect of each finger) to the floor is not just to make the handprint on the floor a little neater, but is key to generating the proper action in the rib cage!

With the scapula in a depressed position and the humeral head being rotated laterally, the offset of the humeral head by the nonzero length of the humeral neck also results in the scapula being pressed forward onto the rib cage from behind to lift and open the chest. However, I feel that this action is only synergistic to chest opening, with the prime mover being subscapularis contraction stabilized by lateral rotation of the humerus. Though this is obviously a complex situation, our poor understanding of the mechanism need not stand in the way of using it at every opportunity to further lift and open the chest.

Returning to *adho mukha svanasana* for a moment, the simple actions of the thumbs and index fingers on the floor results in tangible consequences for the action of the scapulae on the rib cage. This action is further enhanced if the hands are set on the mat with the fingers turned inward (medially), for this gives strength to the disrotatory action of the upper arms, turning the eyes of the elbows forward.[6] Resistive/anchoring actions of this sort are discussed in more detail in Subsection 11.F, page 468.

This action, stretching from the fingertips to

the scapulae while in *adho mukha svanasana*, Box 11.A-5, page 424, involves what has been called the "brachial muscular chain" by some body workers [105] and also the "deep front arm line" by Myers [603]. In the latter, it has been proposed that various muscles in the body are connected through their myofascia and may act in concert to exert stress at points far from the originating (prime mover) muscle. A path of muscles, bones, and connective tissue that work together (even though they are joined only by their connective tissue) is called an anatomy train [603].

Scapular Positions

Yogasana students will be familiar with the scapulae lifted to the ears by contraction of the upper trapezius muscles and the neutral position where the trapezius is relaxed; however, what is needed in order to lift and open the chest using the thumbs is activation of the lower trapezius muscles (figure 10.A-2**b**), so as to pull the scapulae even lower than the neutral position. Lowering the scapulae can be practiced by interlacing the fingers at the small of the back while standing and then pulling the knuckles toward the floor. The strength necessary to lower the scapulae also can be attained by doing chair dips with the arms straight and the shoulders alternately lifting and falling.

Though it is clear that we must lift and expand the chest by pressing it from the rear with the scapulae, it is also the case that the scapulae must be in the proper position on the posterior rib cage in order to achieve the desired results. So, for example, if the scapulae are lifted toward the ears and then pressed forward, the result will be a collapse of the chest rather than an expansion! Test this while standing, or better still, lie down with a block placed at various positions along the spine, and note which position gives the most lift to the chest; you will find that the optimal position for chest opening places the center of the block just opposite the center of the sternum and that placing the block closer to the base of the neck lifts the anterior chest in a way that closes it rather than the reverse. It appears that the scapulae will often need to be lowered in the *yogasanas*

---

6 I may be wrong about this, but it seems to me that the pressure of the scapulae against the rib cage when in *adho mukha svanasana* is stronger if the inward hand rotation is followed by the upper-arm shoulder rotation, in contrast to activating them in the reverse order.

but that they are never too low. Calais-Germain [101] mentions that when the scapulae are depressed, they hug the rib cage more tightly.

We often lift our arms to the ceiling, as in *urdhva hastasana, virabhadrasana I*, etc., and in doing so, we tend to pull the scapulae up to the ears. If, in this position, one tries to then press the scapulae onto the rib cage by lateral rotation of the humerus, the result often is an increased collapse of the chest, as the scapulae are at the level of the clavicles rather than at the level of the sternal center. This collapse occurs because the pressure of the scapulae is being applied to the very top of the thorax and so fails to lift the sternum. It is as if the two actions, lifting the fingertips maximally to the ceiling and using the scapulae to open the chest maximally, are mutually exclusive. If you need maximal opening of the chest in these positions, you must lower the scapulae so that they are at the level of the sternum and then press the scapulae onto the ribs by laterally rotating the biceps and medially rotating the hands. A similar situation holds in the case of arms that are overextended forward. Thus, in the case of *paschimottanasana*, for example, a student may overreach in stretching the fingertips to the feet and so bring the scapulae close to the ears, where they are of little or no value in keeping the chest lifted and open. As with the arms-over-head position when standing, the solution here is to lower the scapulae and so be able to engage the sternal lift, using the scapulae from the rear, with the biceps again rotated laterally and the hands rotated medially. When extending the arms and lifting the chest are at odds with one another, it is the latter that must be given priority.

Similarly, the placement of the hands in *sarvangasana* is a factor in opening the chest; if the hands are placed close to the hips, the posture is more like that of *ardha navasana* as performed by beginners or like *viparita karani*, with the chest more or less collapsed and the lowest ribs approaching the frontal pelvic bones. However, if they are placed on the rib cage close to the scapulae when in *sarvangasana*, the posture is more like that of *tadasana*, and the chest opening that results from the pressure of the hands on the rib cage is

apparent. The positive effect of lateral humeral rotation is also apparent in *pincha mayurasana*, where the classical palms-to-the-floor setup with a block between the index fingers, the thumbs on the front edges of the block, and the upper arms turned out through the use of a belt at the elbows results in a strong lift of the chest via the scapulae and a more vertical alignment of the upper arms. Though doing *pincha mayurasana* with the backs of the hands on the floor is possible, it lacks the scapular pressure so useful as when the palms face down, because it has the lower arms in a supinate rather than pronate position.

The scapulae also tend to move toward the ears when in *prasarita padottanasana*, and in this case the proper action can be obtained by pushing the hands forward on the floor with the biceps rotated laterally. This action brings the scapulae into the proper position on the rib cage and presses them toward the sternum, and it also acts to close the angle between the upper and lower body at the lower hinge (Subsection 9.B, page 319).

Scapular Conformance to the Rib Cage

Namaste with the arms behind the back (*paschima namaskarasana, parsvottanasana*, etc.) can involve not only medial rotation of the biceps rather than a lateral rotation, but also contraction of the pectoralis minor muscles rather than their elongation. As such, it can work to emphasize a collapse of the chest, since the actions are opposite to those for chest opening. When in this chest-closing position, the scapulae no longer lie flat against the rib cage, but instead, the medial edges lift off the rib cage and protrude backward to form "chicken wings," (also called "winged scapulae") again opposite to their orientation when opening the chest. This backward protrusion of the medial edges of the scapulae arises when the shoulders and the elbows are pointing forward and is in conflict with the forward pressure of the medial edges, which maximizes the pressure of the scapulae on the rib cage. In such a case, the biceps of the upper arms must again be rotated laterally so as to bring the hands and thumbs fully onto one another, thereby opening the chest and so releasing the scapulae onto the rib cage. This action is aided considerably by the anterior serratus muscles, which act to pull the medial edges of the scapulae onto the rib cage while moving the scapulae away from the spine [306]. Working in this way forces the scapulae to conform properly to the rib cage and helps to press it forward and upward.

Pressing the palms of the hands fully onto one another in *paschima namaskarasana* (with the little fingers on the spine) often leaves one with sore wrists, whereas this is not the case when the hands are pressed together in *namaskarasana* (with the thumbs on the sternum). In the former case, the wrist strain is a result of asking the wrists to make up a deficit incurred by a lack of openness in the shoulders, just as knee pain in *padmasana* is the result of asking the knees to make up the deficit incurred by a lack of openness in the hips. Working to open the shoulders with the arms behind the back, as with "rope 1," eases the wrist pain of *paschima namaskarasana*.

The chest lifting and opening that comes from placing the hands on the upper back in *sarvangasana* is present as well in various seated postures if the hands can be placed against a chair seat placed to the rear. Thus, for example, sit with the pelvis just beneath the front edge of a chair placed against the wall. With the legs separated and the arms forward, fold forward into *upavistha konasana* and note the inevitable kyphosis of the thoracic and lumbar spines. Repeat now with the hands on the front edge of the chair seat and, as you bend forward, press the hands against the chair seat so as to fully straighten the arms at the elbows. The result will be a deeper bend at the lower hinge and a lifting and opening of the chest at the same time. This highly desirable effect of the arms on the chest can easily be obtained in any and all of the seated forward bends by using a chair as described here for *upavistha konasana*.

Opposable-Toe Yoga

Given the strong similarity between how humeral rotation can dictate the motion of the rib cage (this chapter, page 328) and femoral rotation can dictate the motion of the pelvis (this chapter, page 342), one wonders how disrotatory or conrotatory actions within the leg might influence pelvic orientation. That is, does lateral rotation of the anterior thigh of the right leg, for example, depend upon whether the right foot is in conrotatory or disrotatory action? By comparison with the situation in the arm/shoulder, one expects the leg to function as a coupling of lower leg, upper leg, and pelvis such that when the upper leg is rotated, only the foot rotates if it is free to do so, but if the foot is constrained, then the rotation of the upper leg will act to reorient the pelvis.

To test this, first come into *savasana*, left and right inner legs in contact and hands resting on the groins. From this position, fully roll the anterior femurs laterally, letting the feet follow in the conrotatory sense (little toes laterally toward the floor) and note any changes of the pelvic orientation sensed by the hands. Next, repeat this action, but first cross the legs at the ankles so that the feet can not follow the rotation of the femurs. With the feet locked in the toes-up position, the lateral rotation of the femurs then can work against the pelvis and lift it toward the ceiling.

Similarly, when in *setu bandha sarvangasana* with the legs bent and heels just under the knees, lateral rotation of the femurs will press the knees out to the sides; however, if the knee motions are blocked by having a partner hold the performer's knees at hip width by standing with her knees on the outside of the performer's knees and pressing them inward, then the lateral rotation of the femurs will be noticeably more effective in lifting the pelvis. As applied to *urdhva dhanurasana*, the lifting of the groins comes about by a lateral rotation of the anterior thighs; however, as with the arms, if the feet are not anchored to the ground, this action results in the lateral rotation of the knees and feet rather than in the lifting of the groins. However, if the feet and knees are rotated inward, so that the big toes are firmly pressed to the floor, then the lateral rotation of the thighs becomes disrotatory and the groins are lifted, as desired.[7]

---

7   Note that the action to lift the groins by disrotatory action of the legs in *urdhva dhanurasana* depends upon a lateral rotation of the anterior thighs whereas

With the above in mind, now test the significance of disrotatory leg action while in *anantasana*, right leg vertical and right hand to right foot. In general, in this posture the right groin is pressed backward so that the right buttock is not aligned directly over the left buttock. On rotating the anterior right femur laterally and allowing the right foot to rotate in a conrotatory way with respect to the femur, note that the effect is minimal in regard to realigning the buttocks. Instead, hold tightly to the big toe on the right foot so that its action is disrotatory with respect to the lateral femoral rotation. In this case, the result will be the formation of an anchor at the right foot against which the femur can work in order to press the right groin forward and so pull the right buttock over the left.

When in *trikonasana* to the right, the right foot is pinned to the floor and so offers an anchor against which the right femur again can work to pull the posture into a more two-dimensional form. Can you find the opposable-toe action aligning the lumbar spine when rotating the legs in a disrotatory way in *dandasana*?

The Elbow Joint

The distal end of the humerus is joined to two bones in the forearm, the ulna and the radius. Of these, the ulna is more strongly bound to the epicondyles of the humerus, whereas the radius is the bone more strongly bound to the carpal bones of the wrist (figure 10.A-4c). In fact, the ulna is not a participant in the wrist joint at all; however, it is bound to the radius along its length by an interosseous membrane.

It is the protrusion of the olecranon process of the ulna that is sensed as the knob of the back

---

the standard backbend instruction involves the **medial** rotation of the anterior thighs; though this is troublesome, it is where the working-against-the-anchors approach (Section 11.F, page 468) leads one, provided the inward rotation of the feet and knees is a stronger torque than is that of the outward rotation of the thighs. That is to say, the rotation of the thighs in this is more of an action than a movement (Section 11.A, page 406).

of the elbow, which is placed on or close to the floor when in *sarvangasana,* and it is the bone-on-bone contact of the olecranon with its fossa in the elbow that prevents hyperextension of the elbow. Entrapment of the ulnar nerve within the elbow joint is discussed in Section 3.E, page 60.

The Carrying Angle

Notice that when the arm is pronate, the centers of the shoulder, elbow, and wrist joints are collinear, whereas when the arm is supinate, the elbow is deviated inward (medially) from this line as the medial epicondyle of the humerus is pulled toward the center line of the body; with the arm in the supinate position, the angle between the shoulder, elbow, and wrist on the lateral side of the arm is termed the "carrying angle" or the "cubitus valgus" (figure 10.A-4c). This angle is most obvious after carrying a heavy load for a long time, as this tends to stretch the tissue binding the elbow joint, making the joint temporarily more mobile. The carrying angle is often assessed by having the student place the palms upward with the outer edges of the little fingers touching, and then straightening the arms horizontally. A large percentage of students (almost always women) will display such large deviations from 180° that their inner elbows will touch when the arms "straighten"! This deviation from linearity is the arm's analog of knock-knees in the legs. The carrying angle in women is said to be 165° on average, whereas the corresponding angle in men is 175°.

The excessively large carrying angle is often seen in the arms of those performing *adho mukha svanasana* (in which case the elbows are displaced toward the floor) and *adho mukha vrksasana* (in which case the elbows drop in a direction opposite to that in which the fingers point). In these cases, the forearms must be pressed into place mechanically using blocks, etc., in an effort to straighten the arms at the elbows.

The dropping of the elbows in these postures can be rationalized in the following way. Note first that the radius of the forearm is adjacent to the lateral side of the elbow, but in the pronated position, it is crossed over the ulna so as to appear on the medial side of the wrist (figures 10.A-4**a** and 10.A-4**b**). If the elbow joints in such students are only loosely bound, when the hands are pronated, the crossing of the distal end of the radius, placing it on the medial side of the wrist, results in the ulna being pushed backward and downward by the overlying radius. The combination of this backward push of the ulna and the loose binding of the elbow joint results in the upper end of the ulna dropping toward the floor when the hands are strongly placed in pronation when in postures such as *adho mukha svanasana* and *adho mukha vrksasana*. It also may be that the curvature of the radius is less in these people, and so its pressure on the ulna will be stronger when the forearm is pronated. If this is the case, there should be little or no dropping of the elbows when the hands are placed with fingers fully out to the sides with wrists toward each other in *adho mukha svanasana* or *adho mukha vrksasana*, for this near-supinate hand position largely avoids the crossing of the ulna and radius bones.

The Wrists and Hands

The Wrists

When standing upright with the hands hanging down at the sides with palms facing inward in the neutral anatomic position (figure 10.A-1**a**), the ulna and radius are more or less crossed over one another. In fact, these two bones of the forearm can be rotated with respect to one another by more than 180° [429] and in large part, independently of any rotation of the humerus. With the arms pendant, the radius and ulna are fully crossed when the palms are facing backward (pronate) and are fully parallel when the palms face forward, or supinate (figure 10.A-4**c**); the radius is curved so that it can curl about the ulna without making strong bone-on-bone contact with it in the crossed-bones position (however, see the subsection above in regard to dropping of the elbows in *adho mukha svanasana*, etc.). When shoulder rotation is added to forearm rotation, more than 360° of rotation of the hand around the long axis of the arm can be achieved with the arms hanging

down, but only 270° may be achieved when the arms are extended overhead [429]. The difference here is again due to the bone-on-bone contact between the greater tubercle and the glenoid cavity when the arm is lifted (Section 10.A, page 323).

Hand Yoga

There is an ancient form of hand and finger yoga known as *mudra,* in which the positions of the hands and digits are used to access and alter one's emotional states [728]. It is hypothesized [728] that performing or witnessing the *mudras* promotes emotional shifts via the mirror neurons (Subsection 4.G, page 142) associated with Broca's area in the left cerebral hemisphere.

The relaxed position of the hand in *savasana* has equal tension in all of the muscles and is rotated midway between pronation and supination; the fingers and thumbs are slightly flexed, reflecting the superior strength of the flexional grasping muscles of the fingers. Just as with the foot (figure 10.B-7**c**), the nervous system of the hand is divided into two major components: the ulnar branch, controlling the fourth and fifth metacarpals; and the radial branch, controlling the first three metacarpals. Compression of these nerves leads to a feeling of pins and needles in the hand and arm.

As with the discussion of the legs and hip joints, Kapandji also has written an exhaustive volume on the arm and shoulder [429], and the interested reader is referred to this book and to [101] for in-depth discussions.

Section 10.B: The Legs and Feet

The bones of the leg are rather like those of the arm, up to a point. Corresponding to the humerus of the upper arm, one has the femur of the upper leg; however, the hip joint joining the leg to the pelvis is rather different in both structure and function from the shoulder joint joining the arm to the rib cage. Unlike the shoulder, where several bones have joined together to form the glenoid fossa (into which the head of the humerus

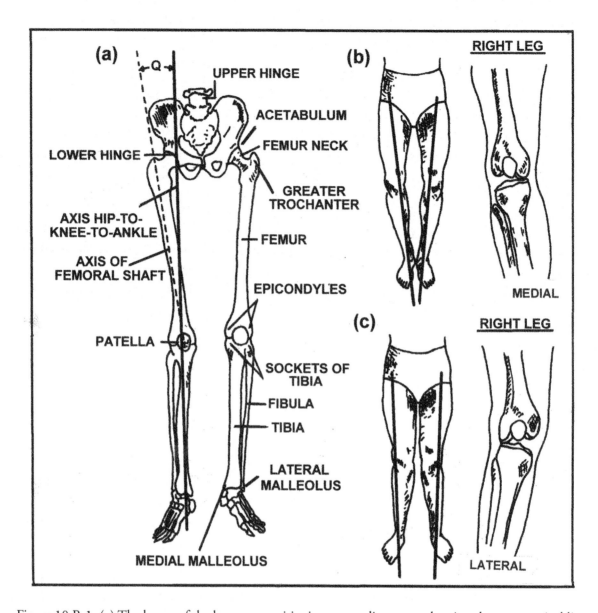

Figure 10.B-1. (**a**) The bones of the lower extremities in proper alignment, showing the near-vertical line passing through the center of the acetabulum, the knee joint, and the ankle joint on the right leg, as seen from the front. (**b**) In the case of bowed legs, the centers of the knee joints lie outside the lines connecting the hip sockets to the ankles, resulting in an articulation of the femur and the tibia at the knee joint that is heavy on the medial femoral condyle, as shown for the right leg. (**c**) In the case of knock-knees, the centers of the knee joints lie inside the lines connecting the hip sockets to the ankles, resulting in an articulation of the femur and tibia at the knee joint that is heavy on the lateral femoral condyle, as shown for the right leg.

will fit), the corresponding cavity into which the hemispherical head of the femur will fit (figures 8.B-7 and 10.B-1a) consists of a single bone in the adult, though it is formed by the fusion of several bones when the infant begins to walk. A second difference between the arms and the legs rests in the fact that both can be imagined to be derived from the limbs of four-legged reptiles in which "knees" and "elbows" point to the sides, whereas in humans, the upper limbs have been rotated so that the elbows point backward when the arms are bent, and the lower limbs have been rotated oppositely so that the knees point forward when the legs are bent. The basic functions of the hip joints are to support the body weight and to allow leg actions for locomotion.

Bones and Joints of the Upper Leg

The Femurs

The femur or thigh bone of the leg is the longest and heaviest bone in the body and is a very mobile bone mechanically, having both a two-dimensional ball joint at the hip allowing 360° angular motion and a one-dimensional curved surface at the knee for extension and flexion. The combined motion around these two joints allows a wide range for positioning the leg (figure 10.A-3b).

As shown in figure 10.B-1a, when standing in *tadasana,* the femur is angled outward from the knee, and at the point of the greater trochanter, it abruptly turns inward to form the joint with the pelvis. The transverse section, known as the fermoral neck, is terminated by the hemispherical femur head, which in turn fits into the hemispherical socket of the acetabulum in the pelvis. Taken together, the acetabulum and the head of the femur form the ball-and-socket hip joint.

There is a rather unexpected geometry of the femur close to the point at which it connects to the hip joint. When standing in proper alignment, there is a near-vertical plumb line between the centers of the hip joint, the knee joint, and the ankle joint; however, the largest part of the femur lies well to the outside of this plumb line (figure 10.B-1a) and then turns sharply inward at the upper end to enter the hip joint.

Though it is often mistaken for a geometric angle of the pelvis, the most lateral point of the femur (called the greater trochanter, figure 10.B-1a) is the bony point on which we lie when performing *anantasana;* in the elderly, it is a common situation that the femoral neck weakens and fractures easily, due to its relatively sharp angle with respect to the femoral shaft.

The Hip Joints

The average arrangement of femur and pelvis allows an approach of the neck of the femur at an angle of 125° with respect to the vertical [430], which in turn allows the pelvis to swing front to back between the femoral necks, like a bucket swinging between the ends of its handles [632] or like a seesaw (Subsection 9.B, page 318). However, natural variations of the femoral geometry occur with great frequency, with the femurs in some having a long neck, a head consisting of two-thirds of a sphere, and an angle between neck and femoral shaft of 125°; whereas in others, the neck is short, the head consists of only a hemisphere, and the angle between neck and shaft is only 115°.

The femur bone also is in a state of partial torsion, with the line of the neck rotated with respect to the left-to-right line through the condyles at the lower end of the bone. The first of these variations (long neck) has a torsional angle of 25° and favors speed of movement, whereas the second (short neck) has a torsional angle of only 10° and is built for strength. The ranges of structural parameters for the femur will be reflected in the apparent strengths and flexibilities shown by your *yogasana* students. As compared with the shoulder joint (figure 10.A-3a), movement of the femur in the hip joint in regard to circumduction (figure 10.A-3b) is rather limited, but this leg movement often can be assisted by movement within the lumbar vertebral column.

Bone-on-Bone Interaction in Trikonasana

The unique shape of the femur allows for some exceptional yogic positions, and at the same time, this shape can be a hindrance. For example, the range of motion of lateral bending at the hip joint can be limited by the pressure of the rim of the acetabulum on the upper surface of the femoral neck, and if this is the case, no further progress in regard to lateral bending is possible. You can test your range of motion as regards bone-on-bone contact in the hip joint in the following way. Prepare for *trikonasana* by first coming into *tadasana* with the spine straight and the back of the body on the wall. In this position, the relative positions of femur and pelvis, with feet together and parallel to one another but perpendicular to the wall, are as shown in figure 10.B-2a. Now sep-

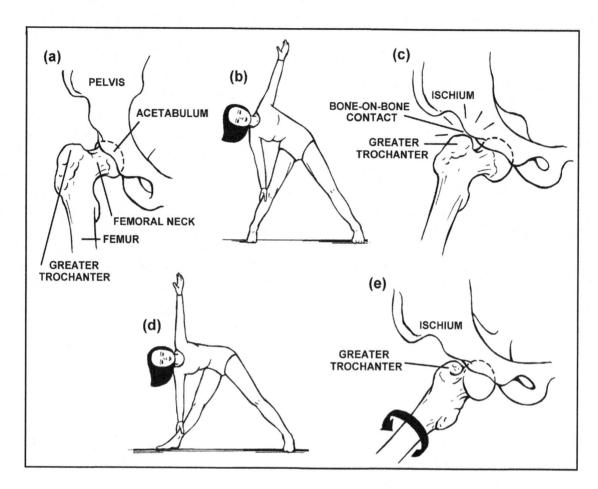

Figure 10.B-2. (**a**) Relative orientation of the of the femoral head and the acetabulum of the pelvis when standing in *tadasana*. (**b**) *Trikonasana* to the right, as performed with the medial lines of the feet parallel to one another. (**c**) With the legs rotated as for (**b**), the congestion within the right hip joint due to the collision of the upper outer rim of the acetabulum/ischium with the greater trochanter of the right femur. (**d**) Anterior portion of the right leg rotated laterally so as to set the right foot perpendicular to the left foot, the conventional alignment for this posture. (**e**) Release of the congestion in the right hip joint as the femur is rotated to the rear, so that there is minimal interaction between the greater trochanter and the rim of the acetabulum.

arate the feet to *trikonasana* width, keep the feet parallel (as when in *tadasana)*, and bend to the right side at the hip joint, closing the lower hinge but keeping the upper hinge open (Subsection 9.B, page 319). Keeping the back of the body on the wall and the feet parallel, slide the right hand down the right thigh and note how far down it goes with respect to the knee (figure 10.B-2b). When in this position, limited bending to the right results, due to the greater trochanter of the right femur colliding with the upper outer rim of the acetabulum on that side (figure 10.B-2c). How deeply one can go into *trikonasana* when done in

this way will depend in large part on the particulars of bone structure in the hip joint rather than upon flexibility of the muscles in the upper leg; i.e., the larger is the angle between femoral neck and femoral shaft, the deeper one can bend in the posture shown in figure 10.B-2**b**.

Next, return to the upright position and then rotate the right leg laterally to the right, setting the right foot perpendicular to the left foot. Keeping the back of the body on the wall, once again bend to the right, closing the lower hinge while keeping the upper hinge open, and slide the right hand down the right leg as far as it will go (figure 10.B-2**d**); note the hand-on-leg placement as compared with that in figure 10.B-2**b**. In general, the hand in the position of figure 10.B-2**d** will be further down the leg than in the position of figure 10.B-2**b**. How does this increased range of motion come about? Stand in *tadasana,* and place the fingers of the right hand on the greater trochanter of the right leg. Then rotate on the right heel so as to send the right foot fully to the right, and note how this lateral rotation of the anterior thigh takes the greater trochanter backward (figure10.B-2**e**). In regard to lateral bending in *trikonasana,* the femoral neck is rotated backward by lateral rotation of the femoral shaft, and being rotated out of the path of the descending acetabulum as it rotates over the head of the femur, the rotation allows a deeper bend to the right side. The desired femoral rotation to the right involves contraction of the sartorius and gluteus muscles and the relaxation of the psoas muscle on the right side of the body. If the femur is not rotated as in figure 10.B-2**e**, then the beginner will be tempted to reach further down the right leg by bending at the upper hinge, but this is to be discouraged, for obvious reasons.[8]

One can think of the situation described in figure 10.B-2 as first involving the compressive stress of bone-on-bone contact, which, through a muscular action, then removes the contact between the bones, and in doing so, converts the compressive stress of the bones into a tensile stress of the muscles and connective tissue (Section 7.F, page 252).

When bending to the side in any of the standing postures, the femur of the leg toward which

one bends always should be rotated laterally, so that there is adequate clearance between femoral shaft and acetabulum. As pointed out by Grilley [298], the length of the femoral neck also will be a determining factor in lateral stretches of this sort. Note that a similar collision between the humerus and the scapular acromion of the shoulder joint necessitates a lateral rotation of the humerus in certain *yogasana* positions, in order to avoid bone-on-bone contact (Subsection 10.A, page 323).

When the anterior femur is rotated laterally in *trikonasana,* three significant things happen in the pelvic area: (1) the femoral neck and greater trochanter are rotated backward; (2) as the greater trochanter is rotated backward, the femoral head presses the right groin forward and so places the hip joint on that side in extension; and (3) with the femoral neck out of the way, the deep bend to the right is unencumbered by bone-on-bone contact and so is transformed from bone-on-bone compression into muscle and connective tissue stretching. Similar benefits when rotating the anterior femur of the forward leg laterally in *parighasana, parsvakonasana,* and *ardha chandrasana* are to be noted.

Anantasana

It was discussed in Subsection 10.A (page 328) that the lateral rotation of the humerus can move the scapulae, provided the lower end of the limb is rotated in the disrotatory mode (figure 8.B-8**b**) by pinning it to the floor. Similarly, lateral rotation of the femur in *trikonasana* can press the groin forward, because the foot of the leg is restricted in its motion, so that rotating the femur must rotate the pelvis. (See Subsection 7.D, page 241, for more on the effects of pinning the end of a moveable bone.) However, it is different when in *anantasana,* because the leg is not bound at both ends, and so the leg and foot can turn without forcing the pelvis to move. Thus, rotation of the femur easily can be effected so as to avoid collision with the acetabulum in *anantasana.* Nonetheless, it is far more difficult to bring the groin forward into the plane of the body in *anantasana* than in *trikonasana,* because the rotation of the thigh only rotates the lower leg

---

8   Alternatively, the effect of the bone-on-bone interference within the hip joint when bending laterally is obvious if one begins lying on one's side body, as if to begin *anantasana.* From this point, lift the upper leg to the full *anantasana* position, first keeping the foot of the raised leg pointed forward and parallel to the dorsiflexed foot of the leg on the floor. Compare this angle of elevation with that achieved when the upper anterior thigh is then rotated laterally so that the foot of the raised leg points toward the shoulder on that side, thereby releasing the bone-on-bone contact within the hip joint.

rather than the pelvis when the lower leg is free to move. Admittedly, this solves the problem of the bone-on-bone contact in *anantasana*, but still leaves the problem of pressing the groin forward in this posture, unless the foot on the upper leg is immobilized, i.e., turned in disrotation.

Backbending

The integrity of the hip joint throughout the range of motion of the femur is enforced by several ligaments binding the femoral neck to the pelvis, as shown in (figure 10.B-3a). For our purposes, the most significant of these ligaments are those between the femoral neck and the ischium of the pelvis (the ischiofemoral ligament or ISF), between the femoral neck and the ilium of the pelvis (the iliofemoral ligament or ILF), and the pubofemoral (PF), an internal ligament otherwise not shown in the figure. If one could look along the femoral neck from the greater trochanter to the center of the acetabulum while standing erect in *tadasana*, these three ligaments connecting the pelvis to the femoral neck would be in a state of modest tension, as depicted in figure 10.B-3b. Note, however, that on going from *tadasana* to *uttanasana*, tension on the ligaments of the hip joints changes significantly (figure 10.B-3c). In this case of pelvic flexion, the tensile stress on the ligaments is considerably decreased, as evidenced by their shorter lengths. If extension at the hip joints is incurred by going from *tadasana* to *urdhva dhanurasana*, the ligaments follow by further increasing their lengths; i.e., by increases of the tensile stress (figure 10.B-3d).

I interpret this in the following way. Our early ancestors assumed the quadrupedal posture, in which they were fully flexed at the hips, and the ligaments in the region were positioned to accommodate this posture with minimum tension (figure 10.B-3b). However, when our ancestors made the transformation five million years ago to a standing bipedal posture (i.e., going from a flexional to a more extensional pelvic posture), the femoral head rotated by 90° within the acetabulum, and the ligaments were stretched and wrapped round the femoral neck in a spiral sense (figure 10.B-3b). If the spinal extension is contin-

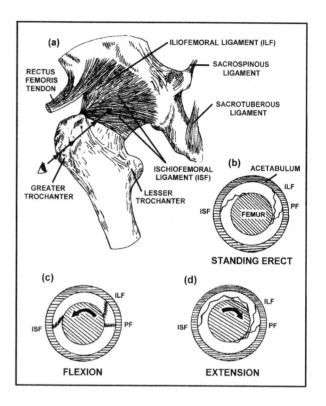

Figure 10.B-3. (a) The various ligaments holding the head of the femur in the acetabulum of the pelvis. Note that the pubofemoral ligament (PF) lies behind the ischiofemoral ligament (ISF) in this anterior view and so is not visible in the drawing. It does appear when viewed looking down the axis of the femoral neck. (b) The orientations of the ischiofemoral (ISF), iliofemoral (ILF), and pubofemoral (PF) ligaments connecting femur to acetabulum when standing in *tadasana*, as viewed axially along the sight line shown by the arrows in (a). (c) The orientations of the ISF, ILF, and PF ligaments connecting the femur to the acetabulum when bending forward in *uttanasana*, as viewed axially along the sight line shown in (a). (d) The orientations of the ISF, ILF, and PF ligaments connecting the femur to the acetabulum when bending backward in *urdhva dhanurasana*, as viewed axially along the sight line shown in (a).

ued so as to place one in *urdhva dhanurasana*, the tensile stress on the ligaments of the hip joint is increased yet further (figure 10.B-3d).

Consequently, when the hip joint is in flexion, the ligaments of the hip joint are fully relaxed and the hip joint is least stable; whereas when the pelvis is in extension, the ligaments are tightly wound about the femoral neck, pulling the femur head deeper into the acetabulum. Should the extension be extreme, as it would be when performing *urdhva dhanurasana,* the resistance to further winding of the ligaments within the hip joints would offer considerable resistance to achieving the posture. In contrast, when the hip joint is flexed and the legs are crossed, as is the case when performing *gomukhasana or maricyasana III,* the ligaments binding the femur to the acetabulum are relaxed, and so the hip joints are maximally unstable in regard subluxation. A similar statement can be made in regard to the glenoid fossa of the shoulder joint (page 323).

Regardless of the reasoning behind the effects shown in figure 10.B-3, it is clear that the ligaments that bind the hip joints will be relaxed in forward bends, somewhat tense in erect postures, and severely stressed in a tensile sense when in backbends. When these ligaments are tight in the student, they will work to hinder backbending by keeping the hip joints more or less closed in flexion.

With one leg rotated outward (i.e., anterior femur rotated laterally, with the foot on the floor), the groin on that side is pressed forward. With both legs rotated outward, the entire pelvis is pressed forward, and the lumbar spine tends to become lordotic as a consequence. In this way, it is seen that when backbending, the "natural" action of the body is to outwardly rotate the feet, knees, and anterior thighs in order to increase lumbar lordosis; this again is a consequence of the length of the femoral neck and its angle with the femoral shaft, as well as the peculiar way in which the psoas is connected to both the lumbar spine and the inner femurs (figure 9.B-2**b**). Note that this natural lateral rotation of the thighs and the consequent lordotic compression of the lumbar spine when yogic backbending traditionally is overcome by deliberate medial rotation of the anterior thighs. This lateral natural rotation of the thighs in backbends also closes the sacroiliac joint; however, the medial rotation of the anterior thighs not only will open it again (as with forward

bends), but it will also reduce lumbar compression while increasing the tensile stress on the quadriceps muscles (see Section 10.A, page 337, for an alternate view of this aspect of backbending).

Soft Tissue of the Upper Legs

Hamstrings

Some muscles act only to change the angle at the hip, some only at the knee, and some, like the hamstrings, at both places. Because the hamstrings cross both the hip and the knee, with origins at the ischial tuberosity and insertions at the tibia, they are prime movers of both hip extension and knee flexion; i.e., if the hip is fixed in the extended position, then hamstring contraction leads to knee flexion, and if the knee is fixed and extended, then hamstring contraction leads to hip extension (backbending).

The hamstrings are made of three components: the biceps femoris, which is the lateral component, and two others that act together as medial components (figure 11.A-2). All three have their origins at the ischial tuberosity of the pelvis, with the biceps femoris having its insertion on the lateral edge of the fibula (and so having an element of lateral rotation of the anterior thigh) and the other two having insertions on the medial side of the tibia (and so having elements of medial rotation of the anterior thigh) [101].

The resistance to reaching the fingertips to the floor in *uttanasana* is due to hamstring tightness, and such tight muscles also will force the lumbar curve into concavity when this student is sitting in *dandasana.* That is to say, tight hamstrings will force the student to bend at the upper hinge instead of at the lower hinge (Subsection 9.B, page 319).

Because the myofascial tissue that is so resistant to stretching is three times thicker on the lateral line of the thigh than it is on the medial line [857a], it is no surprise that the lateral hamstring is often tighter than the medial ones. Because the lateral hamstring is stretched preferentially when in *paschimottanasana,* whereas it is the medial hamstring that is stretched in *upavistha konasana,* one generally can go deeper in the latter posture than the former. For this reason, the stress of hamstring stretching in *janu sirsasana,* for example, can be focused on the lateral component by working with the extended leg at an angle smaller than 90° with respect to the left-right axis of the pelvis; i.e., assume the standard position for *janu sirsasana,* and then move the straight leg toward the bent leg. Similarly, if the goal is to stretch the medial component of the hamstrings, then again take *janu sirsasana,* but keep the legs well separated.

All manner of hip flexion stretches the hamstrings, provided that the legs are kept straight (*paschimottanasana, virabhadrasana III, dandasana* in *sirsasana,* etc.); however, once the knees become bent, as in *utkatasana, bhekasana,* or *garudasana,* the tensile stretch on the hamstrings is released.

Quadriceps

Being the antagonist muscles of the hamstrings, the quadriceps of the leg (figure 11.A-1) work to open the knee joint and so straighten the leg. Of the four quadriceps muscles, the rectus femoris has its origin at the frontal pelvic bone, whereas the other three components have their origins at the femur neck. Consequently, in quadriceps stretches such as *supta virasana,* in which the pelvis is rotated so as to bring the lumbar spine closer to the floor, the rectus femoris will be stretched to a far greater extent than the other three components. This is also true in backbends, in which the lumbar curvature is minimized by pulling the back rim of the pelvis toward the knees. The quadriceps are stretched in all straight-leg postures having an element of backbending in them, such as *hanumanasana, setu bandha sarvangasana,* and *purvottanasana,* and in bent-leg postures where the heels are strongly folded or pulled toward the buttocks, as in *supta virasana, bhekasana,* and *dhanurasana.* When all four components of the quadriceps muscle group work together (rectus femoris, vastus lateralis, vastus medialis, and vastus intermedius; figure 11.A-1), they become the strongest muscle in the body.

The rectus femoris of the quadriceps can be stretched only if the hip is in extension and the knee is in flexion, as when in *supta virasana,* etc. When stretching the rectus femoris, placing the knee in a weight-bearing position on the floor (*parighasana,* for example) risks damaging the articular cartilage surfaces between the patella and the femur by compression. For the same reason, do not do the upright *virasana* stretches while standing directly on the patellas (as required by *virasana* performed with the back body and lower legs on a supporting wall) unless there is sufficient padding between the knee and the floor. However, upward-facing *virasana* quadriceps stretches (such as *supta virasana* and *ustrasana*) and downward-facing quadriceps stretches (such as *bhekasana*) performed on a bare floor are more acceptable, as the body weight is more widely distributed in these postures, and so less is focused at the knee. Unlike the situation with rectus femoris, the three vastus muscles of the quadriceps can be stretched when in full flexion of both hip and knee; i.e., as when in *malasana* or *garbhasana.*

Both the vastus lateralis and the vastus medialis muscles of the upper leg (figure 11.A-1) have tendons that engage the patella at the knee, with the former tending to pull the patella to the lateral side of the knee, and the latter pulling it to the medial side of the knee. Because the patella functions best when it moves so as to be aligned with the groove in the connective tissue lying parallel to the femoral axis, imbalance in the muscle tones of the vastus lateralis and vastus medialis results in the patella painfully scraping against this groove when the leg bends [410a].

Other Muscles

The adductor muscles of the upper leg move the thighs toward the center line and encompass the magnus, longus, brevis, pectineus, and the gracilis. The last of these, the gracilis, is not only an adductor but spans two joints: the knee and the hip. For this reason, the gracilis is stretched in *trikonasana* but not in *parsvakonasana,* where the knee is bent. The tensor fascia lata is inserted into the tibia by the iliotibial band and acts to rotate the upper leg medially. This action works to pin the hips in all postures and to press the thigh onto the arms in *bakasana.*

Lateral Dominance

It is clear that where there are two organs or limbs placed left and right symmetrically in the body, one of the two is always dominant. Because this lateral dominance in the body extends to the legs, one leg will be dominant over the other; i.e., it will be stronger, longer, more flexible, etc. To the hiker lost in the woods or the desert without any markers to steer by, this right-leg dominance means that the uneven stride and uneven strength of the two legs will tend to propel him on a counterclockwise circular course, even as he tries to walk a straight path. Applied to the *yogasana* student, this means that unless the dominance is very weak, one will notice a number of differences in the abilities of the two legs when working both symmetric and asymmetric postures. As it is the right leg that most often is dominant and stronger, one might find that the right leg is stronger in *parsvakonasana*-to-the-right than is the left leg in *parsvakonasana*-to-the-left, for example. Even though leg asymmetry is inherently natural, one should work the *yogasanas* so that the asymmetry is not accentuated [402].

Thanks to the ever-present pull of gravity on the body, the legs are built so as to support the body endlessly; this is why the legs are always larger and stronger than the arms in humans. However, in the end, the leg muscles fatigue and shorten through overuse, so that stretching must be instituted if their normal lengths are to be maintained through old age.

The Knees

Together with the fibula, the two longest bones of the body, the femur and the tibia, meet to form the knee joint. The lower end of the femur bone forms two hemispheres (condyles), side by side (figure 10.B-1), and correspondingly, the upper end of the tibia (the major bone of the lower leg) has two shallow sockets that can accept the hemispheric condyles of the femur in forming the knee joint (figure 10.B-4a), the largest joint in the body. However, as the shapes of the condyles and the top of the tibia are rather incongruent,

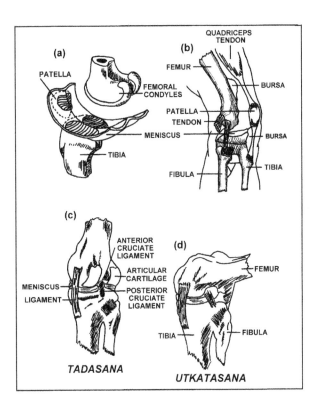

Figure 10.B-4. (**a**) Schematic structure of the knee joint, showing how the femoral condyles mate with the upper end of the tibia, with the supervening meniscus accommodating for the mismatch. (**b**) The internal structure of the knee, as seen laterally. In this area, four bones come together (femur, tibia, fibula, and patella), with over a half dozen cartilaginous pads (menisci) and cushions (bursae) to protect the epiphyses from rubbing against one another, synovial fluid to keep the apparatus lubricated, and ligaments to hold the structure in place, while allowing a certain mobility of the joint. Structures of the knee joint when standing erect in *tadasana* (**c**) and when the knee is bent, as in *utkatasana* (**d**). In *tadasana*, one stands on the bottoms of the condyles of the femurs, whereas in *utkatasana*, the condyles roll within the discs of the menisci and slide forward as well, so that one stands on the back of the condyles of the femur, with the meniscus pressed forward.

considerable stress would be applied to their point of contact were it not for the meniscal discs that separate them, lubricate them, and act as shock absorbers. As the knee is flexed and extended, the femoral heads roll and glide across the top of the tibia, and the intervening menisci deform to accommodate the stress. Internal to the knee joint, there also are crossed ligaments connecting the condyles to the tibial sockets (the cruciate ligaments), and the whole is surrounded by a synovial joint capsule (Subsection 7.D, page 239).

The knee joint functions best as a hinge joint, tolerant of both flexion and extension but intolerant of any appreciable rotation of the lower leg with respect to the upper leg. In turn, the knee is vulnerable to injury if it bends laterally or medially while the toes face forward or if it is subject to rotational stresses (in this regard, see Box 10.B-1, page 352). Even when the leg is straight and in proper alignment (toes and kneecap facing forward, with the latter on the line between hip and ankle), the plane of the upper end of the tibia and the plane of the lower end of the femur are canted with respect to one another by 15°. Should the straight-leg's foot go into pronation (i.e., the inner ankle drops toward the floor, making a flat foot, while the knee moves medially with respect to the line between the hip and ankle so as to form knock-knees), then the angle of mismatch at the knee is increased to 30° when the sole of the foot is braced on the floor. Additionally, being flat-footed exerts an abnormal pull on the quadriceps muscles. Simple misalignments like these can result in functional problems, such as inflammation and pain without any noticeable tearing of tissues in the joint. In order to walk normally, one needs to be able to bend the knees through an angle of 65° from the straight-leg position, through 95° in order to climb stairs, and 110° in order to easily rise from a seated position.

The Patella

The knee joint is protected from outside forces by the patella, or kneecap (figure 10.B-1a). Kneecaps form as cartilaginous pads in about the fourth month after delivery and only begin to show signs of ossification at about three years in females and four to five years in males (Subsection 7.A, page 225).

The patellar bone is free-floating but is embedded in the tendon that binds the four quad-

riceps muscles to the lower leg. Unlike the other bones of the leg, the patella does not bear any weight in standing postures but does so in kneeling postures such as *ustrasana* and *parighasana*. Because the patella is inserted in the tendon of the quadriceps, firming of the quadriceps noticeably lifts the patella toward the pelvis as the muscle contracts. Awareness of the lifting of the kneecap as the quadriceps straighten the leg can be of great help to the beginning student trying to find the leg-straightening action in the *yogasanas*.[9]

Inserted as it is in the tendon of the quadriceps, the patella increases the mechanical efficiency of that muscle and keeps the tendon from rubbing against the femoral condyles [884]. As shown in figure V.B-2, the torque of a muscle action (T) is equal to the linear force exerted by the muscle (Q) times the lever arm (R) over which it acts; that is, $T = QR$. In the case of quadriceps contraction extending the bent knee, the effect of the patella is essentially to lengthen the lever arm (R), so that with the knee flexed at 120°, the patella increases the quadriceps torque about the knee by 10 percent, as compared to the case where the patella has been removed. In this leg-straightening action, the patella acts as an anatomic pulley (Subsection 11.A, page 406), increasing the torque with which the quadriceps works to straighten the leg; this torque advantage increases to 30 percent when the leg is very nearly straight. Of course, in acting as a pulley, there is great pressure on the patella applied by the contracting quadriceps. In response to this,

---

9   In theory, the leg also can be straightened by pressing the kneecap straight back; however, this can lead to two negative situations. First, pressing the knee back without lengthening the leg results in a compaction of the knee joint, which is not good. Second, if the leg is loosely jointed, then pressing the knee back can readily lead to hyperextension of the knee joint. Again, this is not good.

If, instead, the kneecap is lifted toward the hip while the heel is stretched forward along the line of the leg, then the overall lengthening of the leg leads to a straight leg, an open knee joint, and no risk of becoming hyperextended, regardless of however strong the action might be.

the posterior surface of the patella is covered by a 3-millimeter- (0.1-inch-) thick layer of cartilage, among the thickest in the body [61a].

Allowed Motions of the Knee

Thanks to the structure of the joint at the knee, only flexion and extension of the leg at the knee are allowed formally. Other actions at the knee, such as axial rotation of the lower leg with respect to the upper leg (*mulabandhasana* or *padmasana,* for example) may overstretch the ligamentous structure at the knee, and so they should be practiced with great care. See Subsection 10.B, page 352, for a discussion of how to avoid knee damage in performing *padmasana.* If the ligaments and tendons at the knee do become overstretched, then the knee can be easily hyperextended posteriorly (pressed backward so that the center of the knee joint lies **behind** the plumb line of figure 10.B-1**a**) or medially (pressed to the inner side of the plumb line). In that case, the ligaments do not reach the level of tension necessary for supporting the joint, and the students end up "hanging on their joints," further stretching them, as often happens, for example, on the forward leg in *trikonasana,* where medial rotation of the anterior thigh is common. The backward destabilization of the knee that expresses itself as hyperextension also is known historically as "genu recurvatum."

The fact that the femoral shaft is angled with respect to the vertical line of the lower leg (figure 10.B-1**a**) implies that the knee joint will be subject to several types of mechanical stress due to motions at the hip joint. Indeed, of the eleven muscles that cross the knee, seven of them also cross the hip joint (three hamstring and four quadriceps), thus coupling hip and knee actions [833].

As can be seen from figure 10.B-1**a**, the tibia by far is the larger of the two bones in the lower leg and carries most of the load between the foot and the femur. In fact, the fibula, being the slenderest of the long bones in the body, is relatively weak and of not much use; because there is little or no relative movement between tibia and fibula (unlike the relationship between the comparable bones, the ulna and the radius in the forearm;

see figure 10.A-4), a disrotatory action of the leg (Subsection 8.B, page 298) is far more subtle than in the arm.

Meniscus Injury

The knee joint is one of the largest, most fragile, and most abused joints in the body, being stressed from above by one's weight and from below by the impact of walking, jumping, etc. The fragility of the knee joint arises from the fact that the epiphyses of the three long bones (femur, tibia, and fibula) that meet at the knee, along with the patella (figure 10.B-4), are in relatively poor contact. The joint is held together instead by four ligaments: the cruciate ligaments at the back of the knee and at the patella, and two collateral ligaments at the sides of the knee joint. The medial and lateral collateral ligaments connect the femur to the tibia and to the fibula, respectively, and strongly limit sideways motion; whereas the anterior and posterior cruciate ligaments lie deep within the joint and connect the femur to the tibia, limiting rotation and forward motion of the tibia (figure 10.B-4**c**). The lower leg can be rotated axially only when the knee is flexed.

The ends of the two bones forming a joint generally have the hills and valleys on one end matching the valleys and hills of the other; i.e., they are more or less congruent, as is the case with the ball-and-socket joint of the hip, for example. When the ends of two bones meeting in a joint are spatially congruent, then the cartilage separating and lubricating them can be very thin. Conversely, in the knee, where the congruency of the femur and tibia is weak, the meniscal cartilage is much thicker and is deeply dimpled so as to accommodate the two condyles of the femur. On knee flexion, as in *utkatasana* (figure 10.B-4**d**), the femoral condyle glides forward and acts to crush the meniscus. Perhaps this is why opening of the knee joint with a soft towel placed behind the flexed knee often reduces knee pain, by pulling the tibial and femoral bones apart at the knee joint. Healthy cartilage rebounds after being deformed, if one rests, but if the load is heavy and constant, then there can be an irreversible deformation of the cartilage due to viscoelastic flow.

Just as with the intervertebral discs within the spine during rest (Section 8.C, page 303), when the loading on the menisci of the knees is relaxed by lying down, the menisci flow back into their unstressed shapes. Many of the therapeutic *yogasana* approaches to knee pain involve placing a passive element (rolled towel, mat, ropes, etc.) behind the knee and then bending the knee, heel to buttock as in *triangamukhaikapada paschimottanasana* [825]. This procedure allows the quadriceps muscle to stretch while keeping the knee joint open, so that the meniscus is not crushed in the process. Improper action at the knee joint can destroy the meniscus that otherwise keeps the femur and tibia from rubbing directly against one another. Should a meniscus become frayed, particles of tissue may float freely within the joint and then become painfully enmeshed between the bones of the joint, inhibiting motion at that place. This seems to be a rather common injury among those who insist on pulling the legs into *padmasana*-type postures while stiff in the pelvic area (see Box 10.B-1, page 352). When the femoral condyle rubs on the iliotibial band (a long tendon running from the iliac crest to the lateral edge of the tibia), as when the angle at the knee changes, there can be a resultant pain at the knee due to friction between the band and the knee joint. There is a predisposition toward this in the bowlegged, in those with a tight iliotibial band, and in those who do not warm up properly. The iliotibial band is stretched in *maricyasana III*. A strong and chronic contraction of the psoas results in a chronic stretching of the gluteus maximus, and this in turn can stress the femoral-tibial joint, leading to patellar tendinitis.

When abnormal rotations of the lower leg, as in *padmasana, mulabandhasana*, etc., act to tear the menisci in the knees, most often it is the medial meniscus that is injured [884], because it is less able to move. The risk for such knee injuries is much lower when the knee does not bear weight when torqued in such maneuvers. Bursitis of the knee is promoted by standing on the knees on a hard floor (as when in *ustrasana, adho mukha virasana*, or *parighasana)* without padding. Because the joints are not highly vascularized, they are cooler than surrounding muscular tissue. As this is especially true of the knee joint [415], a knee joint that feels as warm as the surrounding muscles is inflamed.

Support on a Bent Leg

When in the standing postures with one leg flexed at the knee (such as *parsvakonasana* and *virabhadrasanas I* and *II*), the bent leg most easily supports the body weight if the knee of the bent leg is just over the ankle of that leg, for in this position, the tibia is vertical and the skeleton is ideally positioned for supporting the body weight, just as is the case when standing on straight legs in *tadasana* (figure 9.B-4c). In these postures, it is largely the skeleton that supports the weight, whereas the muscles have the less demanding job of holding the bones in place. If, instead, the knee is allowed to move forward of the ankle, then the roles of muscles and bones are reversed, with the muscles having the larger responsibility of holding the posture in place. Because the muscles are weaker than the bones, the duration over which one can manage to hold these positions having one leg bent is least if the knee is forward of the ankle (as when in *utkatasana)*; even when the ankle and knee are in vertical alignment, the task is easier if one slightly lifts the toes and takes considerably more of the weight of the posture onto the heel of the forward leg, thereby insuring that the tibia is in parallel alignment with the gravitational field, Section V.B, page 884.

Gender Effects on Knee Injuries

In regard to anatomy, the patella slides in a groove in the femur, and the tibia and the femur are separated by the medial and lateral menisci. Ideally, the condyles of the femur rest squarely upon the head of the corresponding tibia. If, however, there is a left-right imbalance or a front-to-back imbalance, then there will be an uneven load on the articulating surfaces and on the ligaments and/or an uneven stress on the menisci between the bones of the upper and lower legs. These menisci are easily injured by twisting the knee or even by deep knee bending. The cruciate ligaments connect the tibia and the femur and crisscross within the knee joint. These too are easily injured by rapid twisting [331]. Among collegiate athletes, women have four to eight times more knee injuries involving the anterior cruciate ligament than do men, the causes being poor exercise training and/or hormonal imbalances as they pass through the menstrual cycle [900, 901].

In women, their wider pelvis increases the Q angle at which the femoral head meets the tibia (figure 10.B-1a) and so increases the load and stress on the lateral sides of the knee joints. The larger the Q angle, the stronger is the lateral force on the patella, leading to knee pain. In turn, this off-center loading affects the anterior cruciate ligament, which then wears and more readily tears. Moreover, in women, the quadriceps are generally stronger than the hamstrings, whereas in men, they are more nearly equal. The inequality of the quadriceps and hamstring strengths in women also strains the anterior cruciate ligament, which could be put yet further in danger by menstruation, which acts to loosen ligaments at that time.

In contrast to the situation at the elbow, the possibility of the corresponding forward-backward hyperextension of the knee is controlled in part by the tension in the joint capsule and by the ligaments and tendons surrounding the joint, and so it is much more frequently a problem for women, as when in *trikonasana,* for example [430]. The anterior cruciate ligament limits the extension of the leg and lengthens yet more when the leg is put into hyperextension; it tears more easily than the posterior cruciate ligament. Note also the adverse effect on the knees of wearing high-heeled shoes (page 347).

The Q Angle

The angle between the shafts of the femur and the tibia, called the Q angle (figure 10.B-1a), is about 50 percent larger in women than in men, due to the generally wider hips in the former. The Q angle is a measure of the nonlinearity of the bones in the upper and lower leg, just as the carrying angle in the arm is a measure of the nonlinearity of the bones of the upper and lower arm (figure 10.A-4c). The large Q angle in the legs of women (approximately 16°) aggravates

tendencies toward tearing the anterior cruciate ligament, patellofemoral pain, pronated ankles, and fallen arches. Additionally, one might expect large Q angles to lead to the eventual weakness in the pelvic floor and misalignment or imbalance of the higher muscles of the deep front line [603] (Section 9.A, page 312).

Nonlinear Legs

Considering the plumb line between the center of the ankle and the center of the hip joint when standing with the legs straight, the centers of the knee joints can fall either on this line, to the inside of the line, or to the outside of the line, leading to straight and aligned legs, bowed legs, or knock-kneed legs, respectively (figures 10.B-1a, 10.B-1b, and 10.B-1c). The latter two conditions can arise when there is an insufficiency of vitamin D in the diet in the early years, so that the long bones of the legs, being overly flexible, bend either outward or inward under the compressive stress of gravity [878]. As shown for the right leg in figure 10.B-1b, in bowed legs, the knee joint bears unbalanced stress on the medial aspect; the lateral aspect of the knee joint bears the stress in the case of knock-knees (figure 10.B-1c). Unless the knee joints can be brought back into alignment, the asymmetrical stress shown in the figure can be an open door to osteoarthritis at the points of stress. Legs that have been formed in the bowed configuration (figure 10.B-1b) have a "natural" lateral rotation of the anterior femur bone, which can be an advantage in *baddha konasana* but a disadvantage in *urdhva dhanurasana*. Legs that have been formed in the knock-kneed configuration (figure 10.B-1c) have a "natural" medial rotation of the anterior femur bone, which can be an advantage in *virasana*, but a disadvantage in *tadasana*.

Lubrication

As the primary task of the ligaments in the knee is to bind the joint and keep it stable, there is no elastic tissue in these ligaments, and they cannot be stretched without consequences [833]. The ends of the bones not only are covered in smooth-sliding cartilage, but they are also separated in part by thick, cushioning cartilaginous pads

Box 10.B-1: A Safe Way to Practice and Teach *Padmasana*

Located as they are at either end of the femur, the knee and hip joints are intimately interdependent, with injury to the knee joint occurring more frequently than to any other joint in the body. The following prescription will take a student toward full *padmasana* by loosening the hip joints without endangering the knee joints due to unnecessary torque. The scheme is based on the idea that putting the first leg into *ardha padmasana* is relatively safe and that injuries arise from bending the second leg and then trying to lift its foot high enough to rest on the thigh of the first. It is this lift and rotation that should come totally from the outward rotation of the anterior femur and of the femoral head in the hip joint but often involves too much improper rotation at the knee joint and so puts it at risk [146, 391]. Students interested in finding a safe way to approach *padmasana* should consider the scheme given below, moving through the steps in order and only moving on when they have mastered the previous steps.

1. Start in *dandasana*, and bend the right knee toward the right shoulder, pulling the right heel to the right buttock. Keeping the deep flexure at the knee, roll the knee to the right, and holding the ankle from below, position the bent leg so that the right heel rests high on the left thigh, with the right heel in the left groin *(ardha padmasana)*. If you are unable to do this, sit on a block and practice going into and coming out of *ardha padmasana*.

2. Now bend the left leg, and let the full length of the left shin, ankle to knee, rest on a bolster.

3. With the left knee held above the floor by the thickness of the bolster, can you release the right groin, rotate the anterior femur laterally, and take up the slack by contraction in the right buttock, so as to bring the right knee to a level **below** that of the left foot? If so, then …

4. *Padmasana* is achieved without risk to the knees by first depressing the thigh of the bent leg in *ardha padmasana*, so that the second shin does not have to be lifted to be put in place. With this in mind, slide the left foot **horizontally** into its place on the right thigh without lifting its ankle with respect to its knee. Adjust the feet so as to keep the knees as close as possible to one another; tip back momentarily, and push the bolster away, so that both thighs can rest on the ground. Because the hip joint is so much more robust than the knee joint, the former must always defer to the latter in questions of alignment and risk [146].

5. When in the *padmasana* position, bring the two feet into the dorsiflexed position, soles of the feet oriented laterally rather than facing upward. If the feet are sickled upward, the ligaments of the ankle can be overstretched, and the setting of the head of the fibula near the knee joint also can be disturbed [146]. This strong-foot action in *padmasana* can make the posture less compact top to bottom, but this is worth tolerating, as it does protect the knee.

6. Once in *padmasana,* the top shin often presses strongly on the bottom shin, so that when coming out of the posture, it is tempting to first lift the top shin. Resist this temptation, for it will torque the knee in the manner we are trying to avoid.

Instead, slide each knee **sideways** so that there is no upward motion of the top shin. Exiting in this way, the posture ends in a cross-legged sitting position looking much like *swastikasana*.

An intermediate position that helps to loosen the relevant muscles of the pelvis without threatening the knee is a useful preparation for full *padmasana*. From a seated position, bend the right leg so that the shin is parallel to the front edge of the mat. Place the left ankle at the right knee, and then slowly depress the left knee toward the right ankle, using the leg and hip action appropriate to *baddha konasana*. Eventually, the shins will come to rest one over the other, and the legs will form an equilateral triangle with 60° angles at each of the three joints: right knee, left knee, and pubic symphysis. An approach closely related to that presented here for teaching *padmasana* in a safe way is presented by Farhi [237], along with appropriate warm-up *yogasanas* to loosen the hips in preparation for lifting the second leg into place.

When the legs are placed in *padmasana,* each of the ankles presses inward on the upper inner thigh of the opposite leg; i.e., upon the femoral artery of that leg (figure 14.C-2**a**). This pressure on a major artery is thought to restrict the flow of blood to the lower body and thereby to alter the flow of blood throughout the body. The well-known meditative state of mind induced by this posture may well be related to the altered course of blood flow induced by the placement of the ankles on the femoral arteries. Note that *padmasana* would be contraindicated in someone with preexisting circulation problems in the legs, such as varicosities (Subsection 14.C, page 561).

Unfortunately, placing the feet as described above also puts pressure on the sciatic nerves running from the lower spine to the toes of each leg. The case of a meditator who fell asleep for more than three hours in *padmasana* (Subsection II.B, page 835) is instructive: there was eventual loss of nervous sensation in the right lateral femoral cutaneous nerve (tingling became numbness), as evidenced by the loss of sensitivity to pinprick, temperature, and light touch on the skin on the inside of the right thigh [546]. A similar report of a meditating student in *muktasana* for two hours showed that the compression on the medial components of the sciatic nerve (right leg) caused demyelination and axonal degeneration of this nerve, leading to foot drop [876]. Unfortunately, in neither case was it reported which leg was placed over the other. In any event, one must be wary of remaining for a matter of hours in any of the *yogasanas* or of falling asleep in them, especially if there is any pressure on the nerves.

(the menisci), and the entire structure is bathed by the synovial fluid within the joint capsule. Up to a dozen bursae also contribute to protecting the knee from the high pressures, repetitive movements, and rubbing experienced by this joint.

The momentary load on the knee joint when the foot strikes the ground while walking is four times the body weight, and this increases to eight times the body weight when running. Done to excess, these activities can break down or irritate the cartilage of the knee and lessen the extent of lubrication, possibly leading to arthritis (see below) and/or bursitis in and around the joint.

Protecting the Knee

It is of prime importance to *yogasana* students and their teachers that they understand that the knee is constructed to bend like a hinge; rota-

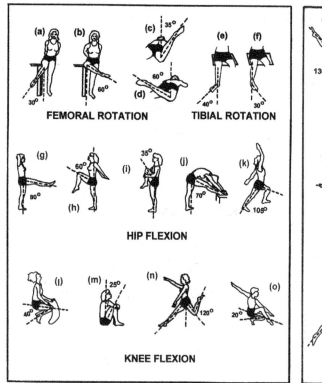

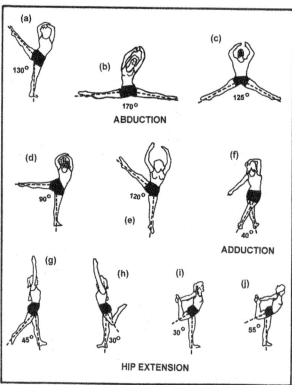

Figures 10.B-5 and 10.B-6. Angles of the legs, as found by Kapandji for normal, untrained subjects in various dance positions [430].

tion around any axis other than the hinge axis risks damage to the ligaments and the menisci. Realization of this limitation on the motion permissible around the knee joint is of special importance when performing a posture such as *padmasana*, where tightness in the hip joint can force the knee into a risky position if force is used to cross the legs. (See Box 10.B-1, above, for a discussion of a safe way to approach *padmasana*.)

Synopsis of Leg Actions

Kapandji [430] gives an exhaustively complete discussion of the various actions of the muscles, bones, ligaments, and tendons in the legs; as only a brief synopsis of this information is given here, the student interested in a deeper discussion is referred to that encyclopedic work and to the book of Calais-Germain [101]. Figures 10.B-5 and 10.B-6 from Kapandji show the ranges of motion typical for the legs of those who do not

practice *yogasana* or ballet and so give*s yogasana* teachers a rough guide as to what their beginning students will be capable of doing. For example, outward rotation of the bent-leg thigh in beginners, as seen from the front, will be about twice as large as the inward rotation, etc. The ranges of angular motion for action of the leg at the hip joint are summarized in figure 10.A-3b.

Bones of the Lower Leg

Allowed Motions

Just below the knee joint, one has the tibia, the straightest bone of the body, connecting the knee joint to the talus bone of the foot (figure 10.B-1a) [101, 430, 863]. The second bone of the lower leg, the fibula (figure 10.B-1a), does not articulate with the femur but lies parallel to the tibia and is connected to it by a web of inelastic, interosseous connective tissue, which helps to

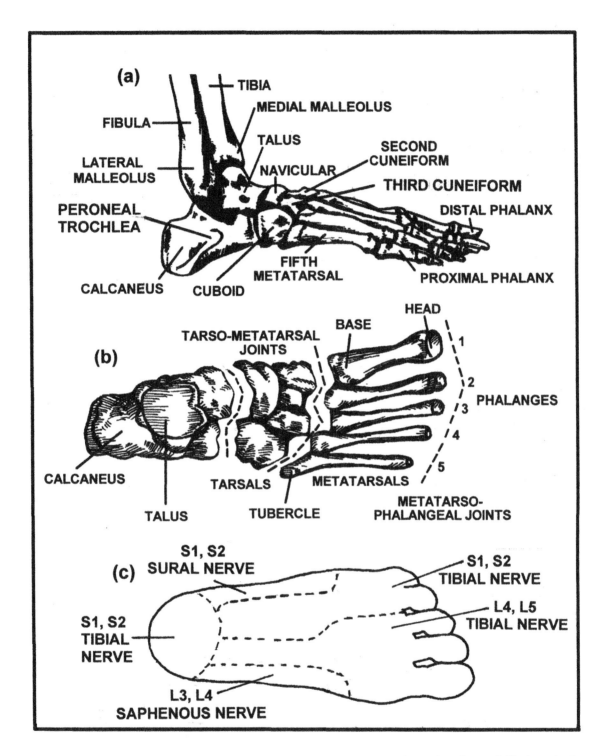

Figure 10.B-7. (a) The bones of the lower leg and the foot, showing how the tibia and fibula articulate with the talus of the right foot, as seen from the right. (b) Superior view of the bones of the right foot, as separated into the regions of the calcaneus and talus bones, the anterior tarsal bones, the tarsometatarsal joint separating the tarsal bones from the metatarsal bones, and the metatarsophalangeal joints between the metatarsals and the phalanges (not shown here, but appearing in panel a). (c) The zones of cutaneous neural innervation of the sole of the left foot by tibial, sural, and saphenous branches of the sciatic nerve, also showing the nerve rootlets involved.

support the leg and to control rotation of the two bones as the foot moves [764]. Being the thinnest bone in the body in relation to its length, the fibula carries only 10 percent of the weight pressing on the knees from above [61a]. The lower ends of the fibula and tibia meet at the talus to form the ankle joint (figures 10.B-7**a** and 10.B-8**b**).

The Ankle Joint

As discussed above, the proximal ends of the tibia and fibula mate rather poorly with the distal end of the femur bone above them, forming a knee joint of relative instability. In a similar way, the two distal ends of the tibia and fibula meet at the talus to form the ankle joint. Though there are no condyles in this case, the distal ends of the tibia and fibula nonetheless are flared so as to form a crude cup, into which the talus fits. The limiting edges of this cup appear as the lateral malleolus of the fibula and the medial malleolus of the tibia (figure 10.B-1**a**). Again, as with the knee joint, the ankle joint is relatively unstable due to the low congruency of the bones involved. Though there are neither muscular origins or insertions on the talus, the talus rests upon the calcaneus and can be moved indirectly by the surrounding muscles and bones. The connection of the foot to the tibia and fibula of the lower leg is through the talus, using a joint that allows limited motion in almost all directions (figure 10.B-7**a**). The talus is supported by the action of the metatarsal heads on the floor, with the front of the talus most supported by the downward action of the metatarsal heads of the innermost three toes; the back of the talus is supported by the downward action of the metatarsal heads of the outermost two toes (see figure 10.B-7**c** for innervation of these segments of the foot). Thus, when standing in *tadasana* with the heads of all five metatarsals of each foot actively engaged with the floor, both the front and the back edges of the talus are being lifted upward.

Dorsiflexion and Plantar Flexion

When the foot is in dorsiflexion, the foot rotates about the ankle joint so that the dorsal (upper) surfaces of the foot and the toes move toward the knee, whereas the heel moves away from

the knee, as for the back foot in *parsvottanasana*. In contrast, when the foot is in plantar flexion, the plantar surface of the foot (the sole) and the toes move away from the knee, and the heel moves toward the knee, as in *purvottanasana*. The structure being flexed when the foot is in plantar flexion is a broad, thick aponeurosis lying between the muscles and skin of the sole of the foot; it is anchored at one end to the calcaneus and to the balls of the foot at the other.

We speak here of dorsiflexion as involving the flexion of the ankle and not of the toes, yet the toes too can be either dorsiflexed (toes lifted toward shins) or plantar flexed (toes curled toward soles). Moreover, note that one can place the ankle in plantar flexion and the toes in dorsiflexion simultaneously, as when standing on tiptoes. It can be confusing to the student if we speak of "dorsiflexion" and "plantar flexion" and do not explain whether we are speaking of the toes, the ankles, or both.

Muscles of the Lower Leg

Triceps Surae and Dorsiflexion

The gastrocnemius or calf muscle (figure 11.A-2) is most interesting in that it spans two joints, the knee and the ankle, much as the hamstring spans both the hip joint and the knee; the gastrocnemius can act on either joint separately but not on both simultaneously. The gastrocnemius muscle (with two heads) and the soleus (with one head) are often considered as one muscle, the triceps surae. As discussed in Subsection 11.A, page 411, the gastrocnemius and soleus muscles of the lower leg are of distinctly different muscle-twitch types.

When the ankle is in plantar flexion, the joint is in fact extended, but the knee joint at the same time tends to be flexed; whereas when the foot is dorsiflexed at the ankle, knee flexion is inhibited (Subsection 10.B, page 360) [788]. In virtually all of the *yogasanas*, the extension of the inner heel and the base of the big toe (the head of the first metatarsal) are basic to straightening the leg and to spreading the toes laterally. Also, in most *yogasana* postures, the foot is held at such an angle that there is equal tension in the calcaneal (Achilles) tendon (Subsection 7.D, page 244) at the back of the ankle and in the extensor hallucis longus tendon at the front of the ankle.

The range of dorsiflexion of the ankle is larger when the knee is bent and the gastrocnemius is relaxed. This ankle flexion is of great value in straightening the leg; as Kapandji [430] states, the rectus femoris of the quadriceps is not strong enough by itself to fully extend the leg. On the other hand, the quadriceps muscles are said to be twice as strong as the hamstrings [833]. The triceps surae, which drives plantar flexion of the ankle, is about four times stronger than the muscles that drive dorsiflexion.

When the leg is straight, the entire triceps surae is stretched as when in *ardha uttanasana* and so tends to pull the heel of the foot toward the knee; however, when the leg is bent, as in *utkatasana,* the gastrocnemius is partially relaxed, and only the soleus is fully stretched. Note too that when in *utkatasana,* the combined vectorial addition of the tensile forces on the tendons at the knee upon simultaneous partial contraction of the gastrocnemius and the hamstrings acts to straighten the leg; in contrast, if the foot is not bearing weight, each of these contractions flexes the knee [101]. For this reason, students in *utkatasana* must be encouraged continuously to bend deeper into the posture.

Dorsiflexion and Straight Legs

As mentioned by Cole [146], contraction of the gastrocnemius both places the foot into plantar flexion and tends to flex the knee. Consequently, in order to stretch the gastrocnemius, one must both dorsiflex the foot and extend the heel so as to straighten the leg; a bent-knee calf stretch with a bending angle of 15–20° at the knee stretches only the soleus.

The tendon of peroneus longus inserts on the first metatarsal head, while the origin is contiguous with the tendon of the biceps femoris of the hamstrings at its lower end, the two meeting at the head of the fibula [603]. Moreover, the biceps femoris winds from the outside of the knee and is bound to the ischium of the pelvis; the combination of the peroneus longus, the biceps femoris, and their tendons, taken together, form a foot-to-pelvis path that Myers [603] describes as a part of the "spiral line anatomy train." Inasmuch as the biceps femoris of the upper leg originates on the ischium of the pelvis, this spiral line path may lie behind the tendency of the collapse of the medial arch of the foot (between points **1** and **3** in figure 10.B-8c) to promote collapse of the lumbar spine and thence lower-back pain [517].

Bones of the Foot

Though the anatomies of the hand and the foot superficially are very similar, the hand (with twenty-six bones and thirty-three joints) is constructed so as to have maximum flexibility and maneuverability, whereas the foot (also with twenty-six bones and thirty-three joints), being stiffer and stronger than the hand, is constructed to provide maximum support and cushioning. As with the hand, the foot also has a cutaneous nervous system innervated by the tibialis nerve, a branch of the sciatic nerve, which is divided into four major components on the sole of the foot; one component serves the fourth and fifth phalanges and their metatarsals, and another serves the first through third phalanges and their metatarsals (figure 10.B-7c). This pattern of innervation on the sole of the foot leads to a local autonomy of contraction of individual muscles of the foot, so that various combinations of muscle contraction are available in aid of maintaining the left-right balance while standing on the foot.

Motions

Motion of the ankle at the joint between the bones of the lower leg and the talus allows only dorsiflexion and plantar flexion, but these two motions have large ranges; other apparent motions of the ankle involve bones of the foot other than the talus. For example, the foot can be rocked into the inversion and eversion postures (figure V.B-1b) due to the condyle-like features of the lower calcaneus rocking within the mat-

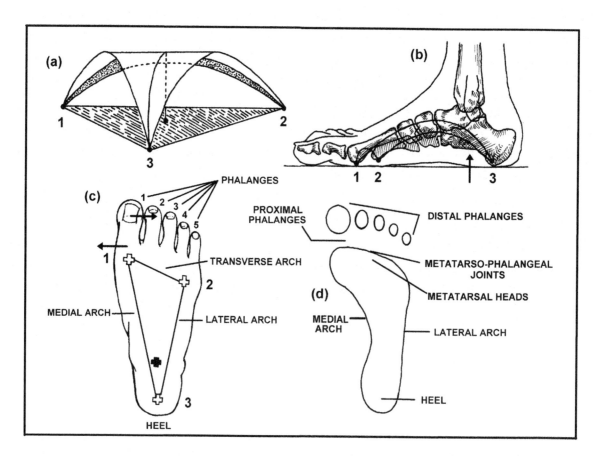

Figure 10.B-8. (a) A systematic display of the three arches of the foot between points 1–2, 1–3, and 2–3, with the point of applied pressure (where the body weight comes into the foot) represented by the vertical dashed line. (b) The three arches of the foot, as drawn appropriate to the anatomy of the foot. The arrow represents the position of the talus, this being where the weight of the body presses on the sole of the foot most directly. (c) The dorsal plan of the foot, with the open crosses showing the lowest points of the three arches and the filled cross marking the point of application of the body weight when standing in *tadasana* [430]. The two horizontal arrows represent the movement of the proximal and distal ends of the first phalanx when contorted by hallux valgus so as to form a bunion. (d) The footprint of the right foot, showing that only certain parts of the foot are in contact with the floor (the distal parts of the phalanges, the metatarsal heads, the lateral arch, and the heel) and others (the proximal phalanges and the medial arch) are not.

ing structures of the cuboid and navicular bones (figure 10.B-7a).

The range of motion for dorsiflexion of the ankle is larger when the knee is bent, for in this case, the flexion does not involve having to stretch the gastrocnemius. Similarly, the talus is gripped more strongly when the foot is dorsiflexed, and so the joint is more stable than when in plantar flexion.

Because dorsiflexion of the ankle is assisted by contraction of the gastrocnemius muscle, if the knee is bent, the gastrocnemius is relaxed, and

therewith, the dorsiflexion of the ankle is relaxed in part. Correspondingly, it is more difficult to dorsiflex the ankle when the leg is straight. When sitting in a chair with the foot of the bent leg on the floor, the foot may be turned inward or outward; however, this is not an allowed movement of the ankle, for the rotation is around the lower leg. When the leg is straight, as for *dandasana*, the rotation then occurs in the upper leg, again with no help from the ankle. Inversion of the foot as in *padmasana* involves both adduction and plantar flexion at the ankle, whereas eversion as when in *tadasana* involves both abduction and dorsiflexion at the ankle.

The Arches

Kapandji [430] describes the foot as "the plantar vault," consisting of three arches connected by strong but elastic muscles and ligaments (figure 10.B-8a), the combination serving as an efficient shock-absorbing system. The three arches span the distance between the heel (3) and the metatarsal head of the big toe (1) (first phalanx); between the heel (3) and the metatarsal head of the little toe (2) (fifth phalanx); and between the metatarsal heads of the big toe (1) and that of the little toe (2). The first of these (called the medial arch) is the longest and highest of the three, yet it is not the strongest, being supported only by plantar tissues and being highly prone to collapse. In contrast, the transverse arch between points 1 and 2 is the strongest, being supported by the cuneiform bones. The third arch, the lateral arch, lies between points 2 and 3 and is rather inconspicuous, as its curvature is not obvious when viewed externally.

When the weight of the body in *tadasana* presses into the talus, the weight is distributed among the three points 1, 2, and 3 of figures 10.B-8a and 10.B-8b, with point 3 bearing the most weight and point 2 the least. Pressure on the sole of the standing foot is distributed among the three arches between the points 1, 2, and 3, with the largest part of the weight being born by the medial arch between points 1 and 3 (figure 10.B-8c). In supporting the weight of the body, the arches are flattened somewhat and broadened.

The heights of the arches are sustained by ligaments and muscles in the sole of the foot and in the lower leg (tibialis and peroneus, etc.), with the ligaments handling short-term compression of the arches, as when the foot strikes the ground while jumping from *tadasana* into a straddle-leg position in preparation for *prasarita padottanasana;* the muscles handle long-term compression, as when standing for long periods of time in *trikonasana*. When not carried to excess, practice of the standing postures strengthens the feet. In general, the lateral arch is involved with weight bearing,

the transverse arch is involved with propulsion (walking, running, jumping), and the medial arch is involved with both weight bearing and shock absorption. The primary arch of the foot, the medial arch 1–3 in figure 10.B-8b, is lifted by several muscles, the strongest of which is the tibialis anterior, the antagonist to peroneus longus (see below).

In general, the foot, when bearing weight on the floor (as when in *tadasana*), should make a pattern like that of the wet footprint, being light on the distal phalanges, heavier on the metatarsal heads and the lateral arch, and heaviest on the heel, at the point shown by the arrow in figure 10.B-8b. The phalanges in this case are extended forward but do not grip the floor, and the medial arch is lifted away from the floor. Five small and relatively immobile bones in the middle of the foot form the anterior tarsal or instep section of the foot.

Alden [5a] presents a concise discussion of how to use *yogasana* practice to develop the arches of the feet, provided the problem of flat feet is functional rather than structural; i.e., provided the arches can be lifted, but that out of habit, they are allowed to fall.

The Metatarsals

Just forward of the anterior tarsal bones of the foot lie five near-parallel bones known as the metatarsals. The proximal ends of the metatarsals (the bases) are partners with the anterior tarsals in forming the relatively immobile tarsometatarsal joints (figure 10.B-7b), whereas the distal ends of the metacarpals (the heads) form highly mobile joints with the phalanges (toes) of the foot.

The distal end of each metatarsal (the metatarsal head) forms the "toe mound" associated with each toe (figure 10.B-7b). It is this part of the foot that we activate in order make the foot strong, among other things, to lift the medial arch (1–3 in figure 10.B-8b) from the floor. Notice that the fifth metatarsal has a prominent tubercle on the lateral edge; it is this bony prominence that presses the floor lightly in *anantasana* but supports significant weight (approximately 30 percent of full body weight) in *vasisthasana* (figure IV.D-2).

The Phalanges

The proximal ends of the phalanges (toes) form the tarsometatarsal joints with the distal ends of the metatarsals (figure 10.B-7**b**). In the second to fifth phalanges, the proximal and distal phalanx in each is separated by the middle phalanx; however, this is missing in phalanx 1 (the big toe). Regarding the movement of the toes, they can be dorsiflexed (as in *mulabandhasana*) and plantar flexed (as in *bhekasana*). Phalangeal dorsiflexion has a wider range of motion than does plantar flexion, and the muscles driving this dorsiflexion are stronger than those for plantar flexion, thanks to years of walking and running. Additionally, there is a weak adduction and abduction of the phalanges possible, which is experienced by respectively closing or opening the space between the toes, using the interossei muscles.

The Heels

The calcaneus bone is the heel of the foot. As seen in figure 10.B-8**b**, it contacts the floor at point **3**, somewhat behind the point at which the medial arch contacts the floor. The Achilles tendon of the triceps surae has its insertion on the calcaneus, and so contraction of the triceps surae muscle pulls the heel toward the back of the knee, and so puts the foot into plantar flexion.

When standing in *tadasana,* the weight of the body falls fully on the talus bone of the ankle and then is distributed among other points on the sole of the foot. The largest part of this weight falls at point **3** when fully erect in the posture, whereas to have equal weight on the three points **1**, **2**, and **3** of the foot implies a strong forward lean of the body.

The combination of the three terminal points of the arches of the foot when standing on the floor (**1**, **2**, and **3**) and the center point of the ankle joint forms a tetrahedron of unusual strength (figure 10.B-8**a**), provided the vertices of the tetrahedron are in their proper positions [438a].

Extrinsic Muscles and Foot Action

In our discussion of the muscular structure of the eye (Section 17.A, page 657), a clear distinction was drawn between those muscles outside of the eyeball, which act to point it, and those within the eyeball, which act to control various optical parameters of the eye (focus, pupillary diameter, etc.). Exactly the same distinction must be drawn in regard to the muscles of the lower leg and foot. That is, there are intrinsic muscles totally within the foot that control the posture and certain movements of the foot's components, and there are extrinsic muscles with origins outside the foot but with insertions within the foot, which are also important in the foot's posture and movement. It is important to make this distinction between intrinsic and extrinsic muscles clear when thinking about the lower leg and foot.

Peroneus Longus and Peroneus Brevis

The peroneus longus muscle (figure 11.A-1) is very interesting and pertinent to the *yogasana* student. It has its origin just below the knee on the fibular head, runs parallel to and on the outside of the lower leg to the ankle, crosses over the bottom of the foot, and inserts at the head of metatarsal 1. As the ligament of peroneus longus crosses the calcaneus of the foot, it is hooked at a small prominence on the lateral side of the calcaneus, called the peroneal trochlea. This protuberance (figure 10.B-7**a**) serves as an anatomic pulley, turning the direction of ligament stress from parallel to the tibia to perpendicular as the ligament crosses the sole of the foot. It performs a similar action for the ligament of peroneus brevis.

The entire peroneus longus muscle appears to be about 25 percent contractive tissue and 75 percent tendonous connective tissue. When the peroneus longus is contracted so as to form a "racing stripe" on the lateral area of the calf, the metatarsal head of the big toe on the underside of the foot is pulled toward the metatarsal head of the little toe, and the foot is plantar flexed. This plantar flexion of the foot is assisted by two other muscles in the lower leg. The peroneus brevis muscle follows the course of peroneus longus on the lateral side of the lower leg, lying just beneath it. However, its insertion at the bottom of the foot is on the head of the fifth metatarsal, whereas that for the peroneus longus is on the head of the first metatarsal. When in *dandasana,* for example, co-contraction of these two muscles will press the head of the first metatarsal forward and pin it in space, while the head of the fifth metatarsal is pulled backward and away from the first metatarsal. The net result is that the foot is pulled toward the strong *yogasana* everted position, even though it remains in plantar flexion.[10] The action of the peroneus longus also flattens the transverse arch of the foot (arch **1–2** in figure 10.B-8c).

This action of the peroneus muscles is independent of the angle at the knee, since the muscles do not cross the knee joint, unlike the situation when the gastrocnemius muscle is used for plantar flexion of the ankle.

Anterior Tibialis

The antagonist to the peroneus longus is the anterior tibialis [302, 613], running from its origin on the lateral side of the upper tibia to its insertion on the upper surface of the base of the first phalanx. Contraction of anterior tibialis is evident as a noticeable thickening of the tissue at midshin on the lateral side of the tibia when the ankle is dorsiflexed. This muscle is the strongest ankle dorsiflexor in the leg; however, because it inserts in part on the upper surface of the base of metatarsal 1, it tends to place the foot in inversion as well. Though contraction of this muscle tends to pull the foot into inversion, its simultaneous contraction with the peroneus longus puts the dorsiflexed foot into eversion. Co-contraction of the peroneus longus, peroneus brevis, and anterior tibialis results in dorsiflexion at the ankle,

phalangeal abduction, eversion of the foot, the lifting of the medial arch, and the full assumption of the *yogasana* strong foot (Subsection 10.B, page 362).

When the hamstrings are contracted with the leg straight or bent, contraction of the peroneus longus not only dorsiflexes the foot but also rolls the anterior aspect of the knee inward. This explains why we strongly dorsiflex the feet using the peroneus longus when in *bakasana* or other such leg-on-arm balances, for this presses the knees against the arms and so stabilizes the posture [276].

The peroneus longus and anterior tibialis muscles, together with peroneus brevis, are very active in maintaining balance in the left to right direction (Subsection V.B, page 878) while standing on one foot. Balance in the front to back direction on one or two feet is aided by contraction of the muscles flexor hallucis longus and flexor digitorum longus, which place the phalanges and their metatarsals into plantar flexion against the floor. The peroneus longus and the tibialis posterior muscles crossing at the bottom of the foot form a sling that is crucial in supporting the medial and lateral arches.

Intrinsic Muscles and Foot Action

Whereas the external muscles of the foot have their origins on the tibia and fibula of the lower legs and insert on the bones of the foot, the intrinsic/internal muscles of the foot connect one foot bone to another and are found largely between the metatarsal bones and the sole of the foot.

Interossei

There are four layers of muscles lying between the sole of the foot and the metatarsal bones. The deepest of the four muscular layers contains the four interossei muscles connecting each of the metatarsals to its neighbors by bipennate muscles (figure 11.A-13c). Because either of the two sides of the bipennate interossei muscle can be contracted independently of the other side, contractions of the sides of the bipennate muscles that are closer to the first phalanx will pull phalanges

---

10   When the foot is moved from the anatomic position so that the mound of the little toe is pressed away from the hip on its side, while that of the big toe in pulled closer to the hip, the action is termed inversion; whereas when the mound of the little toe is pulled toward the hip and that of the big toe is pushed away, then the action is termed eversion (figure V.B-1b) [613].

2–5 toward phalanx 1, whereas contraction of the sides of the interossei muscles closer to phalanx 5 will spread phalanges 2–5 toward phalanx 5 and lower the height of the transverse arch **1–2** (figure 10.B-8c). Spreading of the interossei of the foot reflexively tends to straighten the legs.

Innervation

According to Netter [613], there are several dermatome systems innervating the skin on the sole of the foot (figure 10.B-7c). On the lateral side, the dermatome (Section 13.D, page 530) covering the fourth and fifth phalanges has its dorsal roots at S1 and S2. The skin covering the first three phalanges has its own dermatome at dorsal root L4, and receptors in the skin on the central portion of the foot report to L5. The very high density of pressure sensors, specifically in the skin of the first phalanx (figure 13.B-2a), is likely related to this specific L4 innervation. The peroneus longus and brevis muscles are innervated by the superficial peroneal nerves, and the anterior tibialis is innervated by the deep peroneal nerve.

Plantar Fascia

The fibrous plantar fascial tissue on the bottom of the foot (the plantar aponeurosis) stretches from heel to toe and acts as a bowstring for the formation of the medial arch and so helps to keep the arch from collapsing. Pressure on the bottom of the foot can lengthen the plantar fascia, thereby leading to a painful condition known as plantar fasciitis. On occasion, the pull of the plantar fascia on the bottom of the foot is so strong that the periosteum normally covering the heel bone (calcaneus) is pulled away from it. In that case, the void between the calcaneus and the periosteum is filled by the action of the osteoblasts (Subsection 7.C, page 235), with the resultant formation of painful bony projections called heel spurs.

The strong-foot position of Iyengar yoga (figure 10.B-9c) stretches the plantar fascia ligaments at the bottom of the foot and so eases the pain of plantar fasciitis. For an intense stretch of the muscles of the lower leg and foot, take *parsvot-tanasana* with the front foot up the wall and the back heel on the floor.

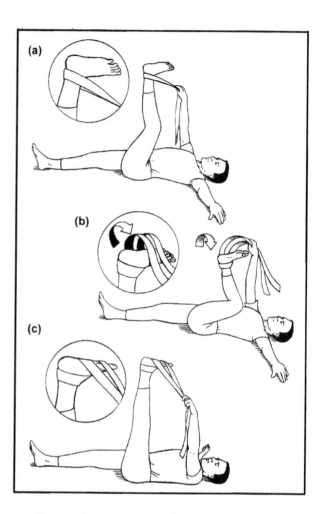

Figure 10.B-9. Using a belt to simulate the action of the peroneus longus, peroneus brevis, and anterior tibialis muscles on the left leg. (a) With the left leg bent somewhat, encircle the ankle of the left foot with the belt, and hold the ends of the belt in the right hand. (b) With the left leg fully bent, take the belt over the sole of the foot, moving it in the counter-clockwise direction, and (c) holding the belt in the left hand with a slight downward pull, straighten the left leg.

Three Steps to Strong *Yogasana* Feet

External Actions

The feet of the beginning student in repose generally will be more or less in inversion, plantar flexed, and with the toes crowded together, whereas the strong feet appropriate to *yogasana* practice should be more or less everted, dorsiflexed, and with the toes spread wide. This strengthening of the feet can be attained in three simple steps, framed in terms of the muscles described above. As a specific example, imagine the student in *dandasana* with feet inverted, plantar flexed, and toes pressed together.

1. Dorsiflex the foot by contraction of the anterior tibialis muscle. This will bring the sole of the foot into a vertical plane but somewhat inverted at the ankle (figure V.B-1**b**); i.e., the sole of the foot will be rotated to face somewhat medially.
2. With the anterior tibialis activated, co-contract the peroneus longus and peroneus brevis as well, in order to rotate the foot into eversion (figure V.B-1**b**), with the head of the first metatarsal pressed forward and that of the fifth metatarsal pulled backward, toward the hip.
3. Maintaining the contractions in the previous step, activate the interossei muscles lying between the metatarsals on the sole of the foot, in order to separate the second to fifth phalanges from each other and from the first phalanx.

These steps can be used irrespective of whether the foot is in the air or must stay strong in order to resist gravitational collapse of the arches when on the ground.

The strong-foot action developed in steps 1–3 above also can be achieved in the beginner by wrapping a belt, as shown in figures 10.B-9**a** to 10.B-9**c**. Once wrapped as in the figure, pulling down on the belt simulates the pull of the peroneus longus, anterior tibialis, and peroneus brevis and everts the foot. Though demonstrated in the figure for *supta padangusthasana*, the three-step belt technique works regardless of the posture.

These three steps to a strong *yogasana* foot are appropriate to virtually every one of the *yogasana* postures one might perform at the beginner and intermediate level, irrespective of whether the leg is bent or flexed. Note here that the feet are properly in plantar flexion in *purvottanasana* and are strongly in inversion when in *padmasana*, but

there otherwise will be relatively few exceptions to the three-step suggestion given above.

Spreading the Toes

When the sole of the foot is on the floor, the toes can be spread by hooking the flesh of the first phalanx by everting the foot on the floor (figure V.B-1**b**) and then pulling the remaining phalanges laterally away. In many students, the action that separates the toes seems to work subconsciously but in sympathy with the action that separates the fingers. Thus, in some students, the spreading of the toes is aided by consciously spreading the fingers.

If one insists on wearing tight shoes that leave no room for the toes, then one can look forward to the painful formation of bunions on the big toes. In this deformity, there is a partial dislocation of the big toe (the first phalanx), with the proximal phalanx being displaced medially and the distal phalanx displaced laterally so as to overlap the second phalanx (arrows in figure 10.B-8**c**), all of which induces bone spurs and inflammation of the bursae in this area. This bunion condition of the big toe is called hallux valgus.

If the interossei muscles that spread the toes are weak while the flexor digitorum brevis is strong, the result is a claw foot, in which the middle and proximal phalanges are so strongly flexed toward the floor that the tips of these toes press the floor when standing. Such claw feet are often seen in beginners performing the standing postures. This foot posture stands in strong contrast to the desired posture, in which the toes are extended forward and lie on the floor without gripping it.

Since humans no longer climb trees, we have become the only primate species that does not have a grasping first phalange on the foot. Those among us who do not wear shoes still retain certain prehensile abilities in regard to using the toes for useful tasks, but this is lost to those of us who were raised wearing shoes [61a].

Balancing on the Foot

Our primate ancestors assumed a bipedal stance about five million years ago. Being bipedal animals, we connect to the earth through feet having many pressure sensors (see Box V.F-1, page 916). These pressure sensors, especially those associated with the big toes (first phalanges), contribute significantly to the input data from which the body's proprioceptive map is constructed, especially in regard to balancing on the feet.

As long as we continue to walk on smooth, horizontal surfaces, the pressure on the soles of the feet will be concentrated on a few local spots, which will tend to become stressed. On the other hand, if the surface is uneven, as with a cobblestone street, the increased muscle action involved in walking significantly increases the pumping of venous blood back to the heart (Subsection 14.C, page 569), significantly improves the sense of balance, and avoids local stresses. Working to balance in *vrksasana* while on a soft, rolled mat will undoubtedly work in the same way to improve balance, though it is generally not recommended that difficult balancing postures be performed on such soft surfaces (Subsection V.C, page 894).

In regard to balancing in *vrksasana,* contraction of the muscle group peroneus longus/ peroneus brevis triggered by pressure sensors in dermatome L4 results in eversion of the foot and so will be useful in countering a medial falling torque (figure V.B-1**b**), whereas contraction of the anterior tibialis muscle triggered by pressure sensors in dermatome S1 results in the inversion of the foot and so will be useful in countering a lateral falling torque in this balancing posture.

11

The Skeletal Muscles

Section 11.A: Structure and Function of Skeletal Muscle

Physical Structure

Gross Structure and Function

Skeletal muscle is both the most abundant tissue type and the most adaptable tissue in the human body, undergoing large changes of plasticity through either specific use or general disuse. Thus, at one end of the muscle-plasticity spectrum, we have the body builder, who is able to rapidly build muscle bulk by lifting weights; whereas at the other end, there is the muscular weakness and atrophy that accompany bed rest or disuse. The primary functions of muscles are to move specific parts of the body with respect to one another, to maintain a rather static posture, to help in circulation of the body fluids, and to generate body heat. In the particular case of skeletal muscles, the movement involves the bones to which the muscles are attached, whereas with cardiac and vascular-wall muscles, it is blood that is moved, and for the smooth muscles of the viscera, it is the contents of the intestines that are moved.

In contrast to the cardiac muscle and the smooth muscles of the viscera, the skeletal muscles are largely under voluntary control of the central nervous system. Note, however, that even though the skeletal muscles may be claimed to be largely

under voluntary control, in fact, *yogasana* practice shows that the "control" is often coarse and that decades of daily practice are required to gain fine control over these tissues. Of the three general types of muscle tissue, this section deals only with striated skeletal muscle; discussion of the cardiac muscle can be found in Subsection 14.A, page 536 and that for visceral (smooth) muscle is found in Chapter 19, page 704.

Our focus in this chapter will be on the detailed mechanism by which a skeletal muscle contracts, the neural circuits that activate the muscle on both the conscious and subconscious levels, how the contraction of certain muscles can be used to stretch other muscles and move the attached bones, how muscles sense when to stop stretching, and how the practice of the *yogasanas* leads to refinement of the postures, all the while increasing our awareness of who we are and how our bodies function (*svadhyaya*).

Muscles and Joints

Because the two ends of a skeletal muscle generally are attached to adjacent bones that form a joint, contraction of the muscle spanning the joint (known as the prime mover) closes the angle at the joint and so sets a part of the body in motion. Moreover, there often is a second muscle spanning the joint in question, which acts in opposition to the action of the first-mentioned muscle, so that activation of the second muscle acts to open the joint. Thus, one has, for example, the opposing actions of the quadriceps and the hamstring muscles at the knee, the first opening the angle at the knee joint by straightening the leg, and the second closing it by bending the leg. For each of these prime movers, there also may be secondary muscle synergists, which also participate in the action. Yet other muscles are joined to bones that are not in bone-to-bone contact, as, for example, the upper trapezius muscle, which is joined to the cervical vertebrae at one end and to the top rim of the scapulae (the shoulder blades) at the other. Contraction of this muscle acts to pull the scapulae toward the neck, without changing any meaningful joint angle in the process. Furthermore, the respiratory diaphragm is a skeletal muscle anchored to bone at only one end, its periphery; and in the skull, the bony plates are capable of movement with respect to the sutures, but there are no muscles in place to move them. Thus, there are multiplicities of joint/muscle combinations active in the body. Some muscles span two joints, so that both joints must be fully open in order to stretch such a muscle; this applies, for example, to the gastrocnemius muscle, which spans both the knee and the ankle and is stretched only when the knee is extended and the ankle is dorsiflexed.

In regard to *yogasana* practice, the skeletal muscles are used for (1) moving the bones in order to attain a new posture, (2) moving the bones in the new posture in order to open certain joints, and (3) holding the bones in place so that the bones support the body against the pull of gravity. In cold weather, the skeletal muscles also are used for lubricating the joints and for generating body heat through shivering. When activated in the course of *yogasana* practice, a muscle can respond in one or more of three ways: it can shorten; it can develop a force against a resistance while retaining its length; and it can elongate, but then contract if the elongation is too rapid.

In general, a "muscle movement" in *yogasana* practice involves many muscles acting simultaneously. Though muscles have anatomic individuality, they usually do not function individually in beginners [422]. However, with the body control gained through the practice of the *yogasanas*, one not only can coordinate muscle actions, but also can separate and individualize muscle movements on a very fine scale. With *yogasana* practice, these muscles also can be lengthened in ways that are

either passive or active, depending upon the circumstances.

On average, each of us has between 600 and 700 distinct muscles, which together account for 42 percent of our body weight in the case of males, and 38 percent in the case of females. The distinct muscles of the body outnumber the bones of the body by more than three to one. In the course of our evolutionary development, certain muscles have become more or less vestigial, with some of them (plantaris at the back of the knee, subclavius in the shoulder, the extrinsic ear muscles, the pyramidalis muscle of the pelvis, and the palmaris in the forearm) having disappeared altogether in substantial numbers of people, but not in all [769].

Naming the Muscles

Given that most joints consist of two bones in contact and are spanned by a muscle, when one bone moves with respect to the other on contraction of the muscle, the end of the muscle on the bone that is stationary is called the muscle's origin, and the end of the muscle on the bone that moves is called the muscle's insertion. On contraction, the insertions move toward the origins. Muscles may have more than one origin, or "head," indicated by the suffix *-ceps* in the Latin name; the triceps muscle has three origins, and the biceps has two.

Discussion of muscle movement in the context of the *yogasanas* would be most difficult without a map of the body's muscles and their identification according to their Latin names. The names and locations of the major muscles of the front body that are of interest to teachers of *yogasana* are given in figure 11.A-1; those for the back body are given in figure 11.A-2. These muscles are shown again in figure 11.A-3 but labeled in regard to their modes of action. In the discussion of muscles, we use the anatomic nomenclature of Netter [613] throughout this work. One sees clearly from the labels shown in figure 11.A-3, the opposing relationships between the placement of the flexors (muscles that fold the body and close the angles at the joints; e.g., the hamstrings in regard to the knee joint) and their antagonist oppo-

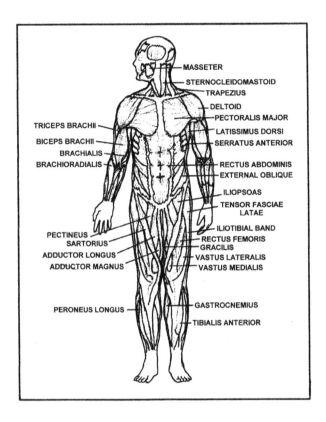

Figure 11.A-1. Illustration of the major muscles of the front body.

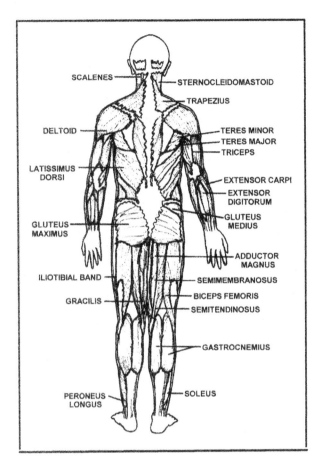

Figure 11.A-2. Illustration of the major muscles of the back body.

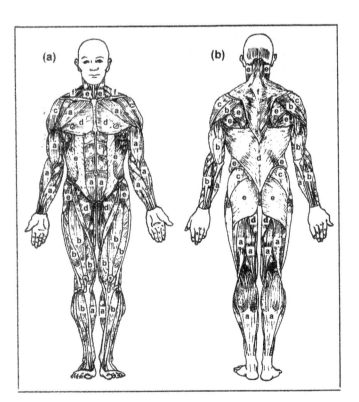

Figure 11.A-3. The muscles of the body as related to their modes of action: the flexors are labeled **a**, the extensors are labeled **b**, the abductors are labeled **c**, the adductors are labeled **d**, rotators are labeled **e**, and the scapula stabilizers are labeled **f** [431].

nents, the extensors (muscles that open the angles at the joints and work to keep one upright against the pull of gravity; e.g., the quadriceps in regard to the knee joint), and between the placement of the abductors (muscles that lift the limbs away from the center line) and the adductors (muscles that pull the limbs toward the center line). Among the rotators, there are those that rotate the forward aspect of the bone toward the midline of the body (medial rotators) and those that rotate this aspect away from the midline (lateral rotators). Pairs of muscles that work in opposition to one another such as those shown in figure 11.A-3 are discussed further below (Subsection 11.A, page 420).

The adductors and medial rotators are both more plentiful and stronger than are the abductors and the external rotators; reptiles such as the crocodile and the lizard do not even have muscles that will externally rotate the legs, and for this reason, they are able to walk forward but not backward. It is also true that the normal effect of gravity on the body is to fold it flexionally so that the joints are closed. Considering that one of the goals of *yogasana* practice at the physical level is to "open the joints," it is understandable that the emphasis of such a practice is more on extension, abduction, and lateral rotation than on flexion, adduction, and medial rotation.

Connective Tissue

Though the contractile parts of the muscle fibers congregate toward the belly of the muscle proper, the non-contractile connective tissue that envelops the muscle (the epimysium) extends beyond the ends of the contractile muscle bundles to become woven into the fabric of the periosteum covering on the adjacent bones (figure 11.A-4a and Sections 7.D, page 244, and 12.B, page 490). The bundle of connective tissue that connects the contractile part of the muscle to the bone is the muscle's tendon. The properties of tendons and a related tissue, the ligaments, as well as the joints themselves, are discussed further in Section 7.D, page 244. Deep within the muscle fibers, immobile connective tissue is found again, forming the anchors against which the microscopic contractile tissues pull (Subsection 11.A, page 381).

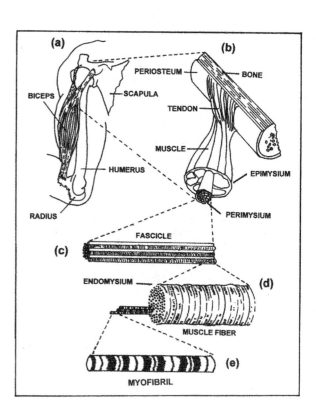

Figure 11.A-4. (a) The insertion of the biceps muscle is anchored to the radius bone of the forearm, whereas its origin is on the scapula; it thereby spans both the elbow and the shoulder joints. (b) Looking more closely, the connective tissue within and around the muscle forms a thick band of tendon at each end of the muscle, which in turn becomes an integral part of the periosteum covering the bone to which the muscle is attached. (c) A cross section of the belly of the muscle shows a parallel array of large bundles, the fascicles (d). Each cylindrical fascicle is filled with parallel skeletal muscle fibers; each muscle fiber in turn is filled with banded myofibrils (e).

Extension versus Flexion

In regard to the relative strengths of the extensor muscles and their antagonist flexor muscles, the extensors often are the stronger of the two in regard to contraction. Thus, in accidental electrocution in which the electric current is sufficiently large to contract all of the muscles in the body, the net effect is to open the body and throw it across the room in extension rather than to freeze it in a folded, flexional position. If, on the other hand, one has a stroke on one side of the brain, so that there is essentially no cerebral inhibition of the contraction of the muscles, the posture of the relevant arm is severely flexional, whereas that of the leg on the same side is severely extensional. It appears from this that the extensional quadriceps are stronger than the antagonist hamstrings, whereas the relative strengths of biceps flexion and triceps extension depend upon the circumstances. However, when the body is at rest, the muscle tone generally is stronger for flexion than it is for extension.

In *yogasana* practice, virtually all of the work is aimed toward strengthening the extensor muscles and stretching the flexors, as we move away from the fetal position and toward the spinal extension of backbends [147]. Regarding the arm, at rest, the flexors are about 50 percent stronger than the corresponding extensors, so that when the arm is in its relaxed state, it is slightly flexed. Moreover, the maximum strength of the flexors in the arm can be 40 percent larger than that in the extensors; however, this difference depends upon the rotational orientation of the arm with respect to the gravitational field (figure 11.A-5). As shown in the figure, the relative strengths of the flexors and extensors are also dependent on the abduction/adduction orientations. It follows that strength built at a particular angle does not translate easily to other angles; i.e., the shoulder strength developed by moving from *chaturanga dandasana* to the straight-arm *chaturanga dandasana* position is not necessarily useful in straightening the arms when coming into *urdhva dhanurasana* from lying on one's back.

The Motor Unit, Neural Sensitivity, and Muscular Finesse

Motor Unit Defined

Every skeletal-muscle fiber of the body is innervated by an α-motor neuron having its cell body in the spinal cord or in the brainstem; an efferent signal along the axon of such a neuron stretching from the central nervous system to the most distant muscle stimulates the muscle

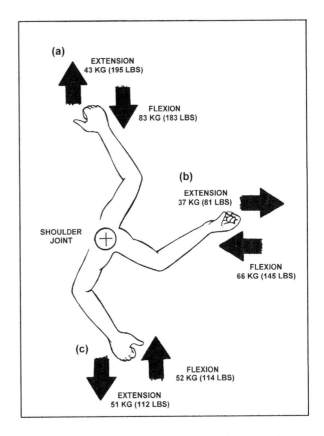

Figure 11.A-5. The relative muscle strengths for extension and flexion of the arm as a function of its orientation with respect to the shoulder [288].

to contract. However, though every muscle fiber must have an innervating neural axon if it is to contract, the number of fibers within any muscle is far larger than the number of neural axons innervating it. That is to say, every muscle fiber has a corresponding neuron connected to it for contractile excitation; however, not every muscle fiber receives a unique neural signal, for each α-motor neuron from the central nervous system branches into between ten and 2,000 sub-branches, connecting to between ten and 2,000 muscle fibers. Each of the fibers in a muscle-fiber group connected to a common α-neuron cell body (called a "motor unit" when the muscle-fiber group is considered together with its activating/branching α-motor neuron) receives the same excitation signal and at the same time, so that all muscle fibers within a motor unit contract or relax in unison.

Muscle-activation signals can originate not

Table 11.A-1: Average Characteristics of α-Motor Units in Human Muscle[a] [549]

Muscle	Location	Number of Motor Units	Number of Fibers	Fibers/Motor Unit
External rectus	Eye	2,970	27,000	9
Platysma	Face	1,096	27,000	25
First lumbrical	Hand	96	10,250	110
First dorsal interosseous	Hand	119	40,500	340
Thenar group	Hand	203	-	-
Extensor digitorum brevis	Foot	143	-	-
Biceps brachii	Upper arm	109	-	-
Brachioradialis	Forearm	333	129,500	390
Anterior tibialis	Lower leg	445	271,000	560
Gastrocnemius medial	Lower leg	579	1,030,000	1,930
Soleus	Lower leg	960	-	-
Vastus lateralis	Leg	220	-	-

a Most, but not all, of the muscles listed in this table are shown in figures 11.A-1, 11.A-2, and/or 11.A-3.

only at the spinal cord and brainstem, but at centers in the brain higher than the brainstem, i.e., at the basal ganglia, the thalamus, the reticular formation, the cerebellum, the cranial nerves, and the cerebral cortex. Neurons from these higher centers synapse in the spinal cord and brainstem with the α-motor neurons, which then extend their axons to the muscles. Muscle actions driven by signals originating in the cerebral motor cortex are conscious actions, whereas those that originate at centers in the brainstem or spinal cord are subconscious actions; actions originating in the thalamus (figure 4.B-1) are only weakly present in the conscious sphere.

Most muscles are composed of at least a hundred to as many as several thousand motor units, and all of the body motions encountered in our *yogasana* practice involve motor-unit excitations as directed by the central nervous system (Chapter 4, page 67). Table 11.A-1 lists general properties of the motor units in representative muscles in humans. In the case of small muscles with fine movement, such as the ciliary muscles of the eyes, one α-motor neuron serves to activate fewer than ten muscle fibers; whereas in the large but coarse

muscles of the leg, the ratio is more like 500 to 2,000 muscle fibers served by a single α-motor neuron [229].

Note that the values in table 11.A-1 are mean values for each muscle as measured in subjects less than sixty years in age, and that within each of the listed muscles, there can be a very large spread of motor-unit sizes. Thus, in the extensor digitorum brevis of the foot, for example, the observed motor-unit sizes range over a thirty-fold variation, with the number of large units being relatively small.

In the postural muscles, such as the erector spinae paralleling the spine, the iliopsoas, and muscles of that sort (figures 11.A-1 and 11.A-2), in which an extended action of low intensity is required but there normally is no need for fine-tuning of muscle action, each of the motor units can at some time relax and refresh itself while other motor units become active, thus retaining the posture for long periods of time without undue overall muscle fatigue or interruption of the support. Motor units in other muscles are best suited to intense contraction for a short time, and when coordinated with the contraction of other muscles, a more global contraction can be formed, intense but short-lived.

The numbers quoted in table 11.A-1 are general, for it is known that among humans, some individuals have more motor units than the average, throughout the entire musculature. It is generally held that the larger the number of motor units within a muscle, the finer is the finesse with which that muscle ultimately can be controlled. Perhaps B. K. S. Iyengar is one of those born with a superabundance of motor units, allowing him special sensitivities in control of his muscles; more likely, his intense practice to refine muscle control in the *yogasanas,* carried out over decades, has resulted in smaller but more numerous motor units in each of his muscles. Indeed, it seems that such fine α-motor-unit resolution as Iyengar apparently has developed is a learned condition, for the practice of anything (*yogasana,* violin, juggling, etc.) is known to result in an expansion of the area of the motor cortex devoted to that practice; i.e., it results in an expansion of the number of α-motor neurons (and consequently the number of motor units) committed to the relevant muscle [710].

α-Motor-Unit Math

Due to the strong divergence of the α-motor neural system (figure 3.C-2**a**) as it divides to activate the muscle fibers, all muscular actions as driven by the central nervous system involve the basic quantum unit of muscular activation and control, the motor unit, rather than individual muscle fibers. The number of motor units in a muscle equals the number of efferent α-neurons originating in the cortex and committed to that muscle. On average, there are about 150 muscle fibers per motor unit (table 11.A-1); i.e., on average, a single efferent α-motor neural axon originating in the central nervous system has about 150 axonal branches. Though the measurement of the number of fibers per motor unit is difficult and subject to large errors, it is still clear from the work of those who perform such measurements that there is a significant variation in this number among individuals who are in all other ways quite comparable. Furthermore, this fact appears to be general for all of the muscles of the body;

i.e., those with more motor units in a particular muscle generally will have more of them in all of the muscles of the body.

The degree of conscious control over a motor unit is apparent when one considers that the α-motor neuron connected to a hundred or so muscle fibers within a motor unit is itself part of a web of neurons in the spinal cord totaling approximately 600 nearest neighbors on average, with each of the 600 neighbors inputting its excitatory or inhibitory contribution to the transmembrane potential on the α-motor neuron. These higher-level neurons in turn are connected directly or indirectly to approximately ten billion other neurons within a cerebral hemisphere, all of which again contribute in their own way to the voltage potentials on the intermediate 600 [94]! One sees from this that the brain operates by mutual consensus, there being a multitude of inputs competing for expression in the action of the brain to control a muscle.

Finesse

In fine-motor actions such as the blinking of an eyelid, motor units are employed in which there are relatively few muscle fibers (fewer than ten muscle fibers control eye movement, and only two or three fibers per motor axon are involved in the muscles of the larynx); whereas for coarse motor actions, the number of fibers in the relevant motor units will be much larger (for example, 1,000 to 2,000 muscle fibers per motor axon in the gastrocnemius muscle of the calf). In general, those α-motor axons innervating less than a hundred or so muscle fibers per motor unit usually energize muscles that are used for fine movements, whereas those innervating a motor unit containing many hundreds (or even thousands) of muscle fibers usually energize muscles used for gross movements, as with the postural muscles of the back. On the other hand, the larger the number of α-motor units within a muscle, the larger is the number of neurons committed to its excitation, and the finer is the muscular control and dexterity of that muscle. The external rectus muscle of the eye contains almost 3,000 motor units, with an average of only nine fibers per unit. This situation within the eye leads to rapid and accurate visual tracking of the surroundings. On the other hand, the bulkiest muscles have the largest motor-unit size but the smallest number of motor units. For example, the gastrocnemius muscle contains only 580 motor units, but with almost 2,000 fibers in each. Such a muscle is built for efficient jumping but not for high-resolution muscle movement. Many other muscles have about equal numbers of motor units and fibers per unit.

Comparison of α-motor-unit data of the human (table 11.A-1) with that of lower mammals shows that the muscles of our hands are relatively rich in the number of motor units, thus allowing our exceptional development of manual skills, as expected from the motor-cortex homunculus (figure 4.C-5).

Assuming that the number of motor units within a particular muscle is a direct measure of the fine-control that one can exert over that muscle—a muscle with a large number of motor units can perform tasks with much more finesse than an equally large muscle with a smaller number of motor units—we see that there may be an inborn neurological factor that will favor one beginning *yogasana* student over another in regard to muscle control. What is most tantalizing is the thought that through the practice of *yogasana,* one increases the number of motor units within relevant muscles through re-innervation [549] and thereby increases one's level of finesse in using the muscle. In fact, the known growth of a particular area of the motor cortex with practice of a particular activity (Subsection 4.C, page 94, and Subsection 18.A, page 691) assures that the number of α-motor axons controlled by that area will increase, and it follows from this that the number of motor units within the muscle served by that area of the motor cortex also must increase by the same amount.

One way to think about the advantages of having a large number of motor units that can be used in *yogasana* practice is to imagine the simple tunes that can be played on a child's piano having just eight keys and to compare this to the music one can make with a keyboard having eighty-eight keys; similarly, compare the quality of the art painted with a paint box having just six colors and that of the artist whose pallet consists of an almost infinite number of color combinations. In the same way, the *yogasana* artist will be able to construct a more refined work of art if more motor units and combinations of motor units are available to her and are under her control.

Graded Response to Load

It is one of our eventual goals in *yogasana* practice to minimize the size of the motor units engaged in performing the postures, while making sure that those muscle units that are engaged are the appropriate ones. Within this framework, *yogasana* beginners may be defined as those who work with maximum effort and the largest motor units while achieving minimum resolution of muscle action, whereas advanced students work with minimum effort and the smallest motor units while achieving maximum resolution of muscle action [644]!

As mentioned above, the larger the number of motor units within a muscle, the finer and more precise is the control over which motor units will be activated in performing a muscular task. In turn, having a large number of motor units from which one can choose sooner or later reveals just which ones are needed to optimize the efficiency of the action. The ability to use only that part of the muscle needed to do the job and no more (i.e., to show a graded response to the task at hand) is clearly energy-saving, provided that one has a variety of motor units from which to choose. In a large muscle with only a few motor units, the degree of activation of the muscle is strongly limited, whereas for a muscle with many more motor units, the degree of activation is much more refined and delicate. The question of the order of recruitment of the various motor units within a muscle is discussed in this subsection, page 373.

Delocalization of Motor-Unit Structure

Experiments show that the fibers of different α-motor units within a muscle are randomly intermixed; which is to say, two fibers of the same motor unit generally do not lie next to one another, and the fibers of a large motor unit may be positioned over the entire cross-sectional area of the belly of the muscle. It appears that during the formation of the neural network energizing a motor unit, there is a discrimination against the formation of clusters of fibers of the same motor unit on a fine scale, though there may be clustering of individual fibers on a much coarser scale. Moreover, in long muscles, a particular motor unit may span only a small portion of the muscle's length, leading to the possibility of being able to contract the belly of a long muscle without contracting fibers closer to the ends of the muscle, or of contracting the motor units at one end of a muscle but not at the other.

Because the various fibers of a single motor unit are dispersed throughout the muscle, no distinct "motor unit" can be discerned anatomically. This somewhat global distribution of fibers within a motor unit leads to a somewhat global contraction of the muscle on neural excitation [877]. This globalization of the components of the motor units means that one can activate a particular portion of a muscle only to the extent that its motor-unit components are localized within that particular portion of the muscle. When the distribution of the muscle fibers of a particular motor unit is random, one cannot hope to excite only a specific portion of a large muscle, for even if only one motor unit is excited (the best one can hope for), it will involve fibers spread throughout a large volume of the muscle. However, by activating a particular combination of motor units, it still may be possible to localize the muscle action. Also possible, but not in any way demonstrated to date, is the spatial aggregation of fibers of a specific motor unit through *yogasana* practice.

There is a distinct advantage to be gained by the spatial dispersion of the fibers of a particular motor unit: picture a single motor unit with component fibers grouped locally at a point within the muscle. All of its muscle fibers contract simultaneously on being excited, and therewith, the high tensile stress in the motor unit leads to immediate ischemia, hypoxia, and fatigue if the fibers are adjacent. On the other hand, if the motor-unit muscle fibers are placed randomly among fibers of other motor units within a muscle, when the particular motor unit is energized, the surrounding fibers of other motor units remain relaxed and so will allow an unimpeded flow of fresh blood through the muscle (Subsection 11.A, page 375).

Motor-Unit Excitation in Time

Within a large muscle, there can be many independent motor units, with little coordination of their excitations in time; however, with practice, the contraction and relaxation of multiple motor units can be orchestrated so as to provide a smooth muscle action of long duration, whereas the simultaneous excitation of all motor units would result in one jerky movement that could be sustained for only a few seconds. Furthermore, by avoiding energizing all of the motor units at once, one achieves a graded response appropriate to the task at hand; i.e., when a large muscle is contracted, the smaller motor units within it are the first to fire, and if that is not sufficient for the task, then larger and stronger units will be brought into play. Because several motor units will share a common muscle tendon, even the random excitation in time of such motor units will be smoothed out at the tendon and so appear as a steady tensile stress on this tissue.

During isometric contractions of the sort encountered in *yogasana* practice, all of the motor units can be contracted simultaneously in some muscles, whereas only portions are contracted in others. Thus, activation is complete in the small muscles of the hands, the dorsiflexors of the ankle, the quadriceps, and the diaphragm, but not in the triceps surae and the short extensors of the toes. It appears that there is also an orderly recruitment of motor units in the stretch reflexes. The order of motor-unit recruitment is fixed, as long as the task is identical in repeated trials, as when repeatedly doing *uttanasana*, for example.

Single Motor-Unit Excitation

Basmajian and coworkers (summarized in [94]) report on some amazing experimental results, showing that the mind can readily control the firing of a specific motor unit, energizing it (and other motor units as well) at any chosen time. This series of experiments involved making the motor-unit excitation either visible or audible through suitable electronics, in which case each motor unit displays its own characteristic voltage pattern in time when it fires. With a little practice, the subject of the experiment can mentally induce the appearance or disappearance of any one of a number of characteristic motor-unit discharge patterns at a time of his or her choosing. This type of biofeedback training requires only about fifteen to twenty minutes, after which the control "just happens" without any specific mental effort of the controller beyond thinking of the desired result. After twenty minutes or so of practicing single motor-unit control, the controllers report feeling exhausted, with a stiffness and soreness in the controlled muscles. Note that the learning taking place here is very different from the control of muscles as guided by the proprioceptive signals of tension and position that we normally use when practicing *yogasana* (Section 11.C, page 441). However, that is not to say that one cannot achieve conscious control over single motor units while practicing the *yogasanas*.

The easiest motor units to control consciously are those of the muscles consciously used most often (fingers, arms, etc.), while the most difficult to control are those of the muscles consciously used least often, such as those in the back or chest for non-yogis. The degree of difficulty most likely correlates with the relative size of muscles and organs in the somatic motor-cortex homunculus (figure 4.C-5). Within a large muscle, the smaller motor units are more easily brought under conscious control.

There is a certain resonance between Basmajian's experimental results and Iyengar's statement [391] about bringing every cell of the body under conscious control and of having an awareness that penetrates to the deepest level of the body. Possibly, without external electronics, B. K. S. Iyengar is able to consciously control individual motor units within a muscle and control their relative levels of excitation in a way parallel to the control shown in Basmajian's experiments!

Muscle-Fiber Types

As described in more detail in Subsection 11.A, page 411, muscle fibers can be grouped into three general classes called types 1, 2, and 3. All of the fibers within a single α-motor unit will be of the same fiber type; however within a single muscle, the different motor units of different fiber types form a well-mixed mosaic.

In general, for weak or moderately strong contractions of an extended or repetitive nature, it is the type-1 slow-twitch motor units that are called upon first, and at the highest levels of exertion, the type-3 fast-twitch motor units are activated as well. However, when the action has to be very rapid, the type-3 units appear to have the lower threshold as compared with type-1 units and so are recruited first. The larger motor units, which are called upon to do the heavy lifting (type 1), are energized at a frequency of 50–100 hertz or so, and at this high frequency, they hardly relax before they are excited again. This means that the motor units are contracting essentially continuously, even though the neural excitation is intermittent, i.e., pulsatile. When we enter this region of high workload, the recruitment of type-2 fibers becomes prominent and helps to carry the load.

Other Neurons within Muscles

In addition to the efferent α-motor neurons that energize skeletal muscle, the muscles also contain sensors that relay many types of muscle-related information back to the central nervous system via afferent neural systems. These sensors themselves contain yet smaller muscles, which are innervated by the γ-motor neurons. Though there can be a strong element of voluntary control of the skeletal muscles (or so it seems), even when fully conscious and at rest, there is an involuntary excitation of the muscles that maintains a certain nonzero level of contraction, called "resting muscle tone" or "tonus." This muscle tone is intimately involved with excitation of the γ-motor neurons, as discussed further in Subsection 11.B, page 436.

Especially interesting to us are those sensors called mechanoreceptors, which measure the state of tension within the muscle bundle (see Section 11.B, page 428), since the afferent neural signals from the mechanoreceptors form the basis by which the body controls the degree of muscle stretching or contraction and evaluates the positions of all of the body parts. Clearly, in our quest for both alignment and opening of the body in the *yogasanas,* the mechanoreceptors play a major role.

Vascularization

In response to either neural or hormonal stimulation, skeletal muscle tissue can contract actively by up to 30 percent of its resting length, and because of the high demand for oxygen and glucose by its mitochondria when the muscle is so strongly contracted, it is highly vascularized with blood vessels carrying a variety of substances into and away from the working muscle. The mitochondria within muscle fibers consume oxygen and use this to oxidize fuel to produce chemical energy in the form of adenosine triphosphate (ATP). Continuous muscular work requires a steady flow of oxygen and glucose into the muscle tissue, a steady outward flow of carbon dioxide and other metabolic products, and the continuous production of ATP.

The cardiovascular system of the body—consisting of the heart, arteries, veins, and intermediate vessels (Chapter 14, page 535) and the blood coursing through them—provides the muscles with all they need metabolically in order to function. The smallest of these blood vessels, the capillaries, formally are not part of the muscle but serve to connect the muscle fibers to the cardiovascular system.

When exercising, blood flow through a muscle may increase tenfold, as the relevant arteries dilate, possibly due to the effects of circulating epinephrine. Due to the strong need for the removal of lactic acid from an actively working muscle, there are five to ten capillaries serving each muscle fiber [288]. On the other hand, inactive muscles are not supplied with such an abundant capillary network.

Muscle tissue appears red in part because of the extensive vascularization present in order to serve such a hard-working structure. The heavy vascularization leads in turn to excellent circulation, and so accounts for the fact that injuries to muscles heal much faster than those to less vascularized tissue, such as ligaments [52]. One of the many health benefits of *yogasana* practice is that the muscle contraction taking place during the practice promotes the formation of new capillaries, which increase circulation in the contracted region. This increased circulation can speed healing and strengthens the region against future injury or disease.

Mitochondria

Mitochondria are organelles dispersed throughout the cytoplasm of all cells. Chemical reactions take place in the mitochondria (the oxidation of glucose by oxygen), supplying the energy to drive the cell's metabolic processes. Mitochondria are the power sources for processes in the brain, muscles, visceral organs, the visual system, etc., as they carry the DNA for producing the enzymes needed for energy production. Mitochondria multiply independently within the cell, not needing to wait for the cell itself to divide. When sperm unites with egg, the mitochondria of the sperm are absorbed and then destroyed by the egg, and so the mitochondria of all cells come only from the mother's side of the union [865]. In muscle tissue, the mitochondria are found in the sarcoplasm adjacent to the myofibrils, ready to provide ATP when it is needed.

While the mitochondria are generating ATP for use in doing work, a byproduct of this reaction in the mitochondria is the free radical known as the superoxide ion (O_2^-). This highly reactive chemical species is converted by the enzyme superoxide dismutase into hydrogen peroxide (H_2O_2), which then is destroyed by the enzyme catalase. In spite of these enzymes, a certain amount of superoxide ion escapes destruction by this route and then attacks the DNA in both the mitochondria and the cell nucleus; being indiscriminately reactive, the superoxide ion also degrades cell proteins and membranes. The degradation initiated by superoxide ions in the mitochondria is cumulative and is felt to lead to the various health problems of old age. It has not been determined whether diets high in antioxidants are of value in battling the deleterious effects of superoxide ions. The roles of the mitochondria in the aging process are discussed further in Subsection 24.A, page 810.

Vascular Diameter and Flow

As discussed in Section 14.C, page 561, the pipe-like elements of the vascular system that serve the muscles have their own smooth muscles within the pipe walls, and these muscles control the vascular diameters and thus their flow rates. Autonomic control (Chapter 5, page 157) of the vascular diameters locally can effectively readjust the relative amounts of blood flowing to the muscles, the visceral organs, and the skin. When a muscle is being used in a vigorous way, stimulation of the sympathetic nervous system reroutes blood from the digestive organs to the muscles. However, when a muscle is strongly contracted, the action tends more or less to clamp down on the vascular system within it and to throttle the flow of blood into and out of the muscle. Even when contracted strongly, the muscle cells continue their metabolism, so that carbon dioxide and organic acids accumulate. Once the muscle tension resulting from contraction is released, the accumulated metabolic products produce a dilation of the vascular system, and in a feedback loop, the accelerated blood flow restores homeostasis as rapidly as possible [528] (Subsection 14.C, page 561).

In general, contraction of a muscle lowers the blood flow through it in proportion to the extent of contraction, with blood flow through the contracted muscle being much less in the inner core of the muscle than through the muscle's periphery. On the other hand, stretching a muscle significantly lowers its consumption of oxygen and also slows the blood flow; however, on releasing the stretch, blood flow then speeds up considerably [7].

Vascularization does much in support of the muscles, and muscles return the favor. Venous blood and lymph in the lower extremities are slow to travel upward against gravity, but the contrac-

tion and relaxation of the muscles in the extremities acts to pump this sluggish venous blood and lymph back to the heart (Subsection 14.C, page 569).

Ischemia and Hypoxia

It occasionally happens that when we practice certain *yogasanas,* a joint is closed in such a way that vascular circulation is impaired; for example, this happens with circulation below the knees when sitting in *vajrasana.* As regards circulation in such a compressed system, though the arterial side of the vascular system is strong-walled and does not easily collapse under pressure, the same cannot be said for the venous side. Thus, when the muscle is pressurized by compression, blood may be able to enter the compressed area, but it cannot leave through collapsed veins, leading to a condition called ischemia. In ischemia, the oxygen in the blood is consumed locally but not replaced, leading in time to a condition in which the oxygen level is severely diminished (hypoxia). Ischemia and hypoxia adversely affect muscles, as they become starved for oxygen and cannot rid themselves of metabolic wastes.

Even when not being compressed from the outside, a similar ischemia ensues when a muscle is strongly contracted; i.e., the blood flow through it is impeded, and the muscle suffers not only from lack of oxygen and ATP, but from increasing levels of waste metabolites as well. In response to this, the endothelial cells lining the insides of the blood vessels release nitric oxide (NO), a material which strongly promotes relaxation of the muscular layer within the vascular walls, thereby leading to vasodilation. This increase of vascular diameters stimulates the flow of blood through the muscle, in spite of its contraction. Vasodilation results in the relevant muscle becoming engorged with fresh blood, so that it feels hot and "pumped."

It is difficult to detail the situation in regard to nerves in a strongly contracted muscle (Subsection 3.E, page 60) but they also suffer oxygen depletion; moreover, they are soft mechanically and are strongly dependent upon material transport down their axons by microtubules (Subsection 3.A, page 35) in order to function. When pressured, the axons become poor conductors of neural signals (if they conduct them at all), and so the muscles so innervated by these nerves may not be excitable; this situation may be further complicated by ischemia and the concomitant hypoxia. Clearly, when a muscle is either ischemic or hypoxic, the aerobic route to ATP production is no longer an option (Subsection 11.A, page 391), and the muscle will tire rapidly once the anaerobic-glycolysis phase of ATP production is exhausted.

Innervation Activates Muscles

Neuromuscular Apoptosis

Just as occurs in the brain, there is a surplus of neural synapses connecting the central nervous system to the muscle fibers at birth; i.e., there is more than one neuron joined to each muscle fiber. However, with use, large numbers of such neuromuscular junctions are deemed redundant and so are pared away by apoptosis. In this way, the muscle reaches a state of lesser but more efficient innervation in the adult, abandoning those circuits used infrequently in favor of those used often. In moving toward adulthood, the number of neuromuscular junctions decreases with maturity, but the strengths of the remaining junctions increase. If this paring away of the excess neurons does not occur, then the muscle will contain an unusually large number of motor units, for each surviving nerve will innervate its own muscle fiber [549]. A similar reduction in the number of synapses as one approaches adulthood is observed in the autonomic ganglia and among the Purkinje cells in the cerebellum (Subsection 4.B, page 73).

α-Motor Neurons

A muscle fiber can contribute force to a contracting muscle only if it is recruited to do so by the central nervous system, either consciously by the higher centers of the brain or reflexively by the spinal cord or brainstem.[1] Skeletal-muscle contraction is initiated only by electrical (neural)

impulses that flow to the muscle via the α-motor and the γ-motor neurons. The rapidly contracting skeletal muscles are innervated by the swiftest afferent and efferent fibers in the body (Section 3.B, page 41). High conduction velocity in these neurons is assured by their oligodendrocyte or Schwann-cell myelination. The α-motor system originates in the cortex of the brain and is used both for the voluntary control of the muscles by higher centers in the brain and the reflexive control of the same muscles by lower centers, whereas the γ-motor system is largely for the involuntary control of the muscles by lower centers in the brain (Section 11.A, page 377).

Axons originating in the motor cortex pass downward through the thalamus and thence into the midbrain of the brainstem. At the medulla oblongata, they decussate from the left to the right and then enter the spinal cord to exit at the appropriate vertebral foramina. This particular myelinated path, from cortex to muscle without the intervention of any synapses, is known as the "pyramidal tract," is found only in mammals, and reaches its greatest development in humans [671a]. Not only does the pyramidal tract carry efferent α- and γ-motor commands from the brain, but it also carries delicate proprioceptive afferent signals from the fingers, hands, and toes upward to the sensory cortex. As shown in figure 11.A-7**b**, there are other tracts from the cortex to the spinal cord; however, it is the pyramidal tract that is of primary importance when rapid, isolated, discrete movements are required.

Chronic activation of the γ-motor system by excitations within the sympathetic branch of the autonomic nervous system (as might be the case if one has chronic stress in one's life) is responsible for high resting-state muscle tone. Depending upon the muscle-fiber type (Subsection 11.A, page 411), some muscles are rapidly contracting and some are slowly contracting. Those that contract rapidly (type 3) are innervated by α-neurons of specific A types, whereas those that are slowly contracting (type 1) are innervated by slowly con-

---

1   Actually, muscle contraction is also possible through external means, via the application of an elec-

trical voltage directly to the muscle, as when stimulated by the galvanic response or by electrocution.

ducting C-type neurons (table 3.B-2). The interesting question of what the relative timing might be in regard to when one decides to contract a muscle and when it actually contracts is discussed in Subsection 4.C, page 96.

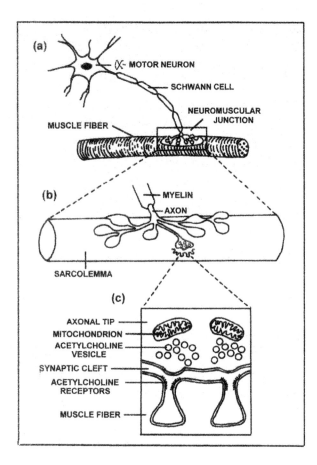

Figure 11.A-6. Progressive enlargements of the junction between the α-motor neuron and the muscle fiber to be energized by it, showing (**a**) the attachment of the motor neuron's axon to the receptor sites on the muscle fiber, (**b**) detailed view of the neuromuscular junction, and (**c**) the relative positions of the acetylcholine-filled vesicles in the axonal tip of the motor neuron and the acetylcholine receptors within the muscle fiber, the axonal tip and the muscle fiber being separated by the synaptic cleft [360].

The Neuromuscular Junction

The originating α-neural axon in the cortex branches between three and 2,000 times and then forms neuromuscular junctions with between three and 2,000 muscle fibers simultaneously within the appropriate motor unit. As shown for a single such muscle fiber in figure 11.A-6, the axonal branch of the efferent α-motor neuron terminates in an end plate that contacts the skeletal-muscle fiber at the neuromuscular junction. The axon of a given α-motor neuron driving a motor unit may receive up to 30,000 inputs from other afferent and efferent fibers; however, if the neuromuscular junction to a muscle fiber malfunctions, the muscle fiber is rendered inert.

Action Potentials

The contraction of skeletal muscle begins with an action potential (voltage spike) moving through the central nervous system and down the axon of the α-motor neuron toward the neuromuscular junction, where it will initiate a contraction in the muscle fiber lasting for between five and fifty milliseconds, after which time the fiber relaxes to its original condition. In this relatively short time, the fiber realizes only a fraction of its total possible contraction.

In most cases, the action potential (Subsection 3.B, page 42) that stimulates muscle contraction is not a single voltage stimulus at the neuromuscular junction, but consists instead of a series of spikes of equal voltage having a frequency (spikes per second) that expresses the intensity of the α-neural signal. Because the muscle fibers are signaled to contract and relax with each voltage spike they receive, the larger the number of voltage spikes per second in the α-neural signal, the more often per second the muscle fibers will be jolted into contraction. When sustained muscle action for a second or so is required, the frequency of the signal in the α-motor neuron will be sufficiently high that the associated muscle fibers will be repeatedly jolted into action before they can fully relax again. These repeated contractions accumulate so as to produce a much larger contractile force than that achievable with only a single neural firing.

On the other hand, if the muscle contraction frequency is too high, it cannot relax between excitations, and the muscle becomes locked in contraction (called tetany), the blood supply to the

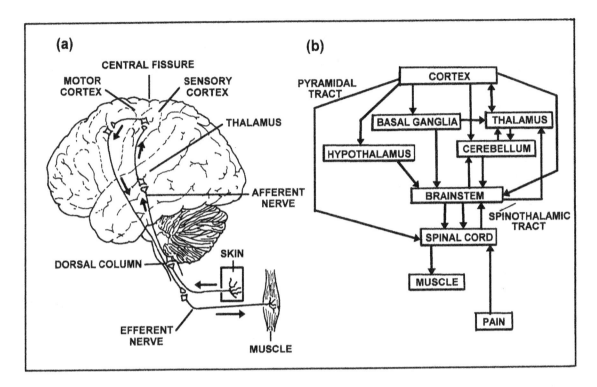

Figure 11.A-7. (a) Sketch of the neural pathway connecting an initial pain sensation in the skin to the sensory cortex; the sensory signal then moves across the central fissure to the motor cortex and then down the α-motor neuron to the relevant muscle. (b) Interconnections between several centers in the brain, which can contribute to the final signal exiting the spinal cord via the α-motor neuron [360] or to the transmission of a pain signal to the thalamus.

muscle is curtailed, and reduced efficiency of the muscle follows. However, if the tetany is less than complete, then there are moments of relaxation, which allow blood to flow through the muscle and so forestall fatigue.

The activation of a muscle fiber is an all-or-nothing affair, rather like a neural action potential (Section 3.B, page 39); i.e., it is either relaxed or contracted for a period of about fifty milliseconds. However, a muscle fiber can be more or less contracted on average over a longer period of time, depending on the rate at which it is excited, relaxed, excited again, relaxed again, etc. Though a particular muscle fiber is either activated or not, in an aggregate of such fibers that are not part of a common motor unit, any degree of activation of the aggregate is possible, depending upon just how many of the fibers are activated simultaneously and how often per second they are activated. In this way, a large muscle can be smoothly energized to whatever level is appropriate to the

task it is to perform, and being asynchronous, the active motor units are able to rest for short times while others carry the load. See Subsection 11.A, page 373, for more on this topic.

Multiple Activation Interactions

In the mature adult, the neural impulses that drive muscle action originate in the central nervous system (Chapter 4, page 67), a hierarchical structure built of lower centers, which control involuntary body functions (including muscle contraction), and the higher centers of the brain, which direct the conscious actions of our bodies. The higher and lower centers within the central nervous system activate muscles in response to afferent signals sent to them from the sensors at the body's periphery. The afferent nerves connecting the sensors to the central nervous system converge upon the spinal cord in order to send their information along the ascending pathway sequentially to the cerebellum, to the thalamus, and possibly to the ultimate center, the cerebral sensory cortex (figure 11.A-7a).

In the deliberate act of contracting the biceps muscle, for example, tensile sensations originating at the biceps muscle (as from the muscle spindles) travel via the afferent neuron to the posterior horn of the spinal cord at C5 and then to the relevant center within the sensory cortex (figure 11.A-7a). Once the afferent signal is processed, the consequent efferent (out-going) signal then descends either from the cerebral α-motor cortex, the brainstem, or the spinal cord, to eventually activate the appropriate muscles, but with many feedback loops for close control at many points in the descent (figure 11.A-7b). The pyramidal tract is the largest of the descending pathways, originating in the cerebral cortices of each of the hemispheres, decussating at the medulla oblongata, and terminating on the opposite sides of the spinal cord. Many axons in both the ascending and the descending pathways intercept the fibers entering and leaving at C5 and so can inhibit or modulate the transmission of the afferent signal to higher centers.

The multiple interactions along and between the ascending and descending pathways of the central nervous system are important for practitioners of *yogasana,* as they allow the subconscious actions to be sensed and altered by the conscious mind and vice versa; i.e., the interaction of higher and lower centers in the central nervous system is the mechanism whereby we can increase our awareness and conscious control of the body at the most subtle levels (and vice versa).

Neural signals traveling the pyramidal tract activate muscles without interference from any of the lower brain centers other than those within the spinal cord.[2]

---

2   In a typical voluntary muscle action, such as a *yogasana* that previously has been practiced, the train of neural pulses would be schematically as follows. The motivational system in the cortex consciously decides on the *yogasana* to be performed *(bakasana,* for example) and sends this information to the cerebellum and the basal ganglia, these being subconscious centers that orchestrate the various muscle contractions and their timing as is necessary for the posture.

Synchronous Activation

It is interesting and amusing to see how certain muscles in the body are activated in synchrony but to no useful end. Thus, for example, when your students are in *tadasana,* and you encourage them to spread their toes, notice how many students will comply by spreading their fingers as well! Also when in *tadasana,* pressing the base of the big toe to the floor often will result in a gripping of the floor with the tips of the other toes, and that gripping the floor with the toes often is accompanied by a clenching of the jaw. In a similar way, have your students sit and then rotate their right foot in a clockwise direction. While the foot is in clockwise motion, have them take the right hand in the air and inscribe the number

---

Having been practiced repeatedly before, the neural circuitry for the performance of *bakasana* is well defined and in place in the subconscious. This master plan is then sent upward to the thalamus and from there to the premotor and motor cortices in the frontal lobes of the cerebrum. Taking the corticospinal tract, neurons descend from the motor cortex to the base of the brainstem. At this point, 90 percent of the fibers decussate (left-to-right crossover) and travel down the white matter of the lateral funiculus as part of the lateral corticospinal tract. At the appropriate spinal level, the nerves go from the region of white matter into the gray region and there synapse with α-motor neurons. These α-motor neurons have their cell bodies in the spinal cord but extend their axons beyond one meter (three feet) to reach the appropriate muscles. Thus, the α-motor neurons relay the plan of action via the corticospinal tract to the appropriate muscles, at the appropriate intensities, and at the appropriate times. With this, the posture appears! The traversal of this neural loop is more easily accomplished the more the posture is practiced by the student, for by practice, the strengths of the relevant synapses are increased.

After a short time, the student voluntarily releases from the posture, sensing that the strength of the muscles can no longer support it; however, this is not necessarily the case, for it might just as well be that the muscles are not fatigued but that the nerves and the synapses that are involved in the muscle contraction instead have lost their strength. Indeed, practice of the *yogasanas* builds strength in both the muscular and the nervous systems.

"6"; this counterclockwise motion of the hand immediately reverses the rotational direction of the foot [563]!

Maps

As the afferent fibers in a nerve bundle ascend the spinal cord, the component fibers have a very specific spatial relationship to one another, and at every level of the spinal cord, the relationship is maintained. This bundle terminates at the sensory cortex, so that a spatial map of the body parts is imprinted on the cortex, though not necessarily in the "real" proportions. Many such body maps are laid down, not only in other areas of the central nervous system (the cerebellum, the basal ganglia, the red nucleus, and the reticular formation) [308], but in the sole of the foot, the eye, and the palm of the hand too; however, in these cases, there is no clear relationship of the locations of the real body parts and their locations in such maps, in contrast to the situations shown in figures 4.C-5 and 4.C-6.

Stimulation of specific areas of the right cerebral motor cortex (figure 4.C-5) has been found experimentally by Penfield and Rasmussen [651] to correlate uniquely with the excitation of specific skeletal muscles. Thanks to this unique one-to-one correspondence, a "homunculus" can be drawn, with each body part of the homunculus drawn in proportion to the fractional amount of the motor cortex dedicated to excitation of the muscles in that part. It is no surprise that in humans, the parts of the motor cortex dedicated to moving the hand and the muscles of speech are disproportionately large in the motor homunculus. A related type of homunculus can be drawn for the sensory cortex (an adjacent area in the cortex, Subsection 4.C, page 92), showing the relative numbers of neural sensors in each of the body parts (figure 4.C-6). The motor and sensory homunculi are seen to be qualitatively similar.

Muscle-Nerve Codependence

Muscle tissue is not only activated by nerve impulses but is metabolically dependent upon nerve action for its health; if the nerve to a muscle is cut, then the muscle atrophies in a few months, leaving only the tendonous material behind. The muscle then dies in one to two years, eventually to be replaced by scar tissue [431]. Re-innervation reverses this process if it can be accomplished within a two-month window following the cut. The intact nerve destined to serve for re-innervation seeks out the muscle in need of repair and connects only to it [877]. Similarly, nerves have a short lifetime when they are removed from the vicinity of their target organs [427].

It follows from this that a muscle and its activating and sensing nerves that are only occasionally utilized cannot remain healthy indefinitely. In fact, the nerve-impulse patterns sent to the muscles are thought to be responsible for the muscles' characteristic bulk and strength; indeed, these properties, together with speed and endurance, are readily changed by changing the pattern of nerve impulses driving the muscle [549]. Because nerves do not usually regenerate but instead tend to die off with increasing age (in the cortex, the number of cells decreases by 40 percent on going from age twenty years to age seventy-five years; see Subsection 4.E, page 119), muscle fibers slowly but inexorably must lose their innervation. As mentioned above, a muscle without its nerve will slowly die. Thus, as we go into old age, muscles begin to thin as their muscle fibers die off from lack of innervation, especially in the legs [621]. It is thought that the legs are most vulnerable, because the nerves to the legs are the longest and so are most at risk for a break, even when in normal use.

Microscopic Muscle Contraction

Internal Structure

At the cellular level, muscle consists of elongated muscle-fiber cells containing various cell nuclei and mitochondria (Subsection 11.A, page 365), each bound by a fibrous-tissue membrane; the connective tissue involved in holding the muscle fibers together is discussed further in Section 12.A, page 486. The connective tissue not only allows the blood vessels and nerves to penetrate deep into the muscle in order to reach the inner-most muscle fibers within a fascicle, but it also offers mechanical resistance to stretching of the muscle.

A muscle fiber is a single cell, cylindrical, elongated, and up to 30 centimeters (twelve inches) long in some muscles (the sartorius in the upper leg, for example), whereas most cells in the human body are about 0.01 millimeters (0.003 inches) in length. Muscle fibers are almost as long as neurons but are only 0.01 to 0.1 millimeters (0.003 to 0.03 inches) in diameter. A large cell, such as that in a long muscle, is supplied with many cell nuclei, usually arranged along the periphery of the fiber.

The mechanism of muscle action becomes clear if we consider a typical muscle at levels of increasing magnification. A cross section of such a muscle, taken through its belly, shows it to consist of parallel bundles of muscle fasciculi, each within its own sheath of connective tissue called perimysium (figure 11.A-4c). A closer look at the structure of a fascicle bundle shows it to be composed in turn of up to 200 long, cylindrical muscle-fiber cells of 5–100 μ diameter (a human hair has a diameter of approximately 75 μ), with each such cell surrounded by an endomysium fascial sheath and the entire fascicle bundle surrounded by an epimysium fascial sheath.

Within each of the muscle fibers are bundles of yet finer fibers called myofibrils (figures 11.A-4e and 11.A-4f), with each myofibril composed of identical units called sarcomeres, and joined end to end. In turn, each sarcomere is filled with equal numbers of two distinct types of myofilaments running parallel to one another over the entire length of the cell. It is these microscopic myofilaments, called myosin (about 150 angstroms in diameter) and actin (about 50 angstroms in diameter), that contain the molecular machinery that drives large-scale muscle contraction. Additionally, there are noncontractive proteins, such as troponin, titin and α-actinin that contribute to muscle action.

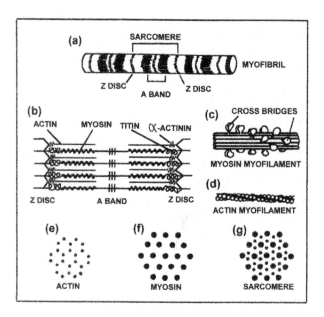

Figure 11.A-8. (a) The banded structure of a typical skeletal myofibril, as seen from the side. The myofibrils fill the sarcolemma sheath surrounding the muscle fiber; each myofibril in turn is filled with myofilaments of the proteins actin and myosin. (b) A schematic picture showing the interdigitation of the actin and myosin myofilaments within a myofibril. (c) Simplified molecular structures of the myosin myofilament with its cross bridges. (d) Molecular structure of the actin myofilament. (e) End-on view of the packing of actin myofilaments within the myofibril. (f) End-on view of the packing of myosin myofilaments within the myofibril. (g) End-on view of the myofibril, showing the relative placement and regularity of the packing of myofilaments of the proteins actin (thin) and myosin (thick).

Myofibrils

Being a single cell, a muscle fiber is the smallest complete contractile fiber possible. As shown in figures 11.A-4e and 11.A-8a, the inner part of a muscle fiber consists largely of parallel lengths of myofibril; each myofibril is 1–2 μ in diameter, and there may be as many as 8,000 myofibrils in a muscle fiber. Electron microscopy of the internal structure of a myofibril (figure 11.A-8b) shows that it contains two types of myofilament, one

Table 11.A-2: The Number of Muscle Fibers and the Number of Sarcomeres per Fiber According to Muscle Type in Various Human Muscles [549]

Muscle	Location	Number of Fibers	Sarcomeres per Fiber		
			Type 1	Type 2	Type 3
First lumbrical	Hand	10,250	-	-	-
External rectus	Eye	27,000	-	-	-
Platysma	Jaw to shoulder	27,000	-	-	-
First dorsal interosseous	Hand	40,500	-	-	-
Sartorius	Upper leg	128,000	153,000	174,000	135,000
Brachioradialis	Forearm	129,000	-	-	-
Anterior tibialis	Lower leg	271,000	-	-	-
Posterior tibialis	Lower leg	-	11,000	15,000	8,000
Medial gastrocnemius	Lower leg	1,030,000	16,000	15,000	15,000
Soleus	Lower leg	-	14,000	-	-
Semitendinosus	Upper leg	-	58,000	66,000	-
Gracilis	Upper leg	-	81,000	93,000	84,000

thin and one thick, each running parallel to the main fiber axis (or inclined to this axis in pennate muscles; Section 11.A, page 397). The thicker myofilament is a polymer of the protein myosin, and the thinner one is a polymer of the protein actin. These myofibrils are constructed internally so that the actin myofilaments are interdigitated with the myosin myofilaments, with a packing pattern in which each myosin myofilament is surrounded by six actin myofilaments and carries appendages (cross bridges) that project toward all six actin neighbors (figures 11.A-8c to 11.A-8g). Each actin myofilament is surrounded in turn by its three myosin-myofilament nearest neighbors (figure 11.A-8g). Over the length of the myofibril, a pattern of myosin/actin interdigitation is successively repeated, with each longitudinal repeat unit (the sarcomere, a subunit within the sheath of the sarcolemma with a length of 1.6–2.2 µ when the muscle is at its resting length, figure 11.A-8a) terminated at both ends by rigid end plates called Z discs. The numbers of sarcomeres in the myofibers of typical human muscles are given in table 11.A-2.

In a given muscle, it appears that where it has been measured, the type-2 fiber is the longest and the length of type-1 fibers may be slightly larger than that of type 3.

Muscle Growth

As with many other cell types, the number of muscle cells in the body is fixed at birth and does not grow as the body grows. Instead, muscles grow by packing more and more myofilaments of actin and myosin into the existing number of myofibrils, so as to become both thicker and longer [422]. Though the number of muscle fibers in a muscle is fixed early in life, the strength and mass of a muscle can increase, because the thickness, length, and strength of each muscle fiber increases, as does the mass of the connective tissue (the epimysium and perimysium, figure 11.A-4c) involved in holding the muscle together. Though muscle tissue has become so specialized in its function that it has lost the ability to divide and reproduce, new muscle cells can grow in small numbers from stem cells within the muscle tissue. Details of muscle growth appear in Subsection 11.A, page 404.

Sarcomeres

Within the myofibril, the distance from Z disc to Z disc is the sarcomere unit length, amounting to 1.35 to 3.6 µ (0.000053 to 0.00014 inches), depending upon the level of muscular tension; the sarcomeres are aligned end to end over the length of the fiber. In a myofibril within a large muscle such as the medial gastrocnemius, for example, there are about 15,000 sarcomeres of each type lined up end to end. The larger the number of sarcomeres, the larger the range of motion of a muscle and the quicker will be its action [877]. In very long strap muscles, such as the very long sartorius muscle in the upper leg, there is a very high sarcomere count; however, the sarcomere chains do not extend from end to end but are broken up into smaller lengths, with separations by transverse knots of fibrous tissue known as inscriptions [549]. When stretched, each of the sarcomeres within a myofibril can attain a length of 3.6 µ, but at this length, the myofibril has lost all capacity to generate a contractive force, due to a lack of myosin-actin interaction.

t-Tubules

In the resting state of a myofibril, most of the actin myofilaments within the sarcomeres are covered by a protein coat of troponin and so cannot engage the myosin myofilaments (figure 11.A-9a); those few that are so engaged in maintaining the resting-state muscle tone use the breakdown products of fatty acids as the energy source.

When a nerve initiates the contraction of a muscle fiber, it initiates an avalanche of ion transport (Na^+, K^+, and Ca^{2+}) across the sarcolemma, the surface membrane of the muscle fiber. The fiber itself contains a three-dimensional structure called the sarcoplasmic reticulum, which is a highly organized signaling system connecting the muscle-cell surface electrically with each of the internal myofibrils at the Z discs via radially oriented tubes called t-tubules. Using these t-tubules, Ca^{2+} ions are transported, upon excitation, to the interior of the muscle fiber, where they combine with the troponin covering the myofibrils. Contact with the Ca^{2+} ions induces a con-

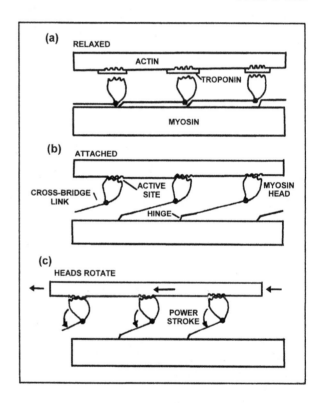

Figure 11.A-9. Showing details of the three stages of cross-bridge interaction between actin and myosin in muscle. (a) In the relaxed state, the cross bridges of the myosin do not engage the active sites of the actin myofilament, because the latter are covered with the protein troponin. (b) When the muscle is energized, the troponin covering is shed at the actin sites, and the actin-myosin cross bridges become engaged. (c) The heads of the cross bridges then rotate counterclockwise, thus moving the actin filament from right to left with respect to the immobile myosin.

formational change of troponin so as to uncover the active sites on the actin myofilaments and thereby allow the engagement of the actin-myosin cross bridges (figure 11.A-9**b**) [549]. The Ca^{2+} ion current propagating inward from the muscle-cell surface through the t-tubules to the myofibrils within stimulates all of the myofibrils to contract simultaneously when so signaled. Once triggered, a depolarized signal then propagates down the length of the muscle fiber, much as with the action potential in the nerve fiber (Section 3.B, page 42), but with much higher initial voltage, so that no amplification is needed.

Muscle Contraction

In the act of muscle contraction, neither the myosin nor the actin actually contracts; the relative motion of the actin myofilaments with respect to the myosin myofilaments leads to the overall contraction of the distance between adjacent Z discs in the sarcomeres. When muscle contracts, the myofilaments slide along one another without shortening, thickening, or bending. A similar statement holds for the case of the muscle being stretched; i.e., when stretching, it is the relative motion of the actin and myosin myofilaments disengaging that leads to an increased distance between the Z discs and hence to an increase in muscle length. This "sliding-filament theory" of muscle action was first proposed by Huxley in 1954.

Cross-Bridge Actions

As shown in figures 11.A-8**c** and 11.A-9, the thick myosin myofilaments have numerous cross bridges, each of which consists of two joints and a head. When the muscle is relaxed, the angles at the joints of the cross bridges are such that there is no contact between the myosin heads and the corresponding attraction sites on the nearby actin chains, which are otherwise covered by the protective protein troponin (figure 11.A-9**a**).

Once the Ca^{2+} ions delivered by the t-tubules remove the troponin covering the actin active sites, electrically depolarized signals propagate within the muscle, the joint angles at the cross bridge heads increase, and the myosin heads are brought

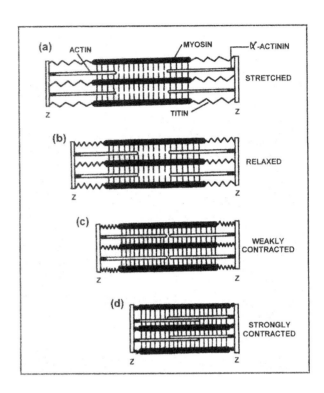

Figure 11.A-10. The internal structure of a sarcomere, showing the relative positions of the thin actin filaments, the thicker myosin filaments, and the Z discs (**a**) in the stretched, (**b**) relaxed, (**c**) partially-contracted, and (**d**) fully-contracted states of a skeletal muscle fiber.

into contact with the corresponding active sites in the actin myofilaments (figure 11.A-9**b**). Having established the myosin-actin contact, the angle at the neck of the cross bridge decreases (the power stroke), thus pulling the Z discs bound to the ends of the actin chains toward one another (figure 11.A-9**c**). Each power stroke of a cross bridge within a muscle fiber moves the actin relative to the myosin by 40–100 angstroms.

The various cross bridges work independently of one another, so that at any one moment, some are detached, some are in contact, and some are ratcheting their way down the actin chain. The net result of this is a smooth, continuous pulling of the actin myofilaments deeper into the spaces between the myosin myofilaments; i.e., a shorter spacing between the Z discs of the sarcomere and overall shortening of the muscle (figure 11.A-10). In the case of the fully contracted muscle, the thin actin chains become so jammed that they are

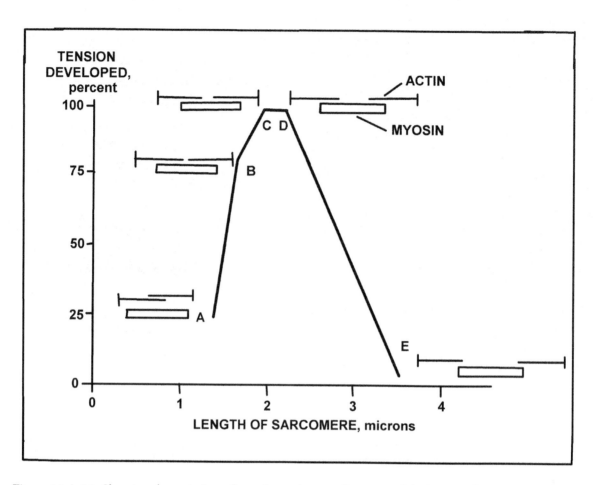

Figure 11.A-11. Showing the variation of muscle tension as a function of the length of the sarcomere. Also shown are the relevant lengths of the actin (thin rods carrying Z discs) with respect to the myosin (heavier bars) in the sarcomere at points A through E in the length-tension curve.

forced to overlap one another (figure 11.A-10**d**). The chemistry driving the action of the cross bridges is described in the following Subsection, page 391.

The strength of a muscle contraction is determined in part by the number of cross-bridge interactions between the two types of myofilament. A muscle is at its most powerful in the resting state (figure 11.A-10**b**), because at this length, there is an optimum overlap of contractive proteins and maximum shortening of the muscle on excitation (figure 11.A-11). Further, if a muscle is immobilized at its resting length for a time, as when confined to bed rest, this slack state promotes the shedding of sarcomeres from the ends of the fibers and an eventual shortening of the muscle. Correspondingly, placing the muscle under tensile stress by stretching it adds

sarcomeres to the muscle-fiber length. This may be the mechanism whereby *yogasana* stretching eventually lengthens the muscle [549, 877]! If, through exercise, a muscle is able to change its resting length, then it is strongest at the new length [450].

As the number of muscle fibers in a muscle is essentially constant, the growth of a muscle involves the radial expansion of each muscle fiber by filling with more and more of the myofibril contractile muscle proteins, and possibly the lengthening of the sarcomere chains. If held momentarily at longer or shorter lengths, the tension that can be developed by contraction is less than at the resting length. The relevance of the curve shown in figure 11.A-11 to *yogasana* practice is discussed in Box 11.A-2, page 401.

Relaxation

When a contracted muscle relaxes, Ca^{2+} ions are pumped from the sarcomeres through the t-tubules into the sarcoplasmic reticulum, again through the action of ATP; with the Ca^{2+} ions no longer available, the troponin again separates the actin and myosin myofilaments so as to inhibit the sliding-filament contraction. However, though a muscle is contracted by the action of the cross bridges (figure 11.A-10), it cannot relax by the reverse process because the cross-bridge action does not run backward. In fact, as muscle fibers contract and experience a compressive stress, elastic energy is stored in the surrounding connective tissues as tensile stress; i.e., the muscle fibers are shortened during contraction, but the connective tissues at the ends of the fibers and sarcomeres are lengthened. Once the myofilaments within the contracted muscle fibers relax their grip on one another through the action of troponin, there is a release of the tensile stress on the connective tissue, which acts both to shorten the stretched connective tissue and return the muscle to its original length. Tentatively, it appears that the tensile stress on a muscle acts in an adaptive way to add sarcomeres to the ends of its muscle fibers, thereby making the muscle longer. Added to this, of course, will be the inelastic (viscoelastic) stretching of the connective tissue.

Titin and α-Actinin

The protein called titin is the largest protein in the body, constituting 10 percent of the muscle mass and forming a web that holds the myosin myofilaments in place with respect to the Z discs as the myofilaments of actin slide in and out (figure 11.A-8b) [877]. Recent experiments show that titin is a chain-like molecule having several tangles along its length. As it is stretched, the tangles release, so that a tangled molecule can increase its length (about 2.2 μ) by almost 50 percent. Titin regulates the flexibility and springiness of contracting muscle and so may be considered to be part of the connective tissue. Just as titin binds the myosin myofilaments to the Z disc, the protein α-actinin binds the actin myofilament to the Z disc (figures 11.A-8b and 11.A-10).

Changing Myofibril Length

When a joint is immobilized by being in a cast for six weeks or so, several changes in muscle structure follow, depending upon the details of the static position of the joint. If the joint is immobilized so that the length of the relevant muscle is shortened with respect to the resting state, then the end result will be a general loss of the number of sarcomeres in the muscle activating the joint. Because the muscle fibers atrophy at a faster rate than do the connective tissues, such immobility implies an increase in the ratio of connective tissue to muscle fiber and results in reduced range of motion and abnormal movement patterns.

If the static position of the joint in the cast stretches the relevant muscle so that it is longer than the resting length, then the effect of the immobilization will be an increase in the number of sarcomeres in the muscle and a decrease in the ratio of connective tissue to muscle fiber. Quantitatively, myofibril-length reductions of 40 percent have been reported for muscles immobilized short, and increases of 20 percent have been reported for muscles immobilized long [117].

If the tensile stretch of a muscle is maintained for a long period, it results in the addition of sarcomeres to the myofibrils; however, when the work is intermittent, as when stretching in isometric or eccentric exercise, the result is the synthesis of new myofilaments (hypertrophy) but no increase in the number of sarcomeres [549]. It is very tempting to imagine that in our *yogasana* practice, carried out daily for decades, the flexibility that results is due partly to increases in the number of sarcomeres incurred through the cumulative stretching over decades of practice. In terms of accumulated time, six weeks in a hip-flexing immobilizing cast is equal in time to being in a *yogasana* posture such as *paschimottanasana* for a total of ten minutes every day for sixteen and a half years. The corresponding time interval will be considerably shorter if the practitioner is allowed to increase the stretch from one week to the next as the flexibility develops. This sounds

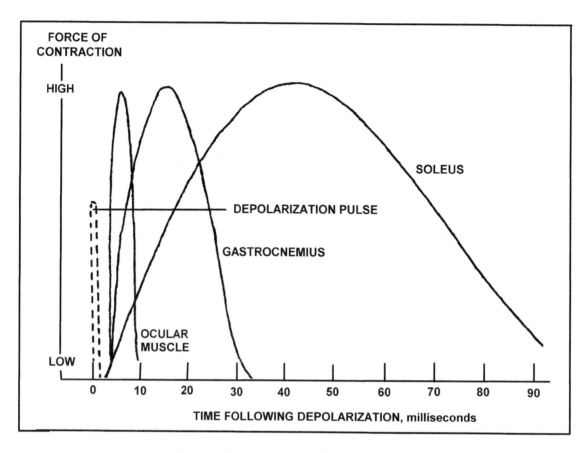

Figure 11.A-12. Showing the latency and contraction times of various muscles (in milliseconds) required to reach their maximum force of contraction after excitation with a brief depolarization pulse.

about right for a 20-percent lengthening of the hamstrings through serious *yogasana* practice. But one must not forget the viscoelastic flow of the connective tissue (Subsection 11.E, page 464) as contributing to positive changes in range of motion.

Muscle Action through Time

In human skeletal muscles and in the nerves, there is a refractory period following an excitation pulse, during which no further excitation is possible, regardless of the voltage stimulating the muscle. This refractory period varies from 2.2 to 4.6 milliseconds in most muscles, and that for the largest and most rapidly conducting α-motor neuron is 0.4 milliseconds. In general, the refractory periods for muscle contraction are somewhat larger than the corresponding values for neural transmission (tables 3.B-2 and 3.B-3) [549].

Muscles also differ in their response in time to a narrow activating pulse (figure 11.A-12). Thus, as shown in the figure, a sharp depolarization pulse applied to an ocular muscle results in a force of contraction that remains at zero level for a few milliseconds (the latency time), rises to a peak in about five milliseconds (the contraction time), and falls to zero again ten milliseconds after the initiating pulse. Applying the same depolarization pulse to the soleus muscle in the lower leg results in a response requiring about 100 milliseconds to go through the cycle; in contrast to this, excitation of the gastrocnemius is complete in just thirty milliseconds. These displays of the contraction time following a brief neural excitation lead logically to the classification of skeletal muscles as fast-twitch (ocular), slow-twitch (soleus), and intermediate-twitch (gastrocnemius); Subsection 11.A, page 411. Though the latency period is only about five milliseconds in skeletal muscle, it is 300 milliseconds in cardiac muscle, thereby allowing sufficient time for refilling following cardiac contraction.

A muscle that shortens its length by about 10 percent of its value when contracted requires between ten and 100 milliseconds to do so. As a general rule, the faster a muscle contracts, the weaker is the force that it can exert but the larger is the peak power (energy expended per unit time) generated over that short time [877].

Muscle Shape on Contraction

It is clear from the above discussion how the muscle contracts and shortens on a microscopic scale in order to do work. In contrast, on the macroscopic scale, we observe that as a muscle is shortened, its belly becomes larger in cross section, but this does not follow necessarily from what has been said up to this point. I postulate that in the relaxed state, with the actin not filling the myosin channels, the channels are otherwise filled with an extracellular fluid. On contraction, the actin moves into the channel, and at the same time, the fluid flows laterally out of the channel into surrounding areas. It is this fluid pressed out of the myosin channels that expands a contracting muscle in directions perpendicular to the direction of shortening. Looked at this way, the muscle is seen to be an organ of constant volume, and if it gets shorter, then it must get thicker in order to maintain its volume. This concept also arises when we consider how to lift the chest in the *yogasanas* (Subsection 10.A, page 328). The thickening of only the belly of the muscle follows from the fact that the contractile tissue resides in the center of the muscle, the ends being reserved for the non-contractile tendons.

Postural Muscles

As discussed in Subsection 11.A, page 411, certain motor units contract slowly but can remain contracted for a long time without fatigue, which characteristics identify them as type 1; whereas those motor units that contract rapidly but can maintain this state for only a short time are identified as type 3 (table 11.A-4). Muscles rich in type-1 motor units are called antigravity or postural muscles, for they are the ones that work continuously to keep the body erect in the gravitational field; whereas the fast-twitch, type-3 motor units are called phasic muscles, reflecting the short-lived nature of their contractions. Though a muscle in general is of a mixed muscle-fiber type, a motor unit is composed of a single muscle-fiber type.

The body's postural (tonic) motor units are of an older embryonic origin, whereas the phasic motor units are of a more recent origin; most muscles in the body are of mixed postural/phasic character. When we are in a *yogasana* posture, it may require that certain of the phasic muscles assume postural status for the length of the posture. For example, in *virabhadrasana II*, keeping the arms extended horizontally requires that the deltoids not only raise them to horizontal but also maintain them in this position for minutes at a time; in such a situation, the deltoids are functioning as postural muscles. With the deltoids acting in a postural mode, there will be recruitment of and then relaxation of individual motor units at a rate sufficient to hold the arms up for an extended time, but not at such a high rate as to lift them above horizontal. Alternatively, it may be that in a muscle having mixed postural and phasic content, the phasic aspect is excited in order to bring a limb into position, and then the postural component holds it there. In our example, the level of excitation must be guided ultimately by those proprioceptors and mechanoreceptors in the deltoid muscles and shoulder joints that monitor the angle of the arms and then call forth the requisite effort.

Muscle Tremor

When a muscle is excited at a frequency of one contraction per second, the result is a single muscle motor-unit twitch. At five to ten contractions per second, there will be no fusion of twitches in fast-twitch muscles and a more significant fusion of twitches, called clonus, in the slow-twitch muscles. In the *yogasanas*, this clonus is due to the muscle first contracting and then reflexively relaxing, followed by another cycle of contraction and relaxing, followed by more such cycles, and so will appear as a low-frequency (5–10 hertz) tremor of the slow-twitch muscle. When in a state of clonus, the strength of a skeletal muscle contraction increases significantly with each contraction for the first five contractions or so, and is constant from that point on; proper warm-up (Subsection 11.E, page 467) quickly brings one's muscles to peak contraction.

Unlike clonus, should the excitation frequency rise to fifty to 100 contractions per second, then successive excitations occur before any appreciable relaxation can take place, even in fast-twitch muscles. In this case, one observes the smooth, sustained contraction of the muscle called tetany. Clonus and tetany are possible since the period of contraction and relaxation are longer than the refractory period during which no action potentials can be launched (Subsection 3.B, page 42). Muscles usually go into tetany for brief periods when used normally.

When the level of muscular effort is maximal, most (if not all) of the fibers are recruited for action, and in that case, an entrainment process takes place that coordinates the excitation-relaxation cycles of the muscle fibers in most motor units and so can lead to tremors as they excite and relax in unison. Most often, the fraction of the fibers in a muscle that can be excited simultaneously is a fixed and inviolable quantity; however, in extreme circumstances, this can be violated, thereby increasing the strength momentarily and the risk of injury. Thus, one has the case of the superhuman "hysterical strength" of a mother lifting an auto off of her child, etc.

In a clever experiment designed to reveal the effects of yoga practice on muscle tremor in the outstretched arm [853], it was found that a group of college students, following ten days of intense yoga training, were able to reduce the amplitude of tremors during fifteen-second intervals by about 20 percent, at least part of which was attributable to increased fine-motor control.

Even when at rest, a muscle will be in a state of partial contraction, called tonus, which is maintained by successive weak contractions of muscles overlapping in time [450]. During weak contractions, the muscle involved contracts at a steady rate of 8–12 hertz; in the slow-twitch soleus muscle (figure 11.A-12), a steady contraction is maintained with a firing rate of only 11 hertz, whereas for the biceps brachii, the rate when at rest is more like 30 hertz. However, at the start of a strong contraction in a slow-twitch muscle, the rate of contraction will be 100 hertz or more. As the contraction continues and the muscle fatigues, its contraction rate slows noticeably, because the muscle stays contracted, thanks to an intrinsically slower relaxation rate in the fatigued state [549].

Other tremors occur only when at rest, as with the 3-hertz tremor of the Parkinson's condition, but they cease on intentional movement in this case. Tremors also can occur when performing or following intentional actions and are related to malfunctions in the cerebellum, that otherwise controls balance and muscle coordination. These intentional tremors also appear when first attempting a muscular *yogasana* with which the neuromuscular apparatus is not familiar; these tremors pass very quickly with practice.

I have often wondered about the seeming contradiction involving the super-athlete weight-lifter and the frail senior citizen, each doing *adho mukha svanasana* for the first time and each trembling with the effort. I first assumed the super-athlete was strong but muscularly tight and so trembled from the effort, whereas the frail senior citizen was weak and trembled from the effort. But how would two totally different bodies display the same physical tremor?

I believe that because the two students are each new to the practice, in their desire to perform at their best, they put everything they have into performing. In muscular activities requiring an unusual amount of contraction, it is possible to bring all of the motor units into a lockstep contraction-and-relaxation cycle, with the result being a global shaking of the muscle at the contraction frequency.

Tremors of lower frequency also will be seen in the novice, due to the clumsy neural activation and release of various motor units in the muscles in an uncoordinated manner, regardless of how active or muscular the performer may appear to be from the outside. With time and practice, the frail senior citizen and the super-athlete will stop shaking as they subconsciously develop more efficient plans of motor-unit utilization; i.e., the appropriate neural patterning develops, and the trembling ceases.

Muscle Chemistry and Energy

ATP and ADP

The overall chemistry of muscle movement is complex, but it is sufficient for our purpose to state that the energy required for contraction involves the dephosphorylation of the important molecule adenosine triphosphate (ATP), as catalyzed by the enzyme ATPase to form adenosine diphosphate (ADP). The depolarization of the neuromuscular-junction voltage and the propagation of the action potential down the length of the muscle fiber initially involve ion channels in the cell membranes allowing the transport of Na^+, K^+ and Ca^{2+} ions into and out of the cell during the contraction process [427]. Once initiated, the ATP comes into play.

ATP, the fuel for muscle action, is a key product of the mitochondrial organelles within every muscle cell. Following the formation of ADP in a contracting muscle fiber, there are several other chemical processes that serve to re-phosphorylate the ADP to re-form ATP, which lives again to help drive another actin myofilament down its myosin channel.

Once the body is asked to do muscular work, the circulating catecholamine levels in the blood rise with consequent rises in the heart rate, breathing rate, and depth of the breath; the blood vessels surrounding the relevant muscles dilate; and glucose and fatty acids are released as fuel for the reformation of ATP from ADP.

ATP Drives Cross-Bridge Motion

ATP is bound to the head of the myosin cross bridges, but on approach to the newly uncovered active sites on the actin myofilaments (figure 11.A-9b), the ATP is cleaved into ADP plus phosphate ion, both of which leave the cross-bridge head as it binds to the actin. Once this simple chemical reaction is accomplished with the help of the enzyme ATPase, there is a strong mechanical movement of the cross-bridge head (the power stroke, figure 11.A-9c), which is translated into actin-myofilament motion. The presence of fresh ATP in the cellular fluid surrounding the myofilaments encourages the head of the cross bridge to disengage from the actin following the power stroke and bind again to any ATP in its neighborhood, thus preparing it for another stroke.

As long as there is Ca^{2+} and ATP in the cell, the heads of the cross bridges will continue to convert ATP into ADP and to pull the actin myofilaments from the Z discs toward the centers of the sarcomeres. Initially, this process occurs about ten to fifty times per second but is limited by the amount of ATP available in the cell for reattachment to the cross-bridge heads.

In a dead body, where the mitochondria no longer function, there is little or no ATP to recharge the cross-bridge heads, the contractile machinery is essentially frozen, and rigor mortis sets in, as discussed in Box 11.A-1 below.

Body Heat

It is estimated that up to 85 percent of the body's total heat is generated by contraction of the skeletal muscles. Part of this muscular heat is generated by the cleavage of the high-energy phosphate chemical bond in ATP; because only 25 percent of the phosphate bond energy in ATP is available for work, the other 75 percent appears as heat (or entropy). Heat is also liberated when the elastic parts of the contracted muscle, the myofasciae, return to their resting lengths. Because the heat generated in using a muscle acts to soften the resistance of the connective tissue to stretching, this heat can be much appreciated when practicing *yogasana* on a cold morning! Heat stress in over-exercising adults has been shown to reduce $\dot{V}O_2$ by reducing blood flow from the heart and the availability of oxygen to the contracting muscles [283].

Box 11.A-1: Muscular Life after Death

Once the heart and the brain become quiescent, the body can then be said to have died physiologically. However, even in this state of death, there still remains a small quantity of ATP in the muscle fibers, and given an electrical stimulus from outside the body, the muscles can still be made to contract until the ATP within them finally is exhausted.[1] This muscle action in the dead can be stimulated for up to two hours after death. Once the ATP in a dead body is exhausted, muscle action stops, leaving the actin-myosin machinery frozen in a state of partial contraction (figure 11.A-10c), with bridge heads in contact but not able to either ratchet forward or relax backward. Muscles in this condition are said to be in the state of "rigor mortis."

Relaxation of a muscle in a state of rigor mortis requires yet more ATP to pump the Ca^{2+} away from its complex with troponin, in which case the troponin then could do its job of separating the actin and myosin myofilaments, and the muscle could return to its resting state. However, because this additional ATP is not available after death, no muscle motion is possible. Rigor mortis begins with the muscles of the face and proceeds in steps toward the toes; the state of rigor mortis lasts for up to twelve hours and then relaxes from that point as the muscle proteins decompose [716]. Once the cells start to die, the immune system collapses, and bacterial decay begins. Smooth muscle does not show rigor mortis following death.

This scenario for the relaxation of dead skeletal muscle is quite different from that of live but contracted muscle. In the latter case, there is enough ATP available to force the Ca^{2+} back through the t-tubules and into the sarcoplasmic reticulum, so that the troponin again separates the actin and myosin myofilaments. From this point, the compressive stress in the titin and the elastic strain in the muscle's connective tissue and tendons are released, and the contracted muscle lengthens therewith.

---

1   Brain cells die when deprived of oxygen for longer than three minutes, whereas muscle cells will live for several hours without oxygen, and bone and skin cells will survive for several days.

Contraction and Heat Production

When a muscle contracts against a load in the gravitational field, not only is energy expended in the contraction of the sarcomeres, but energy also is expended in stretching and reconfiguring the connective tissue and tendons associated with the muscle. Of the energy involved in muscle contraction, only 20–25 percent is used for movement, and the remainder is involved in overcoming the viscous resistance of the connective tissues and the frictional resistance of blood flow through the vascular system. In addition to these resistive sources of heat, various chemical reactions driving muscle metabolism also produce heat.

If a muscle is first stretched and then used to perform work, the work so done is larger than if the muscle were not pre-stretched, because stretching stores elastic energy for a short time in the stretched muscle, and this is recovered during contraction. Muscle power is increased if the sarcomere length is increased prior to doing work. This is a telling example of the importance of a stretching warm-up before any strength competition [822].

Sources of ATP

The energy demands of muscle action are that it be plentiful, readily available, and easily renewable. ATP is needed not only to remove the myosin cross bridges from the actin myofilaments, thus allowing the bridges to move to a new position on the actin myofilaments, but ATP is also required in the many energy-demanding processes that pump Na^+, K^+, H^+, and Ca^{2+} ions across membranes. The Na^+, K^+, and Ca^{2+} transmembrane ion pumps, when working in muscles, will consume at least one-third of all of the ATP consumed in the muscle action. ATP also has functions beyond the muscular. When ATP is released from damaged tissue, it can elicit pain, and when ATP is released from the walls of the urinary bladder, it signals that the bladder needs emptying. Most anabolic reactions—the conversion of amino acids into proteins, the conversion of nucleotides into DNA, the synthesis of polysacharrides, and the synthesis of fats—are driven by ATP. Add to this list both the active transport of molecules and ions and ATP's roles in nerve impulses and sensing taste.

There are three sources of ATP. (1) Creatine phosphate reacts with ADP to reform ATP. The muscle cells contain about ten times as much creatine phosphate as ATP. (2) Skeletal muscle is about 1 percent glycogen (a polymer of glucose), and each glucose molecule within glycogen can be converted into two molecules of ATP and two of lactic acid in the process called glycolysis. Because this process is anaerobic, there is still a need to continue deep breathing following anaerobic exercise, in order to regenerate glycogen from the lactic acid generated by glycolysis; i.e., we must repay the oxygen debt. (3) Cellular respiration creates ATP. On prolonged exercise, the need for ATP is fulfilled by the oxidation of glucose or other fuel by oxygen to produce carbon dioxide and water within the mitochondria [450].

Creatine Phosphate

All muscle cells use ATP to fuel the work of the cell, but the cell at rest contains only enough ATP to fuel intense muscle activity for about five

or six seconds. Obviously, this is not enough to sustain the more general needs of life, and so other indirect sources of ATP may be called upon in times of need. As ATP is consumed by dephosphorylation and its decomposition product ADP is formed, the latter is readily re-phosphorylated by the creatine phosphate (also called phosphocreatine) in the cell to reform ATP. Normally, there is enough creatine phosphate in the cell to extend the cell's working period to twenty to twenty-five seconds or so, but it then requires several minutes to replenish itself. Because this process does not produce lactic acid or require oxygen, it has been described as alactic anaerobic oxidation. It is activated during brief but intense muscular actions, as with *chaturanga dandasana* or *pincha mayurasana* held for times between fifteen and thirty seconds.

Anaerobic Oxidation

For periods of time beyond twenty-five seconds, the muscle cell relies instead on the anaerobic oxidation of fats and glucose (or glycogen, a polymerized form of glucose) to help in reforming ATP. In low-energy exercise or when at rest, oxidation of fats is the main source of energy, and in this slow-twitch mode, the rate of accumulation of lactic acid is slower than the rate at which it is being removed. However, with increasing muscular effort, type-2 fibers are recruited and the rates of lactic-acid production and removal become comparable. At that point, the metabolism switches from oxidizing fats for energy to oxidizing sugars instead. Glycogen is called upon only with increasing muscular effort. Glycogen may be thought of as animal starch, as it is the major carbohydrate stored in animal tissue. Most of the carbohydrate oxidized for energy in the mitochondria is stored first as glycogen in the liver and is available for energy only when liver enzymes (such as glucagon) degrade the glycogen to glucose. Hormones from the brain activate these enzymes whenever we begin to exercise or even begin to think of exercising. Thus, warming up not only loosens the muscles but also gets the glucose flowing, so as to keep the muscles well fueled.

Lactic Acid

With sustained contractions of the muscle and concomitant ischemia of the muscle (due to the systolic arterial pressure being less than the rise of internal pressure in the belly of the contracting muscle), the glycolytic pathway to more ATP becomes very important, as it does not require oxygen for its completion; i.e., it is anaerobic. Said differently, if the level of muscle work requires a level of oxygen that the cardiovascular system cannot meet, then the mitochondria turn to an anaerobic means of refreshing the ATP supply. Receptors on the surface of the muscle-cell membranes are specific for epinephrine, and when so stimulated, they trigger a long chain of chemical events leading to the eventual hydrolysis of glycogen into glucose. Under these conditions, the pyruvic acid that is formed in glycolysis is converted to lactic acid ($CH_3CHOHCO_2H$), which accumulates in the cell and lowers its pH, eventually limiting its activity as the lactic acid buildup leads to muscle fatigue. This acid-induced muscle fatigue is a safety measure, as it protects us from harmful overuse of the muscle. Fast-twitch muscles (Subsection 11.A, page 411), when overused, take the glycolysis route in order to remain functioning. The fast-twitch muscle fibers within the large motor units are well suited to an efficient and rapid switch to anaerobic glycogen metabolism, because they have large stores of glycogen and glycolytic enzymes of high activity within them.

The level of lactic acid produced reaches a limiting value after about three minutes of intense exercise, whereas the glycogen store will last for over sixty minutes of heavy exercise. Once the period of extreme exercise has passed and sufficient oxygen then becomes available, the excess lactic acid is oxidized back to pyruvic acid, and aerobic oxidation again dominates.[3]

3   Realizing that lactic acid buildup was a negative factor in high-intensity exercise, athletes have turned to ingesting large amounts of sodium bicarbonate (as found in Alka-Seltzer); as hoped, the acid-buffering action of this antacid compound has demonstrably improved performance [618]. In no way can one rec-

Aerobic Oxidation and Lipolysis

Anaerobic glycolysis in humans can be active for only about three minutes, at which point, aerobic metabolism takes over. When one is exercising in the aerobic regime, the level of glucose in the blood falls, and in response to this, the glucostat in the hypothalamus activates the sympathetic nervous system, so that both the catecholamines and cortisol are released from the adrenal glands (Section 5.C, page 170). The epinephrine component of the catecholamines increases the mobilization of fatty acids by releasing them from their bound form as triglycerides in a chemical process called lipolysis. However, this lipolysis of the triglycerides by epinephrine is not possible in the absence of cortisol. Thus, when exercising, the sympathetic nervous system is activated and body fat is burned away through the intermediary action of the adrenal hormones [432]. Fat is the most abundant energy source for the muscles of the body; however, lipolysis does not become active until anaerobic glycolysis is first exhausted. Moreover, lipolysis, though energetic, is a slow process. The importance of various energy sources having potential use in fueling muscles are listed in table 11.A-3.

One sees from the table that the body's glycogen stores can sustain one through about a quarter of a day if one is working in a *yogasana* practice that is energetically equivalent to walking, and that fatty acids and proteins are present

ommend "soda loading" to students of *yogasana*, but it might be possible to eat an alkaline diet [473], which would then tend to neutralize the lactic acid produced by prolonged work of the muscles in *yogasanas*, were that a problem. In fact, in slow-twitch type-1 fibers, where there are multitudes of mitochondria, the pyruvic acid is preferentially oxidized to sidestep production of lactic acid and instead promotes high levels of ATP production. As *yogasana* practice is a strongly type-1 activity, it generally does not lead to the problem of lactic acid accumulation. In any event, lactic acid does not accumulate for long periods, as it is rapidly metabolized, and it is not the cause of long-term post-exercise muscle soreness (Subsection 11.G, page 476).

Table 11.A-3: Potential Energy Sources in the Body for Fueling Muscle Action [910]

Tissue Fuel Store	Weight of Reserves (grams)	Days of Walking Supported by This Store
Triglycerides in adipose tissue	9,000	10.8
Liver glycogen	90	0.05
Muscle glycogen	350	0.2
Blood and extracellular glycogen	20	0.01
Protein	8,800	4.8

in abundance, but they are called upon only after the glycogen is consumed, and then they deliver a lower energy output. After three hours of exercise, the amounts of epinephrine and norepinephrine in the blood have risen by factors of seven and four, respectively, the glucagon level has risen by a factor of 2.5, and the level of insulin has dropped by a factor of 0.5 [910].

The aerobic process also uses glucose and fatty acids as fuel for generating more ATP, "burning" them instead using the oxygen carried to the muscle fiber's mitochondria by the hemoglobin in the blood. In this case, ATP is produced, but without the lactic-acid penalty. Once into the aerobic regime, the muscle cell can work with moderate intensity until the supplies of glucose, fatty acids, and oxygen are exhausted. The body's store of glycogen will be exhausted after twenty to thirty minutes of work, and then the body turns to the oxidation of fats as a source of energy for work. Because the average body has an almost limitless supply of fat, it can work at this moderate level of exercise for a very long time, using fat to produce the necessary ATP. It is this process that reduces the level of body fat through exercise.

Yogasana and ATP

Aerobic exercise basically pumps up the cardiovascular system, thus allowing greater volumes of blood to circulate through the body; whereas anaerobic exercise tones the muscles and sets the basic metabolic rate, the rate at which calories are burned. Anaerobic exercise works the muscles and bones and accelerates the metabolism as it increases the ratio of muscle to fat in the body.

The shift into aerobic oxidation after two or three minutes of heavy exercise is evident as the athlete's "second wind." Yoga students benefit from this second wind when performing aerobic jumping routines such as *surya namaskar,* the "salute to the sun," but are otherwise working in the anaerobic regime. When *yogasana* practice is working in the aerobic regime, it increases $\dot{V}O_{2max}$ (the highest rate at which oxygen can be supplied during exercise) and promotes the transformation of fast-twitch into slow-twitch fibers [15] (Subsection 11.A, page 419). Because the amount of work that a muscle can do is strictly limited by the amount of oxygen that can be delivered to the mitochondria of its cells by the bloodstream, $\dot{V}O_{2max}$ is seen to be a measure of the body's ability to do work.

Because muscle tissue cannot work without a flow of blood through the muscle, fatigue will set in after about three minutes of work. In this situation, the muscle responds by the release of nitric oxide from the endothelial cells lining the vascular structures, thereby leading to larger arterial diameters; the muscle is then engorged with fresh blood and is "pumped up."

General Adaptation Syndrome

Muscle cells are constantly repairing themselves from within, as exercise not only uses up certain cell constituents, but also does specific damage to some cells. Therefore, immediately following exercise, you are somewhat injured and weaker than before! The effect of the "general adaptation syndrome" [772] is to repair the damage and to shift the cells' metabolism so that the same stress in the future will have a smaller negative impact; this subject also is discussed in Subsection 5.E, pages 186 and 188. Thus, if we deplete glycogen by a lengthy workout, this triggers a rebound restoration of glycogen to a level higher than the original one. If we sweat excessively, the adjustment will be made to sweat more, but to lose less salt in the process. If the stress is too weak, then there is no adaptive growth, nor is there growth if the stress is too large. Some cellular adaptations to exercise have rapid response rates; plasma volume increases in a matter of a week following hard training, whereas the promotion of capillary growth may require years to complete itself. Exercise at a level below that which stimulates the adaptation response is still of great value, as it helps to maintain previous gains and gives the body a chance to recuperate.

The effects of long-term exercise are even more interesting than those of short-term work. When the exercise is chronic rather than acute, as with an intense daily *yogasana* practice, $\dot{V}O_{2max}$ increases, while the resting heart rate, the rise in blood lactate, and the concentration of catecholamines in the blood (Subsection 5.E, page 188) are lower when exercising. Moreover, there is an almost 100-percent increase in the number of blood capillaries per muscle fiber [169, 618], and in the muscle cells themselves, the myoglobin and enzyme contents increase, as does the size of the mitochondria. On prolonged, chronic exercise, the levels of stored glycogen and triglycerides increase, and more fatty acids than carbohydrates are burned for energy, both of which lead to less glycogen being depleted, less lactic acid being formed, less soreness, less muscle fatigue, and increased endurance.

Physical Limits

There are three physiological variables that limit the speed of your physical performance. (1) There is a limited rate of oxygen consumption in the working muscles, due to limited rates of delivery of oxygenated blood by the arteries. When at this limit, the heart appears to be remodeled, with the formation of larger ventricles, but this positive factor plateaus after a few months at about 15–20 percent improvement. (2) At the lactic acid threshold, lactic pain starts to diminish the ability to work. Limiting factors here are capillary development and density, fatty-acid enzyme levels, and the mitochondrial density within the working muscles. The lactic acid factor comes into play after the oxygenation issue. The ability to work with high lactate levels may plateau after six months of regular training. (3) The efficiency of the process of changing physiological work into movement is the last to respond to training, as neural efficiency improves slowly. As discussed by B. K. S. Iyengar [395], his aging has lessened his strength, but by constant practice, he continues to increase his efficiency and so maintains his level of performance (Subsection 4.G, page 149).

Isotonic Metabolism

An interesting study has been published, in which the relative effects of eccentric and concentric isotonic exercise were compared [334]. The exercise in question involved walking uphill (concentric exercise) versus walking downhill (eccentric exercise). It was found that triglyceride levels were reduced only by uphill walking, whereas walking downhill was twice as effective as uphill walking in removing blood sugars and improving glucose tolerance. Note too that downhill walking places twice the load on the knee joints as does uphill walking, and this difference may apply to the hip joints as well. These aspects should be kept in mind as one moves isotonically into and out of isometric *yogasanas*.

Macroscopic Muscle Contraction

Though the same muscle may be used to lift a one-ounce pencil or to lift a ten-pound sack of sugar, clearly the work performed by that muscle will be very different in the two cases. This is reasonable from two points of view. First, because the number of motor units recruited to a task can be varied to suit the job, lifting a pencil requires only a small percentage of the motor units available in a large muscle, whereas lifting a heavier sack can require a larger percentage. Second, the rate of motor-unit excitation can be varied to suit the job. It is a specific benefit of *yogasana* practice that one can fine-tune not only how many and which of the motor units in a large muscle are called into action, but their contraction frequencies as well. Further, one can balance the effect of agonist contraction by simultaneously activating the antagonist muscle groups (Subsection 11.A, page 422). With such muscular discrimination available, the *yogasana* student not only has precise control of body movement but also uses the body's resources in the most efficient way possible.

Pennate Muscles

The basic contractive unit within a muscle is the muscle fiber. As a muscle fiber can run the full length of a long, thin muscle, the muscle-fiber axis in this case can run parallel to the direction of movement that it initiates. Such a muscle is called fusiform. However, fusiform muscles (the sartorius, for example, figure 11.A-13a) are relatively weak as compared to those muscles in which there is a central tendon to which the muscle-fiber bundles (fascicles) are set on one side only, usually at an angle (up to 30°) to the long axis (figure 11.A-13b). Such muscle-fiber arrangements are called unipennate. This type of fascicle arrangement effectively increases the cross-sectional area of the muscle and so increases the force that can be generated by that muscle, all the while using a relatively small range of motion [549]. So, for example, we have as unipennate muscles the masseters of the jaw, the long flexors of the thumbs, and the deltoids of the shoulders.

In bipennate muscles (figure 11.A-13c) such as the rectus femoris in the thighs, there are two rows of inclined fascicles attached to the central tendon. The small interossei muscles between the metacarpals of the hands and the metatarsals of the feet are bipennate muscles with independent excitation on each side of the central tendon. Depending on which side of the bipennate

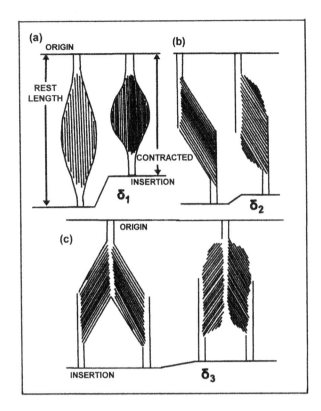

Figure 11.A-13. The various types of fascicle arrangements: fusiform, pennate, and bipennate. Fusiform muscles (**a**) have large changes of length (δ_1) on contraction but are relatively weak, whereas unipennate (**b**) and bipennate muscles (**c**) have much smaller changes of length (δ_2) and (δ_3), respectively but are relatively much stronger than the fusiform variety [877].

interossei muscle is contracted, the action is to pull the phalanges together or to separate them (Subsection 10.B, page 361). Multipennate muscles consist of many bipennate units, while a circular array of fascicles is found in the circular sphincters of the body.

Fusiform muscles, consisting largely of parallel fascicles but lacking a central tendon, have low power but large ranges of motion (δ_1), whereas those that contain large numbers of the pennate structures are much stronger but more restricted in their ranges of motion (δ_2 and δ_3). The oblique pennate muscle structure is the most important in regard to endurance and steadiness in the *yogasanas,* whereas the parallel-fascicle arrangement of fusiform muscles is a strong contributor to elongation of the muscle.

Variation of Muscle Dimensions

There are three factors to consider when discussing muscle size: (1) the diameter increases immediately on contraction, due to the radial displacement of extracellular fluid when the muscle contracts axially; (2) there are long-term increases in diameter, due to packing of the myofibrils with extra myofilaments (hypertrophy); and (3) there can be long-term changes in length, due to added or excised sarcomeres, as discussed above (page 387). Permanent lengthening is most favored by low-force, long-duration stretching done at high temperature [822]. Similarly, muscles that are shortened by injury or lack of exercise are shortened by excision of sarcomere units from their ends; one study showed a loss of 40 percent of the sarcomeres in a muscle held in prolonged flexion when immobilized by a cast.

The effects of exercise on muscle dimension are manifold. As the strength of the muscle increases, so does its cross section, but not necessarily in young children (Subsection 4.G, page 140). At puberty in males, there is a dramatic surge in muscle strength, which is attributable to the anabolic effects of testosterone.

The long-term increased size of an exercised muscle in an adult comes from the larger diameter of the muscle fibers, as their number stays constant. (However, see Subsection 11.A, page 405.) Practice of the *yogasanas* necessarily involves a certain amount of strength training, during which the strengths, resting lengths, and diameters of the muscles increase. This increase in the size of a muscle with *yogasana* strength training again is due to an increase in the diameters of the muscle's fibers, and not due to an increase in their number. However, as the fibers increase in girth, there is a corresponding increase in the amount of connective tissue binding them together [169]. Work such as weightlifting, which increases the bulk of a muscle but does little to stretch its connective tissue, results in a large muscle that can move through only a small range of motion. It is largely for this anatomic

fact that a counterbalancing *yogasana* practice is so important to weightlifters. On the other hand, if a muscle is not used at all, it will atrophy as the individual muscle cells progressively lose their myofibrils [549]; this includes the heart. (However, also see Subsection 14.A, page 556, and Subsection 24.A, page 812.)

When muscle fibers contract, there is no shortening, thickening, or folding of the individual filaments; they just slide past one another. This is in spite of the obvious shortening and thickening of the muscle as observed macroscopically from the outside. Several experiments have shown that the contraction of a muscle (or of all muscles simultaneously) does not change the volume of the muscle (or muscles) [878]. As the channels of the myosin are filled with extracellular fluid in the resting state, this fluid is pressed radially to the outside of the channels as the actin moves axially into the channels. In this way, the macroscopic volume of the muscle stays constant during a contraction.

The mechanical concept that a muscle has a constant volume, regardless of its state of extension or contraction, leads naturally to the expectation that if a muscle is shortened by contraction, it must increase in girth in the perpendicular directions; however, if it is instead put into a tensile stretch along its axis, it will experience compression in directions perpendicular thereto. Thus, stretching, as in *yogasana* practice, works to pull the centers of gravity of the muscles onto the bone, and contraction works to move their centers of gravity away from the bone. With this in mind, we see that the admonition to "contract the muscle so as to pull the muscle onto the bone" often given by *yogasana* teachers is not possible anatomically, but it can be achieved with muscles that are being stretched isometrically. Furthermore, if by "contraction" it is meant that the volume of a muscle decreases, then muscles do not contract, being organs of constant volume, irrespective of the state of contraction.

As applied to the spine, the lengthening of the spine from the coccyx to the crown of the head, as is always the case in *yogasana* practice, is possible only if the girth of the torso decreases radially; i.e., only if the abdomen is gently pulled in toward the spine. As applied to the tongue, it can be shot forward by contracting the muscles that lie transverse to its axis; i.e., if the volume of the tongue is to be kept constant while its width decreases, then the length must increase. Conversely, a relaxed tongue in *savasana* is broad and relatively short.

Tensile Stress on Contraction

On the microscopic scale, a muscle fiber at a given moment is either at rest or fully contracted; there is no middle ground. On the other hand, a graded muscle response is possible, in which the intensity of macroscopic muscle contraction increases as the number of contracting muscle fibers increases, and as the frequency of excitation increases.

The tensile stress that a muscle can develop on contraction is determined largely by its cross-sectional area, being between 2.5 to 3.5 kilograms per square centimeter (35–43 pounds per square inch). If we assign the quadriceps muscle a diameter of 10 centimeters (four inches), at maximum contraction, the load on the patellar tendon will be more than 250 kilograms (550 pounds), which is large enough to tear the tendon from the bone or to separate the tendon itself. Similar forces are applied to the joint surfaces and to the ligaments binding the joint. If a muscle is maximally contracted, then the force necessary to stretch it while in the contracted state (eccentric contraction) is another 40 percent larger still, resulting in a load on the patellar tendon, for example, that is as large as 350 kilograms (770 pounds)!

Muscle Strength

The strength of a muscle—the force that it can exert when contracting—depends on many factors. First, the muscle fibers are activated by signals from the attached neurons. With practice, these neural signals are refined so that the contraction of the relevant muscle fibers is more synchronous and more efficient, whereas inhibiting contractions are reduced or removed with practice. This neural repatterning is reinforced when one practices the contraction with many repetitions at low

load.[4] In addition to the cross-sectional size of the muscle and the sizes of the muscle fibers of which it is composed, the strength of muscle contraction also is dependent on the difference between its resting and fully contracted lengths, the amplitude and frequency of the action potential driving its contraction, and the resistance of the muscle fascia to further increases of the tensile stress.

The concept of "muscle strength" is rather ambiguous, in the sense that a muscle may be considered as "strong" because it can generate a large force over a short time, or it may be considered as "strong" because it can be used continuously at moderate force without fatigue. As discussed more fully in Subsection 11.A, page 412, at the extremes, a muscle may be composed predominantly either of type-3 fibers (which are strong for a short time, but which then fatigue easily) or of type-1 fibers (which are not able to generate a high momentary force but do not fatigue, even when contracted for long times, table 11.A-3). The two extreme muscle types are mutually exclusive, in the sense that a muscle of high endurance (type 1) can never be maximally strong for short periods of time, and a muscle of maximum strength on a short time scale (type 3) can never have high endurance over time [827].

Graded Response

The action potential necessary to excite contraction in a muscle fiber is smaller for the smaller (weaker) fibers in a motor unit. Thus, at low action potential, only the small fibers of a muscle are excited. If the impulses are of such a low frequency that the time between impulses (longer

---

4   The energy expended by a yoga beginner and a yoga master of the same weight when performing the same posture will be identical if the efficiency with which their bodies are put into action is the same. The advantage of the yoga master lies in that training rapidly increases his or her capacity for yogic work via a higher anaerobic threshold, whereas efficiency only slowly increases strength. A higher anaerobic threshold means that the work is well tolerated for extended periods, whereas when the anaerobic threshold is crossed, work is unsustainable, as one becomes strongly distressed.

than fifty milliseconds if the frequency is below 20 hertz) is longer than the muscle-fiber twitch time (five to fifty milliseconds), then the muscle contraction will appear as a tremor, because the number of excited fibers is minimal, and its number oscillates in time, as motor-unit excitations are random. If the neural signal strength is raised, then so too is the action potential; in that case, both small and large fibers are excited, and contraction is then strong and continuous in time; i.e., the tremor disappears as the nervous system is strengthened.

Increasing Strength through Yoga

Cole states that stretching does not make a *yogasana* student weaker, but if the exercise offers no contraction of the muscles against resistance (such as gravity), then weakness will follow [147]. That is to say, our muscles become stronger only by working to overcome resistance to our motions. Low-resistance work done over a long period offers only a minimal benefit in regard to the strength of the average muscle; time spent in *savasana* and *garbhasana* is relaxing but does not do anything for strengthening the muscles. If the goal is only to strengthen a muscle, then the more certain route to success is to do a minimum number of repetitions of the appropriate strength-building exercise, but to do it at the highest resistance.

Two intrinsic factors are relevant to the strengthening of a muscle to be used maximally but on a short-term basis: increasing the muscle mass through enlargement of the muscle cells (hypertrophy), and the optimization of the neural patterning driving the relevant muscle contractions. Hypertrophy involves the formation of more contractive proteins within the muscle, whereas neural patterning involves the simultaneous recruitment of more motor units to the task at hand. The unpracticed muscle will employ an asynchronous excitation of the muscle fibers, whereas for a momentary test of strength, a maximum synchronization of muscle-fiber recruitment is necessary. Both aspects of muscle strengthening are optimized by repeated practice of the appropriate exercises at high load.

Muscular strength of the sort needed in *yogas-*

ana practice is developed through exercises that are low in regard to the load being moved but that are high in duration or in repetition, promoting the formation of type-1 muscle fiber; the muscular strength in this case is largely a strengthening of the neural system that energizes or activates the muscles in question. In contrast, the muscular girth (and therefore strength) that is developed by exercising at maximum load, but with a minimum duration or number of repetitions, promotes the formation of type-2 and type-3 muscle fibers. *Yogasana* practice deals largely with the development of a type-1 body, but it may involve the development of some of the type-2 or type-3 muscle fibers as well.

As Lasater [498] has so eloquently pointed out, *yogasana* practice is involved not only with the strength of the muscles, but also with the inner strength that one demonstrates in one's commitment to practicing what may be difficult. This is the motivational factor mentioned in Box 2.D-1, page 27, and in Subsection 4.G, pages 135 and 146.

Strength and Length

The ability of the muscle to contract and so exert a force on an object depends on the length of the muscle in a very specific way:- it is strongest in this regard when the muscle is at its resting length, and the closer it approaches its limiting lengths, as when stretched or contracted, the weaker it becomes. This is discussed in Box 11.A-2 below.

Muscles at their Limits

A muscle feels taut at either end of the length-tension curve (figure 11.A-11). When contracted totally, the muscle maintains constant volume, as the effective length of the sarcomeres shorten, but the fluid within the myosin channels is expelled outward, perpendicular to the muscle's long axis. At the other end, the muscle is again taut, in this case due to the viscoelastic components being stretched to their limits, both within and outside the sarcomere.

When a muscle is in a weakened condition, as when at either points A or E of figure 11.A-11, it

Box 11.A-2: Muscle Strength versus Muscle Length

Muscle strength—the maximum tension that a muscle can develop—is maximal at the resting length of the muscle but drops to 50 percent of its maximal value when the muscle length is either shortened to 70 percent of the resting length or extended to 130 percent of that length (figure 11.A-11) [432]. The curve of generated tension versus muscle length is highly asymmetric, for when fully contracted, the muscle length is 35 percent shorter than when in the resting state, but when elongated, the muscle is 60 percent longer than the resting length (figure 11.A-11). Considering the variation of muscle strength with muscle length, as in the figure, the strength is seen to be largest at the resting length (B and C) and least when extremely long (D) or extremely short (A). When a muscle is fully stretched (figure 11.A-10a), the overlap of the actin and myosin myofilaments is minimal, and so only a minimum contractive force can be developed. Similarly, when the muscle is tightly contracted (figure 11.A-10d), the actin myofilaments are so severely jammed into the channels of the myosin myofilaments that the actin myofilaments overlap each other, and only a weak contractile force is possible. Muscle action is strongest when the muscle is at a length where all possible cross bridges can be realized but there is still room within the sarcomeres for large-scale movement of the actin myofilaments. This occurs when the muscle is at its resting length, as shown in figure 11.A-10b. The images shown in figure 11.A-11 most likely represent the muscles of *yogasana* practitioners or contortionists in a general sense, but not in detail.

The variation of muscle strength with muscle length can be confirmed by the *yogasana* student in a simple way, as shown in figure 11.A-14. The muscles of the inner forearm (flexor digitorum) flex the fingertips into the palm of the hand; when the wrist is flexed so as to bring the fingertips toward the inner elbow, as in figure 11.A-14a, the flexor muscles in question are at minimal length; when the wrist is extended so that the fingertips move toward the outer elbow (figure 11.A-14b), the flexors are at maximal length. On the other hand, when the wrist is neither flexed nor extended, as in figure 11.A-14c, the flexors are at their resting lengths. With the wrist held successively in each of the positions shown in figures 11.A-14a, 11.A-14b, and 11.A-14c, note how much more strongly one can pull the fingertips into the palm of the hand so as to make a fist when in the neutral position (figure 11.A-14c) as compared to the situations when the same flexor muscles are used to make a fist while at either their shortest (figure 11.A-14a, wrist flexed) or longest (11.A-14b, wrist extended) lengths.

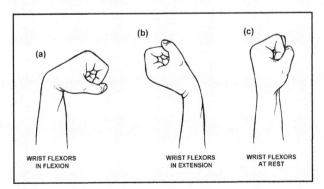

Figure 11.A-14. Comparison of the force of muscle contraction when making a fist of the fingers when the wrist is in the flexed position (**a**), in the extended position (**b**), and in the neutral position (**c**).

will be more subject to injury if asked to do heavy lifting than when in the stronger configurations C or D. The first instance, configuration A, in which a muscle is fully flexed and then put under tensile stress, results in severe damage, as this is eccentric isotonic contraction (Subsection 11.A, page 407). At the other end, configuration D, one is again facing injury if a muscle is weakened, due to its fully extended condition, and then becomes involved in movements requiring great strength. This second is the situation most appropriate to *yogasana* practice.

Often we err as teachers when we give explicit instruction to students on how to enter a posture and how to remain in a posture but are largely silent when we bring them out of the posture. This encourages the students to relax their alignment when coming out of the posture, thereby putting them at risk for straining muscles that have been called into service on a job for which they are unsuited. Even when in perfect alignment throughout, the possibility remains that beginning students can injure themselves when recovering from a strenuous posture using muscles weakened due to the poor myofilament overlap inherent in their stretched conditions.

Two examples are relevant here. When in *trikonasana*-to-the-right, if the left ribs are arched upward by the collapse of the ribs on the right side, then the quadratus lumborum muscles on the left side are stretched maximally. If, in this weakened condition on the left side, the beginning student attempts to return to the upright position, these muscles are being asked to lift the upper body while in a stretched condition and so could be injured through overwork. Similarly, if the back is rounded in *uttanasana* so that the erector spinae of the back are stretched (figure 8.A-4**b**), then when coming up from this position to *tadasana,* the weakened erector spinae can be injured by the implied overwork. Injuries such as these can be avoided by coming out of the postures either by placing the hands on the legs and using arm strength to assist recovery, or by maintaining a more symmetric alignment on coming out of the posture, with the stretch more symmetrically distributed left and right in *trikonasana,* for

example, rather than being totally flexed on one side and totally extended on the other.

The tension that can be generated by a muscle is essentially zero once the muscle is fully contracted. From this, one sees that the very straight arm is relatively weak muscularly, for its biceps is totally extended and so has poor myofilament overlap, whereas the triceps is totally contracted and so suffers from jamming of the myofilaments. For this reason, full-arm balance (*adho mukha vrksasana*) would be much more exhausting if it were not for the bones of the arms supporting the weight of the body in the inverted position, provided they have been placed vertically, with the humerus directly above the radius and ulna.

One also can understand the difficulty students might have in pressing up into *urdhva dhanurasana* from the lying position. With back on the floor and hands in position, the triceps are in an elongated condition, implying minimal contact of cross bridges between myosin and actin in its muscle fibers. Thus, not enough mechanical force can be generated by contraction of the triceps in order to start the shoulders moving away from the wrists. If the student is given a gentle lift at the shoulders at this point so as to help shorten the triceps, the contact between the sliding myofilaments of the triceps increases, the arms begin to straighten on their own, and the chest and pelvis start to elevate. As the arm approaches the straight attitude, the triceps more nearly approaches the resting length, the triceps strength increases, and the lifting becomes easier.

Complete contraction of the triceps in *urdhva dhanurasana* brings the body into the fully extended position; however, once in this position, the triceps are fully contracted and so suffer a loss of force due to jamming of the myofilaments within the sarcomeres. Because the bones have been put into place to support the posture against the pull of gravity at this point, the only triceps action required is that to keep the bones of the arms in their proper places. As one presses up into *urdhva dhanurasana*, a set of actions that are similar to those undergone by the triceps of the upper arms also takes place in the quadriceps muscles of the thighs.

Postural Adjustments

Applying the principle inherent in figure 11.A-11 to our *yogasana* training in another way, it is seen that the muscles are at their weakest when one is trying to make a muscular adjustment while at the limit of the range of motion. For example, it is most challenging to make a postural adjustment of the rib cage in *trikonasana* when the hand is closest to the floor; however, if you will open the posture so that the supporting hand is placed further up the leg, then the rib cage can be more easily adjusted, and following this, the supporting hand can move toward the floor. In general, the longer are the muscle fibers, the larger is their functional range of motion; the closer we are to our limit of range of motion in a posture, the more difficult it can be to make further adjustments, due to poor myofilament overlap.

Doing Work

Because the "strength" of a muscle can be taken as the maximum force that it can exert when contracting (i.e., the weight it can lift against the pull of gravity or some other resistance), strength is proportional to the cross-sectional area of the muscle. Thus, for reasons of size, the biceps muscle is stronger than the muscle that lifts the eyelid. The strength of a muscle lies in its size, its contractive quality, and its resistance to tensile stress; whereas the strength of a bone lies in its resistance to compressive stress.

Technically, the strength of a muscle is different from its ability to do "work," a quantity defined as the product of the force exerted on a load and the distance the load is moved against an external resistance. As such, the ability of a muscle to do work is dependent not only on the microscopic details of the interaction between its myofilaments to generate a force, as discussed above, but also on the range-of-motion factor: if the muscle at rest is already strongly contracted (i.e., if it has a short rest length, as is often seen in the weightlifting physique), then the muscle has a shorter range of motion through which it can move and so is relatively impotent in regard to doing work with respect to the same muscle

having a longer rest length and a correspondingly larger range of motion.

The ideal would seem to be the musculature of the *yogasana* student, for this type of work leads to muscles that are both forceful and supple, having large ranges of motion but minimum bulk. Ruiz [726] presents an interesting discussion of the beneficial interaction of weightlifting and *yogasana* practice, pointing out that if combined, they should be performed in the order weightlifting followed by stretching. Experience shows that if instead, one first opens the body with a long session of yogic stretching and then engages in heavy work (such as weightlifting, rowing, or digging in the garden), then the chances for injury appear to be much higher.

Certain skeletal muscles are constructed so as to be fit for rapid, short-term contractions (the biceps muscles of the upper arms, for example), whereas others are constructed so as to work best during slowly developing, long-term contractions (the erector spinae of the back body, for example). In the case of a long, thin muscle, it will have a large range of motion and a higher velocity as well; however, due to its smaller cross section, the force it will develop on contraction is minimal, and it cannot do much work. In contrast, the thick, short muscle is the more forceful by virtue of its larger cross section. Muscles, in general, are either long and fast or thick and forceful, but not maximally both [549].

Muscle force is proportional to the muscle's cross-sectional area and the muscle velocity (a factor of no relevance to *yogasana* practice, which is isometric) is proportional to muscle-fiber length. When a muscle is exerting 35 percent of its maximal force, the endurance time shortens to about two minutes, and when the exertion is 100 percent of maximum, the endurance time is only ten to fifteen seconds, just the lifetime of the creatine phosphate in the muscle. A large part of this difference may be due to the deleterious effects of ischemia following exhaustion of the creatine phosphate as in the latter case (Subsection 11.A, page 393).

In our *yogasana* practice, we are obliged to move into a postural position, and this requires work against gravity to move bones, tissue, etc. Thus, to start in *tadasana* with arms at the sides, and to then lift them to horizontal, requires that work be done against gravity; however, though holding them horizontal requires energy, no work is done in holding them there, as there is no further movement. In general, we do work going into and coming out of the *yogasanas,* but no work is done in staying motionless in the postures, though considerable energy may be expended in doing so. That energy is being expended is obvious from the fact that if it were not, the arms could be held up indefinitely! However, this energy expenditure can be minimized by using the skeleton to support the posture, with minimal involvement of the muscles other than to position the bones, as in *tadasana.*

Muscle Power

Power (measured in watts) equals the amount of work that can be done per second, or equivalently, the lifting force times the distance moved per second, or the force times the velocity. The peak power of a contracting muscle occurs at approximately 30 percent of the maximum shortening velocity. In theory, a 70-kilogram (150-pound) person of 40 percent muscle mass can generate a power of 5,400 watts for a short time. In fact, we can do nothing approaching this, even in the short term, because of the practical limitations on the availability of oxygen and fuel and the limits on the dissipation of waste products and heat [877].

High muscle tension and considerable heat are generated in holding the isometric positions achieved in *yogasana* practice, even though no work is being performed to further shorten the muscles, and no power is being generated. Because the practice of the *yogasanas* works to the advantage of the slow-twitch muscle fibers (see Subsection 11.A, page 412), the work done by contraction of these muscles may be high or low, but the power expended will be uniformly low, because *yogasana*-trained muscles are inherently slow-moving.

Hypertrophy

When a muscle becomes fully packed with contractile proteins, as is often the case with the bodybuilder physique, it is said to be hypertrophied; in this condition, it has less room for mitochondria and so suffers from mitochondrial dilution. The effect of this dilution is to decrease the endurance of the hypertrophied muscle. The loss of endurance in the bodybuilder physique also involves the extra mass of larger muscles and their attendant connective tissues and their lower lactic acid threshold. Because the strength of a muscle increases by the square of its length but its weight goes up by the cube of its length, a hypertrophied muscle that is growing larger becomes heavier faster than it becomes stronger, and so it is difficult to make lasting gains vis-à-vis strength when working in this way.

Muscle fibers can grow by the accumulation of more myofilaments of actin and myosin, the active proteins in contracting muscle, provided there is adequate protein in the diet and there are periods of rest. Such muscle hypertrophy is promoted by exercising at low repetitions but with high load. Regarding growth and development, as a muscle fiber grows in length and girth, it eventually reaches 50 µ in diameter. This long-term hypertrophy differs from the immediate effects of exercise to make the muscles swell in size by "pumping them up"; this latter effect involves the incomplete relaxation of the muscle following heavy work and its becoming engorged with blood. Initial strength gains in younger students occur largely by a neural mechanism (Subsection 4.G, page 140), and only slowly and much later does the hypertrophy mechanism become significant.

Endurance athletes have a higher density of mitochondria and a higher efficiency for oxygen consumption than do sedentary humans of similar age. In endurance athletes (and possibly *yogasana* students with a vigorous practice), the atrophy of white, fast fibers is balanced largely by the hypertrophy of the slow, red fibers. The endurance runner's extended effort against a small load results in muscle hypertrophy, but of the heart, not the skeletal muscles! On the other hand, brief but high-intensity exercise works to increase skeletal muscle bulk, but not that of the heart [877]. As applied to *yogasana* practice, our work carries us in the direction of the endurance athlete in regard to muscle type; however, our strength in the *yogasanas* also can be rapidly improved by short bouts of intense muscular effort. In this, one may focus on performing a few prone bench presses at high weight in order to build shoulder strength for *chaturanga dandasana,* but do not bother with biceps curls, because biceps strength is not very often called for in *yogasana* practice. If one feels the need for such weight training, similar positive strengthening effects will follow from performance of the *yogasanas* while carrying sandbags or iron plates appropriately strapped to the body.

Hyperplasia

J. Antonio [827a] argues that subjecting a muscle to high tensile overload leads to muscle-fiber injury and DOMS (Subsection 11.G, page 476), but that regeneration then leads to an increase in the number of muscle fibers. This claim stands in opposition to the long-held idea that the number of muscle fibers is constant through life. Antonio claims that an increase in the number of fibers results from the activation of muscle stem cells that go on to grow as new fibers once the original fibers have been injured. This process of new fiber growth is called hyperplasia, whereas the growth of existing fibers is called hypertrophy. The best exercises for promoting hyperplasia involve eccentric contraction, as this maximizes the chances for muscle tearing. In the hyperplasia scenario, the sort of micro-tears that the muscles may suffer when overstretched (and thereby dehydrated) recruits the release of various proteins that are triggers for the transport of stem cells from long distances to the sites of injury. These stem cells regenerate muscle tissue, repair the damage, and then turn themselves off, it is said. In the process of tearing the muscle tissues, endorphins are released, and these provide the "feel-good" sense that exercise generates.

Note too that many workers in the weightlifting and bodybuilding fields also claim (along with

Antonio) that no change in the shape or strength of the body can take place unless tissue first has been damaged and then healed; i.e., remodeled. This approach to remodeling appears to be closely allied to the physical-therapy practice of "muscle scraping," in which injured muscles that have not healed properly are vigorously scraped so as to re-injure the tissue and thus give it a second chance to heal properly.

A question for the future: if weightlifting can injure a muscle and then guide muscle growth and repair so as to create the short, knotty muscles that Westerners seem to want, is it not possible that stretching in *yogasana* practice can injure a muscle and that the growth and repair of this muscle then occurs in a way that makes it longer, stronger, and more flexible? Or is it possible that hyperplasia injures muscle fibers and that in healing, these form micro-adhesions that make the muscle overall low-flexibility and knotty?

Gender and Muscle Function

The basic physiologies of muscle action in men and women are essentially the same, the differences being quantitative at best. Measurements of muscle strength, muscle mass, cardiac output, etc., in men and women show that women's quantities are about 60–75 percent of those of men of comparable age and state of health, the differences being due largely to different levels of circulating estrogen and testosterone in the two genders. In women, the high levels of estrogen promote higher levels of body fat; whereas in men, the high levels of testosterone promote a larger muscle mass.

Movement versus Action

Students of the art of *yogasana* make a distinction between a muscular movement and a muscular action. In the former, muscles are contracted, pull on the bones, and move them in particular directions. In contrast, when performing a muscular action, the muscles are contracted, but there is very little or no motion associated with the contraction. Thus, raising the arms overhead in *urdhva hastasana* is a muscular movement, whereas the lifting of the fingertips yet more upward in this posture while lowering the shoulder blades is a muscular action. To the outside observer, it appears that nothing is happening during a muscular action, but the *yogasana* performer knows that the posture is actually very dynamic but balanced, with considerable muscle activity taking place in spite of the apparent lack of motion. In a sense, a muscle movement involves work against an external resistance, gravity, whereas in a muscle action, the resistance is supplied not by gravity but internally, by other muscles and bones within the body. See Subsection 10.A, pages 331 and 337, for significant examples of muscle action. As will be discussed more fully in Subsection 11.A, page 407, a muscular movement can be defined as an isotonic use of the muscles, whereas a muscular action is an isometric use of the muscles.

Ezraty further discusses the distinction between movement and action, assigning "movements" to the larger muscle groups and "actions" to the more subtle conscious control of smaller, more refined muscles [230].

Anatomic Pulleys

A pulley is a mechanical device for changing the direction of a force. For example, imagine a rope tied to a bale of hay on the floor; if you pull on the rope, the bale will move horizontally across the floor. If, instead, the rope is first passed through an overhead pulley and then pulled, the bale will move upward (vertically), even though there is no upward vertical force on the part of the rope being pulled; i.e., the pulley has altered the direction of the force. Pulleys also can alter the length of the lever arm over which a force is exerted, thereby changing the magnitude of the work done and the power expended in that work.

Within the body, there are several such pulleys. For example, the trochlea of the eye is a pulley consisting of a loop of connective tissue external to the eye; it functions as a pulley with regard to the tendon of the superior oblique muscle. This pulley action reverses the direction of contraction of the superior oblique muscle, so that its contraction has the effect of pulling the eyeball forward, and its relaxation allows the eyeball to fall back into the eye socket (figure 17.A-1c).

In a similar way, the peroneus longus muscle

of the lower leg, when it contracts, pulls the base of the little toe toward the knee but pushes the base of the big toe away from the knee, the pulley here being a bony prominence on the lateral surface of the calcaneus (heel) bone (figure 10.B-7a and Subsection 10.B, page 360). In a sense, both the triceps of the upper arm and the quadriceps of the upper leg work in such a way that contraction of the muscle moves the center of gravity of the limb away from that of the muscle due to the pulley action at the elbow and the knee joint, respectively.

An obvious pulley within the body involves the psoas muscle (figure 9.B-2b), where the origin of the muscle is at the lower lumbar vertebrae and the insertion is at the medial side of the upper femur. In its course downward, the psoas passes over the anterior portion of the acetabulum, which acts as the pulley; the pulley action of the psoas is most evident when in upward-facing *supta baddha konasana*. In this posture, when the knees are pressed down, the psoas is stretched, and in the process, the lumbar spine is lifted off the floor. As a corollary to this action in *supta baddha konasana*, when the lumbar is lifted upward in *urdhva dhanurasana* and similar backbends, there is a strong tendency for the anterior thighs to roll laterally, again due to the pulley action of the psoas on the lesser trochanters of the femurs (figure 9.B-2b).

The action of the patella within the knee joint (Subsection 10.B, page 348) functions as an anatomic pulley in a way that increases the force of the quadriceps contraction acting on the tibia in order to straighten the leg.[5] Anatomic pulleys are discussed further in the footnote to Subsection 11.A, page 426.

Lubricating Muscles

Because muscles move with respect to the bones, there is a need for lubrication, just as there is when one bone moves with respect to another (Subsection 7.D, page 239). To this end, where tissue moves over bone, the body has positioned

---

5   I thank Karin Eisen for bringing this point to my attention.

about 150 pancake-shaped, fluid-filled sacs called bursae in order to lubricate and assist the motion. As pointed out by Tortora [863], the bursae are rather like joint capsules, being composed of connective-tissue capsules filled with a synovial-like fluid. They are located between skin and bone where skin rubs on bone, between tendon and bone, between muscle and bone, and between ligament and bone. When one sits in *virasana,* the ischial tuberosities of the pelvis (figure 8.B-7) are protected from the hard floor by bursae, while there are other bursae between the ischium itself and the gluteus muscles. There also are bursae within the tendons of the knees (figure 10.B-4**b**), both above and below the patella, which act to lubricate the bending mechanism. Overuse of the bursae or unusual pressure on the bursae (as, for example, when doing *ustrasana* or *parighasana* without adequate padding under the knees) can lead to swelling, inflammation, and bursitis. The most common sites for bursitis are the elbow, hip, knee, and shoulder.

Types of Muscle Contraction

Speaking in the most general terms in regard to muscle contraction or elongation, there are four types to be considered:- under neural excitation, the muscle may either (i) stay the same length, (ii) shorten, or (iii) lengthen; whereas without neural excitation, (iv) the muscle again lengthens. Each of these four situations is discussed below [618]. Note, however, that only rarely (if ever) does one experience a single muscle action; rather, we have concerted actions involving many muscles. Among those muscles involved is the prime mover, assisted by several other synergistic muscles, as when an anatomy train (Subsection 11.A, page 424) is activated. Because a real muscle is more than just a collection of muscle fibers, when speaking of muscle contraction, one must also consider not only the synergists but all of the collateral structures (such as tendons, connective tissue, and cross bridges) that have their own mechanical properties. Antagonists to both the prime mover and the synergists also may be factors in the contraction process.

Isometric Contraction

Isometric contraction involves working a muscle against a fixed, unmoving object, as when one stands in front of a desk with the hands below it and, with biceps brachii at the resting length, tries to lift the desk off the floor. The desk does not move, and though the muscles involved (the biceps brachii as prime mover, in this example) are straining intensely, they do not shorten appreciably, nor do they do any work (see subsection above), though they do generate heat by their actions. This is case (i) as outlined above, and it is called an isometric contraction of the muscle.

In the context of muscle action in the gravitational field, a muscle that is strong enough on contraction to overcome the gravitational resistance of the load can shorten or lengthen, depending upon its strength and the weight of the load against which it is pitted. Viewed from this perspective, the intermediate situation where the muscle tension is just equal to the load on it results in no motion; i.e., the muscle action is an isometric one, with no change of muscle length, no motion of the load, and no work or power (but considerable energy) expended in keeping the load suspended.

When muscle fibers contract to shorten the muscle, the Z discs are pulled toward one another, but attached collateral tissues such as titin, α-actinin and the relevant tendons and myofascia are stretched. If the load on a muscle is very large, then the lengthening of the collateral structures may just balance or slightly exceed the contraction of the sarcomeres, with the result that though the sarcomeres are contracted, there is no overall movement of the bones connected to such muscles. This is the microscopic situation in an isometric contraction of a muscle, and in such a situation, the resistance to movement is partly due to the effects of gravity and partly due to the resistance of the connective tissues to lengthening as the belly of the muscle contracts. There is no relative movement of the actin-myosin cross bridges in those muscles held in isometric contraction when in a *yogasana* posture.

The isometric contraction of the body's muscles is especially relevant to *yogasana* practice, for the relative immobility of the postures implies the wide use of such isometric contractions. Such contractions are found in the shoulders holding the arms horizontal in *virabhadrasana II*, in both the abdomen holding the pelvis off the floor and the shoulders holding the chest off the floor in *chaturanga dandasana,* in the lumbar spine holding the upper body horizontal in *ardha uttanasana,* etc. In fact, virtually every *yogasana* posture more elevated than *savasana* that is held steady will eventually involve the isometric contraction of many of the body's muscles; only *savasana* is devoid of isometric contraction and so offers the maximum relaxation.

When the arm is bent and one tries to straighten it by contraction of the triceps, the load against which the triceps works in part is the inflexibility of the antagonist biceps muscle. In general, the connective tissue within the antagonist of an agonist/antagonist pair supplies part of the load against which the agonist (Subsection 11.A, page 420) must work in achieving and holding an isometric elongation (Subsection 11.F, page 468).

When isometric contraction is used to build strength, it should be done at several different joint angles, because the strengthening benefits earned at one angle do not transfer very effectively to other angles. That is, working isometrically with the elbow at 45° does little good for strengthening the arm when the elbow is to be used at an angle of, say, 85°.

When working the *yogasanas* with beginners, the static, isometric nature of the postures encourages such students to hold their breath and so raise their blood pressure [160]. This holding of the breath by students so as to increase their strength is known as the Valsalva maneuver (Subsection 15.C, page 616). As this maneuver is an inappropriate action for students, they must be encouraged to keep the breath moving in the *yogasanas,* even though the skeletal muscles appear not to move.

Isotonic Contraction

In the course of moving from one posture into another, muscle actions other than the iso-

metric will be called upon, because the transitions between postures are no longer static. If the load on a muscle is slight, the contractile force of the sarcomeres is stronger than the forces that resist extending the tendons and collateral tissues, and motion of the load ensues; this is case (ii) above, and the muscle action is called isotonic contraction. When a muscle contracts isotonically, its length changes appreciably when the load on the muscle is put into motion, as, for example, the contraction of the triceps when straightening the arms overhead in *urdhva hastasana*. Note that in the isotonic case, the load may move either with or in opposition to the resistance to movement, but the magnitude of the load is constant. If the muscle-length change in an isotonic contraction is a shortening (figure 11.A-15**b**), then the isotonic movement is said to be concentric; whereas if the change is a lengthening of the working muscle (figure 11.A-15**c**), then the isotonic movement is said to be eccentric, this being case (iii) above.

As an example of the differences between concentric isotonic and eccentric isotonic actions, the lifting of straight legs from the floor into *sirsasana I* involves an isotonic concentric action of the muscles of the lower back (gluteus medius, quadratus lumborum, etc.); whereas the slow lowering of the legs from *sirsasana I* to the floor involves isotonic eccentric actions of the same muscles. Throughout these motions, if the feet are kept broad and dorsiflexed at the ankles, then they are involved in isometric contraction.

In our *yogasana* work, we can generalize the situation to say that the muscles that lift a body part further from the floor are undergoing concentric isotonic contraction (they contract as the load is lifted), whereas those that are used to slowly lower a body part closer to the floor are undergoing eccentric isotonic contraction (they are being stretched longer as the load is lowered). In the former case, the muscle tension required to move the load is at or is less than the maximum that the muscle can generate; whereas in the latter, the muscle tension is less than the maximum that can be generated. In both cases, the muscle is doing work in order to control the relevant motion of the load.

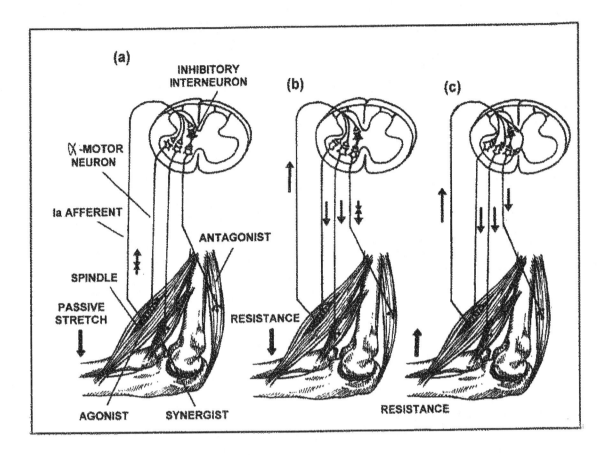

Figure 11.A-15. Neural connections of the muscle spindle of the agonist brachialis to the spinal cord and thence to its agonist, synergist, and antagonist muscles. (a) Under a slow, passive stretch such as traction, the muscle spindle sends its signal to the spine without a reflex reaction; this is case (iv). (b) When working to lift a load, the α-motor neuron from the spinal cord to the brachialis is energized, but not the muscle spindle; the synergist is also activated, but the antagonist muscle is inhibited by the spinal interneuron. This is a case (ii) isotonic concentric action. (c) When working to lower a load, as in a case (iii) isotonic eccentric action, the agonist and the antagonist are co-contracted, but with the agonist more strongly so than the antagonist muscle.

In the course of a concentric contraction, the sarcomeres move from the myofilament configuration depicted in figure 11.A-10b to that in figure 11.A-10d; whereas during an eccentric elongation, the sarcomeres move from the configuration in figure 11.A-10d to that in figure 11.A-10b. During the static isometric holding of a posture, the sarcomeres in a given muscle are in one of the states shown in figure 11.A-10 and do not change as long as the position is stationary.

In eccentric contraction, the muscle involved is stretched as it performs its work; however, fewer muscle fibers are involved in the work of eccentric contraction as compared to concentric contraction. Though eccentric contraction requires 40 percent more force than the corresponding concentric contraction, it not only strengthens the muscle more quickly but also places a much larger stress on the fibers involved while restricting blood flow to the muscle, and so opens the door to excessive muscle soreness and injury [7] (Subsection II.B, page 841).

Interestingly, a recent study has found that the metabolism that fuels the muscles when walking uphill (concentric isotonic exercise) is different from that fueling the muscles when walking downhill (eccentric isotonic exercise). In particular, the concentric mode is driven by the consumption of glucose, whereas the eccentric mode is driven by the oxidation of fatty triglycerides [312]. Extrapolating these results to *yogasana* practice, one expects that repeatedly pressing up into *chaturanga dandasana* from a lying position (a concentric isotonic motion) requires the consumption of glucose, whereas lowering into the position from the straight-arm *chaturanga dandasana* position (an eccentric isotonic motion) is more dependent on the oxidation of triglyceride fats.

Isokinetic Contraction

Isokinetic contraction is done at constant velocity of the load being moved, regardless of the differences in the strength of the muscle at different angles, which can be appreciable; for example, the biceps are strongest at an angle of 120° at the elbow and least strong at 30°. Isokinetic contraction is of no consequence for *yogasana* students, as we make no particular effort to keep an isotonic motion moving at a constant velocity.

Titin, α-Actinin, and Passive Stretching

It is obvious that even in a case (iv) passively stretched muscle (figure 11.A-15a), there is an internal resistance to the stretching that must be overcome in order to take the muscle to an even longer length. For many years, it was thought that the source of this resistance was in the connective tissue residing outside the myofibrils; i.e., in the periosteum, epimysium, and perimysium (figure 11.A-4). However, that view has changed, as new experiments have shown that the resistance to a passive stretch is present in full force in myofibrils shorn of all such connective tissue. The series-resistive elastic element of skeletal muscle is now thought to reside largely in the huge protein called titin, which is found within each of the muscle fibers (figure 11.A-10a). Titin fibers bridge the space between the ends of the myosin myofilaments and the Z discs, thereby stabilizing the myosin, holding it in place, and changing its length and tension as the Z discs move away from one another during any lengthening of the muscle

[549]. Viewed from this perspective, a stretched muscle returns to its resting length due to the release of the tensile stress stored in the muscle's titin during the stretch. This is discussed further in Box 11.A-3 below. In a similar way, α-actinin is the protein keeping the ends of the actin myofibrils attached to the Z discs (figure 11.A-10a), and it is likely that it too is a contributor to the internal resistance to stretching.

Muscle Growth

According to Tortora [863], isometric work such as *yogasana* practice promotes slow-twitch fibers but does not promote any significant increase in muscle mass or short-term strength, for this happens only when one does the type of work (weightlifting) that promotes fast-twitch muscles. Thus, we come to see that the physique of the Eastern yoga athlete is rather different from that of the weightlifting Western athlete, because they have inherently different muscle types: type-1 slow-twitch for the Eastern yoga athlete and type-3 fast-twitch for the Western weightlifting athlete (see the following Subsection for a discussion of muscle types). Typical bodies of the Eastern and Western athletic types, as shown in figures 11.A-16a and 11.A-16b, reflect the different types of muscle tissue promoted by the two activities.

Viewed globally, there are three common human body types, based on their general morphology: the ectomorph (thin and fragile), the endomorph (round and soft), and the mesomorph (muscular and athletic). The idealized Eastern male body is that of the endomorph (figure 11.A-16a), and the idealized Western male body is that of the mesomorph (figure 11.A-16b). It is a goal of *yogasana* practice to train the body so that the postures are achieved with submaximal muscle contraction, so that the body and mind stay soft and relaxed; the muscles do not gather to make knots, but instead, the skin and subdermal muscles remain relatively smooth and lacking in definition, as in figure 11.A-16a. This work on the body and mind is undertaken by the *yogasana* student with the eventual aim of conquering the Self, and in doing so, avoiding the pain associated with the *kleshas* within us [388]; whereas the goal

Box 11.A-3: What Really Stretches when a Muscle Is Stretched, and Why Does It Stop Stretching?

In the contraction of a muscle fiber, the action potential that drives the contraction is triggered by a change in the permeability of the sarcomere membrane to specific ions, and the subsequent movement of the actin within the myosin channels. If the contraction is taken to the limit, the actin is fully driven into the myosin channels, and no further muscle shortening is possible. In contrast, if the same fiber is being stretched, the fiber is relaxed, and the cross-bridge heads are disengaged. In this scenario, it is easily imaginable that continued stretching could pull the actin chain fully out of the myosin channel; were this to happen, the sarcomere could not be reconstituted, because the actin ends would no longer be in register with the channels of the myosin. In this situation, the stretch would have succeeded in essentially severing the muscle fiber, having separated the actin from the myosin.

It is clear from the above that there must be a brake on the stretching of muscle fibers if they are to survive *yogasana* work. Fortunately, there are three mechanisms that serve this purpose. First, as described above, the connective tissues bonded to the sarcomere (the sarcolemma) and within the sarcomere offer significant resistance to lengthening of the muscle fiber and so act to hold the actin and myosin together. Remember that 30 percent of a muscle's bulk is connective tissue. Though an individual muscle fiber can be stretched to 150 percent of its resting length before tearing, the tendon attaching that muscle fiber to the bone can only stretch 4–8 percent before it fails, and so it too will offer considerable resistance to stretching. The lack of elasticity in the tendon is compensated by its very high tensile strength. Ligaments can be stretched only slightly more than can tendons [725]. Second, as is discussed in Section 11.B, page 432, there are mechanoreceptors called muscle spindles within muscles that trigger a muscle contraction if the extent or rate of muscle stretching exceeds certain limits. Finally, as can be seen in figure 11.A-10a, the resistance of the titin holding the two ends of a myosin myofilament to the respective Z discs at a certain point will become resistive toward further stretching of the sarcomere, presumably before the actin is disengaged.

Viewed in this way, we see that how "flexible" a person is depends upon the flexibility of their connective tissue (including titin), the sensitivity of their muscle spindles to stretch, the extent of their motivation to stretch, their willfulness in stretching too rapidly or too far, and their willingness to move slowly into the stretch. As discussed in Subsection 12.A, page 483, there is a strong hereditary factor dictating the flexibility of our connective tissue, making some of us contortionists and some of us inherently as stiff as flagpoles. The important question of how to overcome the resistance that muscle spindles invoke toward muscle stretching is discussed in Section 11.B, Sensors, page 433.

of the bodybuilder appears to be the extreme public expression of his or her self-importance, lack of humility, attitude that only he or she is wise and strong, and thirst for the opportunity to show the superiority of his or her physique.

Muscle-Fiber Types

Composition and Characteristics

There are three distinct types of skeletal mus-

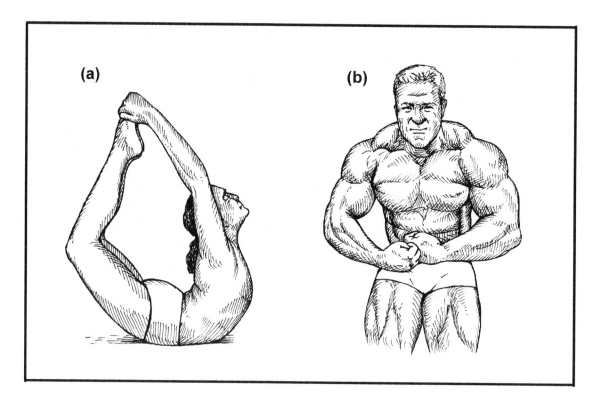

Figure 11.A-16. (**a**) The epitome of Eastern isometric training of the body and (**b**) the epitome of Western isotonic/isokinetic training of the body. Note the obvious differences in the tone and texture of the muscles as each of the body types has been trained specifically to perform in accord with very different objectives.

cle fiber, with every muscle in the body being a particular combination of the three types. Each of the three fiber types (types 1, 2, and 3) is characterized by the unique molecular form of its myosin filaments. Because each of the fiber types has its own advantages and disadvantages, and because the proportions of the three fiber types within a muscle can be changed depending upon the type and intensity of one's exercise, the muscular composition can be altered so as to optimize one's performance or practice over time.

Muscle-fiber types 1, 2, and 3 are also popularly known as slow-twitch, intermediate, and fast-twitch fibers, respectively, for reasons that are obvious from figure 11.A-12. The muscles that contract the slowest (slow twitch; the soleus muscle, for example, in figure 11.A-12) are postural, and their use is appropriate when the load on the muscle has substantial inertia or the muscle is needed for the sustained support of the body. Muscles that contract rapidly and fade just as fast (fast twitch; the ocular muscle, for example,

in figure 11.A-12) are employed intermittently and are appropriate when loads are large and the movements are to be rapid. As shown in figure 11.A-12, the gastrocnemius muscle is an example of a type-2, intermediate-twitch muscle, on the basis of the speed with which it contracts.[6]

In regard to contraction speed, the muscles of the face are the fastest, the muscles of the lower leg the slowest, and the hands and feet are intermediate. Within a given human muscle, the fast and slow fibers are intermingled so as to form a mosaic pattern, with a preponderance of slow-twitch fibers in type-1 muscles and fast-twitch fibers in type-3 muscles. Consider the properties of the three muscle-fiber types in table 11.A-4. Other

---

6   The division of muscles into one of three types is not clear-cut, so that the gastrocnemius muscle is cited by some as type 2 or by others as type 3. Though the threefold division is used here, it should be remembered that the most meaningful distinction is that between type-1 and -3 muscle fibers.

Table 11.A-4: Characteristics of the Three Skeletal Muscle Types [9, 229, 432, 884]

Property	Type 1	Type 2	Type 3
Color	Red-brown	Red	White
Twitch speed	Slow	Intermediate	Fast
Twitch force	Small	Intermediate	Large
Activation threshold	Low	Moderate	High
Contraction time, milliseconds	100–120	40–45	10–45
Mitochondrial density	High	-	Low
Myoglobin content	High	Very high	Low
Innervation ratio	Low	Moderate	High
Type of neural efferent	B	A	A
Capillary density	High	High	Low
Muscle tension	Low	Medium	High
Duration of force	Prolonged	Prolonged	Intermittent
Resistance to fatigue	Very high	High	Low
Order of recruitment	First	Second	Last
Fiber diameter	Small	Medium	Large
Z-line spacing	Intermediate	Wide	Narrow
Muscles high in this type	Postural muscles in back body	Gastrocnemius	Biceps
Type of ATP production	Oxidative phosphorylation/ lipolysis of fats	Oxidative phosphorylation	Anaerobic glycolysis
Glycolytic capacity	Low	Moderate	High
Oxidative capacity	High	Moderate	Low
Alkaline ATPase	Low	High	High
Acid ATPase	High	Low	Moderate
Glycogen stores	High	Moderate	Low
Rate of Ca^{2+} supply	Slow	-	Rapid

classification schemes have been proposed, many having larger numbers of subcategories; however, it is sufficient for us to hold to the simple scheme given in the table above. As can be seen in the table above, the fiber types can be distinguished by their color, speed of contraction, diameter, resistance to fatigue, and many other qualities. The different muscle-fiber types are largely dependent upon different molecular myosin isoforms, but there are other factors at work differentiating each type from the other two.

Type-1 Slow-Twitch Fibers

Type-1 muscle fiber has a red-brown coloration due to its high content of myoglobin (a molecule much like hemoglobin, but noncirculating), which strongly binds oxygen, for eventual oxidation of the fuel in the muscle. These red-brown fibers contract relatively slowly (the maximum velocity of contraction can be only one-tenth as fast as that for type-3 fibers) and so are more numerous in muscles that do not require a rapid response; e.g., the postural muscles in the back body. The postural muscles are often called the "antigravity muscles," because they work continuously for hours on end to keep the joints and other body parts in alignment while opposing the forces of gravity. For example, the masseter muscles of the jaw are type-1 antigravity muscles, because they keep the mouth closed, even while gravity tends to pull it open.

The capillary networks serving the slow-twitch fibers are dense in order to supply abundant oxygen to the muscle in their extended period of work, and these type-1 fibers have relatively small diameters, so as to favor the rapid diffusive exchange of metabolic products with the capillaries. Myoglobin is a red pigment that is found among (but not within) the capillaries of muscle types 1 and 2. Like hemoglobin, myoglobin binds oxygen, but more tightly, so that it is available to a working muscle only slowly, but over a longer period of time. As such, myoglobin is best suited for type-1 muscles, as they expend their energy slowly over a long time. Inasmuch as muscle action is initiated by the transport of Ca^{2+} ions through the t-tubule system (Subsection 11.A, page 384), it is understandable that the rate of supply of this ion is slow in type-1 muscles and rapid in type-3 muscles.

The presence of slow-twitch type-1 fiber in a muscle is enhanced in the sort of isometric contractions met with in the *yogasanas,* and otherwise is most prominent in the postural muscles of the upper body. Actually, when doing *yogasanas,* all of the muscles become postural in a sense (at least for a short time)!

Type-3 Fast-Twitch Fibers

At the opposite end of the muscle-fiber spectrum, there are the type-3 white fibers, which are most abundant in muscles, such as the biceps, that are able to contract rapidly, but for only a short time. In these fast-twitch fibers, there is no myoglobin, for ATP production is via an anaerobic mechanism (Subsection 11.A, page 393); which is to say, the oxygen for combustion is stripped from glucose rather than absorbed as oxygen from the blood, for absorption would be too slow a process for the needs of these rapidly contracting fibers. Type-3 fibers are most often involved in muscle injury, due to the rapidity of their actions.

Fast-twitch muscles are powered by the glycolytic oxidation of sugar in the mitochondria, whereas the slow-twitch fibers depend upon the aerobic oxidation of fats in the mitochondria as their primary source of energy. As might have been expected, the fast-twitch type-3 fibers are energized by those efferent nerves with the fastest conduction velocity, the A_α motor neurons, whereas the type-1 slow fibers are innervated by the slower type A_β neurons (table 3.B-2). The A_α neurons are capable of delivering action potentials at a rate of up to sixty per second to the neuromuscular junction, whereas the figure for the A_β-type neurons is only about ten to twenty per second [427]. Thus, type-3 muscle fibers are more powerful, since their fibers can be excited many more times in a second, but this can be maintained for only a few seconds. Such a rapid but short-lived muscular response occasionally may be advantageous, as when jumping from *uttanasana* into *chaturanga dandasana,* but is not often called upon when performing most *yogasanas.*

Type-2 Intermediate-Twitch Fibers

The intermediate fiber, type 2, is red and fairly fast-twitch and is found in those muscles where both speed and endurance are factors such as in those muscles of the legs used for running.

Mixed-Fiber Types

All of the muscle fibers within a particular motor unit have the same fiber type, and all three types use acetylcholine as their neurotransmitter. The fiber-type composition of a motor unit will be homogeneous, because the nerve type (table 3.B-2) innervating it will be of one type only. However, across the entire muscle, neither the nerve type nor the muscle-fiber type will be homogeneous; i.e., within the muscle, the various muscle-fiber types are simultaneously present and so strongly mixed that one cannot define a particular region as being of any one type.

One must realize how large the individual variation of the ratio of fast-twitch to slow-twitch muscles might be in a random group of seemingly identical people. Thus, a study of muscle biopsies of the vastus lateralis muscle in a group of 418 randomly chosen subjects gave percentage values of type-1 slow fibers ranging from 15 percent to 85 percent.

One sees in figure 11.A-17 that there is an imperfect but suggestive correlation between contraction times and the percentage of type-1 fiber in a muscle of the sort one might expect, if the contraction time is longer when the percentage of type-1 slow-twitch fiber in the muscle is higher. The value of 9 percent slow-twitch fiber content for the rectus muscle of the eye, point 11, is extrapolated on the assumption that it fits the best-fit line and has an observed contraction time of ten milliseconds. The external ocular muscles are very fast, because they are used to move the eyeball when tracking rapidly moving objects.

In the legs of sprinters, the muscle fibers are 75 percent type 3, whereas in the legs of endurance runners, the muscle fibers are 90 percent mixed types 1 and 2. Interesting new evidence [132] demonstrates that there is a strong genetic component to being blessed with either running speed or running endurance. Those who are born sprinters are found to have received an allele from each parent that manufactures the protein α-actinin within the type-3, fast muscle fibers; the function of α-actinin is to attach the actin myofilaments to the Z discs (figure 11.A-10a). On the

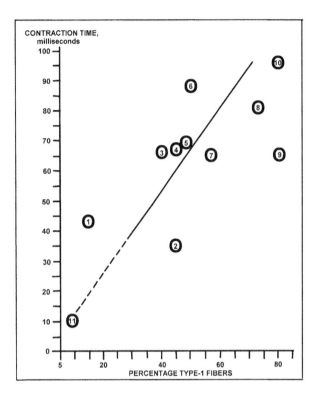

Figure 11.A-17. A plot of the contraction times for various muscles versus the percentage of the fibers in these muscles that are type 1. The muscles plotted here are (1) orbicularis oculi, upper eyelid; (2) lateral gastrocnemius, lower leg; (3) biceps brachii, upper arm; (4) vastus lateralis, upper leg; (5) extensor digitorum brevis, foot; (6) diaphragm, mid-torso; (7) first dorsal interosseous, finger; (8) tibialis anterior, lower leg; (9) adductor pollicis, hand; (10) soleus, lower leg; and (11) rectus, eye.

other hand, the endurance runners show a strong tendency toward either having just a single allele producing α-actinin or none at all. The situation in regard to muscle-fiber types among various vertebrates is presented in Box 11.A-4 below.

Power

Gram for gram and integrated over a long time period, the fast-twitch and slow-twitch muscle types produce the same amount of work but differ in the instantaneous power (the rate of change-of-force production) that they can provide. The slow-twitch fibers do not have the advantage of lightning speed and so are not very

Box 11.A-4: Muscle-Fiber Types among Vertebrates

As shown in figure 11.A-18, the average couch potato has approximately equal amounts of the three types of fiber in the quadriceps muscles of the legs. By comparison, sprinters have four times as much fast-twitch fiber (types 2 and 3) as slow-twitch fiber (type 1) in their quadriceps, whereas marathon runners have twenty times as much slow-twitch fiber as the faster types [9]. In the case of extreme disuse, as for a person with paralysis of the legs, the muscles shrink, ironically leaving behind a preponderance of type-3 fast-twitch fibers. Chronic exercise of the ordinary variety leads to an increase in the diameters of the slow-twitch fibers. See Section 24.A, page 808, for the effects of aging on the proportions of muscle-fiber types in the body.

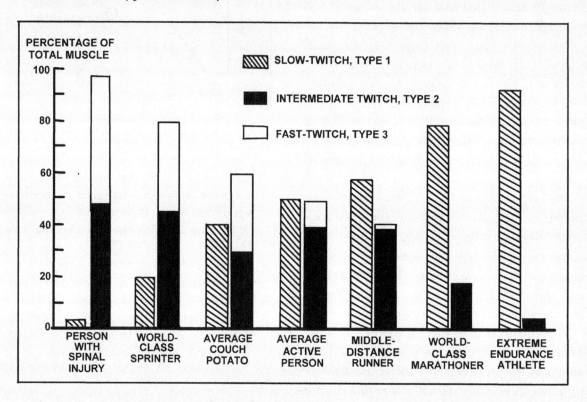

Figure 11.A-18. The relative proportions of the three muscle-fiber types in the quadriceps of people with various athletic skills or none at all. *Yogasana* students are closer to the right-hand side in this diagram.

The muscle-fiber types described in table 11.A-4 may be more familiar to the reader when referred to poultry. In this case, the white breast meat of chicken, for example, is largely the myoglobin-free, type-3 fast-twitch fiber. As might be expected for a flightless bird, this muscle fatigues rapidly. The chicken does do a lot of walking, however, and so the muscle of chicken legs is dark, being loaded with myoglobin and not easily fatigued, as appropriate for type-1 muscle. On the other hand, in the duck, being a bird that both walks and flies, the muscles of both the breast and the leg are rich in the slow-twitch, high-myoglobin, red-brown fiber.

In the restaurant, it is easy to distinguish squab (a young pigeon that is a strong flyer) from Cornish game hen (a midget chicken) by the color of the breast meat, this being much darker in the squab. Diving birds such as cormorants must have large amounts of dark meat (myoglobin) in order to store oxygen for their dives and whales and penguins have more oxygen capacity in their myoglobin than in their hemoglobin [877].

Turning from poultry to fish, salmon is red partly because of the large quantity of myoglobin in its tissues, needed for its long migratory ordeal; whereas in salmon raised in closed pens, the flesh is very pale and must be artificially colored in order to be salable.[1] As would be expected, in a nonmigratory fish such as sole, the flesh again is white, as it is in the flounder, this being a relatively inactive fish. In contrast, a cruising fish such as mackerel has a much larger proportion of dark flesh, and so too is the tuna's flesh colored a deep red, for it cruises for thousands of miles in a year and so carries a large load of myoglobin. Thus, it is seen that the type-1 red-brown tissues in vertebrates are needed for stamina, and the type-3 white tissues in vertebrates are used for short bursts of speed [345].

---

1   Can you now rationalize why the flesh of veal is a pale color as compared to that of beef steak?

proficient in generating power; however, they are excellent performers in regard to resistance to fatigue. They contain large numbers of mitochondria and have an excess of capillaries surrounding the muscle fiber in order to bring oxygen for the production of ATP without accumulation of lactic acid, all in support of repeated muscle contraction. The fast-twitch muscles are able to develop their force in a short time and so have a momentary high power; however, over a longer time period, their integrated power is no higher than that of the slower fibers.

Yogasana and Fiber Types

The soleus muscle lies just forward of the gastrocnemius muscle in the lower leg and would seem to perform the same function as the gastrocnemius. However, the soleus is composed of 80 percent slow-twitch fiber, with a contraction twitch time of about seventy milliseconds (table 11.A-4 and figure 11.A-12), whereas the gastrocnemius is only 49 percent slow-twitch fiber, with a twitch time of only thirty milliseconds. Thus, the soleus is used to lift the heel when walking, whereas the gastrocnemius is used when jumping. The 80 percent figure for the slow-twitch, type-1 fiber of the soleus would be appropriate to the

quadriceps of a world-class marathon runner, and the 49 percent figure for slow-twitch, type-1 fiber of the gastrocnemius would be appropriate to the quadriceps of an average active person (figure 11.A-18).

We shift from the soleus to the gastrocnemius when we shift from walking to running, or when shifting from standing on the sole of the foot to standing on the toes or jumping. Because the gastrocnemius has a short contraction time, it is used to jump, a rapid motion that directly measures the amount of fast-twitch fiber in the lower leg; whereas the soleus is not used in jumping, because it is a postural muscle instead [308]. The ability to move quickly, as in the vertical jump, depends upon the amount of fast-twitch fibers in the legs; in fact, the simple jump-and-reach test can be used to determine the amount of fast fibers in the quadriceps and gastrocnemius.

In contrast to the soleus muscle in the lower leg, which is composed almost totally of slow-twitch muscle fiber, those muscles controlling the blinking of the eye are made up only of fast-twitch fibers. (If they were slow fibers, we would not use the expression "in the blink of an eye" to denote speed.) The majority of locomotor muscles in humans are about 50 percent fast-twitch and 50 percent slow-twitch fibers, but with significant variation among individuals and among the muscles within an individual [827].

In a study that considered the numbers of type 1, 2, and 3 fibers in the vastus lateralis, deltoids, and external intercostal muscles in males between the ages of twenty and eighty years, it was found that with increasing age, the percentage of type 1 fibers increased and that of type 2 decreased, with the vastus lateralis most affected. It was concluded that age-related muscle atrophy is not a general phenomenon, as it does not affect all muscles equally [617]. Practicing the rapid eccentric contraction of the biceps brachii leads to a significant decrease in the number of type-1 fibers and a large increase in type-2 fibers, whereas there is no such change for the slow eccentric contraction of the same muscles [641]. Extrapolating from experimental results such as these, it would be most interesting to compare the muscle-type compositions of Iyengar students (which we conclude are heavily type 1) with those of students who practice the flowing *vinyasa* style of Patabbi Jois et al., which is far more aerobic and rapidly moving.

Order of Recruitment

Muscle force is increased by both increasing the frequency of motor-unit excitation and by the recruitment of additional motor units. The relative importance of these two mechanisms is not clear. Smaller motor units do have lower excitation thresholds than the larger ones and so are recruited before larger ones.[7] It is also true that the motor units having type-1 fibers with the lon-

gest contraction times also have the highest resistance to fatigue and are called upon first when the workload is light.

Muscle-fiber type also is an important factor in regard to the order of recruitment, for there is a preference in regard to which of the various muscle-fiber types is the first to be recruited in a muscle contraction and which is the last to be recruited, except in an emergency situation, where all types are recruited at once [229].

Muscle-fiber type is controlled by the motor nerve that innervates the muscle. Slow-twitch muscles will have low-velocity, type-A_β efferent neurons for their innervation. The smaller motor units in a muscle have smaller neurons and a lower threshold for activation and are recruited first when a muscle is activated. These usually are the slower motor units; however, see the eyelid muscles orbicularis oculi. If these do not have enough force to get the job done, then larger motor units are brought into play. The total force a motor unit can contribute also will depend upon its limited contraction frequency. In fact, the smaller motor units are not able to contract as frequently as can the larger motor units, and this too will limit their possible force-per-unit-time (power) factor. On the other hand, as when in *a yogasana* posture, these smaller motor units can work continuously for a long time, but when they finally fatigue, the fast-twitch units are called upon, and though they help for a short time, their load of lactic acid soon initiates an even stronger fatigue in the muscle [827].

Yogasana Slowing

As the *yogasana* postures are largely isometric in nature, and isometric contraction encourages type-1 slow-twitch fibers, one can only conclude that *yogasana* practice, in essence, slows our internal clocks, re-tuning the muscles to a slower, more energy-efficient mode, as appropriate for reaching higher meditative states. The fatigue felt by the student in a *yogasana* posture held for a long time is less of a factor when the muscle fibers

---

7   It is a general principle of motor-unit physiology that the various motor units within a muscle are recruited in a particular order depending upon the relative sizes of the motor units. This principle holds whether the muscle contraction is that involved with a deliberate action intended to change the angle at a specific joint, or is involved as when the same muscle is being stretched too rapidly in a particular *yogasana* and then is reflexively contracted. However, exceptions to this are known, where the order partly is dependent upon the specific task the muscle is called upon to perform, and moreover, the principle does not apply to

the random recruitment of motor units that occurs in order to avoid long-time fatigue in postural muscles.

in question are the slow-twitch type, for muscles of this type are more economical energetically and so require less fresh blood to function than do fast-twitch fibers [878]; they also are more highly vascularized. Note too that as the percentage of slow-twitch fibers increases in a muscle, its demand for oxygen decreases, so that the relaxed state is promoted (slower heart rate, lower blood pressure, mind's external awareness relaxed, etc.); whereas the energized state is discouraged, and we become more laid back. Said differently, the nervous system moves from sympathetic to parasympathetic dominance (Chapter 5, page 160) as the *yogasana* practice re-tunes muscle fibers away from type 3 and toward type 1.

As *yogasana* students working the slow-twitch fibers, there will be no explosive, all-or-none activation of the motor units, but a slow, asynchronous turning on and off of various motor units, yielding a smooth, continuous contraction in time. The building of "strength" will be much more a nervous system reeducation (Subsection 4.G, page 141) than a bulking up of the muscle per se.

An experimental study supports these suppositions regarding *yogasana* and muscle-fiber type [35]. With *yogasana* practice, it was found that aerobic power, or $\dot{V}O_{2max}$, increased significantly, whereas anaerobic power decreased significantly. These shifts are interpreted as indicating the transformation of fast-twitch, anaerobic glycolic fibers into slow-twitch, oxidative fibers (table 11.A-4) as one practices the *yogasanas*.

Fiber-Type Interconversion

As mentioned above, the slow-twitch muscle fibers are innervated by neural fibers having low conduction velocities whereas the fast-twitch fibers are innervated by neural fibers of high conduction velocities (table 11.A-4). Interestingly, if the neural connectivity of the motor neurons is reversed so that a red slow-twitch muscle fiber is innervated by a rapidly conducting neuron or vice versa, then the slow-twitch fiber slowly becomes fast-twitch or the white fast-twitch fiber slowly becomes slow-twitch [427]. This illustrates the plasticity of the muscle type and its dependence

upon the characteristics of the neural signal driving it. These changes of muscle characteristics are paralleled by changes in the muscle's biochemistry and morphology, implying that if the higher levels of consciousness that control muscle action dictate a new role for a muscle and so change the frequency of its excitation, then its responsiveness, chemistry, and morphology all will change in sympathy with the new demands made upon it by the altered neural signal activating it [157]. In this way, a *yogasana* practice that encourages the dominance of the parasympathetic branch of the autonomic nervous system, for example, changes the muscular form and responses of the body, moving it away from the Western body/mind type (figure 11.A-16b) and toward the Eastern body/mind type (figure 11.A-16a).

As with the brain, when we are first born, the muscle types are essentially undifferentiated. In infancy, weight bearing can induce the conversion of type-2 fibers into type-1. However, as the muscles are used and the frequencies of the activating neurons are either fast or slow, the muscle type adjusts to the neural frequency, becoming either fast-twitch or slow-twitch. In the young child, a particular pattern of energizing pulses, either from the nervous system or applied externally, will direct the protein synthesis within a muscle, leading to the formation of either fast-twitch or slow-twitch muscles. For this reason, the best training for a task is doing it or tasks similar to it [877].

Indeed, several recent experiments have shown that muscle-fiber types 2 and 3 can be readily interconverted, within a period of a month or so, by the appropriate type of exercise [9]. Evidence for the conversions of the fast-twitch types into slow-twitch type-1 fiber or the reverse is on less solid footing, but it seems likely on a longer time scale. It is postulated, for example, that if fast fibers suffer nerve death, the muscles could be re-innervated by the slow fibers nearby, thereby converting the fiber from the fast type to the slow type.

Surgeons now perform an operation called "dynamic cardiomyoplasty," in which a portion of the latissimus dorsi muscle is wrapped around a weakly beating heart so as to enhance the contractility of the ventricles. However, because the heart is a red, slow-twitch muscle (type 1) and the latissimus is a white, fast-twitch muscle (type 3), the latissimus muscle type must be changed to match that of the heart. This change of type from fast-twitch to slow-twitch is accomplished in a few months by retraining the latissimus to respond to a series of low-frequency electrical pulses applied externally. This change of neuromuscular frequency is sufficient to change the latissimus muscle characteristics from fast, white type 3 to slow, red type 1 [877]. Similar changes in muscle character are possible through *yogasana* practice, but probably over the period of decades rather than months.

Reciprocal Inhibition and Agonist/ Antagonist Muscle Pairs

Agonist/Antagonist Interaction

Almost all muscles in the human body are paired so that for almost every agonist muscle action at a joint, there is an opposing antagonist muscle action possible, which allows the motion at the joint to be reversed and thus controlled. It is not necessary that the agonist and the antagonist are each a specific muscle, for often the agonist is a combination consisting of a major muscle called the prime mover and several lesser muscles called synergists. Another such combination of a different prime mover and its synergists assumes the role of antagonist [877]. See figure 11.A-3 for a display of prime-mover muscle pairs having such opposing agonist/antagonist actions. Judicious excitation of these opposing agonist/antagonist muscle pairs allows for fine-tuning of skeletal motions and the reversal of motions. For example, the biceps brachii muscle, which flexes the arm at the elbow, has the triceps brachii muscle as its antagonist, which acts to straighten it. Working together, they allow a careful and graceful movement of the arm at the elbow, as when bowing a violin. In general, the agonist/antagonist muscle pairs control the motion of the joined bones in a single plane, whereas for a complex joint, such as the shoulder (Subsection 10.A, page 323), there

are several pairs acting to make the allowed motion more spherical than planar.

There is a general state of mild contraction (the so-called resting muscle tone (Subsection 11.B, page 436) at all times in all of the muscles of the body. Even when the body appears to be doing nothing, as when standing, many muscles nonetheless play an active role in keeping the body upright, supporting it against gravitational collapse. If, in this state, the intention of the brain is to change the angle at a joint quickly, as by flexion of the arm to swat a fly on the nose, for example, then the instantaneous contraction of the flexor agonist musculature will be resisted by the ever-present muscle tone in the corresponding extensor antagonist musculature. In this case of sudden movement, the nervous system provides a mechanism whereby the antagonist muscle is relaxed by inhibiting its neural signal entirely, while the agonist is flexed quickly and maximally.

Called reciprocal inhibition, this neuromuscular mechanism also is evident in the patellar knee-jerk reflex (figure 11.D-1). In the case of reflex actions, the reflexive contraction of one of the muscles in response to a stimulus elicits a simultaneous relaxation of its antagonist muscle; i.e., there is a reciprocal inhibition of muscle action. In a modified form, reciprocal inhibition also is a factor in the performance of many *yogasanas*. The fact of reciprocal inhibition is of great importance to *yogasana* students, for if there were no reciprocal inhibition, any attempt to voluntarily close a joint by rapid contraction of the relevant flexor muscle might be frustrated by the reflexive contraction of the antagonist extensor muscle as it was being stretched.

Many muscles, when presented in simple diagrammatic form such as shown in figure 11.A-1, appear to be unitary. However, they are in fact composed of separately innervated but adjacent muscles. Excitation within such a "compound muscle" can result in a strongly localized contraction, in contrast to the situation in which a muscle is composed of several motor units, the fibers (and the contraction) of which are delocalized within the muscle. Thus, what is normally thought of as "the deltoid" in the shoulder, in fact, consists of three adjacent muscles, the anterior, lateral, and posterior deltoids, each capable of independent action. In such a triplet, the anterior deltoid that acts to pull the shoulder forward and the posterior deltoid that acts to pull the shoulder backward form an agonist/antagonist pair. Another compound muscle-triplet that contains within itself pairs of agonist/antagonist pairs is the trapezius in which the upper trapezius and the lower trapezius play these roles (figure 10.A-2**b**). Note, however, that it is an open question as to whether these pairs are innervated so as to produce reciprocal inhibition.

Neural Inhibition versus Excitation

Among the neural systems of the human body, inhibition appears to be even more important than excitation, for inhibition is the more common situation in biological systems ranging from genes to brains and muscles. In a practical sense, this global inhibition is thought to promote the avoidance of the myriad wrong responses possible in complex neural systems and promote the correct response. Failure to inhibit biological processes leads to the risk of responses ranging from convulsions to cancer [877], much as a car in motion runs wild if the braking system fails.

Nature manages to selectively activate one element of an agonist/antagonist muscle pair by bifurcating the afferent nerve signal and sending each branch simultaneously to the efferent α-motor neurons of the two muscles in the pair (figures 11.A-15 and 11.A-19). The route to one of the muscles is direct and excitatory, whereas the other one synapses with an interneuron, the sole function of which is inhibitory (Subsection 3.C, page 51). In this case, the inhibition is the result of raising the transmembrane voltage so that a threshold negative voltage cannot be attained. Thus, by interposing an interneuron in the synaptic gap of one of the muscles but not in the other, only the first is contracted, while contraction in the second is inhibited. Of course, agonist/antagonist inhibition works the other way as well; if it is the second muscle that is excited, then excitation of the first will be inhibited.

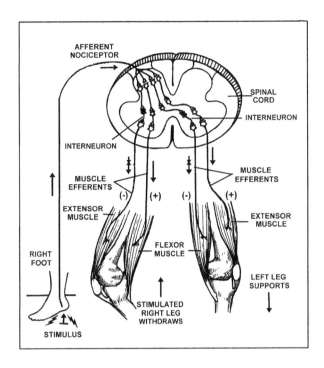

Figure 11.A-19. When the right foot steps on a sharp object, the pain signal travels up the afferent nerve fiber from the nociceptor into the spinal cord. Simultaneously, the flexor muscle (the hamstring) of the right leg is contracted so as to draw the foot upward, whereas the contraction of the extensor (quadriceps) on that leg is inhibited by the interposed interneuron. Meanwhile, to keep from falling with one leg lifted, the opposite scenario is being played out on the left leg, where the extensor is contracted to support the body, while the flexor is inhibited, again by the appropriately placed interneuron.

Other muscles respond as well in this reflexive action. Thus, when the right leg lifts reflexively, as in figure 11.A-19, the gluteus medius (with its origin at the iliac crest and insertion onto the greater trochanter of the femur) on the left also contracts reflexively, so as to support the pelvis and keep it from dropping when the support of the right leg is no longer present. This interplay of excitation and inhibition within an agonist/antagonist muscle pair characterizes the situation regarding reflex actions, as described in Section 11.D, page 448.

The mechanism described above also works

much in the same way when the muscle action is voluntary and slow rather than reflexive and fast; i.e., when a muscle is activated voluntarily, its antagonist often is inhibited synaptically in support of the desired movement. For example, in *uttanasana,* one seeks to stretch the hamstrings. The hamstring stretching can be facilitated by contracting the hamstring's antagonist, the quadriceps, as the reflexive reaction to quadriceps contraction is inhibition of the hamstring contraction; i.e., relaxation and lengthening. That is to say, when the agonist contracts, the antagonist relaxes and stretches. In the stretched state, the antagonist's forcefulness is very much reduced due to poor overlap of its sliding myofilaments (figure 11.A-11 and Subsection 11.A, page 401), and so it cannot generate much force to oppose the desired action (full contraction of the agonist) [288]. In rapid but controlled motion, the antagonist muscles come into play in order to modulate the motion. If, however, the cerebellar component of the stretch reflex is faulty, the antagonist muscle is not activated when the agonist is brought into play, resulting in an excessive movement of the limb called "rebound."

Co-Contraction

The mutual inhibition within the agonist/antagonist pair is of great value for beginners, but when practicing the *yogasanas* at a higher level, both muscle groups of a pair are often worked simultaneously, as the inhibition can be overridden by influences from higher centers. The simultaneous activation of both partners of an agonist/antagonist pair is called co-contraction. Though less energy efficient than reciprocal inhibition, co-contraction does allow for finer control of small movements by balancing the opposition of two active muscles rather than having one active muscle balanced against little or no resistance, as in reciprocal inhibition. The practice of *yogasana* allows for a sophisticated interaction of the agonist and antagonist muscles in a pair. Co-contraction of the muscles in an agonist/antagonist pair also can be used to immobilize a bone or joint for reasons of stability. For example, both the biceps and the triceps are active in *chaturanga dandasana* in

order to stabilize the elbows. Chandra points out how important co-contraction of various muscle pairs is while in *sirsasana,* for without it, the body is not sufficiently monolithic to maintain the inverted but erect posture [112a].

It is interesting to note that outside of *yogasana* practice, co-contraction is held by sports authorities to be inappropriate and to be a characteristic of unskilled movements in infants and children! In fact, we in the *yogasana* field often employ co-contraction as a source of internal resistance against which we work in order to achieve an increased opening of the joints (Subsection 7.D, page 239, and Section 11.F, page 468).

It is occasionally the case that due to a loose arrangement of tissue around a joint, it may easily be hyperextended, thereby exacerbating the looseness and taking the joint out of alignment. This problem may be dealt with by co-contraction of the muscles around the relevant joint, thus stabilizing it.

Sensor Adaptation

We have opposable systems in the body, such as the green/purple consciousness in the neurons of the visual system and the agonist/antagonist stretch receptors in the muscles. When one component of such a pair is activated continuously, the magnitude of its afferent signal tends to fade, in contrast to the signal from the other component. Thus, for example, the brain compares the spindle signals from the agonist flexor and the antagonist extensor muscles (Subsection 11.C, page 441) and then compares their relative magnitudes so as to deduce the limb position in space. However, Haseltine [344] states, "Stretch receptors in opposing muscles can give rise to ghostly after-images when one set of receptors fatigues more than the other. As time passes, the excitation transmitted from an overstretched flexor gradually declines even though the length of the flexor stretch sensor never changes. This neural fatigue causes the stretch receptor to under-report the true length of the muscle." The possibility of distortion of the body image through this phenomenon of asymmetric neural fatigue should be kept in mind when practicing.

On the other hand, as we stretch, we may be inhibited by the signal coming from the stretched muscle spindles, but with time, these signals slowly adapt toward zero (Subsection 13.B, page 506), so that as the stretch signal diminishes, we can then increase the stretch until a newly inhibiting stretch signal arises. Thus, by staying in the posture, we slowly stretch the muscle to longer and longer lengths. If true, this fading effect will reveal itself by a sensation of the elongation and shift of the limb position. Yet another factor in stretching is that there is slow viscoelastic flow of the connective tissue, which, over time, tends to reduce the tension on the muscle and so allows the muscle to lengthen without tripping the muscle-spindle alarm. See also the discussion below on the effects of the Golgi tendon organ and autogenic inhibition on muscle spindles.

Muscle Imbalance across a Joint

Optimal functioning of a joint requires that the two prime movers responsible for opening and closing the joint be in reasonable balance. Muscular imbalance between the agonist and antagonist muscles can result from postural stresses, repetitive movements, low technical skill in movement, lack of core strength, aging, or immobilization. Once out of balance, the weaker component of the two prime movers may delegate its role of prime mover to its synergist muscles, which then must be used in ways for which they are not meant. For example, if the psoas is hypertonic, then the antagonist gluteus maximus, by reciprocal inhibition, eventually will be weakened, and its synergist muscles (the hamstrings, the erector spinae, and the piriformis) will consequently become overactive; i.e., synergistically dominant. This dominance by synergists in turn leads to inefficient muscle action, tissue fatigue, reciprocal inhibition, and decreased neuromuscular control over the actions of the joint. Examples of the use of synergistic muscles in *yogasana* postures are presented in the following subsection (this page) and in Box 11.A-5, page 424.

Joint Structure and Movement in *Yogasana*

When a muscle contracts, the two bones spanned by the muscle generally move toward one another; however, other muscles often come into play, immobilizing one of the bones but not the other. In such a case, that part of the relevant muscle tendon attached to the stationary bone is called the origin, and that part of the tendon attached to the mobile bone is called the insertion. In the limbs, the origins are usually proximal and the insertions distal. Note too that when a muscle that spans a joint contracts, there is a rotational moment that develops around the center of the joint (the rotational force) and simultaneously a second force, which pulls the articulating ends of the joints toward one another, acting to close the joint (the stabilizing force); there is no possible action involving two bones and the contracting muscle that connects them that opens the joint! However, it is possible that on relaxation of a muscle, the relevant joint can open somewhat, due to the inherent elasticity of the connective tissues and other elements that otherwise resist the resting muscle tone.

In our *yogasana* practice, we work to open the distance between the two ends of a joint that are normally in contact, which is an action normally not met with in body mechanics. This sort of joint opening generally results in a larger range of motion of the joint, whatever its function.

One goal in *yogasana* practice, from the point of view of the muscles, is to use them in a way that leads to an expansion of a joint or joints, even though an individual muscle cannot actively extend but can only contract, and contraction leads to closing of the joint. How, then, can contracting muscles lead to expanding joints? As with almost everything in *yogasana* science, the answer is indirect and paradoxical. Consider first the process of inhalation. On inhalation, the diaphragm contracts, and with its outer edge connected firmly to the lowermost rib (T12), one would reasonably expect the lowest ribs to move inward upon contraction of the attached diaphragm as when inhaling. Now take a deep breath with your at-

Box 11.A-5: The Hands Help Wag the Scapulae in *Adho Mukha Svanasana*, Possibly as in an Anatomy Train

It is an interesting question as to how a specific joint may be pulled open using muscles that can only be used actively to pull joints closed. With the idea of the anatomy train [603] in mind, let us see if there is a reasonable way of connecting thumb action in the pronated hand to movement of the rib cage.[1] There are two muscles in the upper arm that work to flex the arm at the elbow: the brachialis and the biceps brachii. The former has its origin on the lower half of the humeral shaft, with insertion on the ulna of the forearm; whereas in the latter, the origin is on the scapula, with insertion on the radius of the forearm (figures 11.A-20**a** and 11.A-20**b**). In *adho mukha svanasana,* one wants the triceps of the beginning student to contract so as to straighten the arms at the elbows, and correspondingly, the biceps brachii and brachialis should be released, to allow the triceps to pull the bones of the arms into alignment. That is to say, one is looking for the reciprocal inhibition of the arm flexors by the arm extensors. Now, relaxation of the biceps brachii comes from pronation of the forearm; i.e., pressing downward through the base of the thumb and index finger. When the hand is worked in this way in *adho mukha svanasana* (and in other postures, such as *adho mukha vrksasana),* then (a) the biceps are relaxed, (b) the triceps then can contract with the greatest effect, and (c) the tug of the biceps on the scapulae pulling them toward the nape of the neck is released, so that the scapulae can more easily be pulled down the back by the lower trapezius and latissimus dorsi muscles. With the scapulae in this depressed position, they can then be pressed into the rib cage so as to lift and open the chest (see Subsection 10.A, pages 328 and 331, for further discussions on the effects of

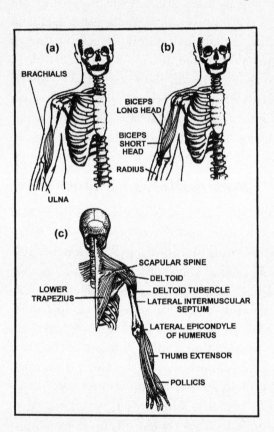

Figure 11.A-20. (**a**) The origin (lower humeral shaft) and insertion (ulna) of the brachialis muscle on the arm. (**b**) The origin (scapula) and insertion (radius) of the biceps muscle on the arm. (**c**) A possible anatomy train [603] from the pollicis muscle of the thumb to the muscles in the rotator cuff.

---

1   This scenario is meant to be illustrative of the concept of the anatomy train, but it is not meant to imply that this mechanism is of major importance when performing *adho mukha svanasana*. In fact, I feel that hand action in this posture is important, as it serves as an anchor against which the disrotatory action of the humerus can work (Subsection 10.A, page 328), whereas the action described here serves more as a synergist than as a prime mover in this posture.

arm and thumb actions on the chest). This action, stretching from the fingertips to the scapulae, figure 11.A-20c, involves what has been called the "brachial muscular chain" by some body workers [105] and the "anatomy train" by others [603].

Performed in this way, the simple actions of the thumbs and index fingers on the floor in *adho mukha svanasana* result in tangible consequences for the action of the scapulae on the rib cage. In fact, this action is enhanced considerably if the student sets the hands on the mat with the fingers turned slightly inward (medially), for this gives strength to the disrotatory action of the upper arms, so as to turn the eyes of the elbows forward.

As discussed in Section 10.A, page 328, the muscular chain extending from the thumb to the rib cage is important not only in *adho mukha svanasana*, but is also virtually universal in *yogasana* practice, for the lifting and opening of the chest promoted by this action is a key part of all *yogasanas* performed in the Iyengar way, except for *savasana*. Only in this case does one forego activation of the sympathetic nervous system in order to activate the parasympathetic nervous system.

tention on the lowest ribs, and you will see that in fact, the lowest ribs move **outward** on inhalation! In order for the diaphragm to function properly on inhalation, the points of attachment cannot move inward, for if they did, then the low pressure external to the lungs would not develop, and the lungs would not inflate.

In fact, the inward movement of the lowest ribs during inhalation is resisted by the actions of the anterior serratus (intercostal) muscles (figure 10.A-2a) that bind the outer surface of each of the lower ribs to the one above it; contraction of the anterior serratus, acting as synergist to the diaphragm, flares the lowest ribs outward, and the diaphragmatic contraction works against this to inflate the lungs. Thus, it is seen that the action of the diaphragm is to pull the lowest ribs on the two sides of the chest toward one another, but that inhalation also involves the top-to-bottom contraction of the muscles pulling up the outer edges of the T12 and higher ribs so as to expand the lower ribs laterally. In this way, we see how the contraction of muscles secondary to those spanning the bones in question might act to counter the natural movement of these bones. This scenario is but another example of how we use internal resistances within the body in order to achieve a particular muscular movement (Section 11.F, page 468). Another example of the roles of syner-

gist muscles in *yogasana* postures is presented in Box 11.A-5 above.

Linear Joint Opening

To simplify the discussion of joint opening, consider next how, with the arms held parallel to the floor and out to the sides, one might contract the muscles so that the fingertips on the left hand move away from the fingertips on the right, i.e., how one can open the shoulder joint. Let us assume that only the humerus and the scapula meet at the shoulder and form the shoulder joint. As the deltoid spans the shoulder joint, it clearly should be relaxed if the two bones forming the joint are to move apart. But now, if contraction of the latissimus dorsi and rhomboid muscles pull the scapulae closer to the spine, while at the same time the muscles of the forearm (brachioradialis and the triceps) pull the humerus toward the wrist when the arms are straight, then the bones that meet at the shoulder will move **away** from one another; i.e., the shoulder joint opens because the more distant joints are pulled closed. This general method for the linear opening of a joint is shown diagrammatically in figure 11.A-21.

Imagine a train of alternating muscles and bones (figure 11.A-21), the leftmost of which (bone B4) is to be moved to the right. Contraction of prime-mover muscle M4 will move bone B4 to

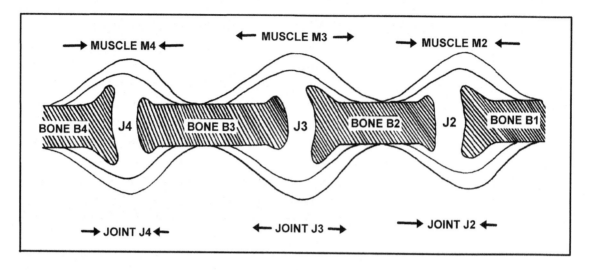

Figure 11.A-21. The mechanics of a simple linear anatomy train. In order to open joint J3 between bones B3 and B2, muscle M3 must first be relaxed, thereby lessening the resting muscle tone and opening the joint somewhat. However, it is the **closing** of adjacent joint J4 (between bones B3 and B4) and joint J2 (between bones B2 and B1) by contraction of muscles M4 and M2, respectively, that substantially **increases** the distance between bones B3 and B4; i.e., opens joint J3.

the right; however, there will also be a movement of bone B3 to the left as joint J4 closes. If B3 is also pulled to the right by contraction of synergist muscle M3, then B3 will remain stationary and B4 will be moved even more to the right. The effectiveness of the contraction of M3 in turn will be heightened by the contraction of its synergist muscle M2, which will pull B2 to the right, and with it, B3 and B4. Finally, bone B1 is pulled to the left as joint J2 closes, and the result is that B4 and B1 are pulled toward each other, though there is no muscle that directly connects bone B4 to B1. Alternately, if muscle M4 contracts and so pulls bone B3 to the left, whereas muscle M2 contracts and pulls bone B2 to the right, then these contractions lead to a separation of bones B3 and B2 with an opening of joint J3. In effect, these scenarios lead to the idea of an anatomy train consisting of bone, muscle, and fascia connecting distant points and leading to a linear opening of a joint.

It would appear from the above picture that all of the active joint openings in the body involve selective joint closing at nearby joints so that the joint in question is pulled open. Looked at in this way, it would appear that there is a zero-sum game operating here, with joints opening in one place only if joints in another place close. In this model, elongation in the *yogasanas* involves the interplay of muscles at a joint that is to open and the closing of those at and around the joints adjacent to the joint in question; it does not seem possible to actively open all joints simultaneously. That is not to say that all joints cannot be opened somewhat by relaxation in *savasana* or by anesthesia, but these are passive openings, and we are here discussing the **active** opening of joints.[8]

---

8   Another possible approach to how contracting muscles can lead to an opening of the associated joint comes to us from studying the extrinsic musculature of the eye (figure 17.A-1). Note that in the superior oblique muscles of the eye, the muscle initiating oblique motion is attached toward the rear of the eyeball, but that its tendon passes through a loop of tissue called the trochlea, which is forward of the eyeball. The function of the trochlea is to serve as a pulley, which acts to change the direction of the muscular tension. Thus, when the oblique muscle of the eye contracts, seemingly to pull the eyeball deeper within the eye socket, the trochlear pulley reverses this direction so that muscular tension on the superior oblique pulls the eyeball forward instead of backward! "Relaxing

Attachment of the Tendons

In the case of the reciprocal inhibition of an agonist muscle and its antagonist, the two muscles are attached to opposite sides of the joint and work oppositely in regard to opening or closing it. A somewhat similar condition can exist at a joint at which two muscles (types A and B) span the same joint but are placed on the same side of the joint; in this case, the two have different ranges of motion and power. In such a muscle pair, contraction of the type A muscle results in a large angular range of motion but with low average power over time, whereas contraction of the type B muscle results in a small angular range of motion but with high average power over time. The differences result from different muscle-lever configurations, i.e., where the muscles insert on the bone being moved. In a type A muscle, the tendon is inserted close to the joint and the muscle is largely fusiform and fast-twitch type 3, whereas in a type B muscle, the insertion is farther from the joint and the muscle is often bipennate and slow-twitch type 1 [288].[9]

the eyes," in large part, means relaxing tension in the oblique muscles so that the eyeballs can fall back into the eye sockets.

In principle, this arrangement could function around a joint, with contraction of an attached muscle leading to an opposite movement of the bone, provided there is some sort of a pulley to redirect the muscular force. The action of peroneus longus on the head of the first metatarsal (Subsection 10.B, page 360) may be another example of the anatomic pulley function in the body. The pulley option is discussed further in Subsection 11.A, page 406.

9   The anatomy of the muscle dictates whether it will function best as an aid to power or as an aid to speed. In this discussion, "speed" refers to angular rate of change (degrees/second) at the joint. If the fibers are long and parallel to the mechanical axis, then the muscle will be fast but low power; i.e., it is type A. However, if the muscle is pennated (see figures 11.A-13a and -13b), as is the case for type-B muscles, the muscle cross-section is larger, the fibers are shorter and not parallel to the line between origin and insertion, there is a smaller change of length upon contraction,

Many joints have components of both A and B types simultaneously; e.g., the elbow joint is spanned by both the biceps muscle for speed (type A) and the brachialis muscle for strength and endurance (type B), and the back of the knee is spanned both by the biceps femoris for instant speed (type A) and the slow-moving inner hamstrings for strength and endurance (type B). Within this framework, we may classify the gastrocnemius of the lower leg as the type-A component and the soleus as the type-B component of the triceps surae musculature that plantar flexes the ankle (Subsection 10.B, page 356).

When the muscle attachment is close to the joint, as it is in a B-type muscle, the contraction of the muscle acts largely to "stabilize" (immobilize) the joint, whereas when the attachment takes the geometry characteristic of an A-type muscle, the result is rotatory motion around the joint center. This leads to the idea that type-B muscles are better for maintaining position, balance, and stability, as appropriate to isometric contractions while in the *yogasanas*. Classification of the muscles as types A or B closely resembles the type-3 (fast-twitch) and type-1 (slow-twitch) classification of muscle types, respectively, as described above.

Biarticular Muscles

Certain muscles within the body span two joints rather than just one. For example, the biceps femoris, running from the ischium to the tibia, spans both the hip and the knee joints at the back of the legs, whereas the quadriceps spans the same joints at the front of the legs; the gastrocnemius also is biarticular, as it runs from the femur to the calcaneus and spans both the knee and the ankle joints. If the gastrocnemius is contracted, the ankle bends in plantar flexion (heel toward the back of the knee) and the knee also bends. If instead it is one's intention to keep the leg straight, then one must point the heel, i.e., place the foot in dorsi-

and the movement is slow but powerful. If the muscle attachments in both A and B are at the same place on the moving bone and muscles A and B have equal volumes, then they will perform with equal average power.

flexion by contraction of the anterior tibialis in the lower leg (Subsection 10.B, page 361), relax the gastrocnemius, and tighten the quadriceps. This action both straightens the leg and stretches the gastrocnemius. In a similar way, if it is desired to stretch the hamstrings, it will be necessary to keep the leg straight at the knee (for bending the knee relaxes the hamstrings) while putting the hip joint into flexion so as to pull the ischium bones away from the knees, as in *uttanasana*.

Tensile Strength

It is interesting to see just where muscle stands with respect to other materials in regard to tensile strength. A steel cable has a tensile strength of more than 3,500 kilograms per square centimeter (50,000 pounds per square inch); this means that a cable having a cross section of 6.45 square centimeters (one square inch) will separate only when carrying a load larger than 22,700 kilograms (50,000 pounds). For tendons, the tensile strength is 1,100 kilograms per square centimeter (15,000 pounds per square inch) and for muscle, it is only 1–10 kilograms per square centimeter (15–140 pounds per square inch). Because bone has a tensile strength somewhat lower than that of tendon, the bone often separates before the tendon breaks when the tendon and its attachment to bone are under a tensile stress of more than 1,100 kilograms per square centimeter (15,000 pounds per square inch). Note, however, that the cross section of the belly of a muscle is often 100 times larger than that of its tendon, thus putting it in the same range as tendon in regard to the tensile load it will bear before separating [877]. In effect, the muscle is able to bear a large tensile load by distributing the stress over the very large cross section of its belly, and conversely, the small cross section of the tendon translates into a very large tensile burden.

Mechanism aside, one should realize that it is the muscles that support the skeleton in an erect position, whereas in the *yogasana* postures, one comes to realize that the favor is returned many times over, with the bones playing key roles in maintaining posture. Though Juhan has stated [422] that "Stability of the joints is maintained above all by the activity of the surrounding muscles. Ligaments also play a part but they will stretch under the constant strain when muscles are weak or paralyzed," the major effect of skeletal support is obvious when one compares the time one can spend comfortably in *tadasana* versus that in *utkatasana*. Unfortunately, our muscle strength is at a maximum at about age twenty-five years and then declines with further aging. Still, regardless of age, movement improves all aspects of joint function when the joint is in good health. With increasing age, the loss of muscle strength is most apparent, followed by the loss of precision in movement, and finally the loss of speed [288].

Section 11.B: Sensors: The Mechanoreceptors

The Mechanoreceptors in Skeletal Muscle

There are huge numbers of sensors both within and upon the body called mechanoreceptors, that are readily distinguished from one another, but which nonetheless operate in very similar ways. All mechanoreceptors are activated by mechanical stimuli; i.e., by mechanical distortions of the sensors due to pressure. The term "mechanoreceptors" refers to structures as varied as the muscle spindles within muscles that respond to stretch and rate of stretch of muscle fibers, and the baroreceptors within the heart that respond to changes of arterial blood pressure, again through mechanical deformation. In all of these receptors, the mechanical distortion is first transformed into a DC voltage, which is transformed a second time into the frequency realm (Section 3.F, page 65) and sent along an afferent neuron to the central nervous system. The end result of this process is that the degree of mechanical stress sensed by a mechanoreceptor is translated into an electrical wave in the nervous system having a frequency proportional to the stress: large distortions sensed by mechanoreceptors generate high-frequency electrical signals, and small distortions generate low-frequency signals.

Stretch Receptors

There are five general types of mechanoreceptors associated with muscle tension: (1) muscle spindles (concerned with muscle length and the rate of change of muscle length); (2) Golgi tendon organs (concerned with forces developed within the muscle tendon); (3) Pacinian corpuscles (which play a minor role in muscle but are important in skin); (4) Ruffini corpuscles (sensitive to skin deformation); and (5) free nerve endings (the nociceptors that respond to muscle injury following trauma or overstretching, among other things) [549]. Each of the first four mechanoreceptor types is a factor in sensing both consciously and subconsciously where the body is in space (Subsection 11.C, page 441), what the degree of tension is in each of the skeletal muscles, and how these are changing with time as we stretch.

Stretch receptors also are found in the viscera, and in the bronchi, bronchioles, and alveoli of the lungs. During the breathing cycle, stretch receptors in the lungs are alternately activated and relaxed and report their levels of mechanical stress to the brain, using the afferents of the right vagus nerve (cranial nerve X). In response to this, heart action and blood pressure shift appropriately throughout the breathing cycle (Subsection 15.C, page 619). These mechanoreceptors in the lungs are the signaling centers for interoception (Subsection 11.C, page 444). The mechanoreceptors in the lungs and those that monitor blood pressure and blood volume within the cardiovascular system are of great importance to *yogasana* students.

Notice that the sensory signals from the various mechanoreceptors mentioned above are fundamentally identical. In every case, the sensory signal that is sent upward consists of a series of action potentials of constant voltage, but with frequencies that reflect the intensity of the stimulus. It is significant, then, that each sensory signal travels on a neural track dedicated to it alone (an afferent neuron) and heading to a specific point in the nervous system. The look-alike signals from different

receptors are kept separate until they reach their appropriate destinations at higher centers, where they then can contribute to the competition for attention among all of the sensory-information inputs. (However, see also Subsection 3.B, page 47, and Section 13.D, page 530.)

Structure of Muscle Spindles

Our muscles are able to propel various body parts in various directions while other muscles can work to reverse these motions (see Subsection 11.A, page 368). These two actions can be thought of as being the accelerator and brake of an automobile. The two opposing actions must work in concert in the automobile if the ride is to be a smooth one, and so it is in the graceful movements of the *yogasana* student as well. As a more pedestrian example, certain muscles propel the fork into one's mouth, while other muscles on the opposite sides of the relevant joints limit the motion so that the fork does not jab the back of the throat. By what means are these muscle actions coordinated so that not only is the movement graceful, but its extent does not risk injury, either to the muscles involved or to nearby muscles? And while we are in a questioning mood, let us also ask, "Does a muscle itself have anything to say in regard to how far or how fast it is to be stretched or contracted, or is this under the jurisdiction of higher centers in the central nervous system?"

The answers to questions such as those posed above lie, in part, in the actions of receptors in the muscles and tendons that are interspersed throughout both the contractile and noncontractile parts of all skeletal muscles and that monitor muscle length, muscle tension, and the rates at which these quantities are changing. Such receptors are found not only in the largest muscles of the leg but also in the smallest muscles of the eyelid and in all others in between.

There are so many receptors in so many muscle fibers, constantly sending their messages upward, that if they were able to make their way to the conscious level of the nervous system, the system would be totally overwhelmed. In fact, much of the afferent data stream is handled by lower centers in the subconscious domain, with very little of it penetrating into our conscious awareness. Through *yogasana* practice, we can elect to bring a small fraction of this mass of real-time data into our consciousness and also to lower its intensity by relaxing the muscle tone (Subsection 11.B, page 436). Among the most important of such stretch receptors are the muscle spindles found within the body's skeletal muscles, serving both to keep the muscles from overstretching and to report proprioceptively on the state of muscle tension.

Muscle-Spindle Structure

The muscle spindles are elongate, fluid-filled capsules up to 10 millimeters (half an inch) long in some muscles. A muscle spindle will contain between three and ten stretch-sensitive fibers, with each spindle being much shorter than the muscle cells that surround it. There are three types of sensor fibers within the muscle spindles: the static and dynamic nuclear-bag fibers, so called because the nuclei are gathered at the center of the cell; and the nuclear-chain fibers, so called because the nuclei are strung out as in a chain (figure 11.B-1). Surprisingly, there are also muscle fibers within a spindle; these are known as "intrafusal," to distinguish them from the fibers outside the spindle, which are called "extrafusal." The intrafusal fibers contain stretch-sensitive structures wrapped helically around each of their central parts, whereas the ends of the intrafusal fibers consist of more ordinary, striated contractile muscle innervated by γ-motor neurons operating through the actin-myosin interaction.

Innervation

The contractile ends of the intrafusal fibers within the spindle capsule are innervated by the γ-motor neurons issuing from the ventral horn of the spinal cord, just as the extrafusal muscle fibers outside the spindle's capsule are activated by the α-motor neurons from the ventral horn. The α and γ systems are efferent-motor systems, with the α system generally controlling the skeletal muscles while itself being under the control

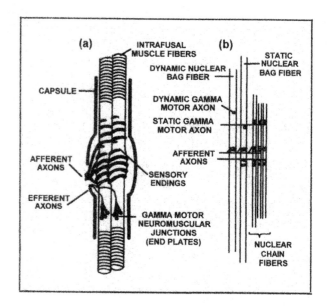

Figure 11.B-1. A muscle spindle is shown, as it would appear under the microscope (**a**), and as drawn schematically, (**b**). There are three types of stretch sensors within the muscle spindle: the dynamic nuclear-bag sensors, the static nuclear-bag sensors, and the nuclear-chain sensors. All of the stretch sensors are connected to afferent neurons. Additionally, each of the intrafusal muscles is innervated by an efferent γ-motor neuron that adjusts the tension within the intrafusal spindle fiber by relaxing or contracting.

of the central nervous system, whereas the γ system is energized by subconscious centers in the brainstem and controls the intrafusal fiber tension within the skeletal-muscle spindles. Among other functions, these spindles dictate the levels of resting-muscle tone.

Of all the motor neurons in the body connected to the vast number of muscle fibers, fully one third of them are hidden from our awareness as γ-motor neurons [422]. The central portion of the spindle is innervated by a fast, type Ia afferent neural axon, whereas the myofilaments at the ends of the spindles are innervated by the slower type II afferent fibers of the γ-neural system. The type Ia fibers are large in diameter and rapidly conducting, whereas those of type II are of a smaller diameter and conduct more slowly (table 3.B-3). Note, however, that there are cross con-

Table 11.B-1: Spindle Numbers and Densities in Various Human Muscles [549]

Muscle	Muscle Location	Number of Spindles	Muscle Weight, Grams	Density, Spindles/Gram
Obliquus capitis superior	Neck	141	3.3	42.7
Rectus capitis posterior minor	Neck	122	4	30.5
Masseter, deep portion	Jaw	42	3.8	11.2
Abductor pollis brevis	Hand	80	2.7	29.3
First lumbrical	Hand	51	3.1	16.5
First lumbrical	Foot	36	1.7	21
Biceps brachii	Upper arm	320	164	2
Triceps brachii	Upper arm	520	364	1.4
Pectoralis major	Upper torso	450	296	1.5
Latissimus dorsi	Back	368	246	1.4
Teres major	Back	44	123	0.4

nections, with a few type Ia fibers terminating at the nuclear-chain fibers and a few type II fibers also terminating at nuclear-bag fibers.

Spindle Densities

The muscle spindles described here operate in two extremely important ways. First, they monitor the intensity of a muscle stretch and so are able to convert stretching into contraction if the stretch becomes too deep or too fast. Moreover, the signals that the muscle spindles report also are used for constructing a map of the body in space, based largely on the levels of muscle tension throughout the body. This map reveals, in real time, any imbalance in the body and so is an integral part of our balancing.

The densities of muscle spindles are not uniform throughout the body, as is clear from the data in table 11.B-1. It is interesting to note that the highest density of muscle spindles (number of spindles per gram of muscle tissue) is to be found in the rectus capitis posterior minor and the obliquus capitis superior, these being quite small muscles within the back of the neck, con-

necting the occiput to the spinous process of C1 and to the transverse processes of C1, respectively, in left-right pairs (figure V.C-1). In contrast, the lowest densities so far measured are for the large muscles of the arms and back. In general, a high density reflects the muscle's ability to move quickly and accurately; with respect to the back of the neck, this relates to the need to keep the head in balance. That is, spindles in the capitis muscles supply high-resolution proprioceptive signals to the brain as regards the state of extension of the neck and left-right tilting of the head. In this case, comparison of the proprioceptive signals from the stretch receptors in the left and right capitis muscles work in support of those head-orienting signals otherwise generated by the saccules of the vestibular system (Subsection 18.B, page 696; however, also see Section V.C, page 893). The simple fact of the high density of muscle spindles in the rectus capitis posterior minor and obliquus capitis superior muscles within the neck unavoidably leads to the idea that head position will be an important factor in any posture requiring balance (Section V.D, page 907).

Function of Muscle Spindles

Stretch Limiters

As the nuclear-chain and nuclear-bag intrafusal fibers are connected to the ends of the muscle spindle's capsule, which itself is nested firmly within the extrafusal fibers of the muscle tissue, any change in the length of the extrafusal muscle fibers is followed by a parallel change in the length of the intrafusal fibers. That is to say, the length of the intrafusal fibers increases as the muscle in question stretches, and decreases again when it relaxes or contracts. Referring to figure 11.B-1, the sensory ending spiraling around each of the three types of fiber functions much like the spring in a sensitive spring balance. When a muscle is stretched, the intrafusal fibers within the spindles are stretched as well, thereby lengthening the spiral springs attached to them. The lengthening of the spring-like sensors is then transduced into an electrical signal that propagates along the afferent axons to the central nervous system; in this way, the muscle spindles function as stretch sensors.

Rates of Change

Though the three types of intrafusal fibers share certain afferent pathways (figure 11.B-1), it appears that the function of the nuclear-chain fibers is to measure the static length changes attendant to muscle stretching, whereas the faster nuclear-bag fibers monitor the more dynamic rates of change of muscle lengthening. It is known that the nuclear-bag fibers are distinctly viscoelastic in their response to stretch [549] (Subsection 11.E, page 462).

The response of the dynamic-stretch sensors within the nuclear-bag fibers adapts to zero in a time less than a second; however, the static-stretch reflex, as sensed by the nuclear-chain fibers, can be continued indefinitely once the dynamic sensor has done its work. The function of the static-stretch reflex when in a *yogasana* position is discussed on page 432.

As with other sensors (Section 14.E, page 580, for example), the muscle spindle encodes its information as a series of nerve impulses, the frequency of which increases as the intensity of the stimulus increases. In the simplest case, the afferent motor neurons from the intrafusal fibers have a single synapse within the spinal cord, the efferent end of which is the α-motor neuron activating the motor unit in question, as in figure 11.D-1, for example. If the muscle is being stretched too far or too fast so that the mechanical integrity of the muscle fibers is at risk, the high frequency of the muscle-spindle afferent signal then acts to stimulate the appropriate efferent α-motor neuron so that the motor unit contracts, thereby releasing the tensile stress on the muscle fibers. Operating in this way, the muscle spindles are able to regulate the amount a muscle is stretched and its rate of stretch, always keeping it in the "safe" range. In addition to acting as stretch limiters, the muscle spindles are still active, even when in their more normal state of resting muscle tone, for they also report this tension due to resting-muscle tone to the subconscious, to be interpreted there as contributing to the proprioceptive map of body position in space (Subsection 11.C, page 441).

It seems reasonable that the nuclear-bag fibers are the first line of defense for a muscle being stretched. If the initial rate of stretch is too large for a cold muscle, then this too-fast stretch alarm will sound, and the muscle will be thrown into contraction to slow the rate of stretching. On the other hand, if the rate of stretch is reasonably slow, then the nuclear-bag fibers are not excited, and the nuclear-chain fibers monitor the slow stretch to see that even when done slowly, it does not proceed too far.

But even this level of protection against overstretching is not enough. Joints generally are crossed by more than one muscle, so that if a muscle acts to open the angle at the joint, another one on the opposite side of the joint will act to close it. Such oppositely acting pairs of muscles, called agonists and antagonists (Section 11.A, page 420), play an important role in muscle stretching; when the spindles of a muscle motor unit signal that the stretching has gone too far, its mono-synapse to the α-motor neuron is energized, causing the muscle to contract; however, part of the afferent signal also is diverted through an inhibitory interneuron, which then synapses with the α-motor neuron of the antagonist muscle, as in figure 11.A-19. Through this dual action, the overly stretched (or too-rapidly stretched) muscle will begin to contract, and the contraction in the antagonist muscle that was originally driving the stretch will then relax in sympathy with the need to return the stretched muscle to its resting length. This mechanism, called reciprocal inhibition (Subsection 11.A, page 420) is discussed from the point of view of reflex action in Section 11.D, page 448.

Reciprocal inhibition is met not only in the case of excessive tension on the muscle spindles, but also in the case of a noxious stimulus to the body from outside the body. Thus, the neural diagrams in figures 11.A-19 and 11.D-1 look very much alike, as both involve reciprocal inhibition, but it should be noticed that in the former case, the stimulus for the reflex arc is a pain receptor lying outside the neural arcs of the relevant muscles, whereas in the latter, the initiating receptor is not a pain receptor but a muscle spindle within the muscle it eventually will cause to contract.

It is an open question in the Western medical community as to whether signals from muscle mechanoreceptors are totally subconscious or can be sensed consciously. In regard to this question, McComas [549] includes several paragraphs in his book *Skeletal Muscle: Form and Function,* in a section entitled "Do Signals from Muscle Receptors Reach Consciousness?" He concludes that the answer as to whether these muscle-spindle signals actually reach as high as the thalamus and cortex is still uncertain as yet; however, I would guess that among *yogasana* adepts, the answer is definitely yes! Note too the discussion in Subsection 1.B, pages 12 and 15.

Adaptation

As shown in figure 13.B-1 [308], there is a range of adaptation (Subsection 13.B, page 506) in various types of receptors. That is, if the stress due to muscle extension is constant in time, the spindle signal nonetheless decreases with time, tending toward zero. Thus, the Pacinian corpuscle at constant pressure has a signal that adapts to

zero in about 0.1 second, and the signal of a bent-hair receptor adapts to zero in about one second. In contrast, the muscle-spindle signal adapts to only 10 percent of its sensitivity in thirty seconds and drops very little from that point. The joint-capsule sensors (Subsection 11.B, pages 438 and 440) are even slower in their adaptation than the muscle spindles. With respect to *yogasana,* this adaptation of the muscle sensors means that if we are patient and move slowly, we can attain extreme positions of the body without tripping any stretch alarms. Without adaptation, the muscles would contract as soon as the stretch went beyond the level set by the spindles. On the other hand, the slow adaptation of the muscle receptors means that they are essentially constantly aware of the body position but slowly decreasing in sensitivity, guaranteeing that they will stay below the threshold if we stretch slowly.

Silencing the Spindle Alarm

The problem for the student of *yogasana* is how to achieve a deep stretch if the muscle spindles always react to contract the muscle whenever the stretch tries to lengthen it. The solution to this puzzle is not at all clear on this key point of *yogasana* physiology, but it is likely to involve the following. Over a period of many seconds of constant elongation, the afferent spindle frequency drops to a lower constant level, as the system resets the spindle tension by lowering the frequency of the γ-motor efferent signal through adaptation. Behaving in this way, the spindles are said to be slowly adapting receptors (see Subsection 13.B, page 506), as are the mechanoreceptors for joint position [432]. The adaptation of the spindles may be due to a viscous flow of the intrafusal spindle materials, or there may be a lessening of the γ-motor action-potential frequency prompted from above. This γ-motor frequency is known to be under the control of centers superior to the brainstem and is readily changed by various emotions, psychological attitudes, and body perceptions [422] (see Subsection 11.B, page 437).

It seems likely that a significant factor in the relaxation of the γ-motor tension on the muscle spindles is the conscious relaxation of global body tension through conscious release and through relaxation of the breath. Given the thirty-second time interval for a muscle spindle to lower its sensitivity by 90 percent, one can guess that one should stay in a slow stretch for many tens of seconds in order to achieve a deep stretch. Iyengar [388] recommends times to hold the *yogasanas* as between thirty seconds (just the time interval necessary to insure autogenic relaxation; Subsection 11.B, page 439) and fifteen minutes in order to get the optimum benefits of the stretch; Cole [147] points out that the duration of the stretch is important in regard to flexibility, whereas strength is promoted by repetitions of the posture at high intensity.

As movements and limb positions become more familiar and are held for a longer time, the stretch receptors' sensitivities decrease through adaptation, and the movements and positions cease to impress us as much as they did on first meeting them [632]. At the same time, this allows for more and more elongation of the extrafusal muscle fibers without triggering the intrafusal fibers of the muscle spindles.

γ-Motor Neurons and Temperature

The γ-motor neurons within muscle spindles are stimulated by the cold center within the pre-optic area of the anterior hypothalamus, which acts to lower the body's temperature; conversely, these neurons are inhibited by the posterior hypothalamus, which acts to generate and conserve heat [427, 471] (table 5.B-1).[10] As tension in the γ-motor sensors is higher when the body is cold, it is more difficult to stretch at this time, whereas when the body is warm, tension in the spindles is inhibited, and stretching is easier. As the anterior hypothalamus is also the center for pain, anxiety, and fear, these emotions also can stimulate the γ-motor neurons and so make stretching more

---

10   One might at first think that this connection between the thermal center in the brain and the γ-motor center is odd; however, when we are feeling cold, it may be the constant momentary excitation of the intrafusal-muscle fibers that jolts the muscle into contraction and so promotes shivering and warming.

difficult, especially in backbends (Box 11.D-1, page 453). The effects of temperature on muscle viscosity are discussed further in Subsection 11.E, page 468.

Muscle Tone

There are really two muscle tones in a working muscle: that of the contractile muscle fibers and that within the muscle spindles. According to Kurz [471], there exists a compensatory mechanism, in which the spindle tone tends to increase when the muscle tone decreases, which means that the muscle is least able to experience stretch without initiating a contraction when it is most passive and at rest. Kurz claims that it is for this reason that we wake up stiff in the morning, as the contractile machinery has relaxed, but the muscle spindles have tightened in response to this. Based upon this idea, there is a simple (but non-yogic) technique that can work to overcome the spindle blockade of overstretched muscles. Called PNF, it is described in Box 11.B-1, below.

Proprioceptors and Pain

The signals from muscle spindles [427] in combination with other mechanoreceptor organs are used by the body to determine static and dynamic limb position. These spindle receptor signals, together with those from the joints and skin, form the sensory net of the proprioceptive system (Subsection 11.C, page 441).

Sensory signals from the muscle mechanoreceptors do not easily work their way high enough to register in the conscious sphere, as they are more in the realm of subconscious reflex action. Thus, they are not the carriers of pain signals sent by our muscles when we overstretch. These instead involve pain receptors (nociceptors) lying deep within the tissue (Section 13.C, page 518), responding to damages wrought upon the muscle tissue by stretching.

Hyperflexibility

It is interesting to contemplate for a moment what the muscle-spindle situation might be in the hyperflexible body. Presumably, this type of body

Box 11.B-1: PNF—Contracting in Order to Lengthen

In some situations, as one works to extend a stretch, the muscle spindles may become over-stressed and signal instead for contraction of the muscle in question as a means of self-protection. In this situation, stretching can continue if the spindles can be momentarily convinced that the stretch has ended and so relax their grip on the muscle. This is the basic philosophy behind the proprioceptive neuromuscular facilitation (PNF) method of stretching [7, 618, 725]. Of course, PNF will be of no value if the stiffness is due to inelasticity in the muscle components rather than to highly excited muscle spindles.

By way of example of PNF stretching, stand with your back to the wall, and let your partner raise your straight right leg to the horizontal position, stretching the hamstring on that leg as in *hasta padangusthasana*. With your partner firmly holding the leg by the heel in this position, press the leg **down** isometrically by contracting the hamstrings and thereby releasing the tensile stress in the hamstring spindles (but increasing the tension in the Golgi tendon organs; Subsection 11.B, page 428). Wait thirty seconds in this position, with the leg elevated but the hamstrings contracted. With the spindle signals turned off by the apparent relaxation of the hamstrings, next have your partner quickly raise the relaxed leg to a new height, and engage the antagonist quadriceps muscles. It is known that after strong voluntary contraction, the resistance to stretching drops significantly; the resistance is minimal one second after the PNF release and is still 30 percent less than normal five seconds after release [471]. Repeat the hamstring release again at the new height, followed by renewed elevation, slowly ratcheting your way toward placing your shin on your forehead. Blood pressure does not rise appreciably during PNF stretching, as long as the stressful positions are not held for more than ten seconds at a time [160a]. The longer the contraction time, the greater the increase in flexibility. There is a certain obvious relationship between the PNF technique and the autogenic reflex (Subsection 11.B, page 439), but they also differ in significant ways.

When practicing PNF without a partner, take the stretch to a submaximal position, and then, holding that position, deliberately contract the muscle for thirty seconds rather than stretching it. With the spindles relaxed due to the contraction, quickly shift into stretching mode, and go deeper into the stretch. It must be pointed out that though the PNF technique is interesting and often effective, it is just stretching for stretching's sake and is not yoga. Furthermore, as explained in Subsection 11.E, page 462, simultaneous stretching and contraction of a muscle relieves stress on the belly of the muscle but transfers it to the tendons, which may tear or pull away from the bone in the process.

PNF is essentially a negative-stretch reflex. If a muscle is taut and the stretch reflex is active, then rapid release of the stretch tension results in inhibition of the stretch reflex for a short time. Thus, this negative-stretch reflex can inhibit shortening of the muscle in exactly the same way that the positive-stretch reflex can inhibit lengthening of the muscle [308].

has very extendable collagen; which is to say, a small stress yields a large displacement (strain). As the hyperflexible student stretches, there is a relatively large lengthening of the relevant muscle, yet there apparently is no inhibiting signal from the muscle spindles. It must be that hyperflexible practitioners can stretch so far without triggering the spindle warning signals because the highly flexible collagen of their extrafusal muscle fibers is also incorporated into the intrafusal spindle apparatus, so that it too is able to stretch abnormally without too large an increase in tension. This could result from the muscle components having a larger than normal amount of viscous matter in their viscoelastic makeup (see Subsection 11.E, page 462), with strain on the spindle being released by viscous flow. In any event, the intrafusal fibers of the muscle spindles must be at least as flexible as the extrafusal fibers, or the muscles would be in a constant spasm driven by the over-extended spindle fibers. Alternatively, the alarm points in the spindles may be set very high in these practitioners. In any event, the general feeling [490] is that the hyperflexible student is also hypermobile and can be easily injured by overstretching.

Resting Muscle Tone

In regard to resting muscle tone, this is a reflex action and so could as well appear in Section 11.D on reflex actions; also see the discussion on antigravity muscle tension in Subsection IV.D, page 857.

Neural Noise

As with all physical measuring systems, the nervous system is subject to certain levels of noise; i.e., not only sporadic bursts of brief but random electrical activity not associated with any specific sensation, but also steady levels of useless neural activity associated with stress in the body or mind. Given this unavoidable level of noise (like the static in a radio), meaningful neural signals, such as those from the proprioceptive sensors (Section 11.C, page 441), can be detected only if their amplitudes are significantly larger than the noise level. (However, see Subsections V.D, page 895, and 3.F, page 66, in regard to noise in systems operating with threshold requirements.) Neural static is important to *yogasana* practice, because the more we are able to reduce the level of the background noise in the nervous system, the more easily we can become attuned to the weak signals characteristic of subconscious inner awareness. In the same way, it would be difficult to sense the

effect of a lit candle in a room ablaze with bright lights, whereas in a dark room, the same candle becomes a beacon of light for the eyes.

One of the sources of the background noise in the nervous system arises from the ever-present tension in the muscles and the neural current that maintains this resting tension (tone) by energizing both the intrafusal and extrafusal components of the muscles (Subsection 11.B, page 434). The mechanism leading to a nonzero muscle tone is discussed below.

Source of Tone

When there is a source of mental or physical stress in the body, the sympathetic branch of the autonomic nervous system is activated, and one consequence (among many) is that there is a neural stimulation of the γ-motor systems within the body's skeletal muscles. External activation of the γ-motor neurons stimulates contraction of the intrafusal muscle fibers within the spindles and the consequent elongation of the intrafusal sensors, just as they are elongated when in a *yogasana* posture. However, simulated stretch of the muscle spindles by the γ-neural system then stimulates the myotatic stretch reflex (Subsection 11.D, page 450), which works to contract the extrafusal muscles that appear to be stretching too far or too fast. The end result is that the stress or anxiety, via the sympathetic nervous system, has promoted a tonic but global low-level **contraction** of the skeletal muscles, otherwise known as the "resting muscle tone." See also the discussion of the antigravity muscle tension in Subsection IV.D, page 856, and the relaxation of resting muscle tone by autogenic inhibition as discussed in Subsection 11.B, page 439.

Excessive resting-muscle tension tends to decrease one's proprioceptive sensitivity and raise one's blood pressure. Interestingly, when a person who is very stiff due to a high resting muscle tone is given general anesthesia, the result is a body of significantly higher flexibility. This implies that stiff people can achieve a lower level of muscle tone if they can relax their γ-motor excitation. Indeed, it is known that a contracted muscle is more difficult to stretch than is a relaxed muscle.

In any case, the larger the current in the γ system that one must contend with, the higher the tension in the muscles served by the γ-motor system and the more difficult it will be to consciously sense the proprioceptive signals buried within these spurious neural currents.

Contracture

Partial contraction as found in the resting muscle tone is called contracture. Chronic contracture shortens muscles, making them less supple, less strong, and less resilient to the shock and stress of various muscle movements. This leads to thick but excessively short muscles, as in figure 11.A-16**b**. Indeed, if a muscle were to be cut off from the bone, the central nervous system, and all surrounding structures, its resting length would be 10 percent longer than its *in situ* resting length [7]. It has been found that exercise is more effective than meditation in reducing muscular tension, in turn leading to longer resting-muscle lengths [7].

The resting muscle tone implies a certain muscle tension and with it, a certain stiffness due to the engagement of the cross bridges. This stiffness is increased by time at rest and decreased by movement. Thus it is that we have a strong "feel-good" sensation when we stretch or engage in various forms of physiotherapy, for this relieves us of the sense of tension and stiffness inherent in the contracture of the resting-muscle tone (see also the role of the endorphins in the feel-good process, Subsection 13.C, page 521).

Ischemia

Additionally, muscles that do not receive their proper circulation, as when the resting-state muscle tone is too high, suffer from ischemia. The cold feet that one often observes in extended inversions is a temporary form of ischemia, as is the situation when the upper arm is pressed against the upper leg in *maricyasana III*. Even the more modest muscle contraction that characterizes the normal, resting-state muscle tone works in a significant way to reduce circulation. This can be especially significant because resting-state muscle tone is a twenty-four-hour, seven-day-a-

week stress on the system, wasting considerable amounts of both oxygen and energy in an activity that produces no useful work. Remember: "The more a skill is practiced correctly, the better the athlete learns to use only the muscles involved in performing this particular skill. The athlete thereby reduces the amount of energy necessary to perform a given amount of work" [169]. This also applies to *yogasana* students and their associated resting muscle tone.

Sympathetic Nervous System

Inasmuch as a positive muscle tone is a consequence of sympathetic activation of the autonomic nervous system (Section 5.C, page 170), which in turn is subject to intervention by higher brain centers, through *yogasana* practice and stimulation of the parasympathetic nervous system, one can consciously influence the intrafusal spindle tension, even in the resting state, thereby lessening the muscle tone and achieving ever deeper levels of relaxation. That is to say, through *yogasana*, one can reduce stress in the body, even when it is part of a tonic reflex such as the resting-muscle tone; relaxing *yogasanas* that release mental anxiety thereby can make one looser in a muscular sense [157]. Working in this way can lead one from *yogasana* into higher-level meditative states. This is discussed more fully in Section 5.E, page 190, and Section 5.F, page 193. On the other hand, extreme stress can produce so much resting-muscle tension that the subtle signals from the kinesthetic and proprioceptive sensors so necessary for *yogasana* practice are swamped by the tension signals, and one has no hope of going to deeper levels of awareness [169]. Muscles that are habitually tense are energetically inefficient and so are often fatigued and even can be in pain.

Role of Emotions

Sarno [745] takes a somewhat different approach to excessive muscle tone. He feels that repressed emotions also result in muscle tension and that pain may follow from the ischemia in the regions of chronic tension. Most often the muscles so involved are the slow-twitch postural muscles of the back of the neck and the shoulders, the entire back (especially the lumbar), and the buttocks. The muscles that are responsible for posture eighteen hours a day become painfully tense when the body is tied in emotional knots and is starved for oxygen due to poor local circulation. Accordingly, Sarno claims the cure for this painful muscular condition is psychological rather than physiological. Of course, *yogasana* is both psychological and physiological (Section 5.F, page 193) and so is consistent with Sarno's ideas. Further experimental support for Sarno's theory of chronic lower-back pain is presented in Subsection 13.C, page 519.

The Golgi Tendon Organs

Structure

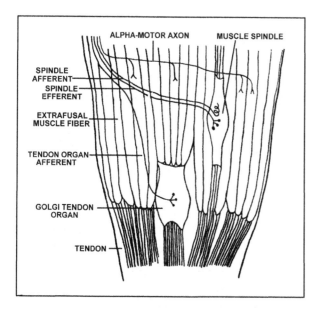

Figure 11.B-2. Situation of the Golgi tendon organ within the tendon of a muscle. Note the relative size and position of the Golgi tendon organ with respect to a muscle spindle, and note that the tendon organ has no neural efferent for readjustment of the tension on the organ.

A second type of mechanoreceptor, the Golgi tendon organ, is found as a capsule embedded in the collagenous tissue of the muscle tendon (figure 11.B-2), at a point very close to where the contractive tissue and the tendon meet. The Golgi organ's function is to monitor the tensile stress along the tendon of a contracting muscle, and the rate of change of the tensile stress. The Golgi organ also functions as a proprioceptive sensor and is a key element in reflexive muscle relaxation.

As shown in the figure, the Golgi tendon organs are situated in the muscle rather differently than are the muscle spindles, for the afferent neurons of these receptors are intimately intertwined with the braids of the surrounding tendon-fiber bundles. When the muscle contracts, the tendon-organ sensors are compressed by the intertwined and elongated tendons and so transmit a signal along a myelinated type Ib afferent having a frequency proportional to the tension in the muscle tendon. In the course of changing the tension of the tendon, the signal varies wildly but contains data that can be interpreted in regard to how rapidly the muscle is contracting. The tendon organ's information is processed in the brainstem in tandem with that from the stretch receptors within the muscle spindles, in order to coordinate complex reflex movements [360, 427].

The Golgi tendon organs are far more common in the tendons of extensor muscles than in the flexors, implying that the tensile stress is higher in the tendons of extensors than in the tendons of flexors. The primary beds of the Golgi tendon organs are in the vicinities of the talus joints of the ankles, the hip joints, the spine, and the atlanto-axoid joint between C1 and C2 [168]. There are between ten and fifteen muscle fibers driving the signal in a Golgi tendon organ.

Function

Just as one of the functions of the muscle spindle is to protect the muscle tissue from harm, one of those of the Golgi tendon organ is to protect the bones onto which such muscles are attached. That is to say, it is known that a muscle can contract with such force that its tendon is pulled from the bone, taking part of the bone with it. Remember now that when a muscle contracts, the tendon binding this muscle to the adjacent bone is being stretched. If the tension becomes too high, the Golgi tendon organ in the relevant muscle initiates a reflex arc that terminates with the muscle unit being relaxed and the antagonist muscle contracting instead. Activation of the Golgi organ then leads to a decreased pull of the muscle's tendon on the bone to which it is anchored.

The Golgi organs and the muscle spindles are alike in several ways and very different in others. Both receptors have alarm levels that are set by supraspinal feedback loops, both are readily reset by emotional factors, and both function as sensors in the proprioceptive system of the body. On the other hand, one receptor monitors muscle contraction, and the other monitors muscle elongation. Furthermore, one is adjustable in regard to its alarm level, and the other is not.

The tension on the tendon of an active muscle generally increases as the muscle attempts to move against a certain resistance, usually a weight being lifted against gravity; the heavier the weight, the larger the resistance and the larger the tension. Thus, for the heavier body moving from lying on the floor into *urdhva dhanurasana,* for example, there will be more tensile stress on the tendons of the triceps as the student lifts into the final position. If the lifting is too rapid (I admit this is unlikely) in a heavy student, the triceps may avoid pulling the humerus apart by relaxing on signal from the Golgi tendon organs within. In other *yogasanas,* the situation is more like one muscle working to overcome the resistance of another to stretching (for example, the action of the forward arm against the forward leg to turn the upper body in *parivrtta trikonasana).* In all of these situations, we must be aware of the fact that while certain muscles are being stretched and tend to react to this by contracting, other muscles in the body are being contracted and tend to react to this by relaxing.

Considering the protective actions of the muscle spindles in regard to stretching and the protective action of the Golgi organs in regard to contraction, it is a wonder that we can move at all! As Juhan points out [422], it is one of the fundamental jobs of the muscles' sensory system to resist any **sudden** change, using the muscles'

automatic reflexes. Fortunately for *yogasana* students, there are ways around these roadblocks (Subsection 11.E, page 461). It is important to point out that muscle health also is dependent upon the health of the ligaments, and there also are mechanoreceptors in the body that monitor the degree of tensile stress in the ligaments.

Autogenic Inhibition

The Golgi tendon organs also play a role in the development of the flexibility sought in *yogasana* practice. When we rapidly stretch a muscle, the muscle-spindle alarm is sounded, and there follows a reflexive contraction of the muscle being stretched; i.e., the myotatic stretch reflex. Even when at rest, there is a residual tone to all of the muscles, i.e., the resting muscle tone (Subsection 11.B, page 436). In this case, stress in the body has the effect of energizing the γ-neural system within the muscle spindles, and these then set the level of the resting tone by stimulating the corresponding α-motor neurons to activate low-level muscle contraction. If, on the other hand, the stretch is more moderate, so that the muscle spindles are not activated, and the stretch is held for about thirty seconds, then there is an inhibitory action of the relevant Golgi tendon organ on the intrafusal fibers of the muscle spindles, the effect on the α-motor fibers being to relax them. The inhibitory reflex action of the Golgi signal on the intrafusal fibers of the muscle spindles is known as autogenic inhibition [117], an action wholly within a single muscle, in distinction to reciprocal inhibition (Subsection 11.A, page 420) involving an agonist/antagonist pair of muscles. This little trick of releasing muscle tension nonetheless is closely related to that described as PNF in Box 11.B-1, page 435. The importance of autogenic inhibition to stretching in the *yogasanas* should be obvious to the reader.

Workers in the field quote the time interval necessary for the autogenic release of muscle tension as being from six to twenty seconds, and so thirty seconds is seen to be a conservative value. In essence, the tension on the Golgi tendon organ when stretching slowly inhibits the spindle alarm signal and so allows the sarcomeres and associated connective tissue to lengthen. In particular, a type Ib afferent neuron (table 3.B-3) within the Golgi tendon organ synapses with an interneuron in the spine, which in turn is inhibitory with respect to the α-motor neuron appropriate to that muscle. In this way, the Golgi signal hyperpolarizes the α-motor neuron, and relaxation follows. Yet another branch of the Golgi tendon organ afferent is sent to the cerebellum, where it participates in the formation of the proprioceptive map of the body.

Though autogenic and reciprocal inhibitions are distinctly different, achieving a full stretch in the *yogasanas* involves the simultaneous activation of both types of inhibition. Once a muscle has been relaxed by autogenic inhibition, it will tend to slowly contract again to its original length; however, the largest increase in length can be obtained by stretching it using autogenic inhibition once every four hours. The autogenic inhibition originating with the Golgi tendon organs is also effective in releasing the tension in those muscles that are synergists to the prime mover.

In addition to the position and motion sensors in the tendons, there are complementary mechanoreceptor sensors in the ligaments and joint capsules (see the discussion on Ruffini corpuscles below), which not only serve to monitor and limit the mechanical stresses at those places but also contribute to the proprioceptive sense.

The Ruffini Corpuscles

The Ruffini corpuscle consists of a spray of unmyelinated deformation sensors attached to neural branches, which in turn synapse to a parent myelinated sensory axon terminating in the spinal cord; the sensors are found both in the skin (figure 13.A-1) and within the joint capsules of the body. The Ruffini corpuscle resembles the Golgi tendon organ in structure but is only 20 percent as large.

In Joint Capsules

The spray endings of the Ruffini corpuscles within the joint capsules are three-dimensional and respond to the mechanical stress within the capsule, as when the joint angle is changed and therewith induces a deformation in the tissue of the joint capsule [708]. The afferent nerve serving the Ruffini corpuscle in the joint capsule transmits a series of electrical pulses to the spinal cord, having frequencies that are characteristic of the joint angle. Within a particular joint, there are several Ruffini corpuscles, each with a different angular range of sensitivity. In parallel with the high density of muscle spindles in the capitis muscles of the neck, there is also said to be a high density of joint-capsule sensors between C1 and C2 in the cervical spine.

Once the afferent Ruffini signal has been calibrated, the brain can easily and quickly deduce the relevant joint angle from the joint-capsule frequency. On moving from one joint angle to another, there is an exaggerated change of frequency, so that several seconds may be required before the joint-angle signal settles down to its new static value, even though the joint motion is over in less than one second. The transient excursion of the frequency of the joint-angle signal also is significant, for it too is analyzed and yields information to the brain on how rapidly the joint angle is changing. This latter type of information is useful as the information from which a feedforward response (Subsection V.F, page 917) will be initiated if the size of the angular change is to be restricted. The lower centers of the brain are able to continuously synthesize a global map of all of the joint angles and velocities representing the geometry of the body's skeleton in space.

In The Skin

The Ruffini corpuscles also respond to slow, steady stretching of the skin (Section 13.B, page 508). The Ruffini sensors are subcutaneous, residing in the dermis, below the epidermal layers. Though the Ruffini corpuscles are skin sensors, they are discussed in the Section on muscular mechanoreceptors because they are quite responsive to the contractions of the muscles lying below the skin. As muscle is extended or contracted, the overlying dermis is extended or contracted along with the muscle, and the length of the muscle is indirectly sensed by the degree of dermal stretching of the Ruffini corpuscles. Ruffini corpuscles are slowly adapting (Subsection 13.B, page 508) and have a large sensing field. Most interestingly, they can detect not only the degree of skin tension, but the direction of stretch as well. The stretching of the skin when a muscle is either flexed or in extension is also a source of resistance to movement and must be overcome in order to get a maximum response of the muscle action. The relation of the Ruffini corpuscles to the contraction of muscles underlying the skin is discussed further in Box 13.A-1, page 504.

The Ruffini corpuscles most likely are involved in Iyengar's sense of the "stretching of the skin" in the *yogasanas* [391]. It appears once again that Iyengar, through *yogasana,* has mastered the process of making conscious what is otherwise buried in the subconscious mind.

Section 11.C: Proprioception and Interoception

Proprioception

All sensations come into consciousness through our sense receptors and then elicit an emotional response. Thus, a painting sensed by the retina can be a visual delight, to use the ear to hear a song sung can be an auditory delight, to receive a massage can be a tactile delight, to eat a great meal can be a gustatory delight, and to feel a cool breeze on the skin on a hot day can be a thermosensory delight. Moreover, the more discriminating these senses become, the deeper is the delight that we can feel through them.

Question: Which sense is delighted when we do *yogasana?* Answer: The pleasure of doing *yogasana* must come from the appreciation of the kinesthetic and proprioceptive sensors in the body that monitor the limb positions, motions, and tensions within the muscles, joints, etc. These sensors also assess the recruitment needs of the muscles in a specific task and then call upon the appropriate number of motor units to perform

the task. Going a little deeper, we perform the *yogasanas* with very specific intentions as to alignment and elongation, and these kinesthetic and proprioceptive sensors are the measures of our actions. When these two factors, intention and action, are compared in the cerebellum (Subsection 4.B, page 73) and are found to be in strong accord, then the level of delight is high. As with the other senses, our delight of doing *yogasana* increases with increasing discrimination and sophistication in the practice. The pleasure felt during and after *yogasana* practice is discussed further in Section 13.C, page 522.

The fact that we can perform *yogasana* in total darkness strongly suggests that we do have some "sixth sense" that reports on the motions and positions of our body parts even though we cannot see them. This sixth sense, in fact, is the positional sense called proprioception, in which the muscle spindles and other mechanoreceptors (Section 11.B, page 428) combine with the central nervous system to form a subsystem capable of knowing not only where all of the body parts are at any time, but also of knowing the velocities and directions of their movements. This is the proprioceptive system; though the majority of the body's proprioceptors are in the head and neck [632], they extend from there to the soles of the feet as well.

The word "proprioception" comes from *proprius,* meaning "one's own," as in the word "proprietor." It is one's own muscles, tendons, and joints that contain the receptors necessary for receiving proprioceptive sensations [877]. Subconscious signals resembling those of the proprioceptors of the muscles, joints, etc., also originate in the internal organs of the body; however, they are concerned with the health of the organs rather than with their positions and velocities; these are termed "interoceptive" signals. The existence of the proprioceptive sense can be demonstrated readily, as described below in Box 11.C-1.

Though the mechanism behind the proprioceptive sense is not well understood, one can still gain an appreciation of its effect by sitting in *virasana* for a lengthy time, so that the nerves of the legs have become anoxic from lack of circulation,

Box 11.C-1: Confirming the Presence of the Proprioceptive Sixth Sense

One readily can assure oneself of the reality of the proprioceptive sense by the following simple experiments. First, with the eyes tightly closed, bring the right index fingertip to the nose. The finger will be guided unerringly to the nose by the proprioceptive sensors in the upper body, without input from any other sensory system. However, if the cerebellum is damaged, then this task cannot be accomplished, for one cannot coordinate muscle action with the proprioceptive sense in this case. Most interestingly, those with dyslexia are thought to have problems with sequencing actions in the cerebellum, and they often are unable to perform the finger-to-nose test with the eyes closed. However, their dyslexia can be overcome by practicing balancing *yogasanas* (Subsection 18.B, page 701). The same proprioceptive system is at work when we subconsciously bring our finger to the itching spot on the body in order to scratch it, which is fortunate, because we may not be able to locate the itching spot with our eyes.

Somewhat more challenging, but still possible, is to bring the tips of the left and right index fingers together in front of the face, again with the eyes closed. Next, try to repeat this with the hands held behind the back. Finally, with the hands behind the back, bring the index finger of the right hand far to the left, and then bring the tip of the index finger of the left hand to meet that of the right, using only the proprioceptive sense. Those who cannot succeed in these simple tests, even after practicing them, will have difficulty balancing proprioceptively in the *yogasanas* (Subsection V.C, page 886).

The series of proprioceptive tasks given above are a graded series of increasing difficulty, due to the fact that touching the finger to the nose is very closely related to bringing the hand to the nose as when blowing it or guiding the spoon into our mouths when we eat. Because we have practiced these actions since an early age, the proprioceptive sensors are well exercised, and the aim is unerring. On the other hand, touching finger to finger with the eyes closed is not something that we practice very often, and so the proprioceptive aim is not yet very well developed, and even less so when trying to do this behind the back and off to the side. These proprioceptive senses will be more or less active in the *yogasanas,* positioning the limbs or the pelvis even though they are out of our view, and the accuracy of their placement will increase with practice. Eventually, one subconsciously can sense proprioceptively when the position of the body is correct, as when lifting the leg just so as to be aligned with the thorax in *ikapada adho mukha svanasana* without being able to see it.

When we perform *virasana* with the fingers interlaced overhead (*parvatasana*), the feeling in the hands is very different than when the registration of the fingers is reversed in this posture; i.e., instead of beginning to interlace with the right index finger over the left, begin instead with the left over the right. With the fingers interlaced in the reversed registration, it feels as if we are holding someone else's hand, because we have trained the proprioceptive system to always interlace in one way (the "comfortable" way; Section 1.B, page 8), and so we get a very strange proprioceptive sensation when interlocked in a different way. With practice, this feeling of strangeness passes, and both grips come to feel equally comfortable. There is little question that holding the arms (or legs) out to the sides so as to form balancing poles (Subsection V.D, page 905) is of great value to balancing (try this in *vrksasana* or *virabhadrasana III*); perhaps this advantage comes from proprioceptive signals in the outstretched shoulders, which give one a clue as to imbalance in the position of the upper body.

and then noting how difficult it is to use the legs in a coordinated way on trying to stand up. In this case, we are trying to walk without proprioceptive feedback [450]. Those who lack a sense of proprioception, called autotopagnosia, often have suffered brain tumors or strokes, cannot distinguish left from right, and have few or no sensations of the placement of their limbs.

Such sensory information, as deduced by proprioception, is absolutely essential to the student performing *yogasana*, especially as regards balance, degree of muscle tension, and correctness of alignment. Unfortunately, there is not much agreement as to how proprioception works, for the proprioceptive sense has a very short history by comparison with the other senses, being discussed first only in the early 1900s. Moreover, there is no unanimity as to just which mechanoreceptors are active in proprioceptive sensing. My own taste in this is to include the muscle spindles and various joint and tendon sensors as functional in proprioception, but the pressure sensors (Section 13.B, page 506) are in a class by themselves, outside of proprioception.

Balancing

The neural conduction velocities and muscle reaction times conspire to make proprioceptive response times rather long, up to 100 milliseconds. Thus, when we perform rapid movements such as swinging a baseball bat, the trajectory of the limbs is ballistic, and there is no proprioceptive control of the limb involved until the event has passed [877]. A second path to higher centers, using swift Ia and Ib neural conductors (table 3.B-3), is found in humans and primates and does carry the information concerning precise localization of touch sensations, pressure, vibration, and proprioception. The fibers of this more modern system run uninterrupted along the length of the

spinal cord until they synapse in the medulla oblongata [432].

In many balancing situations, we use the vestibular apparatus in the inner ears for balance, trying to keep the head in an up-right, balanced position and then correcting the body position with respect to this reference plane. It is the proprioceptive muscle spindles and Golgi tendon organs in the muscles in the back of one's neck (spindles that are present in very high proportions in this area, as dense as in the hands and fingers; see table 11.B-1) that are responsible for this action. The strong implication of the muscle spindles and tendon organs in the back of the neck in balancing the vestibular system may be the connection between neck extension and dizziness and nausea often noted by beginners, in addition to the complication of the interference of the blood flow to the brain (Subsection 4.E, page 118). If so, then this problem, as a form of seasickness, possibly may be treated with Dramamine, which might distinguish between vestibular upset due to changing head position and cervical arterial blockage as the cause of the effect.

Static and Dynamic Proprioception

It is agreed that there are two general types of proprioceptive sense: that of static limb position and that of limb movement about joints, called kinesthesia [427, 432]. The proprioceptors for kinesthesia appear to be the slowly adapting muscle spindles and Golgi tendon organs (Section 11.B, page 438), whereas limb position is assessed from joint angles, as deduced in turn from the levels of muscle-spindle and Golgi tendon organ excitation. Experiments show that the accuracy of the proprioceptive signal is higher for limbs on the left side of the body, as appropriate for the superiority of the right cerebral hemisphere in handling proprioceptive, muscle memory, and kinesthetic information [470] (see Section 4.D, page 99). As the construction of a body map that is accurate in both space and time requires the simultaneous integration of information from many different sensors, the proprioceptive map is generated first in the right hemisphere of the brain, for it specializes in the parallel processing of sensory information [470, 635].

Because *yogasanas* are more static than dynamic, the kinesthetic mechanism of proprioception has less relevance for *yogasana* students, though it would be a factor in coming into and releasing from the *yogasanas*. Surprisingly, the joint-capsule sensors seem not to play a major role in sensing static limb position. However, they may be more important in signaling when at the extremes of limb position (as is often appropriate to *yogasana)* and also may signal pressure changes within the joint capsules. A contrary view has been put forth [432], in which it is postulated that proprioceptors are special organs and do not involve either muscle spindles or pressure sensors in the skin.

Innervation

Afferent fibers from the proprioceptors (type Ia, large-diameter, myelinated, and fast) are bundled with those for vibration sensing, fine touch, and pressure in the human nervous system [432]. As these proprioceptive fibers ascend the dorsal column of the spinal cord, they leave the bundle at different levels [432, 632], as described below.

Those afferent fibers of the proprioceptive system that synapse with efferent fibers at the same level in the spinal cord may serve as elements of reflex arcs (Section 11.D, page 448), such as the patellar knee jerk.

Other fibers travel via the anterior and posterior cerebrospinal tracts to synapse on the cortex of the cerebellum. This leads to more complex subconscious reflex acts, such as the shifting of posture to relieve muscular tension while sitting, but not falling off the chair in the process. A continuously updated proprioceptive body map is on file in the cerebellum.

Yet other mechanoreceptor afferents move upward via the medial lemniscus and synapse instead in the thalamus; their activation regis-

ters consciously as tension in specific areas of the body.

The highest level of proprioceptive awareness arises from those fibers that synapse at the thalamus and then ascend to the postcentral gyrus of the cerebral cortex. In the sensory cortex, the information supplied by the proprioceptors in the skin, bones, muscles, ligaments, and joints is synthesized into a body map of position and movement [270]. Stimulation at the level of the sensory cortex results in a clear, conscious sense of body position and movement, with strong reference to earlier experiences. When in this state, the mind is acutely aware of the physical orientations of the distant parts of the body and how they interact.

In addition to the proprioceptors mentioned above, two others are very important for sensing body position and rates of movement in space. Closely associated with the hearing apparatus and located within the inner ear are the balancing organs of the vestibular system (Section 18.B, page 696). The special sensitivities of the vestibular organs serve to sense the static and dynamic positions of the head and so contribute valuable information for the formation of the proprioceptive body map. The first of these vestibular organs works on the basis of gravitational attraction and the second on the basis of inertia, in each case using pressure-sensitive hairs within the organs as sensors of head position. As discussed further in Subsection V.C, page 886, the vestibular organs are critical to balancing, as are the visual sense and that of skin pressure.

Interoception

Internal Senses

Even more recent than the recognition of the proprioceptive sense is that of interoception [173], in which one constructs a mental representation of the **inner** states of glandular and visceral physiology, rather than of the outer states of the muscles and joints, as with proprioception.[11] This

---

11   The Eastern approach has long regarded as separate and distinguishable the *karmendriyas* (the organs

sense of the internal state of the body is accomplished by processing afferent signals from the inner organs involved with respiratory, gastrointestinal, and neuromuscular processes.

Particular interoceptive functions monitored by specific receptors include arterial blood pressure, central venous blood pressure, blood temperature in the head, blood oxygen content, cerebrospinal fluid pH, plasma osmotic pressure, glucose-concentration differences between artery and vein, extent of lung inflation, extent of urinary bladder stretch, and stomach fullness. With proper training, a deliberate mental focus on interoceptive signals can be used to control the level of autonomic excitation, whereas unbalanced disturbances in the interoceptive system can lead to problems such as anorexia and distorted body image. Interoceptive signals also contribute to the affective sense of pleasure in performing *yogasanas* (Subsection 13.C, page 522) [220].

Interoception also is an integral part of the process of homeostasis used to monitor internal physiological conditions within the body. The afferent system that provides a direct cortical "image" of the internal state of one's body also has connections to feelings of emotion, mood, motivation, and consciousness [173]. Though interoceptive signals are more diffuse, less well localized, and usually below the threshold of perception (figure 1.B-1), *yogasana* students having a sharp interoceptive sense are easily aware of their heartbeats (especially when in a quiet state, such as that of *savasana*), the need to urinate when inverted, the sense of hunger, etc. Sensations of pain and temperature also are parts of the interoceptive system. In accomplished *yogasana* masters such as B. K. S. Iyengar, it is the interoceptive system that allows them to sense the level of CSF within the spinal canal, the craniosacral pulse, the tension in

the skin and bones, etc., and so it becomes an important component of their conscious awareness.

Proprioception, Interoception, and *Yogasana*

Note how similar are the above physiological concepts of proprioception and interoception and the statements of B. K. S. Iyengar [391], whose impressions are derived not by Western scientific study, but by closely watching the internal and external response of his own body while perfecting the *yogasanas*:

As you work, you may experience discomfort because of the inaccuracy of your posture. Then you have to learn and digest it. You have to make an effort of understanding and observation: "Why am I getting pain at this moment? Why do I not get the pain at another moment or with another movement? What have I to do with this part of my body? What have I to do with that part? How can I get rid of the pain? Why am I feeling this pressure? Why is this side painful? How are the muscles behaving on this side and how are they behaving on the other side?"

You should go on analyzing and by analysis you will come to understand. Analysis in action is required in yoga. Consider again the example of pain after performing *paschimottanasana*. After finishing the pose you experience pain, but the muscles were sending messages while you were in the pose. How is it that you did not feel them? You have to see what messages come from the fibers, the muscles, the nerves and the skin of the body while you are doing the pose. Then you can learn. It is not good enough to experience today and analyze tomorrow. That way you have no chance.

Analysis and experimentation have to go together and at tomorrow's practice you have to think again, "Am I doing the old pose, or is there a new feeling? Can I

of action, such as the muscles and the organs of excretion), the *jnanendriyas* (the organs of external sensation, such as hearing, sight, and proprioception), and the *antarindriyas* (the organs of internal perception); it is the last of these that correlates with the Western concept of interoception.

extend this new feeling a little more? If I cannot extend it, what is missing?"

A similar point of view can be found in reference [632]: "The more developed and thorough our capacities for receiving and responding to sensory information, the more choices we have about movement coordinations and body functioning."

We see that the proprioceptive and interoceptive senses are bridges between the doing of the *yogasanas* and the awareness that comes from doing the *yogasanas*. Without the proprioceptive and interoceptive sensations, it is impossible to refine the *yogasanas*, and it is difficult, if not impossible, to take pleasure in going deeper into the postures.

Proprioception and Stretching

As we stretch in the *yogasanas*, the resting length of the muscle gets longer. Thus, after practice, the muscle tension in the spindles and other receptors must be less than before practice, meaning that the relationship between muscle tension and limb position must change as the muscle resting length changes. This recalibration of the muscle-tension versus geometric-position relationship is important in constructing the proprioceptive map and must happen subconsciously in order to accommodate yogic transformations.

Repetition of the *yogasanas* through dedicated practice results in a more facile transfer of the mechanoreceptor signals to the higher centers of the brain (Section 4.G, page 135), yielding, in turn, more conscious awareness of where the body parts have been placed in the *yogasana*, where the muscle tension is, where the skin is being stretched, whether or not we are in balance or falling, the internal states of the organs, compositions of the body fluids, etc.

Proprioceptive sensors are not the only tools we use to sense movement of the body; experiments show that we perceive a sense of movement and posture when the motor neurons that would activate such a movement are activated, even though there is no physical movement due to an external restraint [922].

One must be aware (and be amazed) by the propensity of the brain to synthesize a completely seamless picture in space and time even though the sensations at the moment that drive the sensation are incomplete. Thus, for example, our view of the world is not interrupted by occasional blinks, nor do we perceive a black spot representing that part of the visual field that falls on the optic nerve, for in each case, the brain "knows" how to handle the interruption and successfully smooths it over with interpolated information (Section 17.B, page 668). Perhaps there is such a smooth operation at work within the assembly of the proprioceptive map. Should a conflict ever arise between the picture assembled proprioceptively by the mechanoreceptors and that assembled by the visual system, it is the latter that is judged to be stronger and therefore more correct [352].

Section 11.D: Reflex Actions

Reflex actions involving the muscles are important, as they are always with us, sometimes working to our advantage and sometimes not. Such reflexes usually operate in the realm of the subconscious and can have profound effects on our bodies, within and beyond *yogasana* practice. However, through attentive *yogasana* practice, reflex actions eventually become amenable to conscious control from higher brain centers, just as our bodies are controlled by reflex actions as infants, and we then learn how to gain more conscious control of many of them as we mature.

Reflex versus Habit

We are born with our reflexes, though we may consciously overcome them through the agency of higher mental functions. Habits, on the other hand, have the outward appearance of being reflexive, but they are learned responses to situations rather than being inborn. It is said that a process can be learned after ten repetitions, but that one must repeat the process every day for three months in order to establish a habit; in neither case is it a reflex. Learned subconscious processes such as habits are understandable in terms of the actions of the neuromodulators (Subsection 3.D, page 59). Note too that when a *yogasana* expert performs, for the thousandth time, a one-arm handstand with immense skill and a highly conscious awareness of the actions necessary to maintain balance, the performance is too deliberate and conscious to be called a habit.

Phasic Reflex

General Definition

There are, in general, two types of muscular reflex. The first is a phasic reflex, in which a fast-twitch fiber is energized in a rapid, momentary action; e.g., step on a tack and withdraw the foot (figure 11.A-19). The second is a tonic reflex, in which certain slow-twitch postural muscles are activated by proprioceptors in order to establish a long-lasting postural balance (Subsection 11.A, page 414). In both cases, the muscular responses to the aggravating stimuli are largely subconscious ones, and in both cases, a simple neurological scheme can be put forth to "explain" the reflex. However, it is also clear that all of the simple neurological reflexes actually take place within a web of complexity, as all such neurons involved in reflexes are directly or indirectly connected to all others. Note too that there are neurological reflexes that involve the visual and auditory systems, for example (Subsection 17.B, page 668, and Subsection 18.A, page 690), and that are totally outside the muscular system.

A phasic reflex is a pre-programmed, hard-wired reaction in response to noxious or painful stimuli in the muscles, joints, or skin. A phasic reflex is at work when we jump on hearing a loud but unexpected noise. Being preprogrammed and hard-wired into the central nervous system, the possibility of a phasic reflex is with us at all times and, as will be shown, can have a profound effect on how we perform the *yogasanas*. There are five basic steps involved in a phasic reflex action:

1. A receptor receives a stimulus, which may be pain, pressure, chemical, thermal, acoustic, rate of stretch, etc. If the stimulus is strong enough,

2. An afferent fiber carries the stimulus signal directly to the spinal cord and indirectly to higher cerebral centers.

3. The reflex center in the central nervous system acts swiftly and appropriately on the stimulus signal.

4. Via one or more synapses, an efferent neuron is activated, and

5. An effector organ (skeletal muscle, visceral organ, etc.) is then energized. In general, a phasic reflex is rapid, brief, and involves an intense muscular contraction. A monosynaptic reflex is the fastest reflex known, having a delay of only one millisecond at the synapse. In contrast to this, a tonic reflex is long-lived and of a low muscular intensity.

By the criteria given above, the responses of the muscle spindles and the Golgi tendon organs to rapid muscle elongation and muscle contraction, respectively, (Section 11.B, page 428), qualify as phasic reflexes. Note too, that by these criteria, reflex reactions bypass the higher brain centers, having a trajectory from the sensor to the spinal column and back to the region of sensation. Only after the entire reflex arc has been traversed might an awareness of it appear in the consciousness.

Controlling Reflexes

The above description of the reflex arc is most relevant in the new-born infant, but on maturation, control of the reflexes by higher cerebral centers becomes more and more possible. Thus, for example, when the stretch receptors in the bladder signal fullness, the infant urinates reflexively, whereas the adult can delay the release for a more convenient time and place. With practice of the *yogasanas,* more and more of the purely reflexive actions of the body, phasic and tonic, come under the control of the more conscious centers of the brain.

Control Mechanism

The mechanism for bringing a reflex under control is straightforward. In general, an α-motor neuron may synapse simultaneously with several afferents, so that the overall signal at the neuron is an algebraic sum of the action potentials coming from the reflex stimulus, the inhibitory interneurons, and the descending fibers originating at the supraspinal centers. Other combinations also are possible, in which the descending fibers synapse with the interneuron and modulate its effect on the α-motor neuron, for example. Given connections of this sort, it is possible then to interrupt and redirect the reflex arc using conscious signals (willpower) from the higher centers, providing their action potentials are large enough to compete with those originating at the lower centers, and provided they can be activated quickly enough to compete with the more subconscious tendencies. Thus, if our finger is being burned by a candle, we reflexively move the finger without thinking what motion must be undertaken. However, as an act of willpower, one can consciously use the higher cerebral centers to keep the finger in the flame, in spite of how intense the pain becomes.

"Voluntary" Movements

Note that the ideas of "reflexive action" and "voluntary movement" are not mutually exclusive in practice, for there is a strong element of reflexive action even in a voluntary movement. Thus, deliberately moving into *trikonasana* with great awareness still involves considerable reflexive action, as many agonist/antagonist pairs adjust their muscle tones accordingly, but with little or no conscious control. As a corollary to the above, the line between "conscious" and "subconscious" also becomes blurred as we practice our *yogasanas* (figures 1.B-1 and 1.B-2). Moreover, the reflexive excitation of a muscle also may reflexively excite its synergist muscles. Thus, for example, reflexive excitation of the biceps-muscle efferents not only drives the biceps contraction but also can drive contraction of the brachialis muscle and its synergists.

The Myotatic Stretch Reflex

The Patellar Reflex

As its name implies, the "myotatic" stretch reflex involves a muscular stretch induced by a tactile stimulus and the phasic response to this stimulus. In the most famous example of the myotatic stretch reflex, the classical knee-jerk (patellar) reaction [801] (also known as the deep-tendon reflex), the reflex is excited by striking the patellar tendon of the knee with a rubber-tipped hammer just below the quadriceps in the relaxed bent leg (figure 11.D-1a). The impulsive blow acts to rapidly stretch the quadriceps muscle, and in response to the resultant shock wave, virtually all of the muscle spindles at the top of the knee

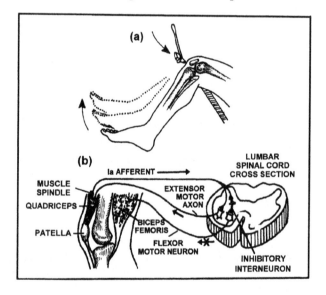

Figure 11.D-1. (a) The patellar tap that initiates the patellar (knee-jerk) reflex. (b) The Ia afferent axon from the dynamic nuclear-bag fiber of the muscle spindle within the quadriceps (rectus femoris) muscle is too rapidly stretched by the tendon tap. The neural signal from this muscle spindle enters the spinal cord via the dorsal-root ganglion in the lumbar region and separates into two branches, one of which synapses with the efferent quadriceps α-motor neuron and the other of which synapses with an inhibitory interneuron synapsing in turn with the efferent α-motor neuron leading to the biceps femoris (the hamstrings), the antagonist to the rectus femoris (figures 11.A-1, 11.A-2, and 11.A-3).

sense a stretch that is developing too rapidly and so send distress signals along afferent neurons terminating in the L3-L4 region in the lumbar spine. The neural alarm is sounded, because the stretching is occurring at such a rapid rate that if it were to continue at that rate, the muscle would be overstretched and possibly injured. To prevent this from happening, the afferent signal takes the quickest route and, using synapses in the region of the gray matter of the lumbar vertebrae, sends an efferent signal via an α-motor neuron to contract the quadriceps and straighten the leg (figure 11.D-1**b**). At the same time, relaxation of the hamstring muscles by reciprocal inhibition aids the straightening of the leg. The reflex does not occur if either the Ia afferent or the quadriceps α-motor neuron is severed [574], and it is minimal in those who are in a depressed mental state [626].

Simultaneous with the contraction of the quadriceps, a branch of the quadriceps afferent bundle also goes to the region of L5 in the spinal cord, where it synapses with an inhibitory interneuron, the purpose of which is to inhibit the contraction of the hamstrings (biceps femoris), which would otherwise tend to bend the leg and stretch the quadriceps even more. The net result of such a simultaneous excitation and inhibition is that the leg is immediately straightened without any resistance from the hamstrings and apparently without any input from the supraspinal centers. Similar stretch-reflex arcs are observed when rapidly extending the biceps tendon, the styloid process of the radius, the triceps tendon, and the Achilles tendon. A reflex similar to that of the patellar tendon also is observed for the hamstrings; if the student rests on his back with the leg partially bent and supported by the teacher's hand, then rapping the hamstring tendons at the back of the knee will result in the leg flexing further at the knee as it tries reflexively to lessen the tension on the tendons. The myotatic stretch reflex is stronger in the extensor muscles than in the flexors, because the extensors are on almost constant duty in regard to resisting the pull of gravity.

In the case of the knee-jerk reflex, it is observed that if the brain is injured so that inhibition does not take place from higher centers, then the reflex is clearly exaggerated. This is interpreted as showing that higher centers actually do contribute in an inhibitory way to reflex arcs normally thought to be localized in the spinal cord [621]. Indeed, it is known that there is a second reflex path that is slower and longer lasting, which sends the initial signal as high as the cerebellum and then down to the γ fibers of the muscle spindles [308]. The knee-jerk response should be essentially the same on both legs, and if it is significantly different, this is evidence of a neurological problem.

Muscle-Spindle Reflex

The myotatic stretch reflex in the above example is stimulated by an external factor (the hammer) that causes an unacceptable stretch to a particular muscle or tendon. There is no essential difference between this reflex arc and that precipitated in *supta virasana,* for example, where rapid stretching of the quadriceps muscle by virtue of the body position induces it to contract and the antagonist to relax. Thus, we see that the discussion of muscle-spindle action given in Subsection 11.B, page 432, in many ways is equivalent to the myotatic stretch reflex.

Because the myotatic stretch reflex is a primary means by which all muscles resist stretching, all efforts at elongation in the *yogasanas* must deal with this reflex. Being strongest in the extensor muscles and weakest in the flexors, the stretch reflex is of special importance in *yogasana* work focused on opening the body. Activation of the stretch reflex, thereby impeding the stretch, may incorrectly be attributed to a lack of strength in the *yogasana* student, but a lack of control over the muscle spindles may be closer to the truth. The yogic method for overcoming the myotatic reflex is discussed in Subsection 11.E, page 461.

Returning to the knee-jerk reflex for a moment, note that the reflexive jump of the lower leg does not occur when the hammer is pressed slowly but firmly into the patellar tendon. In this case, the muscle attached to the tendon is stretched so slowly that the relevant muscle spindles are able to re-set the muscle-spindle tension via the γ neurons (and autogenic inhibition of contraction), so that the overstretching alarm signal is never sounded (Section 11.B, page 433). This, then, is the secret to stretching in the *yogasanas* without resistance from either the muscle in question or its antagonist muscle:

Move slowly into the stretch, so that the Golgi tendon organs sense the stretch and act by autogenic inhibition to relax it, while the muscle-spindle sensors do not raise their alarms. In this way, the tension in the γ system is relaxed by autogenic inhibition, followed by the release of the tensile stress in the relevant muscle and its spindles without suffering a reflexive contraction. In this way, the muscle spindle's reflex arc is not triggered but the Golgi's arc remains active in relaxing both intrafusal and extrafusal muscle tension.

If the stretching is too rapid, as when stretching ballistically, the spindle alarm will be sounded and reflexive contraction rather than reflexive stretching will follow.

Though the above prescription will lead one to an increasing length of the stretched muscle, once the stretch is relaxed, the muscle will return to its original length because, up to this point, the muscle has been assumed to be purely an elastic structure with perfect memory of its resting state. In order to get a **permanent** increase in the resting length of a stretched muscle, one also has to introduce the concept of viscoelasticity, as in Subsection 11.E, page 464.

Emotional Factors

Yet another variety of myotatic reflex is driven by mental or emotional factors, rather than external or internal muscle stretching. For example, in the normal course of life, we experience a certain amount of unavoidable anxiety. Because activation of the γ-motor neurons by the sympathetic nervous system can be induced by emotions, anxiety can drive the sympathetic nervous system to stimulate increased γ-system discharge that leads to a general tightening of the muscles; i.e., a shortening of their resting lengths (Subsection 11.B, page 437). In this way, anxiety, acting reflexively through the sympathetic nervous system, really can make one feel "uptight." The nonzero tension

of the skeletal muscles in the body when at rest is a tonic reflex reaction rather than phasic, in that it is long-lived and of low intensity. In the *yogasana* postures, we work slowly so as to minimize the sympathetic excitation and thereby minimize the γ-excitation that leads to shorter, stiffer muscles.

The Flexional Tonic Reflex

The flexional tonic reflex is an especially interesting one, with many ramifications [164, 360]. In general, in this reflex, the limbs draw rapidly away from the noxious stimulus and in toward the body. As expressed in the full-body muscle tone, the tonic flexional reflex tends to fold the knees into the chest, heels to buttocks, forehead onto the knees, and arms around the shins, in this way protecting all the vulnerable places in the body from attack from the outside. This reflex, like all others, is spinal, not cerebral, so that even a brain-dead animal can show the flexional/withdrawal reflex.

When the flexional reflex is more local (lifting the bare foot off of a sharp stone, for example), there is an associated extensor reflex on the opposite side of the body in aid of keeping postural balance (figure 11.A-19). As seen in the figure, the reflex arc goes no higher than the relevant vertebrae in the spine and involves the interplay of the excitation of certain muscles and the inhibition of others. Note that in the myotatic reflex example given in the subsection above, the initial stimulus came from the muscle spindle and resulted in the leg being reflexively bent; whereas in the case of the flexional reflex described here, the stimulus is from a subcutaneous pain receptor in one leg, and the reflexive response is to bend that leg and straighten the other.

Born Flexional

The flexional reflex begins in utero, as the fetus assumes this shape in order to conform to the shape of its container. Babies born prematurely can more or less miss this phase of neurological development and, as adults, may show a tendency toward lumbar hyperextension (lordosis) in backbending and chronic lower-back pain as a consequence. The psychology and physiology of the fetal state can be regained in *karnapidasana* [235].

A person with a strong flexional reflex will have generally stronger muscle tone in the front body than in the back. In this case, it is easier to fold forward into a ball but more difficult to extend the front body, as in backbends. Consider too that spinal extension implies action in the back body, a mysterious and little-known region for the beginner.

Symptoms

Those who display the flexional reflex may have one or more of the following physiological symptoms [640]: incontinence and impotence, increased heart rate and cardiac output, internal organ dysfunction, lower-back pain, abdominal tension, anal contraction, rounded shoulders, hyperkyphosis (dowager's hump, figure 8.A-3**b**), or a pelvis with the pubic symphysis rotated forward (figure 9.B-4**b**). The assumption of the flexional reflex posture in adults may be the result of trauma, disease, or repetitive motions or the result of emotional states such as depression or fear [640]. Understandably, a student who has such a reflexive posture would work on those postures that open and stretch the muscles of the front body while strengthening the muscles of the back body.

Emotional Response

In keeping with the yogic union of body, mind, and spirit, the self-protective flexional reflex is also present more or less in response to grief, fear, emotional pain, and sadness [164]; when we experience these psychological states, the tendency is for the body to fold inward in an act of self-preservation and self-protection. Put in *yogasana* terms, the body prefers supported forward bending to backward bending when in these emotional situations. Since the bridge between spirit and body can be crossed in both directions, it is possible that not only do the emotions listed above inhibit backbending but that backbending can elicit the negative feelings associated with the flexional reflex. To open up

in backbends can be frightening, because one is then instinctively vulnerable in all of those soft places otherwise protected in the reflex: the face, the throat, the breasts for women, the abdomen, and the genitals. Moreover, to lean backward into a backbending position is to fall into a dark and scary place, going in a direction in which the eyes are of little use and into a place about which one knows little or nothing. No wonder that backbending can be so frightening and counter to the instinctive reflex. No wonder that forward bends cool the body and mind (soft parts protected and parasympathetic nervous system activated), whereas backbends are arousing and warming (soft parts unprotected and vulnerable, with the sympathetic nervous system activated as a defense against the unknown; see Box 11.D-1, page 453). From this, the meanings of the phrases "You've got me over a barrel" to express a vulnerable position or "I am bending over backward to help you" to express maximum effort, difficulty, and stress [487] are obvious! In *yogasana* practice, the goal eventually is to try to remain as cool in backbends as one is in forward bends (or even *savasana*).

For some students, the flexion reflex is so intense that even *savasana* might feel like a backbend! In this case, a relative level of relaxation can be experienced in *savasana* only by bending the knees, resting the hands on the abdomen, and slightly raising the back of the head [164]; i.e., by assuming a weakly flexional posture. It is interesting that in spastic paralysis of the lower extremities, the flexional reflex is hyperactive. In this case, passive flexion of the big toe drives the full-body flexion reflex even harder. In the *yogasanas*, we would seem to be working oppositely, often stressing dorsiflexion of the big toe in aid of opening the body, and so avoiding the flexional reflex.

In opposition to the tonic reflex of the flexional case discussed above, one has the situation shown in figure 9.B-4a, where the tightness is in the back body rather than in the front. In this case, the posture is associated with neck and back pain, sciatica, and headaches [640]. The tension here is such as to make the top of the pelvis roll forward, creating lordosis in the lumbar spine. Given muscle tension in the back body, the *yogasana* therapy will involve considerable forward bending to stretch the back body and to strengthen the front so as to bring the muscle tone in the front and back of the body into balance.

In Love with Backbends

What, then, of those *yogasana* students who love to do backbends from the very beginning? It could be that they also feel the same vulnerability, but being thrill seekers, they enjoy the threat rather than run from it. These are the same people who ride motorcycles, hang glide, do headstands on elevated surfaces, etc., claiming that the action makes them feel "more alive." Both dopamine and norepinephrine in the limbic regions are active in stimulating a sense of heightened awareness in regard to danger and are promoted in the excited states reached in the above activities. Because the sleep centers in the brainstem may react to the release of the dopamine and norepinephrine aroused by backbending and become so energized that they later interfere with having a restful night's sleep, it is wise to follow backbends with spinal twists in order to release any muscular or neurological tensions in the spine.

It also appears that backbending can be sexually stimulating; perhaps some students enjoy the sexual self-stimulation that backbends can provide (front body open, genitals pressed forward) or use it instead as a substitute for sex [438]. The arguments for why backbends might elicit the reactions that they do are discussed in Box 11.D-1 below.

A Reflection on the Cervical Flexion Reflex

As explained above, when the front body is put into the open, vulnerable position characteristic of backbends, the reflexive response is excitation of the sympathetic nervous system in anticipation of any threat that may appear while vulnerable and exposed. In all of the *yogasanas* that elicit the extensional response, the head is thrown back, and the eyes turn inward and upward toward the

eyebrows. The head posture that is counter to that associated with backbending is that in which the chest and forehead move toward one another so as to protect the vulnerable area of the throat [649]. In this position (*jalandhara bandha,* figure 11.D-2), the head is dropped forward, and the eyes look down to the heart. Once in the safe and protected position, what then is the tonic reflex response, if any?

Jalandhara Bandha

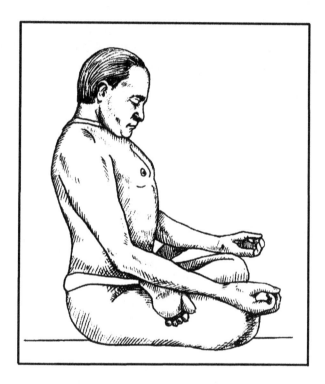

Figure 11.D-2. B. K. S. Iyengar sitting in *jalandhara bandha* [394].

Experience shows that postures done passively with the chin pulled into the sternal notch, as in *jalandhara bandha* (figure 11.D-2), with the eyes looking toward the heart, are calming and so probably excite the parasympathetic nervous system. Indeed, contraction of the inferior recti muscles of the eyes (figure 17.A-1**b**), which act to turn the eyes downward and outward, is driven by excitation of cranial-nerve III, a branch of the parasympathetic nervous system. As might have been expected, the eye's upward-and-inward action, as when backbending, strongly involves the superior recti muscles of the eyes, actions not

Box 11.D-1: Why Are Backbends Energizing?

From the Ayurvedic perspective, the center of our fear complexes rests at the core of the body, at the level of the solar plexus in front and at the level of the kidneys in back [449] (table 1.A-1). According to Kilmurray [449], fear and anxiety manifest themselves not only as muscular tension in the region of the solar plexus and kidneys but as tight breathing as well. Indeed, Ezraty points out the close connection between backbending and how critical it is to keep the breath free as opposed to holding the breath and thereby tightening the body and the mind [231].

As we attempt to open the region between the collar bones and the kidneys in *yogasanas* such as *urdhva dhanurasana* and its variations, we are forced to come face to face with our inner fears. When one is in a fearful state such as this, the breath, the organs, and the muscles of the body and mind contract. That is to say, the reflex reaction to such a situation is the flexional reflex described above. By what physiological or psychological mechanism does this come about?

Let us hypothesize that many beginners show what appears to be an innate fear of backbends (references [437, 449] among many others), that the rise in energy level is related to the release of the catecholamines into the bloodstream from the adrenal glands (Section 3.D, page 54), and that the immediate effects of backbends can be reversed by appropriate *yogasanas*. Let us discuss three possible mechanisms by which these backbending "facts" might come about.

1: Squeezing a Sponge

Perhaps the backbend action simply squeezes the adrenal glands on top of the kidneys to release the catecholamines. Without doubt, backbend action is certain to increase fluid circulation in the area of the kidneys, which will have a long-term benefit, but this is not the way endocrine glands themselves work in the short term. Endocrine glands are not wet sponges waiting to be wrung out by a squeezing action, but instead they are activated by either neural or hormonal signals (Chapter 6, page 207, and figure 5.E-1). On receiving such a neural or hormonal signal, the gland releases vesicles filled with hormones to the surface of the gland, and the hormones within the vesicles then are released into the extracellular fluid in much the same way as is the case for neurotransmitter release into the synapse [107] (figure 3.C-1).

Moreover, it is questionable as to whether the adrenal glands are really squeezed when in a backbend. When backbending, there is a rotation of the lumbar vertebrae, which compresses the spinal processes at the back of the vertebrae onto one another, whereas the more forward parts of the lumbar vertebrae are placed in tension rather than compression (figure 8.A-6b). Because the kidneys reside just forward of the portion of the vertebrae that are in tension, it is possible that they too are in tension rather than in compression. From this anatomic point of view, it seems more likely that the adrenal glands will be squeezed or compressed in forward bends rather than in backbends!

It is also relevant that in Iyengar's latest book on yoga therapy [398], in which the benefits of each of the therapeutic postures is listed, those for *urdhva dhanurasana* and *ustrasana* do not even mention the adrenal glands, whereas each lists an increased circulation of the blood in the lumbar region as a benefit.

2: Squeezing a Nerve

Perhaps the nerves that stimulate the release of the catecholamines from the adrenal glands on the kidneys are somehow activated by the compression in the kidney area. But the nerves in question are efferent nerves, and the general effect of compression on an efferent nerve is to weaken its signal or shut it off all together (Section 3.E, page 60, and Subsection II.B, page 835). Moreover, if mechanical pressure in the lower back were the determining factor, as in argument *1*, then spinal twisting would be expected to have the same energizing effect, whereas spinal twists are antidotal for the stimulating effects of backbending.

Furthermore, if backbending pressure on the adrenal glands can activate them, then in *sarvangasana,* the pressure on the thyroid gland should activate it as well. Because thyroid secretions promote increased metabolism, the heart rate should be raised and/or become irregular, and *sarvangasana* should increase body heat and accelerate the heart, whereas this posture is generally held to be cooling and globally relaxing [388]. The benefit of *sarvangasana* in regard to the thyroid likely is that it increases circulation to the area, but it does not necessarily initiate an immediate glandular secretion (Subsection 6.B, page 215). A similar statement should apply to *urdhva dhanurasana* and the lumbar area.

3: Fear and Flexion

If one accepts the catecholamines as being responsible for the energizing effects of backbends, then one is talking about stimulation of the sympathetic nervous system (Section 5.C, page 170). As noted in the discussion above, the sympathetic nervous system can be activated by the flexional reflex, which is essentially a fear reflex in which the more vulnerable parts of the body are shielded from attack from the outside by a full-body anterior flexion, whereas backbending places one in full-body anterior extension.

It seems more likely that the primary reason backbends are so stimulating is that there is a **psychological** fear of opening the front body, and in response to this, the sympathetic nervous system is activated, and epinephrine and norepinephrine flood the bloodstream. As with all sympathetic excitations, all of the standard consequences then follow; i.e., increased heart rate and respiration, redirection of the blood supply to the muscles, sweating, etc. (Section 5.C, page 173). That the characteristic physiological consequences of backbending are related to fear is supported by the fact that in many cases, the consequences appear even before the backbending is begun. Iyengar discusses this fear of backbending in a lecture given in 1990 [400]. In a recent paper, Shapiro and Cline [781] report that backbending is more energizing mentally than are standing postures or forward bends.

Leaving the Body

Yet another possible factor in backbending is that the position most often involves tipping the head and eyes up and back. However, the eyes-up position is a well-known one among hypnotherapists for promoting a dissociation in which the subject feels that he or she is leaving the body [507]. This may be a contributing factor to the element of fear among some students when in this type of *yogasana.*

Fighting Fear

With practice of the backbends, it is also true that the panic felt by many of us in *urdhva dhanurasana,* for example, can be considerably reduced by relaxing the muscles of the face and front body and by **consciously** relaxing the breath. This strongly implies a conscious control and reining in of the sympathetic nervous response and a corresponding heightening of the parasympathetic influence. With practice, the fear aspect decreases, and so the level of sympathetic response decreases as well. These ideas do not resonate well with scenarios *1* and *2* but they do agree with scenario *3*. Moreover, with practice, the fear and discomfort of backbending can be moderated, as learning and control by the more conscious centers of the brain gain dominance over the purely reflexive. Finally, with relaxation following the backbending practice, the parasympathetic system has a chance to exert its strength and so brings one back into hormonal and emotional balance in a matter of ten to twenty minutes, just the time it takes for the catecholamines to clear the body.

Backbending at the Sistine Chapel

Independent evidence for pain while backbending comes to us from one of the world's most famous backbenders, Michelangelo, who painted the Sistine Chapel standing on a scaffold while bending backward and looking upward [452]. In a comical sonnet, Michelangelo wrote (in part) in the early sixteenth century:

> I got myself a goiter from this strain
> As water gives the cats in Lombardy
> Or maybe it is in some other country,
> My belly's pushed by force beneath my chin
> My beard toward Heaven, I feel the back of my brain
> Upon my neck, I grow the breast of a Harpy;
> My brush, above my face continually,
> Makes a splendid floor by dripping down.
> My loins have penetrated to my paunch,
> My rump's a crupper, as a counterweight,
> and pointless the unseeing steps I go.
> In front of me my skin is being stretched
> While it folds up behind me and forms a knot,
> and I am bending like a Syrian bow.

Iyengar could have been of great help to Michelangelo and his lower-back pain, but for their separation in time and space by almost 500 years and 4,000 miles.

Supported Backbends

In view of the discussion above, it is interesting then to consider that in Lasater's book, *Relax and Renew: Restful Yoga for Stressful Times* [491], many of the relaxing, renewing, and restful postures are backbend variations! Though seemingly at odds with what has been said in this subsection, note two things about her suggestions. First, the backbending is very gentle, being only a lift of the thoracic chest. Second, the backbending is always **sup-**

ported. Thus, it must be that in this case, the phasic aspects of flexional reflex are minimized when the backbending is minimal, and the vertebrae are supported comfortably from below. If it were otherwise, relaxation would not follow. It would appear reasonable to assume here that the stimulation of the deep-pressure sensors in the skin and muscles of the back when supported in a backbending position (Subsection 13.B, page 511) in some way inhibits the triggering of the fearful flexional reflex. It is also relevant that in almost all of the upward-facing postures in Lasater's book, the head is supported so that the eyes are tipped downward toward the heart. As explained in the following subsection, this *jalandhara-bandha* position of the head and eyes is another posture promoting reflexive parasympathetic relaxation.

coordinated by the parasympathetic system. We might call the relaxation that comes with tipping the head forward and turning the eyes outward and downward the "cervical flexion reflex." Consider the following examples:

1. In *savasana*, if the head is tipped backward so that the chin is further from the floor than the brow, then there is a strong excitation of extraneous mental processes, which interfere with the relaxation. It is best to place a folded blanket under the head so as to adjust the head toward *jalandhara bandha* [394], thereby allowing the brain to relax.

2. Lifting the chest and hips somewhat with respect to the head, while the legs are up the wall, as in *viparita karani*, leads to both the relaxing effect of having the chin and chest in the *jalandhara bandha* position and the calming effects of the semi-inversion (head below heart, Subsection 14.F, page 590).

3. The *jalandhara bandha* action appears with increasing prominence in the passive, supported versions of *setu bandha sarvangasana, sarvangasana,* and *halasana*.

4. When the seated forward bends are done passively with head support, then the *jalandhara bandha* reflex stimulation of the parasympathetic system is reinforced by the ocular-vagal heart-slowing reflex action that follows when the weight of the

head rests on the forehead (Subsection 11.D, page 457).

5. To the list given above must be added the meditative seated postures in which full *jalandhara bandha* plays a large part (figure 11.D-2, for example).

In all of the examples quoted above, the parasympathetic system will express itself only if the conscious will does not enter the picture. Though the head and neck are in the *jalandhara-bandha* position in *ardha navasana,* for example, the posture is quite strenuous and so activates the sympathetic system much more than the parasympathetic.

Chin-Lock Physiology

According to Iyengar [394], the *jalandhara bandha* position is stimulating to several centers below the chin but the chin-lock aspect of the posture keeps the energy and pressure from rising into the head, where they might otherwise cause dizziness and tension. From the Western medical perspective, it is likely that when the chin is dropped into the sternal notch, there is a local pressurization of the baroreceptors in the carotid sinuses (Subsection 14.E, page 581), and the body's response to this is to regain homeostasis by lowering the heart rate and blood pressure. This chain of events makes *sarvangasana* a much more relaxing posture than is *sirsasana I,* though both are fully inverted; in this way, cervical flexion can be a welcome accessory to any posture otherwise intended to be relaxing.

The physiological effects of *jalandhara bandha* have been studied [286] when done with breath retention *(khumbaka)* and so are not relevant to a posture such as *sarvangasana.* Still, with *khumbaka,* no change in carotid pulse was observed. However, there was reported to be easy venous drainage through the neck whereas our argument assumes a blockage of the blood vessels in the neck when in this posture.

Yet a different aspect of the cervical flexion possibly involves the extraordinary number of muscle spindles in the capitis muscles in the back of the neck (table 11.B-1). When in the *jalandhara-bandha* position, these muscle spindles will be activated, and this may in some way induce a parasympathetic relaxation response.

Other Reflex Actions

Non-Muscular Reflex

The word "reflex" refers to a flexing of a muscle driven by neural signals that do not originate at the higher cortical centers. However, not all reflexive actions in the body involve muscles. See, for example, Subsection 17.B, page 669, where a purely visual "reflex" known as blindsight is described involving the eyes and certain visual centers in the brain. Auditory reflexes related to blindsight also are known (Subsection 18.A, page 691). In a similar way, hearing a particular sound or smelling a particular odor can trigger a reflexive fear response originating in the amygdala (Subsection 4.C, page 82), and decision making can be subconscious and reflexive as well as deliberate and conscious (Subsection 4.G, page 136).

Ocular-Vagal Heart Slowing

Cole [143] mentions a rather interesting and pertinent reflex: when pressure is applied to the forehead or the orbits of the eyes, a parasympathetic vagal heart-slowing reflex becomes operative. Thus, when infants and small children rub their eyes with the backs of their hands, the pressure applied to the rectus muscles of the eyes (Subsection 17.A, page 658) stimulates the vagus nerve to slow the heartbeat and thus prepare the

infant for sleep. In order to activate the ocular-vagal reflex in preparation for *yogasana* practice, set the head down on a solid surface so that the skin of the forehead is pulled toward the bridge of the nose rather than toward the hairline. It is likely that the ocular-vagal heart-slowing reflex and the cervical flexion reflex are closely related, as both involve a triggering of the relaxation response by increasing the blood pressure sensed by baroreceptors within the neck or about the orbits of the eyes.

The ocular-vagal reflexive slowing of the heart rate is of special usefulness in several *yogasanas,* as for example, in *sirsasana I:* if one rests with the forehead on the floor for a few minutes before inverting in this *yogasana,* the lower heart rate so induced will keep pressure from building up too rapidly behind the eyes. Many other *yogasanas* that are downward-facing, when performed in a passive way, are done with the weight of the head supported on the brow of the forehead [491]; presumably, the ocular-vagal heart-slowing reflex is at work in these postures. The reduced tension felt in child's pose *(garbhasana)* also may be attributed to this reflex. It is said that just the weight of the eye bag in *savasana* is an aid to relaxation, again due to the ocular-vagal reflex [143].

Approximately 90 percent of headaches are of the "tension" variety, and many of these involve an expansion of the arteries of the brain due to dilation of the arterial walls (Subsection 4.E, page 114). Often, the vasodilation can be released by placing weight on the forehead and/or the orbits of the eyes, either by letting them rest on a hard surface in a downward-facing posture *(adho mukha svanasana* with the head on a wooden block, for example) or resting a weight on these features, as with a wooden block balanced on the forehead and shading the eyes while in *savasana.* In either case, one is taking advantage of the ocular-vagal heart-slowing reflex in order to lower the blood pressure and so reduce arterial expansion (Subsection 14.D, page 579).

Tonic Neck Reflex

Yet another reflex of interest to the *yogasana* practitioner comes to the fore in postures that are left-right asymmetric. When the head is tipped to one side, the reflex reaction to this is to straighten the leg and arm on that side but to bend the arm and leg on the opposite side [427]. As such reflex actions are most apparent in beginner students, their tendency in *trikonasana*, for example, would be to drop the head toward the floor, and in doing so, the upward-pointing arm and the back leg would be encouraged to bend! Moreover, as the head drops toward the floor in *parsvakonasana* to the left, the tendency of this reflex would be to encourage straightening of the left leg and the bending of the right arm, whereas just the opposite is the goal. This reflex, known as the tonic neck reflex, is rather primitive and so may be more active in children and less so in adults. Higher centers will inhibit such reflexes in the more practiced student.

Foot Reflex

It is amazing to see how many reflexes there are that act on the foot to flex the big toe and spread the toes away from one another [863]. All of these can be found in the infant but are active in the adult only when there are neurological problems. How strange that we focus so strongly on this foot posture in our *yogasana* practice (Subsection 10.B, page 362)!

When we get out of bed in the morning and first place the soles of the feet on the floor, the foot broadens, the interosseus tissues (Subsection 10.B, page 361) are stretched, and a reflex action is triggered that acts to contract the quadriceps muscles, strengthening the legs so that we do not fall. The same reflex is active when lying on the floor in *supta padangusthasana* and helps to straighten both of the legs if the sole of the foot of the horizontal leg is pressed into the wall while the sole of the foot of the vertical leg is belted (Subsection 10.B, page 362).

Startle

When the body experiences a sudden, unexpected shock, there follows a phasic closing of the eyes, rapid increases of breathing and heart rates, a clenching of the fists, and a general tightening of hundreds of muscles from neck to stomach.

This startle reflex stands in strong contrast to the myotatic stretch reflex, as demonstrated by the patellar reflex (Subsection 11.D, page 448), for example, in which only the quadriceps muscle of the upper leg reacts to the stimulus. The global startle reflex is triggered whenever a person is exposed to an unexpected stimulus, as when struck from behind or upon hearing a loud noise. The stiffening of the body initiated by the startle reflex is thought to protect the softer parts of the body against any attack, and indeed, all of the consequences of the startle stimulus are in accord with the fight or flight reaction; i.e., excitation of the sympathetic branch of the autonomic nervous system (Subsection 5.C, page 170, and table 5.A-2). Auto drivers who are unprepared for an instantaneous rear-end collision experience the strongest startle reflex and are most likely to suffer from whiplash (Subsection 8.A, page 266) as compared with those who are able to sense beforehand that the collision is upon them. A more innocent example of the startle reflex can be observed when a student stands in *tadasana* and is pushed forward from behind.

Transverse Pressure

Contraction of a muscle acts to make the belly of the muscle thicker, and it will come as no surprise that if this thickening is resisted in some mechanical way, then the contraction responds by relaxing. Thus, in many situations, the application of sharp pressure in a direction perpendicular to the fibers of a muscle in contraction will act to release its tension [644]. This is most apparent in a posture such as *ardha baddha padma paschimottanasana*, where the shin of the bent leg presses crosswise on the belly of the quadriceps of the straight leg. In this case, it takes a great effort of the will to keep the quadriceps activated, as the reflexive response to this pressure is to release the contraction of the muscle being pressed. Using the pressure of a judiciously placed pole, this reflex action can be used to great advantage in releasing stubborn contractions in large muscles [644]. A similar effect is at work when we relax the brow by stroking it with the fingertips from side to side. Nonetheless, there are cautions that should be kept in mind in this type of relaxation.

Cautions

When working with a pole, one should be aware that if the pole is pressed perpendicular to the line of the muscle fibers at the belly of the muscle, the neuromuscular junctions are located on the midline of the muscle fibers and so are just beneath the pole. Consequently, the muscular relaxation that results from the pressure of the pole at this point may well be due to momentary strangulation of the α-motor neurons otherwise responsible for the contraction, with the effects on these neurons being at least ischemia, hypoxia, or both. This is a violation of *ahimsa*, a *yama* calling for nonviolence [388], especially when one considers that if an efferent neuron is injured and dies, the motor unit dies with it.

The sharp local pressure generated by pressing a pole into muscle tissue also endangers the vascular system, in that it can promote the formation of blood clots (Subsection II.B, page 838) if it is intense enough to injure the endothelial layers within the blood vessels. Thus, it is better to use a soft foam roller rather than a wooden stick, even if the stick is wrapped with a yoga mat. Should a tender spot be located using the soft foam roller, stay on the sensitive spot for twenty to thirty seconds, so as to give the Golgi tendon organ time to create an autogenic inhibition (Subsection 11.B, page 439) and so allow muscle tension to release [117].

Laughter

The effects of emotions on muscle tone and reflexes are well known. Thus, for example, when the tibial nerve is stimulated, there is a monosynaptic reflex lifting of the heel as the soleus muscle contracts; however, this reflex action disappears almost completely when the subject has been told a joke and is laughing [639]. This is related perhaps to the state of cataplexy, a sudden state of bilateral muscle weakness brought on by strong emotional feelings, as when laughing; of course, if the emotion is strong and negative, the cataplexy may result in fainting (see also Box 14.F-3, page 594).

Nasal Laterality

The results of a study aimed at the effects of asymmetric exercise on nasal obstruction are instructive and relevant to *yogasana* practice, inasmuch as such asymmetric obstruction is intimately related to autonomic balance (Section 15.E, page 629). In particular, the isometric exercise studied was a five-minute hand grip at 30 percent of maximum effort. This study [894] showed that such asymmetric exercise performed isometrically leads to nasal obstruction, and that both the afferent and the efferent branches of the reflex are side-specific (Section 15.E, page 629). When the isometric exercise was performed to one side, the nasal resistance increased in the nostril on that side while decreasing in the other. Switching hands for the exercise switched the resistance among the nostrils. In this context, see Sandra Anderson's article in regard to the subtle effects of nasal laterality on the *yogasanas* [11].

Smooth-Muscle Reflex

A muscular reflex occurs in a rather unexpected place. When the intestine is pressurized from within by filling it with food, the smooth muscles of the gastrointestinal tract reflexively begin to contract, so as to push the food mass from the oral toward the anal end of the intestine (Subsection 19.A, page 711). This action is observed in sections of gut that are totally severed from any connection to the central nervous system, showing that the gastrointestinal system has a self-contained nervous system of its own and can function without control from the central nervous system [268].

Yogasana and the Conscious Control of Reflex Action

Both the intrafusal and the extrafusal fibers within and surrounding the muscle spindles are contractile (Subsection 11.B, page 432), with subconscious activation by the γ-motor system adjusting the intrafusal spindle sensitivity, while conscious activation of the α-motor system contracts the extrafusal muscle fibers. This implies that

---

Box 11.D-2: Conscious Action Pays Off in *Yogasana*

Try this experiment put forth by Coulter [165]. After warming up, sit in *baddha kona-sana,* and then press down sharply and heavily on the knees, and release as quickly. Done in this way, the knees spring up reflexively, as the rate of stretch is just too great to allow the stretching to continue. If, instead, the knees are depressed slowly, deliberately, and consciously and then released, they stay down. In this case, the rate of stretch is both consciously controlled and acceptably slow, so that the reflexive contraction does not materialize.

The point here is that if the stretch is not done too rapidly, there will be a constant resetting of the spindle trigger point, which allows an on-going stretching without triggering a reflexive contraction. Thus, it is possible, through conscious action, to redirect or modulate reflex actions through the spindle response to stress (Subsection 11.D, page 459).

As another example of the impact of consciousness on stretching, the knee-jerk reflex appears only if the leg is relaxed and there is the conscious will to let the reflex happen. In a similar way, the reciprocal contraction/relaxation, activation/inhibition action between agonist/antagonist muscles that occurs reflexively can be augmented in the *yogasanas* by a willful action that will contract both muscles simultaneously (Subsection 11.A, page 422).

As mentioned in Box 11.A-2, page 401, the ability of a muscle to contract is least when it is at the limit of its range of motion. Thus, when fully into a *yogasana* posture, one can place the fully stretched but weakened muscle at risk of injury when asking it to contract in order to release from the posture. Especially when working with beginners, one should be conscious of the strain on stretched muscles when coming up from a stretched position, and so find ways to support and recover without further stress.

Performing the balancing *yogasanas* requires an especially sharp focusing of one's conscious awareness on what is needed to preserve balance (Subsection V.H, page 930). Finally, the most obvious control of the body's physiology by conscious control of the breath (Section 15.F, page 637) must be mentioned again.

γ-neuron activation can cause spindle length and tension to be set independently of the extrafusal length and tension in the muscle fibers. However, because there are several neural connections between the α and γ systems, interactions of the α (the conscious) and γ (the subconscious) systems is possible; i.e., the higher centers of consciousness can influence the sensitivity and response of the spindles. Since the α and γ systems do co-activate, the linkage between them is flexible and allows for independent α and γ excitation as well. As with the autonomic situation, higher centers can be brought into play, thus bringing the automatic reflex under more conscious control. As shown in

figure 11.A-7, if the muscle-spindle afferent goes as high as the thalamus, there are then many opportunities for conscious cortical influence on the efferent that finally reaches the spinal cord (see Box 11.D-2, above).

In the case of reflexive actions, the afferent signals go only as far as the spinal cord and then return via efferent motor fibers to the appropriate muscles (figure 11.D-1). Note, however, that the several inputs to the spinal cord from higher centers such as the cerebellum, basal ganglia, and brainstem extend all the way from the cerebral cortex. These centers can encourage, moderate, modulate, or inhibit the efferent signal originating in the spinal cord and so add an element of conscious choice to the muscle action.

At this point, it must be mentioned that some reflexes do go directly into the brain, where decisions are made as to what motor neurons are to be activated reflexively [432]. Thus, when falling, for example, the accelerations of the fall stimulate the vestibular organs (Section 18.B, page 696), and their afferent signals are sent directly to the cerebellum, where a plan of action is computed and the proper motor neurons are excited to preserve balance. All of this is done with a speed close to that of the knee-jerk reflex. Application of conscious action in *yogasana* practice is reviewed in Box 11.D-2 above.

Coulter [165] acknowledges the importance of conscious action in the *yogasanas* when he states that we "can read the record of past traumas in the rawness of our flexion reflexes. This is best done in the course of a regular hatha yoga practice carried out with an attitude of self-study and non-attachment. In this attitude, we can separate past from present and can re-program our nervous systems to meet our current needs rather than continue to live as though we were still in danger of being visited by ancient traumas."

Section 11.E: Microscopic Resistance to Muscle Stretching and Contraction

Relaxation

If there is no signal transmitted from the α-motor neurons to the muscle fibers of a motor unit, then the actin-myosin cross bridges remain disengaged, and the motor unit is relaxed. In this case, the actin-myosin myofilaments will readily slide past one another as the sarcomere is stretched. If, on the other hand, there is a significant muscle tone to the motor unit, this implies that the cross bridges are more or less engaged and that the toned muscle will show

significant resistance to sliding the actin-myosin myofilaments past one another. Thus, it is seen in this simple way that a relaxed muscle at the resting length will show less resistance to stretching than will a toned muscle at its resting length. When a relaxed muscle is contracted, the muscle fibers contract; however, a number of structural elements of the muscle will bear tensile stress on contraction. Thus, on contraction, the tensile stress in the axial direction rises in the tendons of the muscle and in the epimysium surrounding the belly of the muscle as it expands radially while contracting axially; however, there is no such stress in the titin and α-actinin within the sarcomeres.

Connective Tissue

As discussed above, a realistic picture of muscle must consider the endomysium connective tissue binding each muscle fiber to its neighbors. With this picture in mind, even in a relaxed muscle in which the cross bridges are disengaged, muscle stretching sooner or later runs up against the resistance of the connective tissue and possibly that of certain noncontractive proteins (Section 12.A, page 481). It is the nature of many intramuscular proteins and tissues that they are only slightly extendable; i.e., they can be strained only slightly (by only a few percent) before breaking. Given the make-up of relaxed muscle tissue as a composite of an easily stretched material inhibited by its wrapping of a largely inextensible material, how then can one practice the *yogasanas* and effect a permanent change in the structures of the relevant muscles? A possible answer to this important question is provided below.

When Stretching, Time Matters, and Time Is on Your Side

How have we come to regard time as our enemy? Why do we need to "kill time" or "hold back the tide of time" or "beat the best time" in everything we do? Whether we can answer this or not, it is still good to know that in the *yogasanas*, time is our friend and time spent soaking in the *yogasanas* is time well spent. In this subsection, we will consider the more useful aspects of time in regard to *yogasana* practice and how this can lead to longer muscles.

Viscoelasticity

The stretching of a "muscle" is readily seen to be a complex affair, for muscle is far more than the myofilaments on which we have been fixated for the previous 100 pages. It is the connective tissue between the muscle fibers and the noncontractive proteins within the sarcomeres that both limit the extent of stretch of a relaxed muscle and allow the muscle in its resting state to lengthen. Because mild stretching of the muscle and its associated connective tissues is essentially elastic and does not change the numbers of sarcomeres in the muscle, it will not lead to a permanently lengthened muscle unless there is either an actual lengthening of the muscle fiber through the addition of sarcomeres or an element of viscous compliance either within or external to the muscle fiber. The former option is discussed in Subsection 11.A, page 387, and the latter will be discussed here.

In fact, real muscle is viscoelastic, meaning that for short-term stretches, it behaves as an elastic band and, though it does not show any permanent lengthening once the stretch is released, when the stretch is extended in time, the noncontractive elements of the muscle flow in a viscous manner and this will result in a permanent positive change of length once the stretch is released. With the admission of a viscoelastic flow after a long-term holding of a *yogasana,* the muscle is no longer elastic in regard to the original length, and the muscle will be elongated for the long term. In this way, it is seen that spending a prolonged time in the *yogasanas* works both to disarm the muscle spindles and to allow viscous flow of the connective tissue to occur, again leading to a lengthened muscle in the long term.

A Model of Viscoelasticity

The viscoelastic character of a material can be thought of as a result of its being a mixture of solid and liquid components. For example, the liver is such a viscoelastic composite structure. If an area on the liver is slowly compressed, the water component simply moves to regions of lower pressure; however, if the same pressure is applied instantaneously, the water is not able to move quickly enough to reduce the strain, and the result will be the shattering of the organ, as if it were a rigid solid.

Though muscle is a complex mixture of different entities, each with its own mechanical properties, for ease of discussion, let us assume that each of the relevant elements of a muscle is either elastic or viscous, that elements of like property can be grouped together, and that the two types of element are in series in a muscle, as in figure 11.E-1. We can model a real muscle containing both elastic and viscous elements, as shown in figure 11.E-1a, wherein the viscous element is represented by a piston within a cylinder, with the piston filled with a viscous liquid (say, honey) and connected to the cylinder by a small hole. A spring is connected to the cylinder and represents the elastic element in our viscoelastic composite. When a load is applied to the end of the spring (figure 11.E-1b), the spring responds immediately and lengthens, while the viscous element shows no response. Were the load to be disconnected at this point, the spring, being elastic and having perfect memory, would quickly return to its original length. However, were the spring in figure 11.E-1a very stiff, then after a long time in the loaded state, the viscous element will have leaked honey from the inner to the outer cylinder, thereby lengthening the muscle (figure 11.E-1c). When the load is released in this case, there is no return to the original condition, as the viscous deformation has no memory whatsoever. When both the elastic and viscous elements are active simultaneously (figure 11.E-1d), there will be full recoil of the elastic part, but no recoil of the viscous part.

Thus, when a muscle is stretched ballistically, as when bouncing, it has an elastic resistance to stretching; whereas when the muscle is stretched slowly, the resistance to stretching changes to viscous compliance. In the latter case, the tissue fibers lengthen without returning to their original length because they are without biomechanical memory. Thus, if the stress on the muscle is held

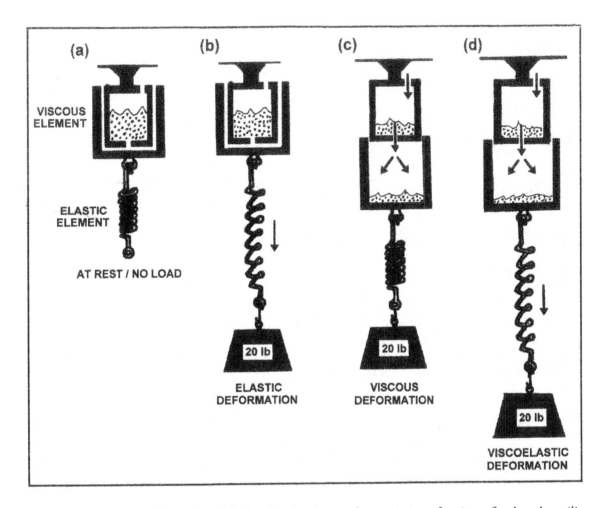

Figure 11.E-1. (**a**) A mechanical model of a viscoelastic muscle, consisting of a piston fixed to the ceiling and filled with a viscous fluid in series with a cylinder surrounding the piston and an elastic spring with no load. (**b**) A load is rapidly applied to the spring, and only the spring responds, by lengthening. (**c**) If the spring is very stiff, then after a long time, the viscous part of the structure will have responded to the load by lengthening, and on release of the load, there will little or no tendency to return to the original length, condition (**a**). (**d**) In the more realistic case of both elastic and viscous behavior simultaneously, in the short time under load, the spring will stretch and then return to its original length; whereas if under load for a long time, the elastic component will return to its original length when the load is removed, but the viscous response to the load results in a permanent lengthening.

for a sufficiently long time so as to allow viscous flow, then the change in length will be permanent; moreover, a relaxed muscle can change its length more easily than a tense muscle [871], as mentioned above. If a stretch is held for only a short time so that the there is no viscous flow, even in this case there will be benefits to circulation, neural patterning, etc., though there will be no permanent change in length.

In the case of muscles being stretched, our goal is to affect an overall lengthening of the muscle, with little or no return to the initial length; i.e., we want to stretch the muscle in a way that accentuates its viscous properties and minimizes its elastic properties. To this end, yogic stretching should be done in a slow way and the final position maintained for a reasonably long time, so that the viscous elements within the muscle have every opportunity to reach their maximal length. On releasing from this stretch, the muscle will have a longer resting length. The effects of stretching on muscle and tendons are discussed quantitatively below (Subsection 11.E, page 462).

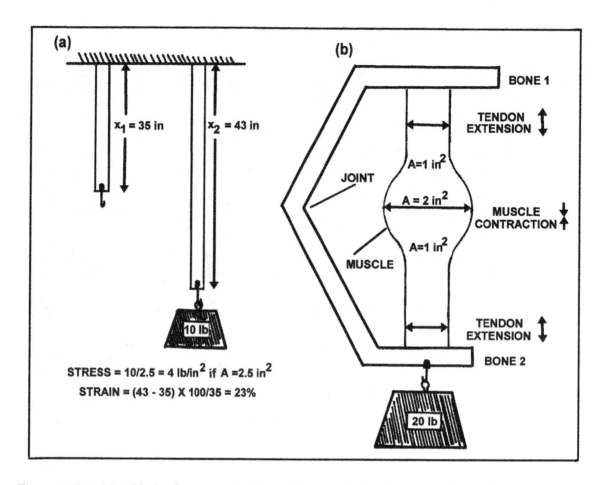

Figure 11.E-2. (**a**) A block of cross-sectional area 2.5 square inches increases its length from 35 inches to 43 inches when a 10-pound weight is hung from it. The stress on the sample is 4 pounds per square inch, and the strain is 23 percent. (**b**) An idealized muscle with a cross-sectional area of two square inches at the belly and one square inch at the tendons is stretched by a 20-pound weight. The muscle lies between two bones joined at the point labeled "JOINT." Though the muscle is stretched by the 20-pound weight it is also contracting isometrically.

Stress and Strain in an Elastic Material

The concepts of physical stress and physical strain are relevant to a discussion of muscles, but in general, these concepts are often either confused with one another or are thought to be synonymous. Let us look at the situation first from a purely didactic point of view, and then consider the case of stress and strain in a real muscle.

In figure 11.E-2**a**, a block of material of length X_1 inches and cross-sectional area A square inches is left to hang under its own weight. When a 10-pound weight is then hung from the block, it is stretched elastically to length X_2 inches. In this situation, the material is under a stress defined as 10/A (pounds per square inch). For concreteness, let the area of the block be 2.5 square inches, so that the stress then is 10/2.5 = 4 pounds per square inch. Because $(X_2 - X_1)$ is positive in this example, the two ends move away from one another; i.e., the stress is a tensile stress. Were the ends to move toward one another, then the stress would be a compressive stress. In response to the 4-pound-per-square-inch tensile stress, assume the length increases from 35 inches to 43 inches. The strain is then defined as the percentage increase in length due to the stress; i.e., (43–35) x 100/35 = 23 percent. Thus, it is seen that though stress causes strain, they are very different quantities. Furthermore, were the material under discussion here viscoelastic, then the concepts of stress and strain would be time-dependent and therefore beyond this simple discussion.

The tensile strength of a material is defined as the smallest tensile strain that is sufficient to break the material. For most tendons, the material in question is essentially collagen, which breaks when the strain typically reaches 4–8 percent [6]. However, this figure is variable, for tendons may contain more or less of the material elastin (Subsection 12.A, page 484), which has a strong positive effect on the tendon's strain. For example, the ligamentum nuchae that spans the cervical vertebrae in the neck can be strained by up to 200 percent, as when in *sarvangasana*, due to its high elastin content.

Consider now an even more realistic model of muscle, figure 11.E-2**b**. In this case, the two tendons of the muscle in the resting state are attached to the two bones forming the joint and have cross sections of A = 1 square inch, whereas the cross section at the belly of the muscle is A = 2 square inches. As a source of stress, we pull on one of the bones with a weight of 20 pounds as we try to stretch the muscle isometrically. At this point, the weight on the muscle and on the tendons is 20 pounds, but the stress on the muscle is 10 pounds per square inch, and that on the tendons is 20 pounds per square inch. The stress is much higher in the tendons than in the belly of the muscle because of the smaller cross-sectional area of tendon versus muscle (see figure 11.A-4**b**, for example).

It is often said by *yogasana* teachers that in an ideal stretch of a muscle, the "strain" is localized in the belly of the muscle, and little or none appears in the tendons. This would appear to be a situation over which we have no control, for both the muscle and the tendons experience the 20-pound tug of the external weight, and the stress each experiences (as pounds per square inch) depends upon their cross-sectional areas, which are beyond our control.[12]

Though we often think of "a muscle" as contracting when active, only the belly of the muscle contracts, whereas the tendons of the muscle are being pulled longer as the belly shortens! It is this pull of the tendons on the bones that not only helps build bone density (Subsection 7.G, page 254) but puts us at risk for tendon or bone damage. This is shown quantitatively using the model in figure 11.E-2**b**.

If the muscle in figure 11.E-2**b** contracts isotonically in the concentric manner, the tensile stress on the belly of the muscle would appear to drop below ten pounds per square inch as the myofilaments of the muscle overlap more strongly and the cross section at the belly appears to increase (figure 11.A-10). This increase in cross section of the contracted muscle is due to the pumping of fluid from the actin channels into the extracellular space, and because this trapped fluid can support weight in the extracellular space, it makes a nonzero contribution to the effective cross section of the belly of the muscle. The distribution of stress on a muscle in the resting state is determined by the cross sectional areas of the different parts of the muscle; contraction alters this distribution even though the contracted muscle may not appear to have changed its diameter.

In the case of a muscle being eccentrically contracted, i.e., a muscle being contracted while it is in the act of being stretched, the two forces of contraction and stretching work together to put the tendons under tremendous stress, perhaps exceeding the tensile strength of either the tendons or the bones to which they are attached. Should a tendon be torn by such an action, it can be very slow to heal due to the poor vascularization of such tissue, and it may require surgical repair.

---

12   The situation described here in regard to purposely changing the ratio of the load borne by the muscle and its tendon while both are under identical tensile stress is exactly like that discussed in Subsection

IV.B, page 854, in which one tries to isolate the effect of gravity on the body by pressing the feet harder into the floor. That is to say, you cannot press your feet into the floor while standing on it in *tadasana*, nor can you hold a twenty-pound sandbag in one hand and change the proportion of the weight on the biceps muscle and on its tendons, regardless of instructions to the contrary.

Even if a muscle and its tendons are only slightly toned, if they are stretched too rapidly, as in a reflex motion, then the tendon may tear before the spindle's reflex arc is active, just because the tendon has a relatively small cross-sectional area with which to bear the stress generated by the contraction. However, if the stretching is carried out slowly, so that the muscle spindles can reset their alarms, thereby allowing time for viscous flow, then the muscle can be lengthened without putting undue stress on the tendons. Said differently, we stretch slowly and without bouncing so as to reduce the stress of the tensile stretch on the tendons.

Each spike of the activating voltage for a muscle will excite it, and then the muscle will relax. If the frequency of the excitation is low (below 15 hertz), then the excitation will be a jerky on-off affair; but if it is sufficiently high (50 hertz or more), then the contractive pulses meld into a smooth, sustained contraction called tetany. When at tetany, a muscle can generate a tension of about fifty pounds per square inch at the resting length, meaning that in a quadriceps with a cross section of sixteen square inches, the patellar tendon can experience a load of 800 pounds (364 kilograms), thus showing all too clearly why and how the tendons can be pulled away from the bone.

Though there is no quantitative meaning to stress and strain in the emotional or mental spheres, the terms stress and strain still can be used. There are stressors in our lives that place us under stress (job, relationships, money, time, etc.), and if these stresses change our mental or physical states, then the changes are the strains under which we work and live. They are the true cost of living.

Muscle-Fiber Interconversion

When we take our time in stretching the muscles, moving slowly and staying longer, the fast-twitch fibers are transformed into slow-twitch fibers (Subsection 11.A, page 419), with the result that our internal clock is slowed. Once in the *yogasana* habit, we have no need to rush impetuously nor do we have the feeling of having

to move for no reason. When done in this way and coordinated with the breath, the *yogasanas* thus form a natural bridge to the more meditative aspects of *yoga* practice.

Bouncing

In contrast to the situation where one stretches slowly, rapidly moving in and out of position (as when bouncing) in the stretch will generate warmth as the muscles contract and relax repeatedly, but the only thing being stretched will be the elastic elements of the muscle, and these, by definition, return to their original lengths once the exercise is finished. When bouncing, the stress does not last long enough for the viscous component to contribute to a permanent deformation, and the impact of rapid motion will trigger the muscle spindles, which then throw the muscle into contraction rather than extension. The heat generated by bouncing can warm the muscle and increase its extendibility, but this will disappear once the muscle cools unless the warming/bouncing is followed by autogenic inhibition. Note that Kurz [471] presents an opposite opinion in regard to the flexibility advantages of ballistic stretching.

Physical Stretching Can Lead to Mental Stretching

Our willingness at the mental level to go into uncomfortable places on the physical plane eases the discomfort, allowing us to go more willingly into other uncomfortable places, whether physical or otherwise. If we can profit and learn from the initial discomfort of beginner's *yogasana* practice, we may be able to extrapolate to uncomfortable positions in the social, emotional, and spiritual spaces of our lives, believing that there too, something interesting can be learned about ourselves if we will bear the discomfort and seek its source within ourselves. Tias Little has expressed this concept beautifully in terms of *yogasana* practice releasing fixations that bind us with self-absorption and fear, which ultimately are paralyzing or crippling [518].

As we learn to broaden our bodies, we learn

to broaden our minds as well. At the same time, stretching physically calms and strengthens the nervous system and in doing so, makes us less likely to react impetuously to unexpected events. Thus, for example, *halasana* not only defuses anger in the present, but doing *halasana* now will make anger a less likely response to unexpected events in the future [724].

Complementing these effects of the body on the emotions, there are similar effects of the emotions on the body. Thus, for example, when the mind is occupied with thoughts that are sad and depressing, the muscle strength at that time is lessened, whereas if the thoughts are switched from sadness to joyous and positive, the muscles are strengthened again [649]. See Box 17.E-1, page 684, for a demonstration on this point. One can assume from this that if *yogasana* students are met at the door with a few happy words from their teacher, they may be put into a mood more conducive to working their *yogasanas* with energy, purpose, and strength. The emotional component of stretching is implied in B. K. S. Iyengar's comment, "selfishness means rigidity; selflessness means pliability" [389].

Warming Up

Certain aspects of *yogasana* practice more or less conform to the normal understanding of exercise physiology, and this is especially true in regard to warming up in order to avoid injury. Peterson [655] lists ten good reasons for fast-twitch athletes to warm up before more vigorous exercise, and these will apply more or less to the slow-twitch *yogasana* student as well.

1. To increase the decomposition of oxyhemoglobin, the oxygen-carrying molecule in the blood. When oxyhemoglobin decomposes, the oxygen set free is more available to the exercising muscle.

2. To increase the body's temperature without becoming fatigued, and to reduce the risks for injuries to the otherwise cold skeletal muscles and connective tissue; an intense stretch while the body is cold read-

ily can lead to injury. If we stress joints and muscles that are cold because there is little or no flow of warm blood through them, then small-muscle tears and muscle spasms will be the result. When cold, one must begin a *yogasana* practice with light work, so as not to excessively load the muscles while they are in a state of minimal circulation; i.e., work the large muscle groups, but with low ranges of motion. In this way, agonist muscles will be prepared for work, and their antagonists will relax more completely. Similar thinking applies to working the *yogasanas* just after arising from bed, at which time the muscles are relatively inactive. The benefits of warming up will fade to zero after forty-five minutes of a cool-down.

3. To increase blood flow to the muscles to be exercised, thereby bringing glucose and fatty acids where they are needed for exercise. The elasticities of muscle, tendon, and ligament depend upon the muscle's level of blood saturation; cold muscles have a low blood saturation level.

4. To increase the flow of blood to the heart, thus reducing the risks of exercise-induced cardiac abnormalities.

5. To decrease the viscosity of the synovial fluid in the joints and the muscles, thereby making their actions more efficient and powerful. Without the warmth of flowing blood, the elasticity of the connective tissue will be inhibited. Warming up shifts the tension from the muscle attachments to the belly of the muscle and also increases the ease of muscle-fiber recruitment.

6. To promote early sweating, so as to cool the body before heavier exercise.

7. To increase the speed of nerve impulses, so that neuromuscular patterns are activated.

8. To increase the blood saturation of the muscles, thus making them warmer and more elastic for stretching.

9. To increase the supply of oxygen to the muscles, thereby bringing the cardiovas-

cular system up to speed for the tasks that lie ahead.

10. To ease into more strenuous work, so that muscle soreness is minimized.

All of the ten points above are reasonable factors for the *yogasana* student to consider when ready to begin the daily practice, however, to the ten points listed above, one should add

11. To increase lubrication of the joints prior to moving them to the limits of their ranges of motion, and

12. To enhance the activity of muscle enzymes.

These twelve points are most effectively taken advantage of by the *yogasana* student when he or she moves from side to side (for example, *trikonasana*-to-the-right, *trikonasana*-to-the-left, *trikonasana* to-the-right, etc., with only slight pauses "in the position" [644]) or moves between postures, as in *surya namaskar*, with slowly increasing speed.

There is also possible a neurological warm-up, which is practiced by performance athletes. If the actions to be used in the competition are rehearsed in the imagination while sitting passively, the result is a warm-up of the neurological system that will be used later to activate the muscles implicated in the actual event. This warming up of the neurological system beforehand allows one to perform optimally the first time one is called upon to do so (Subsection 4.G, page 141).

Surya Namaskar

Douillard [211] has presented a list of long-term and short-term benefits to be derived from the practice of *surya namaskar* as either a warm-up or a regular part of *yogasana* work. It deeply massages internal organs; takes the spine through its full range of motion, if spinal flexion and twists are added [275]; breaks adhesions in the rib cage that inhibit deep breathing; coordinates movement and breath to send *prana* to every cell; increases strength, flexibility, and endurance of every major muscle group; reproduces PNF natu-

rally (Box 11.B-1, page 435); and improves one's circulation, energy, and vitality.

Body Temperature

It is best to warm up the muscles before engaging in a *yogasana* practice, as this will increase the temperature of the tissues and increase the blood flow while lowering the viscosity of the extracellular fluids. Attempting a difficult *yogasana* without proper warm-up, while the relevant muscles are cold and immobile, will result in unnecessary microtears of the tissues.

It has been found that artificially raising the temperature of a muscle increases its power significantly, by 8–10 percent per degree centigrade. This is superior to traditional warm-up of the sort described above for fast-twitch athletes, because the muscles are warmed without the expenditure of any energy or risk of fatigue; perhaps this is more relevant to fast-twitch, high-power athletes than to slow-twitch postural athletes, as found in *yogasana* practice [696]. Muscles can be warmed while passive by irradiating them with a short-wave diathermy unit [212], with ultrasound, or by the application of a moist-heat pack [257]; in each case, significant increases of stretching flexibility of either the hamstrings or the plantar flexors were reported following such heating.

Section 11.F: Macroscopic Resistance in Support of Muscle Stretching

Rationale

Consider a limp, wrinkled yoga belt, one end of which is held in the right hand and the other in the left hand. If the end of the belt in the right hand is pulled to the right but the other end of the belt and the left hand simply follow the movement to the right, then the result is a motion of the belt to the right, but no change of belt dimension or tension. In contrast, if the right hand gripping the belt moves to the right but this is resisted by the left hand gripping the opposite end of the belt and moving to the left, then these two seemingly contradictory but simultaneous left-and-right actions result in maximum elongation and straightening of the belt. This discussion applies not only to a wrinkled belt, but also to the active stretching of the muscles in all of the *yogasanas*, where some part of the body functions as an anchor against which some muscles contract in order to stretch or twist yet other muscles that are relaxed.

Simply put, for every *yogasana* in which some muscle is to be stretched in the x direction, one end of the muscle must be moved in the +x direction while the opposite end of the muscle must be moved in the -x direction; in this way, the muscle is stretched maximally along the x line. For every *yogasana* in which a body part is rotated in a clockwise direction, another body part must resist by rotating in the counterclockwise direction around the same axis in order to maximize the rotation. (Note, however, the risks involved in this disrotatory action, Subsection 8.B, page 298.) Activation of the multiple resistances within a *yogasana* will maximize the degrees of stretching and/or rotation attained in the posture. However, be aware of the risks for beginner students in going too deeply into the postures.

The resistance necessary for stretching is not always found within the body, for sometimes it is the action of the foot against the floor, as when balancing (Subsection V.B, page 878), or a hand against the wall, as when twisting. The resistance to a yogic movement or action may be internal (bone on bone, bone on muscle, muscle on muscle) or external (body parts on floor, wall, chair, pole, partner, etc.). Nonetheless, there will always be some resistance, an internal or external anchor, against which one can work in order to increase the depth of the posture. What is here called "macroscopic resistance in support of muscle stretching" is called "internal traction" by Williams et al. [897, 897a]. There also is an obvious close relation between finding an internal resistance against which to work and the practice of co-contraction (Subsection 11.A, page 422).

Note that the macroscopic resistance of interest here is between the action of one muscle against another, or between one muscle and a bone, and is different from that occurring within a muscle, where the stretching of the muscle fibers is resisted by that of the muscle fascia in the same muscle (Subsection 12.B, page 486).

Yogasana Examples

In the following examples, the instructions are minimal, because I feel that the principles of the resisting action are easily sensed if one just keeps one's awareness open, sharp, and on the lesson. With your years of experience in doing these postures, you will find many pairs of resisting motions in each of the postures given below, which can be of use to your beginning students as they work to open the postures. I recommend that you prepare a class for your beginning students based on this simple idea and see how generally useful and effective the use of macroscopic resistance can be. See Subsection 7.A, page 232, for several examples of the resistance principle in action. In addition, consider the following.

Tadasana: (a) Rotate the front thighs medially, and press the front of the thighs toward the back of the thighs, making the lumbar spine lordotic (figure 9.B-4**a**). (b) At the same time, pull the centers of the buttocks toward the heels, making the lumbar spine convex. Work these two opposing actions (a and b) against one another in order to lift the pelvis off the femurs and to lift the chest. Students may need more of (a) than (b), or the reverse.

Trikonasana-to-the-right: (a) Bending to the right, stretch the right arm and the right ribs to the right. (b) At the same time, move the hips to the left, increasing the bending at the right lower hinge (Subsection 9.B, page 319). (c) Rotate the right leg backward, from front to back (figure 10.B-2**e**). (d) At the same time, resist rotating the left frontal pelvic bone to the right by pressing the left thigh from the front to the back. (e) Stretch the fingers of the left hand upward. (f) At the same time, reach more strongly toward the floor through the fingers of the right hand. The three opposing-action pairs are a) versus b); c) versus d); and e) versus f).

Uttanasana: (a) Lift the inner ankles by rolling the weight onto the little-toe edge of each foot. (b) At the same time, press the base of each big toe to the floor, thus activating the arches of the feet. (c) Contract the quadriceps muscles. (d) At the same time, pull the hamstrings onto the femur bones. (e) Tilt the pelvis so that the anal mouth points to the ceiling. (f) At the same time, reach the crown of the head toward the floor.

Dandasana: (a) Press the thighs toward the floor. (b) At the same time, lift the crown of the head away from the floor. (c) Press the thumbs into the floor. (d) At the same time, lift the side ribs. (e) Work the hands on the floor, rolling the thumb and index finger inward so that the inner, upper armpits move back. (f) At the same time, roll the upper arms in disrotation to the hand action, thereby pressing the scapulae forward onto the rib cage in order to lift and open it (Subsection10.A, page 328).

Opposable-thumb yoga: Sit in *dandasana* with the fingers interlaced behind the back and the knuckles pulling backward. Press the hands against the front edge of a chair seat placed behind you and against the wall, so that the scapulae are pressed forward, as in *dandasana*. Consider a second example of the use of macroscopic resistance: with the hands and head in place for *sirsasana I,* contract the biceps, and at the same time, roll the biceps laterally, but with the hands immobilized; this will act both to press the scapulae onto the rib cage (Subsection 10.A, page 331) and to immobilize the shoulders in support of balance.

Adho mukha svanasana: Work the feet, thighs, and hamstrings as in *uttanasana* above. Work the hands, arms, shoulders, scapulae, and rib cage as in *dandasana.* Tilt the pelvis as in *uttanasana* and in *tadasana.* Or (a) place the thighs within the wall ropes, and pin the feet to the sticky mat and the pelvis to the ropes. (b) At the same time, walk the hands on the floor away from the feet, in order to lengthen and straighten the spine.

Chair *bharadvajasana:* (a) Sit on the edge of the chair seat, and turn only the upper body to face the chair back. Push and pull with the appropriate hands on the chair back so that the closer shoulder moves away from the chair back and the farther shoulder moves toward the chair back. (b) At the same time that the farther shoulder moves toward the chair back, pull the femur on that side into the hip socket, so that the pelvis and shoulders are rotated in a disrotatory sense.

Pasasana **at the wall:** The application of macroscopic resistance in regard to twisting while sitting cross-legged and while in chair *bharadvajasana* I have been described in Subsection 7.A, page 232, but it is mentioned here again in regard to *pasasana* for the sake of completeness. (a) Setting the sticky mat aside, place a blanket on the floor next to the wall, and come into *malasana* with the right shoulder at the wall. Turn toward the wall, and press the right hand into the wall, in order to increase the spinal torsion. The result of this will be a rotation of the entire body with respect to the floor, because there is no resistance offered by the feet when they rest on the slippery blanket on the floor. (b) Repeat the entire action, with the blanket replaced by the sticky mat. In this case, the rotation of the shoulders around the spine is resisted by the friction of the feet on the sticky mat inhibiting the rotation of the pelvis, and increased twisting results. Thinking along the same lines, it is clear that one uses the pressure of the arm against the leg in both *parivrtta trikonasana* and in *parivrtta janu sirsasana* in order to increase the amount of spinal rotation by macroscopic resistance via disrotatory action.

Inhaling the breath: The action of the external intercostal muscles of the rib cage during inhalation is a good example of the internal resistance offered to diaphragmatic contraction while breathing in the thoracic mode. In particular, because the rib T1 is effectively fixed and immobile, contraction of the external intercostal muscle between T1 and T2 lifts the plane of T2 into a more horizontal position. T2 in turn becomes an anchor for lifting of the rib T3 by contraction of the next intercostal. In this way, the planes of all of the ribs are lifted upward toward the horizontal plane; this increases the effective side-to-side dimensions of the rib cage, and as the diaphragm pulls downward against the active lifting of the rib cage, thereby increasing the volume of the rib cage, an inhalation is begun (figure 15.B-1c). In this train of action, rib T1 moves least and rib T12 moves most, and the acute angle that the sternum makes with the vertical increases by 5° or so; i.e., it is less steeply inclined at the peak of the inhalation, due to the greater lift of the lower ribs against the action of the diaphragm.

Baddha konasana in *sarvangasana*: In this posture, there is no external resistance against which the legs and pelvis can work to bring the legs into the plane of the upper body. The feeling is very different from that felt when doing *baddha konasana* seated on the floor.

Balancing in general: See Box V.D-1, page 910, on resistive balancing.

It is an exercise for the reader to find the sources of the binary resistance in postures such as *parivrtta trikonasana, prasarita padottanasana, pincha mayurasana* (see Subsection V.G, page 927), *ardha chandrasana, maricyasana III, parivrtta janu sirsasana*, etc.

Section 11.G: Aspects of Muscle Training, Distress, and Injury

Yogasana Detraining and Overtraining

Losing It

The most meaningful benefits of *yogasana* practice are hard won, and once they are in hand, we begin to worry about losing them if we skip a few practice sessions. It is of interest, then, what the effects might be of going from a moderate, regular practice to an irregular practice or to no practice at all. Moreover, if we stop practicing (detraining) and then start again, will we continue to learn as quickly as when we were practicing? Is it possible to practice too often or too intensely? Answers to questions such as these are not known with any certainty in regard to *yogasana* practice, but they should not be too different from those

referring to resistance exercise in general, and answers abound in this case [90].

For young children, it has been observed that their strength increases with physical training, but without any noticeable increase in the size of their muscles, and it is thought that the effect involves a more complete and efficient use of the nerves driving the muscles; i.e., muscle memory (Subsection 4.G, page 140). There is a general inhibition of the α-motor nerve pulses from the brain, but with exercise, more motor units can be activated on demand, and there is a better integration of the work patterns of the motor units. One can think of all of this as a long-term warm-up benefit, comparable to those listed by Peterson [655] for short-term exercise (Subsection 11.E, page 467); however, the gains of long-term exercise are lost through lack of activity about as fast as they were gained.

Muscle-Protein Turnover

As mentioned above, in the untrained, one can make rapid progress in increasing the apparent strength of the muscle in a very short time, but this is due largely to muscle learning and neural repatterning. However, with continued exercise, there is both a repatterning of the neural proteins and the addition of new contractile proteins entering existing muscle fibers. The proteins within a muscle fiber undergo continuous breakdown and re-synthesis; in an adult human, about 1–2 percent of the muscle mass is involved in this cycle at any one time. All of the protein will turn over in about two months. With a lack of exercise, the breakdown will be a little more rapid than the re-synthesis, and the muscle will slowly atrophy; whereas when exercising regularly, the re-synthesis will be a little faster than the breakdown, and the muscle will grow [877]. This process involving the muscles sounds much like the remodeling going on in bones (Section 7.C, page 237), but at a much faster rate in the muscles.

As we age, there is a natural loss of skeletal muscle mass (called muscle wasting) and as a consequence, we grow frail as we grow older. In skeletal-muscle wasting, a genetic trigger first promotes the labeling of the myofilament proteins with ubiquitin as "unnecessary"; these proteins are then fed into the proteasomes within the muscle cells. In turn, the proteasomes digest all proteins so labeled, turning them into their constituent amino acids for reuse. In this process, the number of muscle cells remains constant but the cells become thinner, whereas in muscular dystrophy, the cells thin and die [896a]. This wasting can be slowed by eating regularly and exercising. However, once we get sick and are unable to eat and exercise properly, the wasting cycle takes the upper hand and we slide further into frailty [896a].

One guesses that protein remodeling in muscles can heal injured tissue but that the collagen in muscle tissue would remodel at a much slower rate than the contractive protein in the belly of the muscle, because the fluid circulation within the connective tissue is so much slower than in the belly of the muscle. Perhaps this is the reason that the turnover time for "intercostal muscle" is quoted to be as long as 15.9 years (table 24.A-1).

Long-term growth of a muscle's girth does not take place without substantial effort, for essentially no enlargement occurs in an adult muscle unless the exercise involves contraction of the muscle to within 75 percent of its maximum [308]. On the other hand, as we in *yogasana* practice know, long practice of milder exercise does result in increased muscle endurance, better circulation, and more efficient neural patterning, all of which make us stronger in ways that go beyond the merits of simple muscle girth.

Strength versus Memory

In an activity such as *yogasana* practice, muscle strength increases not only from structural changes in the muscles, but also from the learning process, in which motor units become selectively involved in the work, and various muscles learn how best to work with one another in the postures. It is the case with beginners that the strength increase is largely due to the "muscle education" process (Subsection 4.G, page 140). Interestingly, a large part of the muscle weakness induced by disuse is attributable to a lack of motor-unit stimulation, with the nervous system essentially having "forgotten" how to properly energize the muscles!

Because a significant amount of the strength gain from *yogasana* practice comes from the education of the muscles and from muscle memory, strength is maintained for a significant period after quitting practice. Thus, young people can retain the full strength developed in their resistance exercise for up to five weeks after quitting; however, noticeable weakening occurs for those over sixty years old after only two weeks of detraining. For young people, 30–60 percent of the strength gain will have vanished by twelve to thirty weeks, but even after thirty weeks of detraining, they will still be stronger than they were before training was started. One hundred percent of top strength can be maintained for twenty weeks with a once-a-week practice that is as intense as those leading up to detraining. Breaks from *yogasana* practice of five weeks or less will leave a student largely where they were before the break.

Muscle Wasting

The effects of detraining are, in part, just opposite to those of training. Another important factor in this regard is the loss of muscle mass and strength, due largely to the lack of gravitational loading. The effects of zero gravity in space can be simulated on earth by going near-horizontal for thirty days of bed rest, with the head tipped "downward" by 6°. Muscle fibers that have been disabled in this way are smaller, more easily fatigued, and weaker, and innervation also may be affected. The quadriceps show particularly rapid deterioration with disuse, becoming weak and wasted after only a few days of neglect; however, the effects of disuse are reversible [549].

Limb immobilization, such as having the leg in a cast, promotes rapid wasting, most rapidly in the first three days, and then more slowly; due to a lack of neural excitation, a muscle can atrophy to about half its size if confined to a cast for a month [308]. Wasting is always more severe in the postural antigravity muscles than in their antagonists. Thus, wasting of the quadriceps is faster than that of the hamstrings on immobilizing the leg. If, while immobilized, a certain amount of isometric action is performed, as with the simpler *yogasana* postures, this will better maintain the slow-twitch postural muscles than the fast-twitch muscles.

The effects of immobilization depend on the length of the muscle at immobilization, so that if the knee is immobilized with the leg in the elongated position (so that the quadriceps is short), its sarcomeres will be absorbed during the immobilization to keep the muscle short. It appears that the changing length of a muscle fiber is due to the addition or subtraction of sarcomeres to the ends of the fibers, the sarcomere being the quantum unit of muscle length (Subsection 11.A, page 384). On the other hand, if the leg is immobilized with the heel touching the buttocks (so that the quadriceps is lengthened), sarcomeres will be added to it, making the muscle longer but not stronger. That is to say, the change in the muscle is such as to accommodate whatever the long-term stress might be, just as in *yogasana* practice.

Cardiorespiratory Effects

As we undertake exercise, the stroke volume of the heart increases, and so then does $\dot{V}O_{2max}$. However, as we age, the heart rate drops (or stays constant over shorter time periods), but the stroke volume makes up for it, and the heart does its work with higher efficiency. This increase in stroke volume happens rather quickly as we begin training, but it is also lost rapidly when we stop training—even within days [827].

It is also known that in spite of regular and intense exercise when young, what you did as a young person is of little or no value regarding sickness and long life if it is not continued into old age. (However, see Section 7.G, page 254, for a counterexample.) On the other hand, even if one did no exercise when young, beginning in old age still can add years of good health. It is never too late to start *yogasana* practice!

Overtraining

In some sports, it is possible to train so intensely that the effects on the body are overall negative rather than positive. Such overtraining results in the generation of chronically high levels of cortisol and growth hormone, leading to muscle wasting, loss of bone, stress fractures, and a suppressed im-

mune system that is unable to fight even minor infections. Compare this situation with the statement of Samantha Dunn in regard to the gift of moderate *yogasana* training: "If I did any kind of exercise too much, my immune system would crash and I would get sick. Yoga was the only thing I could do that would not make me sick [214]."

Adaptation

If muscular contractions are intense and repeated at a high rate, then the body tends to adapt, as if it is anticipating work of this sort in the future. Thus, if the work is forceful and requires close to maximum strength, then the adaptation will be toward making the relevant muscle more forceful and stronger. If the work is such as to require high levels of endurance, then the adaptation will be toward muscles that do not fatigue very easily. If the work is to extend the resting length of a muscle, then the adaptation will be toward a longer length of this muscle. This is the general adaptation syndrome (GAS) of Selye (Subsection 11.A, page 395). Training for strength and muscle mass involves high-intensity, near-maximum loads worked for a small number of times. In this type of work, the fast-twitch fibers increase in size much more rapidly than do the slow-twitch fibers and have a larger increase in the number of mitochondria when compared to the slow-twitch fibers.

It does appear that the number of muscle fibers in a muscle is determined genetically and is not increased by strength training (however, see below). Note too that weight training can yield a large improvement in the isotonic ability to lift weights, while the isometric strength of the same muscle hardly improves at all. This illustrates the specificity of the training response. McComas [549] feels that the large difference here is due to neural adaptations. All of this suggests that weight training may be of use in that part of *yogasana* practice involving isotonic work, but not for isometric positions. If this is correct, then prone presses on a bench may help develop the upper-arm strength needed to move into *chaturanga dandasana* from the supine position, for example, but only *yogasana* practice in the posture can build the stamina to remain there.

Cross-Training

Cross-training does not work, except to sell shoes. The benefits of any particular exercise rarely transfer very far into another mode of exercise. It is also possible that the cross-training will actually interfere with the primary skill (a very specific pattern of joint and muscle coordination) being worked on. On the other hand, a little cross-training can help to add spice to one's exercise life. It also can be useful to promote a more balanced strength in the body, so as to better avoid injury while engaged in the primary-focus activity. For example, many football injuries could be avoided if the players had more flexibility training. In *yogasana* practice, cross-training will not be a benefit in general, as the body is strengthened in all modes by the activity, so that no supplement is needed; however, there may be something to be gained by lifting weights [726].

Muscle Fatigue

Muscle fatigue is partly due to several physiological effects. When in the arena of anaerobic oxidation (Subsection 11.A, page 393), fatigue is the consequence of the accumulation of lactic acid in the muscle, which impedes further contraction. The lactic acid concentration in the fatigued muscle may be ten to fifteen times as high as in the resting state and interferes with the functioning of the neuromuscular junctions. When fatigued, more muscle fibers contract in synchrony, seeming more like a spasm, and trembling may be visible. To continue working while fatigued, muscles require more effort, and the task is done with less precision when in this state [288]. Indeed, experiments show that long bouts of tiring physical work are accomplished most quickly if they are broken up to allow for short rests. Fatigue also can be due to the lack of fuel, to impaired neuromuscular nerve transmission, or to ischemia and hypoxia. Once the muscles are fatigued, their proprioceptive accuracy and efficiency are reduced. A tired muscle relaxes more slowly than does one that is not fatigued [822].

It is most interesting—and quite possibly worth remembering—that in the case of chronic fatigue syndrome, the cause presently is held to be in the central nervous system (possibly due to a viral infection among the microglia) and not in the muscles themselves.

Under-Performance

It will come as no surprise to *yogasana* students that there is also a prominent mental component to muscle fatigue. It has been shown that when we become overly exercised, the level of interleukin-6 in the blood rises by a factor of sixty or more over normal; this chemical works to make the body feel tired, even if the muscles themselves are fresh. The result of high levels of interleukin-6 in the blood has been given the name "under-performance syndrome." It is proposed that, like the muscle-stretch reflex (Subsection 11.D, page 448), under-performance syndrome acts to protect the muscles from overexertion and injury [697].

Muscle Cramping, Spasm, and Tremor

In the contraction of a muscle doing work—the biceps, for example—the various motor units are energized in a random way, so that as one motor unit relaxes, another begins to contract, with the result that the overall contraction is smooth and sustainable over a long time. If, however, the neural connection stimulates the contraction of many of the motor units simultaneously, then the result is a painful muscle cramp or spasm that may last for a day or more.

There are undoubtedly several mechanisms responsible for muscle cramps and spasms. In the case of heavy exercise, the prime cause of cramping would seem to be the buildup of metabolic waste products in the over-worked tissue. This may result from insufficient blood flow into and out of the muscle due to the intense contraction it undergoes in doing its work. If, for example, the arterial blood supply to the heart is inadequate, painful signals (angina) are sent to the brain as the cardiac muscle spasms, until either the workload on the heart is lowered or the blood supply is returned [562]. Dehydration and electrolyte imbalance also can raise the risk of cramping [555], especially if one is on diuretic drugs, which can upset electrolyte balance.

Leg and Foot Cramp

Claudication is the severe pain attending cramping of a muscle during exercise; it is the result of significant arterial blockage to the lower extremities, as to the foot when in *virasana*. In *yogasana* practice with beginners, the most frequent cramp seems to be that of the foot in postures such as *urdhva mukha svanasana, virasana,* or *vajrasana*. In this case, it is likely that the cramp is a reflexive response to the contraction of the muscles in the soles of the feet; however, the cramping certainly is not helped by the acute angle at the knees when in the sitting postures, which acts as a tourniquet to keep circulation from passing beyond the knees. Leg cramps also are more frequent in smokers, who generally have poorer peripheral circulation.

Cramp Release

Given a muscle cramp in the body, one can often release its grip by breathing so that the exhalation is sent mentally to the point of cramping, so that the mental-relaxation sensation of the exhalation can nullify the mental-pain sensation of the cramp. This allows one to stay in the posture while working on the cramp. If this is not effective, then coming out of the posture to allow more blood circulation, and massaging the cramped area so as to overload the neural circuitry in that area with skin sensations (Section 13.C, page 523), can be of short-term help [555]. Cramps also can be relieved by the passive stretching of the affected muscle, by active contraction of the antagonist muscle, or by the ingestion of quinine.

It is conjectured that a systematic program of stretching will prevent cramps from occurring [7], and I have found this to be true in my *yogasana* practice. It is said, for example, that regular stretching of the pelvic area by *baddha konasana, upavistha konasana, supta virasana,* etc. in women reduces or eliminates the pain of menstrual cramping associated with dysmenorrhea [404].

Spasms

Spasms may occur in muscles as an automatic and protective response to an injury in a related part of the body [52]. The spasm is triggered when a movement in the body threatens to impinge upon an already injured structure. Most often, the injuries that can trigger a spasm involve torn muscles, ligaments, or tendons; a disc pressing upon a nerve; irritation within a joint; or an infected organ [52]. Thus, for example, if one sleeps in an awkward position that strains the ligaments of the neck, one might awaken with spasms in the neck muscles, which act to immobilize the neck and so protect the ligaments from further stretch. The phenomenon of muscle tremor is discussed in Subsection 11.A, page 389.

Paying the Price for Stretching Too Far, Too Fast, or When Misaligned

As a muscle is stretched, signals are sent by the various mechanoreceptors in the muscle about its length, tension, and rate of lengthening. As long as these quantities are within reasonable bounds, the conscious sensation is only that of stretching; i.e., muscle tension. However, done too far or too fast, reflex signals are sent to the spinal cord, which in turn activates the stretched muscle, leading to a contraction (Subsection 11.D, page 448). Nonetheless, through willpower or sheer speed of action, one can continue to stretch in spite of the reflex attempting to inhibit further muscle lengthening, and this deliberate action can lead to torn muscle fibers. Once torn, a second type of muscle sensor will be activated, the nociceptor, sensitive to injury and signaling pain. Details of how injury leads to a pain signal and the neural pathways open to this signal are discussed in Section 13.C, page 515. At the same time that the injury initiates a pain signal, it also initiates a local chemical process that leads to inflammation of the injury site. It is argued by many that changes in muscle morphology and action can occur only after the relevant tissue has been injured and then reformed.

Muscle Injury

Muscles can be injured by two different mechanisms. First, the capacity of the muscle to contract may be considerably less than required by the load being moved, with the result that the orderly alignment of the myofilaments within the sarcomere chains is disrupted. This is especially likely if the muscle is already in the weakened condition shown in figure 11.A-10a or shown by point E in figure 11.A-11. This situation can come about during a rapid intentional movement, or during a fall in which there is a rapid stretching of the muscle; this leads to inflammation, muscle soreness, and the triggering of repair mechanisms. Even a motor unit of very few fibers and low loading can be injured, since the load is being carried by such a small number of fibers.

Second, the muscle may be asked to work into the region of strong fatigue and so overexert itself. Again, the result will be a disruption of the close interaction between actin and myosin myofilaments. After injury, satellite cells proliferate to repair muscle damage; however, there are fewer such cells in the aged, and so recovery is slower.

Though both the force and the power of a muscle decrease with age, we are lucky as *yogasana* students, for it is muscle force that we need in our practice, whereas it is muscle power that decreases more rapidly. Reduced blood flow through a muscle is another factor predisposing it to injury. The blood flow is reduced by internal or external pressures on the muscle, which easily can exceed the systolic pressure in the relevant artery and so reduce arterial flow to zero.

Once soft tissue in the body suffers a traumatic injury, the stage is set for the initiation of the cumulative injury cycle, as described in Subsection 11.G, page 478, and in figure 11.G-1, page 479.

Muscle Stiffness

Muscles tend to stiffen with time if there is no movement, leading to a state of stationary rigidity wherein blood flow and oxygen concentration in the blood decrease while the concentrations of carbon dioxide and metabolic products increase. If a limb is immobilized for longer than four weeks, the sarcomeres begin to degenerate, and their number falls; fibrous connective tissue and fatty tissue become larger parts of the inactive muscle; and the prime movers in the affected area become secondary to their synergistic muscles. In contrast, the squeeze/flood cycle of stretching in the *yogasanas* brings fresh blood to the muscles and with that, a strong "feel-good" sensation.

In our quest for the feel-good sensation, we can overindulge in our *yogasana* work, and the result is often stiffness or muscle soreness. Excess physical work can lead to cross-linking of the collagen in muscles, making them stiff. Muscle stiffness in general is lessened by raising the temperature of the muscle, either by external means or as a by-product of muscle action.

As with most every other body function, muscle stiffness too seems to follow a circadian rhythm, for body stiffness is reported to be least at 2:00 PM. This can be rationalized as a consequence of the parasympathetic relaxation that is operative in the noon-to-6:00 PM time interval, table 23.B-3.

Prompt and Delayed Muscle Soreness

Prompt Soreness

There are two types of muscle soreness: prompt and delayed. In prompt soreness (also called acute soreness), physical work engorges the relevant muscle so that blood flow is impeded, and lactic acid and K^+ accumulate in the muscle tissue. The excess of these materials in the tissue stimulates pain receptors (Subsection 13.C, pages 515 and 519) during and immediately after exercise; however this pain usually passes in a few minutes. The prompt-pain signal induced by ischemia of specific muscle tissues is of great relevance to the *yogasana* practitioner.

Delayed Onset of Muscle Soreness

More likely for *yogasana* students is delayed onset soreness due to torn muscle, torn connective tissue, or spasm [7]. Whereas prompt muscle soreness occurs during or immediately after the exercise, delayed onset of muscle soreness (DOMS) only appears on the following day or the day after that and can then last for four or five days beyond the initial event [618]. It is most intense for two days after exercise, and it is caused by extensive but microscopic tearing of muscle fibers due to excessive tensile stress. This soreness is most intense following eccentric contractions, for example, when slowly lowering into *malasana* or *utkatasana* from *tadasana,* or coming into *chaturanga dandasana* from the straight-arm *chaturanga dandasana* position. The tissue tearing may also be accompanied by swelling.

DOMS and Yogasana

Predisposing factors for DOMS include poor physical condition, insufficient warm-up (Subsection 11.E, page 467), and the performance of eccentric isotonic contractions (Subsection 11.A, page 408). DOMS is often the result of over-vigorous exercise for someone unaccustomed to its intensity, and it can be avoided by making only gradual changes in the types and intensities of the normal practice patterns. If *yogasana* students are to avoid the distress of DOMS, they must warm up thoroughly and make no sudden increases in physical activity; they are not to avoid difficult postures but must ease into them over time, using props and learning to perform different aspects of the posture one at a time.

When we are young, progress in *yogasana* practice is made by damage of the muscle tissue and subsequent recovery. However, because recovery is more difficult in an older body, this type of hard work is less appropriate. In the older body, one should work to maintain and to refine but not to advance in the way appropriate to the younger body [407].

A study shows that for a given eccentric hamstring stretch, the least flexible athletes have the strongest DOMS reaction and lose isometric strength in the process [56]. It is suggested that because muscle-fiber damage is caused by the strain of lengthening stiff muscles during eccentric contraction, the more flexible you are, the longer and harder you can work without suffering DOMS. Indeed, when one trains regularly so that the body is in good *yogasana* condition, the body

adapts to the practice, and the occurrence and severity of DOMS becomes less of a problem.

For *yogasana* students, most practice sessions will not drive the physiology into the region in which excess lactic acid is produced in the muscles, and so this is not likely to be a source of soreness. Moreover, the pain of lactic acid accumulation is immediate, whereas the pain of a DOMS injury appears only twenty-four to forty-eight hours later. A study of the intensity of DOMS discomfort following eccentric exercise reveals that when followed by *yogasana* stretching, the peak level of discomfort is significantly reduced, and *yogasana* stretching has been recommended to coaches, athletes, and the exercising public for this purpose [87].

DOMS-type damage occurs most often during isotonic eccentric movements; i.e., when muscles produce force while lengthening, during which blood flow is restricted, as, for example, when slowly lowering from *adho mukha svanasana* into *chaturanga dandasana*. DOMS soreness that persists for days after the exercise is due to damage of the sarcolemma membranes surrounding the muscle fibers (figure 11.A-6), allowing cell contents to leak out and extracellular fluid to leak in. Microscopically, in this type of exercise, the actin filaments are being pulled in a direction opposite to that normally experienced in the concentric muscular contraction, with the result that some of the sarcomeres in the middle of the muscle fibers are severely overstretched in the process. When this occurs in an untrained student, the result is DOMS, with special discomfort when repeating the offending motion one or more days later. When in the DOMS state, the injury is so severe that scar tissue is formed during the healing, and the attempt to stretch this newly formed scar tissue is responsible for the delayed-pain response. Specifically, when overstretched so as to produce DOMS, the eccentric contraction has promoted inflammatory and degenerative changes in the muscles [549]. Repeated eccentric contraction can lead to severe muscle damage.[13]

---

13   Set up two bicycles in a head-to-head configuration, with the sprockets connected by a common chain. Let the first cyclist pedal in the normal way, by

A sudden or violent stretch may lead to ligament or tendon damage around a joint. A mechanical definition of strain is given on page 464; however, the word is used in a less quantitative way in regard to muscle injury; a strain in this context is an overstretching of a muscle. This differs from a sprain, which involves the overstretching of the structures around a joint due to wrenching or twisting at the joint. The latter may involve damage to blood vessels, muscles, tendons, ligaments, and nerves, leading to considerable swelling and discoloration. Joint sprain is more often observed in those involved in percussive actions, as with the inflammation of the lateral epicondyle of the elbow of the racquet arm of tennis players or the medial epicondyle of the elbow in golfers. Tissue injuries of this sort are discussed further in Subsections 11.B, page 434, and 11.G, page 471, and Section 13.C, page 515.

Ischemia

Restricted Blood Flow

Extended ischemia of muscles that are under extended contraction can generate either local or delocalized pain signals due to decreased blood flow. This is especially true for students who

quadriceps extension, but let the second cyclist pedal backward so as to resist the motion of the first by quadriceps flexion. In this case, the first cyclist is carrying out a concentric isotonic action with the quadriceps, whereas the second is carrying out an eccentric isotonic action with the quadriceps. Which rider does more work, and which feels the distress of hard work on the following day(s)? Surprisingly, it is the first rider pedaling in quadriceps extension who uses more oxygen (370 percent more), but it will be the second rider who will suffer from DOMS!

The eccentric quadriceps action is more efficient and more forceful than the corresponding concentric action. Whenever we contract a muscle in a concentric way, the corresponding antagonist is being stretched in an eccentric way, as it resists the action of the first. This will be the case with the second cyclist who was pedaling to resist the efforts of the first. In this case, the agonist is doing positive work, and the antagonist is doing negative work [877].

might have peripheral blood-vessel disease; i.e., for those in whom blood flow is already low for reasons other than severe contraction. If blood flow into and out of a particular muscle is impeded mechanically, there will be a painful reaction in a very short time if the muscle is undergoing work at the time, or somewhat longer thereafter if the muscle is passive; in either case, the muscle becomes starved for oxygen and at the same time cannot get rid of its metabolic waste. For example, if the inner upper arm is pressed against the tibia in *maricyasana III*, and the hands are clasped loosely behind the back using a belt, then the blood flow into and out of the forearms may be impeded, and pain in the forearms may be felt after a few minutes in this position. If, instead, the hands are clasped so that the muscles of the forearms are working hard as well, then the more intensely working muscles of the forearms become painful in only tens of seconds due to the ischemic production of pain-causing chemicals within the working muscles (Subsection 3.E, page 61).

Muscle spasm is also a cause of pain in the ischemic area, because the muscle is so fully contracted that blood flow in and out of the affected muscle is severely reduced (the pressure due to the contraction of the muscle is larger than the systolic blood pressure trying to force blood into the muscle), and the muscle in spasm cries out for release from the strangulation. Some measure of relief follows from increased blood pressure, due to increased sympathetic tone in the muscle and due to vasodilating metabolites that accumulate in the muscle.

The Cyclical Nature of Injury

One aspect of injury of which the *yogasana* practitioner must be aware involves recurrent injury. As shown in figure 11.G-1, an injury may begin with tissue trauma, but this may be only the first step in a long series of physiological responses ending with further injury to the tissue in question. Thus, the original injury is accompanied by inflammation, tissue hypoxia, and pain, to be followed by protective muscle spasms, muscle stiffness, and eventual changes in neuromuscular control. Being unaccustomed to working in the new way, the muscles then react improperly, and the original tissue injury reoccurs. This can be the first cycle in an ongoing process called the "cumulative injury cycle" [117], unless one finds a way directed toward healing rather than toward re-injury.

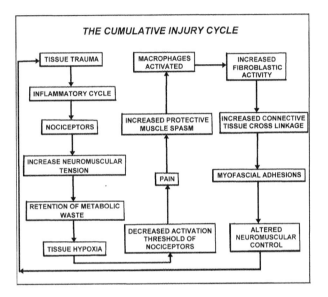

Figure 11.G-1. The cyclic nature of injury, according to Clark [117]. The cycle begins with an initial muscle trauma and moves on to the inflammatory cycle, activation of the nociceptors, hypoxia, pain, and on to muscular problems, which lead eventually to further tissue damage at the original site. This renewed damage initiates a new cycle of injury.

Healing Muscular Injuries

RICE

Musculoskeletal injuries are usually best handled in the short term by the RICE protocol, where RICE stands for:

Rest: This allows time for the injury to heal and is most important just after an injury.

Ice: Cooling the injury site numbs the pain and reduces swelling by vasoconstriction. After intermittent icing for twenty-four to forty-eight hours, begin to alternate icing with the application of heat.

Compression: Mild pressure, as with a elastic bandage, on the injury site can help in reducing swelling.

Elevation: Lifting the injured limb appropriately will aid vascular circulation in the injured area and will speed recovery. For example, with a leg injury, *viparita karani* promotes healing.

Immediately after an injury is signaled by sharp, piercing pain, one should turn to RICE [52]. The pain of musculoskeletal injury can be eased by binding the area so as to control edema and swelling, while periodically cooling the affected area with ice. Heat is to be avoided in the first day or two, as it promotes hemorrhaging and the inflammatory response [618]. If you rub or gently massage a DOMS injury that is not swollen or inflamed, the action can act to stimulate a flood of touch-sensor signals that act to drown out the pain signal, and so it offers some immediate pain relief (Subsection 13.C, page 523).

Rest

In treating a DOMS-type *yogasana* injury, it is best to allow for a rest period, so that tissue can recover and rebuild [281]. As shown in table 11.G-1, there are specific time intervals recommended for the rest period, depending upon the injury. The rest phase of recovery can be as short as one day for a minor muscle pull, and as long as eight weeks for a lower-back strain with complications of a herniated disc. Most importantly, once the times stated in the table have elapsed, one should then begin an activity phase, in which the affected muscle is brought back into use. To begin exercising in the active phase can be painful, but this pain is in part emotional (Section 13.C, page 516), is secondary to the original injury, and is a healthy part of the recovery process. If one allows the resting phase of the healing to go much beyond the times quoted in the table, then the affected area starts to atrophy, the muscles shorten and stiffen, and even more pain is in store once the area is activated. On the other hand, once rehabilitation has commenced, it is wise not to work directly on the site of the injury, but to work peripherally.

Table 11.G-1: Recommended Resting Intervals for Various Muscle Injuries [281]

Injury	Rest Period Prior to Active Phase
Minor muscle strain	One to ten days
Upper-back, shoulder, or neck muscle strain	Up to seven days
Lower-back strain	One to fourteen days
Lower-back strain with complications	Two to eight weeks
Torn muscle	Three to four weeks

If a muscle is injured but re-innervates within a few months after trauma, it can regain its full size and strength; however, if the re-innervation is not complete by this time, it is less and less likely to respond thereafter. If a muscle is so injured that it is denervated, the muscle begins immediately to atrophy, and this process can continue for several years, until all muscle has been converted to fat and inflexible fibrous tissue.

When faced with a case of DOMS, consider a light practice to reduce stiffness and pain, abetted by gentle massage and vitamin C, but do not directly challenge the sore spot by stretching it directly. Once healing is well underway, mild stretching is advised, as it acts to break up adhesions in the muscle tissue (especially common in the abdomen following surgery) that can lead to inflexible scar tissue.

Adhesions

In a muscle that has never been injured, all of the fibers run parallel to the line between the insertion and the origin if the muscle is fusiform, or at least parallel to one another if not fusiform (Subsection 11.A, page 397). However, once some of the fibers have become separated from the others by overstretching or by some other mechanism, the healing process often joins the loose ends of torn fibers to neighboring fibers in a haphazard way. The result is scar tissue, or an adhesion, in which the fiber axes within the scar are no longer parallel to those of the uninjured fibers. The scar is then a point of *yogasana* weakness that often is the site of further tearing and scarring. Most often, there is more scarring in the tendons and ligaments than in the bellies of the muscles [52]. This is understandable in terms of the higher stresses on the tendons (as displayed in figure 11.E-2) and the low extendibility of the tendons. Needless to say, inelastic scar tissue and adhesions formed within muscles by overstretching will inhibit them from stretching fully.

Connective and Supporting Tissues

12

Section 12.A: Connective Tissues

The Body's Glue

Connective tissue is the body's glue. In its different forms, it works to keep various organs in place; to bind groups of cells together to form organs, plexuses, etc.; to surround and cushion every cell in the body; and ultimately to define the overall shape of the body [714]. The tendons, ligaments, and fascia of the body are different forms of connective tissue. The supporting tissues are closely related to the connective tissues, but they are constructed so that they can help support the weight of the body.

Connective tissue in muscle not only holds a muscle together, but is also largely responsible for the gross shape and consistency of that muscle. Because the connective tissue in muscles is somewhat resistant to stretching, it distributes tensile stress evenly among many muscle constituents, thereby reducing the chances of injury. Once muscle contraction has relaxed, the elasticity of the connective tissue helps to return the muscle to its resting length, warming it at the same time [549].

Fibroblasts

Unlike the situation in muscles and nerves, where there are dense concentrations of the relevant cells, in connective tissue one finds relatively

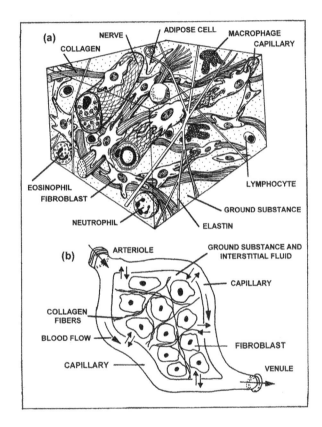

Figure 12.A-1. (a) Section of body tissue and (b) details of the chemical exchange routes within the vascular system encompassing ground substance, collagen, and fibroblasts.

few cells (called fibroblasts) otherwise present in a large excess of noncellular components: large numbers of collagen fibers, elastin fibers, and a semi-fluid gel called ground substance (figure 12.A-1a). These three noncellular components (collagen, elastin, and ground substance) are produced by the connective-tissue fibroblasts floating in the interstitial fluid and the wide variety

Table 12.A-1: Biological Building Materials [603]

Tissue Type	Cell	Fiber Types	Surrounding Ground Substance
Bone	Osteoblasts, osteoclasts	Collagen	Replaced by mineral salts
Cartilage	Chondrocyte	Collagen, elastin	Chondroitin sulfate
Ligament	Fibroblast	Collagen	Minimal proteoglycan
Tendon	Fibroblast	Collagen	Minimal proteoglycan
Aponeurosis	Fibroblast	Collagen mat	Some proteoglycans
Fat	Adipose	Collagen	More proteoglycans
Areolar	Fibroblasts, white blood cells, adipose	Collagen and elastin	Significant proteoglycans
Blood	Red and white blood cells	Fibrinogen	Plasma

of mechanical properties found within this tissue type is the direct result of the various proportions of these three components. The fibroblasts of the connective tissue are a major class of cells in the body, being one of the four major cell types in the body, along with the muscle, nerve, and epithelial cells.

As pointed out by Schultz and Feitis [764], "connective tissue is alive in the sense that it responds to stimulus," and one might add that it also responds to a lack of stimulus. For example, in the embryo, internal pressures develop that stimulate the production, aggregation, and orientation of collagen fibers to form connective tissue. As the bones begin to grow, they too exert pressures on the amorphous tissue, converting it into tendons and ligaments. The muscles then form, enfolded within the tendonous tissue spanning the gaps between adjacent bones. On the other hand, in the adult, if the connective tissue is not exercised, it can harden and thicken in response to the lack of movement. The pattern of collagen fibers in the adult body is a history of the uses and misuses to which the body has been subjected; if compacted, stretching of these collagen fibers in the *yogasanas* can release a flood of the emotions associated with the events pre-

cipitating the trauma of compression (Subsection 11.D, page 459).

Compositions

Though the connective tissues form a continuous web throughout the body, the proportions of ground substance, collagen, and elastin may vary widely from point to point, depending upon the tasks they are to perform locally. Thus, connective tissue that is subject to strong tensile loading but that nonetheless should stretch only slightly, as is the case for tendons, will be high in collagen, a molecule that is strong in tension but rather inextensible (Subsection 7.B, page 233, and this subsection, page 483). Other areas of the body may require much more flexibility in the connective tissue, as is the case for muscle fascia, and so will be high in elastin instead. In yet other connective tissues, it will be the ground substance that predominates. In general, connective tissue functions as a binder for other tissues; as the medium for the intercellular exchange of cell metabolites, nutrients, wastes, etc.; and as a lubricant [884]. Because the connective tissues of the body contain stem cells, the connective tissues may develop in various directions depending upon conditions; i.e., into fat cells, fibroblasts, white blood cells, etc.

The chemical makeup of several different tissue types are compared in table 12.A-1, where it can be seen that the basic formula of these building materials is a mixture of (a) hydrophilic (water-loving, fat-phobic) proteoglycan (mucopolysaccharide) ground substances ranging from very fluid to glue-like and solid and of (b) hydrophobic (fat-loving, water-phobic) fibers of collagen and elastin intermixed with the proteoglycan, all taken in various proportions in order to satisfy the needs of mechanical support and/or flexibility.

Details of the characteristics of the three basic components of connective tissue are presented below.

Collagen

Collagen, in its various forms, can be found in the transparent cornea of the eye, the tendons connecting the muscles to the bones, the ligaments that bind bones to one another, the spongy tissue of the lungs, in the teeth and bones, and within the delicate membranes encasing the brain [603].

Types

Collagen is not only a major component of connective tissue; it is the most abundant protein in the animal world. Molecularly, collagen is a long-chain polypeptide (protein), with the chains wrapped three at a time into triple helices (Subsection 7.B, page 233). Presently, nineteen types of collagen have been identified; relatively thick type I collagen is the most common type in the cartilage, fascia, skin, bones, ligaments, and tendons. The primary forms of collagen found in the connective tissues are described below [450].

» **Type I:** Found in tendon, ligament, and bone. Mutations here lead to Ehlers-Danlos syndrome (see below).
» **Type II:** Cartilage.
» **Type III:** Forms the walls of hollow structures such as arteries, intestines, the uterus, etc. Mutations here lead to a type of Ehlers-Danlos condition specific to intestines and arteries.

» **Type IV:** Forms the meshwork that filters blood in the capillaries and the kidneys.
» **Type IX:** Genetic errors here lead to herniated discs and sciatica.

In all nineteen types, the triple helices of the collagen molecule are bound together to form collagen fibrils, and the fibrils are bundled to form fibers. When properly aligned, connective tissues formed with a high percentage of collagen fibers have very high tensile strength but relatively low extensibility and so are able to resist strong pulling (tensile) forces. The manufacture of collagen fibers by fibroblasts within the connective tissue is aided considerably by vitamin C in the diet.

The collagen strands within the triple helix are joined not only by the relatively weak hydrogen bonds between amino acids on adjacent strands, but also by stronger cross-links that are chemical in nature. The cross-links between collagen strands resemble somewhat the cross bridges between the actin and myosin of muscle fibers (figure 11.A-9); however, in the case of connective tissue, the immobile cross-links prevent the relative motions of the strands rather than promote it, as with muscles.

Because the collagen strands, even though chemically cross-linked, are still mostly wavy and crimped, there is a certain limited elasticity to them, as the waves and crimps are ironed out upon elongation. Motions involving short excursions of length are elastic; i.e., when the stress is relieved, the tissue returns to its original length, and the induced strain is zero (Subsection 11.E, page 462).

Once the strain in collagen under elongation reaches 10 percent beyond the original length (Subsection 11.E, page 462), further elongation requires work against the cross-links that inhibit motion, and this is hard work indeed. In fact, attempts to increase the length of collagen by more than about 10 percent often results in rupture of the fibers. The more the collagen chains are cross-linked, the more rigid they become and the harder one must work to elongate them. It appears that the cross-linking of the body's collagen chains with glucose is an important factor in the loss of flexibility with aging (Subsection 24.A, page 809).

The viscosity of soft tissue is time-dependent, so that the faster one tries to stretch it, the greater is the resistance to elongation. On the other hand, if the stress is applied slowly and for a long period of time, then the deformation is viscoelastic, the strain will be permanent, and the deformation is plastic, but not elastic. This plastic deformation occurs when the tissue is lengthened by about 3–5 percent of its resting length; if the deformation extends to 6–10 percent of the total length, then the tissue is overloaded, microtears of the tissue occur, and this leads to the initiation of the cumulative injury cycle (figure 11.G-1). This cycle begins with a trauma to the connective tissue, followed by the release of compounds promoting inflammation and activation of the nociceptor pain signals. In addition to inflammation and pain, the release of the prostaglandins also promotes the formation of fibrous adhesions about three days after the initial injury. The fibrous adhesions act locally to form an inelastic matrix of connective tissue, which is resistant to any further extension. The local immobility of a soft-tissue injury leads to the consequences of poor circulation, higher sensitivity to pain, accentuation of the adhesion factor, and finally, altered neuromuscular control [117]. Flexibility training, such as *yogasana* practice, results in a permanent lengthening of the connective tissue due to plastic deformation.

Skin

When animal flesh or bone is boiled with acidified water, the collagen helices unwind to give a solution of polymer chains that are randomly intertwined. On cooling, this solution forms a semisolid gel called gelatin (or Jell-O, commercially). When the collagen of our skin is present as triple helices, the skin itself is vibrant and resilient; however, on aging, the helices again tend to unwind. The skin, in effect, "gelatinizes" and so sags under the pull of gravity.

If, on the other hand, the fibroblasts run wild and generate excess collagen, then the result will be skin that is extremely tough and inflexible (a condition known as scleroderma), in addition to

ligaments that pull the joints out of alignment. This condition would clearly pose great problems for the *yogasana* student. By far the stiffest and strongest form of collagen-based connective tissue is bone, a composite material formed from collagen (30 percent) and bone minerals (70 percent). This tissue is discussed in detail in Section 7.B, page 233.

Among the many different types of collagen, there is one that is "normal," one that is unusually stiff, and one that is unusually elastic [7, 927]. These distinctions are largely hereditary. Those who inherit the very loose form of collagen can become contortionists and more or less show the Ehlers-Danlos syndrome, in which the flexibility of the collagen is so extreme that joints easily become dislocated, skin is very elastic but very fragile, wounds are slow to heal, and the internal organs and blood vessels tend to collapse from lack of support. Both nutritional and hereditary flaws in collagen biosynthesis can lead to Ehlers-Danlos symptoms without involving any change in the elastin content of the tissue. Related hereditary collagen disorders involve hyperextension of the joints (Subsection 7.D, page 248), Marfan syndrome, and osteogenesis imperfecta.

Elastin

Elastin is another fibrous material found in connective and supportive tissues. It has the ability to deform to a large extent and then return to its former size and shape. Collagen fibers are white, whereas those of elastin are yellow, due to their content of bile pigments. Elastin is also highly resilient: when it is stretched, it stores energy, and when the stretch is released, a large fraction of the stored energy is returned as heat. The generation of heat when connective tissue is stretched and then released can be of great importance to *yogasana* students, for the elongation of such tissue is strongly temperature-dependent, being much larger when the tissue is warmed. Though the structure and composition of elastin fibers are not well understood, they are thought to consist of long protein chains formed into random sections of coils with occasional interchain bridges. When placed under tensile stress, the coils within elastin unwind and so allow the strain to reach 200 percent before the fibers separate, whereas the corresponding figure for collagen is only about 10 percent. Moreover, when the elongation of elastin under tensile stress is released, the coils form again and the fibers return to their original, pre-stressed length. This allows tissues containing elastin (such as blood vessels) to regain their shapes after being deformed by muscle actions. The most extendable ligaments in the human body are found in the upper spine and in the feet; in general, women have more elasticity in their ligaments than do men.

The connective tissues of the body are variable blends of the collagen and elastin fibers. Those structures that are overwhelmingly collagenous, such as the tendons, are strong and rigid; whereas those that are overwhelmingly made of elastin, such as the ligamentum flavum of the cervical vertebrae (figure 8.A-5), are supple and extendable. All connective-tissue structures are blends of these two extremes. Because of its extreme elastic property, tissue high in elastin is found surrounding those sites in the body where expansion is of utmost importance; i.e., in the walls of arteries and veins, the air cells of the lungs, the vocal folds, some ligaments, and erectile tissue.

As a person ages, the elasticity of the muscle fascia tends to decrease, so that range of motion decreases as well, especially when one is inactive physically. If and when a ligament is damaged by overstretching, healing will require from eight to twelve weeks, during which time the affected joint must be immobilized.

Ground Substance

Ground substance is a viscous gel (possibly liquid crystalline) forming the matrix within which the collagen, elastin, and cells function. Being somewhat fluid, ground substance serves largely as the agent for intercellular transfer of various cellular materials, as the connective tissues otherwise are without any of the blood vessels that normally serve this function. This transfer of cellular materials, however, can be slow due to the high viscosity of the gel in which they are suspended and through which they diffuse. It is the gel-like nature of the ground substance that keeps the water suspended as well, for without it, all of the interstitial fluid of the body would simply pool in the legs in a matter of minutes! Retention of excess fluids in the ground substance results in edema.

Being glue-like, ground substance serves both to separate adjacent cells and to bind cells together in muscles, etc.; connective tissues high in ground substance are flexible and binding but offer very little support against outside mechanical loads. Ground substance may also function as a lubricant within moving muscle, as when *yogasana* postures are held for several minutes [725]. In those parts of the body that are "frozen," the ground substance becomes more viscid, holding on to cell metabolites and toxins (see Box 7.B-1). Ground substance that is low in water content is thicker, more viscous, harder, and more resistant to motion on both the microscopic and macroscopic scales [637]. This, no doubt, is what Iyengar speaks of when he talks of practicing the *yogasanas* so that the muscles and joints stay moist and juicy (Section VI.D, page 940) and when he speaks about the stiffness that can come with old age when the sternum dries out [395]. Large amounts of ground substance are found in the synovial fluid of the joints and the aqueous humor of the eye [603].

Immobilization of a joint, among other things, results in a loss of ground substance. This in turn is expressed as a loss of connective-tissue lubrication, shrinkage of the connective tissue, decreased diffusion of nutrients through the ground substance, and a weakening of the mechanical barrier against bacteria. In view of the importance of a properly functioning ground substance, the role of proper body hydration is clear.

In most connective tissues, the basic component of the ground substance is a proteoglycan (table 12.A-1), a huge molecular complex between a protein, a sugar, and a considerable percentage of water. When proteoglycan is combined with collagen or elastin, the result is a range of substances called cartilage. Cartilage is a tough, rubbery material that is not only strong in tension, as are the regular connective tissues based on collagen, but that also can be strong in compression, shear, and bending, unlike regular connective tissues (Section 12.C, page 498).

Section 12.B: Fascia

Fascia is the tough connective tissue that holds us together, enveloping all structures of the body, from the tiniest blood vessel to the largest bone. Meaning "band" or "bandage," the fasciae most often occur as membranous sheets, dividing the body into compartments. The totality of the fasciae in the entire body is a single system, for one can travel from any point in the body to any other point without ever having to leave the fascial highway. Because all body parts are interconnected by fasciae, any tension or stretch in one part of the pattern will be rapidly transmitted from the point of application to further parts, as in figure 12.B-1. One must bear in mind that all of the mechanical interactions in the body between distant points are mediated by the intervening connective tissue [603]. Soft tissue, such as fascial tissue and tendons, will remodel along the lines of stress, just as with bone.

The Three Layers of the Skin

As discussed in Chapter 13, page 502, the tissue lying just below the skin is composed of three layers, the uppermost of which is the superficial fascia consisting of fatty, fibrous tissue supporting blood vessels and nerves. The superficial layer is strongly bonded to the overlying skin and serves as a shock absorber, as a fat storehouse, and as a thermal insulator [857a]. Just below the superficial layer lies the myofascial layer (also called the deep layer), in which compartments are developed to accommodate the muscles and to anchor them to the periosteum of the bones in a way that is mutually efficient for all concerned elements. The adhesion of the superficial layer to the myofascial layer is highly variable. It is only weakly adherent

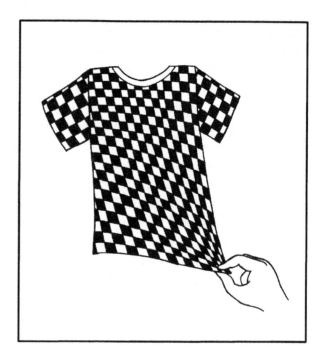

Figure 12.B-1. An elastic medium, when pulled at one point, as with the hand and shirt shown above, transmits the strain to distant parts of the system. A similar distortion-at-a-distance is produced by stress in the fascial system of the body.

at the back of the hand, but it is strongly adherent in the lumbar back and the lower rib cage, where it works to support the muscles in those areas [857a]. A far more internal layer (the serous fascia) lies below the deep layer and acts to hold the viscera in place.

Myofascia

Our focus here is on the myofascial layer covering the muscles, muscle fibers, bones, and blood vessels [7]. Approximately 30 percent of the muscle mass is attributed to the connective tissue around and within the muscle. In such dense fibrous myofascial connective tissue, the relative amount of collagen is very high, with the fibers packed tightly around the fibroblasts in an orderly parallel array when the load on the muscle is high. In general, the myofascia of the body has its fibers oriented longitudinally (parallel to the long axis of the body); however, the orientation in some places is transverse, where it acts as a flexible support (as with the thoracic and pelvic diaphragms) to control lateral spreading. Should the load on the muscle be relatively light, then the collagen fibers of the myofascial tissue are set at 45° to the muscle axis and are readily displaced when the muscle contracts. In certain muscles, the fascial elements are oriented perpendicular to the long axis of the muscle, and for this reason, the myofascia is often very tight and in pain when the muscle is contracted [857a].

When packed in the parallel arrangement, myofascial tissue has a very high tensile strength and so is found in most ligaments and tendons. In the tendons, the connective tissue blends smoothly and seamlessly into the various layers of the myofascial connective-tissue sheaths surrounding the muscle fibers (see Section 7.D, page 244). Yet other fasciae may be randomly oriented. The fasciae have some mobility and elasticity, as witnessed by any ballet performance; however, wherever the myofascia is under constant positive stress due to muscle contraction, there is an eventual hardening and thickening of the tissue. Over the course of a lifetime, the myofascial sheaths readily accommodate postural distortions, becoming dehydrated and losing their elasticity in the process. Even if the muscles are strongly exercised, they may outgrow their myofascial sheaths, leading to herniation of the sheaths or to very restricted ranges of motion. It is only with a comprehensive daily *yogasana* practice that the totality of the myofascial apparatus can be engaged and then coaxed into a more flexible, efficient form.

As with bone (Subsection 7.C, page 238), continuous stress on the myofascia, as when the resting length of a muscle is shortened by muscle tension, leads to the piezoelectric charging of the tissue; nearby firbroblasts then exude collagen fibers, which are attracted to the charged area, align themselves with the pattern of charges, and are deposited, thereby making the tissue thicker and more resistant to strain in the stressed areas. As stated by Myers [603], the result of such thickening of the myofascia is reduced functioning (stiffness), pain, weakness, and the restricted movement of metabolites. In this way, as the size of an exercised muscle increases, so too does the mass of its associated connective tissue.

Most interestingly, Myers states that the opposite also holds true: that through the long-term lessening of the myofascial stress resulting from *yogasana* practice (stretching), the thickening can be reversed through the reabsorption of the excess myofascial tissue, with the restoration of the full function of the muscle. A similar mechanism may be active in the healing of wounds. Myers's hypothesis implies that the proportion of myofascia is less in *yogasana*-stretched muscles as compared with exercise-pumped, contracted muscles. If true, this would explain why *yogasana*-trained muscles have longer resting lengths than do the weight-lifter types (figure 11.A-16).

With respect to muscles, myofasciae perform four functions [7, 857a]:

» They bind the muscle fibers together and orient them in a common direction, along with the blood vessels and nerves serving the muscle. At the same time, they serve to separate the muscles from surrounding structures.

» Should the muscle be less than totally contracted, the myofascial connective tissue serves to spread whatever stress results from the muscle action over a large area, and so offers a safety factor for the muscles.

» They serve to lubricate the muscle internally, so that the component parts can move easily with respect to one another when the muscle changes shape.

» Being of low extensibility, the myofasciae more or less support the muscles they envelop. Thus, for example, there are very thick myofascial bands running down the lateral edges of the thighs, which act to support the large muscles of the thighs when standing vertically.

Layered Structure

The connective tissues associated with muscles (figure 11.A-4) are organized at three levels:

1. The epimysium is a tough tissue of collagen fibers covering the entire surface of a muscle, thereby separating it from adjacent muscles.

2. Within the muscle, thinner layers of collagen called perimysium divide the muscle into groups of fibers, each group being called a muscle fasciculus or fascicle. The perimysium is a softer tissue and so allows the entry of soft structures such as blood vessels and nerves into the muscle interior.

3. Within the muscle fasciculus, each muscle fiber is surrounded by the collagenous endomysium. As muscle fibers approach their tendons, the muscle-fiber diameters narrow considerably, some by as much as 90 percent. It is the tissue of the endomysium that transfers a large part of the contractive force of the muscle fibers to the associated tendons.

Though microscopic in scale, the epimysium, perimysium, and endomysium connective tissues are directly connected to the macroscopic connective tissues (tendon and periosteum) that bind the muscle to the bone and to the microscopic cytoskeletal structures within the individual cells themselves (see below). At the level of the sarcomere within the muscle fiber, the molecules titin and α-actinin in effect play the role of connective tissue, as they attach the actin and myosin myofilaments, respectively, to the mobile Z discs (Subsection 11.A, page 384).

Stretching

As discussed in the case of muscles (Subsection 11.E, page 462), connective tissue is a viscoelastic material. That is to say, it has properties of both the ideal viscous and elastic materials. When the myofascia is weakly stretched and then relaxed, the original length of the tissue is fully recovered, as appropriate for an elastic material. In contrast, when the stretching is done slowly and held for a long time, on release of the tension, the material is permanently elongated, as appropriate for a viscous material. If muscle were only elastic, one could never change its length by stretching it, as a purely elastic material will always return to its original length after the stress on it is released. On the other hand, the ability of a viscous material to flow under stress allows it to be permanently lengthened following a tensile stretch and release. It is this latter characteristic of the viscoelastic muscle, leading to a permanent lengthening, that we exploit in *yogasana* practice, provided the muscle or its myofascia is not injured in the process, and provided that the sarcomere length (Subsection 11.A, page 387) increases accordingly. Note too that on lengthening a muscle, a number of sarcomeres are added to the fiber length, thereby making the stretched muscle longer.

Viscoelasticity is not the only material property of interest to *yogasana* students, for if the stretch is done both deeply and swiftly, then the fascia may behave as a stiff and brittle substance that is easily broken. Obviously, this aspect of the myofascial tissue is to be avoided in our practice.

As students of *yogasana,* it is most interesting to note that in a relaxed muscle being slightly stretched, the resistance to stretching can be apportioned as follows: 47 percent to the connective tissue (ligaments) in the joint capsule, 41 percent to resistance from the fascia and titin, 10 percent to resistance by the tendon, and 2 percent to resistance from the skin overlying the muscle.[1] A very significant portion of the energy required to stretch a relaxed muscle is expended in stretching the myofascia surrounding the muscle as a whole, and each of the muscle fibers as well. Furthermore, when a muscle is exercised and the muscle grows in girth, the amount of fascial tissue also increases, so that the muscle becomes yet more difficult to

---

1   Because these various factors in muscle stretching can change in different ways as the stretch proceeds (figure 12.B-2), these figures apply only to very modest stretching and can be very different as the stretch proceeds to fullness. In particular, I feel that the assignment of only 2 percent to the stretching of the overlying skin is significantly underestimated in the case of *yogasana* students at the limits of their stretches. In any event, note that there is no assignment of resistance to the lengthening of the sarcomeres themselves!

Box 12.B-1: What Price Myofascia?

In the meat market, the prices on the various cuts of muscle vary inversely as to the proportion of myofascia in the cut; i.e., the most expensive cut of meat has the least amount of myofascia and so is the tenderest. In the cow, this honor falls to the filet mignon, which is the psoas muscle of the animal (Subsection 9.B, page 317). In bipeds, this muscle is depended upon for erect posture, much more so than in quadrupeds, so our psoas may not be as myofascia-free and tender as the cow's. Meat in general is considered to be most tender after the muscular cross bridges formed during rigor mortis (Box 11.A-1, page 392) have relaxed.

Because muscle fibers are not too strong mechanically, they depend upon the connective tissue and surroundings for protection from external trauma. Thus, we find that the amount of connective tissue involved with a particular muscle depends upon the muscle's susceptibility to traumatic injury from the outside [877]. Because the psoas is a highly internalized structure, with the vertebrae protecting it from the back and the abdominal organs from the front, it apparently is so well protected that it can afford to have minimal connective tissue.

stretch, unless equal time is given to this end. As explained in Box 12.B-1, above, there is an economic aspect to the myofascia as well as a yogic one.

When a material such as connective tissue is stressed in one dimension, a one-dimensional deformation (strain) is induced in its shape. These two quantities, stress and strain, can be plotted against one another as in figure 12.B-2 for various body tissues; the slopes of these lines reflect the stiffness of the body parts. Thus, it is seen that in the range 0–10 percent elongation, the fascia and tendon are very stiff compared with the cornea, skin, aorta, and ligamentum nuchae. Furthermore, the data on the fascia and tendon do not extend beyond 10 percent elongation, because they break at that point, unlike the softer tissues, some of which (aorta and ligamentum nuchae) can be elongated by 50 percent or more. Obviously, these tissues differ from one another, as they are tailored to do very different jobs, with properties that can change depending upon the extent of the stress; i.e., a soft structure can become stiff when stretched impulsively. These curves show that the elongation for a given stress is not a constant and there is an unspoken assumption that there is no

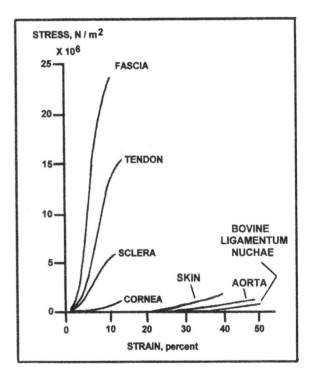

Figure 12.B-2. Stress-strain curves for various connective tissues. The stiffness of the tissues is defined as the slope of the stress-strain curve; at between 0 and 10 percent strain, myofascia is seen to be stiffer than tendon, and both are far stiffer than skin or the aorta.

viscous-flow component to the observed elongation.

The resistance of a tissue to moderate tensile stress is a measure of safety, for truly stiff structures are not easily injured. On the other hand, very stiff structures at high tensile stress will snap, whereas the softer tissues will continue to stretch without breaking. Stiff students in *yogasana* practice may not feel that they are stretching very far, but they rarely sprain a ligament or strain a muscle, whereas the hypermobile students have very soft tissue, can easily over-extend, and so can be more easily injured by their stretching (Subsection 7.D, page 248).

How far should one then stretch in the *yogasanas*? Speaking physiologically and psychologically, the answer, as given by Alter [7], is to stretch to the point of pain but not beyond it. However, as discussed in Section 13.C, page 516, pain is a very subjective sensation, so Alter's answer to the question will have a different meaning for different students. Furthermore, if one is already injured, stretching to the point of pain may be going too far and so can cause further injury. Iyengar [390] also answers this question, stating, "When practicing *asanas,* go beyond thoughts of pleasure and pain…. When you feel that you have obtained the maximum stretch, go beyond it. Break the barrier to go further." From the physiological point of view, it is held by many that in order to attain a lasting elongation of a muscle, it is necessary to stretch it to the point where fibers are injured, and that their healing then results in elongation (Subsection 11.A, page 405).

Time and Temperature

What is somewhat more certain, with regard to stretching connective tissue, is that the time factor can be very important, as can the temperature. If a stretch is held at a constant elongation, with time, the tensile stress will relax by itself. Similarly, if the stretch is conducted at constant stress, then the elongation (called "creep" when done at constant stress) takes place naturally as one waits. It is also known that a strong stretch held for a short time yields largely an elastic deformation, whereas a more shallow stretch held

for a longer time will result in a viscous lengthening of the muscle that is more or less permanent. When working with beginners, it is better to place the accent on the duration of the postures rather than on their depth. High temperatures encourage myofascial elongation, especially if the muscle is heated while stretched and is then cooled while in the stretched condition [7].

Muscle strength is yet another factor to consider. When a muscle is stretched strongly at a low temperature but for a short time, the loss of strength on relaxing is larger than when the stretch is softer and held longer, especially when done at a higher temperature. It is admittedly difficult to apply these facts gathered from isolated muscles in a science lab to living students in the yoga studio, but it strongly suggests that not-too-deep stretches held for long times are the most effective at stretching connective tissue, especially if the room is warm.

Ligaments and Tendons

Composition

Collagen predominates in the connective tissues that require great mechanical strength. Tendons, ligaments, and joint capsules consist almost totally of parallel bundles of collagen fibers interspersed with the fibroblasts that produce the collagen. Such collagen-rich structures will be very strong in regard to tensile stress but will be very stiff. In a ligament, the collagen bundles are very much parallel and suspended in a ground substance; whereas in a tendon, the collagen bundles are more randomly oriented. As it is now known that there are both sex hormone and neurotransmitter receptors in myofascial tissues, tendons and ligaments apparently respond to more than mechanical stress; clearly, they are more complex structures than previously thought.

Molecular Stretching

The collagen polymers that form the ligaments and tendons are in a pleated form in the resting state, but when stressed positively, the pleats are ironed out and the tissues extend. This elongation is accompanied by the generation of a significant amount of heat, which in turn acts to further soften the tissue [483]. However, because ligaments contain a higher percentage of elastin (see below) than do tendons [471], less heat is generated on stretching ligaments than tendons, so ligaments have a higher resistance to prolonged stretch and resume their normal pleated configuration more quickly than do tendons. Some ligaments can be stretched 25–30 percent of their resting length (that is, the strain equals 25–30 percent; see Subsection 11.E, page 462), and some in the cervical spine can be elongated to 200 percent [483] to allow flexion of the neck (see the stress-strain data on the ligamentum nuchae in figure 12.B-2)! In contrast, the ligaments that bind the knee, for example, have little or no elastin content, and stretching them leaves them permanently loose and ineffective in stabilizing the knee (Subsection 10.B, page 347). In general, there is no need to stretch the ligaments in the *yogasanas,* because stretching them can destabilize the associated joint. Consequently, if a joint feels warm, it may be taken as a possible sign of inflammation, as there should be very little or no thermal effect from the ligaments at the joints when stretching.

Tendons are composed almost totally of collagen, because they are not meant to stretch, but instead function to transmit the muscle force to the relevant bone in order to move it. Though resistant to elongation, tendons have a very high tensile strength, larger than those of either the muscle or the bone to which they are attached. This means that when under high tensile stress, either the muscle will tear, or the bone will pull apart before the tendon connecting them will fail. In growing children, it occasionally happens that the bones grow longer and faster than the muscles attached to them, so that tightness about such joints occurs, followed by a loss of range of motion [822].

Connective-Tissue Injuries

Ligaments, tendons, and joint capsules are among those connective tissues that are very high

in collagen, that are naturally stiff, and that serve the body as essentially inextensible substances. The fascia, ligaments, and tendons are all very strong in the young body. In such a body, the tendon has a central artery, but this disappears at about age thirty years or so, and after that, the tendon is nourished only by diffusion [288]. If, in our *yogasana* work, we adults mistakenly take these connective tissues beyond their mechanical limits, the results will be torn tissue that is extremely slow to heal and unstable joints that can readily cascade into misalignment.

Overstretching

The primary function of the tendon is to transmit force from muscle to bone. In simple use, the tendon is stretched uniaxially in the direction of the muscle fibers; however, in the awkward or extreme postures often met in *yogasana* practice, the risks for transverse forces that tend to shear the tendon increase, especially in the hand and wrist. The ultimate strength of tendons and ligaments is somewhat larger than that of the bones to which they are attached; however, if they are overstretched, they can rupture at lower stress. Tendons deformed by exceeding the limits of elastic strain will show viscous flow in part, and there will be a tearing of tissue and swelling, all of which are part of the formation of a "sprain."

"Tendinitis" is a catch-all category for a wide variety of injuries to the tendons involving pain and swelling, usually brought on by overuse. Restoration of function of an injured tendon may be very slow and time-consuming (up to two years for the knee), and premature exercise of a deformed, devascularized, or inflamed tendon will provoke further injury, pain, and loss of mobility. There is considerable conjecture as to whether the effects of hormones are a significant factor in tendon and ligament injuries in younger women (Subsection 10.B, page 350).

The grip of certain ligaments and tendons on the bones of a joint may be compromised through overstretching, hormonal shifts during pregnancy, through hyperelasticity due to genetic factors, or for other reasons. When one or more of these is the case, there is reduced stability of the joint, which places a stress on the remaining ligament and tendon fibers and on the highly sensitive nerve fibers within the periosteum covering the bone (figure 7.A-2). The intense joint pain resulting from this condition has been treated with great success by the injection into the joint of innocuous solutions of dextrose, using a technique known as prolotherapy, which strongly promotes new cell growth in ligamentous tissue, thereby tightening it [232].

The Cumulative-Injury Cycle

As shown in figure 11.G-1, a repeating cycle of injury to tissue is possible, beginning with an initial tissue trauma and leading eventually to an inappropriate neuromuscular action, which then acts to injure further the site of initial trauma, so that the cycles continue and eventually compound the consequences of the initial injury. The cycle also involves the accumulation of myofascial adhesions that strongly limit flexibility [117].

The connective-tissue sheaths that surround the peripheral nerves are innervated in turn by the nervi nervorum; i.e., the nerves themselves are self-innervated. Injury, compression, or inflammation of the nervi nervorum within the connective-tissue sheaths surrounding the peripheral nerves will be painful, as these systems are very reactive and readily transmit neuropathic pain signals.

Muscle Fatigue

Yet another cause of connective-tissue injury is muscle fatigue (Subsection 11.G, page 474). For example, the cruciate ligaments of the knee can be damaged by fatigue of the thigh muscles, which have failed to keep the knee joint open and in alignment. This fatigue of the thigh muscles (as a beginner might experience in the standing postures) places too much weight on the cruciate ligaments, and as they fatigue, they slowly tear [52]. Moving into and out of *padmasana* also can stretch and weaken these ligaments, which makes them even more vulnerable to this type of injury from fatigue of the thigh muscles. Once damaged in this way, one must forego all forms of *padmasana* and any sort of deep knee bend for a long while. However, see Box 10.B-1 (page 352) for a

relatively safe way to learn, to approach learning, and to teach *padmasana*.

Myofascial coverings of the muscles serve to separate the muscles and to ease the movement of one muscle past another. Myofasciae are not meant to bear weight indefinitely, so, for example, if the feet tire in standing postures and the arches of the feet collapse, then the plantar fascia across the bottoms of the feet needlessly bear the body's weight, and a painful case of plantar fasciitis results [52]. Stretching the gastrocnemius muscle, as when dorsiflexing the heel away from the knee in straight-leg postures, aggravates plantar fasciitis, and obesity too can be a negative factor here.

Skin Wounds

When the integrity of the skin is breached due to a cut of any sort, the healing process involves the activation of fibroblasts and the generation of a tangled web of collagen fibers at the site as a skin patch. Because scar collagen has a molecular form different from that of the collagen in normal skin, it will not die in order to be replaced by new collagen, as with unscarred skin. In this way, scars become a permanent decoration of the skin. If a hypertrophic scar is formed at the site of tissue injury, thickening the skin at that point, it is at great cost to the local flexibility of the skin. If the injury is deep enough to have severed muscles as well, the collagenous binding of the muscle tissues and fasciae, as they heal, will result in a significant tightening of the muscle, as the internal scar (adhesion) will impede the relative motions of the muscle fibers with respect to one another. Most often, when a muscle is torn, it is the ligaments and/or tendons that have suffered the injury and that must therefore bear the scars [52].

The Cytoskeleton and Tensegrity

That the connective tissue of the body is a continuous sheath running from the top of the head to the bottom of the feet, from the skin to the innermost organs, is by now an accepted concept among Westerners and Easterners alike [409, 603, 637, 764]. Less well known is the fact that the connective tissue also penetrates each

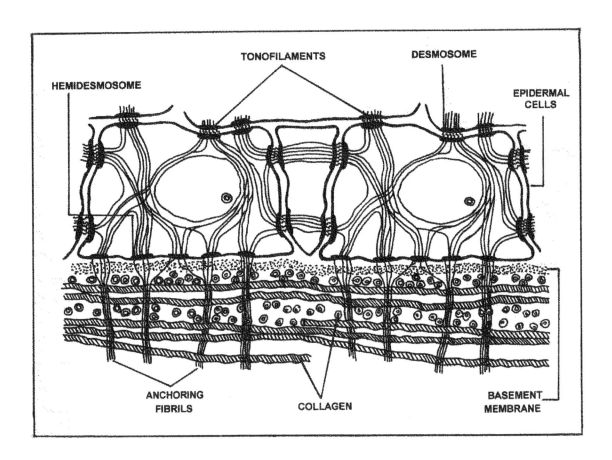

Figure 12.B-3. Details of the fascia in the upper layers of the skin, showing how the epidermal cells are connected through tonofilaments to one another and to deeper collagen layers of the skin through anchoring fibrils [637].

and every cell of the body, in effect coupling the contents of every cell in the body to the contents of every other cell in the body. As shown in figure 12.B-3, some of the collagen fibers outside the cell walls (called tonofilaments) in the skin actually penetrate the cell membranes, passing through the hemidesmosomes, to form a distinct structure within each cell, called the cytoskeleton. The tonofilaments of the cytoskeleton connect the extracellular connective tissue with the intracellular connective tissue.

The cytoplasm of a cell consists of all of the material lying between the cell nucleus and the cell membrane; the cytoskeleton is one component of the cytoplasm. The cytoskeleton of a cell in turn is composed of several distinct components, each on the submicroscopic scale of tens of nanometers. Key among these structures are the microfilaments and microtubules; the first of

these is composed of the muscular proteins actin and myosin (Subsection 11.A, page 382), which are used not only to move cells about, but also to move components within the cell. Microfilaments also act as semi-rigid supports within the cell, giving the cell its characteristic external shape. Microtubules are thought to serve as conduits for material transfer within the cells, especially along neural axons (Subsection 3.A, page 35). Other molecules called integrins act as adhesives to bind adjacent cells together. Experiments show that mechanical forces are readily transmitted from cell to cell through the adhesive integrin molecules that bind neighboring cells to one another.

From this, it is seen that the living matrix of the body is not only macroscopically global but is microscopically global as well, with the inner components of every cell contributing to the global net. It follows from this that the internal conditions of the body and the health of the internal body are reflected in the look and feel of the skin and flesh, as B. K. S. Iyengar states so often [391]. As might have been expected, the connections within the living web of connective tissue are sufficiently mobile and dynamic so as to respond to changing conditions, with structures retracting, dissolving, and reforming, allowing cells to move within the body when necessary, as when the leukocytes move to areas of infection (Section 16.B, page 642).

It recently has been demonstrated [186] that when two cells of the immune system trade molecular information, they first join to form a neural-like synapse, and the cytoskeletons of the cells then are used to swap molecular fragments (called cytokines) between the cells. A similar cytochemical drive is used by viruses to infiltrate their DNA into the benign cells of the body (Subsection 16.D, page 650).

Tensegrity and Cell Shape

The particular shape of a cell in a given situation is determined by the balance of compressive and tensile stresses that are external and internal to the cell. The architectural principle behind this, known as tensegrity, involves a basic combination of two structural elements, one of which is strong in compression and the other of which is strong in tension. Tensegrity structures (figure 12.B-4) can be built using rigid sticks as compressive elements and flexible rubber bands as tensile elements. An interesting feature of such a tensegrity system, when in mechanical balance, is that the tension in the structure is transmitted uniformly across all structural members, so that a tensile force originating at one end of the structure will be felt undiminished at the other end and at all intermediate points as well, with mechanical balance being maintained by the compressive elements of the structure, each of which is compressed locally. Thus, as Buckminster Fuller has pointed out, the tensegrity structure is one having a uniform tension throughout but balanced by local compressions [387]. The elements of a tensegrity structure are placed so as to offer the maximum amount of strength in resistance to mechanical stress and

allow structures to sustain ever larger mechanical stresses without disintegrating.

In regard to the relation between tensegrity and the cytoskeleton, it is implied that there is a plasticity in the cytoskeleton. Indeed, the microtubules forming the cytoskeleton constantly form and dissolve, growing in all directions in a random way. This allows the cell to assume an external shape that eventually is the most useful to it in a particular circumstance. Nerves and blood vessel systems seem to form in the same random way. Thus, the ability of the human body to adapt mechanically or geometrically to its environment is operating at the deepest levels within the cytoskeleton of each cell.

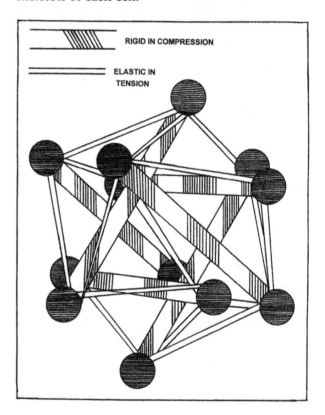

Figure 12.B-4. (a) A toy model with a tensegrity structure and held together by tensegrity forces; i.e., compressive stress in the sticks and tensile stress in the rubber bands connecting them.

As *yogasana* students, our interest in such tensegrity structures comes from the fact that virtually every structure of the body, regardless of scale, is a tensegrity structure. On the grossest scale, the body's bones are the compressive elements, whereas the roles of the tensile elements are played by muscle, tendons, and ligaments. This combination of compressive and tensile elements gives us our shape on both the micro and macro scales. When in balance, the tensegrity structure of muscles and bones forms the basis of our physical mobility and offers maximum strength for a given amount of material.

On the finest scale, the internal components of each and every cell of the body are a tensegrity structure made of the components of the cytoskeleton. Within the cell, the microfilaments are contractile and so exert tensional forces within the cell, whereas the microtubules serve to add a compressive element to the cell, and intermediate filaments connect the microfilaments and the microtubules to one another and to the other cellular components, such as the nucleus and the cell walls. These structures serve to stiffen cells and give them their characteristic shapes (see figure 3.A-1, for example). As a tensegrity structure in mechanical equilibrium, it follows that supposed "local" stresses in the human body in fact are felt throughout the body, from deep within each cell out to the largest organ!

Most interestingly, if one changes the shape of a cell by applying an external force, then one actually influences the chemical and even genetic functions of the cell. Thus, in experimental tissues in which the cells are forced to spread into a flat configuration, the cells divide more frequently, as if there were a tear of the tissue and more cells were required to heal the supposed wound. On the other hand, cells that are restrained to a spherical shape without spreading activate their voluntary death program (Subsection 3.A, page 32), as if there were a surplus of cells causing the crowding and some cells must be sacrificed so as to reduce the crowding. Cells that are neither too extended nor too compressed neither divide nor die but instead become tissue-specific cell types: heart cells, muscle cells, etc.

Elegant microforce experiments on individual human cells reveal that tugging on the cell walls promotes the formation of proteins that increase the longevity of the cell when in the presence of infectious organisms [97]. Given this context, it is easy to imagine physicochemical cell transformations driven by the stretches and compressions of *yogasana* practice especially, that muscle stretching might promote both muscle-cell division and resistance to infection, and that contraction might promote muscle-cell apoptosis. In regard to the former, see the discussion on sarcomere length in stretched muscle (Subsection 11.A, page 387).

Cell Vibrations

Using the atomic-force microscope, cells of Baker's yeast have been found to vibrate at room temperature at a frequency of 800–1600 hertz, due to the rumbling of the internal machinery driving the microtubule transport of chemical components within the cell [650]. Metabolic inhibitors reduce the vibrational amplitude completely. Vibrations of this sort may well be active in the perineural system of the human body, in which case, the vibration will show up as a fluctuating electric field on the outside of the cell, assuming the cell wall is piezoelectric.

Intracellular Water

As each and every cell in the body is filled with microfilaments, microtubules, and trabecular struts, with very little room for aqueous solution, virtually all of the water in the cell is bound in specific ways to the rigid elements of the cytoskeleton. The enzymes in the cell that catalyze so many reactions are not in true solution, as was previously thought, but are bound to these many solid-state cytoskeletal struts within the cell. In turn, the cytoskeleton forms a scaffold that acts mechanically to give the cell a specific shape and a particular rigidity, all the while being connected to the external structures of the connective tissue. The connection runs from the external connective tissue, through each cell membrane, to connect to the cell contents and thence to the genetic material within the cell nucleus. It is inescapable that whenever we stretch a muscle in the *yogasanas,* the physiological impact extends not only all the way down to the genetic material in the cells being stretched, but also into the genetic material of all other cells connected to them through the seamless web of connective tissue. Indeed, recent research [421] shows quite clearly how disuse of a muscle on the macro scale affects the expression of specific genes on the micro scale that regulate the extent of atrophy of the muscle and/or its regeneration.

The living matrix described above is a supramolecular network consisting of a nuclear/genetic matrix within a cellular matrix within a connective-tissue matrix, so that the effects of any disturbance originating in any one part of the body is transmitted to all parts of the body. The global nature of the tensegrity model on the micro scale leads naturally to the notion of anatomy trains (Subsection 11.A, page 424) on the macro scale and to Iyengar's claim to have realized the connection of his intelligence and awareness to every cell in the body!

Sensors

It is important to note that mechanical deformations will act on the various components of the living web to generate either piezoelectric charging of the materials (Subsection 7.C, page 237) or else electrical potentials called "streaming potentials," which develop in response to the flow of ionic fluids. The piezoelectric and streaming electric potentials are mutually interactive algebraically. It is hypothesized that such charging patterns within the connective web represent information that can be used to control various body processes. For example, mechanical stress on bone results in piezoelectric surface charging, which then acts to stimulate either the bone-building osteoblasts or the bone-destroying osteoclasts, depending on the polarity of the charge (Subsection 7.C, page 237). Inasmuch as the mechanical stresses are readily transmitted throughout the connective-tissue web, one has a mechanism then for the subconscious transmission of electrical signals concerning tensile and compressive stresses, tissue movements, and flow conditions over a very long distance within the web, all the way down to the level of the organelles of a single cell! Moreover, it appears that the signaling can be both electrical and magnetic, as the flow of a piezoelectric charging current is always accompanied by the

development of a magnetic field, according to Oresteds Law. Again, one's mind leaps from this immediately to the repeated comments of B. K. S. Iyengar in regard to extending one's awareness down to the levels of each of the single cells in the body while in the *yogasanas*.

This sensory system within the web of connective tissue (including the perineural system, page 26) is more or less independent of the more conventional neural and hormonal sensory systems described in Chapter 3, page 29, and Chapter 6, page 207, and is genetically far older than these systems. Therapies that operate largely or solely within the connective-tissue system include acupuncture, polarity therapy, Reiki, magnet therapy, and yoga. That hormonal changes within the body can be expressed as changing voltages on the associated connective tissue is shown in figure 12.B-5, where it is seen that the voltage appearing spontaneously between fingers on the two hands during the ovulation/menstruation cycle in a human female displays a peak voltage of +75 millivolts on the day of ovulation, to be compared with a voltage of -50 millivolts two weeks before and two weeks after the peak event [637]. This voltage is presumed to be the result of mechanical stresses on the perineural system, which are generated in response to the chemical changes within the body attendant to ovulation. It would be fascinating to see how such voltages appear on the body while in the various *yogasanas*!

In a more hypothetical vein, though it is apparent that if there is an electrical charging pattern associated with stress in the body and that this can exist on a very small scale, there is no evidence that there are specific sensors in the body that can read this pattern and act upon it. However, are such sensors present or even necessary? Do the well-documented actions of the osteoclasts and osteoblasts in regard to the charging patterns in remodeling bone (Section 7.C, page 237) imply that such things can happen vis-à-vis other body tissues? Are the charging patterns of various body tissues involved in the phenomenon of interoception (Subsection 11.C, page 444), in which the state of health of the various organs and tissues are subconsciously sensed? We await the answers

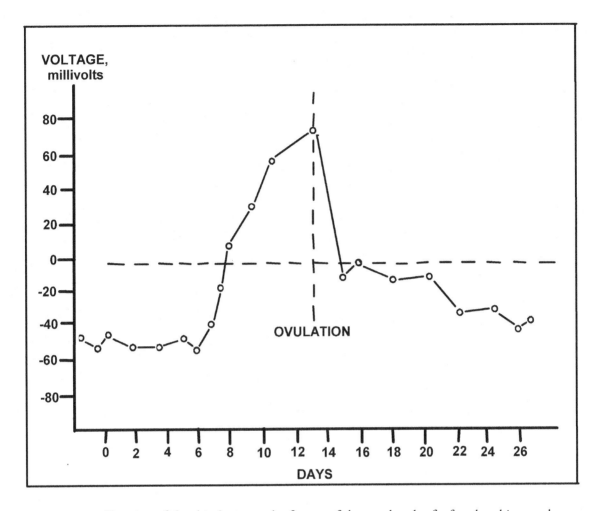

Figure 12.B-5. Charging of the skin between the fingers of the two hands of a female subject as she goes through ovulation [637].

to questions of this sort, of so much interest to *yogasana* practitioners.

Energy Blockage

Massage therapists [226a] also report that their clients may experience an emotional release as their tissues are massaged, perhaps not unlike the emotional release experienced by some *yogasana* students when in *savasana* (Section 20.C, page 723). However, they report that this is a phenomenon of "tissue memory," which does not involve the central nervous system but is a matter of stress in the tissue stored as energy, forming an "energy cyst." The cyst is formed as a result of a traumatic injury, and when the injury site is massaged, the emotional consequences of the injury appear, without any intervention of the traditional mem-

ory of the brain. This damming of the energy following trauma may involve the perineural system, since communication along the connective-tissue web may be interrupted by flaws in the system that block energy and information flow in either the electrical or vibratory aspects of the system. If the flaw is the faulty pinning of the tissue (or ground substance) at a certain point in the body, then flow of electric potential or of mechanical stress can be impeded at that point.

From this point of view, therapy consists of unblocking the blockage, by yogic stretching, massage, or any of the other manifold Eastern therapies, either hands-on or at a distance. Healing of the blockage will be in part dependent on the plasticity of the web; i.e., the ability of the components to readily change their form, position, tension, composition, electric charge, etc. Again, from the Iyengar perspective, one can imagine that overcoming such barriers to the flow of information through the practice of the *yogasanas* corresponds to his admonition to work the *yogasanas* so as to extend the intelligence of the body to distances further and further from the source, or head (see Section VI.A, page 937).

Other Connective-Tissue Types

Following Kapit et al. [431], a few of the other relevant connective-tissue types are described here. In loose connective tissue, the viscous ground substance forms the organic matrix within which several different cell types float, along with a loose tangle of collagen fibrils and a few elastin strands. Loose connective tissue is found under the skin as superficial fascia and allows the skin to roll back and forth over the deeper myofascial layers.

In adipose tissue, the cells of the tissue are largely fat cells, clumped together, with only a scant amount of collagenous fibers present. Adipose tissue usually is found under the skin and covering the surfaces of some of the viscera. As with most other cells in the body, fat cells profit from having a well-developed capillary system to supply nourishment needs, and they promote this using the same angiogenesis factors that tumors use to speed their growth (Subsection 16.D, page 647). Correspondingly, the anti-tumor drugs that work by strangling a tumor's blood supply also are effective in weight reduction in the obese!

Aging Effects on Connective Tissue

The effects of age on collagen and elastin appear to be the same. In both, the amount of cross-linking between chains increases with increasing age, resulting in a loss of flexibility. Simultaneous with this, the ground substance loses water with age (ground substance is 85 percent water in infants' tendons versus 70 percent in adults) and becomes more viscous. Immobilization of a joint also leads to connective-tissue cross-linking and

rigidity in the vicinity of the joint. The major changes in the body in regard to flexibility as one ages (in order of their relative importance) are muscle atrophy with an accompanying increase in fibrous, fatty connective tissue; neural atrophy; hypertrophy of connective tissue; increased tissue stiffness; and dehydration [117]. As one might hope, it appears that exercise and regular use of the joints decreases cross-linking in the associated connective tissue while maintaining hydration and so increases flexibility. It is at this point that *yogasana* practice can become a very important factor in one's quality of life as one ages.

Not only do our bodies stiffen with age if we do nothing to resist such a fate, but so too do the internal elements of the cytoskeleton within the epidermal layer of the skin. Experiments have shown that with age, the epithelial cells become more dense as they fill with protein fibers, with the result that the cells are two to ten times stiffer than the corresponding cells of younger skin [376].

Section 12.C: Cartilage

Properties

Cartilage plays a dual role in the body. It is a rather stiff material capable of helping to support the weight of the body (as with the intervertebral discs; see Section 8.C, page 303), and it serves as lubricant at the points where bone meets bone (as in the knee joint; see Subsection 10.B, page 347). In regard to stiffness (technically, the ratio of the stress to the strain in a structure; see Subsection 11.E, page 462), cartilage is more stiff than regular connective tissue and less stiff than bone. A rather lax form of cartilage is found in the external ear but is of no significance to *yogasana* practice. Cartilage is a more primitive tissue than bone [582], as one might guess from reading Box 8.A-1, page 270, and the fact that bone springs from cartilage and not the reverse.

Transformation to Bone

The weight-supporting tissues (cartilage) are dense tissues of great strength and high water content. In hyaline cartilage, one has collagen fibers embedded in a gelatinous matrix, the whole being rather solid yet flexible. Such hyaline cartilage is found capping the epiphysial ends of bones (figure 7.A-2) and also is prominent in the rib cage (figure 15.A-3c). The sliding of one hyaline-covered bone with respect to another is eased by the lubricating synovial fluid exuded within the joint capsule. In joints of relatively low mobility, there also are cartilaginous connections between bones that function as ligaments. Thus, the intervertebral discs are largely cartilage and function as ligaments, and there is a cartilaginous ligament within each hip joint, binding the femoral head to the acetabulum.

The early fetus is composed largely of hyaline cartilage, allowing high fetal flexibility and a safe delivery for both mother and child. This cartilaginous skeleton of the neonate at first resembles the cartilaginous skeletons of sharks and rays [878] (Box 8.A-1, page 270) but is then slowly transformed into the bony skeleton of the infant as it is vascularized. As described in Section 7.A, page 225, the cartilage of the infant is the model for the later formation of the bones. The fetal cells known as chondrocytes (or chondroblasts) generate cartilage so as to form the model skeleton. Once this is penetrated by the vascular system, bone-growth proteins become active, and the chondrocytes are transformed into osteoblasts, which excrete the inorganic salts that mineralize and further stiffen the cartilage, turning it into bone [422]. In the adult, the remaining hyaline cartilage covers the moving ends of bones, connects the ribs to the sternum, and supports the nose and throat; even this cartilage tends to harden in advanced age.

Like bone, cartilage is piezoelectric and so is able to display the momentary pattern of mechanical stresses on it as a pattern of voltages. However, though bone has an extensive system of blood vessels and nerves, neither of these is found in cartilage. Not being vascularized means that if the cartilage is in some way injured, there will be very little support for healing and repair. Injuries to cartilage (and to avascular ligaments and tendons) are very slow to heal.

Fibrocartilage

As with the regular forms of connective tissue, different forms of cartilage can have differing amounts of collagen, elastin, and ground substance, and the resulting composite can have widely varying properties, depending on the proportions of the three components. A second form of cartilage, known as fibrocartilage, is much like dense regular connective tissue but with the parallel collagen bundles interspersed with chondroitin sulfate and parallel bundles of matrix-producing cells, the chondrocytes. This tissue, the strongest of the cartilage types, is intermediate in strength between regular cartilage and bone, forms the outer casing (annulus fibrosus) of the intervertebral discs (Section 8.C, page 303), and also is found in the areas of the joint capsules and ligaments. The pubic symphysis is formed of fibrocartilage.

Lubrication

When the cartilage-covered surfaces of the bones in contact at a joint are sliding well, the forces are compressive only. However, if the surface becomes sticky, then there is a tendency for the forces to become more shearing in nature, and the result can be ripped cartilage [52, 878]. This happens most easily to the cartilaginous meniscus of the knee when in *padmasana* or when twisting the knee while it is bearing weight, as in *mulabandhasana.*[2] If injured, this avascular cartilage is nourished only by diffusion of nutrients via the synovial fluid. However, this diffusion can be aided greatly by repeated cartilage compression and release of the joint [7, 878], for this pumps the surrounding fluids in and out of the

---

2   This suggests that, for safety reasons, postures such as *mulabandhasana* should be learned while sitting in a chair, so that there is little or no weight on the knee as it is being twisted and bent.

pore spaces of the tissue, just as with the diurnal compression and elongation of the intervertebral discs (see Section 8.C, page 309).

Viscoelastic Deformation

When cartilage is kept under a constant load, it suffers viscoelastic creep to a region of lower compressive stress, is permanently deformed, and suffers from poor nutrition. Looking at the mis-aligned knee joints in figure 10.B-1b, one would expect the cartilage covering of the bones to be chronically thinner at the points of contact and therefore to be less well nourished at those points. Should this covering of cartilage wear away so

that the epiphyses of the bones forming the joint become rough and pitted, one is then looking at a case of osteoarthritis (Section 7.D, page 249). On the other hand, cartilage health is maintained by a dynamic compression that first compresses and then releases the cartilage without tearing or shearing it.

All tissues in the body need stress to stay healthy, as the stress remodels the tissue in accord with the lines of stress. If the weight bearing in a joint is uneven, then the part of the articular cartilage that is under-stressed will weaken and atrophy, whereas the part that is over-stressed will wear away prematurely, leading to a degeneration of the cartilage [117].

The Skin 13

The paradox of the skin is that it is both a barrier between one's Self and the outer world, and at the same time, it is one's window into the world that lies within the Self [422]. As the former, it is the key to keeping all sorts of toxins and microscopic predatory species from entering the body, and it is the key to keeping the life-sustaining chemicals within the body in their places. Not only is the skin largely waterproof in both directions and tough enough in most situations to be puncture-proof, but it is also able to repair itself when cut or damaged. Skin is an important element of the body's temperature-regulation apparatus, an organ of purification, and an organ of metabolism. Moreover, though it is a gland of sorts, for vitamin D is manufactured in the skin when it is exposed to sunlight, it also filters out potentially harmful ultraviolet rays.

Though it is not widely realized, "the skin" does not stop at the entrances to the body's orifices. Skin continues over the lips and into the mouth, goes down the throat into the stomach, through the intestines, and to the anus. All of our "insides" in fact are firmly and seamlessly attached to the outside skin, but with modifications to suit particular functions. This chapter deals with what we can consider to be the "outer skin", whereas the "inner skin" is considered in Chapter 19, page 703.

The skin also serves as the interface to our experiences of the outer world beyond the skin, thanks to the large numbers and many types of sensors located within it. In this chapter, the many aspects of the skin's function will be discussed, along with the special properties of its sensors and how they relate to the practice of *yogasana*.

Section 13.A: Properties of the Skin

Structure of the Skin

The skin is one of the largest organs within the body, composed of about 300 million cells in an adult, weighing about 4 kilograms (eight pounds), and spanning an area of 2 square meters (eighteen square feet). At the lowest magnification, skin is seen in cross-section to consist of three distinct layers: the epidermis, the dermis, and the subcutaneous layer (figure 13.A-1a). The outermost layer of the skin, the epidermis, is an avascular layer consisting of a lower layer of living cells (the basal cell layer) covered by an upper layer of dried, scaly cells (the horny layer). These two layers of the epidermis are separated by a third layer of maturing cells, the squamous layer. Cells of the horny layer contain a large amount of the protein keratin and constantly are being sloughed off as dead skin and replenished from below. Within and through the epidermis grow the nails, hairs, and various superficial glands of the body. On average, there are ten hairs, 100 sweat glands, and 1 meter (three feet) of vascular plumbing in each 6.5 square centimeters (one square inch) of skin.

Glabrous skin is thick and hairless, and is found where there is movement and abrasion, as on the soles of the feet and the palms of the hands (figure 13.A-1b). The thickness of the epidermis is largest in those places that bear the

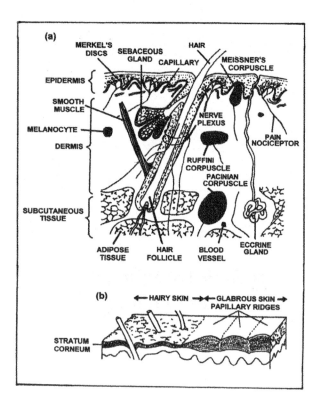

Figure 13.A-1. (a) A cross-section of skin, showing the three layers, (the epidermis, the dermis, and the subcutaneous layer), together with some of the other structures found in these layers [422]. (b) Note the structural differences in the upper layers of hairy skin (as on the outer portions of the arms) and glabrous skin (as on the palms of the hands).

most weight (the soles of the feet and palms of the hands) and varies from about 4 millimeters (0.16 inches) in the sole of the foot to about 0.1 millimeters (0.004 inches) in the eyelids. Ridges in the epidermal layers of the skin on the palms of the hands and the soles of the feet aid in gripping the sticky mat in postures such as *adho mukha svanasana*. In contrast to glabrous skin, thin skin is hairy, is composed of one fewer layers than is glabrous skin, figure 13.A-1b, and is found on the outer surfaces of the arms, for example.

Epidermis

A closer study of the epidermal layer shows it to consist of at least four layers, the deepest of which, the Malpighian layer, gives birth to epidermal cells that diffuse upward as they mature, to eventually become the dead, scaly cells of the horny layer (the stratum corneum in figure 13.A-1b). As the horny layer sloughs off—more than a million dead cells are cast off every hour—new cells are being produced at the same rate in the deepest layer. Formation of a new cell in the Malpighian layer requires only about two hours, and such a new-born cell has an average lifetime of about twenty-seven days [422] before it is cast off; the entire epidermis replaces itself every seventy-five days or so. With a lifetime of only seventy-five days, a seventy-year-old person will have made and discarded approximately 310 skins in a lifetime, together weighing more than 16 kilograms (thirty-six pounds) overall!

Dermis and Subcutaneous Layers

The dermis is vascularized, and being made largely of connective tissue (collagen and elastin; Subsection 12.A, page 481), it functions largely as the skin's supportive layer. This basal layer of the skin is the thickest and contains vessels for both blood and lymph, as well as nerve endings sensitive to touch, pressure, pain, heat, vibration, etc. The vascularization of the dermis plays a strong role in the regulation of the body's temperature, whereas the connective tissue within it works to hold the upper layers of the skin in strong contact with the deeper layers of fat and muscle.

The dermis also contains the melanocytes (figure 13.A-1a), pigment-bearing cells that can give skin the outward appearance of being pink, yellow, brown, or black, depending upon the quality and quantity of the pigment. Tattoos are formed when artificial colorants are inserted into the skin; they are permanent when the colorant is injected into the dermis, but not when injected into the epidermis, for in the latter case, epidermal exfoliation quickly releases the colorant to the outside. More relevant to *yogasana* teachers is the color change of the skin as a result of both vascular changes and changes in the degree of oxygenation of the blood while in the *yogasanas* (see below). Below the dermis lies the third layer, a subcutaneous tissue which is both muscular and the storehouse for the body's fat, which serves as fuel, as thermal insulation, and as cushioning.

On the molecular level, the two chief structural components giving skin both its strength and its resiliency are collagen and elastin, two proteinaceous substances (Subsection 12.A, page 481). Exposure of skin to sunlight not only results in the formation of vitamin D but unfortunately also weakens these proteins. As we age, the skin loses water, connective tissue becomes more dense and less elastic as it loses elastin (two layers below the uppermost stratum corneum in the epidermis), and the skin loses about 30 percent of its thickness as it becomes dried, wrinkled, and flaccid. Because skin in this aged state can be easily bruised, teachers of *yogasana* must use special care in adjusting aging students.

Skin Stretching

The ability to move deeply into a *yogasana* depends in part upon the resistance to stretching of the skin overlaying the muscles being stretched. This resistance of the skin to stretching is smallest in students with large, round bodies and largest in students who are thin. In both cases, the stretching of the muscles and overlaying skin will be sensed in the former by the muscle spindles (figure 11.B-1) and in the latter by the Ruffini corpuscles (figure 13.A-1**a**).

This stretching of the skin in *yogasana* offers an external signal to the *yogasana* teacher and an internal signal to the alert student as to what is happening in deeper layers of the student's body. As a superficial muscle is stretched in a *yogasana,* the skin just above the muscle, being bonded to it, will be stretched as well; i.e., when we stretch a muscle, we also must stretch the skin over that muscle. Thus, it is seen that muscle stretching involves overcoming the resistances to elongation in both the muscle and in the overlaying skin. With this in mind, two techniques that can be used to aid muscle stretching by pre-stressing the skin in concert with the muscles of the torso are presented in Box 13.A-1, page 504.

Scars

When the skin is injured, the pattern of electrical charges within the skin is altered, and in response to this local disturbance of the trans-

membrane voltage pattern, genetic processes are turned on, and repair cells are attracted to the region. Scars in the skin are formed when the skin is cut, and the cut edges are then bridged by a protein known as fibrin, which traps a certain number of red blood cells and platelets within itself; this matrix contracts to pull together the two sides of the wound (Subsection 12.B, page 492). Fibrin is the most stretchable natural fiber known, stretching elastically to a strain of 280 percent and finally breaking only at a strain of 430 percent. Scar tissue is the remnant of the collagen that eventually bridges the wound, and can severely impede the stretching of the skin in the vicinity of the wound and the muscles beneath the injured skin. Scars that form totally below the surface of the epidermis are known as adhesions (Subsection 11.G, page 480).

Skin Color and Trauma

On occasion, the pressure of a bone on muscle while in a *yogasana* posture results in the breaking of small capillaries under the skin and the release of blood between layers of connective tissue. Because the connective-tissue sheaths that trap the blood spilled from a bruise may conduct it far from the site of damage, a bruised coloration may appear at a distance from the point of injury. It is the hemoglobin in the released blood that gives the bruise its red-brown color. White blood cells, which are called into the damaged area to digest the spilled blood, form smaller hemoglobin fragments that are first green (biliverdin) and then yellow (bilirubin) [633]. As the trauma heals, coloration at the site of the bruise passes through brown, green, and yellow. Where there is an excess of bilirubin in the body, as when jaundiced, the skin again assumes a yellow color, however, this fades to normal skin tone as the excess is cleared.

Pressure on the skin that is so intense as to produce a wheal involves the sympathetic nervous system in the case of white wheals, and parasympathetic vagal hyperactivity in the case of red wheals [583]. White wheals immediately result from deep pressure on the skin, for at this time, blood is absent from the tissue, as super-

Box 13.A-1: Muscle Stretching Means Skin Stretching

It is simple to demonstrate the truth behind the idea that because the skin is bonded to the underlying muscle through the dermis, the skin is necessarily stretched when the overlaying muscle is stretched during *yogasana* practice. For example, lie on your back with both legs bent and with the right ankle resting on the left knee. With the thumb and index finger of the right hand, gently grasp the skin over the hamstrings at the back of the right thigh, and casually assess how loose it is. Then straighten the right leg, stretching its hamstrings, and note how little loose skin there is in the same place on the back of the thigh once the hamstrings are in extension. The work expended in extending the hamstrings of the right leg includes a contribution from that required to stretch the skin over the hamstrings. A similar relationship holds for a muscle in contraction and the skin over it, but perhaps to a lesser extent in most cases. This unavoidable relation of hamstring stretching and overlaying-skin stretching also applies to all of the other superficial muscles of the body. For those sensitive to stretching sensations in the skin, these signals originate with Ruffini corpuscles in the skin, which respond to the stretching of the underlying muscles (Subsection 11.B, page 440).

Overcoming Skin Resistance

A similar stretching penalty must be paid if the muscle being stretched is bound by tight clothing. For example, while wearing a tight T-shirt, twist far to the right in a seated, crossed-leg position, and note again how the fabric of the shirt appears bonded to the underlying skin and so only reluctantly follows the twist. While at the limit of the range of twisting motion, then grasp the left side of the shirt with the right hand, rotate it to the right, and note the increase in twist angle that results from the conrotatory (Subsection 8.B, page 298) action of skin and garment moving in the same direction.

Though adjustment of one's T-shirt is less practical in a posture such as *trikonasana*, for example, a prop can be used to the same end.[1] Cut an old six-foot-long yoga mat lengthwise into strips about 20 centimeters (eight inches) wide, and have a partner partially wrap it from left to right around your lower rib cage while you are standing in *tadasana*, leaving an upwardly projecting "pigtail" at the navel and taking care not to bind the breasts. Move then from *tadasana* to *trikonasana*-to-the-left as the partner pulls upward on the "pigtail" so as to encourage a conrotatory rotation of the mat along with that of the thoracic skin and muscles gripped by the mat. A student so aided in their spinal rotation while in *trikonasana* will see the ceiling as they never have seen it before!

A similar aid to linear stretching rather than spinal rotation is obtained with the student in *adho mukha svanasana*, thumbs and index fingers to the wall; a partner then stands with back to the wall, and placing a foot at the small of the back of the student, presses the foot upward and backward so as to stretch both the erector spinae and the skin over these muscles in the head-to-tail direction.

---

1   I am indebted to my teacher Judy Freedman for showing me this aid to spinal twisting. It is of great help in every *yogasana* requiring a depth of spinal twisting, and it is also useful when applied to rotating the upper arm (for example, *gomukhasana)* or leg (for example, the thigh of the bent leg in *parsvakonasana).*

ficial blood vessels contract in expectation of a large letting of blood to the outside. However, after about seven seconds, blood does flow to the injury site, and it becomes red and swollen as fluids leak from the affected cells, forming a red wheal [716].

Skin Color and Yogasana

Iyengar repeatedly has drawn our attention to monitoring the skin color of our students while they are in the *yogasanas* [391]. Much of the skin color is due to the nature of the blood just beneath the skin. Thus, when the skin is hot and is flushed with arterial blood, the color is red. On the other hand, if the skin is cold and the flow of blood through the skin is sluggish, then the oxygen in the blood will be consumed by the tissue, and the color will be that of deoxygenated blood; i.e., it will have a bluish cast, as it does in the veins. If, instead, there is a severe constriction of the vascular system and blood is lacking in the area, then the skin will have an ashen-white pallor [308].

Skin Rhythms

Several of the skin functions operate on twenty-four-hour cycles, known as circadian rhythms (Subsection 23.B, page 774). Thus, skin cells damaged by ultraviolet light during the day are repaired in the evening, the repair rate being largest at midnight and least at noon. On the other hand, the sebaceous glands, which keep the skin well oiled and supple, are most active at noon and least active at between 2:00 and 4:00 AM. The skin sweats most in the late afternoon, just when body temperature, muscle flexibility, and coordination are at their peaks.

As with many medications (Subsection 23.B, page 774), those absorbed through the skin are best applied at specific times for best results. Thus, most such medications work best when applied in the afternoon, when skin temperature is highest and the skin is most porous; an injection or topical rub of lidocaine, a pain killer, is twice as effective when applied at 4:00 PM as when applied at 8:00 AM. Many skin disorders, such as psoriasis and skin cancer, as well as the results of allergy

and tuberculosis testing, show cyclic patterns of activity in time [804].

Hair and Nails

Hair Growth

Hairs on the body surface are simple extensions of the epidermis, as are the fingernails and toenails. Hairs grow from structures within the skin called follicles; once a hair reaches maturity, it forms a club at the follicle base, which firmly anchors it in the skin (figure 13.A-1a). When a new hair then begins to grow at the base of the follicle, the old hair sooner or later drops out. Hair is constantly being shed in this way, at the rate of 50 to 150 per day. The hairs on our heads grow at a rate of 20 to 25 centimeters per year (eight to ten inches per year) and so can reach an overall length of 2 to 3 meters (six to nine feet) in ten years.

The arrector pili muscles, located at the bases of the body's hairs, are the smallest muscles in the body. In response to fear or to cold, contractions of these muscles make the hairs stand up on end; i.e., they are the muscles responsible for "goose pimples."

Hair Color

Aside from sexual attraction, hair (or the lack of it) would seem not to play a major role in the yogi's practice. Nevertheless, a nerve plexus does exist at the base of each hair, so that if and when a hair is moved, an afferent nerve impulse is triggered [431, 432, 878]. These hair receptors are undoubtedly triggered whenever a teacher touches a student's skin in order to make an adjustment, and possibly when the skin is stretched during *yogasana* practice.

Hair color is dictated by pigment cells (melanocytes) at the base of the follicles; when the melanocytes are no longer replaced because the corresponding stem cells no longer function, hair color returns to its natural, unpigmented hue: white. Because the genetic variation that leads to red hair also imparts to redheads a 25 percent higher threshold for pain as compared with blondes and brunettes [899], this aspect of hair color may express itself sooner or later in *yogasana* practice.

Composition

Chemically, hair is composed largely of a piezoelectric fibrous protein called keratin, which is also present in animal hooves, nails, horns, fish scales, silk, and spider webs. Keratin is a highly elastic, helically wound protein with a composition very different from that of collagen (Subsection 7.B, page 233). Though hair is a dead material, its apparent look depends upon secretions from the sebaceous glands, so that with too little secretion, it appears dry and brittle, and with too much, it appears greasy and lifeless. In all cases, hair consists of keratin-filled dead cells, the only live cells being within the follicle embedded in the skin.

The hairs on the heads of Asians are round in cross-section and therefore are straight, whereas hairs on the heads of African blacks are flat in cross-section and therefore are curly, and those of Occidentals are elliptic and thus intermediate in curviness.

The amount of body hair is largely determined by genetics, whereas the texture of the hair changes over a lifetime as the hormonal balances shift; androgens from the adrenal glands convert fine, white hairs into pigmented, stiff hairs and also can shift the relative abundances of hair in different areas of the skin [324].

Nail Growth

As with hair, the nails of the fingers and toes also are made largely of keratin; the growth rate of fingernails is about twice that of toenails, due to the greater rate of blood flow through the fingertips. The nails grow 30 percent more rapidly than normal when a female is pregnant, but when there are circulatory problems, nail growth slows; it is faster in children than in adults and faster in warm weather than in cold. The growth rate is larger in the big toe than in the other toes of the foot, presumably due to a greater rate of blood flow.

Section 13.B: Sensory Receptors in the Skin

There are a variety of sensory receptors populating the skin, with the abilities to record sensations not only of touch and pressure at the surface and at deeper layers, but also superficial sharp pain, deep-tissue pain, heat, cold, and muscle tension. The largest number of receptors sense pain, whereas the fewest sense temperature. There are an estimated fifty receptors in a 1-square-centimeter (0.15-square-inch) area of skin; however, the number is approximately 200 per square centimeter at the tip of the tongue [653], and overall there are between six and ten million such sensors on the skin of the body. It is important to point out that the sensors for light pressure and deep pressure are totally different functionally from the receptors for pain (Section 13.C, page 515) in the same skin areas. Strangely, some blind people have the ability to sense the direction of and distance to objects, which they describe as involving a feeling in the skin of the face (Subsection 17.B, page 669). Before going into the various types of touch sensors in the skin, we will first consider the general phenomenon of sensor adaptation, below.

Receptor Adaptation

You may walk into a yoga studio and sense a strong smell of impurity, yet after a minute or two, the sensation has passed, though the odor is still present. This is an example of the phenomenon known as receptor adaptation, in which there is a constant stimulus, but the receptor response to the stimulus falls toward zero with time. It is as if the sensor rapidly becomes fatigued, and so its output falls toward zero. As shown in figure 13.B-1a, a receptor with a rapid adaptation has an output that falls rapidly to zero, in spite of the constant stimulus, i.e., its response is nonzero only when the stimulus is rapidly changing, as when it is first applied or removed. For example, if you place your fingertip on the lip, there is a momentary sensation as they come into contact, but this fades rapidly to zero because of the rapid adaptation of the touch receptor. On the other hand, the sensation seems to persist as the fingertip is drawn back and forth over the lip, so as to constantly renew the contact.

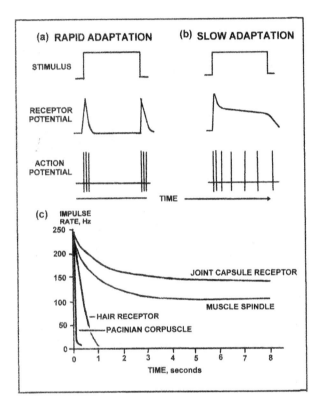

Figure 13.B-1. Comparison of the receptor and action potential responses for (a) a rapidly-adapting receptor and for (b) a slowly adapting receptor, both responding to the same square-wave stimulus. In the latter case, the receptor potential falls only slowly during the stimulus, and the action potential remains above threshold over the full course of the stimulus, but with decreasing frequency. In the former case, the action potential is above threshold only at the rapidly rising and rapidly falling ends of the stimulus, and so the receptor potential is zero at all places except at the points of rise and fall. (c) Variation of the impulse rates of some sensors in the body over time.

In contrast to the rapidly adapting sensor, receptors with slow adaptation (figures 13.B-1**b** and 13.B-1**c**) have outputs that are only slowly decreasing; the frequencies of their receptor potentials fall with time, albeit slowly, even though the stimulus levels are constant. Pain signals adapt very slowly if at all.

Adaptation occurs in most receptors and is useful in that it prevents the nervous system from being bombarded with information that is constant from one instant to the next, while favoring information that is changing in time. That is, a rapidly adapting receptor only gives a momentary signal whenever the stimulus turns on or off, but not in between where it is essentially unchanging (figure 13.B-1**a**). Thus, it is useful in tracking a stimulus that moves rapidly across the skin, but it is ineffective in staying in touch with a constant stimulus. In contrast, a slowly adapting receptor will give a signal of almost constant amplitude for a long period, but it is of no use in tracking a signal that varies rapidly in time or space (figure 13.B-1**b**). The consequences of such slow or rapid adaptations are presented below in the context of the touch receptors of the skin [422, 427].

Phasic Receptors

Skin receptors often are classified as either phasic or tonic, just as with muscle reflexes, (Section 11.D, page 448). The phasic receptors are rapidly adapting and are associated with pressure, touch, and smell, and though these receptors have very rapid responses to stimuli, they adapt to extinction (zero value) equally rapidly, even though the stimulus persists undiminished. The signals from the Pacinian corpuscles adapt to extinction in less than a few hundredths of a second, and hair receptors adapt to extinction in about one second, (figure 13.B-1**c**). Note that the rapidly-adapting phasic sensors do not adapt due to a rapidly-developing fatigue, but that they are constructed to be inherently sensitive only to the changing character of the stimulus and to be insensitive to constancy [107].

The phasic receptors are useful in that they not only offer immediate information as to rapid changes in the stimulus, but they also are rate sensors, and from rate information, one can anticipate what is about to happen and move to avoid it before it happens, if that is advantageous. The phasic receptors are important in that they can respond rapidly to a shift of the balance sensors, as when falling (Subsection V.C, page 886).

Tonic Receptors

Tonic receptors, such as the muscle-spindle fibers (Subsection 11.B, page 432), adapt only very slowly and are associated with the sensations of pain, body position, and certain chemicals in the body fluids. The tonic receptors are useful in that they can supply a long-lasting, ongoing signal that can contribute to the construction of the proprioceptive map. For this, we rely upon the muscle spindles and the Golgi tendon organs. Other slowly-adapting receptors are in the vestibular organs of the inner ear, the pain receptors, the baroreceptors of the arterial system, the chemoreceptors of the carotid and aortic systems, and the Ruffini endings and the Merkel's discs within the skin. There are some tonic receptors that require several days to reach extinction (the carotid and aortic baroreceptors) and some that may never go to extinction [308]. In contrast, the Meissner corpuscles, the hair receptors, and the Pacinian corpuscles are all rapidly adapting phasic receptors [422, 562].

Proprioceptors

As we assume a *yogasana* posture, the proprioceptors (Subsection 11.C, page 441) are actively sending their messages regarding body position and movement to the brain for synthesis into a complete body-posture picture. Because the neural signals adapt toward zero amplitude in time, once in the posture, one's sense of postural alignment fades. However, in the Iyengar approach, one first poses and then reposes [33] by continuously making slight adjustments. This constant readjustment keeps the posture dynamic, and from the proprioceptive point of view, readjustments repeatedly refresh the proprioceptive picture in the subconscious. Rapidly adapting sensors are important in this situation.

On the other hand, in a motionless posture such as *savasana,* many sensors are activated on first lying down, but after a few minutes, most will cease to transmit a signal, due to their rapid adaptation, whereas others may transmit for a long time afterward. Thus, the sensory signal in time may change in amplitude, etc., however, after about five minutes in *savasana,* virtually all of the proprioceptive signals will have reached extinction. Furthermore, while lying in *savasana,* the proprioceptive signals change only slowly with time, and signals that are near-constant in time are largely blocked by the reticular formation before they reach the higher brain centers.

Viewed psychologically, a student's sense of identity is closely tied to the sense of body image (Subsection 4.G, page 147) as reported proprioceptively, and as the proprioceptive signals adapt toward zero in *savasana,* the sense of personal identity fades. As the many small muscular activities that work to keep us locked in our ordinary state of consciousness fade when in *savasana,* the doorway is then opened to altered states of consciousness [848].

Light Touch

Our earliest sense response is to touch; this is present as early as one month of gestation. Though it has long been thought that the sense of touch is independent of the other sensory channels, it has recently been shown, for example, that the pain of a needle prick is enhanced when one looks at the needle and is lessened when one looks away [629]. This may relate to the tendency of beginning students to close their eyes when experiencing discomfort in the *yogasanas.*

Receptors

Several types of touch receptors such as Meissner's corpuscle, Merkel's disc, the Pacinian corpuscle, and the nerve plexus at the hair root occupy the more superficial layers of the skin (figure 13.A-1a). Such tactile sensors are most plentiful in the fingertips, around the mouth, and in the erogenous zones, with Meissner's corpuscles being 25 percent of all sensors in the fingertips.

These sensors are connected to the overlaying epidermis by discrete collagen fibers, so that even the slightest movement of the epidermis disturbs the Meissner's receptor and launches a signal.

The sensitivity of the surface sensors to light touch depends not only upon their depth beneath the skin's surface but also upon the density of touch-sensing units, or equivalently, the reciprocal of the distance of separation (D) between neighboring sensor units, i.e., 1/D. Simple experiments with pins, a ruler, and a willing subject show that the tongue, genitalia, fingertips, and lips have only a 1–3 millimeter (0.04–0.12 inch) separation between sensing units, whereas on the back of the hands, on the back body, and on the legs, the separation between adjacent receptors can be as large as 50–100 millimeters (two to four inches), figure 13.B-2. When expressed in terms of the number of receptors per unit area, the fingertips and tongue may have 100 touch receptors per square centimeter, whereas the back of the hand has only 10 ten per square centimeter. You can verify this difference by feeling the sharp cutting edges of your front teeth as you bite gently into the tip of your tongue and compare that to the relatively dull feeling when you bite gently into the back of your hand [340]. One clearly sees the effect of age on skin-touch sensitivity, because the average number of light-touch Meissner's corpuscles per square millimeter is eighty in the three-year-old, twenty in the young adult, and falls to just four per square millimeter in old age [583]. One should keep in mind the relative lack of skin sensitivity to changing pressure in the older student, especially when balancing on the feet.

Because the density of touch sensors in the fingertip is fifteen times as large as that on the leg, the area in the sensory cortex for finger sensations is far larger than that for leg sensations (figure 13.B-2), even though the legs themselves are by far the larger body part. As a consequence of this variable density of pressure sensors across the body, the skin-sensation map in the cortex is highly distorted compared to the body with which we are familiar. These quantitative differences in the degrees of spatial discrimination are reflected in the proportions of the sensory homunculus of Penfield [431, 651], (figure 4.C-6). This representation of the body is based upon each of the body parts having a spatial representation in proportion to the number of sensors per unit area within the body part. Thus, as with the representation of the motor cortex, the lips, tongue, and hands are quite large, and the back body and legs are quite small relatively. There is no representation of the heart, liver, or kidneys in the sensory homunculus, as sensations from these organs are referred to other skin areas [574] (Section 13.D, page 530).

Meissner's corpuscles are sensitive to very light touch, and though they are especially plentiful on the fingers (twenty-four corpuscles per square millimeter) and lips, they can be found just under the skin on all surfaces of the body, including the sole of the foot (for balance), the forearm, and the tongue. Meissner's corpuscles are very small and function at low frequencies (0.3–3 hertz). Because these receptors are solidly in the rapidly adapting category [422], when lying on the floor in *savasana*, for example, pressure signals from the Meissner's corpuscles are transmitted upward for proprioception, but only for an instant. Such proprioceptive signals can be refreshed in time by slight shifting of the weight on the floor, as when making small adjustments, but such shifts are not likely when in *savasana*. Therefore, when in *savasana,* the most neutral body position, there is a minimum of proprioceptive signaling, and thus it becomes the most relaxing position because it is the least stimulating to the central nervous system.

The Merkel's discs are sensors used to convey the sensations of itch on the skin. Light-touch sensors often are found close to a hair follicle, so that even if the skin is not touched directly, the hair can be moved, and the "touch" is detected.

Neural Routes

The afferent nerves carrying the signals of light touch and pressure utilize type-A fibers, i.e., thick, myelinated, and with rapid signal conduction (about ten meters per second), as is characteristic of the newest biotechnology available to primates and humans (Section 3.B, page 44). The rapidly

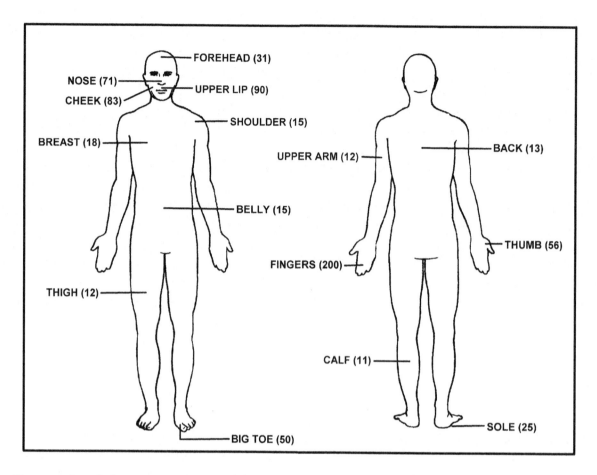

Figure 13.B-2. Relative measurements of the density (number per square centimeter) of receptor cells for surface pressure in the skin of the human body. The highest densities of such receptors are on the fingers, on the big toes, and within and around the mouth, in agreement with the relative proportions of the sensory cortex devoted to these areas (figure 4.C-6).

adapting signals from pressure and touch receptors ascend the spinal cord to the thalamus and then radiate to the postcentral gyrus in the sensory cortex. However, just before entering the spinal cord, the sensory nerves branch, so as to provide collaterals to the α-motor neurons participating in reflex-arc circuits (Section 11.D, page 446). The ascending fibers from the light-touch receptors also send branches to midbrain motor centers and to centers in the reticular formation (Subsection 4.B, page 74) to influence involuntary motor activity. Sensors of the skin often are involved in reflex arcs, as when one steps barefooted on a sharp object and instantly lifts the foot, or when one tries to pick up a hot potato and immediately drops it. See Section 11.D, page 446, for details on the neural circuitry involved in such arcs.

The sensory nerves from different parts of the body are bundled more and more as they ascend, but they still keep their sense of order, with the nerves from the legs on the inside of the spinal cord and those from the arms, neck and face on the outer edge. These packing patterns are then resolved into a coherent picture of the body in the higher centers of the brain.

That signals from the light-touch receptors can be factors in conscious intelligence is shown by Braille reading, wherein one learns to read patterns of raised bumps on paper using the fingertips, and these patterns are then understood by the conscious mind as letters. Other forms of "dermographia" are discussed by Montagu [583]. Perhaps this is a form of the skill developed by Iyengar [391], for whom reading the messages of the skin during *yogasana* practice plays such a large role. One can imagine, in his case, that the muscle tensions generated in the *yogasanas* pull on the skin so as to stimulate the light-pressure and deep-pressure sensors, and that he is consciously aware of the pressure patterns in his skin generated both by the muscles upon the overlaying skin and by the pressure of the floor.

It is worth noting that Iyengar [391] places great stress on the skin as both an organ of perception and as the body's outermost boundary. In the work of the *yogasanas,* he strives to connect the intelligence of the mind to sensations in the skin and the underlying flesh. All the while, he remains relaxed so that the skin is not overstretched to the point of transmitting pain signals, which would swamp the more subtle signals of the pressure sensors. Once the link between skin sensations and the intelligence of the mind is established, one then can begin to move from the skin toward the soul, the innermost level of one's being.

Tickling

In contrast to touching, tickling is a random stimulation of nerve endings, registering as confusion in the cerebellum [419, 632]. It is strange (and meaningful) that you cannot tickle yourself (unless you are schizophrenic), nor can someone tickle you if you dislike them; only someone you like and feel trusting toward can elicit the laughter of tickling [583]. This suggests that in the overabundance of touch signals going upward to the spine, those involving self-touching are discarded as unimportant, whereas those with a stronger emotional content (a lover's caress or an insect crawling up one's leg) register more insistently in the conscious sphere. The anticipation of a tickle, as when approached by someone with wiggly fingers, leads to the same end as a real tickle, perhaps involving the activation of mirror neurons (Subsection 4.G, page 142) and/or spindle cells (Subsection 4.C, page 97) in the brain. Tickling of a very light sort in especially sensitive areas is described as "knismesis," and is pure pleasure, whereas "gargalesis" is a harder type of tickle with sensations of mixed pleasure and pain.

The laughter of tickling is a consequence of

an uneasy feeling due to the physical contact, which leads to tension and a mild state of panic. However, if one can remain calm and relaxed and keep the breath moving when tickled, then just as with the situation when one is trying to tickle oneself or when one is in a *yogasana* posture, one will survive the tickling ordeal in a state of detached solemnity. Laughing when tickled also involves an element of surprise at being touched in that way. The *yogasana* teacher sooner or later will attempt to adjust a new student and find that whenever they place their hand at that innocent spot for adjustment, the student collapses to the floor in a fit of laughter. Unwittingly, the teacher has found a very ticklish spot and so must approach it in the future with slow and firm pressure so as to avoid stimulating the reflex.

The random nature of the stimulation apparently is important in tickling, for a gentle rhythmic stroking of the skin in general is quite relaxing, as are rocking the body at a low frequency and chanting in the lower register.

Laughter as Therapy

During laughter, the muscles of the abdomen, legs, and back momentarily spasm; stress hormones are released by the adrenal medulla; fifteen muscles in the face create a smile; the tear ducts are activated; the concentrations of cells of the immune system rise in the mouth; diaphragmatic spasms force air through the epiglottis and vocal folds and the heart rate, the blood pressure, and the breathing rate increase [419]. The mechanics of the laugh are orchestrated in the brainstem.

Humor is very effective in easing pain. According to N. Cousins, ten minutes of a good belly laugh is equal to at least two hours of pain-free sleep [170]. On the other hand, there really is only a slight physiological difference between laughing and crying (Box 14.F-3, page 594).

Deep Pressure

Pacinian Corpuscles

The Pacinian corpuscles (figure 13.A-1a) are located not only in the deeper layers of the skin but also in the joints and within the internal organs. These corpuscles respond to heavy pressure at those deep layers [432] and are most sensitive for vibrations in the 40–1,000 hertz range. The presence of these sensors within the internal organs may be an important factor in the subconscious interoceptive sense we have of the conditions of such organs (Subsection 11.C, page 444), whereas their large numbers in the soles of the feet allow us to be very sensitive to ground vibrations and to incipient falling when on our feet. The Pacinian corpuscles are most plentiful in the palm of the hand, the sole of the foot, the genitals, and in the joints.

A Pacinian receptor consists of a sensory nerve ending surrounded by a collagenous capsule up to 4 millimeters (0.2 inches) long. When deformed by external pressure, the capsule wall changes its permeability to Na^+ ions, thus leading to a DC voltage change within the capsule that is proportional to the pressure. As with many such mechanoreceptor signals, the DC voltage is transduced into the frequency domain, so that the pressure is proportional to the frequency of the signal rather than to the magnitude of its voltage, and the modulated signal then is sent to the central nervous system. Because the deformation of the Pacinian capsule is quickly relieved by a readjustment of the layers of the capsule, the signals from the Pacinian corpuscles are rapidly adapting, and as such, they produce a signal only when the stimulus is rapidly changing.

Pacinian corpuscles use type-C neural fibers (slow, 1 meter per second), thin, and unmyelinated (table 3.B-2) for afferent transmission, as found in the basic primitive sensory systems of all vertebrates [432]. These type-C fiber bundles synapse at the dorsal spine and then rise as high as the thalamus. As discussed in Section 11.C, page 441, signals from the Pacinian corpuscles may help in constructing an instantaneous proprioceptive map of the body in motion, for the thalamus is known to share information with many parts of the brain involved with construction of such a map. Type-C fibers also have been found to carry light-touch sensations from hairy skin, sending the signals to the region of the ce-

rebral cortex called the insula, this being a region receptive to them and eliciting an emotional response. Such signals are sensed as "pleasant," and they may be responsible for the pleasant feeling one senses on being touched gently by the teacher during *yogasana* practice (Subsection 13.B, page 513) or otherwise caressed or bundled.

It is rather strange that we *yogasana* students spend so much time walking around in bare feet, for one generally hardens the soles of the feet in this way, thereby making them less sensitive to light pressure.

Merkel's Discs

Up to this point, it has been uncertain which sensors are slowly adapting so that they can continue to transmit a pressure signal from the skin on a long-term basis. It would appear to be the Merkel's discs, which are slowly adapting and are sensitive to skin indentation. When the student lies down for *savasana*, there are immediate sensations from the Meissner, Pacinian, and Merkel receptors, with the first two adapting rapidly to zero and only the sensations from the Merkel's discs persisting. After five minutes or so, even the Merkel's disc sensations have adapted, and one totally loses the sensation of the back of the body pressing on the floor, unless the muscles are periodically reactivated. When in postures held for long periods of time, such as *sirsasana*, etc., sensations of pressure from the floor after five minutes or so in the posture may still involve the Merkel's discs, but more likely they arise from the frequent readjustments of the posture, which reactivate these and other pressure sensors.

As discussed in Section 11.B, page 440, the Ruffini corpuscles are subcutaneous sensors, sensitive to both the magnitude and the direction of skin deformation as the muscles below contract and relax. Such slowly adapting and direction-sensitive sensors of skin deformation are assumed to play large roles in the construction of the proprioceptive map and in balancing (Subsection V.C, page 886) and they are no doubt active in Iyengar's perception of the muscular actions sensed through the skin [388, 394].

Thermal Sensors

It is thought that the temperature receptors in the skin are just free nerve endings [432], but they must be more than that, since there are two distinct types: Krause corpuscles for sensing temperatures below 33° C (91.4° F) and Ruffini corpuscles[1] for sensing temperatures above 33° C (91.4° F) [360]. The Krause corpuscles are found within the membranes of certain joints. Both use slow (less than 2.5 meters-per-second conduction velocity) types C and A_δ fibers. As with other skin receptors, the information from the temperature sensors is presented to the brain as a frequency representation. These sensors are intimately involved in thermoregulation of the body (Subsections 14.C, page 573, and 20.D, page 725).

In most parts of the skin, there are about ten times as many cold receptors as hot. In addition to the hot and cold receptors, there are receptors in the skin for burning hot (45–60° C; 113–140° F) and freezing cold (5–15° C; 41–59° F) temperatures; signals from these sensors connect directly to the pain nociceptors. (Nociceptors for sensing pain, Subsection 13.C, page 518, simply are free nerve endings that are excited by exposure to the fluids surrounding injured tissue.) At the extremes of temperature, the sensations are identical, i.e., hot or cold, the sensation is painful. Abrupt changes of skin temperature of 0.01° C are said to be detectable by the hot and cold receptors [308]. As the mid-range thermal receptors are rapidly adapting, we feel much warmer (or colder) when the temperature rises (or falls) abruptly than when the change is more gradual.

In some cases, the rapidly conducting nerves that otherwise would carry sensations of touch have been disabled; however, in this situation, the sensations of a soft caress can be carried by the slowly conducting nerves normally reserved for sensing temperature and pain [279]. Indeed, when a cold object touches the skin, both the rapidly conducting A_α fibers sensitive to cold sensations and the C-type fibers that carry sensations of pain are activated; however, these converge on the same neurons in the spinal cord. It appears that the signal from the A_α fiber gets to the spinal cord sooner and then acts to block the pain signals, so that one senses a strong cold signal but no pain [355].

Emotions and Touching

Given the unquestionable importance of touching and caressing in all infants [583], it is no surprise that tactile stimulation of the skin can be of great importance to an adult's emotional stability. Thus, actions such as scratching the head, rubbing the chin, and rubbing the eyes are self-comforting and help to reduce tension. Because clasping of the hands also releases tension, both facial self-massage and light hand clasping can be recommended when doing *savasana* with beginner students who are tense.

Montagu [583] discusses several examples of how the body may express psychosocial and cultural stress as skin disorders. Thus, soldiers bombarded repeatedly in World War One developed a darkening of the skin called "fear melanosis." In other cases, pent-up anger and frustration precipitate itching that is satisfied only by scratching.

The waxing and waning of many diseases of the body and emotional states are expressed through eruptions through the skin. Thus, stress is held to be a significant factor in profuse sweating, warts, itching, eczema, hives, psoriasis, acne, and herpes, given in order of decreasing importance of the stress component, with stress being 100 percent responsible for profuse sweating but only 36 percent responsible for a herpes outbreak.

Touching by the *Yogasana* Teacher

One can do no better than to read Montagu's monograph on the skin [583] in order to learn how absolutely crucial touching is to the proper

---

1 The temperature-sensitive Ruffini corpuscles in the skin are not to be confused with the other Ruffini corpuscles also within the skin, which function as stretch receptors (Subsection 11.B, page 440). Strangely, the temperature sensors of the tongue are able to bind the capsaicin of chili peppers, and so the hot "taste" of such peppers is a really a stimulation of the Ruffini temperature sensors.

socialization and maturation of the infant. This is true in different cultures, at different times, and in different species. Babies who are cuddled, pressed to a parent's breast, wrestled with, tossed and caught, swaddled, etc., are much more outgoing, sociable, and happy as children and adults than are their touch-deprived brothers and sisters. The sense of touch is the first sense to be developed, appearing in the first month of gestation.

Even as adults, the innocent touch can be a life-affirming gesture for those who are otherwise untouched for whatever reason. This can be especially true for the elderly. To be touched in a sympathetic way by another person is to connect with them, not only on a yogic level, but on a personal level, if they need to feel that. *Yogasana* practice with a teacher offers the opportunity for such touching as a side benefit to proper *yogasana* instruction, but also for its own sake. Similar comforting effects can result when the students hold themselves, as in *pasasana* or *pavan muktasana*.

The object in touching the student in *yogasana* is either to try to reconnect the student's consciousness with the muscular action in a particular region of the body, or to aid a particular motion or action from the outside. If the teacher wants to stress the rolling inward of the upper front thigh, for example, then it is sufficient to use the fingertips to brush the flesh of the thigh in the proper direction, giving a student a clear signal of what is to be done. In this situation, it is the rapidly adapting Meissner's corpuscle that responds to the touch and transmits its sense of movement to the brain.

When placing the hand on a student with the intention of moving a limb, for example, the full length of the hand (fingertips to palm) should be placed on the limb, and the fingers should point in the direction in which you wish the student's flesh to move. The teacher's hands should never press on flesh that is not supported by bone; i.e., never press on the eyes, throat, lower abdomen, etc., and never hold or press at a joint. Instead, apply pressure at the belly of the muscle.

Physiologically, when the pressure sensors in the skin overlaying a muscle is stimulated, the large muscle fibers are activated more quickly and used

more efficiently, leading to an increase of muscle strength [723]. This fact may be relevant to the increased action that results from wrapping the thorax with a yoga mat and then pulling on the mat (and, indirectly, the thoracic skin) in order to induce a deeper spinal twist, (Box 13.A-1, page 504).

When the student is adjusted manually by the teacher and the student is receptive to that touch, then a bond begins to develop between them. This bond can be strengthened if the teacher adjusts his or her breath so as to be in synchronicity with that of the student. In this case, the signal for movement on the student's part is on the exhalation [488]. Experiments have been carried out on women who, when placed under stress by the experimenters and then touched by their husbands, immediately reduced their levels of stress by significant amounts. There was a smaller but noticeable reduction in stress even when touched by a stranger. There must be some element of this touch response when the teacher touches the student while he or she is stressed in an uncomfortable *yogasana* posture.

Unwelcome Touching

In working to move students appropriately, you will find some students who clearly like the touching aspect of the adjustment, or at least like where the adjustment is taking them, as witnessed by their sigh of pleasure. On the other hand, there also will be students who, for whatever reason, do not like to be touched, especially women being touched by a man. Teachers must remain alert to this possibility and respect the student's wish without seeking clarification or further comment. If you are rebuffed, rather than taking it personally, consider instead that the woman may have been abused by a man as a child or as an adult and is not ready to be touched in any way by a person in authority. Many times, demonstration on the teacher's body rather than on that of the student (or use of a prop) will suffice to get the yogic point across without violating a student's personal space. In this regard, there is a general confusion among some students that equates tactile touching with sexual touching. The differences between these two kinds of touching are described very clearly by Juhan [422] and Barrett [40] and should be clear in the minds of *yogasana* teachers, if not in the minds of their students.

Touching and Balance

A rather new and interesting approach to balancing on the foot involves the exquisite sense of touch in the finger, as discussed in Subsection V.D, page 902. In this approach, one stands in *vrksasana,* for example, but near enough to a wall so that the tip of the little finger on one hand is in contact with the wall. As one starts to fall, the sense of the falling in the little finger is immediately relayed to the ankle, and the appropriate action at the ankle is taken so as to restore balance!

Section 13.C: Pain and Pleasure

Delayed Gratification

The subjects of pain and pleasure are so closely related that it is often difficult to separate them, but we will try. In this section, the nonspecific aspects of pain and pleasure in general are discussed, with specific mention of their relevance to *yogasana* practice, whereas the specifics of *yogasana* injuries to muscles and joints that lead to pain are considered in Section 11.G, page 478, and in Appendix II, page 833.

In recent experiments, it has been shown that when the result of a particular action is pleasurable, then delay of the outcome increases the level of pleasure; i.e., "It is worth the wait," and the longer we wait, the deeper is the eventual gratification. It also works in the opposite sense, because the longer we postpone experiencing the outcome of a fearful, negative action, the higher then is the level of pain associated with that experience. Translating this into the *yogasana* realm, one might argue that the longer and deeper is one's *yogasana* practice, the sweeter and more satisfying is the *savasana* that follows, whereas if one is fearful of the discomfort of backbending, then

the longer its practice is delayed, the more painful is the experience. In general, a sense of fear and/or dread heightens the level of pain experienced when finally confronting the object of our dread.

The Physiology of Pain

The yoga practitioner who is committed to teaching often finds herself enmeshed in other people's pain and will quickly come to see how much pain there is in the world and how great are our efforts to avoid pain if we can. Understandably, it may seem that the world would be a much better place if pain could be banished from our lives, however, that view ignores the fact that pain is a **useful** signal, alerting us to something going wrong in the body; those without any sensitivity to pain are at great risk for harming themselves, because they do not sense the alarm signals. Touch a hot object, and the pain of the contact goes immediately to the somatosensory centers in the spine and leads to an immediate withdrawal of the hand before further damage can be done; without the pain signal, the damage to the hand might otherwise be catastrophic. Conversely, pain is not only uncomfortable but often causes muscles to contract and so blocks the responsiveness of the tissues involved. Frequently, there is strong activation of the sympathetic nervous system when we are injured and feeling pain. Because pain sensors are only slowly adapting, if at all (Subsection 13.B, page 506), the sensation of pain can linger for a very long time, even being present long after the wound or injury has healed.

Because pain occurs whenever there is damage being done to the tissues of the body, pain signals are protective unless overridden. Thus, sitting in *padmasana* for an extended period, for example, can lead to a local ischemia of the tissue pinned between the floor and the ischial tuberosities, and this lack of circulation can lead to tissue damage and resulting pain (Subsection II.B, page 835). Normally, we subconsciously sense the onset of such pain and subconsciously shift the weight to restore circulation. However, if one were insensitive to this pain, then one could do serious damage to the body by remaining in the posture without a shift of the weight [308]. Depending on the tissue injured, pain may be cutaneous (skin), somatic (muscle), or visceral (internal organ).

Pain and Muscle Action

Once a muscle is in pain, there is a strong tendency to assume a guarded posture that serves to avoid or minimize the pain, often by transferring the mechanical stress onto other muscles, thereby placing them in spasm (Subsection 11.G, page 474). While in the guarded posture, unused muscles meanwhile lose strength, thereby creating more discomfort. People in this situation of guarding themselves against pain by not moving, will come to feel that any type of physical therapy, including *yogasana* therapy, can be the toughest part of pain treatment [243]. Perhaps we are all more or less like this, with assumed positions that keep our internal pains hidden from ourselves, but which we later have to face in *yogasana* practice. Perhaps it is this aspect of having to face hidden pains that makes *yogasana* practice such an emotional experience, both positive and negative.

Of course, *yogasana* practice can be used in a deliberate way to reduce pain, rather than generate it. So, for example, many stretches are designed to release tension in chronically tense muscles and so give one a sense of relief from pain and discomfort. Elongations also are used to realign the bones of the body, thereby easing the pain at misaligned joints, etc. Mental anguish also can be relieved by *yogasana* practice (Chapter 22, page 766).

In many other places in this work, we speak of how there are often two routes for afferent neural signals, one going rapidly to subconscious centers in the central nervous system, and a second, slower route going to the conscious sphere. It is this way with pain signals as well [105]. Thus, when we sprain an ankle and then try to walk on it, there is a subconscious reflexive action to the attendant pain that shifts the way we walk, so as to minimize the pain. This subconscious, after-the-fact reflex has been called by Mezieres, the "antalgic reflex a posteriori" (ARAP). Unfortunately, when ARAP is in action, it can silence the pain without curing the problem, and so it not only

can postpone the moment of reckoning but can act to transport the problem to another place in the body. I feel that a significant part of the bodily pain and discomfort experienced by the beginner in *yogasana* practice is the result of a simple uncovering of these unimagined ARAP problems lying dormant within all of us.

As we age, we tend to limit our spectrum of bodily responses, so as to be more sensitive to pain and less sensitive to the other aspects of body awareness. Our feelings about pain are strongly colored by our fear of it, and this is second only to our fear of death. It is known that fear, anxiety, and worry make pain worse. It is also relevant that if we hear mentioned a tale of agony, we respond to it with not only an emotional sympathy but also with an autonomic response of the sympathetic branch that often involves either the involuntary lifting of the testicles by the cremaster muscles, or by contraction of the womb. Considerable evidence suggests that men and women use different neural circuitry in sensing pain.

Men and women differ in another way. Though women tend to feel more pain initially, their anxiety falls thereafter with time, whereas the anxiety for men tends to increase with time after the initial sensation. This is important, for the levels of anxiety can have a strong influence on the intensity of the pain sensation.

Two Components of Pain

Because pain is both a sensation and a perception, perhaps more so than with any other sense, pain brings the body and the mind immediately and intimately together at the level of the central nervous system. Pain often has two major components: (**1**) the physiological sensation of pain at the site of physiological damage and (**2**) the emotional and psychological responses to the pain, such as worry, anxiety, and agitation (which can keep the pain gates open) or exercise, relaxation, and understanding the sources of pain (which can keep the pain gates closed). The first component of pain, **1**, involves the somatosensory cortex and reflexive activation of the relevant muscles, whereas the second component, **2**, goes to the limbic system in the brain (Subsection 4.C, page

80), which then adds an emotional component to the sensation.

The physiological component **1** of the pain response eventually is localized in the anterior cingulate cortex, which is stimulated to register pain regardless of whether it is due to bodily injury or to a psychic wound. The pain registered as component-**2** is psychological and so is sensitive to our mood, the perceived pain being damped by good mood and accentuated by bad mood. Similarly, if the level of pain is high, it tends to make us grumpy and high-strung. Those who see everything as a catastrophic calamity are reinforcing a mental habit of thinking that generally maximizes pain sensations.

Pain signals are known to travel from the sensor, through the spinal cord and brainstem, to synapse finally at either the medial or the lateral portions of the thalamus, these two paths being called the paleospinothalamic and the neospinothalamic tracts, respectively (figure 11.A-7**b**). Sharp pain signals are carried rapidly by A_α afferent fibers to the lateral portion of the thalamus, and the location of the pain is well defined and conscious, whereas dull pain signals are more slowly carried by the C-type afferent fibers to the medial portion of the thalamus, where they are diffuse and only weakly in our awareness [671a]. The neospinothalamic tract is phylogenetically much newer than is the paleospinothalamic tract, as one might have guessed from their names; rapid and localized excitation along the former corresponds to component **1** of the pain signal reaching the sensory cortex, while the diffuse pain signal, with its many branches to subcortical nuclei, correlates well with dull, diffuse-pain component **2**, as described above.

When watching another in pain, our response is an empathetic stimulation of our own anterior cingulate cortex, much like the phenomenon of mirror-neuron learning by watching someone else perform a physical act, (Subsection 4.G, page 142). In the context of *yogasana* practice with a fellow student, this empathy can be a hindrance if it is expressed too strongly, for this could encourage a negative mental state in one's partner, if applied injudiciously, and an increased sensation of pain.

Yogasana practice can be of great use in regard to the two aspects of pain, as with practice, one can learn to more or less control the pain, component **1** and to alter one's perception of the meaning of pain, component **2**. One of the lessons of our *yogasana* practice is that some pain is an inescapable part of life and that one can learn how best to handle such times of unavoidable pain by practicing pain control in the *yogasanas,* by learning how to minimize the pain, how to deal with that part of pain that cannot be ignored, and how to get on with one's life.

There are several physiological situations relevant to *yogasana* practitioners that can result in pain:

> » Excessive stimulation of a sensory organ, as when exceeding by far the thresholds of cold, heat, or pressure
> » External pressure on or pinching of a nerve
> » Nerve damage
> » Swelling of an internal organ
> » Extended contraction of a muscle
> » Muscle spasms
> » Low blood flow to a muscle or an organ

Though the topic of pain is discussed under the heading of "The Skin," pain receptors are to be found not only on the skin but also deep within the body, and unlike the situation with pressure and touch sensations, such referred-pain signals are slowly adapting and therefore long-lasting. When pain signals are delivered to the brain, there follows a diffusion of the signal to many different areas simultaneously; i.e., pain involves a highly distributed processing system within the central nervous system. It can be difficult to launch a pain signal unless one is supersensitive, and once launched, it can be difficult to turn off.

Guyton [308] describes the two types of component **1** physiological pain as acute (sharp, fast, and immediate), as when one pricks oneself with a needle, and as slow or chronic, such as the pain accompanying arthritis. Acute pain is rarely felt in the deeper organs but is more or less localized to the skin and is relayed upward using A_α pain fibers, whereas chronic pain is associated with deep-tissue destruction, is not localized to surface structures (as with acute pain), and uses type-C pain fibers for transmission of the sensation (tables 3.B-2 and 3.B-3). Because recognition of the pain signal is so important to the well-being of the body, the chronic pain signals are essentially nonadapting with time (Section 13.C, page 520); and in fact, in some cases, the pain sensation intensifies with time rather than fades, as with the other receptors.

Fetal Pain

It has been argued most recently that because the perception of pain involves neural circuitry that is not yet present in a fetus, and because the fetus in utero is bathed constantly in sleep-inducing hormones, there is little or no chance that pain can be sensed by a fetus in utero. This is in line with the idea that pain is a learned psychological phenomenon, requiring experience and memory of the pain-causing event. Fetuses do not feel pain until the twenty-eighth week of gestation, for it is only in the third trimester that nociceptor signals from the skin actually are transmitted beyond the thalamus and up to the emotional center in the cortex, where they are interpreted as "pain." Previous to that, the higher-level neural machinery is not in place in order for nociceptor signals to be felt consciously, even though the pain receptors are in place after only the eighth week of gestation.

Nociceptors

In all cases, the pain receptors are free nerve endings, but the stimuli responsible for pain may be mechanical, thermal, or chemical. In the latter category, pain is elicited by exposure of the free nerve endings to chemicals like bradykinin, serotonin, histamine, the prostaglandins, K^+ ions, acetylcholine, and proteolytic enzymes, among others. If the free nerve endings have been sensitized by the release of histamine, then a pin prick, for example, in the involved area can cause intense pain.

When one is in pain, both the acute-pain and the chronic-pain signals can be stimulated simultaneously and the pain signals can be sent as high as the thalamus, and thence to the cortex for action and interpretation. In the case of chronic-pain transmission, there is a considerable neural interaction with nuclei in the reticular formation that is absent in the case of the acute-pain transmission. The acute and chronic pathways differ in another regard: the acute pain is sensed to be quite localized at the point of bodily insult, whereas the chronic-pain sensation is much less localized, and the area of affliction can be difficult to pin down.

More or fewer of the fibers in a muscle will be recruited to participate in a muscular action, depending upon the magnitude of the load to be moved. In a similar way, more or fewer neural sensors may be recruited to carry pain signals upward to the cortex, depending on the severity of the pain.

The nociceptors as found on the skin, in the joints and muscles, and in the viscera can be triggered by thermal (both hot and cold), mechanical, and chemical insults to the body tissue. Unlike all of the other mechanoreceptors (Section 11.B, page 428), those for pain are simply the free nerve endings of the pain-conducting nerve fibers (figure 13.A-1). Though some endings are specific for thermal or mechanical pain stimuli, others are polymodal, responding to all forms of pain-generating stimuli.

The nociceptor fibers in general are either the A_α myelinated fibers (Section 3.B, page 44), having high conduction velocity and giving the sensation of sharp, stabbing pain, or the more slowly conducting, unmyelinated C fibers, which are polymodal. It appears that signals of intense pain travel more quickly than those for slight pain [338], and once tissue is injured and the pain signal is sent upward, then inflammation is initiated.

The free nerve endings of the nociceptors have relatively high thresholds for activation, so that those noninjurious stimuli that can strongly excite touch receptors, for example, do not excite the pain receptors. If the stimulation is so intense that the tissue cells are injured, then the affected cells burst and immediately release chemicals into the surrounding tissue. Two of these released chemicals that are of the most interest to us are the prostaglandins and histamine.

Prostaglandins

The prostaglandins (a group of fourteen different substances), when released from injured cells, act to sensitize and to activate the free nerve endings of the nociceptors in the vicinity of the injury. With this sensitization, exposure of the nerve endings to substances at the injury site such as serotonin, bradykinin, or histamine leads immediately to a pain signal being launched along the nociceptor toward the spinal cord. From there, the nociceptor signal may become active in a reflex arc (withdrawal of the foot from a sharp object, say) or may branch upward toward the cortex, to be registered psychologically and consciously as pain.

Prostaglandins not only stimulate uterine contractions during childbirth and during the active phase of the menstrual cycle, but they are also prominent in the brain during headaches at the times of menstruation [201]. Because aspirin and NSAIDS (nonsteroidal anti-inflammatory drugs) inhibit the action of the COX-2 cyclo-oxygenase enzyme (which otherwise produces the prostaglandins), they can lessen pain sensations. The effect of hormones on the perception of pain during the menstrual and pregnancy cycles is discussed in Subsections 21.A, page 742, and 21.B, page 745.

In men, the pain centers most often involve cluster headache, back pain, pancreatic disease, and duodenal ulcer, whereas for women, the most common complaints are for migraine, tension headache, gallbladder disease, arthritis of elbow and knee, irritable bowel syndrome, cystitis, and carpal tunnel disease [561].

Histamine and Inflammation

Histamine acts not only to trigger the pain reaction but also to promote inflammation, the first stage of healing following an injury. Histamine dilates the blood vessels locally, so that the injured tissue is flooded with fresh blood, making the af-

fected area redden and rise in temperature. It also promotes a super-permeability of the vessel walls, so that excess lymph (Section 14.G, page 595) is produced, and swelling appears. The extra blood flow attendant to inflammation also brings immune cells to the area in question, and the cell walls in the inflamed area becomes sticky, so that the immune cells become anchored to the affected area and are not swept away in the blood flow.

Once a tissue site is damaged, the threshold for generating a nociceptor action potential is lowered below that of the initial threshold, i.e., the injured area becomes more sensitive to pain stimuli. Although inflammation speeds the healing of wounds and is antimicrobial, it also seems to be an important causative aspect of arthritis, asthma, atherosclerosis, etc. The inflammatory response is inhibited by cortisone.

Ischemia

There is another aspect of pain production that may be particularly relevant to the student of *yogasana*. When a muscle is either strongly contracted or overstretched, there is a mechanical stress on the local musculature that slows the flow of blood into and out of the muscle. In response to this ischemic condition (low or zero blood flow locally), the stressed cells exude arachidonic acid. In the presence of the enzyme cyclo-oxygenase, arachidonic acid is oxidized to the prostaglandins, and the free nerve endings in the muscle thereby become sensitized to pain [427, 654]. This pain mechanism may be at work while stretching in the *yogasanas,* or afterwards, if there is a residual spasm in the muscle in response to stretching. It might also be responsible for the pain of a herniated vertebral disc, which presses on spinal muscles so that arachidonic acid is released, leading to the production of the prostaglandins (see the work of Sarno [745, 746]).

As one might expect, if there are yogic ways to chemically generate pain, there are also yogic ways to chemically eradicate pain (Subsections 3.D, page 57, and 13.C, pages 523 and 525).

Regardless of the exact physiological mechanism for pain and its relief, it is a good idea not to directly challenge pain through the *yogasanas.*

Thus, for example, if one has a torn hamstring, one should avoid a direct hamstring stretch, such as *uttanasana,* but it would be acceptable to work the hamstring peripherally, as in *dandasana.* Because the connective tissue forms one continuous web throughout the body (Subsection 12.B, page 486), even working to stretch peripheral muscles, nonetheless will have a significant effect on the site of the injury. A timetable for reasonable resting periods following different muscle injuries is given in table 11.G-1.

Chronic Pain

In general, repetitive sensory signals command the brain's attention and are dealt with in one of two ways: the brain either accommodates to the irritation or is sensitized to the irritation. If the signal is only mildly bothersome (as with a loud radio in the next room when one is trying to practice), then the central nervous system becomes habituated to the signal, and the sensation of the annoyance fades with time. In contrast, if the sensation is truly noxious (pain from a stone in the shoe or worse), then the central nervous system becomes sensitized to the signal, and for this reason, it becomes even more painful over time. See Subsection 4.F, page 129, for a further discussion of the effects of sensitization and habituation on neural morphology. In the case of the noxious stimulus, the neural circuitry associated with the action that is persistent over time changes so as to make the neural path easier to traverse. This is called learning (Section 4.G, page 135). Unfortunately, if pain signals are transmitted for a sufficiently long time, the neurons learn this lesson too and then are able to transmit pain spontaneously. Called chronic pain, this condition is often associated with psychological or emotional problems [326]. Chronic pain signals have a way of indiscriminately sensitizing other pain pathways so that they respond to weak stimuli. Moreover, it has been shown that chronic back pain can lead to a physical shrinking of the prefrontal cortex and a corresponding diminution of the ability to make decisions [561a].

In the case of chronic pain, the neural circuits may be cut surgically; however, even severed nociceptors seem to find new paths to the brain and so can re-establish the pain signal. Over time, the nociceptors also can develop resistance to the most powerful opioids.

Neuropathic Pain

The above discussion focuses on nociceptive pain; i.e., the pain arising from tissue injury, which is sensed by the nociceptors in the vicinity of the injury and then transmitted as a pain signal to the central nervous system. In the course of a normal injury to the body, immune cells in the central nervous system are activated by the pain signals incident to the injury, and in turn, these cells provoke other cells to trigger inflammation and other healing processes. Once the healing is underway, the initiating pain signals fade away.

On the other hand, it is also possible to have neuropathic pain, wherein the nerve itself is injured and the pain signal is spontaneous and ongoing, i.e., the nervous system itself is injured and generates its own pain. When the neurons are themselves injured, the associated microglia become hyperexcited, releasing large amounts of cytokines that promote inflammation and hyperexcitation of the nociceptors in the vicinity.

The pain of a herpes zoster flare-up involves the viral infiltration of nerve fibers, and excruciating pain is sensed along those fibers. Even in this case of neuropathic pain, psychology is a large factor in one's response to the pain, since the initiation of a herpes flare-up is dependent in part on the state of mental stress being felt by the person.

In addition to the larger nerves, smaller nerves surround each larger nerve, and arterioles and venules carrying nutrients, oxygen, and metabolic wastes penetrate deeply within the larger nerve bundle. These smaller nerves (called nervi nervorum (Subsection 3.E, page 61) also may be involved in neuropathic pain.

Intercepting Pain

Both the acute-pain and chronic-pain pathways can be intercepted at several points on their upward journeys to the cortex, and the pain signals can be turned off, or at least decreased in intensity, either by electrical suppression of the pain signals or by the release of pain-killing opioids (beta endorphin and the enkephalins) within the central nervous system. Pain signals also can be reduced in intensity if the surrounding tactile receptors are stimulated. This is due to the fact that pain neurons and touch neurons share certain neural pathways in the central nervous system, and a large amount of traffic in the touch neurons can swamp that in the pain neurons (see the discussion of the gate-control theory below). Thus, we rub the skin over painful spots to reduce pain and possibly stimulate such receptors when treating pain by acupuncture. This lessening of the pain by rubbing an affected area is due to an overstimulation of the neural pathways by the rubbing, so that the original pain signal cannot get through to the pain centers in the brain.[2] Rubbing also promotes increased circulation to the site, followed by an immune response that sometimes can remove the initial cause of irritation. When rubbing with a compound that contains a neural stimulant such as capsaicin (the potent ingredient of hot peppers), one is again flooding the area with generalized pain sensations with the hope of drowning out a specific pain sensation. In the same vein, it is reported [844] that pelvic pain in women is blocked for hours by applying gentle pressure on the vagina, but not on the clitoris. A somewhat more detailed description of the neurological dimming of the pain sensation by rubbing the affected area is given in Subsection 13.C, page 523.

Pain messages from the spinal cord and from the peripheral nerves move as high as the thalamus, however, people have been observed to have widely different levels of pain and neural excitation in the prefrontal and the anterior cingulate cortices when exposed to the same pain stimulus [131]. A Yoga Master who claims not to feel pain while meditating [424] showed unusually low electrical activity in the thalamus, the insula, and

the cingulate cortex (figure 4.B-1) while in that state.

The brain itself has no pain receptors [432], however, see Subsection 4.E, page 114, for a discussion on headaches. The alveoli of the lungs also are without pain receptors, but the bronchi are very sensitive to pain. Besides the brain, many internal organs have few or no pain receptors, whereas the skin is acutely sensitive to pain. It also happens that many visceral organs, when in pain, refer the visceral pain signal to the corresponding dermatome in the skin (Section 13.D, page 530).

The Physiology of Pleasure

The flip side of pain is pleasure. The centers for registering both intense pain and intense pleasure are found in the midbrain; however, the mechanism is poorly understood, other than to say that pleasure is a driving force in humans, much like hunger, thirst, sex, or the needs for drugs or music. The centers for pain and pleasure are linked to the motivational system in the limbic area (Box 2.D-1, page 27), and they encourage certain behaviors, rewarding some behaviors with pleasure and discouraging others with pain. When motivationally driven, we can never get enough pleasure. This drive differs from homeostasis (Subsection 5.A, page 158), where there is a driving force only when the system is out of balance [204, 427, 654].

Dopamine

The ingestion of recreational drugs such as cocaine, alcohol, opioids, or amphetamines and the consequent release of endorphins and enkephalins trigger the stimulation of neurons in the ventral tegmental area (VTA) near the base of the brain. These neurons synapse with neurons in the nucleus accumbens in the midbrain, which are activated by the neurotransmitter dopamine, and a deep sense of pleasure follows from there. The release of dopamine in the midbrain also stimulates the dorsal striatum, a center associated with motivation. Thus is an addiction spawned.

As discussed in Subsection 3.D, page 56, the neurotransmitter dopamine plays a key role

---

2   Ask your doctor or dentist to rub the injection site before giving you an injection, and you will notice that the pain attendant to the needle entering the body is far weaker than normal [864].

in pleasures of many kinds. The neural circuitry for pleasure is complicated but appears to use the opioids to produce desire and dopamine to produce pleasure; furthermore, the opioid receptors are spread all over the cortex. Emotional content is also present in the reward of pleasure, involving excitations within both the hippocampus and the amygdala [612]. The question of taking pleasure in the practice of *yogasana* is addressed from the proprioceptive point of view in Subsections 11.C, page 441, and 13.C, page 522.

Mu-Opioid Receptors

Certain cells within the brain bear mu-opioid receptors on their surfaces, which react to the presence of opioids such as heroin, morphine, and the endorphins, causing a feeling of pleasure. The pleasure that comes from learning anything new—intellectual, yogic, or whatever—releases endorphins, which in turn stimulate the mu-opioid receptors, which are especially plentiful in areas that trigger the most memories and that have the strongest personal meanings for a person. The thirst for new knowledge is a primal drive, as strong as those for satisfaction of hunger, sexual union, and the avoidance of harm. The response is especially strong the first time the experience is encountered and then decreases in intensity with repetition. The connection between mu-opioid receptors and the beta-endorphins should be very much obvious in our *yogasana* practice, as they are brought into our consciousness when we are thrilled by learning new aspects of our practice, whereas we suffer the loss of pleasure when the practice becomes routine and unthinking.

The Affective Sense

All teachers and practitioners of *yogasana* are familiar with the pleasurable sense that follows a *yogasana* practice that may have involved several instances of postures performed so intensely as to elicit the comment that it "hurts so good." This seeming oxymoron appears to be based on the physiological pain incurred in challenging the body; i.e., the component **1** "hurts," and the component **2** "so good" emotion that accompanies the

pride one feels in completing a challenging practice. Understanding the physiology of this "hurts so good" sensation is presently very sketchy, but even in its nascent state, it appears that there are some aspects that are relevant to *yogasana* practice [220]. The psychological aspects of the feel-good sensation are discussed below.

Ekkekakis [220] states that positive feelings, (i.e., affective responses), are felt during and immediately after exercise of mild intensity and short duration. On the other hand, if the exercise is moderately vigorous, as with *yogasana* practice, then the affective response during the exercise will be positive for some people but negative for others. Still, regardless of whether the affective response during exercise is positive or negative, the feeling following moderately vigorous exercise will be uniformly positive! In this regard, Ekkekakis states that this phenomenon "seems to transcend modes of exercise, environment, types of participants and measures of affect." If the level of exercise is so strenuous that it approaches one's physical limit, then the physiological stress will impact strongly on the autonomic nervous system during the exercise, and the affective response will be uniformly negative, whereas following moderately vigorous exercise, the affective response nonetheless will be uniformly positive. The criterion separating moderate from vigorous exercise appears to be the strong shift of physiological parameters from the lactate-free, homeostatic, aerobic state at low intensity to the lactate-heavy, homeostatically non-steady-state, anaerobic metabolism at high intensity (Subsection 11.A, page 393). The approach to and passing beyond this transition is sensed by the interoceptive nervous system (Subsection 11.C, page 444). The variety of responses during and after exercise of varying intensity has been explained as depending upon the relative importance of the two factors: the physiological stress felt during the exercise and the pleasure felt when the feeling of stress is overtaken by the effects of the endogenous opiate system on the mu-opioid receptors (Subsection 3.D, page 57).

Extinguishing Pain

Distraction through Overloading

Pain sensations may be eased by creating alternate neural sensations that compete successfully with the pain sensation for our attention, as was mentioned above in regard to rubbing a painful spot on the body. In general, dwelling mentally on pain or distress opens the pain gate, but this can be closed by a more intense counter-stimulus. For example, a patient reports to his doctor that his back pain goes away whenever his teeth start to act up and give him pain. It is surmised that the pain of toothache is more immediate and intense than the back pain, and that in opening up the tooth-pain channel as a counter-stimulus, the gate has been closed to the back pain. If, however, the toothache results in a feeling of strain and distress coming from having to deal with yet another stressor, then the result can easily be intensification of the back pain, along with that of the toothache! Indeed, experiment shows that if one can be absorbed in an activity so that attention has been shifted away from the pain sensation, then the perception of pain is reduced.

Yet another aspect of chronic pain is the sense that its intensity waxes and wanes in a regular way, often being more intense in the evening and less in the beginning of the day. Most often, such effects are related to levels of activity, so that after a night's rest, one feels good enough in the morning to be overly active and then suffers the consequences later in the day. The period may be a matter of a week rather than a day, but the cause is still the same: engaging in a pattern of restful under-activity followed by a pattern of energetic overactivity. A similar pattern may easily develop in the *yogasana* practitioner on recovering from an injury. This roller coaster must be smoothed out by conscious moderation in order for the pain to subside.

Learning and Memory

Pain is closely tied to learning and memory. Without memory, pain would not persist, and without pain, memory perhaps would not have evolved. Neurons in the spinal cord can become hypersensitive for prolonged pain, such that experienced in the chronic pain of arthritis, cancer, and diabetes. But sensitization and learning can become a two-way street as we form pain memories and overactive pain learning can lead to fibromyalgia. After severe pain, there is a rewiring of the nervous system and a reinforcement of the pathways for pain. In fact, curing pain medically may erase all memories [188].

Factors such as the above will be at work more or less in all of the students in *yogasana* class, and the teacher must be open to the wide range of pain responses possible among the uninitiated. As a *yogasana* teacher, one also must be aware of how suggestible our students might be and how open they are to suggestions about "good" pain and "bad" pain. This is discussed further in Subsection 13.C, page 528.

Sarno [746] takes a different approach to the psychological component of pain. He argues that unresolved emotional problems lead to a sympathetic excitation in the nervous system that raises the resting muscle tone (Subsection 11.B, page 437). As a result, there is an ischemic (low blood flow) condition in the soft tissues (muscles, nerves, tendons), and the affected tissue responds to the oxygen deficit with sensations of pain. In his view, the "herniated disc" problem is a nonstarter in regard to lower-back pain, for the problem is emotional rather than mechanical, and the cure is mental rather than surgical. Indeed, recent research has shown that when one suffers chronic lower-back pain, it is an emotional center in the brain (the medial prefrontal cortex) that is energized, whereas if the pain is acute, then the pain signal appears only in the insula, a center dedicated to acute pain signals.

Pain is experienced not only as physical distress but as emotional distress as well. Interestingly, emotional distress can stimulate the same anterior cingulate brain region as that which is stimulated when the pain is physical.

Time of Day

Cortisol is an inflammation-fighting hormone that is released in large amounts when one awakens; once released, it dulls the sensation of pain. As cortisol is otherwise almost totally absent at night, the sensitivity to pain is often found to be higher at night than during the daylight hours. Correspondingly, during the time of high cortisol concentration in the body, external analgesics are less effective than when cortisol levels are low. Thus, in regard to dentistry, it is known that externally delivered pain killers are much more effective in the afternoon than in the early morning, when cortisol levels are at or near their peak. Similarly, post-surgical pain is highest in the early morning, but the effectiveness of aspirin in reducing such pain is higher in the afternoon than in the morning [804]. If *yogasana* practice is painful, then one can hypothesize that cortisol can act to mask this pain best in the early-morning hours, when it is at its highest concentration. However, as explained in Subsection 5.D, page 178, the excessive release of cortisol can have a negative effect on learning and memory.

Endorphins

Not only does the body have its own analgesics against pain (called endogenous opioids; Subsection 3.D, page 57), but, as will be seen below, these drugs are available on demand to the *yogasana* practitioner. Imagine that a pain signal from an outlying nociceptor travels to the dorsal root of the spinal cord. Normally, at this point, it synapses with a spinal nerve fiber, which ascends to the thalamus and beyond to register its painful message in the higher centers (Subsection 4.C, page 85). However, at the level of the dorsal root's synapse with the nociceptor, there is a second synapse involving a descending neuron from the periaqueductal gray nucleus in the midbrain of the limbic system. The periaqueductal gray area within the brainstem has reciprocal connections to the hypothalamus and is known to be intimately connected as well to sensations of pleasure and pain. This second synapse uses endorphin, a neuropeptide, as its neurotransmitter, and when called upon, its effect is inhibitory. Thus, if a signal is sent downward from or through the periaqueductal gray center to the relevant dorsal horn, its effect will be to lessen or cancel completely the

action potential of the ascending pain signal! In this way, the endogenous opioids dull or erase entirely the sensations of pain by effectively changing the threshold for the sensation of pain [427, 654]. This is thought to be the mechanism behind the "runner's high" experienced by distance runners.

Pert [654] also points out that receptors for endorphins are found throughout the central nervous system and that through proper breath control, one can achieve control of the release of endorphins from the periaqueductal gray area. These released neurotransmitters diffuse through the cerebrospinal fluid to receptor sites at many places in the central nervous system, and in this way, they inhibit the upward movement of pain signals. It has been shown that acupuncture also stimulates the release of beta endorphins into the cerebrospinal fluid [20, 654].

The scheme put forward by Pert would fit with the general experience among students of *yogasana* that the discomfort of a challenging posture can be met by focusing one's attention on the qualities of the breath while keeping it moving in a smooth but deliberate way, or by visualizing each of the exhalations to be through the point of discomfort. It is also known that changes in the rate and depth of the breath release a flood of neuropeptides from the brainstem and that many of these are endorphins [654].

It also must be said that a large number of pain-relieving neuropeptides have been identified and that many of them have other functions besides that of analgesia. This may explain why there are receptors for these neurotransmitters throughout the body. Moreover, because the important periaqueductal gray area has many reciprocal neural connections with the hypothalamus, the door also is open for the influence of the autonomic nervous system on pain.

Gender Differences

Both the enkephalins and the endorphins are painkillers, with the latter being almost ten times stronger at reducing pain than is morphine. There also exist strong pain killers called "kappa-opioids," which are very effective for women but which actually increase the pain sensations when given to men! A similar difference exists for the trademarked analgesic ibuprofen, which is far less effective for women than for men. The sense of smell appears also to have an effect on the sensations of pain; women feel less pain from their skin sensors when smelling pleasant odors as compared with men, who report no pain reduction under the same conditions [542].

The ability to sense pain is essential, but this advantage is defeated if the pain becomes chronic and debilitating; in this situation, the sensation of pain is desensitized by the enkephalins, which bind to the same mu-opioid receptors in the brain as does morphine [450].

Neural Mechanisms of Pain Reduction

The neural fibers for nociception enter the spinal cord and then travel upward, some passing through the thalamus and some passing through the reticular formation (Subsection 4.B, page 74) on their way to the cortex. Attempts have been made to map the pain loci in the cortex, as has been done for tactile sensation (figure 4.C-6, for example), however, no such map could be found. It appears that at the conscious level, pain signals are processed in parallel at widely distributed points in the cortex, though the anterior cingulate is known to be especially important.

Sensations originating in the skin and muscles travel into our consciousness using the spinothalamic tracts of the central nervous system, these being nerve bundles in the white matter at each of the two sides of the spinal cord. The tract is bilateral, because the skin and muscles that it serves are bilateral. By contrast, pain signals from the internal organs use the dorsal tract of the spinal cord [792], an area on the posterior side of the cord.

The conclusion that the level of pain perceived is very dependent upon other circumstances (emotional and psychological) is well documented. For example, fear raises the sensitivity to pain, whereas thinking deeply sexual thoughts erases pain. This is rationalized by noting that the nociceptor axons are synapsed with many non-nociceptor neurons (both ascending and descending) in the central nervous system, thus affording ample opportunities for modulation or even blocking of the ascending pain signal through the intervention of inhibitory interneurons (see the discussion on the endogenous opioids in Subsection 3.D, page 57). Because the reticular formation also integrates ascending and descending neural information, it is able to lessen or block totally the nociceptor signal as it attempts to pass upward from that point, just as it suppresses or transmits neural signals from any of the other sensory receptors.

Gate-Control Theory

The gate-control hypothesis of pain control is outlined schematically in figure 13.C-1. In this theory, both the C-fiber nociceptor and some non-nociceptor neuron (A_α for touch, for example) are energized simultaneously, as with a pinprick. Being adjacent in the skin, these afferent nerves are in the same nerve bundle and enter the spinal cord through a common dorsal horn, where they synapse onto an interneuron in the cord. The effect of the interneuron on the nociceptor is assumed to be inhibitory (hyperpolarizing), and the effect of the non-nociceptor is assumed to be excitatory (depolarizing). This interneuron has an inhibitory synapse, in turn, with a projection neuron, to which the nociceptor and the non-nociceptor are also synapsed, with both of these synapses now being excitatory. Should the interneuron shown in figure 13.C-1 be excited, it will act to hyperpolarize the projection interneuron, thus inhibiting it from sending its signal to the cortex. However, the projection neuron also is influenced directly by potentials from the C-fiber nociceptor and from the A_α neural afferent, both of which tend to depolarize the projection neuron. In this circuit, both the C fiber and the skin afferent have an effect on the strength of the eventual signal moving through the projection neuron to the spinothalamic tract, either canceling it, weakening it, or intensifying it. If there is a greater amount of activity in the large nerve fibers than in the small, there will be little or no pain sensation, whereas, if there is more in the small nerve fibers

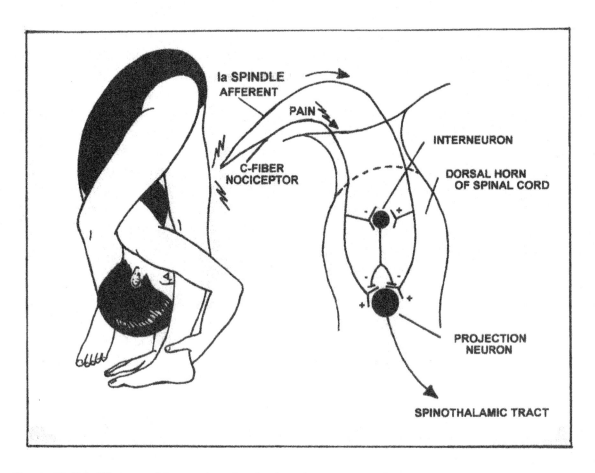

Figure 13.C-1. The neural connections involved in the gate-control theory of pain. See the text for an explanation of how this mechanism can reduce the intensity of pain coming from the peripheral nerves, as when overstretching the biceps femoris in *ruchikasana*.

than in the large, then pain will register. This is in agreement with experiments that show that slapping and rubbing ease pain in the area of the skin so treated. The glutamate ion and the neuropeptides act as neurotransmitters (Section 3.D, page 56) in the nociceptor realm.

An alternate scenario [326] also involves the gate-control theory. Here, the ascending nociceptor nerve has two descending nerves by its side and synapsed to it at several points. Each of these synapses uses either serotonin, norepinephrine, or an endorphin as its neurotransmitter and acts as a gate that can either block the pain, lessen the pain, or increase the pain, depending upon supraspinal decisions, mostly subcortical. Thus, in situations of extreme emergency, one might be totally unaware of the pain of one's own injuries, while consumed with the need to help others who are

injured. In this situation, the gates for ascending pain signals have been closed by cortical actions that sense a higher priority, i.e., helping others in pain. The higher nuclei that might react downward to block the upward passage of pain signals are the periaqueductal gray and the nucleus raphe magnus. On the other hand, there is evidence that the sympathetic nervous system can intensify pain sensations, just as it sharpens certain other senses in time of danger [326].

Using gate-control theory, one can rationalize the situation of pain induced by a herniated intervertebral disc (Subsection 8.C, page 307). In this case, it is assumed that there are no nociceptor free-nerve endings within the spinal cord but that the herniated disc exerts pressure on the spinal muscle afferent and that this pressure impedes the propagation of the action potential along its axon (Section 3.B, page 42). This change in the afferent action potential then influences the potential balance at the projection neuron (figure 13.C-1), thereby allowing the pain signal access to the cortex.

Yogasana, Injury, and Pain

Pain is a graded response to injury, and at the lowest end of the pain scale, it is expressed as discomfort. Feeling a sense of discomfort in a *yogasana* arises as we challenge the psychological and physiological boundaries of our region of postural comfort. As long as one is comfortable in one's posture, there is no reason to change, no incentive for growth, and a general stagnation (Subsection 11.C, page 441). In order to grow and progress in *yogasana* practice, one must learn to push back the boundaries, i.e., to be uncomfortable and to grow in the process. However, it does not follow that there is more growth or more rapid growth when the student goes from discomfort to pain. On the other hand, as discussed in Subsection 11.A, page 405, there are some [827a] who postulate that muscle tissue first must be torn apart in order to be transformed into a form that is more appropriate to the exercise. In this scenario, pain is unavoidable if the desired structural transformation is to be achieved.

As a muscle is stretched in a *yogasana,* many sensations will be sent to the brain for evaluation. At the beginning of the stretch, there is a strong sense of muscle tension from the stretch receptors and a sense of the changing body position from the proprioceptors. The stretch sensation is a dull, delocalized feeling of discomfort that penetrates to the cortex and so is very present in the consciousness. If the stretch is now taken too far or too fast, the myofascial tissue will tear locally under the stress. In this case, the prostaglandin release will precipitate a sharp and stabbing nociceptive pain signal which is qualitatively and quantitatively very different from that of the stretch discomfort. Needless to say, the sensory goal in *yogasana* practice is to stay within the bounds of discomfort and not cross aggressively into the realm of tearing, pain, and inflammation. This is what Joel Kramer

calls "working at the edge," using the breath and the mind to handle the discomfort of going to a new place, all the while honoring *ahimsa* (nonviolence) and remaining conscious of the limits that should not be exceeded. In this context, then, one can speak of "good pain" and "bad pain," depending upon which side of the discomfort-to-pain threshold one is on. Pain in moderation can be a wonderful *yogasana* teacher, and we must learn to welcome it as a friend rather than avoid it as we would an enemy.

Hypnosedation

The efficacy of self-hypnosis in reducing pain during surgery is very well known and documented. Called "hypnosedation," this method of pain reduction has many advantages. During hypnosedation, the subject is conscious and able to cooperate in the procedure, the use of anesthesia is significantly reduced, and recovery times are far shortened due to reduced inflammation. Functional MRI studies of pain perception while hypnosedated show that cortical sensations of pain are much reduced, but that there is a significant increase of neural activities in the anterior cingulate cortex and in the basal ganglia. It would be very revealing to see if such MRI changes occur in the brains of *yogasana* practitioners while in challenging postures. As with many things in medicine, techniques such as hypnosedation at present are viewed as too Worldview I in the minds of many surgeons (Subsection 1.A, page 3); this too will change with time, possibly with help from the yoga community!

If one is suffering from sciatic pain (Subsection 8.C, pages 307 and 308, and Section 21.B, page 747) that radiates more or less down the leg or legs, then those *yogasanas* that tend to centralize the pain (i.e., make the pain move from a more distant location, such as the knee, toward the base of the spine) are beneficial, whereas those that extend the pain yet further away from the base of the spine should be avoided [208].

Women with persistent pain problems for three or more months attended regular Iyengar yoga classes three times per week and reported significantly reduced usage of pain medication, enhanced mood, lessened anxiety, etc. If the pain signal stemming from a *yogasana* injury is not too severe and the site is not inflamed or swollen, a brief but immediate relief of the pain sensation can be had by gently rubbing the affected area or slapping it, so that the pain signal is swamped by the signals coming from the touch receptors in the area [669]. Analgesics and balms that cause a slight irritation of the skin also can be used to mask a more internal pain, and it is possible that acupuncture also works in this way to block pain signals to higher centers. Cold also can be effective as a counterirritant in erasing pain.

In the most recent study of the efficacy of acupuncture, it was found that the application of the needles was very effective in reducing the pain of migraine, but there was no noticeable difference between random placement of the needles and placement at the acupuncture points [785].

The Yogasana Paradox

Philosophers argue that one of our constant goals in life is to behave in a way that avoids pain—in which case, it is strange that we *yogasana* students work voluntarily to increase our sensitivity to sensations in our bodies, pain among them. Moreover, it is generally held by neurologists that repeating a painful act makes the associated pain fibers yet more conductive and so **increases** the pain; and sports doctors argue strongly against "toughing it out" when injured, as this can make the pain chronic and intractable.

On the other hand, it is well documented that the perception of pain is strongly modulated by mental processes (this subsection, page 529). Perhaps the solution to this paradox is that yogis work in the region of discomfort but not pain, and that even when "in pain," the sense of it is very dependent upon one's attitude; if it is considered as "good pain," a welcome sensation that makes one's life worth living, one can overcome pain, survive it, or learn how to either ignore it or even love it!

The Psychology and Memory of Pain

The interaction between the body and the mind is perhaps nowhere more evident than in the area of pain perception, as examples abound of how one person's intense physical pain is unbearable, whereas another person with the same injury but with a different attitude toward it is able to bear the pain with grace and good humor, or perhaps not even be aware of it. Placebos too are famous for their analgesic effects (Subsection 5.F, page 196), even though they operate totally on the psychological level. Box 13.C-1, next page, lists several examples of the factors that influence our perception of pain.

Placebo Statements and Placebo Pills

It must also be mentioned that the swallowing of inert sugar pills dispensed by a doctor figure who tells the person in pain that "these pills will diminish your pain in just a few minutes" can be very effective in easing pain. This is discussed further in Subsection 5.F, page 196. Placebo analgesics operate by dulling the experience of pain in the thalamus and cortical regions. When real pain is reduced by treatment with placebo injections, it is found by PET scans that the receptors for the painkiller endorphins in the pain, stress, reward, and emotional centers have been strongly activated.

Yet another aspect of pain control in the *yogasana* sphere involves placebo-like statements by the teacher, not unlike those of hypnosedation. In the placebo effect (Subsection 5.F, page 196), a person of high authority proclaims a procedure to be physiologically effective in curing a specific problem, and for many of the students, there follows a beneficial physiological shift on hearing the good news. Thus, receptive students might be reassured by hearing that there is a strong pull on the hamstring of the forward leg of *trikonasana,* that it is more or less unavoidable in the beginner, and that it is a "good" pain. This positive statement by the teacher can reduce anxiety on the part of the student and with that, the pain in the forward leg.

Box 13.C-1: Psychological and Cultural Factors in Pain

Abundant evidence exists that the psychological component of pain is huge, that our mental and cultural attitudes toward pain greatly influence the magnitude of the sensation we feel as pain, and that our response to pain is a learned behavior. Listed below are several generalized examples of these aspects of pain, gleaned in large part from a large body of work in this area [266].

» People living in the Mediterranean area tolerate pain poorly.

» A level of heat that Israelis and Italians consider as merely warm is considered by northern Europeans to be intolerable.

» Subjects were asked to hold their hands in ice water until the pain was unbearable; on average, women held their hands in the water for 69 seconds and men tallied 109 seconds. When told the average time period for men and women was 90 seconds, on retesting, the average for women rose to 102 seconds and that for men rose to 112 seconds.

» Jewish women increased their tolerance to a pain stimulus after they were told that Jews have a low tolerance for pain. However, when Protestant women were told that Protestants have a low tolerance for pain, their threshold did not change.

» Jews are big complainers about pain, wondering about its meaning and what the implications might be for their having been chosen to suffer. Italians also are big complainers about pain and wonder how they can gain relief.

» Nepalese porters carry heavy loads to the tops of the world's highest and coldest peaks without complaint. Tests show that these people are just as sensitive to stimuli as Westerners, yet they can endure much higher levels of pain. The Nepalese have been taught by their culture to stoically endure pain levels that Westerners consider unbearable.

» Many recent experiments have shown that two people may receive equally intense pain stimuli on the skin but will register very different levels of discomfort in the brain.

» If an infant sees its parent scream at the slightest pain, that infant will learn and execute similar responses in its own life.

» Chronic pain can generate psychological neuroses; when the pain is relieved, the neuroses vanish.

» People often experience horrific war wounds but rarely complain about the pain, whereas the same sorts of injury incurred in a peacetime situation often involve intense pain and anguish.

» When one is angry and the sympathetic nervous system is activated, one is less sensitive to pain, whereas when one is afraid and anxious, the sensitivity to pain increases [747]. A vicious cycle is set in motion, for pain promotes anxiety, which acts to intensify the pain.

» Pain is often more intense at night, when there are no other distracting influences and we can focus on the sensation (see also the effects of low levels of cortisol in the blood during the evening hours; Subsection 13.C page 523). Rubbing a painful spot can diminish the pain signal by adding many other non-pain signals to the area.

» Men may react more strongly to serious pain than do women because they feel powerless in the face of something society expects them to endure silently and because they resent having to depend upon others for relief.

» *Yogasana* students in India appear to have a mental point of view that allows them to bear significantly higher levels of discomfort than do the corresponding students in America.

» Yoga practitioners understand that "pain is the wisdom of the body speaking in nonverbal terms" [113a] and that we must learn how to pay attention to our pain, try to understand its basis, and to heal ourselves by learning from the pain.

Section 13.D: Dermatomes and Referred Pain

The Skin Dermatomes

The afferent pain fibers (nociceptors) from the skin show a strong convergence (figure 3.C-2b) on the dorsal-horn relay cells, often joining there with nerves from a visceral organ. Due to this convergence of nerves from different locales onto one particular dorsal root, the brain may be confused as to the exact area that is the source of the sensation, often with the result that the specific area is misidentified. This is the basis of the phenomenon of referred pain. As examples, the rapid eating of cold ice cream can lead to a sense of pain in the forehead, even though it is the tongue and throat that are being over-cooled. Similarly, the visual stimulation of viewing a strong light can spill over from the optic nerve into the trigeminal nerve in the nose, leading to a nasal tickling sensation or to a sneeze. Such examples of referred pain can be understood by first considering the thirty-one pairs of segmentally arranged spinal nerves that lead to a segmental organization of the receptive area of the skin into sixty-two distinct local surfaces, each such local surface being served by its own spinal-nerve bundle. The local area of skin innervated by one spinal nerve is called a derma-

tome [360, 427, 431, 432, 574].[3] Specific nerves within the spinal cord receive information from specific dermatomes.

Extensive experimentation has led to the construction of dermatome maps of the sort shown in figures 13.D-1 and 13.D-2. Each dermatome shown there reflects the convergence of all of the superficial afferent nerves in that area onto one dorsal root of a spinal nerve. The edges of the dermatomes actually are not as sharply defined as shown, for in fact, adjacent dermatomes have a large overlap. Note, however, that the visceral organs that contribute to a dorsal-root bundle are not necessarily within the dermatome area as defined by the skin over the organ. That is to say, the area of skin and the visceral organ that shares a dorsal root with that skin may not lie over one another.

Table 13.D-1 shows how the nociceptor nerves in various places on the skin join those of the muscles and organs of the body, and where they converge on the dorsal roots of the spinal column. One sees that the motor neurons of the muscles closely follow the same nerve bundles as the overlaying skin and synapse at about the same place on the spinal cord. Thus, if anesthetic is administered to a particular spot on the spinal cord or is close to that spot on the cord, it will produce an anesthesia in the relevant dermatome converging upon that spot in the cord [320].

---

3   Actually, the first cervical nerve has no dermatome, as it has no dorsal root.

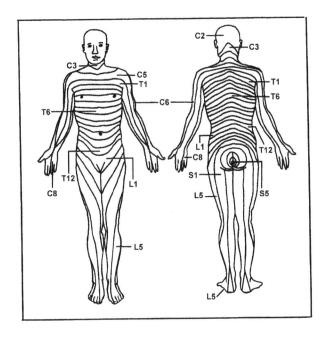

Figure 13.D-1. The dermatome zones on the front body (**a**) and the back body (**b**), each labeled according to the vertebral designation of its dorsal root (figure 4.A-1).

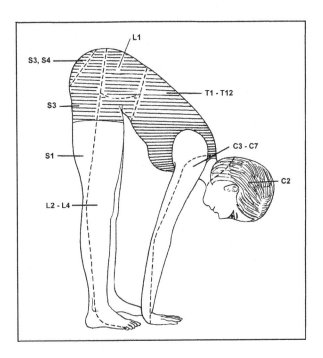

Figure 13.D-2. The approximate positions of the dermatome boundaries corresponding to a few of the dorsal roots, while in *uttanasana*.

Table 13.D-1: Correlation of Dermatomes with Skin and α-Motor Neurons with Muscles [360]

Dermatome Location	Dorsal Root Location	Muscles or Organ
Neck	C1–C4	Neck
	C3–C5	Diaphragm
Deltoid	C5, C6	Biceps
Radial forearm and thumb	C5–C8	Shoulder joint
Ulnar border of hand and little finger	C7–T1	Heart; triceps and forearm
	C8, T1	Hands
	T2–T12	Axial musculature, intervertebral, respiration, abdominals
Groin	L1, L2	Thigh flexors
Knee	L2, L3	Quadriceps femoris
Dorsal side of foot and big toe	L5, S1	Gluteals
Lateral side of foot and little toe	S1, S2	Plantar flexor, ankle
Genito-anal	S3–S5	Pelvic floor, bladder, sphincters, genitals

One sees that the homunculus derived from the study of the sensory cortex, figure 4.C-6, does not show any specific mention of the visceral organs, yet the phenomenon of interception (Section 11.C, page 444) is based upon the visceral sensations that travel to the sensory centers in the brain. There are at least two possible reasons for this. First, the interoceptive signals may not travel as high as the sensory cortex where the measurements leading to figure 4.C-6 were made or the visceral sensory signals may be expressed via their corresponding dermatomes and thereby conflated with the normal superficial-skin signals displayed in the dermatome maps.

Referred Pain

The existence of dermatomes that do not necessarily lie over the visceral organs with which they are paired neurally leads to the phenomenon of "referred pain." In this phenomenon, a visceral, deep-tissue afferent pain fiber synapses simultaneously on the spinal cord with other fibers of some superficial-tissue skin dermatome with a significantly different location on the body. The visceral pain signal from the misplaced organ is eventually sensed in the brain and misinterpreted as a pain in the skin rather than in the organ!

As mentioned above, the visceral organ paired with the skin in a dermatome is not necessarily in close physical proximity to that dermatome. This arises from a lack of correspondence between the position of the skin and the position of the organ due to its migration during both evolutionary and fetal development (see Box 8.A-1, page 270, and figure 13.D-3). In the lower animals from which we have ascended, the correspondence between organs and overlaying skin was more obvious, but evolution has changed this. For example, a heart attack brought on by an inadequate blood supply to the heart often is signaled by pain sensed at the ulnar side of the left arm, because the T1, T2 dermatome for cardiac pain is displaced to the left arm; menstrual discomfort appears as lower back pain via L1–L5 [531]; kidney pain may be sensed as pain in the skin

at dermatomes T10 and T11; whereas pain from the gallbladder appears in the right chest [268]; and inflammation of the pleura appears as pain at the tips of the shoulder blades C3–C5 [360] (figure 13.D-3). In all of these cases (and more), the organ in question and the dermatome share a common spinal-cord segment, but the skin in question does not lie exactly over the affected organ, and the brain cannot distinguish the true location of the stimulus.

The dermatome afferent nerves of the facial skin do not pass through one of the segmental spinal nerves but instead use trigeminal cranial nerve V for access to the central nervous system.

Herpes Zoster

In an attack by the herpes zoster virus (called shingles), a cluster of neurons near the spine that has been harboring the virus for years starts to spread out either to the left or right along a specific nerve pathway, heading toward the area of skin normally served by these nerves. The section of skin associated with the particular nerve pathway infected by the virus then displays a band of rash, blistering, and intense pain. The banded area of attack will be a dermatome of the body (figure 13.D-1), most often on the upper torso, around or below the waist, or in the area of the eyes.

Theoretically, understanding of the dermatomes could be of use in *yogasana* practice, as, for example, over-twisting might generate pain in the kidneys, which is then referred to dermatome areas T10 and T11 and sensed as pain in the umbilicus. Similarly, the blood supply to the heart could be thwarted in an intense spinal twist, and the discomforting signal of the resulting ischemia could appear in the left shoulder! Severe compression of the right lower abdomen (the area of the appendix), as when performing *parivrtta trikonasana,* could lead to the sensation of referred pain on the center line of the body, close to the solar plexus [562], for this internal organ refers pain to this place; however, if the discomfort were in the peritoneum at the position of the appendix, then the pain would be

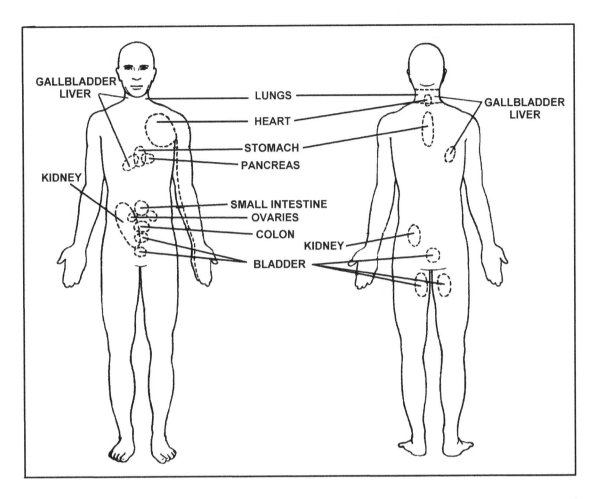

Figure 13.D-3. Visceral pain can manifest as pain in cutaneous layers just outside the organ (stomach, bladder, etc.) or far removed from the site of the organ (heart, diaphragm, etc.), depending on the position of the relevant dermatome to which the pain is referred [360].

sensed at the appendix, because the point of peritoneum innervation, in this case, lies just over the appendix [562].

Something resembling the neural confusion inherent in the dermatome maps of the body, as organs have shifted their locations but kept their neural connections, appears in other instances. Thus, it is common that the signal for gastritis originating within the stomach is misidentified by the brain as either angina or a heart attack, again due to nerve signals from different locations converging on a common nerve root.

A phenomenon known as "referred itch" sounds much like referred pain, but the explanation is not as obvious [228]. In this situation, when an itch is scratched, another itching sensation appears on the same side of the body, usually on the front or back of the upper thorax.

The Heart and Vascular System

14

Circulation and Its Importance

According to the ancient yogis, the heart (the *anahata chakra*) is the seat of the soul and the center for compassion. These yogis placed the body's consciousness (*jivatma*) in the heart, just a few inches to the right of the sternum, just where we now know the pacemaker of the heart to be located [742], suggesting that they possibly were conscious of this electrical stimulator. Though the heart is located at almost the geometric center of the chest, the left ventricle is tilted leftward of center, and because it presses against the ribs on that side during systole, that is where the location of the organ is sensed: to the left and just below the pectoral on that side [827]. According to modern medicine, the heart is the center of the circulatory system, pushing blood to every part of the body through its pumping action so as to deliver the necessary nutrients to the cells and carry away metabolic wastes.

The Vascular System

The heart and the various blood vessels that connect it to all the other parts of the body make up the vascular system. The arteries carry the oxygenated blood from the heart to all of the cells in the body, whereas the veins carry the spent blood back to the heart for recharging with oxygen; the arterial and venous systems are connected to one another by the capillaries. Within the body, not all regions are served equally well by the heart; because the primary task of the heart is to maintain the circulation of the blood through the brain, many areas will be deprived of fresh blood in order to keep the brain well supplied. Of course, the heart itself must be well served by the coronary vascular system if it is to take care of the brain's needs for circulation.

Inadequate Vascular Service

The abilities of our body tissues (muscles, tendons, ligaments, cartilage, nerves, etc.) to perform the *yogasanas* presupposes adequate levels of blood flow, tissue oxygenation, nutrient supply, and the removal of waste products via the circulatory system. Should the circulatory supply be throttled by internal or external factors, then tissue damage may result. With respect to *yogasana* practice [752], assuming a slouched posture day in and day out compresses the multitude of internal organs from the heart to the large intestine as effectively as if they were tied with tourniquets. In this state, the circulation of blood and lymph (Section 14.G, page 595) is impaired, the channels through which they flow tend to collapse, and the hormones and enzymes produced at various sites in the body are not carried promptly to those places where they can do their work. With poor oxygenation of the muscles due to poor circulation, the muscle metabolism tends to shift toward the production of lactic acid, the presence of which in the body can generate a shift in the autonomic balance toward sympathetic excitation and stress. Indeed, it is a key tenet of Iyengar's yoga therapy that the *yogasanas*, done properly, act first to "squeeze" the blood out of a particular organ or muscle, and then, on release of the squeezing, allow the organ or muscle to "soak" in the fresh blood that rushes in. In this way, circu-

535

lation is brought into dull or sluggish areas (such as the collapsed thorax), and healing commences [752]. Continuous motion of the blood is critical as stagnant blood readily begins to clot.

Improved circulation in the sick body implies that the body then can work with higher efficiency, performing the work it needs to do with the expenditure of the minimum amount of energy. For students who are already in good health, practice of the *yogasanas* will avoid any stagnation of the body fluids and so will keep them healthy as they age.

In this chapter, the physiology of circulation and the impact of this on *yogasana* (and vice versa) will be discussed. We will see how the heart pumps blood through the vascular plumbing of the body, how the autonomic nervous system influences this process, and how the internal pressure in the blood vessels is influenced by turning the body more or less upside down.

Section 14.A: Structure and Function of the Heart

The Pumping Chambers of the Heart

The heart is about the size of a closed fist, weighs about 300 grams (eleven ounces) and pumps about 4,000 liters (1,000 gallons) of blood a day through over 96,000 kilometers (60,000 miles) of vascular plumbing. It is surrounded by and held in place by the pericardium, an inflexible tissue of two lubricated layers in close contact with one another but designed to support the heart and to allow room for movement as it beats.

Heart and Lungs

Though the heart formally is a single four-chambered organ, it functions more like two hearts side by side, each with an upper chamber, the atrium, and a lower chamber, the ventricle (figure 14.A-1). Let us call them the right heart and the left heart. The function of the right atrium is

to collect deoxygenated blood from the muscles and organs, using the large veins, and pump it into the right ventricle. Contraction of the right ventricle sends the spent blood, via the pulmonary vein, to the lungs for charging with oxygen (O_2) and stripping of carbon dioxide (CO_2). Once refreshed, the oxygenated blood leaves the lungs and enters the left atrium and then the left ventricle, where a forceful contraction pushes it into the aorta and the arterial system connected to it (Section 14.C, page 561). The left and right hearts are separated by a common wall, the interventricular septum, and share a common system of nerves, which activates the two hearts simultaneously. The circulatory pattern external to the heart is shown somewhat more broadly in figure 14.A-2.[1]

The heart and the lungs are connected in yet a second way, for there are ligaments that connect the pericardium of the heart to the central tendon of the diaphragm; when the diaphragm contracts and then relaxes during the breathing cycle, the heart is pulled downward and then allowed to rise in the thoracic cavity. In this way, the heart may be considered to be massaged by the breath!

Arteries and Veins

The arterial side of the vascular system carries blood from the heart to the muscles, the brain, and the organs, via the aorta. The arteries are noteworthy in being both contractile and elastic, whereas the veins are less contractile but more elastic. As the arteries become more distant from the heart, they branch to form arterioles, and these in turn branch to form the smallest members of the arterial tree, the capillaries. Because an injury to an artery can easily be catastrophic, it is no surprise that nature has placed the arteries

---

1   In the fetal heart, there is a hole (the foramen ovale) within the interventricular septum at the level of the atria. Approximately one third of the blood volume is pumped directly from the right atrium through the interventricular foramen to the left atrium, bypassing the flow resistance of the nonfunctional lungs. Soon after birth, the foramen ovale heals, and normal oxygenation of the blood by the lungs follows.

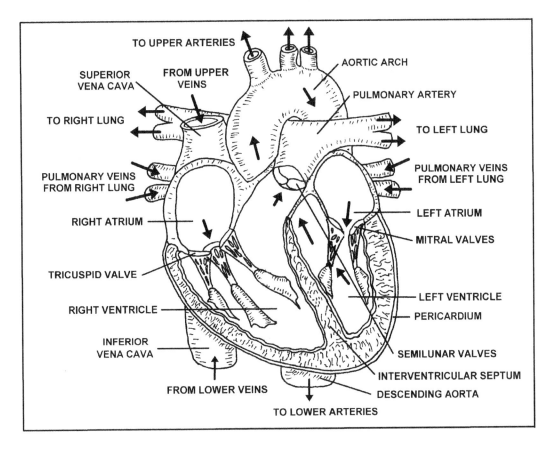

Figure 14.A-1. Cutaway view of the heart and associated vascular plumbing, as seen from the front.

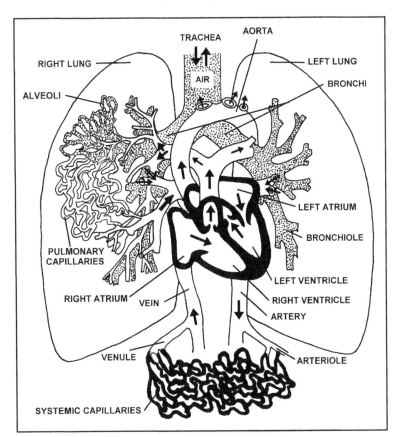

Figure 14.A-2. Circulation of blood in the body follows a circular path, moving from the right heart to the lungs, back to the left heart, and then through the vast network of the body's arteries, arterioles, and capillaries, to return to the right heart via the venous network.

largely on the inner aspects of the limbs where they would be protected by bone from external trauma, and also deep within the musculature. In contrast to this, many veins are superficial in their placements [61a].

The venous system is that part of the vascular net that carries the blood back to the heart, with the vein and the venule being the venous structures corresponding to the artery and arteriole, respectively. The veins of the lower body contain internal valves that direct the flow of venous blood upward to the heart. On the venous side, the return of spent blood to the heart is via three main channels: the superior vena cava, returning blood from above the heart; the inferior vena cava (the largest vein in the body), returning blood from below the heart; and the coronary sinus, which drains the spent blood from the heart and returns it to the right atrium for recirculation (figure 14.A-1). The inferior vena cava has a very short length in the thorax, as it enters the right atrium directly on penetrating the diaphragm, whereas the superior vena cava (the second largest vein in the body) carries spent blood from above the heart to the right atrium and so lies well to the right.

Aortic Pressure

The pressure that the blood exerts on the elastic walls of the aorta is highest at the moment of ventricular contraction; this is called the systolic pressure. However, even when the left ventricle is relaxed while filling, the pressure at the aorta is not zero, because the walls of the aorta balloon outward during each pressure stroke, and even in the relaxed state of the heart, the blood within the arteries continues to press outward on the arterial walls. This pressure in the relaxed state is called the diastolic pressure and is nonzero because at the further reaches of the arterial system, the arterioles offer a high resistance to the peripheral flow of blood and so do not easily allow the diastolic pressure to fall to zero.

At systole, the pressure in the aorta as the blood leaves the left ventricle is five to eight times higher than that of the blood in the right atrium at the point of entry of the superior vena cava (figure 14.A-1). This excess pressurization of the arterioles during the systolic contraction acts both to keep the blood flowing in the arterial system (even while the atria are filling for the next power stroke [742]) and to keep the pressure in the aorta and arteries significantly above zero, long after the contraction of the left ventricle.

Measuring Blood Pressure

Your health-care provider measures your blood pressure by putting a pressure cuff on the arm at the level of the heart and pressurizing it so that no blood can flow through the artery in the arm. Listening then with a stethoscope, the pressure in the cuff is released until the systolic beating is heard; at that point, the pressure in the cuff is equal to that in the artery at systole. Further release of the pressure results eventually in the loss of all sound; at that point, the cuff pressure equals the arterial pressure at diastole.

Blood pressure at the aorta often is reported as A/B, where A is the systolic pressure in millimeters of Hg (mercury) and B is the diastolic pressure in the same units. "Normal" pressure is considered to be 120/80 for young adult males and eight to ten points lower for young adult females; however, see Subsection 14.D, page 575. Vascular tissue is torn apart at pressures above 400/200, and blood will not flow through the vascular system at pressures below 60/30 [68]. A second measure of blood pressure is the mean arterial pressure (MAP), defined as the sum of one-third the systolic pressure plus two-thirds of the diastolic pressure. Should one have a blood pressure of 140/70 measured as A/B, then the mean arterial pressure is (140/3) + 2(70/3) = 93.3 millimeters Hg.

The output of the heart is constant if the arterial pressure is in the range 100–200 millimeters Hg and if the right atrial pressure is in the range 5–6 millimeters Hg. Cardiac output can be increased by 100 percent by either heavy exercise or maximum sympathetic stimulation, whereas parasympathetic stimulation can lower the volume throughput by 20 percent and the heart rate by much more. The volume throughput for the heart ($\dot{Q}$) is 5 liters per minute; with the heart beating at fifty beats per minute, each cardiac

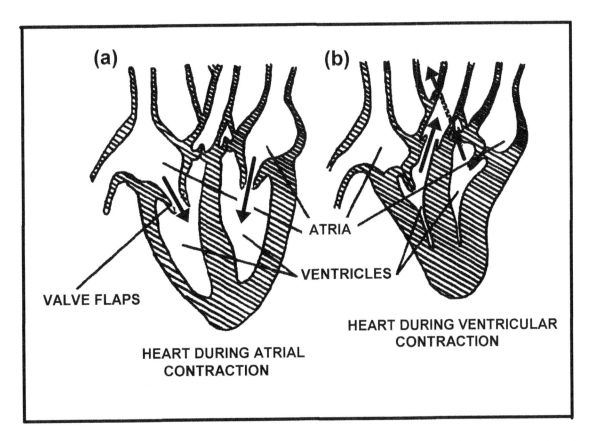

Figure 14.A-3. (**a**) In the heart at rest, the valves between the atria and the ventricles are open, so that the ventricles partially fill with blood. During atrial contraction, the valves within the veins close, but those between the atria and the ventricles remain open, so as to more completely fill the ventricles with blood. (**b**) In the ventricular contraction phase, the valves to the atria are closed, and blood is vigorously pumped through open valves to the lungs by the right ventricle and to the aorta by the left ventricle.

cycle delivers about 100 milliliters (about three fluid ounces) of fresh blood to the muscles and organs. The heart beats thirty-six million times a year, delivering about three million liters (750,000 gallons) of blood in that time.

The diastolic pressure is measured during the passive filling of the atria and so represents a baseline measure of the vascular pressure within the aorta and large arteries. As we shall see, the diastolic pressure reflects the muscular tone of the arteriole walls and thus the level of arteriole excitation (vasoconstriction) by the nervous system (Section 14.C, page 575). By contrast, the systolic pressure is more readily interpreted as showing the strength of the heart's contraction. High readings for either the systolic or diastolic phases of the heartbeat cycle mark one as at risk for heart problems (see Subsection 14.D, page 575).

The Valves within the Heart

The path of blood flow as driven by the heart is strictly one-way: blood enters the heart from the venous system so as to fill the right atrium and right ventricle, is pumped to the lungs, then fills the left atrium and left ventricle and is pumped into the arterial system. The direction of flow is maintained by appropriately placed collagenous flap valves in the heart and in many of the veins. In these valves, the flaps point in the direction of blood flow, so that the flaps are pushed open by blood flow in the desired direction (figure 14.A-3), whereas a counter-flow would act to close them.

During periods of ventricular contraction, the valves between the ventricles and the atria (the tricuspid valve on the right side and the mitral valve on the left side; see figure 14.A-3) are closed so as to force the blood flow out of the heart and into the lungs and aorta, respectively. These valves remain open during atrial contraction, whereas the valves in the vessels feeding blood into the atria are closed at this point in the cardiac cycle.

Opening and closing of the appropriate valves at the appropriate times is partly automatic, in the sense that the valve flaps move with the flow as dictated by the contraction of the heart's chambers; and in part, it is directed by small muscles that are used to pull the flaps into place. If the mitral valve between the left atrium and ventricle is prolapsed, then the flaps do not close tightly on systole but billow back into the atrium, allowing blood to flow in the upstream direction. Semilunar valves are also positioned between the left and right ventricles and the aorta and pulmonary arteries, respectively, so that outwardly pumped blood leaving the heart cannot flow backward into the heart.

The heartbeat (pulse) that one feels in the body during *yogasana* practice is due to the ventricular contraction, whereas the sound one hears through a stethoscope is that of the opening and closing of the valves within the heart [878].

The Timing of Cardiac Contractions and Coordination with Valve Positions

As the actions of the cardiac components are the same on the two sides of the heart, we will discuss that for the left side, with the understanding that the situation is essentially the same on the right side. That is to say, both atria contract together, as do both ventricles. Inasmuch as the heart accepts the venous return of exhausted blood, sends it to the lungs for recharging, accepts the recharged blood, and then sends it out to the furthest reaches of the body, it is no surprise that there is some delicate timing involved between the motions of its parts, if the flow is to be smooth. For example, it is important that the volumes of blood pumped by the two ventricles be equal if the coordinated pumping of the left and right ventricles is to remain in synchrony. Consider the cardiac cycle to consist of four phases, which we describe arbitrarily as specific to the left side of the heart.

Phase 1: With the heart at rest, blood flows into the left atrium from the lungs via the pulmonary vein and from the left atrium into the left ventricle. This passive filling of the atrium is driven by the slight venous pressure in the lungs. This phase requires about 0.1 second, and in this time, 70 percent of the left ventricle is filled in this passive way.

Phase 2: Pumping then begins with the contraction of the left atrium, which acts to close the valves in the pulmonary veins while keeping the valve between the left atrium and its ventricle open. The filling of the ventricle is due in part to the hydraulic pressure of the atrial contraction and in part to the elastic recoil of the ventricular tissue from the previous contraction cycle. Actually, not much blood is moved in this cycle, as much of the filling of the ventricle has already occurred in phase 1.

Phase 3: Once the left ventricular contraction begins, the pressure in that chamber rapidly rises, thus closing the valve between it and the atrium, but at the same time, forcing open the valve to the aorta. Approximately half the blood in the ventricle is forced out in one contraction, and the pressure in the ventricle drops. This phase requires about 0.3 seconds.

Phase 4: Once the left ventricular contraction is exhausted and the ventricular pressure is released through the aorta, the closed valve to the atrium again opens, while that to the aorta closes. Returning to phase 1, the heart rests while the atrium and ventricle are refilled passively, awaiting phase 2 of the next cycle. This phase requires 0.4 seconds. It is to be understood that as the four-phase cycle described above for the left heart is playing out, the right heart is simultaneously going through similar actions with respect to blood received from the cardiac sinus, the inferior vena cava, and the superior vena cava, and then pumped from the ventricle on that side to the right lung via the pulmonary artery on the right side. See Subsection 14.A, page 548, for an experimental display (figure 14.A-6) of the relative timing for contraction of the chambers of the heart.

Timing of Contractions

With a heart rate of seventy-five beats per minute, a complete cardiac cycle requires 0.8 seconds, with the atria in systole for 0.1 second and in diastole for 0.7 seconds; whereas the ventricles are in systole for 0.3 seconds and in diastole for 0.5 seconds. One sees that in the atrial phases, the action is to prime the ventricular pump; in the ventricular phases, one has the power strokes that move the blood throughout the body. At a normal heart rate of seventy-two beats per minute, the systolic phase requires 40 percent of the time for an entire cycle; however, at 215 beats per minute, 65 percent of the period is devoted to systolic action, which does not leave as much time for either diastolic filling or rest.

Details of Cardiac Muscle

The myocardia (heart muscles) of the atria of the heart are relatively thin, as they operate at relatively low pressures. On the other hand, the myocardium of the right ventricle is substantially thicker, as it must pump blood through the lungs, and the myocardium of the left ventricle is thicker still, as it must pump blood through the entire vascular network of arteries, arterioles, and capillaries (figure 14.A-2). The work done by the left ventricle in pumping blood through the arterial tree is about six times that done by the right ventricle in pumping the same quantity of blood through the lungs [308]. Because the myocardium is such a thick muscle, it too has a detailed network of blood vessels to feed the muscle fibers, etc.

Comparison to Other Muscles

Though the myocardial fibers in many ways resemble those of skeletal muscles, they do differ from them in several key respects. As with skeletal-muscle fibers, those of the heart rely upon the actin-myosin interaction for contraction and motion (Subsection 11.A, page 382) and are neurally excited, leading to propagating action potentials (Section 3.B, page 42) along t-tubules [432, 878]; however, the list of dissimilarities between skeletal and cardiac muscles (below) is far longer than the list of similarities:

1. The duration of the action potential in the myocardiac fiber is about 100 times longer than that in skeletal muscle. The long duration of the action potential in cardiac fiber is followed by an anomalously long refractory period, during which time no excitation can take place. Thus, the frequency of cardiac muscle contraction at the highest is only a few hundred contractions per minute, whereas that for skeletal muscle is about a few hundred contractions per second. Unlike skeletal muscle, the refractory period in cardiac muscle is longer than the time of contraction (systole) or relaxation (diastole), and therefore cardiac tetany is not possible in the long term, unless there is a heart attack.

2. Contraction of cardiac muscle is relatively brief, considering that it is followed by a much longer rest period, allowing the ventricles to refill for the next cycle.

3. Because heart cells are smaller in diameter than skeletal muscle cells, all parts of the heart cells are closer to capillaries and mitochondria; i.e., there is a shorter diffusion length for the exchange of gases, nutrients, and metabolites. As one might expect for a muscle that is on duty twenty-four hours a day, the capillaries of the heart are extremely well developed.

4. In the heart, there is practically no fatigue, due to its huge capacity to receive and consume oxygen; however, this fatigue resistance is obtained in exchange for anaerobic capacity, meaning that the heart has only a very small tolerance for deprivation of oxygen, which deprivation otherwise precipitates a heart attack. To meet the high need for ATP, oxygen, and fuel, the mitochondrial density within the heart is very high, being 20–25 percent of the cell volume in adults, and there are high concentrations of enzymes in

the heart that break down fatty acids and allow fragments to enter the mitochondria for oxidation. In terms of muscle-fiber type (Subsection 11.A, page 412), myocardial fibers, with their high content of mitochondrial nuclei and long contraction times, are assigned as type 1 (slow-twitch). Heart cells show a very low production rate of lactic acid, due to special enzymes in the cells; however, because little or no glycogen is used in the heart, anything that interferes with the flow of glucose and oxygenated blood to the heart can lead to cardiac damage or death [450].[2]

5. All of the muscle fibers in the atrial sections on the two sides of the heart are interconnected through high-speed gap junctions (Section 3.C, page 48), so that all atrial fibers at any one time are either excited or are at rest. Cardiac contraction is like a brief muscle spasm. A similar relationship exists among the cardiac fibers within the ventricles. This stands in strong contrast to the situation in type 1 skeletal muscles, wherein motor units within a muscle coordinate their times of contraction and relaxation so as to keep a certain fraction always at work and a certain other fraction always at rest.

6. As discussed in Box 14.A-1, page 545, the action potential driving heart action is intrinsic, so that a heart having all of its neural connections to the central nervous system destroyed will continue to beat at a regular pace. In this regard, it is at odds with the situation in skeletal mus-

cle but not with that in smooth muscle (Subsection 19.A, page 704). The external neural connections to the heart from the central nervous system and the autonomic nervous system modulate the intrinsic heart action, influencing the heart rate and the strength of its contractions, but are not necessary for such intrinsic action.

7. Skeletal muscle cells are long, slender, multinuclear, and shaped to pull on distant bone or tendon; whereas cardiac cells are mononuclear, short, and stubby. The cardiac muscle has cross-striations and terminates at "intercalated discs," which act as separations between the bifurcated ends (Y-shaped split ends) of adjacent fibers. On contraction, the cardiac fibers essentially pull on one another when they pull on the intercalated discs, the net effect being that the circumference of the heart shrinks and the internal volumes of either the atria or the ventricles decrease. See Chapter 24, page 805, for a discussion comparing the enlarged heart of an athlete to the enlarged heart of a hypertensive but inactive person. Further comparisons of the properties of skeletal, cardiac, and smooth muscle appear in table 14.A-1.

Blood Supply to Heart

Of course, the heart muscle itself must be served by its own network of arteries and veins in order to keep the muscle fibers oxygenated, fueled, and free of wastes. The diameters of these coronary vessels are under the control of the autonomic nervous system (Chapter 5, page 157), as the vessel walls carry alpha and beta receptors that are sensitive to hormonal signals stimulated by the sympathetic branch of the autonomic nervous system. Alpha receptors, when activated by the catecholamines, promote vasoconstriction (decreasing diameters of the vessels), whereas stimulation of the alpha receptors by the catecholamines promotes vasodilation (increasing diameters of the vessels). The beta receptors only promote vasodilation [432].

---

2   When internal organs are harvested for transplantation, there is an unavoidable period of ischemia when the organ is without freshly oxygenated blood. Due to this ischemia, even with refrigeration, there is a time limit beyond which the organ is no longer viable for transplantation. These time limits are: heart, four hours; lungs, six to eight hours; liver, twelve hours; pancreas, seventeen hours; and kidney, twenty-four hours. One sees from this the special need of the heart for freshly oxygenated blood.

Table 14.A-1: Comparisons of the Skeletal, Smooth, and Cardiac Muscles [219, 544]

Characteristics	Skeletal	Smooth	Cardiac
Location	Attached to bones	Walls of hollow organs	Heart
Neural-system control	Voluntary, somatic	Involuntary, ANS	Involuntary, ANS
Striations	Yes	No	Yes
T-tubules	Yes	No	Yes
Gap junctions	No	Yes	Yes
Contraction speed	Medium-fast	Very slow	Slow
Modified by hormones	No	Yes	Yes
Triggered by Ca^{2+}	Yes	Yes	Yes
Troponin blocking	Yes	No	Yes
Sliding filament	Yes	Yes	Yes
Myosin/actin	Yes	Yes	Yes
Sarcoplasmic reticulum development	Good	Poor	Moderate
Contraction without nerve input	No	Yes	Yes
Duration of contraction equals duration of action potential	No	Yes	?
Action potential like that of neurons	Yes	-	No
Effect of neural input	Excitatory	Excitatory/inhibitory	Excitatory/inhibitory
Neurotransmitter	Acetylcholine	Serotonin	Acetylcholine or norepinephrine

Interestingly, during systole, when the ventricles are contracted and blood is sent coursing to the furthest parts of the body, the cardiac arteries feeding the heart itself and the aorta are so compressed that no blood can flow through them; instead, the arterial blood feeding the cardiac muscle and the aorta passes through them during the more passive diastole phase. As shown in figure 14.A-4, the coronary artery may first be blocked partially by atherosclerotic plaque and the flow then stopped when the plaque is sufficiently thick to be plugged by a small, circulating blood clot.

Innervation of the Heart: The Cardiac Pacemaker

Innate Heartbeat Frequency

Unlike the situation with skeletal muscle, cardiac-muscle contraction is not driven by a neural impulse from the central nervous system (however, see below). Instead, several cells within the heart are able to launch action potentials without stimulation from the outside, and their innate frequency of excitation becomes the essential

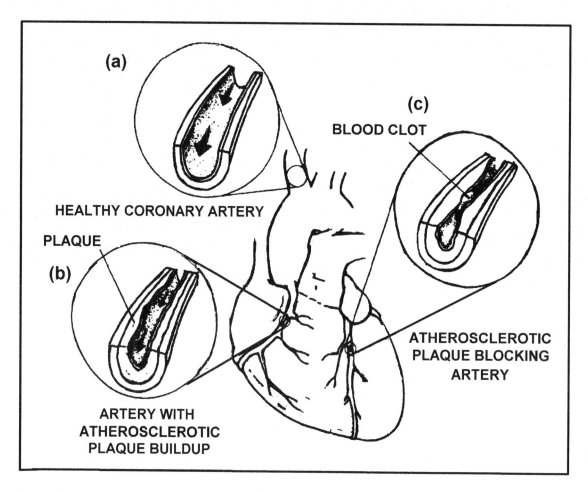

Figure 14.A-4. (a) A cross-section of the healthy coronary artery, (b) the artery partially blocked by atherosclerotic plaque buildup, and (c) a blood clot closing the last remaining opening of the coronary artery partially blocked with atherosclerotic plaque.

heartbeat frequency. The first phase of the cardiac excitation begins in the upper right atrium at a spot called the sinoatrial (SA) node. Even in the resting state, tissue in this area is especially leaky with respect to Na⁺ ions and so has a transmembrane potential that rises spontaneously to eventually initiate a depolarization wave. The cardiac muscle fibers are arranged in a near-parallel latticework, with the fibers dividing, then coming together again and dividing again in an irregular way. Because the muscle cells are so closely bound to one another in the heart, a neural excitation in the SA node rapidly spreads to all of the other cells in the two atria by way of gap junctions (Section 3.C, page 48). In this situation, almost all of the atrial cells are excited virtually simultaneously, resulting in global atrial contraction. See

Box 14.A-1, below, for a discussion of the unique character of the cells in the SA node.

A second node within the right atrium called the atrioventricular (AV) node senses the excitation from the SA node and then sends its own signals to the Purkinje cells of the ventricles. These cells are poor muscle contractors but excellent conductors of neural signals. Again using gap junctions, the Purkinje cells rapidly and coherently excite all of the other cells in the ventricles to contract sequentially from the bottom of the ventricle to the top. In this case, the ion channels of greatest importance are those for the inward flow of Na⁺.

The time delay for the signal transmission from the SA to the AV nodes separates atrial and ventricular contractions in time, as demanded

---

Box 14.A-1: The Cells of the SA Node Share an Electrical Bond

When a heart cell from the SA node is placed in a nutrient solution, it contracts on its own at about forty cycles per minute. A second cell placed in this solution, but not touching the first, also contracts at this frequency, but there is no correlation of the times at which the two cells contract. That is to say, they contract independently of one another. If, however, the two cells are able to touch one another, then the contractions immediately fall into synchronicity! A collection of such contracting cells within the right atrium form the SA node and lead to global timing pulses for atrial contraction, wherein all cells in the atria are contracting at the same moment. The SA node continues its electrical output at approximately forty cycles per minute, without rest, for the entire life of the individual [742]. This frequency can be raised by the cardioaccelerator, a nerve in the sympathetic nervous system, to a level as high as 200 cycles per minute during extreme exercise; however, this acceleration can be canceled by simultaneous excitation by the cardioinhibitor (the parasympathetic vagus nerve), returning the heart rate to a value as low as twenty-five cycles per minute when at rest. In seventy years, the heart beats 2.5 billion times, the rate always being somewhere between twenty-five per minute (*savasana*) and 200 per minute (*surya namaskar*).

---

by the four phases described in Subsection 14.A, page 536. Neural excitation in the ventricles is a very long process, as it is terminated by the slow opening of the K^+ channels, allowing this ion to move out of the muscle fiber (repolarization). Depolarization in cardiac fiber lasts approximately 100 times longer than in skeletal fiber, and concomitant with this, the refractory period is also anomalously long. The long refractory period in the heart allows ample time for the heart to refill with blood before the next heartbeat is initiated in the SA node.

Exceptional acceleration of the heart rate is known as tachycardia, and the exceptional slowing is known as bradycardia. Should the heart go into tachycardia, the heart rate can be slowed by the ocular-vagal reflex; i.e., pressure is applied to the orbits of the eyes to slow the heart via stimulation of the parasympathetic system (the vagus nerve). A similar effect is achieved by placing external pressure on the carotid arteries (Subsection 14.F, page 589). Cooling the face with ice water also acts on the vagus nerve to slow the heartbeat.

For both atrial and ventricular excitation within the heart, it is notable that there is no ran-

dom excitation of muscle units, as is common in skeletal muscle that is to be contracted over a long period; instead, all of the contraction possible is called forth in one burst, short-lived but very strong. If, however, the contraction of the ventricles is arrhythmic or the fibers depolarize not as a group, but randomly as individuals, then the heart is in fibrillation, and a strong DC electrical shock from a defibrillator is necessary to reestablish coherence and rhythm of the contractions; ventricular fibrillation is responsible for 25 percent of all deaths. If the ventricular contraction is not stimulated for some reason, or its timing is off, the heartbeat must be driven externally by an electronic pacemaker. Inasmuch as the heart has its own internal pacemaker, it is somewhat surprising to find that cardiac muscle is innervated externally at several places as well. Cardiac muscle fibers at the SA and AV nodes synapse with the postganglionic neurons from both the sympathetic and parasympathetic nervous systems (Chapter 5, page 157), the neurotransmitter in the former being norepinephrine and in the latter, acetylcholine. Activation of the SA and AV nodes by both neural and hormonal routes by the

Box 14.A-2: Stopping the Heart by Conscious Control of the Vagus Nerve

With constant work on the inner being, adept yoga students are able to gain more and more conscious control over the autonomic nervous system (Subsection 1.B, page 12). In doing this, they are then able to perform many seemingly magical feats with their bodies, such as control of the heart rate, breath, blood flow, or local temperature. Earlier scientific studies regarding yogis' claims to have "stopped the heart" showed that in these cases, there was considerable contraction of the skeletal muscles of the chest and holding of the breath, so that the local contraction closed the venous supply to the heart. With little or no blood being pumped, the heartbeat cannot be heard, and there is little or no pulse to be felt; however, the electrocardiograph shows that the heart in these cases was nonetheless beating electrically [891].

In contrast, Swami Rama et al. [685] present original scientific data from the Menninger Foundation in New York City illustrating some of the Swami's powers over the otherwise autonomic processes in his body. As can be seen in figure 14.A-5a, over a period of 10 minutes, Swami Rama was able to develop and maintain a temperature difference of 10° F between the inner and outer edges of the palm of one hand. One must suppose that in doing this, he was able to dilate the blood vessels in one part of the hand so as to warm the skin in that area, all the while causing the vessels in the opposite part of the hand to constrict and cool the skin (see Sections 14.C, page 573, and 20.D, page 725).

To the amazement and horror of the investigating scientists, Swami Rama then caused his heart to stop pumping blood for over twenty seconds (figure 14.A-5b), at which point they begged him to resume normal heart action. They found that during the period of zero blood flow, the atria were fluttering at a rate of about 300 times per minute, whereas the ventricles had ceased to pump blood. Compare the electrocardiogram of the swami for the first twenty seconds with a normal one (figure 14.A-6). In the context of what has been said in this section, it would appear that he was able to simultane-

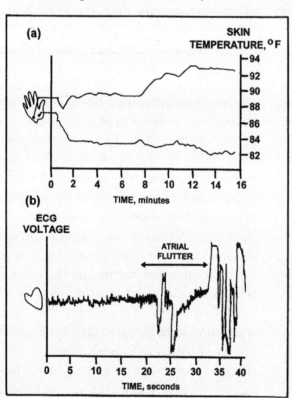

Figure 14.A-5. (a) Generation of a 10° F temperature differential on the surface of the palm, maintained for over a ten-minute period by Swami Rama. (b) Electrocardiogram of Swami Rama, showing no voluntary ventricular output for over twenty seconds [685]; compare it to figure 14.A-6.

ously drive the atrial flutter, using sympathetic excitation, and quench the ventricular contraction totally, using parasympathetic excitation of the vagus nerve. Amazing! Other amazing feats of control of the body's inner states have been reported, but the scientific data is not available to substantiate the claims [65, 178, 371, 463].

sympathetic channel, either through the fight or flight response, through emotional or psychic factors, or by deliberate conscious action increases the heart rate (by up to 200 beats per minute), its contractile force (by up to 100 percent), its stroke volume (by up to 300 percent), and the blood pressure as well.

If, instead, the effect on the heart is parasympathetic activation, all of the significant cardiac functions decrease (table 5.A-2), lowering the heart rate to thirty beats per minute or less, the contractile force by 30 percent, and the volume output by 50 percent, as compared with normal operation [621]. The parasympathetic signals are carried to the heart by the right branch of cranial nerve X (the vagus nerve), using acetylcholine as the neurotransmitter; however, the ventricles are supplied with far more sympathetic fibers than parasympathetic. This modulation of the heart rate and the strength of contraction originate with nerve centers in the medulla oblongata. See Box 14.A-2, above, for a note on how the vagus nerve can be controlled so as to literally stop the heart for a short time.

The effect of norepinephrine on cardiac muscle is to lower the threshold for production of an action potential by increasing the permeability of the cardiac-cell membranes to the inward flow of Ca^{2+}, which speeds the rise of the resting potential. Sympathetic activation also results in the release into the bloodstream of norepinephrine from the adrenal medulla; however, the stimulation of cardiac muscle by norepinephrine is more importantly by the neural route [360]. The action of acetylcholine is to increase the membrane permeability to the outward flow of K^+ thus making the resting potential more negative, and thereby requiring a longer wait for the resting potential to reach threshold. Because the heartbeat is con-

trolled in part by the autonomic nervous system, through its control of the permeability of the cardiac-muscle membrane to Ca^{2+} and K^+ ions, these factors dictate the rate at which the resting potential of the membrane reaches threshold.

Interestingly, there is yet another pacemaker in the body controlling the rhythmic contraction of muscle; see Subsection 19.A, page 711, for a discussion of the pacemaker driving the rhythmic contractions of the smooth muscle of the gut.

The Electrocardiogram

In a way very much parallel to that in which the brain's electrical activity can be measured using external electrodes on the scalp (Section 4.H, page 149), the various electrical phases of the heart action can be followed using external electrodes on the trunk of the body. Called an electrocardiogram (ECG or EKG), this recording shows the relative timing of the phases of the cardiac contraction (figure 14.A-6). One sees in the figure that the cardiac cycle begins with a P wave, the electrical signal initiated at the SA node that contracts the atria and fills the ventricles in the diastolic phase. Signals in the Q, R, S region are initiated in the AV node and correspond to ventricular contraction appropriate to the systolic phase; the Q wave follows the P wave by about 150 milliseconds. The compressed structure of the Q, R, S region reflects the rapid conductivity of the Purkinje cells in the ventricles. Next to appear is a T wave, which serves to reset the voltages on the surfaces of the heart in preparation for the next heartbeat cycle. During the T wave, no further electrical heart action is possible, thus accounting for the long refractory period during which the heart refills with blood for the next heartbeat. On the other hand, if the

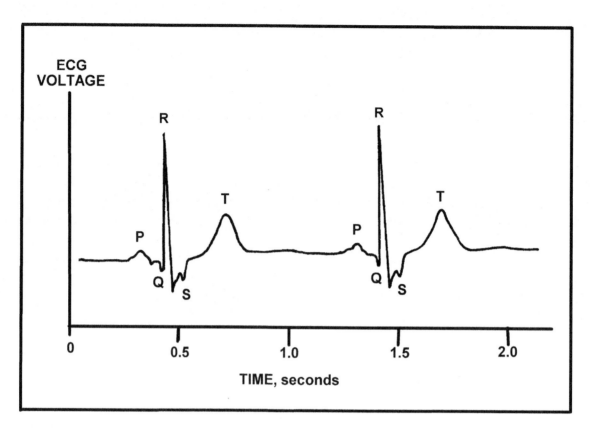

Figure 14.A-6. The author's ECG recorded in the V5 electrode configuration, showing the P, Q, R, S, and T features. The time between R pulses was 1,000–1,200 milliseconds.

left ventricle is struck a modest blow while it is in the T phase, all coherence of ventricular contraction is lost, and the person so struck is dead within minutes.

ECG Variations

Variations in the pattern of cardiac voltages in the ECG are symptomatic for various cardiac malfunctions and are readily diagnosed [432]. For example, the area under the P wave relates to the size of the atrial chambers, lengthening of the P–R interval beyond 200 milliseconds signals inflammation or scarring of the atria and/or of the AV area, an enlarged Q wave is symptomatic for an impending heart attack, and a low or missing T wave signals an ischemic condition in the heart. A variable Q–T interval between heartbeats signals a higher risk for sudden cardiac death.

Magnetocardiogram

The violent contraction of the heart muscle has two associated electromagnetic currents: (a) that associated with the ionic transmembrane neural current exciting the muscle fibers of the heart and (b) that associated with the flow of large numbers of ionic species (H^+, Na^+, Ca^{2+}, Cl^-, HCO_3^-, etc.) within the blood as it flows through the arterial system. These electrical currents are accompanied by associated magnetic fields, as is any current flow, such as that inherent in the contraction of any muscle of the body or that inherent in the current flow along and between neurons in the brain (Subsection 4.H, page 149). In the case of heart contractions, the associated magnetic field has an intensity of about one-thousandth that of the earth's constant field (being the strongest of any biomagnetic field in the body) and yields a magnetocardiogram looking much like that in figure 14.A-6 but which is readily detectable at all

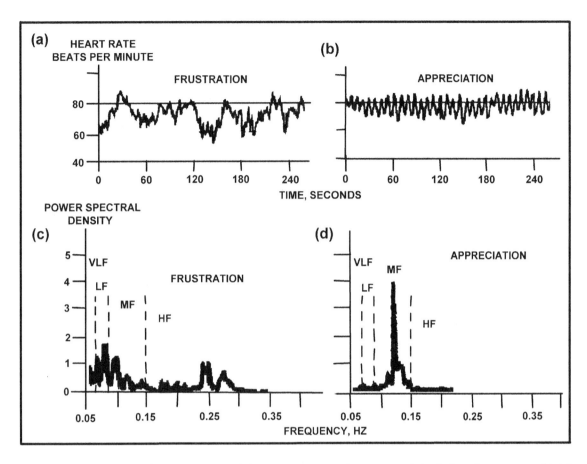

Figure 14.A-7. (a) Plot of the variation of the instantaneous heart rate while feeling frustration. (b) The plot of the heart rate variability while the same subject is concentrating on the notions of love and appreciation. (c) The power spectrum of the variability data while in the frustration mode, and (d) the power spectrum of the variability data while in the love and appreciation mode [550].

points of the arterial tree [637]. The sensation of the heartbeat is an interoceptive one (Subsection 11.C, page 444) and is appropriately sensed within the right cerebral hemisphere [890].

Note that the heartbeat generates the strongest electromagnetic field of any part of the body; the motion of the ions in the blood as it is pumped by the heart results in an external electromagnetic field that is sixty times more intense than is the signal in the electroencephalogram of the brain, and its magnetic filed is 5,000 times stronger than that generated in the brain. The heartbeat is the global internal synchronizing signal in the body.

HR Variability and the Power Spectrum

With all the discussion of the rate of the heartbeat as a fixed number, it is something of a surprise to see that modern work on the ECG

[550] shows a small but significant second-to-second variation of the heart rate, especially in the healthy heart. Furthermore, this variability (or lack of it) is strongly dependent on mental and emotional factors. As shown in figure 14.A-7a, when a person is feeling frustrated, the plot of the **instantaneous** heart rate over a period of four minutes shows variations of over twenty beats per minute over a period of sixty seconds and is otherwise quite irregular. If, however, the subject is consciously thinking of the notions of love or appreciation, then the variability of the heart rate changes to that shown in figure 14.A-7b, wherein the variability is somewhat less but much more regular.

Detailed analysis of an ECG spectrum such as that of figure 14.A-6 shows that the pattern is not exactly repeatable, as the heart rate is not constant

(Subsection 15.C, page 619); it can be deconstructed to show that it is really a combination of several patterns, each of which is perfectly repeatable and has its own characteristic frequency. A plot of these characteristic frequencies versus the amount of that particular frequency contributing to the overall pattern is known as the power spectrum of the initial pattern. The power spectrum of the variability of the heart rate in turn can be divided into four spectral regions, each of which is reflective of a specific neural activity:

1. The very low frequency (VLF) region, 0–0.02 hertz, reflecting neural activity in regard to thermoregulation (Subsection 14.C, page 573).
2. The low frequency (LF) region, 0.02–0.05 hertz, reflecting neural activity in the sympathetic nervous system (Section 5.C, page 170).
3. The medium frequency (MF) region, 0.05–0.15 hertz, reflecting neural activity in regard to the baroreceptors (Section 14.E, page 580, and Subsection 15.C, page 619). Waves in this frequency region are known as "Mayer waves" and are thought to be due to sympathetic excitation within the vascular system.
4. The high frequency (HF) region, 0.15–0.5 hertz, reflecting neural activity in the parasympathetic nervous system (Section 5.D, page 178).

In practice, the regions VLF, LF, and MF are considered together as reflecting sympathetic excitation at the heart, whereas that within the HF region represents the parasympathetic component of the autonomic drive at the heart.

Once the variability of the heart rate is in hand and is transformed into the power spectrum (as in figures 14.A-7c and 14.A-7d), it is a simple act to then measure the relative areas in the sympathetic and parasympathetic regions and thus to arrive at a quantitative measure of the balance between sympathetic and parasympathetic excitation of the heart. Thus, in a demonstration case [550], it was shown that in the normal state, the sympathetic/parasympathetic ratio is 3.15, but when in a deep mental state called "entrained" (figure 14.A-7b), the ratio rises to 17.08. The power spectrum of a yet deeper mental state (that of "internal coherence") has a ratio of only 1.25, implying an almost total lack of sympathetic excitation.

It would be very interesting to apply this technique to yogis in the postures, to see the quantitative effects on the autonomic system. One also wonders if the pulsation at 0.125 hertz so obvious in the power spectrum of the loving heart (figure 12.A-7d), relates in any way to one of the higher mental states achieved in *Ashtanga* yoga. Note that this frequency also is observed in the cranial-sacral pulse and in the pulsation of the capillaries, and that in the "internal coherence" mental state, these oscillators become phase-locked at their common frequency.

Much as is the case with the respiratory sinus arrhythmia (discussed in Subsection 15.C, page 619), subjects with low flexibility in regard to the sympathetic-parasympathetic transition (those who do not cycle easily between sympathetic and parasympathetic dominance) are prone to depression (Subsection 22.A, page 756) and are at heightened risk of sudden cardiac death. That the variability of the heart rate is least at 10:00 AM correlates closely with the hour of maximum risk of heart attack, 9:00 AM (table 23.B-2).

Effects of Western Exercise, *Yogasana*, and the Autonomic Nervous System on the Heart

Cardiac Output

The average cardiac output ($\dot{Q}$) of five liters per minute is determined by the rate of venous return to the right atrium rather than by the pumping capacity of the heart. Thus, lacking any stimulation of the sympathetic nervous system, the pumping capacity of the heart readily can be doubled, and when sympathetically stimulated, as with heavy exercise, $\dot{Q}$ can be as high as thirty-five liters per minute. In this case, the attendant sympathetic stimulation also will act to constrict

Table 14.A-2: Redistribution of Cardiac Output[a] as a Function of the Level of Exercise [308, 618, 851]

Tissue	At Rest	Light Exercise	Moderate Exercise	Maximal Exercise
Liver	1,350 (27%)	1,100 (12%)	600 (3%)	300 (1%)
Kidneys	1,100 (22%)	900 (10%)	600 (3%)	250 (1%)
Brain	700 (14%)	750 (8%)	750 (4%)	750 (3%)
Heart	200 (4%)	350 (4%)	740 (4%)	750 (3%)
Muscle	750 (15%)	4,500 (47%)	12,500 (71%)	22,000 (88%)
Skin[b]	300 (6%)	1,500 (15%)	1,900 (12%)	600 (2%)
Other tissue[c]	600 (12%)	-	-	-
Total cardiac output	5,000	9,500	17,500	25,000

a Given as the amount of blood flow in milliliters per minute and as a percentage of total cardiac output in parentheses.

b On a cool winter day.

c In the resting state, approximately 10 percent or more of the total blood volume resides in the alveoli of the lungs.

blood vessels in muscles that are not working, in order to increase the flow to those that are. In the working muscle, the metabolism of the working muscle and the increased heart rate lead to the muscle's vasodilation and an increased flow of blood through it to the heart.

When the body is inverted, the blood flow to the right atrium increases for no other reason than that of the hydrostatic pressure (Subsection 14.F, page 584). In response to this surge of excess blood, signals from the right atrium act to reduce blood volume by promoting urination and by cutting back on the production of antidiuretic hormone (ADH, vasopressin) from the adrenal glands so that urine production increases.

Effects of Exercise

In general, the body's autonomic response to Western exercise (running, tennis, swimming, etc.) is the same as that appropriate for a fight or flight situation: a general tensing of the body and mind in expectation of an attack from outside. The response begins with the hypothalamus signaling the adrenal medullae to release their catecholamines into the bloodstream. With respect to the heart, this means a sympathetic excitation

that shifts the blood supply away from the viscera and toward the muscles and heart, and an increase of the heart rate, systole strength, and coronary artery diameters (table 14.A-2). In this regard, Nieman [618] presents an interesting discussion, quantitatively detailing just how much blood is diverted from the left ventricle to various body organs as the level of exercise is increased. Thus, at rest, only 15–20 percent of the cardiac output goes to the large muscles, while at the peak of physical exercise, the cardiac output to the large muscles can increase to 88 percent of the total. On going from minimal to maximal exercise, the fraction of the heart's output to the abdominal organs decreases from 12 percent to 1 percent (signaling the cessation of digestion), in the kidneys from 10 percent to 1 percent, in the brain from 8 percent to 3 percent (but maintaining a constant flow rate of 750 milliliters per minute), and in the skin from 15 percent to 2 percent. At the same time, the percentage of blood going to the heart muscle remains constant at 4 percent, but at a rising flow rate, as measured in milliliters per minute. All of these changes are just those expected for strong sympathetic excitation (table 5.A-2). The redirection of the blood flow is accomplished by the appropriate constriction of some blood vessels and the dilation of others.

Note that the brain gets as much blood flow during maximal exercise as it does at rest (700 to 750 milliliters per minute) and that the blood supply to the skin increases somewhat, because the exercise produces heat and circulation within the skin, leading to cooling of the core. During heavy exercise, the blood supplies to the kidneys and to the digestive system are significantly reduced, and this may be part of the reason we get stomach cramps if we try to exercise right after a meal [877]. The constancy of blood flow to the brain regardless of the level of exercise suggests that there is no oxygenation effect on the brain by being in inverted positions. Others have argued that this is not so, because it is known that the rates of flow through certain arteries to the brain are influenced strongly by body posture [503]; however, this may well be just a **redistribution** of flow rather than a change of overall volume of flow. The possible redistribution of blood flow within the brain on inversion could prove to be rejuvenating, even though the overall blood flow through the brain is unchanged [112a, 386, 883].

It is interesting to see just where the blood is to be found in the vascular tree: 59–64 percent of the blood resides in the veins, 13–15 percent in the arteries, 7–9 percent in the heart, 9–12 percent in the lungs, and only 5–7 percent in the capillaries at any one time [308]. That so much more blood is to be found in the venous system than in the arterial system follows from the fact that the pumping of arterial blood toward the veins is so much more efficient than the pumping of blood from the veins toward the arteries. Furthermore, due to the elastic nature of its components, the venous system can function as a rather large blood reservoir; the veins of the abdominal organs (liver and spleen) and the veins of the skin are special in this regard. On average, the flow rates of blood through the arterial and venous systems must be equal if the time-average amounts of blood flowing in and out of the heart are to stay equal.

Once the level of exercise reaches an oxygen consumption rate of $\dot{V}O_{2max}$, it is found that the output from the heart is maximal, whereas the capacity of the respiratory system is only at about 65 percent of its maximum. That is to say, the ability of the muscles to do work is limited by the output of the heart and not by that of the lungs. In old age, the muscle power drops as the cardiac output drops. Experiments on *yogasana* students in *sirsasana* show that the amount of oxygen consumed while in the posture is only 50 percent larger than when in *tadasana* [112a], as expected for light exercise.

Nieman [618] gives an accounting of the oxygen demand during hard exercise (figure 14.A-8). In order to do its work, a muscle may demand 3,000 milliliters of oxygen per minute. With the venous blood containing only five milliliters of oxygen per 100 milliliters and the arterial blood containing twenty milliliters of oxygen per 100 milliliters, the blood flow can deliver only fifteen milliliters of oxygen per 100 milliliters of blood. To meet the needs of the exercise, the heart stroke volume (SV) must go up to 140 milliliters per beat, and the heart rate (HR) must increase to 143 beats per minute. At the same time, the respiration rate increases to forty breaths per minute, with 2.25 liters of air inhaled with each breath. Under these conditions, the muscle will be fed the required amount of oxygen via the capillary arteries and will remove from the muscle the corresponding amounts of carbon dioxide and lactic acid. These parameters of the lungs and heart allow the necessary chemistry (lower part of the figure) to occur in the muscles doing the work. Note too that exercise not only increases circulation, by moving more blood through the vascular system, but actually builds new capillaries as well. The factors influencing the heat balance in the body during intense exercise are presented qualitatively in figure 14.A-9.

The two main effects of vigorous exercise on the heart are:

1. An increase of carbon dioxide in the blood is sensed at the carotid arteries, which generate a signal that is transmitted to the medulla oblongata, resulting in an increased heart rate.

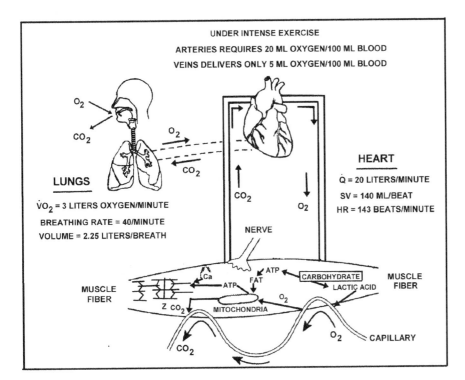

UNDER INTENSE EXERCISE

ARTERIES REQUIRES 20 ML OXYGEN/100 ML BLOOD

VEINS DELIVERS ONLY 5 ML OXYGEN/100 ML BLOOD

O_2

CO_2

LUNGS

$\dot{V}O_2$ = 3 LITERS OXYGEN/MINUTE

BREATHING RATE = 40/MINUTE

VOLUME = 2.25 LITERS/BREATH

O_2

CO_2

CO_2

O_2

HEART

$\dot{Q}$ = 20 LITERS/MINUTE

SV = 140 ML/BEAT

HR = 143 BEATS/MINUTE

NERVE

MUSCLE FIBER

MUSCLE FIBER

ATP

Ca

FAT

ATP

CARBOHYDRATE

LACTIC ACID

O_2

Z CO_2

MITOCHONDRIA

CO_2

O_2

CAPILLARY

Figure 14.A-8. The interactions between the respiratory, cardiac, and muscle systems of the body during intense exercise. See text for explanation.

Figure 14.A-9. Several factors that influence the heat balance within the body are modulated by the skin. In-flowing heat is represented by inward-facing arrows, and out-flowing heat is represented by outward-facing arrows. The heat-loss figures refer to an unclothed performer in air at 60° F [308].

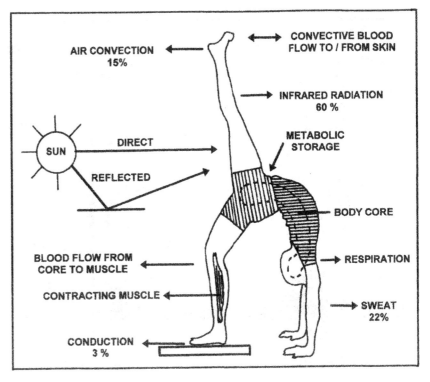

AIR CONVECTION 15%

CONVECTIVE BLOOD FLOW TO / FROM SKIN

INFRARED RADIATION 60 %

METABOLIC STORAGE

SUN

DIRECT

REFLECTED

BODY CORE

RESPIRATION

BLOOD FLOW FROM CORE TO MUSCLE

CONTRACTING MUSCLE

SWEAT 22%

CONDUCTION 3 %

2. The muscle action may pump venous blood so as to fill the right atrium and so activate stretch sensors in the atrium, which in turn signal the medulla to decrease the heart rate [450].

When working the muscles at a high level, the mitochondria are required to produce more ATP from the phosphorylation of ADP; the energy for this reaction is derived in turn from the aerobic oxidation of glucose by oxygen delivered in the bloodstream. As a consequence of this reaction chain, the amount of work that a muscle can do is strictly limited by the amount of oxygen that can be delivered to the mitochondria of its cells by the blood. As noted above, the amount of oxygen that can be delivered to the mitochondria by the bloodstream is a direct measure of the blood-flow rate out of the heart, as the lungs readily can supply the required amounts of oxygen to the blood. In a two-minute race, about 40 percent of the total energy is being supplied anaerobically and this drops to about 20 percent when the race lasts five to seven minutes [827]. Long bouts of *surya namaskar* may take one from the former situation to the latter.

During Western exercise, the systolic pressure will rise with increasing work, climbing to 200 millimeters Hg, and when lifting a heavy weight, the pressure may climb to over 400 millimeters Hg. At the same time, the diastolic pressure will remain constant or even decrease slightly during aerobic exercise, and rises only slightly when weightlifting. Increased systolic pressure in the arteries generated by Western exercise forces lymph out of the capillaries, and this pumps up the muscle while pushing the veins closer to the surface, where they bulge.

If, for any reason, the flow of blood to the heart is impeded, then the heart becomes ischemic, and the stage is set for a heart attack. There are two distinct symptomatic types of cardiac ischemia. In one, there are obvious chest pains of only a few minutes' duration (angina pectoris); in the other, there is no obvious pain, but the episode may last for almost an hour (silent ischemia). Strangely, the angina type of chest pain usually follows physical activity, whereas the silent type follows mental or emotional activity and is most likely to occur in the first six hours after awakening. This latter fact implies that there is an activation of the sympathetic branch of the autonomic nervous system at work here (Subsection 23.B, page 771). Thinking about exercise also can be effective in stimulating the sympathetic nervous system, and this psychic effect can raise $\dot{Q}$ by 50 percent due to increasing heart rate and force of contraction.

Yogasana Effects

In response to the claims that yoga is not sufficiently aerobic [124], consider the study of DiCarlo et al. [202], which compared a thirty-two-minute routine of standing postures in the Iyengar style with a thirty-two-minute treadmill walk at 7 kilometers per hour (four miles per hour). It was found that the *yogasana* routine resulted in a larger increase in heart rate, blood pressure (systolic and diastolic), and rating of perceived exertion than did the treadmill walk, yet it showed a lower metabolic demand. In a similar study aimed at measuring the cardiorespiratory changes during *surya namaskar* [795], it was concluded that this aspect of hatha yoga is an ideal aerobic exercise, as it involves both stretching and optimal stress on the cardiorespiratory system.

Though the effects of all Western exercise on the heart are just those expected for sympathetic excitation of the autonomic nervous system (table 14.A-2), the accomplished student of *yogasana* can control the excitation in the autonomic nervous system through the appropriate choice of *yogasana*. When in *urdhva dhanurasana* or during *yogasana* jumping, for example, there is sympathetic excitation and all of its coronary consequences (increased heart rate and strength of systole, with vasodilation of the coronary arteries); but when in postures such as *sarvangasana* and *janu sirsasana*, it is the parasympathetic branch that moderates, and the response is one of cardiac relaxation instead. In regard to the heart rate, it is interesting to note that the rate can be doubled in about five seconds, given a sufficiently strong activation of the sympathetic nervous sys-

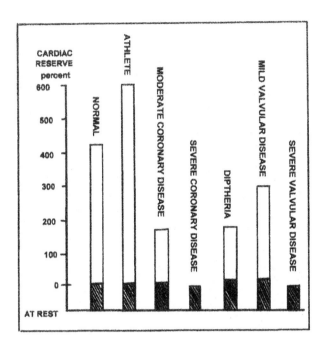

Figure 14.A-10. The cardiac reserve above and beyond the resting state of healthy students, athletes, and those with various medical conditions.

tem, but that it will require ten minutes or more for the parasympathetic nervous system to bring the rate back to normal.

Large and significant differences were reported in the levels of sympathetic excitation while in the *yogasanas* for two groups of practitioners, those new to the practice and those with six months to one year of *yogasana* experience [286]. The steady-state heart-rate level of the trained group was 11 percent lower in *sirsasana I* than that of the novices and 15 percent lower in *adho mukha virasana*. Similar indicators of reduced sympathetic excitation in the trained students were reported for respiratory indicators as well (Subsection 15.D, page 622). The effectiveness of *savasana* as a mode of relaxation has been compared quantitatively to sitting in a chair or simply lying down, by first stressing the body on a treadmill and then noting the rate of return of the heart rate and blood pressure to initial values when in each of the three relaxation modes. Baseline values of these quantities were observed significantly sooner when in *savasana* than when sitting or simply lying down [55].

Cardiac Reserve

The percentage by which the output of the heart can increase beyond its normal output of five liters per minute is known as the cardiac reserve [308] (figure 14.A-10). All of the factors that impact negatively on cardiac performance will lower the cardiac reserve, the immediate consequences being shortness of breath, rapid heart rate, and extreme fatigue. Vigorous practice of the *yogasanas* will result in a cardiac reserve of between 400 and 600 percent if the practitioner is free from cardiac complications, as seen from figure 14.A-10.

Heart Attack

Heart attacks occur with highest frequency between 9:00 and 10:00 AM, with the time between 11:00 PM and midnight being the period of least risk for attack. When we first awaken in the morning, the stress hormones epinephrine, vasopressin, and cortisol are released into the blood, leading to a narrowing of the cardiac arteries and a rise of the blood pressure. This added activity raises the demand by the heart for oxygen by 50 percent. Heart attacks at this early hour result in more damage to the heart than do attacks at later hours, and the risk that a heart attack will prove fatal is highest in the early morning hours. Angina attacks also peak in the morning hours between 10:00 and 11:00.

Even though the general risk for heart attack is highest in the morning, a regular exercise program done daily at the time of greatest risk is found to reduce this risk significantly. Among those who exercise regularly, those few heart attacks that do occur are found to be independent of the time of day. The frequency of heart attack throughout the week is maximal on Mondays, and the number of fatalities is larger in the winter months than in the summer months in the northern hemisphere; the opposite holds in the southern hemisphere.

Anastomoses (Subsection 14.C, page 574) function as alternate paths for blood flow are plentiful in the vascular system within the heart. Thus, collaterals in the heart can take over for a major artery in the heart which is 90 percent blocked, for the heart will function with only 10–15 percent of its normal supply route open if the collateral anastomoses are functioning [863]. If the blood supply to the heart is restricted so that the cells become ischemic but continue to live, then the condition gives rise to the pain of angina pectoris; whereas if the blood supply is so sparse that myocardial tissue dies, then one has a myocardial infarction or heart attack. Aneurysms are most dangerous when in the heart but are most often found in the vascular systems of the legs of older people. Such vascular problems are indicated by a pulsating swelling of the artery in the leg.

Though cardiac cells normally do not reproduce, there are stem cells in the heart that increase in large numbers when the heart muscle is damaged and that can be stimulated to form normal cardiac cells when exposed to growth-stimulating proteins.

Gender Differences

Evidence is rapidly accumulating that the symptoms and causes of heart attacks in men and women are significantly different [39]. As regards heart-attack symptoms, for men it is the classic combination of a tight feeling, pressure, and pain in the chest that is experienced, whereas for women, the symptoms are back pain, nausea or dizziness, lower-chest and/or upper-abdominal pain, disturbed sleep, feelings of fatigue, and shortness of breath. During a heart attack, only one in eight women report chest pain, and even then, it is reported as a pressurization or tightness rather than as pain, as with men.

The wide discrepancy between heart-attack symptoms in men and women reflects the differences in the basic causes behind the symptoms in the two cases. In men, the cause is overwhelmingly the build-up of calcium-based plaque in the coronary arteries, which curtails the flow of blood to the coronary muscles; in women, the cause rests with muscular spasms of the coronary arteries, which similarly deprive the heart muscles of fresh blood. It is emotional stress that is more likely to precipitate a heart attack in women, whereas physical stress is more likely to precipitate a heart attack in men. Interestingly, people

who are impatient and impulsive, (type A personalities) are seven times more likely to suffer heart disease than those who can remain silent and be good listeners. *Yogasana* practice, of course, can help immensely in learning how to control the impulse to act externally.

Heart Changes on Aging

As with any muscle in the body, the more the heart is used to pump blood, the larger and stronger (up to a point) it becomes; contractile proteins make up 60 percent of the volume of cardiac cells. As a corollary to this, the easing of the load on the muscles, as with bed rest or weightlessness in space, quickly leads to atrophy and loss of cardiac muscle mass. In fact, it has been found that in prolonged space flight, the volume of the human heart shrinks by 15 percent! Because one might expect approximately the same shrinkage to take effect in the inactive body, it is surprising to see that the weight of the heart on average **increases** as we age (figure 24.A-1). This can be rationalized in the following way. Because the vascular resistance increases in old age and the diastolic pressure goes up accordingly, the heart must work harder in order to deliver the goods. In response to this extra load, the heart will grow in size; this is a bad sign, because unlike the exercise situation, the load on the heart is ever present, there being no time for cardiac rest and relaxation. This scenario may account for the average weight and volume of the heart increasing as one ages from twenty to sixty-five years. In support of this idea, the diastolic blood pressure also rises from age twenty to sixty-five years (figure 24.A-1). As we age, the maximum heart rate drops, even in super-trained athletes. However, such athletes have a larger stroke volume, to make up for the lowered heart rate [827].

In the course of extended physical exercise, the heart, like any other muscle, will grow in size and its wall thickness will increase. These changes in the heart induce an increase in stroke volume, with a lower heart rate, an increase in total blood volume, and an increase in capillary density, which serves to more easily bring oxygen, glucose, and fatty acids to muscles and carry away waste products. Though there is a large effect of the emotions on the heart rate, chronic exercise tends to decrease heart rate and return it to the resting value more quickly. This suggests that long-term training increases parasympathetic vagal tone. The slower heart rate allows the heart to fill more completely and so to pump more blood per stroke [169]. Through all of this, $\dot{Q}$, the rate of flow, remains unchanged.

The effect of the emotional state on the heart rate during inhalation and exhalation is clear when one compares these quantities while experiencing either appreciation/love or frustration (figure 14.A-7) [550, 764].

Section 14.B: Blood

Chemistry and Function

Blood is the principal extracellular fluid in the body and serves as the messenger service for many different needs [431, 432, 878]. Acting as the body's active distribution system, the blood transports oxygen from the lungs to the tissues and cells and carries the carbon dioxide from these places back to the lungs, all through the agency of hemoglobin. The carbon dioxide bound to hemoglobin is bound at a site different from that which binds oxygen. Blood also transports pathogens from everywhere in the body to sites where they can be deactivated, as well as transporting the agents of the immune system to the site of injury. Moreover, the blood also carries vitamins, electrolytes, and nutrients from the gut to wherever they are needed; transports hormones from their sources to their target organs; and is the pipeline for moving the metabolic wastes from the muscles to the kidneys.

In the average male, the body contains 5.6 liters of blood, about 8 percent of the total body weight; while in the average female, there are 4.5 liters (5.0 liters when pregnant), the difference being due to the male's larger body mass. The heart requires about one minute to pump

five liters of blood through the vascular system when at rest, but under conditions of heavy exercise [528], this time can be reduced to about ten seconds! Via the vascular system, blood is sent to within 20 μ or closer of every cell of the body, except for the cornea, bone, cartilage, middle ear, and testicles.

Myoglobin

The discussion above speaks only of hemoglobin, the circulating, iron-containing protein capable of transporting oxygen and carbon dioxide to and away from working muscles via the bloodstream. This mechanism of fueling muscle action is relevant to fast-twitch, type 3 muscle fibers; i.e., those capable of rapid, high-frequency contraction but which fatigue in a very short time (Subsection 11.A, page 414). A second iron-containing protein that is non-circulating is embedded in the slow-twitch, type 1 muscle fibers; called myoglobin, it too binds and releases oxygen to working muscles (such as the antigravity postural muscles) and makes it possible for such muscles to work for long periods without the need to relax.

Composition

Blood contains both dissolved substances (proteins, salts, organic acids, all in water) forming the blood plasma (55 percent of the blood volume) and suspended blood cells of various sorts and functions. Acid-base balance in the blood is maintained by regulation of its bicarbonate-ion concentration. The acidity (pH) of blood is normally kept within the narrow range of 7.36 to 7.44 by homeostasis, with the lower value more likely for venous blood and the higher value more likely for arterial blood. In any case, the range quoted above is solidly on the basic side, as any acidity above 7.00 is defined as basic. Production of the various types of blood cells (10^{11} per day for an adult) is localized in the marrow of certain bones [450]. The three major types of blood cells are discussed in the subsections below.

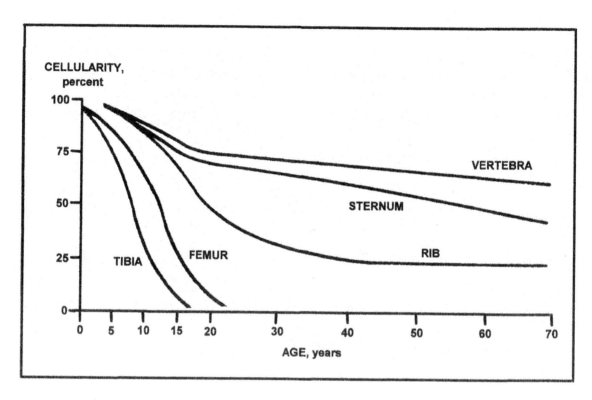

Figure 14.B-1. Fractional decrease of the cells of the bone marrow producing red blood cells as a function of age.

Temperature Regulation

In addition to transporting the chemical species and discrete cell bodies listed above, blood serves another very important function. In general, the temperature of the core of the body is higher than that of the air surrounding it, so that if the heat of the inner body could be brought to the surface, the body could radiate heat into the air and so cool itself. With control from the autonomic nervous system, warm blood can be transferred from deep inside the body to the outer surfaces, with a subsequent return of the cooled blood back to the inner recesses of the body. Just how this is accomplished is considered in Subsection 14.C, page 573.

Erythrocytes: The Red Blood Cells

The erythrocytes (red blood cells) contain all of the hemoglobin to be found in blood, between 200 and 300 molecules of hemoglobin per red blood cell. The structure and function of this important metalloprotein is discussed further in Subsection 15.A, page 609. Red blood cells filled with hemoglobin are manufactured largely in the red marrow of bones, but the liver and spleen are able to generate these cells in an emergency. Many other cells in the body have the DNA required to continuously reproduce the various cellular proteins that make up the red blood cell; however, red blood cells cannot do this, nor can they divide, as they have no nucleus. Thus, they really are not "cells" in the biological sense of the word.

Bone Marrow

Red blood cells die after a few months without reproducing or regenerating themselves [877], after traversing approximately 1,700 kilometers (1,000 miles) of vascular pipeline! Every second, about three million red blood cells die, are degraded into bile pigments by the liver, and are replaced by fresh cells from the bone marrow [450]. The bone marrow within the bones, the birthplace of red blood cells, is a considerably larger organ than one might at first assume, being exceeded in mass only by the liver and the skin. At age five years, the marrow within the tibia, femur, ribs, sternum, and vertebrae are the body's source of red blood cells; however, by age twenty years, the red blood cell productions of the first two of these are essentially zero, and by age seventy years, the vertebrae are down to 60 percent, the sternum to 50 percent, and the ribs to 25 percent of their productions at age five years (figure 14.B-1) [308].

Hemoglobin's sole function is to transport oxygen from the alveoli of the lungs to the tissues and cells (four oxygen molecules per molecule of hemoglobin) and to carry carbon dioxide away from these sites and back to the lungs. If the partial pressure of oxygen is too low in the air being breathed, then hormones are released that accelerate the production of red blood cells, as will also the direct stimulation of the bone marrow by the sympathetic nervous system (table 5.A-2).

Blood Chemistry

Consisting of a very flexible sac packed with hemoglobin but lacking a cell nucleus, the red blood cell is able to fold so as to negotiate the tortuous paths of the capillaries, in order to serve outlying tissue. A red blood cell can leave the heart, travel through the vascular net, and return to the heart in as little as twenty seconds. In an individual, the surfaces of the red blood cells are coated with sugar molecules in one of four ways, leading to the four basic blood types (A, B, AB, and O). These coding systems on the cells' surfaces are intimately involved with immunity and the identification of foreign cells. (See also Subsection 19.A, page 709, for the situation regarding foreign bacteria in the colon.)

When we bring the sympathetic nervous system into dominance by performing vigorous *yogasanas,* one of the many consequences is that the spleen is prompted to release its store of red blood cells, so that more oxygen can be carried by the bloodstream [582]. Yogic training appears to raise both the hemoglobin content of blood and its hematocrit, all the while lowering its ability to coagulate [115]. *Yogasana* students who have an iron deficiency are anemic and will quickly tire

and become breathless during their *yogasana* practice, as the low iron levels imply low red blood cell counts and therefore poor oxygenation of the working tissues. As the viscosity of blood is strongly dependent upon the presence of the red blood cells, anemic blood is very thin, and the heart is only somewhat strained in pumping such blood. On the other hand, when exercising, there is little or no cardiac reserve in the anemic (figure 14.A-10), so that heavy exercise in such students can lead to heart failure.

Platelets

Very large, noncirculating cells in the bone marrow routinely disintegrate, forming platelets by the millions. The normal concentration of platelets in the blood is between 150,000 and 350,000 per milliliter of blood, and the average life of such a cell fragment is about ten days before the spent platelet is scavenged by macrophages in the spleen. Having no nuclei or DNA, the platelets are really not cells but are simply fragments of the larger mother cells; containing serotonin, platelets circulate without effect in the blood until they are called upon to perform their special task.

Blood Clotting

Platelets are responsible for the clotting of the blood when there is an injured blood vessel. Blood in the normal situation does not contact collagen fibers in the body, as the inner layers of the blood vessels are lined with endothelial cells that stand between the blood and the collagen of the blood-vessel walls. However, when the vascular pipeline is cut, the edges of the cut bring blood into contact with the collagen fibrils of the outer layers. As a consequence of this contact, the platelets release their serotonin, which then acts to constrict the bleeding vessel while dilating other intact vessels in the area. Most importantly, the platelets convert fibrinogen into strands of fibrin, which are able to trap red blood cells at the site of a wound and so form a plug that stops the bleeding, if the wound is not too large [716].

This particular initiating event in the formation of a blood clot—the contact between the platelets and collagen—is of special interest to *yogasana* students. In certain *yogasana* positions, there is a pressing of the muscle against bone that can be so severe that the integrity of the endothelial inner layers of blood vessels caught in the squeeze is compromised. In this case, the contact of the platelets in the blood with the collagen within the roughened wall of the traumatized blood vessel can lead to the formation of a blood clot (called a thrombus) at that point. Further work of the same sort can then dislodge the clot, setting the stage for the formation of an embolus further along the circulation route. Such an embolus can lodge in a smaller blood vessel and cause an ischemic attack in the tissues that are normally served by the vessel. See Subsection II.B, page 838, for several case histories relating to this problem.

To the extent that *yogasana* work unavoidably involves a certain amount of forced ischemia in some of the muscles (more so in beginners, less so in more advanced students), it is also relevant that blood that is moving slowly or is at rest is far more likely to coagulate on the spot than is blood that is flowing rapidly through cleared vessels. The formation of such blood clots is guaranteed in organs in which the blood flow is totally blocked for a matter of hours. This gives us an upper limit to the time that one should spend in a *yogasana* if there is an element of ischemia in it [308].

The White Blood Cells

The first line of defense of the body against foreign cells, microbial infections, and toxins is formed by the white blood cells (leukocytes), of which there are a great variety. The white blood cells are less numerous than the red by a factor of 700, have nuclei, protect the body from infection, and consist of lymphocytes, monocytes, and granulocytes [450]. The bones of the skull, spine, and ribs produce ten million white blood cells per minute in a healthy adult [68].

Leukocyte Function

The first leukocyte to attack foreign invaders is the macrophage, which immobilizes them.

Neutrophils then attack if necessary, and should this fail, the monocytes are called into battle. Functionally, the white blood cells may be divided into those that respond to inflammation and tissue injuries but are otherwise of a nonspecific nature, and those that are targeted toward specific intruders. Reactions of the first group are innate, whereas those of the second group are acquired through a previous exposure to a particular pathogen. See Section 16.D, page 650, for the effect of HIV on white blood cells. Leukocytes that fight infectious bacteria in the bloodstream, and their relations to the autonomic nervous system and to *yogasana* practice, are discussed further in Chapter 16, page 641.

The Blood-Brain Barrier

More so than with any other tissue in the body, the delicate neural apparatus within the brain must be protected from fluctuating levels of most of those chemicals released into the bloodstream when we eat or exercise. To this end, nature has devised the blood-brain barrier, which allows glucose, oxygen, and carbon dioxide to pass easily between the blood and the brain, but resists the passage of larger molecules. However, alcohol and nicotine molecules are small enough to get past this barrier and so strongly affect the workings of the brain.

The capillaries in most of the body are neither featureless nor continuous pipes but instead have many small breaks and windows, which aid in the mass transfer of materials (lymph proteins) between the inside and outside of the capillary. This arises because the endothelial cells forming the capillary wall are only loosely packed, and the wall itself is only one or two cells thick. Not so in the brain, however, for here, the endothelial cells are packed so very tightly that the only way material can pass between the blood and the extracellular fluid is by virtue of the microscopic permeability of the intact capillary wall. As the capillary-wall cell membranes within the brain are constructed of tightly packed hydrophobic lipids (figure 3.A-2), they are very selective in what chemical species they will let pass from the blood to the brain. In particular, fat-soluble materials in solution (such as glucose, alcohol, and the small amino acids) find easy passage through the lipid layers, whereas materials that are only water soluble cannot penetrate the lipid barrier; highly charged ions are particularly discriminated against. The capillary walls in the brain thus act as a blood-brain barrier, protecting the neurons of the brain and spinal cord from harm by noxious chemicals and biological substances that might be present in the blood. Very large molecular species are especially discriminated against by the blood-brain barrier; i.e., bacteria, viruses, white blood cells, proteins, and parasites cannot pass through. Because proteins cannot pass the blood-brain barrier, there is no lymphatic system (Section 14.G, page 595) in the brain. Of course, the blood-brain barrier also works between the blood and the cerebrospinal fluid (Section 4.E, page 109), but only in the CSF-to-blood direction. It appears that the hypothalamus is not protected by the blood-brain barrier.

Glucose

The brain's total reliance on glucose for energy is made all the more important by the fact that though the brain is only 2 percent or so of the body's mass, it commands 20 percent of the body's glucose metabolic budget. One can see from this the severity of the problem in those having type 1 diabetes, for example, where glucose can not be transported readily across cell membranes, and mental performance suffers (especially in children).

Barrier Leaks

Certain molecules are not able to pass from the blood to the brain in normal situations, but it has been found that under stress, the blood-brain barrier can become leaky and so can allow these substances to pass through [16]. The blood-brain barrier can be breached when one is suffering from hypertension, infection, trauma or injury, microwave or other electromagnetic irradiation, or high concentrations of transported substances. Note too that there are several places in the barrier where the brain monitors the composition of the blood, and these places also are sites of weakness in regard to trans-capillary transport.

Though the human mouth is home to approximately 500 different bacterial species and approximately 200 normally can be found even in the outer ear, thanks to the blood-brain barrier, the brain itself remains a sterile organ.

Section 14.C: The Vascular System

Architecture

As described in Section 14.A, page 536, the four-chambered heart is much like two hearts side by side (figure 14.A-1). The right side of the heart is filled with deoxygenated, depleted blood, which it then pumps into the lungs for recharging with oxygen and stripping of carbon dioxide (pulmonary circulation); the oxygenated blood from the lungs is then pumped by the left side of the heart to the waiting muscles and organs of the body (systemic circulation). The vessels that carry the blood from outlying reaches of the body to the right heart, from the heart to the lungs and back again, and from the left heart to the furthest extremities, taken together, are known as the vascular system [742]. Reductions or increases in the diameter of the vascular system are known as vasoconstriction or vasodilation, respectively, and are under the control of the vasomotor center in the brainstem.

The activities and health of all of the body's organs are dependent upon receiving an adequate and timely supply of blood. Most often, the blood in motion does not come into direct contact with the cells in the body that it services; however, because almost all cells in the body are no further than 20 μ from a capillary [450], diffusion between cell and capillary can be an efficient means of service. The red blood cells do not diffuse through the surrounding tissue, but the smaller molecules in the blood can diffuse.

Aortas

The ascending aortic arch (figure 14.A-1), in carrying blood away from the left ventricle, branches to form the coronary arteries, the thoracic aorta, and the abdominal aorta. The ascending and descending aortas, as they leave the heart, are conduits with diameters of approximately 2–3 centimeters (approximately 1 inch), running close to and parallel to the spinal column; however, they shortly branch to form smaller arteries, which in turn branch further to form arterioles; these in turn branch to form capillaries. Blood flow through all of these conduits is driven by the pressure of the left-heart ventricular contraction. The general schematic for the flow of blood through the body is given in figure 14.C-1, while the aortas and major arteries of the body are shown in figure 14.C-2a.

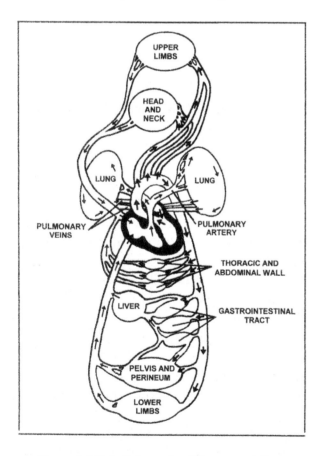

Figure 14.C-1. Schematic of the general flow pattern of blood through the various capillary beds of the vascular system. The heavy and light arrows represent the directions of blood flow at high pressure (arterial) and low pressure (venous), respectively.

Arterial Walls

The aorta is a large-diameter, elastic vessel (see figure 14.A-1) that swells with each beat of the heart and then shrinks as the subsequent blood flow reduces the pressure within. With increasing distance from the heart, the aorta becomes smaller and less elastic but more muscular. This more distant part of the arterial system distributes blood to the muscles and organs in general, but most importantly, the more muscular the artery is, the more its blood flow can be controlled by the autonomic nervous system. As can be seen in figure 14.C-3a, such an artery is composed of several layers, the middle one of which (layer 3) is a cylindrical muscle that when contracted, acts to narrow the artery's diameter. The walls of arteries and veins are constructed of the same five layers, but the veins are constructed of much less smooth muscle and a larger percentage of white fibrous tissue [863].

Constriction of the arterial walls is largely under the control of the sympathetic nervous system, whereas parasympathetic activation leads to the dilation of already constricted vessels. For a given blood vessel at 100 millimeters Hg pressure, the maximal sympathetic vasoconstriction can reduce the arterial blood flow by a factor of four, and the maximum parasympathetic vasodilation can increase it by almost a factor of two, as compared to the resting state. Because the venous walls are so much less muscular than those of the arteries, the latter are far less distensible than are the former; i.e., for a given increase in pressure, the change in diameter will be about twice as large for the veins as compared to the arteries. It is possible with *yogasana* practice to bring control of arterial diameter into the conscious realm.

The relative thickness of the arterial walls changes with their locations in the body. The outer layers of the arteries are thin in those arteries that are internal and therefore well protected behind bone; they are much thicker in the limbs, where they are exposed. A similar shielding by heavy connective tissue occurs for the muscles, depending upon the extent of their exposure to the outside (Box 12.B-1, page 489).

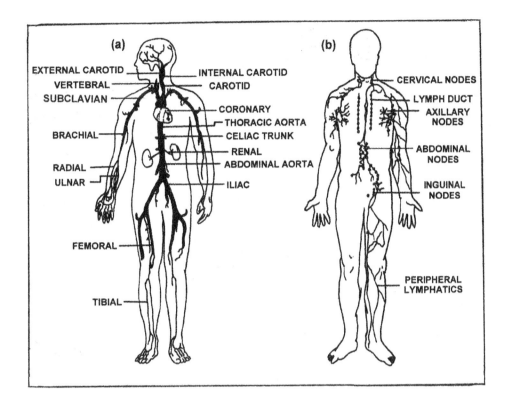

Figure 14.C-2. (a) The major arteries of the body. Because the veins and arteries in the body are often paired, the figure also gives a fairly accurate picture of the locations of the major veins. (b) The lymphatic channels and lymphatic nodes in the body.

Figure 14.C-3. Comparison of the multilayer structures of arteries (a) and veins (b). In an artery, the smooth-muscle layer (3) is much thicker and more powerful than in a vein, whereas the latter has directional valves that are absent in the former [431]. The arrows indicate the directions of blood flow.

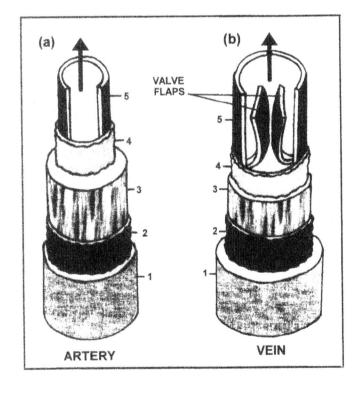

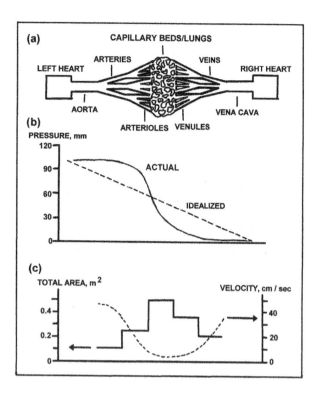

Figure 14.C-4. (a) Schematic display of the branching of the elements within the vascular system, going from the left ventricle to the right atrium. (b) The mean blood pressure at every point in the vascular system, assuming that the resistances to blood flow of all of the elements in (a) above are equal (idealized, dashed line), and the actual pressure profile across the system (solid line). (c) Reciprocal nature of the variation of the cross-sectional areas of each of the vascular elements (full line) and the velocity of blood flow through each (dashed line).

Arterioles

The arterioles are small in diameter (less than 0.5 millimeters or 0.02 inches) and are found just at the entrances to the capillary beds (figure 14.C-4a). They are sufficiently muscular (layer 3) that they can turn off the local blood supply totally, thus redirecting the blood flow to other organs with a greater need for it. Arterioles offer the largest resistance to blood flow, and therefore the largest pressure drop in the vascular system is across the arterioles (figure 14.C-4b). Control of the arteriole diameter is the responsibility of

the sympathetic nervous system, as controlled in turn by the vasomotor center in the medulla oblongata. As sympathetic excitation of an arteriole can only be vasoconstrictive, the vasomotor tone of the arteriole wall depends upon the frequency of the sympathetic neural pulses sent to the arteriole. Parasympathetic relaxation of the arterial diameters can be as large as the sympathetic excitation, but not larger. As is characteristic of smooth muscle (table 14.A-1, page 543), arterial muscle tone is a tonic reflex and so can be retained for a very long time.

Capillaries

The capillaries have very thin walls, only a cell diameter or so thick, and it is here that the exchange of gases, metabolites, waste products, etc. between the vascular system and the extracellular fluids surrounding the muscles and organs occurs most easily. The capillary length is about 0.25 millimeters (0.01 inches) but can reach 1 millimeter (0.04 inches) in muscles [7]; with cell walls only a cell diameter or so thick, it is clear that the capillary walls have a structure very different from the multilayer structures of arteries and veins (figure 14.C-3). On average, a hemoglobin molecule spends only one second within a capillary and must perform all of its gas exchange work in that period. It is now thought that the straining of the blood through the capillary net within the lungs not only serves to aerate the spent blood but also to filter out small, mobile blood clots.

There is an observable pulsation in the capillary beds, which reflects the oxygen content of the blood, but it is only about one-tenth of the frequency of the systolic contraction of the heart driving the 1–2 hertz pulsation frequency in the arterial network. See Subsection 14.A, page 549, for more on this low-frequency (0.15 hertz) oscillation (the Mayer wave) in the ECG power spectrum.

Angiogenesis

Wherever there is an insufficiency of oxygen, angiogenesis factors are released that promote the formation of more capillaries in the vicinity of the oxygen deficit. These are the same capillary-promoting factors that lie behind the growth of malignant tumors (Subsection 16.D, page 647), but in this case, the proliferation of cell growth is activated by the increased demand for oxygen. If the metabolism in a particular tissue increases, as it would during the practice of the *yogasanas,* then the vascularity will increase proportionally in that tissue, within days in the very young body, but only partially, in a matter of years, in the older body. Similarly, if the metabolism decreases in a particular tissue through disuse, the result will be a decrease in vascularity, occurring much faster in the younger body. Thus, in almost all tissues, there is an automatic adjustment of the tissue vascularity to meet the metabolic needs of the tissue, the adjustment being driven by the relative need for oxygen; this adjustment is prompt and exact in the young body and slow and approximate in the aged [308, 877]. The impact of the response of vascularity to exercise is obvious to the *yogasana* teacher or student, as it relates to the muscle soreness felt by *yogasana* students and their teachers (Subsection 11.G, pages 476 and 477) following a sharp increase in the strength of a practice.

Aortic Aneurysm

Systolic pressure in the vascular network is highest in the aorta just above the heart. Though normally only 120 millimeters Hg, it can rise momentarily to well over 300 millimeters in situations where a heavy weight (about 75 percent of body weight or more) is being lifted. In such cases of heavy lifting, it is often advantageous to hold the breath by blocking the glottis and contracting the abdominal and thoracic muscles to pressurize the thorax, thereby stiffening the spine and thorax. Called the Valsalva maneuver (Subsection 15.C, page 616), its application in susceptible persons, such as those with Marfan syndrome, leads to a ballooning of the aorta and the possible formation or bursting of an aortic aneurysm. Moreover, the vascular problems of Valsalva over-pressure when lifting heavy objects also may occur in the nearby carotid or vertebral arteries. Aortic aneurysms are more common in the older athlete, since the flexibility of the aorta decreases with age. Bursting of an aortic aneurysm (aortic dissection) is a very serious condition, often resulting in death [223, 224]. Schievink [759] mentions "yoga practice" as one of the activities that can lead to such dissections, though I cannot find any specific mention of this in the medical literature.

With this in mind, it is interesting to see just how large a proportion of the body weight is being lifted in certain *yogasana* postures (figures IV.D-1 and IV.D-2). To lie on the floor and press up into *urdhva dhanurasana* would appear to be an arm lift of about 50 percent or more of full body weight, and to press from *chaturanga dandasana* into its straight-arm version (classical push-up) or into *adho mukha svanasana* involves lifting up to 75 percent of full body weight. Indeed, Elefteraides [224] reports two cases of aortic dissection in athletes doing push-ups! It appears that such heavy-lifting motions, in *yogasana* practice or otherwise, should not be assisted by the Valsalva maneuver in those who have any history of aortic aneurysm or aortic enlargement, but instead should be done on an exhalation of the breath or not at all. On the other hand, because the Valsalva maneuver does strengthen the spine when lifting, avoiding the maneuver when doing heavy lifting puts one more at risk for injuring the lower back, unless one is able to lift with the legs bent at the knees and the torso bent at the lower hinge (Subsection 9.B, page 319).

Adipose Tissue

Because fat tissue must be served as well as muscles, obese people have several extra miles of capillaries to serve the fat cells in their bodies. And just like muscles and fat cells, the blood vessels themselves require a network of smaller blood vessels to bring them nutrition and oxygen; these are found within the walls of the larger vessel.

If an area of the body is little used, then the capillary net in that area will be only slightly filled with blood; when activated maximally, the capillary net will fill with blood. Tendons and ligaments will have very sparse to nonexistent capillary networks, and the epidermis, cornea of the eye, and cartilage are totally devoid of capillaries, functioning metabolically by diffusion instead.

Venous Structure

The venous and arterial systems differ greatly in that there is no active, dedicated pump for moving venous blood through the system the way the heart moves the arterial blood. This significant difference is reflected in the internal architecture of these two subsystems. Venous and arterial walls each are composed of five distinct layers of tissue (figure 14.C-3), but since the arteries must support a much higher internal pressure,[3] their middle wall of smooth-muscle cells (layer 3 in the figure) is much thicker, and the walls themselves are much less elastic. The elastic veins can easily swell so as to become blood reservoirs, and as a corollary to this, they also can be easily pinched off by any sort of internal pressure (muscle tension, for example) or external pressure (that of the arm against the leg in *maricyasana III*, for example).

Furthermore, the arteries have no valves, whereas the veins below the heart and in the neck have one-way valves that aid in directing deoxygenated blood back to the heart by closing whenever the blood tends to flow backward; i.e., away from the heart. The innermost layers of both arteries and veins (layer 1 in figure 14.C-3) are lined with endothelial cells that act to separate the collagen of the vessel walls from the blood, which would clot were it to come into contact with collagen.

In the venous system, there are many fewer vascular problems (such as occlusions or hemorrhaging) than in the arterial system, due to the many anastomoses (Subsection 14.C, page 574) and the inherently lower blood pressure in the former.

Vascular Smooth Muscle

The smooth muscle in the arteries and veins is activated involuntarily, and unlike skeletal and cardiac muscle, it can maintain its contraction for very long periods of time. In fact, if there is

damage to the wall of a blood vessel, a reflexive vascular spasm occurs that can stem the flow of blood for up to thirty minutes. The arteries operate at high pressure, and if there is a breach of the arterial wall, the loss of blood can be rapid. However, if the rate of loss is not too high, it can be stemmed by this reflexive contraction of the artery, slowing blood flow. As discussed below in Subsection 14.D, page 575, this latter fact is a key to understanding certain aspects of the phenomenon of chronically high blood pressure (hypertension).

Mechanics of Blood Flow and Blood Pressure

Blood Flow

Blood flows through a section of the vascular system only if there is a difference of pressure between the two ends of that system. In particular, the rate of flow of blood through a blood vessel will depend directly upon the difference of pressure at the two ends, and inversely on the resistance the blood vessel offers to flow:

$$\text{Flow} = \text{Pressure} / \text{Resistance}$$

Rate of blood flow can be changed by appropriate changes in either the blood pressure or the resistance to flow, or both. As discussed below, the resistance to flow is controlled by the diameter of the vessel conducting the flow. In every case, the blood flow through any part of the vascular plumbing occurs because there is a pressure gradient across that part; there is no flow from one end of a pipe to the other end if there is no pressure difference (gradient) between the ends. The successive components of the vascular system through which the blood flows (left heart, aorta, arteries, arterioles, capillary beds, venules, veins, vena cava, right heart, lungs) are shown schematically in figure 14.C-4a. Imagine for a moment that each of these elements in the vascular loop offers the same resistance to blood flow. In that case, the change of pressure from the high-pressure end of the system (the left heart, pressure at

---

3   The blood pressure at the right ventricle is only 20–30 millimeters Hg, whereas that at the left ventricle is 100-150 millimeters.

Table 14.C-1: Blood Flow through Various Components
of the Vascular System [432]

Vessel	Velocity, cm/sec	Total area, cm^2
Artery	45	800
Arteriole	10–35	2,500
Capillary	0.5–1	5,000
Venule	5–10	3,500
Vein	10–35	2,000

100 millimeters Hg) to the low-pressure end (the right heart, pressure at 0 millimeters) is shown by the straight dashed line in figure 14.C-4**b**; i.e., there is a constant pressure drop (gradient) of about 10 millimeters Hg across each segment of the system, so that the pressure across an artery, for example, would drop from 80 to 70 millimeters, and the pressure across a venule would drop from 60 to 50 millimeters.

In actuality, the real pressure-drop curve across the vascular system is known to be more like that of the full curve in figure 14.C-4**b**, which differs from the dashed curve of the idealized situation in that the true pressure drop across the arteries is close to zero, while that at the arterioles is 60 millimeters Hg, not 10 millimeters! This means that there is a disproportionately larger resistance to arteriole flow, with the result that the pressure is anomalously high at their input end (about 100 millimeters Hg in the aorta and arteries) and anomalously low on the output side (15–0 millimeters in the capillary beds, venules, veins, and right heart). It is as if the arterioles are acting like an almost-closed faucet, with high pressure behind but low pressure beyond and very little flowing through. The resistance to flow within the arterioles is due largely to the constriction of the smooth muscles in the arteriole walls, which reduces the diameters of the arterioles and so makes blood flow more difficult.

Figure 14.C-4**b** shows that the largest drop of the vascular pressure is across the arterioles and that the venous side of the system supports little or no pressure gradient. On the other hand, though blood flow through the capillaries and venules is very slow, blood does not accumulate behind them, because there are so many more of them to handle the load. Obviously, if the blood circulation is stable in time, the output through the arterial side of the system can be no larger than the input by the return route through the venous side.

The large pressure drop across the arterioles dictates that the pressure drop across the venules and veins is quite small, of the order of a few tens of millimeters Hg, meaning that there is very little resistance to flow. However, resistance to blood flow in the veins can be anomalously high, because in many veins, there is constriction from the outside (due largely to the resting muscle tone), thereby reducing their diameters (Subsection 11.B, page 436); were it otherwise, the veins would offer virtually no resistance to blood flow. Note too that the flow rate of blood through a particular vessel varies as the fourth power of its diameter, meaning that small changes of diameter due to compression or dilation can result in large changes of flow rate.

In table 14.C-1 and figure 14.C-4**c**, certain parameters of blood flow through the various components of the vascular system are listed. One sees from the figure that as expected, the velocity of flow through the arterial side decreases as the diameter of the carrier decreases; whereas on the venous side, the velocity increases as the diameter increases. Every time a vascular pipe bifurcates, the total cross-sectional area increases and the flow velocity through that new pipe increases; whereas should the vascular system converge, the area decreases, and so the velocity drops (figure 14.C-4**c**).

Though capillaries in muscles are generally only about 1 millimeter (0.04 inches) long, there are so many of them that the total area of the capillary walls is six times larger than that of the wide-diameter arteries; if all of the 1-millimeter-long capillaries in the human body were strung together end to end, the chain would be 100,000 kilometers (65,000 miles) long! Given that the capillaries are so short, it is a great advantage that the velocity of blood flow through them is low (about 1 millimeter per second), for this gives a longer residence time (approximately one second) for the diffusive exchange of gases and other cellular materials (see Section 14.B, page 558) with the outside world. No doubt by design, the diameter of a red blood cell (7 μ) is just that of the capillary channel (6–7 μ), and so the red blood cells are just able to squeeze through; placing the cell wall of the red blood cell against the cell wall of the capillary guarantees the shortest possible distance for transfer of oxygen from the red blood cell, through the capillary wall, to the extracellular fluids.

Flow Velocity

Also shown in figure 14.C-4c is the reciprocal relationship between the velocity of flow through a vascular section (flow velocity = flow volume / cross-sectional area of the conductor) and the cross-sectional area of that section. Because there are so many capillaries in the capillary bed, its total cross-sectional area is large, even though the cross-section of just one of them is small. Correspondingly, the flow velocity is low through the capillaries (allowing a maximum time for diffusive gas exchange), whereas in the vena cava and aorta, the total cross-sections are low and the velocity is high.

A further complication of blood flow arises at high heart rates. In this case, the blood flow is turbulent rather than smooth and laminar, and the net effect of the turbulence is to slow the flow, thereby making the heart work even harder to achieve a certain elevated flow rate. On the other hand, blood tends to coagulate if the flow is smooth and laminar, since the blood is actually stagnant at the vascular walls when in laminar

flow. In response to this, the insides of arteries are naturally shaped like a corkscrew, so that blood swirls through the arteries and does not lie stagnant at any place in the arterial system.

Venous and Lymphatic Flow

It is clear from the discussion in this Subsection that the pressure of the blood and lymph are very low in the veins (0 to 10 millimeters Hg) and in the lymphatic channels (Section 14.G, page 595), respectively; as a consequence of this low pressure, venous and lymphatic flow to the heart will be severely retarded by even slight pressures applied from the outside, and the heart will have to beat faster and stronger to make up the difference.[4] This squeezing effect can be important at those places in the body where simple gravitational collapse would significantly impede venous and lymphatic drainage: the neck, the armpits, the abdomen, and the groin. It is for this reason that in the Iyengar protocol, special care is taken to see that these regions do not collapse, but instead are held open.

In the thoracic region, venous and lymphatic flow to the heart can be hindered by the internal pressure exerted by pregnancy, a full urinary bladder or colon, overweight, or a stomach full from having eaten recently. Moreover, such an internal pressure can come from the movement of the lungs, in which case the movements of the *yogasana* must be coordinated as well as possible with the movements of the breathing cycles [851]. Finally, drainage of the spent blood trapped within the veins serving strongly contracted muscles can only occur after the muscles relax. The problems associated with excessively high pressures within the veins (varicosities) and lymphatic channels (edema) are discussed in the following subsection.

---

4   Tension in the muscles reduces the blood flow through them and thereby increases heart action. If we can perform the *yogasanas* with a minimum of such muscle tension, then the heart action too will be minimal, and we can more closely approach Patanjali's ideal as expressed in Sutra II.46 (Subsection II.A, page 834).

Circadian Variation

Blood pressure, as measured at the upper arm, is higher when a person is standing than when lying down, and generally it is higher when a person is active than when passive. In preparation for the activities of the day, blood pressure begins to rise even before one wakes from sleep; it surges beyond that once one arises, and finally peaks in late afternoon. During this period of wakefulness, the systolic and diastolic pressures are 25–30 and 15–20 millimeters Hg higher in the daytime as compared with the nighttime values (Subsection 23.B, page 774). In some, the differences of daytime and nighttime pressures are either very small or very large compared to the norm, or the morning surge is larger than the norm; these are signs of poor cardiovascular health. Cold winter weather and smoking both raise one's blood pressure, leading to increased risk for heart attack (see Subsection 14.A, page 555).

Vascular Blockage

As there is much overdesign of the vascular system, with many parallel paths to the same end, blockages of the smaller arteries are often of no consequence as other vessels take over. However, in *yogasanas* such as *ustrasana,* in which the neck is placed in deep extension, the bending at the neck tends to block the large vertebral arteries (figure 4.E-1), which are threaded through the cervical vertebrae and serve the hindbrain. This blockage can lead to dizziness, nausea, and fainting [162]. Retraction of the scapulae down the back toward the waist using the latissimus dorsi and lower trapezius muscles relieves this blockage and the symptoms that flow from it.

There is a general stagnation of the blood within varicosities, but when the body is inverted, the stagnant blood is flushed out and replaced by fresh healthy blood. This can be important, as the flushing may stimulate the production of anticoagulants, which can forestall clotting [112a].

Shock and Blood Pooling

In the adult, the total volume of the capillary networks in the body is five liters, which also is very nearly the total volume of blood in the body. Clearly, then, not all of the capillary beds will be filled at once, as this would leave no blood for filling the other parts of the vascular system. In an active body, there is a constant transfer of blood between different capillary beds, depending upon need at the moment. However, in a time of high stress, **all** of the capillary beds may open, so as to absorb all of the blood in the body. This pooling of the blood in the capillary beds is called shock and is often fatal if not treated promptly. Because the brain and heart have the highest priority for blood flow, in the case of such blood-draining shock, the first priority is to elevate the legs with respect to the head and chest in order to promote flow to the brain and heart [308]. In cases of severe bleeding, the body may close all capillary beds so that there is enough blood to serve the brain and heart [450]. Working homeostatically, the body can compensate for the loss of up to one liter of blood before it goes into circulatory shock.

Venous Flow against Gravity

When standing upright, how does the venous blood move from the feet upward to the heart if its pressure (figure 14.C-4b) is close to zero? This is especially intriguing, considering that if one is upright and motionless, the first reaction to this simple posture is fainting within an hour, followed eventually by death.[5] The answer is that one does not remain motionless, but by contracting the skeletal muscles, the arterial flow is momentarily turned off to the muscle, while the venous blood inside the venules and veins within the muscle is

_____

5   The death that results from crucifixion is in part due to the loss of blood draining from the brain into the legs [878] and in part due to the suffocation that follows from not being able to exhale when hanging from the arms with the hands widely separated [545, 850]. This latter effect involves the spasm of the exterior intercostal muscles, which otherwise relax to allow exhalation.

squeezed into the uncompressed veins, outward and upward. In fact, the soleus muscle of the lower leg is known as the "second heart" for the high efficiency with which its contraction pumps blood from the lower leg back to the heart [61a]. It is because of soleus contraction that you can walk all day, but will faint after standing motionless for only an hour.

The difference between blood flow in arteries and veins arises from the fact that since the arteries are already at high forward pressure and are stiff, contraction of the muscle cannot force arterial blood to flow backward toward the heart, whereas veins, being the opposite, are easily deformed so that the venous blood leaves the contracting muscle and overfills nearby venous channels.

Venous Collapse

The large veins of the body have almost no resistance to the flow of blood when they are distended; however, the low pressure within the veins means that they are rather easily collapsed by the application of external pressure, throttling the flow. Thus, for example, the axillary veins of the arms are collapsed, as are the subclavian veins as they pass over the first rib; the pressures within the veins of the neck are so low that they are often collapsed, and intra-abdominal pressure is often enough to collapse the inferior vena cava. All of these examples of collapse offer resistance to venous blood flow back to the heart and highlight the consequences of a collapsed posture.

Throttling of the venous return to the heart due to the collapse of the venous diameters is caused by both the resting muscle tone and postural misalignments induced by gravity. In this regard, the focus of Iyengar yoga on activating the body so as to work against gravitational collapse, and to keep the body open and the body fluids moving, is seen to be very much appropriate, as is the accent on reducing the resting muscle tone.

Venous Valves

Moreover, the veins are outfitted with one-way valves that only allow blood to flow toward the heart (figure 14.C-5). The presence of the one-way valves in the veins of the lower body cannot be overemphasized, for without them, the squeezing of the veins would push as much blood away from the heart as toward the heart, making the squeezing totally ineffective. Thanks to the venous valves, the effect of muscle contraction pumps venous blood toward the heart and works best when the contraction and relaxation of the surrounding muscles is rhythmic; in fact, if the muscle is contracted for an extended time or is "pumped up" by heavy exercise, the resulting congestion impedes venous blood flow through the muscle. Surprisingly, the two largest veins in the body, the inferior and superior vena cava, have no valves; whereas the smaller veins below the heart and in the neck have one-way valves that aid in directing deoxygenated blood back to the heart by closing whenever the blood tends to flow backward; i.e., away from the heart.[6]

---

6   Actually, when the muscles in the legs contract, there is a momentary surge of venous blood sent upward to the heart; however, from that point on, there is an increased resistance to venous blood flow through the contracted muscle, and the flow is thereafter diminished. If, on the other hand, the muscles of the legs are alternately flexed and then relaxed in a rhythmic way, one has an efficient pump for continuously moving venous blood to the heart against gravity. We see from this that rhythmic contraction of the muscles will efficiently pump venous blood toward the heart, whereas the resting muscle tone, being tonic and everlasting, only works to throttle this venous flow, acting much as a tourniquet impedes the flow of both blood and *prana*. Similarly, squeezing the abdomen (as when coming into *paripurna navasana*, for example) yields a strong burst of venous blood to the right atrium; however, this flow is only momentary, as the muscle contraction then raises the resistance to blood flow.

The importance of muscle action in pumping blood is graphically demonstrated by experiments in which subjects are leaned against the wall and left in that position **without** any activation of the muscles in their legs; by the end of an hour in this passive position, more than 95 percent of them will have fainted. Without muscle action in the legs, so much blood will pool in the legs that the volume receptor will sense an insufficiency of the filling of the right atrium and will signal the central nervous system to shut down, triggering a faint. This reflex places heart and feet at

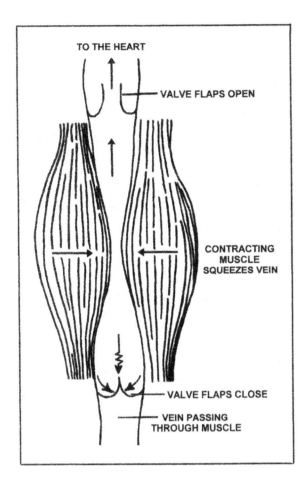

TO THE HEART

VALVE FLAPS OPEN

CONTRACTING
MUSCLE
SQUEEZES VEIN

VALVE FLAPS CLOSE

VEIN PASSING
THROUGH MUSCLE

Figure 14.C-5. As muscles contract, they press against the veins, pressurizing the blood within. The flap valves within the veins are constructed so that the pressure can be relieved in only one way: flow of the blood toward the heart. A similar drawing is appropriate for the pumping of lymph toward the heart by muscle action.

Pneumatic Pumping of Venous Blood

A second important mechanism that returns venous blood and lymph to the heart involves the action of the lungs. In the act of respiration, the downward movement of the diaphragm creates a momentary negative pressure above itself (which is sufficient to draw air into the lungs) and a positive pressure below (Section 15.C, page 613). In combination, these two pressure effects act to help venous blood from below rise to the level of the heart [752, 823], but only because the venous system of the lower body passes through the thoracic chamber on its way to the heart, and only if the abdominal muscles are toned so as to keep the intra-abdominal pressure high on inhalation. The respiratory pumping of blood works because the inhalation brings blood from the legs to the heart, and because the exhalation allows maximum blood flow through the lungs. The pumping of venous blood through the action of respiration is strongest when the breathing is deep and thoracic, with the abdominal muscles toned.

Atherosclerosis

A situation somewhat similar to that in the arterioles may exist in the arteries themselves. If the arteries are open and unclogged, then little or no pressure difference will be measured between points in an artery close to the heart and one distant from the heart, just as with the veins. Hydrostatic effects will be of no consequence here, for reasons discussed in Section 14.F, page 584. If, however, an artery is blocked by atherosclerotic plaque, then, as with the constricted arteriole, there will be a large pressure drop observable between the ends of the artery, as measured in the arm and at the ankle, for example.

In arteriosclerosis, the coronary arteries lose their elasticity and stiffen, thereby limiting blood flow through the heart; whereas in atherosclerosis, fatty deposits (plaques of cholesterol and/or triglycerides) form on the inside of the coronary arteries, thereby limiting the flow of blood through the heart. The coronary arteries are at the point of highest blood pressure in the vascular system. Clearly such plaques reduce the effective diameters of the arteries and reduce blood flow while raising the pressure gradient across the artery, and so require more work of the heart muscle.

Lymph

The blood pressure of 5–10 millimeters Hg or so within the capillaries is sufficient to force

the same height so that gravity no longer impedes the proper filling of the right atrium [140]. Because there are valves in the veins of the limbs, muscle contractions in the arms while in inverted positions such as *sirsasana* also pump blood back to the heart against gravity [431].

some of its water and proteins through the capillary wall into the extracellular space within tissues. However, at the low-pressure end of the capillary, the osmotic pressure of the extracellular fluid then forces some of the fluid back into the capillary. The fluid that remains outside the capillary walls is called lymph and it is loaded with blood proteins. It is the function of the lymphatic system to constantly drain the interstitial spaces between cells of their protein burden and return it to the venous system [450]. See Section 14.G, page 595, for a more complete discussion of the lymphatic system.

Varicosities

The veins of the legs, like all veins, are very flexible and distendable, and when the pressure within is excessive and long lasting, the effect is to balloon the veins. When this happens (often in older people who spend long hours standing up), the diameter of a vein may exceed the sum of the lengths of the valve flaps (figure 14.C-5), with the result that the valves cannot close completely and so will leak blood in the backward direction, away from the heart. The result is a bulging varicose vein. Deep veins may also leak blood, but they do not bulge, due to their support by the surrounding muscle tone.

Should the valves in superficial veins of the lower body fail to close properly and thus fail to hold back the venous tide, the veins below the leaky valve will bulge as varicose veins. In a related way, hemorrhoids are blood vessels in the rectum that sag under the pull of gravity when standing erect. As with lymph edema (Section 14.G, page 596), hemorrhoids and venous varicosities are relieved by rhythmic exercises and inverted *yogasanas,* which help pump or drain body fluids toward the heart. Just as clearly, extended periods of time in postures such as *padmasana* and *virasana,* which impede blood circulation in the legs, are contraindicated if one has varicose veins in that region.

Venous Pressure in Tadasana

That muscle action of the legs is effective in pumping venous blood from the legs to the heart is shown quantitatively by experiments in which pressure sensors were inserted into the saphenous veins of subjects, near their ankles [670]. The average venous ankle pressure when lying down was measured to be 12 millimeters Hg, but this rose to 56 millimeters when sitting upright and to 90 millimeters when standing in *tadasana*. This increase is due to the larger hydrostatic pressure exerted by the blood column when fully erect (Subsection 14.F, page 584). However, upon walking, the venous pressure at the ankle dropped from 90 millimeters to 22 millimeters and then rose again to 90 milllimeters once the subjects stopped walking. Thus, the venous pressure in the ankle is reduced by 75 percent by the simple rhythmic use of the muscles of the leg when walking, as compared with just standing still. A similar type of venous pumping in the *yogasana* standing poses undoubtedly is at work when one uses the approach of Iyengar [33], wherein one makes ongoing adjustments of the muscles, in essence turning them "on" and "off" repeatedly while in the posture; i.e., his concept of "pose and repose" (see also Subsection VI.F, page 943).

All of the veins in the torso of the body and in the legs emptying into the inferior vena cava are equipped with the one-way valves, as are the veins in the arms. However, as one is normally upright rather than inverted, the veins from the head leading to the superior vena cava have no valves. This means that when inverted, either actively or passively, return of venous blood from the head to the heart against the pull of gravity can be aided only by the rhythmic flexing of muscles in the arms and neck [140, 431].

Gravity Effects

When standing, muscle motion in the legs pumps venous blood against the pull of gravity back toward the heart. If the legs are still, then there is a stagnation of body fluids and an insufficiency of the blood supply to the brain, and one faints. What happens when one lies down and is motionless? In this case, there is little or no gravitational effect to be overcome, but the muscles of the legs still are not pumping blood at all. It seems to me that this is where the thoracic pump comes to the fore. On inspiration, the diaphragmatic displacement pulls air into the chest and also blood from the extremities, through the partial vacuum so formed. Thus, when still and horizontal, the diaphragm assumes a more prominent role as the venous pump! It would be interesting to know the relative importance of diaphragmatic and muscle pumping of venous blood to the heart when in various postures.

If one lies on the back with the legs up the wall (*urdhva prasarita padasana*), the arterial pressure is sufficient to pump fresh blood to the feet, and the return of the spent blood is easy, as its return to the heart is assisted by gravity. For this reason, any injury to the leg is bathed in fresh blood when in this posture, and so healing of the injury will occur most readily when the legs are so lifted.

Chronic muscle tension that inhibits free-flowing circulation can lead to constriction of the arteries in the head, leading in turn to headaches (Subsection 4.E, page 110). When this is the case, relief often can be had by promoting vasodilation using the ocular-vagal heart-slowing reflex (Sections 11.D, page 457, and 14.D, page 579).

Relevance of Circulation and *Yogasana* to Healing

Not only is *yogasana* a stimulant to the immune system and thus an aid to healing, but by promoting vascular circulation, it is a double blessing. Tissues of the body that have been injured can be healed in many cases, provided that they are supplied with an abundance of the proper nutrition (protein and vitamins A, B, C, D, E, and K) and are serviced by a strong vascular circulation. This latter factor in tissue repair is of utmost importance, because it is the vascular circulation that will bring the nutrients, antibodies, and oxygen directly to the injury site, as well as carry away deoxygenated blood, cellular debris, foreign bodies such as bacteria, and the spent fluids involved in swelling. Given the primal importance of circulation to healing, it follows then that actions that promote circulation, such as *yogasana* practice, will promote healing [752].

Muscle Tone

The higher the muscle tone, the more resistance there is to the flow of blood through the muscles and the poorer the circulation will be in the stressed muscles and in other body parts located farther from the heart. On the other hand, if the muscle tone can be relaxed, then the resistance to blood flow will decrease, provided the heart rate and stroke volume do not decrease in response to the lowered vascular resistance. That is to say, muscle tension can act as a tourniquet to both blood flow and healing. Furthermore, as the muscles are used in *yogasana* practice, they become infiltrated with an extensive web of capillaries, which promotes a widening of the network that carries blood to injured tissue, where it is most needed. *Yogasana* positions such as inversions can be used to carry more blood to the extremities and so speed healing in those areas, provided the postures can be held for long periods, as with *sirsasana, sarvangasana,* and *viparita karani*.

Avascular Healing

Some tissues, such as cartilage, tendon, and ligament, are inherently avascular, and so injuries to them cannot be attended to by the vascular system, except in a very indirect way. In this case, the injury will be very slow to heal. Nonetheless, healing can be speeded if one performs *yogasanas* that promote circulation over long periods, as, for example, *urdhva prasarita padasana* at the wall for leg injuries. The rate of healing is also very much age dependent, with the advantage going to the young, whose cells metabolize faster, reproduce faster, and generally are in a better state nutritionally than are those of the elderly. Nonetheless, it is wise for the elderly to optimize their circulation as best they can through appropriate *yogasana* practice.

Thermoregulation

The body's vascular system is intimately involved with regulating the flow of heat from the core of the body to the skin, with the aim of keeping the core temperature relatively constant, as measured rectally. That is to say, the core temperature is regulated in part by shifting more or less of the blood from the core to the skin for cooling by contact with the surrounding air by conduction, convection, and radiative loss (figure 14.A-9). Local temperatures are automatically measured by sensors in the skin, spinal cord, hypothalamus, and gut, and all such thermal information is sent to the posterior hypothalamus for review. Additional cooling of the skin and of the core may be obtained by the evaporation of sweat (Subsection 20.D, page 724).

Anastomoses

Throughout the vascular net, one finds two or more arteries serving the same small region; such collaterals are often connected to one another. Due to the connections between these redundant vascular routes (called anastomoses), the blockage of one of the routes can be handled by circulation within the other. Anastomoses between arteries serving different regions also allow for the rapid shift of the blood circulation between these regions.

In addition to the capillary beds of the nutritive system, which connect the arterioles with the venules (1), temperature-controlling pathways (2) also exist in the skin between these two, bypassing the capillary beds. However, these bypasses between anastomoses are generally kept closed by actions of the sympathetic nervous system. The anastomoses are built with strong muscular walls, the contraction of which is driven by the catecholamines released by excitation of sympathetic nerve fibers driving the muscles within the blood-vessel walls [308].

When the body overheats, the sympathetic signals keeping the anastomoses closed decrease in intensity, and warm blood then flows directly from the subsurface arterioles to the superficial venous plexuses of the skin, thereby dissipating the excess heat by radiation, convection, and sweating.

Blood flow through the nutritive system (1) of the skin is only about 10 percent as large as that through the temperature-controlling system (2). When the skin is cold and the vascular system is contracted, the flow through system (2) is as low as 0.05 liters per minute but as high as three liters per minute when hot and vasodilated; under normal conditions, with the body at rest, 70 percent of the body's excess heat in the core is lost by contact with the surrounding air and by radiation into space (figure 14.A-9). The significant diversion of the blood supply from system (1) to system (2) when the core temperature is high can precipitate cardiac failure in those having weak hearts.

Variation of Body Temperature

In each of us, the core temperature varies in a regular way throughout the twenty-four-hour light-dark cycle, with a maximum temperature (38.1° C or 100.6° F) in the late afternoon (4:00 to 5:00 PM, table 23.B-3) and a minimum (36.3° C, 97.3° F) at about 2:00 AM (table 23.B-1). Because these core temperatures are strongly entrained with the rhythm of the rising and setting sun, they are strongly constrained to a twenty-four-hour cycle. However, when shielded from the sun or when in perpetual sunshine (the "free-running condition"), the period of the core-temperature oscillation shows two components, one at 24.8 hours and a second one at 33.5 hours [584] (Subsection 23.B, page 774). The characteristics of the temperature cycling in the human body are only weakly affected by ambient temperature in the range 20–32° C (68–90° F), and exercise raises the body temperature less during the day than during the night.

Skin Temperature

Our skin is an organ that is very responsive to the state of balance in the autonomic nervous system (table 5.A-2). When the sympathetic nervous system is dominant, the blood vessels at the skin surface constrict so as to send the superficial blood to large muscles [360, 431, 582], and with this, the skin temperature drops [143], especially at the fingertips and the toes. When instead, the parasympathetic nervous system becomes more active, the blood vessels in the dermal layer are dilated, the skin temperature rises and the shivering response to cold is inhibited [626]. The skin temperature at the fingertip is often taken as reflecting the relative activities of the sympathetic and parasympathetic nervous systems [143, 626]; the greater the stress (physical or mental), the greater the sympathetic arousal and the colder the fingertip (figure 5.E-2**a**). On the other hand, when the parasympathetic system is active during relaxation, there is significant blood flow to the hands and feet and thus a large radiative-cooling effect. Due to this effect, the hands and feet should be covered while in *savasana* unless it is quite warm in the room.

Section 14.D: Blood Pressure

Vasoconstriction, Vasodilation, and Hypertension

All of the blood vessels of the body except the capillaries are ringed with their own muscular systems (figure 14.C-3) that allow them to change their diameters, and which in turn allow them to control the blood flow. On signals from the involuntary vasomotor center of the brain, the muscles within the vascular system are contracted or relaxed so as to adjust the local blood flow, increasing it here, decreasing it there. Moreover, by judicious transfer of warm blood from the inner core of the body to the outer surfaces of the body, again by vasomotor activation, the temperature profiles of the body can be regulated (Subsection 14.C, page 573).

Though the regulation of the overall flow of blood through the vascular system is primarily under the control of the heart, considerable local control can be exerted through the smooth muscles of the blood vessels themselves. The endothelial cells can discharge certain prostaglandin paracrine hormones (see Chapter 6, page 207) that dilate the blood vessels, and the sympathetic nervous system can activate the smooth-muscle inner sheaths to cause vasoconstriction [432, 878]. It is also now known that the simple molecule nitric oxide (NO) is very effective in inducing vasodilation, increasing the arterial diameter by up to 15 percent by disengaging the contractive actin and myosin filaments within the smooth muscles of the arterial wall [21].

Hormonal Effects

Yet another of the body's mechanisms to raise the blood pressure is hormonal. In this case, when the baroreceptor signals to the brain (Section 14.E, page 580) report a low pressure, the brain directs the kidneys to release renin, which reacts with angiotensinogen circulating in the bloodstream from the liver (Chapter 6, page 221). The product of this reaction, when acted upon by enzymes in the lungs, is angiotensin II, a very powerful vasoconstrictor. Angiotensin II also acts on the adrenal glands to release aldosterone, an antidiuretic compound that acts on the body's salt and water content to increase the blood volume [140, 153, 858] and thereby raise the pressure. The catecholamines released by the adrenal glands (Subsection 6.B, page 217) also are active in raising the blood pressure, with epinephrine causing an increase in heart rate and norepinephrine causing a vasoconstriction of the arterioles.

Clots, Strokes, and Thrombi

When hypertensive, the blood vessels are in a constant state of mild constriction, resulting in a heart that is overworked, enlarged, and eventually weakened. Moreover, the excess pressure on the blood vessels acts to produce small tears in the lining of the arteries in the brain, the kidneys, and the small vessels of the eyes, thus weakening them with regard to hemorrhage [742]. In fact, the two prime areas with high sensitivity to blood pressure are the kidneys and the brain. Low blood pressure lessens the chance of plaque being dislodged from the walls of the vascular system and forming an embolus that might then retard blood flow in a distant part of the vascular system (figure 14.A-4). However, when blood pressure is high, the walls of the arterioles in the kidneys thicken and so resist the flow of blood through this important blood purifier [863]. Because the arteries in the brain are not as resistant to an aneurysm as are those associated with skeletal muscles, the risk for cerebral stroke can be high as a consequence of chronic high blood pressure.

If a blood clot forms in a vessel and sticks to the vessel wall, it is termed a thrombus; if the flow of blood succeeds in breaking the thrombus away from the wall so that it becomes free-floating, it is then an embolus (figure 4.E-2). The embolus circulates until it lodges in a vessel having a diameter smaller than its own. Emboli originating in the left side of the heart or in the large arteries are eventually lodged in the brain, kidneys, or elsewhere; whereas those that originate in the venous system or the right side of the heart usually lodge in the lungs. Clotting of blood is promoted by roughening of the endothelial surfaces of blood vessels (as when pressing a pole across a muscle in order to get it to relax) and by a slow rate of flow, as when blood flow is blocked for a matter of an hour or so in *yogasana* postures held for extended times.

Of the two numbers given as the blood pressure reading (Subsection 14.A, page 538), systolic/diastolic, the first relates to how hard the heart has to work in order to meet the supply for oxygenated blood, whereas the second is a measure of the vascular pressure when the heart is in a resting phase; a high diastolic pressure reading implies a high peripheral resistance in the arterioles due to sympathetic vasoconstriction. As intense emotion and intense exercise will both act to change the heart rate and the resistance of the vascular system, blood pressure readings usually are taken in the relaxed, prone position. Other factors aside, blood pressure increases with age due to increasing inelasticity of the vascular system, and as a person ages, an increase in systolic pressure precedes an increase of the diastolic pressure. Heart rate is somewhat higher in females than in males and drops monotonically with increasing age in both sexes.

Hypertension Defined

Hypertension is an abnormally high blood pressure, but the limits are difficult to define. If one accepts as "normal" a systolic/diastolic pressure ratio of 120/80 (Subsection 14.A, page 538), then the hypertensive label would apply to those with blood pressures in the range 140/90 and above, in three successive readings. However,

blood pressure tends to increase naturally with age [742], with children having a systolic pressure of only 75–90 millimeters Hg, whereas the elderly clock in at 130–150 millimeters. Furthermore, "normal" refers to meat-eating subjects in a stressful, high-tech society. Thus, blood pressure in the range 140/90 is a much more serious situation for a young person than for an older one, and even a "normal" pressure of 120/80 may be far from ideal, considering how unhealthy "normal" might be. External factors also affect our blood pressure readings: everyone's pressure rises when they speak, and correspondingly, the pressure drops when we listen [635].

One would expect that as the body goes into a state of hypertension, the baroreceptors would respond to the increased pressure and thereby moderate the heart and vascular activities so as to reduce the pressure. That this does not happen in the hypertensive person has been traced to a lack of baroreceptor sensitivity [86, 217, 771]. As this sensitivity is posture dependent, one sees immediately that *yogasana* practice can be relevant to dealing with hypertension.

Eighty percent of hypertension cases, called "essential hypertension," are idiopathic, in that they have no known medical cause and can be cured only with the help of yoga and meditation [742], though modern drugs too are effective in reducing the symptoms [458], but without offering a cure.

Hypertension Mechanisms

When the body is gripped by the effects of the fight or flight syndrome, the stimulation of certain centers in the hypothalamus directs the sympathetic nervous system to dilate the blood vessels to the heart and striated muscles, while the blood vessels serving other parts of the body constrict. However, in this redistribution of the blood supply, more blood vessels are constricted than are dilated, with the result that the **net** effect is vascular constriction. This immediately translates into a higher blood pressure and more work for the heart. In figure 5.E-4, the interdependence of the various factors that react so as to form the stress response of sympathetic excitation is shown [751]. Many aspects of this cycle reinforce high blood pressure, both short term and long term. Nonetheless, once the stress has passed, the sympathetic dominance ideally yields to parasympathetic relaxation, the peripheral resistance declines as the arterioles return to their net dilated state and both the blood pressure and heart rate return to normal, as in figure 14.D-1.

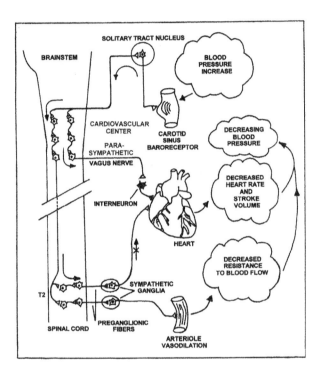

Figure 14.D-1. The carotid-sinus reflex arc, beginning at the carotid-sinus baroreceptor, showing the interneuron between the parasympathetic vagus nerve and the heart (which acts to suppress heart rate), and the inhibition of the ganglionic fibers of the sympathetic nervous system (which inhibition acts to lower the heart rate and the force of contraction), and the dilation of the arterioles so as to reduce the peripheral resistance to blood flow. All of these factors, acting together, lower the blood pressure once the carotid sinus has been pressurized.

Many individuals continue to carry the thought of the stressful event in their conscious mind and continue to replay the event over and over again, without understanding that just the thought of the event is enough to trigger the en-

tire sympathetic display, long after the event itself is past. As a consequence of this repeated replaying of the stressful event and its associated neurological pattern,[7] there is a long-term net vasoconstriction within the vascular system and a long-term net elevation of the blood pressure and heart rate; this is the condition known as hypertension [626, 742]. In this condition, the heart is under a constant strain, and because the circulatory system then functions at reduced efficiency, the organs being served cannot recover readily once they have been used and so rapidly become exhausted. If the state of high-pressure alarm is maintained for a long time, the baroreceptors will slowly reset the alarm level to a higher value, so that the elevated value then becomes "the norm" and hypertension becomes chronic, persistent, and pathologic (figure 5.E-3). When the arterial system is in vasoconstriction so as to result in hypertension, the arteries lose their mechanical flexibility and so do not readily change their diameters to accommodate changes in internal pressure.

Yogasana and Hypertension

Assuming that hypertension is rooted in the excessive stimulation of the sympathetic nervous system [458] that one often encounters when living a fast-paced and stressful lifestyle, it is clear why *yogasana* practice is recommended for the hypertensive student. With the action of *yogasana* on the lungs and its effect on breathing, with the action of *yogasana* on the brain via thought control, and with the action of *yogasana* on the muscles through relaxation (figure 5.E-4), one can reverse the associations that drive high blood pressure. *Yogasanas* performed to reduce the blood pressure at first should be very relaxing and devoid of inversions (see Section 14.F, page 592), with el-

---

7 This mechanism, whereby mentally repeating a scenario encouraging sympathetic excitation results in a chronic vascular hypertension, is not unlike the neural repatterning of muscular actions that results from using the imagination to practice body movements (Subsection 4.G, page 140). However, in the first case, the result is a negative one, as the wrong lesson is being learned, whereas in the second case, it is a positive lesson that is being reinforced.

ements of challenge added only as the tension in the vascular system resides [742].

The efficacy of *yogasana* practice toward relieving hypertension has been demonstrated in several medical studies [183, 742, 771]. Following *yogasana* training, heart rate, respiration rate, metabolism rate, and blood pressure in the resting state were all decreased, while the alpha-wave activity in the EEG increased. All of these changes are consonant with increasing prominence of the parasympathetic nervous system. Of the postures *vajrasana, sirsasana, sarvangasana, viparita karani, setu bandha sarvangasana,* and *savasana,* the last of these was found to be the most effective in lowering the blood pressure. If a student is hypertensive and performs the *yogasanas* with a slight holding of the breath, then parasympathetic balance can be restored by looking down with the eyes [826].

In a study focusing on *savasana* as a treatment for essential hypertension, Datey et al. [183] found that on average, the mean arterial pressure dropped from 134 millimeters Hg to 107 millimeters by daily practice of thirty minutes of *savasana* over several months. For subjects already taking medication for hypertension, *savasana* for several months led to a reduction of their medication by 32 percent while maintaining a mean pressure of 102 millimeters. As expected for hypertension resulting from atherosclerosis, *yogasanas* had no effect for people having this condition.

Datey et al. explain that with slow, rhythmic breathing, the frequencies of the afferent proprioceptive and interoceptive signals sent to the hypothalamus decrease, and because of this, the "normal" homeostatic blood pressure level (as set by the hypothalamus) is reset to a lower level. Similarly encouraging results have been reported for the benefits of relaxation to hypertensive patients in an extensive investigation by Patel and Marmot [648]. In another study of the effects of *yogasana* on essential hypertension, Selvamurthy et al. [771] conclude that *yogasana* practice works to increase the sensitivity of the baroreceptors and thus amplifies the effects of the baroreceptors on the adrenal hormones, as well as on the renin-angiotensin system via the sympathetic nervous system.

Hypertensive students may be taking medications that lower their blood pressure into the "normal" range, but they nonetheless should perform only those *yogasanas* appropriate to those with hypertension [645]; i.e., in a manner that is as restful as possible.

Experiments on middle-aged volunteers having hypertension showed improvement with exercise for those with mild hypertension, but not for those with more severe problems. In spite of evidence of the sort discussed above, certain practitioners of Western medicine, for example [319], still feel that alternative techniques "such as relaxation and biofeedback, though appealing in theory, haven't reduced blood pressure significantly in clinical trials," whereas others are becoming more accepting (see, for example, [274]).

Black Americans

It is known that black Americans suffer a 50 percent greater rate of death by heart disease than do white Americans, and that this difference is strongly related to differences in hypertension [153]. It appears that both black men and women are deficient in the simple molecule NO (nitric oxide), which otherwise is very active in dilating the smooth muscles within the blood vessels, thereby lowering the blood pressures within. That is to say, in times of stress, the blood vessels of blacks are less able to relax than those of whites. Nitric oxide acts as a paracrine or autocrine hormone, as it is chemically reactive and so does not travel far. Because it relaxes smooth muscle in the walls of the arterioles, at each systole, endothelial cells release nitric oxide and so lessen the resistance to blood flow. Nitric oxide release also increases the flow of blood through the kidneys and therefore increases the rate of urine flow. In the body, nitric oxide can be formed by the decomposition of nitroglycerine, which relaxes the walls of the coronary arteries. Nitric oxide also inhibits the aggregation of platelets, thereby insuring that the blood viscosity stays low [450].

Social tensions also may be a contributing factor to hypertension in black Americans [661]. In any case, yogic relaxation should be especially valuable. Note, however, that there are other theories of hypertension, involving the interactions among proteins in the liver, lungs, and kidneys, which make no mention of nitric oxide [153], and the assumed role of the sympathetic nervous system in hypertension also has been questioned by some medical workers [458].

Hypotension

Adults for whom the blood pressure reading is 100/60 or less are termed "hypotensive" or "orthostatic." Their problem largely is postural, with long-term vasodilation leading to pooling of the blood in the extremities and the abdomen, so that not enough blood is delivered to the brain; lightheadedness, fainting, nausea, and weakness are common in those having this condition. These symptoms are most often present when standing up from a sitting or lying position, as when recovering from *uttanasana* or *savasana,* for example. "Postural hypotension" in the elderly is due to failure of the cardiac baroreceptors and the volume receptor in the right atrium to respond to the blood pooling by proper cardiac stimulation and/or reflexive sympathetic action (which speeds the heart and constricts the blood vessels). This leads to a fainting feeling when standing erect [360].

The reflexive lowering of the blood pressure on shifting body position is especially common in older students. Hypotension may not be evident at all when measured in a seated position but then becomes a strong factor when standing upright. In such a situation, students of *yogasana* may find themselves weak and dizzy in the standing postures but have no such problems when seated or lying down. Moving slowly between body postures eases the drop in blood pressure in those showing orthostasis. Hypotensive students may also display the "possum response" (figure 5.E-3), demonstrating a parasympathetic (passive) response when the situation calls for a sympathetic (energized) response instead.

Note too that if the hydrostatic pressure of a blood vessel while in an inversion is of the order of 110 millimeters Hg (Subsection 14.F, page 584), this will be sufficient to collapse the carotid and vertebral arteries in a hypotensive student

having a systolic pressure lower than the hydrostatic pressure.

The Ocular-Vagal Reflex

The left and right common carotid arteries bifurcate as they rise from the aortic arch, with the external carotid branch serving the neck and head, but not the brain or orbits of the eyes, and the internal carotid arteries supplying blood to the brain and to the orbits of the eyes, but not to the head or neck. Moreover, the baroreceptors for high blood pressure are located within the internal carotid arteries. These two facts suggest an explanation for how pressing the orbits of the eyes onto a solid support, as when resting the forehead on the floor in *adho mukha virasana* or when simply taking *savasana* with an eye bag resting upon the eyes, leads to the ocular-vagal heart-slowing reflex.

Just as when the neck is in the *jalandhara bandha* position (Subsection 11.D, page 452), we propose that pressure on the orbits of the eyes increases the pressure within the internal carotid arteries in the vicinity of the orbits of the eyes, and this in turn stimulates the carotid baroreceptors to report an over-pressure. This results in a lower blood pressure due to a slowing of the heart rate and a decrease of the cardiac stroke volume. It appears that this ocular slowing of the heart is closely related to that induced by the effect of *jalandhara bandha* flexion of the neck on the carotid artery (Subsection 11.D, page 452). In the medical literature, this effect is known as the Aschner-Dagnini reflex and is said to occur either when there is traction on the extra-ocular muscles surrounding the eyes, or when there is direct compression of either the eyeball or the carotid artery; something similar may occur when one uses an eye bag or head wrap while in *savasana*.

For students who experience deep reddening of the face and pressure behind bloodshot eyes in *sirsasana,* these effects can be reduced by first resting the weight of the head on the forehead on the floor in *adho mukha virasana* for five minutes and then going inverted without lifting the head off the floor. This action activates the ocular-vagal heart-slowing reflex, which reduces the blood pressure before going into the posture (Sections 11.D, page 457, and 14.D, page 579).

Eye Bags and Baby Fists

Direct pressure on the eyeballs also causes a reflexive slowing of the heart rate, as when one uses an eye bag in *savasana* or a head wrap [144]. Be aware that because the parasympathetic effect of placing an eye bag on the eyes when in *savasana* is to reduce the intraocular pressure as one relaxes, the flaccid eyeball may be somewhat flattened by the weight of the bag, so that the student's vision may be blurred for a few moments on recovering from the posture.

Just before they go to sleep, babies reflexively rub their eyes with their fists, and it is thought that this pressure on the eyeballs is effective in slowing the heart rate and stroke volume, thus promoting the relaxation into sleep.

Section 14.E: Monitoring Blood Pressure with the Baroreceptors

The body's need for homeostasis requires that there be one or more mechanisms available to it for controlling blood pressure within a narrow range. In turn, this implies the existence of sensors that can respond to blood pressure changes, together with afferent nerves from these sensors running to autonomic control centers in the brain and efferent nerves running from there to the various pressure-controlling organs of the body.

The pressure sensors in the cardiovascular system that are responsible for blood pressure homeostasis are known as baroreceptors, these being a special class of sensor within the larger class of mechanoreceptors sensitive to mechanical stress (Section 13.B, page 506). The baroreceptors responding to diastolic blood pressure are located in the walls of all of the larger systemic arteries (figure 14.D-1) and are very important in controlling the arterial pressures. Being stretch receptors, they are active when the artery is over- or under-pressured, and they respond by controlling

the heart rate and arterial diameters via the parasympathetic vagus nerves and the corresponding sympathetic nerves. Baroreceptors are especially abundant in the carotid sinuses and in the wall of the aortic arch, and when active, the response to high arterial pressure is vasodilation and reductions of the heart rate and of the cardiac contractive force. Baroreceptors also can be found in the midbrain of the brainstem, as well as in the walls of the right atrial chamber of the heart.

In response to the baroreceptor signals, the peripheral blood vessels may be dilated or constricted by changing the smooth-muscle tone of the arterial and venous walls, while the heart rate, the blood volume, and the contractile force of the heart also may vary due to changing baroreceptor signals. Moreover, factors other than baroreceptor pressure also may work to alter the characteristics of the heart function; e.g., increased body temperature will act to increase the heart rate, as will feelings such as fear, anger, and anxiety, whereas negative feelings such as depression or grief work to lower this function. These changes in blood pressure are the result of both the changing heart function, as controlled by the cardiac acceleration and inhibition centers in the brainstem, and of the changing smooth-muscle tone of the arterioles, as controlled by the vasomotor center (see below). Clearly, the diastolic blood pressure is controlled by complex interactions, and it is estimated that were the baroreceptor system nonfunctional for whatever reason, this pressure would vary by up to 100 percent in the course of a twenty-four-hour day.

Consider that the cardiac accelerator and decelerator nerves between the brainstem, and the heart and the nerves from the baroreceptors to the brainstem, form a two-way loop connecting the brain to the heart and the heart to the brain. Nevertheless, given this close relation between the heart and the head, it is almost beyond belief that focusing one's thoughts on love and appreciation while imagining the heart leads to very clear and apparently unique effects on the heart function, ECG, and blood pressure (figure 14.A-7) [550]. See also Section 14.A, page 549, on the power spectrum of the ECG for more on this connection and how it can be used to shift the sympathetic/parasympathetic balance through thought.

Sensitivity

Baroreceptor function has a lower limit to its range, being active reflexively only at diastolic pressures above 60 millimeters Hg for the carotid baroreceptors and 90 millimeters for those of the aortic arch. If the arterial pressure is above 60 millimeters in the carotid artery but is still below the normal value of 100 millimeters, the effect of the baroreceptors will be to excite the sympathetic nervous system and so increase the arterial pressure, whereas they will have the reverse effect should the arterial pressure rise significantly above 100 millimeters.

Neurons from the baroreceptors synapse to the cardiovascular center in the brainstem (the medulla oblongata), with afferent and efferent fibers lying side by side. It appears that the baroreceptors can measure not only the changes in peak and average pressures but also the time-rate-of-change of pressure and the heart rate [432]. In regard to receptor adaptation (Subsection 13.B, page 506), the baroreceptors are very slow to adapt, yet they are so rapid in their response that they can easily follow the rise and fall of the pressure during the systole/diastole cardiac cycle, and they are at their most sensitive when the pressure is rapidly changing. Other types of baroreceptors within the heart are sensitive to the degree of filling of the right atrium and to the volume of the blood sent forward by the contraction of the left ventricle.

With increasing age, the functioning of the baroreceptors normally degrades and so diminishes the body's ability to maintain blood pressure homeostasis [162]. The situation for *yogasana* students, however, may be very different, for they regularly exercise the baroreceptor apparatus through the practice of inversions, and so keep the baroreceptors in working condition.

Venous Pressure

The baroreceptors are involved with arterial pressures, which can be substantial, whereas little or no attention is paid to the significantly lower blood pressures on the venous side. One can get a rough measure of venous pressure in the *yogasana* student by noting the distension of the veins in the neck. For a student sitting still, there is no distension of the neck veins, as the atrial pressure is essentially zero; however if the pressure in the right atrium rises to 10 millimeters Hg, the veins in the lower neck are seen to bulge, and at 15 millimeters, all of the veins in the neck are distended. When lying in *savasana,* a measure of the venous pressure is obtained by noting the angle of the arm with respect to the floor at which the blood in the veins in the back of the hand drains to the heart; the higher the arm must be lifted for drainage, the higher is the blood pressure in the right atrium [308]. Any variation of the pressure in the saphenous vein at the ankle that is dependent on the position of the body is due to the hydrostatic pressure of the venous blood, as described in Subsection 14.F, page 584.

The Baroreceptor Reflex Arc

In the body's equilibrium resting state, the cardiac baroreceptors output a steady 0.5–2 hertz modulated electrical signal along the afferent fibers, which synapse at the solitary tract nucleus in the lower medulla oblongata, a brainstem nucleus prominent in autonomic activity. Suppose then that the blood pressure rises and that the need for homeostasis requires a reflexive lowering of the pressure. How can this happen? The answer lies in the baroreceptor reflex arc illustrated in figure 14.D-1. The baroreceptors are embedded in the arterial walls; when the pressure rises, the walls bulge outward somewhat, and the baroreceptors sense this increased mechanical stress. In response, they raise the frequencies of the signals launched up the afferent nerves, in proportion to the amount of mechanical strain induced above that in the resting state. On reaching the solitary tract nucleus, the signal is relayed to the nucleus ambiguus [360, 432], which in turn energizes the parasympathetic neurons, which inhibit cardiac action by slowing the heartbeat via the vagus nerve. At the same time, there is reduced activity in the sympathetic fibers controlling heart rate, force of contraction, and arteriole diameter. The net result is that the heart rate decreases and the flow rate through the arterioles decreases[8] as they dilate, so that the blood pressure drops back into the normal range.

On the other hand, if the pressure becomes too low, the baroreceptor signal frequency drops below 0.5 hertz, and the autonomic nervous system reacts so as to increase the heart rate and constrict the arterioles and veins, thereby resetting the pressure at a higher level. A low blood volume also can give a low-pressure signal at the baroreceptors, and so this stimulates drinking behavior while inhibiting urination [427]; the opposite effects are elicited when inverting (see Box 14.F-3, page 594). If the carotid baroreceptors are failing or not working at all, the cardiac acceleration center receives a constant low-pressure signal, and this results in a state of chronic cardiac stimulation; i.e., a state of hypertension.

Savasana and Hypotension

If a baroreceptor signals an over-pressure in its vicinity, as when first coming into *savasana*, the heart center in the medulla oblongata reports back to the heart via the vagus nerve, and the heart rate and the strength of contraction are both lowered, while the arteriole diameters are relaxed as well. If this reflex is not working properly, then when one goes from *savasana* to sitting erect or from sitting to standing, there is a deficit of arterial pressure in the head and neck and a tendency to dizziness and loss of consciousness. Ideally, on getting up slowly from *savasana,* there should be a rapid baroreceptor-driven stimulation of the sympathetic nervous system and an increased arterial pressure. This should not be a problem, for the baroreceptors usually have such a fast response time that they can even follow the rise and fall of the aortic pressure with each heartbeat. However, this apparently is not the case for the hypotensive student; the consequences of low arterial pressure

follow the same path when hypotensive students try to stand erect too soon after coming down from *sirsasana.*

Carotid Receptors

Conversely, strong mechanical pressure at the neck, as when in *halasana* or *sarvangasana* or from manual massage of the carotid receptors while sitting upright, can increase arterial pressure (locally) so as to stimulate the carotid baroreceptors to slow the heart and dilate the arteries. If the student is older and has atherosclerotic plaque in the carotid arteries, the heart may be slowed so much in *halasana,* for example, that it actually stops beating. In the more normal cases, *yogasana* students will experience generally parasympathetic responses in *halasana* and *sarvangasana,* as appropriate for relaxing postures. Though we purposely assume these *yogasana* postures in order to induce parasympathetic activity, in the nonyogic situation of a tight collar, for instance, the fainting response is known as "cardiac sinus syncope." Cole [141] has observed a rather interesting correlation between baroreceptor stimulation in the carotid sinus and aortic arch with EEG changes signaling sleep or arousal; this is discussed in Section 4.H, page 149.

Inversion

Pressure at the baroreceptors can be raised by tipping the body toward or into an inverted state. As baroreceptor activation requires relatively high over-pressure, it usually does not activate until the body has been tipped about 50–60° from vertical [140]. Because the baroreceptors in both the carotid sinuses and the aortic arch only respond to relatively high pressure, they may not respond in mild inversions such as *viparita karani.* The situation involving a posturally driven increase in blood pressure and the body's response to this are discussed below (Section 14.F, page 584). When inverted, there is a general raising of the muscle tone in the postural muscles of the neck, shoulders, and back, while at the same time, the general non-postural musculature is relaxed [98a].

---

8   But not those to the brain or to the heart, neither of which can afford to have their blood supplies curtailed!

Response Time

Because the response time of functioning carotid baroreceptors ideally is very short, the baroreceptors can follow and respond to the rise and fall of arterial pressure as the heart goes through the diastole-systole cycle; in fact, the carotid baroreceptors are also sensitive to the rate of change of pressure. It is the opinion of medical researchers that because the baroreceptor reflex is a short-term response, it is unimportant for the long-term remediation of elevated arterial blood pressure; i.e., hypertension. On the contrary, the response of the carotid baroreceptor is initiated immediately after a sharp rise in pressure and is at peak effectiveness for about four hours but then falls slowly to reach extinction only after eight days, as long as the stimulating signal remains at full strength [308]. This behavior does not depend upon the rate of response of the baroreceptor but instead on its adaptation (Subsection 13.B, page 506) or lack of same. As *yogasana* practitioners, we can accept this gladly, for it suggests that there can be a substantial long-term decrease in arterial pressure if one exercises the baroreceptors appropriately through daily *yogasana* practice.

Heart Enlargement

If the body is under physical stress so that there is a strong sympathetic activation of the heart, calling for more blood flow, as with endurance runners, then the heart will enlarge in response to this. A similar enlargement occurs when the source of the stress is nonphysical but chronic (see Subsection 24.A, page 812), as with cigarette smokers. The nicotine ingested while cigarette smoking is strongly stimulating to the adrenal glands, which respond by releasing large amounts of aldosterone, epinephrine, and norepinephrine, all of which are strong vasoconstrictors and so function to raise the blood pressure in opposition to the baroreceptor action. As both the blood pressure and the respiration rate are important factors in delivering oxygen to tissues under stress, their autonomic controls are closely coordinated. Indeed, their simultaneous action must be coordinated if the system is to maintain cardiorespiratory homeostasis.

Other Circulatory Sensors

Atrial Volume

There are other sensors in the circulatory system that affect the return of the blood pressure to its resting value. One such sensor within the cardiac wall of the right atrium measures the fractional volume of blood filling the heart in the diastole phase and adjusts the blood flow accordingly, while another measures stroke volume of the expelled blood from the heart, decreasing it when it is too high and increasing it when it is too low. According to Cole [140], the atrial-volume baroreceptor is more sensitive than those in the carotid arteries or in the aorta, both of which are relatively high-pressure sensors. On the venous side, flow rates are controlled in part by the autonomic nervous system through the diameters of the veins, thus limiting (by vasoconstriction) or enhancing (by vasodilation) the flow of blood to the heart.

Chemoreceptors

The relevant baroreceptors in this discussion are located along the aortic arch and very close to the bifurcations of each of the carotid arteries. In very close proximity to these are sets of chemoreceptors that are sensitive to the amounts of oxygen, carbon dioxide, and H^+ ions in the blood and that also send their inputs to the solitary tract nucleus in the autonomic nervous system. As such, they also are factors in regulating the heart rate, blood pressure, and respiration rate [360]. So, for example, if the H^+ and carbon dioxide concentrations rise in the arteries, the ventilation is speeded, and if the oxygen concentration rises in the arteries, it is slowed. Ventilation rate is much more strongly responsive to changes in H^+ and carbon dioxide concentrations than to changes in oxygen concentration.

Carotid bodies in the carotid arteries and aortic bodies in the aortic arch are sensitive to the amounts of oxygen and carbon dioxide in the arterial blood, and when the amount of oxygen is too low or the amount of carbon dioxide is too high, these receptors trigger an increase in the breathing rate, using either the vagus nerve (cranial nerve X) from the aortic arch or the glossopharyngeal nerve (cranial nerve IX) from the carotid arteries [621]. The condition of too little oxygen in the blood is known as hypoxia, and that of too much carbon dioxide in the blood is known as hypercapnia. Because changes in the concentrations of carbon dioxide and H^+ drastically affect the activities of all neurons, the body closely regulates these by controlling vascular diameters and thereby controlling local blood flow.

The autonomic response to the baroreceptor signals outlined above is subject to control by yet higher centers in the brain. Thus, the simple reflex arc of figure 14.D-1 can be overridden by deliberately intense exercise, so that changes in the heart rate, filling volume, blood pressure, and blood chemistry rise to anomalous values and remain there for a time, in spite of the autonomic tendency toward homeostasis.

Hormonal Shift

As the brain receives high-pressure signals from various sensors, it also reacts via the neuroendocrine route to shift hormonal levels so as to reduce blood pressure and volume. Thus, on inversion, the level of norepinephrine drops in the vasoconstricted smooth muscles, leading to vasodilation; plasma renin activity falls, thereby reducing the production of angiotensin II; aldosterone levels fall so as to increase the excretion of Na^+; and vasopressin levels fall so as to increase urination [144]. In anticipation of these aftereffects, it is wise to empty the bladder before performing a long-duration *sirsasana*.

Section 14.F: Blood Pressure in Inverted *Yogasanas*

Relevant Factors

Estimation of "the blood pressure" at a point in the body while in a *yogasana* posture (inverted or not) is fraught with unknown quantities and interlocking complications; all we can do at this point is present some of these and perhaps rank them as to their general importance. The most obvious and most important of these many factors is that in the first approximation, the blood within the body is like the milk in a half-filled bottle: when it is inverted, the fluid runs to the opposite end of the bottle. When one goes from an upright position to a fully inverted position, gravity initially pulls the fluids in the body toward the head rather than toward the feet. This shift of pressure has multiple consequences for the circulatory system and the ultimate blood pressure reached in the head and brain while inverted. The significant factors affecting the blood pressure while inverted are discussed below, whereas the related effects of body orientation on the efficiency of oxygenation of the blood in the lungs are discussed in Section 15.C, page 613.

Hydrostatic Pressure

The question of just what happens to a *yogasana* student's blood pressure when inverting is a fascinating one. Clearly, there is much more to it than the blood simply rushing to the head, for it is known [140, 823] that a practicing yogi can have diastolic blood pressures in *sirsasana* and *sarvangasana* that are **lower** than that when seated! In order to understand the situation in regard to the homeostatic behavior of blood pressure when inverting, it is useful to first consider the concept of hydrostatic pressure.

The pressure at the bottom of a column of liquid is greater than that at the top, because the liquid at the bottom is supporting the weight of all the liquid above it. This pressurization, due to gravity, is called hydrostatic pressure and is only dependent on the height of the liquid column involved and its density. The hydrostatic pressure at the base of a column of liquid, such as blood or cerebrospinal fluid, that stands L millimeters high is L/13.6, in units of millimeters Hg.

In a person of average height in *tadasana*, the height of the column of blood may be taken to be the distance between the sole of the foot and the top of the heart (about 1.2 meters or four feet), and the hydrostatic pressure of the body's blood, as experienced at the ankle, therefore should be about 0.12 atmospheres (90 millimeters Hg; 1.7 pounds per square inch), but it is essentially zero at the level of the heart. This pressure at the level of the ankle, experimentally measured to be 92 millimeters Hg when in *tadasana,* is well below the normal systolic pressure in the arteries and is approximately equal to the diastolic pressure.

Venous Pressure

The pressure throughout the venous system is 0 millimeters Hg, as the pressure drop is almost totally on the arterial side; however, to this must be added the hydrostatic pressure of the blood, the variation of which with height above the floor is as shown in figure 14.F-1**a**. Thus, when standing absolutely still, the total venous pressure in the ankle will be 100 millimeters Hg and close to 10 millimeters Hg at the right atrium of the heart. The total venous pressure due to hydrostatic loading when inverted is shown in figure 14.A-1**b**.

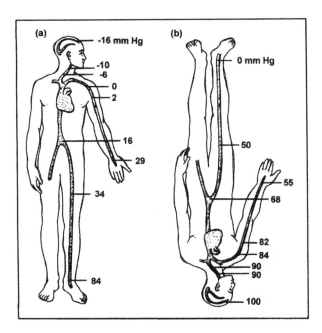

Figure 14.F-1. The hydrostatic pressure within the venous system when standing in *tadasana* (**a**) and when inverted (**b**). The hydrostatic column is assumed to be 1.2 meters (four feet) high and to exert zero hydrostatic pressure at the level of the right atrium of the heart when standing upright.

The same hydrostatic pressure increment described for the venous tree holds for the arterial tree as well, but in this case, the hydrostatic increments must be added to the aortic pressures due to cardiac actions. Thus, hydrostatic loading adds another 90 millimeters Hg to the arterial pressure (about 100 millimeters, the average of the systolic and diastolic pressures) at the ankle, the total coming to almost 200 millimeters. Similarly, on inversion, the sum of the arterial and hydrostatic pressures in the arteries of the brain would be a frightening 200 millimeters Hg in this approximation. Fortunately, this over-pressure in the brain is largely reduced through the actions of various receptors within the vascular system and the hydrostatic counter-pressure of fluids outside the vascular system.

Though there is only a small pressure drop between the ends of an unclogged artery (figure 14.C-4**b**), if there is atherosclerosis present (figure 14.A-4), then the measured pressure will also depend upon just which part of the artery is chosen for measurement.

Aortic Pressure

Pressure at the aorta is equal to that at the exit of the left ventricle but is subject to modulation by various baroreceptors, the emotions, holding of the breath (see the discussion on the Valsalva maneuver, Subsection 15.C, page 616), etc. Inversion when calm and relaxed may lower the aortic pressure, but only in students with a long and continuing practice.

There will be a significant pressure drop between the proximal ends of the arterioles and the distal ends of the venules, so that the pressure in both the anterior tibial vein and at the right atrium will be close to zero. With hydrostatic pressure added in, these values will change considerably and even then will depend upon what actions are taken to return the venous blood to the heart. Thus, as discussed in Subsection 14.E, page 581, the pressure in the saphenous vein at the ankle varies between 12 and 90 millimeters Hg, depending upon posture and muscle actions.

As mentioned above, if the pressure within the vascular system at the level of the beating heart is arbitrarily taken to be zero, then the hydrostatic pressure at the ankle while in a standing posture will be about 0.12 atmospheres (90 millimeters Hg; 1.7 pounds per square inch), and that above the heart will be slightly negative (figure 14.F-1). However, a rhythmic muscular action in the legs reduces the hydrostatic pressure to about 10 millimeters or so at those times between the rhythmic contractions. The complication of the additive effects of aortic and hydrostatic pressure as experienced by the giraffe when drinking and the dinosaur when eating are discussed in Box 14.F-1, below.

As for the effects of hydrostatic pressure while in the inverted *yogasanas,* we consider two possibilities: semi-inversion, where the length of the hydrostatic column is approximately half the body height (as in *halasana* or *uttanasana,* for example); and full inversion, where the hydrostatic column height is the full-body height (as in *sarvangasana,* for example). These are discussed below in terms of the actions of the baroreceptors (Section 14.E, page 580) and the autonomic nervous system (Chapter 5, page 157) working together to return the body to its homeostatic state.

General Effects of Inversion on the Baroreceptors

Sarvangasana

In order to illustrate the many ways in which inversion can affect the circulatory system, consider the schematic shown in figures 5.B-2 and 5.E-4, imagining it to be appropriate to a beginning student trying *sarvangasana* for the first time. The student's first response to being told "We will now attempt to stand upside down on the backs of our heads" is one of fear. The fear of inversion will work at the subconscious level (through the hypothalamus) and at the conscious level (through the cortex). Both of these become inputs to the medulla oblongata housing the cardiovascular center, prompting it to get ready to do battle with an external force; i.e., to activate the sympathetic nervous system. If, as seems likely, the fear element also results in excess muscular effort when

in the posture, this too will become input into the medulla, again promoting an intensified sympathetic response. Finally, fear is known to raise the sensitivity to pain [747], thus intensifying the apprehension factor even more.

Once the sympathetic alarm has been rung, the circulatory consequences when in *sarvangasana* are the constriction of certain of the arterioles, an increased cardiac stroke volume, and an increased heart rate, all of which act to significantly increase the systolic blood pressure. See figure 5.E-5 in this regard.

In addition to the fear reaction, the simple act of inversion leads to two key hydrostatic effects. First, it acts to increase the blood pressure in the neck and chest, and this increased pressure is sensed by the carotid sensors in the aortic arch and in the carotid sinuses. Second, Copeland [154] explains that in inverted postures, there is an "easy" return of venous blood to the heart, thus filling it more than otherwise. In response to this larger filling factor for the right atrium, the heart rate tends to drop as more blood is pumped with each contraction.[9] To the extent that there is no extra muscular effort or extra demand for oxygen when inverting, (*sarvangasana,* for example, performed without undue effort), both the increased pressurization of the carotid baroreceptor and the extra filling and correspondingly larger stroke volume will activate sensors in the heart for these parameters (Subsection 14.A, page 550). In turn, these will be accommodated by a lowering of the heart rate and blood pressure. Indeed, medical students with some experience in doing the inverted *yogasanas* and for whom there is no significant fear factor are reported to have had an average heart rate of sixty-seven beats per minute in the supine position, eighty-four beats per minute upon standing from the supine position, and, in *sirsasana I,* an average heart rate of only sixty-nine beats per minute [256, 431].

---

9   Actually, Cole [140] reports that the right atrial filling is largest when in a 30° head-down position and that inversion beyond 30° tends to drain blood away from the heart and toward the head, provided the head is not lifted.

Box 14.F-1: How the Giraffe and the Dinosaur Gamble When Taking Their First Lunch

For a giraffe (camelopardus), with its long neck, taking its first drink of water with its head between its long legs can be a risky business, just as it must have been for the long-necked but short-legged dinosaur sampling its first taste of leaves from the top of a tall tree. In both cases, there is an important hydrostatic effect that comes into play that will kill the animal if it is not dealt with appropriately.

In the upright giraffe, to the systolic blood pressure at the aorta must be added the hydrostatic pressure of the three-meter (nine-foot) long column of arterial blood that otherwise rests upon the heart. (See [32] for a contrary view.) Fortunately for this animal, the material of the arterial walls at the aorta is strong enough to withstand this combined pressurization from the systolic heartbeat and the hydrostatic effect.[1] Note too that when standing erect, the pressure within the blood vessels in and surrounding the giraffe's brain have no contribution from the hydrostatic effect, as they are at the top of the blood column and so are pressurized only to the systolic pressure at the aorta. This is fortunate, for the blood vessels in the brain are much smaller and weaker than the material forming the aorta.

When the giraffe bends over to take its first drink, placing its long neck between its long legs, head at ground level, the hydrostatic pressure in the arteries surrounding the brain and the arterial pressure from the contraction of the heart reinforce one another, but in this case, the resultant over-pressure occurs in the arteries within the brain and is far higher than the weak blood vessels in this area can withstand. That is to say, the giraffe should suffer a burst artery within the brain the first time it bends over to drink!

That the giraffe does not suffer an aneurysm or stroke is due to two reactions that work to moderate the expected increase in cranial blood pressure when drinking. First, note that the arteries **within** the brain are protected from this over-pressure because they are surrounded by the cerebrospinal fluid, the hydrostatic pressure of which presses inward on the blood vessels, thereby canceling the outward hydrostatic pressure of the blood when the animal's head is down. In this case, the largest effect of the hydrostatic pressure is borne by the skull rather than by the vascular system. However, this cancellation effect is not a factor for the arteries of the head that are not surrounded by cerebrospinal fluid, such as the carotid and vertebral arteries and those within the eyes (see this subsection, page 589).

A second reaction protects the vessels not otherwise protected by the cerebrospinal fluid. The baroreceptors in the animal's heart and neck sense the rapidly increasing pressure as the animal bends forward and correspondingly adjust the heart rate downward, while enlarging the vascular diameters to allow the pressure in the vicinity of the brain to remain in a safe range.

In the case of the herbivorous dinosaurs, it has been thought that these huge animals with their necks of ten meters (thirty feet) or more in length would eat by grazing the tops

---

1   The giraffe's heart is huge, being 10 kilograms (twenty-five pounds) in weight and 65 centimeters (twenty-four inches) in length. The thickest parts of the heart (the ventricles) have walls that are up to 7.5 centimeters (three inches) thick.

of very tall trees. However, this implies a huge hydrostatic pressure at the aorta in addition to the systolic pressure of a column of blood being pumped upward by more than ten meters. Again, no known biological material is strong enough to stand up to the combined pressures (hydrostatic plus systolic) at the aorta that such a situation implies. In this regard, see the pressure for aortic dissection brought on by the Valsalva maneuver in humans while lifting (Subsection 15.C, page 616). In an effort to get around this objection, some have suggested that the dinosaurs had one heart in the chest cavity and then one or more along the length of the neck to act as relay pumping stations, but no evidence for this has been found. It is more likely that these animals had very long necks but never lifted their heads much above their hearts, eating low on the trees and sparing themselves the risk of vascular over-pressure at the aorta [829].

Fortunately, we as upright humans do not have the huge hydrostatic forces that an upright dinosaur or a thirsty giraffe would have to deal with, but we too have mechanisms that can respond to the increased pressure of yogic inversion, albeit not nearly as rapidly (see below).

The long necks of certain dinosaurs raise another interesting question. Breathing through long pipes can be fatal, for the pipe itself is essentially a dead volume, and if the pipe is a long one, the breathing action simply moves dead air back and forth within the pipe, without ever bringing fresh air into the lungs. The mechanisms that the long-necked dinosaurs apparently used (and modern giraffes use today) to avoid dead-air problems are discussed in Box 15.D-1, page 625.

Theoretically, the increased pressure at the baroreceptors in the aorta and carotid arteries will promote a slowing of the heart and a decreased blood pressure in the head upon inversion; however, these receptors at first may be slow to act, and so the student's face becomes very red and flushed, and the eyes may even become blood-shot. These effects can be minimized if one goes into the inverted position in steps and spends time at each step, rather than going too rapidly from upright to inverted [140, 823]. A similar strategy holds for coming out of inversions and not standing up too soon.

Thus, we see that there are several opposing factors acting simultaneously, each trying to dictate to the circulatory system, in an effort to coax the autonomic balance in one direction or the other. The various opposing effects of inversion on the blood pressure are summed at the carotid sensors, and the more important one will then dictate to the medulla the best autonomic balance. Having mechanisms that operate in opposition to one another makes it possible to continuously vary the level of dominance and so prevent a runaway super-excitation of either autonomic branch. Thus, if the sympathetic system is overexcited, then the signal prompting parasympathetic excitation will strengthen, the sympathetic channel will be inhibited, and the blood pressure will drop, along with the smooth-muscle tone in the arterioles.

As the student's expertise increases in *sarvangasana*, the fear factor and the muscular-effort factor become less important, and the ascendance of the parasympathetic channel is more closely approached. Once this happens, *sarvangasana* has been transformed from a fearful, energizing posture into a calm, relaxing one (point B in figure 5.E-5). A systematic study of the effects of this *yogasana* on students who practiced it twice daily for two weeks confirms the parasympathetic effects it can have on cardiovascular function [461].

The throttling of the blood supply to the brain can have both positive and negative consequences in inverted *yogasana* practice. For example, in the head-down positions (flexion), as in *sarvangasana,* etc., there is generally a slowing of the heart, as the baroreceptors in the internal carotid artery within the neck are tricked into reporting a high blood pressure. This is a beneficial effect, as it promotes relaxation. Similarly, if one massages the carotid arteries so as to stretch the baroreceptors, there will be an automatic activation of these receptors and a falling of the blood pressure. On the other hand, when the head is pressed backward (extension) as in *ustrasana,* the blood flow through the vertebral arteries may be inhibited, with the result that the student feels nauseous and/or dizzy from too low a blood flow to the brain.

An interesting reflex also may be a factor in the question of autonomic dominance in *sarvangasana.* Pinching the skin at the back of the neck is known to cause the pupils of the eyes to dilate, indicating sympathetic dominance. With this in mind, it may be beneficial to make sure that both the pad at the back of the neck and the skin of the neck are smooth in *sarvangasana,* so as to avoid any sympathetic involvement due to the pupillary-skin reflex.

Blood Pressure in Semi-Inversion

Halasana

Consider the question of initiating an aneurysm due to increased arterial pressure in the brain by inverting. Lasater [483] has spoken to this point, as has Katz [435a], in refuting an earlier claim that *halasana* (figure 14.F-2c) is dangerous and should not be performed by anyone. In her rebuttal, Lasater points out that on inverting in *halasana,* the hydrostatic pressure of the blood in the brain does increase, tending to push the arterial walls outward. However, with the head lower than the pelvis, there is also the hydrostatic pressure of the cerebrospinal fluid to be considered, for the brain floats in this (Subsection 4.E, page 107), and its hydrostatic action is to press inward on the walls of the arteries it surrounds. Thus, the net result of this *halasana* semi-inversion, from the hydrostatic point of view, is that there is little or no increase

in the net pressure upon the arterial walls in the brain and spinal cord, because the outward hydrostatic pressure of the blood on the arterial wall is opposed by the inward hydrostatic pressure of the cerebrospinal fluid on the arterial wall. Of course, there is an increase in the fluid pressure within the head when inverted, but this pressure is borne by the bones of the skull and not by the arterial walls within the brain. (However, see Subsections 14.F, page 589, and II.B, page 840, for an important exception to this statement.)

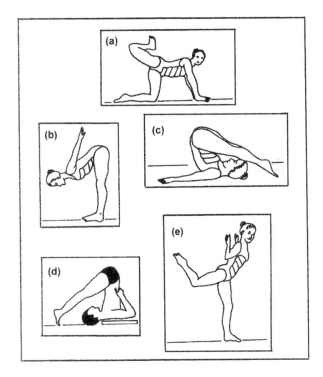

Figure 14.F-2. (c) Demonstration of *halasana* together with a warning about its dangers to the nerves and muscles of the neck and back. If you rotate illustration **c**, you will see how closely the illustrated posture resembles full *paschimottanasana,* but with the back rounded/overstretched and the chin jammed against the chest. (**d**) *Halasana* as it should be practiced, with blankets under the shoulders, the back supported by the arms, and the legs pressed upward so as to protect the neck and back (compare to illustration **c**).

Moreover, with the chin pressed more or less toward the sternum in *halasana,* the baroreceptors of the carotid arteries and the aortic arch will be activated (Sections 11.D, page 452, and 14.E, page 582). In response to this, the activity in the sympathetic nerves driving the heartbeat will be inhibited by the parasympathetic system (Section 5.D, page 178), the heart rate will be slowed, and the arteries will dilate, thus lowering the blood pressure still further. Nonetheless, *halasana* must be done with the neck soft, so that the blood in the head can move as easily as possible through the neck and back toward the heart. The feedback loop described above for *halasana* will be more or less active in all of the inversions, especially for students practicing inversions on a regular basis.

Cole [140] raises another interesting point in regard to inversions. The return of venous blood to the heart from the lower body and the arms is aided by one-way valves in the veins that allow blood to flow only toward the heart (Subsection 14.C, page 570). There are no such valves in the veins of the head, as none are needed for the upright posture, which drains the blood back to the heart by gravity flow. However, when inverted, there appears to be nothing to return blood from the head to the heart. Because of this, working the arms vigorously in the inversions is of great benefit, as the contraction and relaxation of the muscles of the arms helps to pump venous blood from the arms, head, and neck to the heart against the pull of gravity, though not as effectively as when standing upright, where the venous flow is via veins containing valves.

Uttanasana

Uttanasana is particularly interesting [140], in that the head is below the heart, while the feet are on the floor. In this posture, there is much pooling of the blood in the upright legs, while pressure in the carotid arteries (largely hydrostatic) promotes a slower heart rate and vasodilation. The problem with this is that on coming back to *tadasana* from *uttanasana*, with the heart rate low, the blood pooling in the legs, head, and neck, and the blood vessels dilated, there is a great rush of blood **away** from the brain on standing up, and the student can feel very faint. This is especially so if *uttanasana* is a new position for the student or if the student has a sluggish heart-rate response

or a low blood volume. Similar effects can be experienced on just getting up rapidly from a seated position or getting up to urinate in the morning. This latter voiding is driven by parasympathetic excitation, and so is the decreased heart rate and vasodilation. Even if the student is not feeling faint on coming up from *uttanasana*, doing so rapidly can trigger a too-low signal from the baroreceptors, with consequent racing of the heart and vasoconstriction—but not in the heart and brain! This too can be avoided by coming up slowly. Should a person faint from lack of blood to the brain, the situation is self-correcting: in the horizontal position, the blood pressure quickly equalizes, head to toe.

Viparita Karani

In *viparita karani*, the pelvis is positioned so that the abdomen is more or less horizontal, forming a lake into which the blood of the legs can drain [398]. Done in this way, there is no rise in the pressure in the head, while the blood and lymph in the legs have the advantage of a free ride downhill to the abdominal pool. In this way, the blood does not rest on the heart but only gently spills over in that direction. The higher atrial filling factor inherent to *viparita karani* will slow the heart and promote vasodilation.

Full-Body Inversions

In full-body inversions, such as *sirsasana* or *adho mukha vrksasana*, the column of cerebrospinal fluid is only about half as long as the column of blood, and so its pressure acts to counter only about half of the hydrostatic pressure of the blood in the arterioles of the brain. Still, the carotid baroreceptors do their all to reduce pressure, by reducing heart rate and by vasodilation (figure 14.D-1). Again, active use of the muscles of the arms in these postures will aid the return of venous blood to the heart, which in turn will act to reduce the heart rate (typically from eighty per minute to sixty-five per minute for *sirsasana* [112a]) and blood pressure, but the muscular effort expended in the postures also will act to increase the heart rate in opposition to the effect of the baroreceptors. As *sarvangasana* for beginners appears to be a more relaxing posture than does *sirsasana*, one might assume that in the former there is a larger compression of the carotid baroreceptors due to its inherent cervical flexion [863], and to the lesser fear of falling backward in *sarvangasana* as compared to that in *sirsasana*.

Blood pressure while in *sirsasana* has been measured [112a], and it is reported that when inverting, about 500 milliliters of blood flows from the legs toward the head. As a consequence of this translocation of blood, the mean pressure in the leg falls from 200 millimeters Hg to about 10 millimeters (due to loss of both hydrostatic and arterial pressures), whereas in the arm and neck, there is a rise from about 90 millimeters to only 108 millimeters mean arterial pressure. The low blood pressure in the feet while in *sirsasana* implies a lack of circulation of warm blood in that area and cold feet, just as such a weak circulation on sympathetic excitation in the hands leads to a low fingertip temperature (figure 5.E-2**a**). Studying the heart-rate variability following a two-minute *sirsasana*, Manjunath and Telles [534] find the characteristic signs of sympathetic activation, together with a lower heart rate.

Benefits of full-body inversion include improved drainage of body fluids from the legs toward the heart and a different flow of blood through the heart. Regular practice of inversions within a balanced *yogasana* program are said to correct general fatigue or lack of vitality; headache and migraine; loss of hair, or graying hair; bad facial complexion; eye, nose, and throat ailments; indigestion; constipation and diabetes; prolapse of internal organs; sexual malfunction; varicose veins and hemorrhoids; rheumatism; depression; tension and anxiety; insomnia; and general psychological problems [112a, 398, 743].

Provided the baroreceptors are in good working order, the body can readjust the pressure parameters to stay in the safe range as long as the mean arterial pressure remains in the range 60–160 millimeters Hg.

Inversion and Blood Pressure at the Eyes

Intraocular Pressure

In the discussions above, the hydrostatic pressure of the cerebrospinal fluid was described as countering the hydrostatic-pressure rise in the arterioles of the brain and spinal cord when inverted. This counter-pressure is effective because the cerebrospinal fluid completely surrounds the brain and spinal cord. Like the brain, each of the optic nerves and most of each eyeball is surrounded by the dura mater and pia-arachnoid sheaths, and so it is continuous with the meningeal spaces around the brain. Thus, they too are surrounded by an outer layer of CSF, which counters the pressure within the eyes at these places. However, because the cerebrospinal fluid does not completely surround the arterioles of the eyes, any increase in the hydrostatic pressure of the blood in the skull, as when inverting, is transmitted hydrostatically to these arterioles without a compensating pressure from the cerebrospinal fluid. This excess pressure on the central retinal artery when inverting may lead to complications for individuals with a disposition toward bloodshot eyes, glaucoma, or detached retina [140, 823]. It also appears that individuals who are strongly nearsighted are at high risk for retinal detachment when inverted [112a].

The general anxiety felt by many students in inversions leads to a general sympathetic response, which increases arterial and intraocular pressures in the eye. Though the arterial pressure in general is sufficient to bring blood to the eye, the compensating pressure of the cerebrospinal fluid can impede the drainage of both lymph and blood from the retina and so encourage hypertensive retinopathy. This mechanism is exactly parallel to that faced by the uterus during inversions in menstruating women (Section 21.A, page 742) and so argues against such inverted postures in the hypertensive student or in students with eye problems.

Due to a reflex action, inversions cause arteries and veins in the arms and legs to dilate due to both the high pressure sensed by the aortic baroreceptors and to the volume sensors that monitor filling of the right atrium. Furthermore, the heart's output per beat will equal the heart's input per beat in regard to the volume of blood pumped. Because inversion increases the blood input to the heart (thanks to an easier filling of the right atrium), it will also increase the heart's output per beat, and so the heart can afford to beat at a lower rate and still maintain adequate blood flow.

At the other end of the body, in the fully extended inversions, the arterial pressure in the feet rapidly falls to zero, as the heart is not strong enough to pump blood efficiently to the feet against gravity [144, 485, 823] (see Box 14.F-2, below). This lack of circulation in the full inversions leads to very cold feet after many minutes of being inverted. In some students with low blood pressure, these is a loss of blood in the legs and feet while inverted, as described above; however, when they then take a standing position, the rush of blood from the head to the feet is so strong that they feel a sense of fainting. It is best to stand up slowly if one is hypotensive and recovering from an inverted position.

Inversions and Hypertension

There are many different situations that result in chronic hypertension, many of which are not understood. Still, one can present a list of general symptoms for this condition [308]. In the hypertensive:

1. The mean arterial pressure is elevated by 40–50 percent, the left ventricle is significantly enlarged, and the arteries have become sclerotic. These conditions often lead to cerebral and renal failure.
2. The renal blood flow decreases to only 50 percent of normal as the resistance to blood flow through the kidneys increases by three to four times normal.
3. Cardiac output $\dot{Q}$ remains normal.
4. The total arterial resistance increases by 40–50 percent
5. The kidneys fail to excrete Na^+ and water, probably due to decreased renal blood flow.

If the student is hypertensive, then one cannot depend upon the compensating factors of homeostasis to do their job immediately. In this case,

---

Box 14.F-2: Turning Red During and After Inversions

When a muscle is temporarily deprived of its blood supply, the cells within nonetheless continue their metabolism, with the consequent accumulation of carbon dioxide and other acidic products. These metabolites act as local vasodilators, so that when circulation is restored, there is a strong surge of fresh blood into the dilated blood vessels in an attempt to restore normalcy as quickly as possible. This effect is readily observed by hanging head down in an inversion swing for about five minutes. Lack of blood to the feet first cools them, and the veins dilate in expectation of a return of the blood supply. Once out of the swing and on your feet, see how red and warm the feet become as they suck up blood like a dry sponge. Once the metabolites are flushed from the feet, circulation returns to normal, as do the color and temperature of the feet.

One often notes a reddening of the face when a student is in *sarvangasana*. In this case, there is a collapse of the jugular veins draining blood from the head and neck due to too sharp an angle at the throat. This condition is relieved by opening this angle by using more blankets under the shoulders [480], and by leaning backward, so that the weight is heavier on the elbows and lighter on the back of the skull.

mild inversions can be introduced slowly, with great attention paid to their outward effects on the blood pressure. For both normal and hypertensive students, there is great value in doing the appropriate inversions or variations of them, for in doing so, the baroreceptors are thought to eventually reset at a lower level, thus keeping the blood pressure within a lower range of values on a long-term basis [485, 823]. However, the inverted *yogasanas* should not be performed by hypertensive students if the blood pressure rises in the course of their performance [826] or if their blood pressure has been normalized through medication [646, 851].

In accord with the principle of successive approximation in the psychology of learning [781], inversions can be approached rationally by breaking them up into stages and then performing each of the successive stages as a complete *asana* [399]. If one then rests in each stage to allow the body to accommodate to the partial inversion, the fully inverted position eventually may be achieved. For example, first work on *sirsasana* with the knees on the ground. When this can be done without a significant rise in pressure, start straightening the legs in order to elevate the pelvis. Once this is accomplished without a significant rise in pressure, elevate the legs slightly, with the legs straight, and in time, work toward having the legs straight and supported at chair height. Continue working in this way so that students can slowly work toward inversion without risking a precipitous rise in their blood pressure. The idea here is that by performing the intermediate steps of the inversion in a comfortable, nonthreatening manner, the blood pressure will slowly lower and so not be unreasonably out of range when the final inverted position is attempted.

It is thought that by learning to relax while doing inversions that temporarily might raise the blood pressure, the baroreceptors react by resetting their trigger levels in the **downward** direction. This means that following an inversion, one's blood pressure should be lower thereafter, even when sitting passively [823]. This does not mean that inversions are appropriate work for students who are hypertensive! Their blood pressure can be brought down through the use of inversions,

but to do it safely, one must slowly introduce the inversions and incrementally work toward attaining the fully inverted position.

The rush of blood to the brain when inverting can be handled by the homeostatic baroreceptor response, provided the mean blood pressure before inversion is in the range 60–160 millimeters Hg. However, if the systolic pressure is as high as 220 millimeters on inversion, then the mean pressure is above 160 millimeters Hg, and hydrostatic compensation by the CSF will be incomplete.

If a headstand is performed following a *pranayama* practice in which the carbon dioxide level of the blood has been raised by *bhastrika*, the blood vessels dilate in response. When inverted in this condition of cranial vasodilation, blood pours into the brain and can initiate a problem [112a]. However, such a problem can be avoided by practicing *pranayama* **after** *yogasana,* and not the reverse.

Benefits of Inversions

Lymph flows easily from the feet to the heart via the right and left subclavian veins when in inversions, and so inversions can be very helpful in relieving edema in the legs.[10] Inversions also help sluggish venous blood flow at the end of a long day on one's feet, when blood and lymph tend to pool in the lower extremities. Inversions are the standard *yogasana* approach to relieving the pressure in varicose veins and hemorrhoids and also are effective in relieving constipation [404] and promoting urination (Box 14.F-3, below). Note also that the abdominal viscera hang in part from the diaphragm and tend to sag into the pelvic cavity and to even herniate the abdominal tissues under the pull of gravity. Inversion reverses this tendency and so can be therapeutic.

---

10   In edema, there is a localized fluid retention in the legs, which can be relieved by performing *viparita karani*. In this posture, the gravitational pull leads blood and lymph more easily to the heart, and as a result, the brain dilates the blood vessels in the kidneys, which results ultimately in a diuretic-like effect in an effort to lower blood volume in the body [140]; see Box 14.F-3, below.

Box 14.F-3: Inversion (and Laughter) Can Lead to Urination

Whenever one goes inverted, the volume sensors in the atria of the heart sense the increased blood volume, and the brain reflexively dilates the blood vessels in the kidneys, thus transforming more blood into extracellular fluid and urine. By urinating, the blood volume and hence blood pressure are reduced, bringing the body back to a homeostatic condition appropriate to an inverted posture. Of course, once on your feet again, having urinated, the blood pressure and blood volume will then be momentarily low, and long-term homeostasis in the upright posture can then be restored only by the intake of fluids.

It also can happen that if one rises in the middle of the night to urinate, the flow of blood away from the heart toward the feet, along with the parasympathetic action that slows the heart, dilates the blood vessels, and releases the urinary sphincter, are sufficient to cause one to faint while urinating. Being related to parasympathetic relaxation, urination is begun on an exhalation, as with laughter and all *yogasana* postures.

As discussed more fully in Section 7.G, page 254, exercise helps to strengthen bones that bear weight, thus protecting them from osteoporosis. Only yoga offers the opportunity to safely bear weight on the head and so strengthen both the muscles of the neck and the vertebrae in that area. Lasater [491a] mentions that in preliminary research, Cole has found that inverted postures have a strong effect on hormonal levels and reduce brain activity, blood pressure, and fluid retention.

Laughter

Laughing also dilates the blood vessels, lowering the blood pressure. This parasympathetic response might explain, in part, why we tend to pee in our pants when laughing too hard, as urination is also driven by the parasympathetic system (table 5.A-2). See also Subsection 11.D, page 459, for an account of the effects of laughter on muscle tone, and Subsection 13.B, page 511, on the physiology of tickling.

In response to humorous material, brain activity begins in the occipital lobe and then moves to the frontal lobes, where it is recognized as funny. The left frontal lobe analyzes words and structures, and the right lobe does the intellectual analysis required to "get" the joke. Finally, the motor areas are activated in preparation for the laugh.

Laughing activates and exercises the cardiovascular system, so that heart rate and blood pressure increase; following this, the arteries dilate, and the heart rate and blood pressure then decrease. Muscle tension also decreases as we become "weak with laughter," and endorphins are likely generated. Laughter also reduces the production of stress hormones and leads to the production of T cells in the immune system [106]. Both laughing and crying involve an inspiration followed by many short convulsive exhalations, but of somewhat different rhythm. The sounds of laughing and crying can be indistinguishable [863].

Of course, how the blood pressure changes in inversions also can reflect the performer's emotional attitude and fears about being turned upside down, and these psychological effects can compete successfully with the purely physiological ones discussed above. The imagined danger of being in such a precarious position is as potent as any real threat from any source and will be sufficient to excite the sympathetic fight or flight response. Further, anticipation can be more stressful than the real thing.

Weight on the Head

There are a number of interesting aspects to the benefits of inverted postures. If one walks while carrying a load upon the head, one finds that one can carry easily a significant fraction of one's body weight with less heavy breathing, less fatigue, and less back pain than when the same load is carried in any other way [105]. Thus, when hand-carrying a load and walking, the transport is about 65 percent energy efficient, whereas when carrying the same load on the head, the efficiency rises to 80 percent. It also has been found that when supporting a 15-kilogram (thirty-three-pound) weight on the head, in the space of one second, the spine reflexively elongates by approximately 12 millimeters (half an inch) by reducing the spinal curvatures, and one has a feeling of respiratory freedom. On removing the weight from the head, there is a feeling of lightness and spinal elongation. Somewhat the same effects can be sensed by experienced students when performing *sirsasana* with the feet loaded with sandbags.

African women traditionally carry loads on top of their heads amounting to as much as 70 percent of their body weight [105], which would be equivalent to a 46-kilogram (100-pound) *yogasana* student going into *sirsasana* and not working the arms and shoulders so as to reduce the load on the neck (figure V.D-2). If, instead, the female student weighed 70 kilograms (150 pounds) and again did not work the arms in the accepted Iyengar way [388], then the 70 percent passive loading on the neck would be far in excess of what African women safely carry on their heads. For men, the Sherpas of Nepal traditionally carry 66 kilograms (145 pounds) on their heads without incurring neck problems. This suggests that a man weighing significantly more than 77 kilograms (170 pounds), when placed in *sirsasana,* exceeds the limit of what Sherpas carry and therefore is at risk of neck injury unless he is able to shift his weight off the top of his head and onto his forearms and shoulder girdle. Further aspects of loading the head and neck are discussed in Chapter 8, page 265.

Section 14.G: The Lymphatic System

Structure and Function

Thanks to the arteriole pressure applied to their proximal ends, the capillaries tend to leak fluid into the extracellular space surrounding these cells. This interstitial fluid (called lymph) and the channels (known as lymphatics) that transport it form the lymphatic system. Like the vascular system, the lymphatics interconnect so as to form larger and larger conduits for their fluids. However, the lymphatics are not a closed loop like the vascular system, being open-ended at the level of the smallest channels. Lymph flows toward the heart in the same direction as venous blood and eventually drains into the subclavian veins [582] (figure 14.C-2**b**).

Motion pictures of exposed lymphatic vessels show that these vessels contract periodically, with the result that lymph is pumped by these actions toward the heart [308]. This intrinsic action, known as the lymphatic pump, is aided by external contractions (such as that of muscles), by arterial pulsations, and by external compression of body tissues.

The lymph system serving more superficial tissues is rather independent of and disconnected from that part of the system serving the deeper tissues [181, 528]. The largest of the lymphatic vessels drain their contents into the thoracic and right lymph ducts in the vicinity of the upper chest. The lymphatic system does not extend into the brain, spinal cord, bone marrow, or avascular structures such as cartilage and epidermis. Surprisingly, the lymphatic system is an active part of the digestive system (Chapter 19, page 711), for it serves to carry emulsified fats from the small intestine into the bloodstream. The lymphatic system processes two to four liters of lymph per day, whereas the heart pumps five liters of blood per minute.

Composition

The composition of lymph is very much like that of the blood plasma from which it is derived, except for the near absence of blood proteins such as serum albumin, which are too large molecularly to diffuse through the capillary walls. Lymph contains many fragments of cell debris [446], as well as bacteria, etc. In healthy, active muscle tissue, the weight percentage of the lymphatic fluid bathing the cells is about 15 percent of the total weight of the muscle [187].

Lymph Drainage

From one-third to two-thirds of the plasma entering the capillaries passes into the interstitial spaces outside the capillaries and is then picked up by lymph capillaries and carried in the lymphatics. Lymph from the entire left side of the body, the digestive tract, and the right side of the lower body flows into the thoracic duct and then into the left subclavian vein at a rate of about 100 milliliters per hour. Lymph from the right side of the head, neck, and chest flows into the right lymphatic duct and then into the right subclavian vein [450]. Thus, lymph flow is very asymmetric; the possible yogic consequences of this are discussed further in Section 15.E, page 635.

Edema

As the gravitational effects on the body are minimal when the body is horizontal, the lymph volume in the body is minimal and evenly distributed when we get out of bed in the morning. However, in the course of a day spent on our feet or just sitting, the gravitational pull toward the feet is sufficient to promote leakage of lymph preferentially in the lower limbs, and so the legs tend to swell. At this time, the volume of blood is depleted by the amount converted into lymph, and so the low blood volume may promote a faster heart rate in compensation.

In order to prevent swelling of the tissue, it is necessary to somehow pump lymph back to the heart, where it will again join the blood supply in the vascular system. The mechanism for moving lymph to the heart is much like that for moving venous blood; the larger lymph vessels contain one-way valves, so that on compression of the vessels by the action of the surrounding muscles, the low-pressure fluid is pumped in one direction only: toward the subclavian veins (figure 14.C-5). If the lymph system breaks down, or a limb is injured, or one simply is too passive physically, the lymph accumulates in that limb, and swelling of the tissue (edema) ensues. On the other hand, in the case of a blood hemorrhage, the vascular system can draw on the lymphatic system for fluid, as the lymph is reabsorbed into the capillaries. In a student standing motionless in *tadasana,* the hydrostatic pressure in the lymphatic system at the ankle will be 90 millimeters Hg after thirty seconds, and 15–20 percent of the blood volume may be lost from the circulatory system after fifteen minutes in this position; walking reduces this pressure to 25 millimeters [308]. This illustrates how important it is to perform periodic pumping actions with the muscles of the legs when there is no gross movement of the body, as when in *tadasana* and the other standing postures held for long durations, or when bound to a seat on a long trip by airplane.

As the capillaries offer a nonzero resistance to blood flow, they support in part the blood pressure surge on cardiac systole. This periodic pressurization of a relatively weak structure leads to a pulsation of the capillary diameter,[11] which then serves to pump nearby lymph toward the heart [878]. Some of the smaller lymph vessels drain directly into small veins and so contribute to relieving the lymphatic pressure.

It is generally agreed that exercise and inversion are important factors in keeping lymph in circulation. The output of the lymphatic pump increases by a factor of ten to thirty on going from a resting position to one of repeated muscular action. As a

---

11   Interestingly, the capillary pulse also has a frequency (0.1 hertz) that is about one-tenth that of the heartbeat, placing it far below the region of the alpha rhythm of the EEG brain waves (Subsection 4.H, page 151) but squarely in the range of heart-rate variability (Subsection 14.A, page 549) and the cranial-sacral pulse (Subsection 4.E, page 109). This pulsation is known as the Mayer wave.

corollary to this, lymphatic swelling results when a limb is positioned below the heart and is physically inactive. However, the *yogasana* practitioner must use caution in prescribing lymph-activating *yogasanas* for relief of edema in certain situations, for the lymphatic system also can be the pathway for the metastatic spread of cancer cells. A similar caution is in order for students having sinus infections, for inversions can help spread the infection to other sites [446].

The Respiratory Pump

As with the venous supply to the heart, the motion of the diaphragm when breathing will act to pneumatically pump lymph from the feet toward the heart, this being strongest when breathing deeply [752]. As for using upright *yogasanas* to improve lymph circulation, repetitive motions are better than static positions [531]. *Yogasanas* recommended for promoting lymph drainage are given by Schatz [752] and by MacMullen [531].

Lymph Nodes

Though the lymph channels closely resemble the venous system in form and function, they do differ in one very significant way. The lymph vessels, at several points, contain nodal structures of the size of small beans, the purpose of which is to filter the lymph fluid on its way to the heart (figure 14.C-2b). Lymph nodes are most prominent on the underside of the jaw (cervical lymph nodes), in the armpits (axillary lymph nodes), in the inner elbows, and in the groin (inguinal lymph nodes). Over 99 percent of the bacteria in lymphatic fluid are filtered by the lymph nodes, which also manufacture antibodies and lymphocytes [450].

The lymphatic nodal system is a very important part of the body's defense system, as it contains macrophage cells, which intercept and kill foreign bacteria, and lymphocytes, which manufacture antibodies in order to control foreign microorganisms. By our practice of *yogasanas*, we promote the more rapid circulation of the lymph through the nodes and so are performing acts of blood purification in doing so.

In modern man, lymph nodes are colored blue-black due to filtered particles of carbon and dust [582]. The swelling of one of these nodes is obvious whenever the node begins rapid manufacture of lymphocytes in response to an infection. When lymph nodes are removed surgically, as for breast cancer, lymph edema often occurs in the arm or leg closest to the site of removal.

The Thymus and Spleen

Two organs in the body are lymph-node-like in their function: the spleen and the thymus gland. However, there is no afferent lymph supply to the spleen, and so it cannot act as a lymph filter. The spleen does produce B lymphocytes and is a storehouse for red blood cells, whereas the thymus gland, lying just behind the upper part of the sternum and containing several lymphatic nodules, is of marginal value in the adult, for even in the adult, there is only marginal T-cell production by the thymus. The spleen is relatively easily crushed in the course of abdominal trauma and must be removed if it is bleeding profusely.

Respiration 15

Section 15.A: Anatomy of the Respiratory Apparatus

Control of the Breath

For over 5,000 years, mystics and Eastern medical practitioners have claimed that control of the breath and/or modification of the breath can have profound impact on the health and well-being of an individual. Today, medical researchers are confirming these ancient views with studies that show the relation between the way we breathe and our cardiovascular functioning, the circulation to the brain, metabolic and endocrine activities, muscular, visceral, and vascular tones, lymph drainage, arteriole blood flow, blood pH, and autonomic homeostasis [576]. Respiration has been coupled to the central nervous system, both physiologically and psychologically, in several ways and so cannot be considered separately from these connections. In particular, the breath directs the movement of the ribs, the intrathoracic and intra-abdominal pressures, the cyclic change of the spinal muscle tone on inhalation and exhalation, the balance in the autonomic nervous system, the emotions, the heart rate, and the respiratory sinus arrhythmia.

The breath is of the utmost significance to our *yogasana* practice and to our health and well-being. Outside of the yoga community, in general, it is little appreciated that control of the breath is possible and that with control of the breath, there follows control of our mental and somatic states. The first step in controlling the nervous system is modifying the respiration pattern, for the respiration is both the most easily modified of the vital functions [692] and the most subtle in its effects on the body and mind. The link between breathing and the other autonomic functions involves strong interactions between the cortex, the brainstem, and certain hormones. Control of the body through *yogasana* and control of the breath through *pranayama* form the doorway to higher levels of meditation. The terms "inspiration" and "expiration" in reference to breathing are synonymous with "inhalation" and "exhalation," respectively, and are used here interchangeably.

Breathing Modes

The Ayurvedic approach to understanding the functioning of the body divides breathing phenomena into two categories called *langhana* and *brmhana,* meaning "to fast" (as when one goes without eating) and "to expand," respectively. Miller [576] gives a long list demonstrating how these two qualities or principles differ, presented here in an abbreviated form in table 15.A-1. Note how similar this table is to table 1.A-1, describing the two world views given in Subsection 1.A, page 3. According to table 15.A-1, the two ways of breathing, abdominal-diaphragmatic *(langhana)* and thoracic *(brmhana)*, correlate with many aspects of the autonomic nervous system. Some authors consider other modes of breathing than these two to be more basic, and so there is no unanimity as to the "basic" forms, but the differences are not

Table 15.A-1: Comparison of the *Langhana* and *Brmhana* Principles of Ayurvedic Medicine [576]

Langhana	*Brmhana*
Contraction/exhalation	Expansion/inhalation
Abdominal-diaphragmatic breathing	Thoracic breathing
Left-nostril dominance	Right-nostril dominance
Right cerebral dominance	Left cerebral dominance
Apana moves upward	*Prana* moves downward
Located in colon and pelvis	Located in chest and stomach
Forward bends and twisting	Backbends
Catabolic	Anabolic
Female	Male
Parasympathetic	Sympathetic
Afferent nerves	Efferent nerves
Activated by darker colors (brown, violet, etc.)	Activated by lighter colors (red, yellow, etc.)
Positive feelings of love and compassion	Positive feelings of activity and intelligence

large. The two types of Ayurvedic breathing will be discussed in this chapter, along with a few other related types. But first, we must consider the anatomy of the breathing apparatus.

Journey into the Lungs

The Larynx

The respiratory passage begins its downward journey at the nasal cavity, moving then through the pharynx and larynx within the throat and on to the trachea, which is also open to any food swallowed by the oral cavity (figure 15.A-1). Though both air and food travel through the pharynx, the epiglottis (just below the pharynx) will be either closed, to route food down the esophagus, or open, to route air down the larynx on inhalation and up the larynx on exhalation. During swallowing, the larynx is elevated, so that the epiglottis forms a lid over the glottis, the glottis being the space between the vocal folds. When the epiglottis closes the glottis, food is routed into the esophagus and so is kept out of the airways. Should anything other than air pass through the glottis, a cough reflex is stimulated to clear the airway.

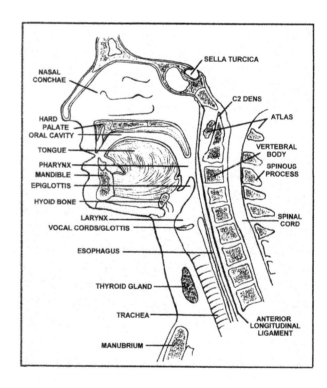

Figure 15.A-1. Sagittal section through the head, showing the common path of the nasal and oral cavities down to the epiglottis, at which point they separate, with air going down the larynx and trachea and food going down the esophagus [431].

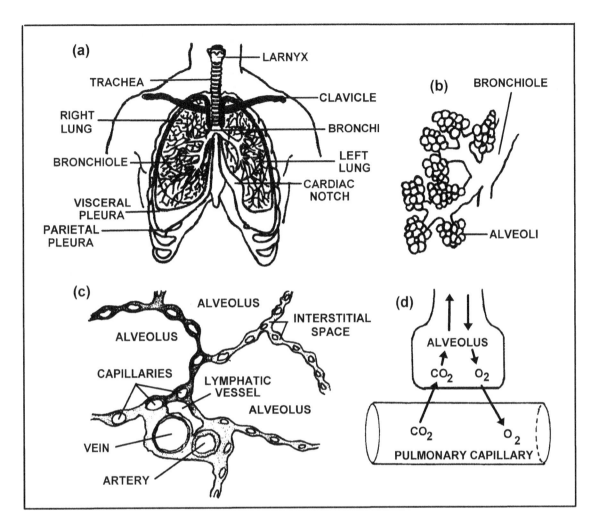

Figure 15.A-2. (a) As the trachea descends, it bifurcates first to form the left and right bronchi, and each of these further branches repeatedly, leading eventually to the grape-like alveoli shown in (b). The empty space depicted as the cardiac notch in fact is occupied by the heart, not shown here [431]. (c) The boundary of the alveoli and the circulatory system within the lungs, showing the intimate contact between the alveoli and the capillaries. (d) Diagram of the exchange of gases between the alveolus and the pulmonary capillary.

When the epiglottis is open, air passing upward through the larynx results in the production of vocal sounds; whereas when the air passes downward through the larynx, it enters the trachea, a pipe of smooth muscle and cartilage [432]. As the trachea descends to enter the chest, it branches at the level of vertebra T4 into two limbs called the bronchi, with each limb going to its respective lung on the left or the right (figure 15.A-2a). The sinuses of the skull are also factors in respiration and are discussed in Subsection 9.A, page 311.

The Trachea and Beyond

Air enters the lungs by passing successively through the trachea, the bronchi, and the bronchioles (figure 15.A-2a), finally to reach the alveoli (figure 15.A-2b). There are cartilaginous plates in the walls of the trachea and bronchi that prevent these airways from collapsing. On the other hand, bronchioles with diameters of less than 2 millimeters (0.1 inches) lack this cartilage and are formed entirely of smooth muscle. The bronchioles are encircled by smooth muscle, which dilates in response to the stimulation of sympathetic beta-receptors and constricts in response to parasympathetic stimulation. On inhalation, the lungs inflate due to the lengthening of the bronchi, and not due to their separation.

Filtering and Heat Exchange

The inner surfaces of the trachea and bronchi are covered with epithelial cells bearing hairlike appendages, which in turn are covered by a thin mucus film that traps any particulate debris in the inspired air (Subsection 20.B, page 723). In addition to trapping foreign particles in the upwardly mobile mucus film, the passage of incoming air through the nose and the trachea warms the air on cold days, using heat from underlying blood vessels, and also raises the humidity of the air before it enters the lungs [431]. On hot days, the nasal heat exchanger can work to reduce the temperature of the blood in the head. The effects of this heat exchange can be sensed in *savasana,* as the air entering the nostrils will feel cool, but the air exhaled will feel warm. These nasal blood vessels are close to the surface and have only a very thin layer of skin between them and the outside air, for obvious reasons of efficient heat transfer; however, one must be careful when putting anything up the nose, as it can easily tear the thin layer and cause a nosebleed.[1] Furthermore, the yogic preference for breathing through the nose rather than the mouth is given credence by the work of Wernitz [721], who showed that the EEG patterns when breathing orally or nasally are quite different.

The Alveoli

The right lung is sculpted into three distinct lobes, whereas the left is separated only into two. Within each lung, the bronchi again bifurcate, first forming secondary bronchi and then form-

ing the bronchioles, which continue to branch until the level of the alveolar sacs is reached (figure 15.A-2b). These sacs at the terminal edges of the bronchial tree appear like clusters of grapes, each "grape" being a sac of approximately 0.3 millimeters (0.01 inches) in diameter. If we assume that such sacs half fill the lung volume of 6 liters when expanded, then the total number of alveoli in the lungs comes to 300 million, a number that implies twenty-eight successive bifurcations; i.e., each bronchial branch divides twenty-eight times. Being as finely divided as they are, the alveoli within the lungs of the average adult, if spread flat, would have an area (50–100 square meters) approximately equal to that of half a tennis court and eighty times the area of his or her skin.

Oxygenation

The membrane forming the alveolar sac has a thickness of only 0.6 μ, just the thickness of a capillary wall. Each of the alveoli is surrounded by a capillary system with which it is in close contact. At any one time, there is a volume of 0.9 liters of blood (approximately 20 percent of the total blood volume) occupying the capillaries surrounding the alveoli of the lungs.

On inhalation, each of the alveoli fills with fresh, oxygen-charged air. Venous, deoxygenated blood from the right side of the heart (the right ventricle, figure 14.A-1) is pumped through the lung's capillary system via the pulmonary arteries, where it absorbs fresh oxygen from the alveoli and releases carbon dioxide into the alveoli. Blood refreshed in this way is sent back via the pulmonary veins to the left atrium of the heart (figure 14.A-1) and then pumped through the left ventricle and the aorta into the arterial system. Though the oxygen–carbon dioxide gas exchange across the walls of both the alveoli and the capillaries within the lungs is by diffusion, it nonetheless can be rapid, because the relevant cell walls are very thin, and the distances involved are very short [432].

Pulmonary Resistance

The transit time for blood within the capillaries of the lungs is 0.8 seconds when the body is at rest but drops to about 0.4 seconds during

---

1   A similar situation is found at the insides of the wrists, where blood runs very close to the surface; when working intensely in the *yogasanas,* running cool water over the wrists will be found to be immediately restorative. On the other hand, if one feels too cool, running warm water over the wrists leads to immediate warming of the body.

heavy exercise. This shortening of the pulmonary residence time during heavy exercise would be even shorter were it not for the fact that during heavy exercise, more capillaries are opened up for circulation, and so there is a smaller pressure drop across any one capillary and therefore a somewhat longer residence time for the blood in transit through the capillary [308].

Because the resistance to flow in the pulmonary venules and in the capillary nets of the lungs is so small, a pulmonary pressure of only one-seventh that at the aorta is necessary to drive blood from the right ventricle through the lungs. It is this small pressure drop from one end of the capillaries to the other within the lungs that translates into the long residence time for venous blood in the lungs and correspondingly offers an increased opportunity for the venous blood to exchange its burden of carbon dioxide for oxygen. Occasionally, the pulmonary resistance within the lungs can be unusually high, leading to pulmonary hypertension, a condition in which oxygenation of the blood is poor and the person suffers fatigue and breathlessness.

Gas Exchange

Over 50 percent of the lung volume is occupied by blood and the blood vessels [431]. It is the large surface area defining the interface between the air in the lungs and the blood in the lungs that makes breathing so efficient that little or no reserve of oxygen is necessary in the body. If the overall area of the alveoli is reduced, or if the alveoli lose their elasticity, as when a person has emphysema, then breathing becomes substantially more difficult. Note that though the lungs are totally involved in the strong muscular action of the breath, there is very little muscle tissue to be found in the lungs, just that within the layers forming the vascular net. The lungs are largely passive organs, the functioning of which is totally dependent upon a complicated mechanism of external musculature and bony levers.

Ventilation-to-Perfusion Ratio

Though the lungs are uniformly filled with the alveoli and the capillary systems intertwined with them, the effect of gravity is to bring the larger portion of the pulmonary blood to the lower regions of the lungs when the person is upright, as in *tadasana*. Because of the pooling of the blood in the lower regions of the lungs, there is less room for air in those lower regions, whereas at the top of the lungs, there is an excess of air and too little blood to take advantage of it. If one were inverted, as in *sirsasana,* then gravity would carry the oxygen-poor blood to just the upper parts of the lungs, forcing the air out of this region and into the lower regions. Only in the middle third of the lung tissue are there more equal volumes of blood and air, and it is here that the most efficient transfer of gases between air and blood takes place [140, 687]. Thus, the optimal ratio of air volume to blood volume (called the ventilation-to-perfusion ratio) is found in the middle third of the lungs. In order to work the other portions of the lungs adequately, one has to tip the rib cage through various angles, as in *trikonasana,* so that the portion of the lung volume having a ventilation-to-perfusion ratio near 1 occupies different parts of the lungs, and then one must breathe while in these nonvertical positions for significant times.

As stated above, in a standing person at rest, blood pools preferentially in the lower part of the lungs, showing nearly zero flow in the upper third of each lung. During exercise, the flow will increase and more blood will perfuse the upper third. Respiration in the lying position is more efficient than when standing, because there is a more complete mixing of the blood and the air in the central zone in the prone position [493].

Heavy Exercise

Remember now that the pressure forcing the blood through the lungs is unusually low, being only about 10 millimeters Hg at diastole and only 20 millimeters at systole. As the pulmonary pressure varies from one part of the cardiac cycle to the next, there will be parts of the lungs where the systolic blood pressure is high enough to allow blood flow but where the diastolic pressure is too low and the same arteries are collapsed. This zone of intermittent blood flow is called zone 2.

In the normal chest, zone 2 starts 7–10 centimeters (three to four inches) above the level of the heart and extends to the very top of the lungs. In zone 3, the pressure is high enough at both cardiac systole and diastole to keep the arteries open; this zone extends from 7–10 centimeters (three to four inches) above the heart to the very bottom of the lungs. When in the prone position, all parts of the lungs are in a zone 3 condition, and when fully inverted, the blood flow to the top of the lung is actually larger than that to the bottom. Similarly, the entire lung is converted to zone 3 behavior under heavy exercise, as the cardiac pressure increases in order to serve the working muscles [308].

Bronchial Diameters

Resistance to the flow of breath is governed in part by the diameters of the airways into the lungs, with the small airways offering more resistance to breathing than do the large airways. The bronchial diameters are controlled by the smooth muscles within their walls, which in turn respond to signals from the autonomic nervous system; in times of crisis, the smooth muscles are relaxed by the catecholamines, the bronchi dilate, and the breath flows more easily; whereas in a more calm environment, it is the acetylcholine of the parasympathetic nervous system that keeps them somewhat contracted (Section 3.D, page 54).

Pressure on the Heart

The heart lies between the lungs, more so on the left side, where there is a cardiac notch in the left lung to accommodate it (figure 15.A-2**a**). One sees from the figure that there is less weight pressing on the heart when resting on the right side than when on the left, which suggests why we turn to the right side when recovering from *savasana*. (However, see Subsection 15.E, page 634, for another reason to come out of this posture by turning onto the right side.) In the case of a pregnant student, she turns to the left when arising from a supine position, in order to avoid pinching off the blood flow from the inferior vena cava to the heart, this being a blood vessel lying

to the right of the spine in order to enter the right atrium.

The Thoracic Diaphragm

Structure and Function

Air that makes its way into the alveoli rapidly would become stagnant were it not replaced forcefully and frequently by fresh air from the outside. This important task falls to the muscles and bones surrounding the lungs, which act so as to repeatedly fill and empty the otherwise passive lungs of their air. A prime mover among these muscles is the diaphragm, a slow-twitch muscle (Subsection 11.A, page 411) unique to mammals [582].

The diaphragm is a large, horizontal, sheet-like muscle that effectively acts as a separator between the ventilation action of the thorax and the digestion action of the abdomen. It is the floor to the chest cavity and the ceiling to the abdominal cavity [105]. Its shape is asymmetric, with the dome on the right being larger than that on the left.

As shown in figure 15.A-3**b**, the diaphragm is anchored to the lowest ribs and to the anterior side of the lumbar and sacral spine and is domed upward in the relaxed position, looking much like an open umbrella. The apex of the dome is the so-called central tendon, which in this case is not connected directly to a second bone forming a conventional joint; rather, it is a tendonous island surrounded by the radially aligned muscle fibers of the diaphragm. As the muscle fibers run radially from the outer edges of the diaphragm to the central tendon, the diaphragmatic area shrinks when the muscle is contracted, the sheet is pulled downward by 1–2 centimeters (0.4–0.8 inches), and the thoracic volume correspondingly increases. This action of thoracic expansion momentarily causes a reduction of the air pressure within the lungs as compared to that outside the lungs, and so air flows into the lungs; i.e., one has inhaled. Viewed somewhat differently, the diaphragm acts like a piston, drawing air into the lungs on the down stroke (diaphragmatic contraction) and releasing the air from the lungs on the up stroke (diaphragmatic relaxation). The motion of the diaphragm when breathing acts to lower the pressure in the thoracic cavity and to raise it in the abdomen; not only does air enter the lungs on inhalation, but venous blood is sucked and pressed upward from the abdomen into the right atrium of the heart during this act [288].

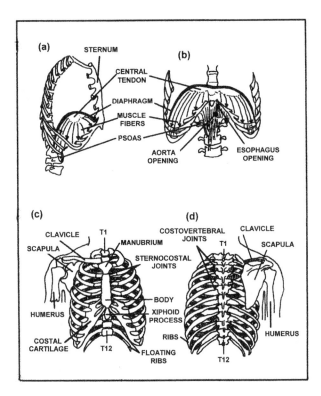

Figure 15.A-3. (a) A lateral view of the diaphragm within the thoracic cavity, showing its central tendon, the radially aligned muscle fibers, attachments to the anterior sides of the lower vertebrae, and the orientation of the tension (arrows) when the diaphragm is contracted. (b) The anterior view of the diaphragm within the thoracic cavity, showing more clearly its attachments to the lumbar vertebrae. Also shown are the openings through which the aorta and the esophagus pass [428]. (c) The attachment of the ribs to the sternum (manubrium, body, and xiphoid process) via the sternocostal joints and the costal cartilage, as seen from the front. (d) The attachment of the ribs to the twelve thoracic vertebrae via the costovertebral joints, as seen from the back.

The lungs rest on the diaphragm (figure 15.A-3), which itself forms a dome over the stomach, liver, and spleen, separating these viscera physically from the heart and lungs. This dome rises higher on the right-hand side in order to accommodate the liver [394]. In fact, the lower surfaces of the lungs are attached to the upper surface of the diaphragm, which in turn is pierced by three openings to allow passage of the esophagus, the descending aorta, and the inferior vena cava. The inferior undersurface of the diaphragm on its right side is molded to accommodate the right lobe of the liver, the right kidney, and the suprarenal gland on that kidney; on the left side, the accommodation is for the left lobe of the liver, the fundus of the stomach, the spleen, and the left kidney and its associated suprarenal gland. Because the lobe of the liver on the right side offers more resistance to compression than does the stomach on the left, the diaphragm is stronger on the right side than on the left [288]. Note too that there are ligaments that connect the pericardial fibers surrounding the heart to the central tendon of the diaphragm, so that with each breath, the heart is lifted and dropped by a few centimeters (about one inch), which is to say, it is massaged by the motions of the breath [61a].

Respiratory Synergists

Together with the iliacus and the psoas muscles (figure 9.B-2), the diaphragm and its partners form an anatomy train [603], the components of which tend to act in unison.[2] Though the diaphragm is the prime mover for inhalation, it is assisted greatly by the external intercostal muscles. Since a muscle cannot push but only can pull, how does the activation of the diaphragm result in an increase in all three dimensions of the chest, as occurs when we inhale? The answer to this lies

---

2   Such a train often will contain a minimum of two biarticular muscles sharing overlapping tendons; for example, the hamstrings and the gastrocnemius form such a muscular chain, overlapping at the back of the knee. The hamstrings are biarticular muscles and as such, are able to extend the hip joint, flex the knee joint, and drive rotation around either of these joints.

in the variable plane of the curved ribs. When relaxed, the ribs hang forward and downward from the costovertebral joints, but when we inhale, the ribs are lifted so that the plane of each rib is more horizontal, and so the circumference increases. This does not involve any great stretching around either the sternal or vertebral joints, only a change of angle of the plane of the rib with respect to the horizontal plane at these joints. It is the external intercostals (assisted by synergist muscles such as the sternocleidomastoid and scalenes) that lift the ribs on inhalation.

The diaphragm is important not only for breathing but also for pumping blood and lymph from the nether regions up to the heart. It is active in vocalization and provides the motive force behind all expulsive actions. It is a universal habit among people to freeze the diaphragm and hold the breath when in painful, fearful, or stressful situations, as one might experience in a challenging *yogasana*. Muscular tension in the diaphragm, as when chronically holding the breath, can result in a reduced flow through the vascular vessels that penetrate the diaphragm, and this reduced circulation can set the stage for varicosities and menstrual problems [105].

The Peritoneum

All of the muscle and visceral organs within the abdominal cavity are surrounded by a smooth, slippery serous lining known as the peritoneum, which acts to keep adjacent organs from adhering to one another. There are serous membranes between the lungs and the thoracic cavity that are filled with fluid, thus easing the relative motions of these during breathing. The high surface tension of this fluid makes the lungs stick to the walls of the chest, and so the lungs will fill when the chest is expanded.

If the peritoneum is cut during surgery, it is very likely that as the wound heals, the cut surfaces of the peritoneum will bond to different internal organs, forming adhesions. These adhesions express themselves as stiffness, in that they will restrict motion of the internal organs in postures such as spinal twists and backbends. Though adhesions can be broken up by follow-up surgery,

such surgery is usually followed by the formation of new adhesions, formed at the sites of the new incisions.

The Ribs, Sternum, and Costal Muscles

The Rib Cage

The ribs are part of a bony cage that not only offers protection to the lungs and heart but also is an active participant in the breathing process. As seen in figures 15.A-3c and 15.A-3d, there are twelve pairs of ribs, connected by hinge joints to vertebrae T1 through T12, the top ten of which are also hinged in the front body.

The volume enclosed by the ribs and their junctures defines the thoracic cavity; the diaphragm is the muscular sheet forming the floor of this cavity. The upper ten pairs of ribs are joined in the front body at the sternum via the sternocostal joints, whereas all twelve pairs of ribs are joined to the vertebral column in the back body through the costovertebral joints. Each of the ribs is thin, flat, and slightly twisted so as to form a helical curve; those ribs anchored in the back body to vertebrae T1–T7 are connected to the sternum in the front body by short lengths of costal cartilage, whereas those anchored to T8–T10 connect to significantly longer pieces of costal cartilage below the sternum, and those anchored at T11 and T12 (the floating ribs) have no front-body anchors but instead are attached to the abdominal muscles [288]. The thorax is widest at the seventh rib, and the xiphoid process (figure 15.A-3c) is attached only to the sternum.

Many muscles of both the arms and the abdomen are attached to the ribs. Because the sternum when young is elastic, it is rarely fractured; however, the middle ribs are the most likely to break, most often in front, at the sharp angle where the curvature is largest. The ribs joined to T1 and T2 are rarely injured, due to their protection by the clavicles and the pectoral muscles; those connected to T11 and T12 are rarely injured, because they are free-floating. In the past, broken ribs were treated by wrapping the chest with adhesive tape, thereby retarding motion of the rib cage during breathing; this is no longer the case, as it is now known that throttling the breath increases the risk for lung infections [105].

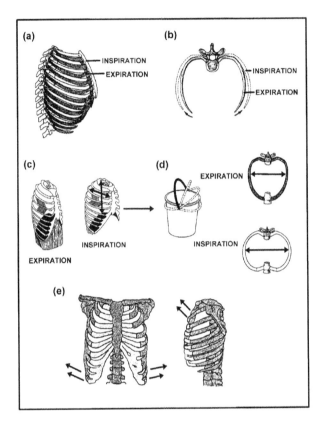

Figure 15.A-4. (a) The variation of the angle of the planes of the ribs, with respect to the horizontal plane, and the rise and fall of the sternum during inspiration and expiration. (b) The change of the circumference of the thorax on inspiration and expiration. (c) The changes of the rib-cage geometry on inspiration and expiration and (d) its relation to that of the movement of a bucket handle. (e) Directions for the movement of the lower ribs and sternum on inhalation.

Taking a Breath

In general, the plane of each rib is inclined downward, but on inspiration, the ribs are lifted and the angle more closely approaches horizontal, while the side-to-side and front-to-back dimensions of the rib cage increase (figure 15.A-4). This clever arrangement of the planes of the ribs allows the volume of the thorax to increase on inhalation, thereby drawing fresh air into the lungs by just changing this angle, without any significant loosening of the sternal or vertebral joints holding the ribs onto the sternum and the spinal column. Because the lowest ribs (T11 and T12) move the most and lack the sternocostal binding, in many postures, such as *urdhva hastasana,* it will be possible (but not desirable) to thrust the floating ribs forward without a corresponding thrust of the other ribs (figure 15.A-4).

Intercostal Muscles

In addition to the joints with the vertebrae and the sternum, each of the ribs is bound to its neighboring ribs through a pair of muscle sheets, the external and internal intercostal muscles. As the muscle-fiber direction in one of the intercostal-muscle sheets is perpendicular to that in the other, these muscle can be thought of as derived from the mutually perpendicular internal and external abdominal oblique muscles. Contraction of the external intercostal muscles pulls the outer surfaces of the ribs toward one another, thereby flaring the ribs outward, whereas contraction of the internal intercostal muscles pulls the ribs more toward the centerline of the thoracic cylinder.

The ribs are lifted first by action of the external intercostals, and finally muscles in the neck lift the ribs to the maximum. The ribs, together with their joints front and back and the muscles between the ribs, collectively form the rib cage. It is the motion of the diaphragm aided by those of the walls of the rib cage and the abdomen that work to pump air in and out of the lungs.

On a deep inhalation, the rib T1 is largely immobilized, and the contraction of the external intercostal lifts T2 toward T1 in a bucket-handle motion. This transforms T2 into an anchor, against which T3 can pull, and in this way, the planes of all of the ribs are raised and the inter-rib distances are increased. At the same time, the angle of the sternum with respect to the horizontal plane decreases by 5° or so. Further lift of the entire rib cage is then initiated by contraction of the sternocleidomastoids and scalenes, with origins on C1–C2 and with insertions on the T1 and T2 ribs. In this action, the contraction of the sternocleidomastoids and the scalenes essentially stabilizes T1 (Subsection 11.F, page 468), and the external intercostals then work against this anchor to lift the rib cage, while the diaphragm contracts downward so as to fill the lungs and stretch the abdominal muscles. The mechanics of the breath are considered more fully in Section 15.C, page 613.

The Abdominal Muscles

The abdominal muscles are closely associated with the spinal column, contribute significantly to the rotation and curvature of the spine at the levels of the thoracic and lumbar vertebrae, and are important in certain breathing modes. Of the four muscle groups in the abdomen (the rectus, the external and internal obliques, and the transversus; see figure 15.C-1), the rectus is the most visible. The roles of these muscles in the breathing process are discussed in Sections 15.B, page 610, and 15.C, page 613. Interestingly, the quadratus lumborum connecting the posterior iliac crest to T12 and the transverse processes of L1 to L4 may be considered as the fifth member of the abdominal group, in effect acting as the antagonist to the rectus abdominis.

As a group, the abdominal muscles protect the vital organs of the lower abdomen from the anterior, posterior, and lateral directions, and with their opposing directions of muscle-fiber orientations and large widths, they strengthen and stabilize this central aspect of the body.

Rectus Abdominis

The rectus abdominis are twin muscles running from the pubis directly upward to the lower ribs; each of the strap-like rectus abdominis muscles has its origin on the pubic bone and its insertion on the sternum and lower ribs. The two vertical muscle sheets are evenly divided left to right by a vertical tendon known as the linea alba, and each is separated into five sections by four horizontal fibrous aponeuroses, which give the abdomen the "six-pack" look, though it really is a ten-pack (figure 10.A-2a).

Contraction of the rectus abdominis muscles pulls the lowest ribs toward the pelvic iliac crests, thereby flattening or even reversing the lumbar curve, as often occurs with beginners when doing *paripurna navasana*. The rectus muscle is sandwiched between the aponeuroses of the internal obliques and the transversus muscles, and in turn, these aponeuroses blend into the linea alba on the center line of the abdomen (figure 10.A-2a). The erector spinae muscles paralleling the spinal column on the back body (figure 10.A-2b) and the quadratus lumborum are the antagonists to the rectus abdominis.

The rectus abdominis is stretched in *urdhva mukha svanasana,* as the iliac crest and the lowest ribs move away from one another in this posture. If one then moves from *urdhva mukha svanasana* to straight-arm *chaturanga dandasana,* the ribs and iliac crests must move again toward one another, and so there is a strong contraction of the rectus abdominis in the latter posture to keep it from falling into the former posture. Consequently, straight-arm *chaturanga dandasana* held for a minute or two or moving between it and *urdhva mukha svanasana* prove to be excellent strengtheners for the rectus abdominis.

Abdominal Obliques

The net of the abdominal muscles forms a girdle around the abdomen. Largely due to the tone of the external abdominal obliques, the abdominal muscles function mostly to hold in the viscera of the abdomen, in opposition to the pull of gravity when standing or sitting. With the points of origin and insertion held fixed, contraction of the abdominal muscles raises the pressure on the abdominal contents and promotes expulsion or a strengthening of the thoracic cylinder. The role of the abdominal muscles in breathing is an important one, as discussed in Section 15.C, page 613.

The tendons of the external abdominal obliques attach to the eight lowest ribs and then run downward and backward so as to insert on the iliac crest and as far inferiorly as the pubic symphysis; each of the two components (left and right) of the muscle has a very large aponeurosis, which covers the entire surface of the belly and lies on top of the rectus abdominis. Acting bilaterally, the external abdominal obliques flex the trunk if the pelvis is immobilized, or tilt the posterior rim of the pelvis backward and downward if the thorax is fixed; both of these actions work to flatten the lumbar curve. If, instead, both the pelvis and the thorax are fixed, then the action of the external abdominal obliques is to compress the abdominal contents so as to produce an energetic expulsion, as during vigorous exhalation, defecation, childbirth, vomiting, or coughing. The end of the gastrointestinal tract at which the expulsive action will be experienced depends on whether the larynx is open or closed at the time of contraction. When the contraction of the external abdominal obliques is unilateral, then the action is to flex the body to that side but rotate it to face the other side, much as the psoas does in *parivrtta janu sirsasana*.

The external abdominal obliques on one side of the body are aligned with the internal abdominal obliques on the other side. The internal abdominal obliques are smaller, thinner, and weaker than the external abdominal obliques, and its fibers are oriented 90° to those of the external obliques, with the origin in the posterior pelvis and insertion on the ribs, the anterior pelvis, and on the linea alba. Their fibers are interwoven with those of the rectus abdominis.

When the abdominal obliques are contracted, they are pulled into a hyperboloid surface that is hollowed and waisted, with the top and bottom drawn away from one another (figure 8.B-4b). If the contraction is forceful and unilateral, then the effect of the abdominal obliques is to twist the body accordingly. In this, the external abdominal oblique on one side contracts to turn the body to face that side, whereas the internal abdominal oblique on the opposite side also contracts to reinforce the initial rotation. In this way, the external abdominal obliques on one side and the internal abdominal obliques on the opposite side work synergistically to turn the body in the same direction around the spinal column (see also Subsection 8.B, page 294). This twisting action of the abdominal obliques is supported as well by intervertebral muscles, such as the rotatores and transversospinalis (figure 8.A-4c).

Transversus Abdominis

Of the five abdominal muscle groups, the transversus abdominis is the deepest. When standing erect, the muscle fibers of the transversus abdominis layer run horizontally, and contraction of the muscle compresses the abdomen onto the spine; it is probably active in *ashwini mudra* and during forced exhalation.

Quadratus Lumborum

Oriented parallel to the erector spinae muscles, the quadratus lumborum is a posterior version of the anterior rectus abdominis, with origin on the posterior iliac crest and insertion on T12 and the transverse processes of L1–L4. When contracted unilaterally, quadratus lumborum tilts the pelvis to that side, and when contracted bilaterally, it elevates the posterior rim of the pelvis while assisting lumbar extension [61a].

The Function of Hemoglobin

Oxyhemoglobin

With each inspiration, the oxygen that we breathe into our lungs dissolves in the blood flowing through them. Eventually, this oxygen is brought to the mitochondria within the body's cells and is used to oxidize the body's fuels (carbohydrates, sugars, fats, etc.) in a chemical chain reaction that leads to the eventual formation of adenosine triphosphate (ATP). It is this high-energy molecule that drives the body's energy-demanding processes (see Subsection 11.A, page 391). A key material in this chemical chain leading from inspired air to ATP is oxyhemoglobin, an iron-containing protein found in the red blood cells.

Oxygen inhaled into the alveolar depths of the lungs crosses the thin (0.6 μ) layers of cells separating the alveolar and capillary tissues and tends then to dissolve in the blood. Were the blood free of hemoglobin, the dissolved oxygen would rise to the level of 0.3 percent within the plasma; however, with a normal amount of hemoglobin in place, the value rises to over 20 percent as the hemoglobin and oxygen react to form oxyhemoglobin.

This increase of almost a factor of seventy in the oxygen-carrying capacity of the blood is directly related to the molecular structure of the hemoglobin molecule within the red blood cells.

The situation for carbon dioxide is rather different from that of oxygen, in that carbon dioxide is very soluble in water without the aid of hemoglobin; when dissolved in water, carbon dioxide first forms carbonic acid (H_2CO_3), which then dissociates to form H^+ cations and bicarbonate anions (HCO_3^-). It is also known that increasing levels of carbon dioxide and of H^+ in the blood lower the ability of the hemoglobin to bind oxygen and vice versa. This is especially important in the capillaries of working muscles and the inner muscle layer of the heart, where hard work is done and there is a high demand for both the presence of oxygen and the removal of carbon dioxide. If all of the carbon dioxide formed by the muscles were to simply dissolve in the blood plasma (via the reaction $CO_2 + H_2O \rightarrow H^+ + HCO_3^-$), the pH would drop to a fatal level of acidity; the binding of the carbon dioxide to hemoglobin keeps the acidity within a more reasonable, safe range. Circulating hemoglobin also carries the molecule nitric oxide (NO) to the medulla oblongata, where it is desorbed. If the oxygen level is low, then the released nitric oxide stimulates sensors in the medulla, which increase the breathing rate and the depth of the breath [450].

Within the hemoglobin molecule, there are four molecular subunits, and each subunit contains a nonprotein heme group having a central divalent iron ion capable of binding oxygen. Each of the heme groups, in turn, is surrounded by a polypeptide web. The arterial blood issuing from the aorta has oxygen bound to 97 percent of the iron at the heme sites; whereas in the oxygen-depleted blood in the pulmonary vein, many of these sites (75 percent in the course of intense physical exercise) have been stripped of their oxygen, and the hemoglobin molecules carry a derivative of carbon dioxide instead.

Oxygen Binding

Studies of the chemistry of hemoglobin show that the strength of the attraction of a heme site for oxygen—and conversely, how easily such a site will give up its oxygen when it is needed—depends upon how many sites in the hemoglobin molecule are occupied. The binding and unbinding of oxygen to hemoglobin is a cooperative process and works best when there are four heme units participating in the binding, since in this case the binding is substantial, yet not so firm that there is any difficulty in removing the oxygen when needed.

Red blood cells containing hemoglobin are manufactured largely within the marrow of the bones (Subsection 14.B, page 558); however, some are produced by the liver and spleen. The bones of the sternum are cancellous and contain red marrow, and so they are part of the red blood cell factory of the adult body.

Yogasana students with iron deficiencies will have low red blood cell counts and consequently will quickly become breathless in their practice due to the low level of oxygen in the blood. Similarly, the carbon monoxide (CO) in cigarette smoke combines strongly with the heme sites in hemoglobin, and so blocks them from carrying oxygen. It requires eight hours for the carbon monoxide from one cigarette to clear the bloodstream.

Section 15.B: The Three Breathing Modes

There are four main muscle groups involved in drawing a breath: the abdominal muscles, the diaphragm, the muscles of the neck, and the intercostal muscles. Though there are many, many ways of breathing, it is logical to divide the breathing types on the basis of which of the four muscle groups is most strongly involved in the breath. This is the approach taken here, based on the earlier work of others [166, 236, 576]. The mechanics behind these modes of breathing are given in the following Section (page 613).

Note that the intimate connection between the breathing pattern and the patterns of sympathetic-parasympathetic switching of the auto-

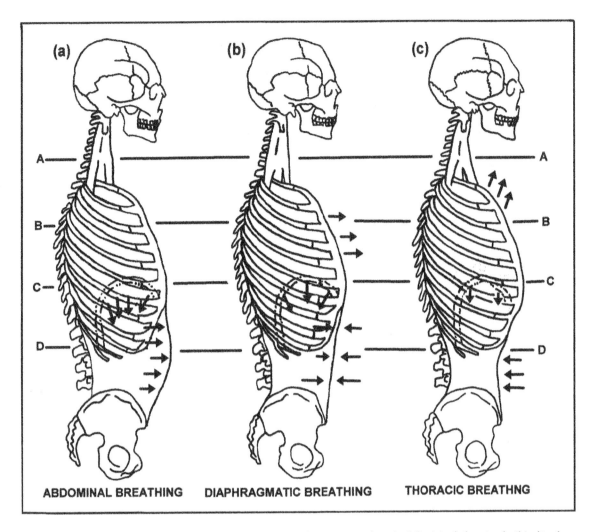

Figure 15.B-1. The three modes of inhalation, according to Coulter [166]: (a) abdominal, (b) diaphragmatic, and (c) thoracic.

nomic dominance suggest that any idiosyncrasy in the breathing pattern will have repercussions on the nervous system and vice versa.

Abdominal Breathing

The movements appropriate to abdominal breathing are shown in figure 15.B-1a; in this case, as the diaphragm descends, there is little or no resistance from the abdomen, which simply pushes forward in response to the downward diaphragmatic pressure. There is little or no involvement of the rib cage in abdominal breathing, and though it strongly involves motion of the abdomen, the abdominal muscles remain relaxed throughout the breath when "belly breath-

ing," with the diaphragm driving both phases of the action. Being the breath of minimal muscular involvement overall, the abdominal breath is a relaxing breath, appropriate to *savasana, viparita karani,* and other relaxing postures of that sort.

Abdominal breathing directly influences the visceral organs lying below. That is to say, on inspiration, the visceral organs below the diaphragm are compressed as the diaphragm descends; conversely, on expiration, the diaphragm rises and so releases the pressure on the viscera. In this way, the breathing action massages the internal organs and promotes blood flow through them, and some say it acts to promote peristalsis [37, 576] (Subsection 19.A, page 711). It also has been proposed that the rhythmic rise and fall of the chest as the lungs fill and empty while breathing also acts to massage the heart and the right and left vagal nerves as they pass through the thorax, and so helps in some unspecified way to control the heart rate [626].

Diaphragmatic Breathing

In diaphragmatic breathing (figure 15.B-1**b**), the movement is again largely that of the diaphragm moving down on inhalation and up on exhalation. However, in this case, there also is a specific involvement of the abdominal muscle wall, which results in lifting and expansion of the lower rib cage on inhalation, because the taut abdominal muscles confine the incompressible viscera as the diaphragm descends. It is the involvement of the muscles of the abdomen and the external intercostals (which flare the lower ribs on inhalation) that distinguishes the diaphragmatic breath from the abdominal breath.

The effect of the diaphragmatic breath is a stimulation of the sympathetic system (a general activation and warming of the body's autonomic systems; see table 5.A-2), and the mental effect is that of clarity and attentiveness. This is clearly the appropriate breath for most of the *yogasanas* and has been recommended as the breathing mode to use when an asthma attack is about to begin [315], because the main characteristic of asthma is the abnormal contraction of the bronchi, leading to the narrowing and blockage of the airway. Through breath control, one often can achieve the same physiological effect (an opening of the airways) as when using bronchodilator medication. However, an intense *yogasana* practice also can precipitate an asthma attack if the air is cold and dry [315].

Thoracic Breathing

In this style of breathing, the action is opposite to that of diaphragmatic breathing; i.e., the upper ribs and upper chest expand maximally on inhalation, with a minimum of diaphragmatic involvement, and the abdominal wall is tightly held [166] (figure 15.B-1**c**). The effect of such a vig-

orous breathing style, also called chest breathing, is stimulation of the sympathetic nervous system and a general arousal of the body's autonomic functions (see table 5.A-2) [626]. Accordingly, the mental state associated with thoracic breathing is arousal and anxiety, as appropriate for an emergency situation; however, thoracic breathing can be a source of ongoing stress if allowed to continue once the emergency has passed. By continuous thoracic breathing, we establish a constant state of sympathetic arousal characterized by a high oxygen level, anxiety, lightheadedness, and hyperventilation [687].

Hyperventilation

If the diaphragm is tense, for whatever reason, as it is in thoracic breathing, then the inspiration is less than adequate to supply the normal demand for oxygen, and the body reciprocates by breathing more rapidly than normal: sixteen to twenty breaths per minute, versus six to eight in the case of diaphragmatic breathing. As a result, one experiences a sense of breathlessness during thoracic breathing, which is acted upon by breathing faster yet. This rapid breathing is called hyperventilation [120, 236, 626]; you are hyperventilating if your breathing rate is significantly above fourteen breaths per minute while resting.

Regardless of the manner in which we breathe, the demands of the body for oxygen are rather constant and will be met by regulation of the breathing rate; if the oxygenation is low per breath, then the breathing rate will be high in compensation. It is interesting that when breathing in the thoracic mode, the hyperventilation associated with this mode requires up to 50 percent more energy than is required for diaphragmatic breathing [626]. The energetic inefficiency of thoracic breathing is a consequence of the fact that when we are upright, gravity pulls the blood in the alveoli into the lower halves of the lungs; whereas in thoracic breathing, the inspired air is held in the upper two-thirds of the lung volume. In contrast, during diaphragmatic breathing, the newly inspired fresh air is sent more to the lower halves of the lungs for higher efficiency in gas exchange [626]; i.e., for a higher ventilation-to-per-fusion ratio.

When the parasympathetic nervous system is ascendant, we breathe abdominally, whereas when we are involved in a challenging *yogasana* practice, we often switch to sympathetically driven thoracic breathing in order to satisfy the demand for more oxygen. Normally, the rise in the body's level of energy is controlled by the demands of the exercise; however, if the sympathetic system is activated when there is no need for it, as when breathing in the thoracic mode while at rest, then the result again is hyperventilation and lighthead-edness.

The direct physiological consequence of hy-perventilation, as when performing thoracic breathing, is a drop in the level of carbon dioxide in the blood and a shift toward alkalinity, which in turn has many ramifications. When the carbon dioxide level is depressed, the arteries to the brain and to the muscles contract (producing headache and cold hands and feet), muscles imbibe too much calcium and become hyperactive (produc-ing muscle tension), the nervous system becomes far more excitable (producing rushed and inap-propriate responses and over-reaction to minor problems), and the hemoglobin is reluctant to exchange its oxygen with tissues (producing yet more breathlessness) [236]. All of the conse-quences of hyperventilation as listed above are opposite to those of the parasympathetic action of diaphragmatic breathing and so most likely have a general sympathetic excitation as their source.

It is also possible to breathe by expanding the chest and contracting the abdominal muscles si-multaneously. Termed "reverse breathing," this mode is pathological and has its cause in emo-tional responses to external events [687].

Factors Affecting the Breath

As infants and young children, we tend strongly to breathe abdominally, for the dia-phragm is the only muscle available for the task; whereas in adults, women tend to breathe more in the upper chest (and more rapidly) and men tend to breathe more in a mixed diaphragm and upper chest mode (and more slowly) [428]. Once we are aged, the accentuated curvature of the tho-racic spine, the ossification of the cartilage in the rib cage, and flabby abdominal muscles all work to make the inspiration more shallow and more abdominal/diaphragmatic, so that eventually we will be breathing again as children—unless we are able to keep the spine in alignment, the cartilage of the ribs supple, and the muscles of the abdo-men toned. Thus, we come to see another benefit of *yogasana* practice: the muscles of the body are conditioned so as to support healthier modes of breathing into old age.

When lying on one's back, the abdominal vis-cera press on the diaphragm and make inhalation difficult. Note, however, as stated above, that in the prone position, there is a more efficient mix-ing of air and blood in the lungs, which will act to slow the heart and respiration rates. Further, when lying on one's side, the lower lung becomes less efficient, and it may develop circulatory prob-lems. The problem of the viscera pressing upon the diaphragm should be yet more important when one becomes inverted, for in this case, one must lift the total weight of the viscera with each diaphragmatic contraction. It is reasonable to as-sume that while inverted, the breathing becomes more thoracic in character, at the expense of the diaphragmatic mode.

Section 15.C: Mechanics of the Breath

Using the Diaphragm, the Abdominal Muscles, and the Ribs

Inhalation

During a quiet inhalation, the diaphragm is pulled down by only 1.5 centimeters (about 0.5 inches), but with deeper breathing, this increases to 6–10 centimeters (two to four inches). Further, excursion of the diaphragm while breathing is de-pendent upon the posture in the following ways.

When lying supine in *savasana* and inhaling in the normal way, the dome of the diaphragm is at its closest to the throat and has its largest excursion toward the feet. In contrast, when standing in *tadasana,* because of gravity, the upper point of the dome is lower and the excursion smaller than when in *savasana.* When sitting in a collapsed position, the central tendon of the diaphragm is at its lowest point in the body, and the respiratory excursion is at its smallest. Motion of the diaphragm is most asymmetric when one lies on the side, for the diaphragm on the lower side of the body drops even lower than when one sits in a slouched posture, and has only a very small movement on inhalation; whereas on the upper side, the diaphragm is raised higher than it is when supine, and it shows large excursions [288].

Even when one takes a slow inhalation, there is nonetheless a significant pressure difference between the lungs and the atmospheric pressure outside the lungs, which continues to drive their expansion. This is due to the air-flow resistance in the medium-sized bronchioles, which only allows the pressure differential to relax slowly. As the inhalation is a muscular action, whereas the exhalation is more passive (in many senses of the word), it is not surprising that in those who do not practice breath control, the complete exhalation can require an almost 50 percent longer time than does inhalation [716]. When resting, exhalation of the inhaled air is a highly passive action, as one merely relaxes the breathing muscles and the lungs, then exhales 0.5 liters of air; in this, the diaphragm expands and rises, and the thoracic volume returns to the initial value.

Expanding the Rib Cage

Were the diaphragm the sole driving force of the inhalation, then the contraction of the diaphragm on inhalation would act to pull the lowest ribs in toward the center of the body. A moment's investigation will show the reader that in fact, it is just the opposite: on an inhalation, the diaphragm attached to the lowest ribs is pulled downward, but at the same time, these lowest ribs to which the diaphragm is attached are moved outward and upward rather than downward and

inward! This seemingly contrary action is shown schematically in figure 15.C-1a and comes about through the agency of the abdominal muscles and the external costal muscles, which bind each rib to its neighbors. In the course of an inhalation, the diaphragm initially is pulled downward but very quickly presses down upon the abdominal contents, which are incompressible if the abdominal muscles are toned. At the same time, contraction of the external intercostals is assisted by contraction of the pectoralis minor, and in doing so, they pull the ribs upward and outward in order to increase the thoracic volume, which otherwise is being expanded by the diaphragm; it is estimated that the external intercostals contribute 10 to 25 percent to the work necessary to inflate the lungs [432], the more so the deeper the breath taken.

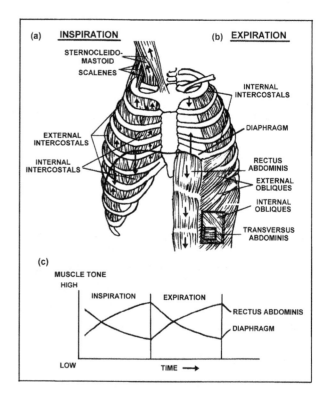

Figure 15.C-1. Motions of the ribs, sternum and thoracic muscles upon inspiration (a) and (b) expiration while breathing in the thoracic mode. Arrows indicate the directions of stress in the thorax during these breathing actions. (c) Variation of the muscle tones in the rectus abdominis and diaphragm muscles during the inspiration and expiration phases of the thoracic breath.

The external and internal intercostal muscles binding adjacent ribs together are oriented in a mutually perpendicular manner; contraction of the externals lifts the ribs upward and outward and contraction of the internals pulls the ribs downward and inward. During inhalation, the pressure of the diaphragm's dome on the viscera is quickly met by the resistance of the abdominal muscles (Section 11.F, page 468). From this point on in the inhalation, the lower ribs are lifted and pressed forward by the external intercostal muscles.

Lifting the Rib Cage

If one inhales deeply in the thoracic mode, there will be considerable diaphragmatic pressure on the viscera unless the rib cage is lifted up, away from the pelvis. This accommodation is accomplished by the scalenus medius and sternocleidomastoid muscles of the neck, which run from the back of the skull forward to the sternum and clavicle (figure 11.A-1). If one breathes in a shallow way, with hands at the throat, there is no muscle action to be felt there; however, if the breathing is deep and diaphragmatic, then as the upper lungs are filled, one can feel the contraction of the sternocleidomastoid muscles in the neck working to lift the sternum on inhalation, whereas the contraction of the scalenes in the neck lifts the upper ribs (T1 and T2). This lifting of the rib cage by the scalene and sternocleidomastoid muscles of the neck releases the tension of the diaphragm on the abdominal contents and so allows the diaphragm to be pulled further down, so that the inhalation becomes deeper. During inspiration, the external intercostals contract, lifting the ribs up and out, and the diaphragm contracts, pulling the central tendon down (figure 15.A-4a). This action, which so closely resembles the lifting of a bucket handle (figure 15.A-4d), involves considerable torsion of the sternocostal joints as the ribs lift. On the other hand, when the ribs relax on the exhalation, the energy stored by sternocostal torsion of the sternal cartilage is used to return the ribs to their original positions, regardless of whether one is standing erect or inverted. Working in this way, the breathing rate is about

fifteen to eighteen breaths per minute, exchanging about 0.5 liters of air per breath. Though the elasticity of the lung tissue drives the exhalation, in a more vigorous exhalation, as when blowing out a candle, the internal intercostals draw the ribs down and inward, and the walls of the abdomen contract so as to push the stomach and liver upward. Under these conditions, an adult male can flush his lungs with about four liters of air per breathing cycle, with 1.2 liters (the dead volume) remaining as residual (Box 15.D-1, page 625).

Exhalation

Exhalation of the breath is based on the lungs assuming their initial volume once the force that fills them is released. Experiments show that about one-third of the contractile force tending to collapse the lungs comes from the elasticity of the lung tissue, but that two-thirds comes from the special material with which the alveoli are bathed. Called a "surfactant," this fluid material acts to increase the surface tension of the alveolar tissue, thereby encouraging it to have the smallest possible surface area; i.e., to contract [432].

The primary expiratory muscles, when breathing deeply, are the internal intercostals; otherwise, exhalation is accomplished largely by the elastic recoil of the lungs and the chest. The energy of inspiration is stored in large part in the elasticity of the muscles and cartilage of the rib cage, so that on expiration, the elasticity of these materials restores the original thoracic position.

When we inhale, the brain moves forward, and when we exhale, the brain moves backward. When we hold our breath in the *yogasanas,* the brain is immobilized and its function is impaired [391]. In *savasana* especially, we allow the brain to relax and fall to the back of the skull. The breathing cycle also has an impact on the heart rate and blood pressure [122]. As the chest expands on an inhalation, blood pools in the lungs, and the blood pressure drops. In compensation for this, parasympathetic excitation along the vagus nerve dims, and the heart rate accelerates. As the chest is compressed on exhalation, blood is squeezed out of the lungs, the blood pressure rises (as does the parasympathetic signal from the vagus nerve to the heart), and the heart rate decelerates. This coupling of the heart rate to the breathing cycle has been studied extensively and yields several clues as to how to determine one's general state of health (Subsection 14.A, page 549, and Subsection 15.C, page 619).

Because we tend to exhale only partially before filling our lungs again when we are tense, an increased level of relaxation in *savasana* can be obtained by deliberately making the exhalation take twice as long as the inhalation [811], but without encouraging the development of any tension.

Given that the exhalation is the breath of relaxation and calm, we use the exhalation as a doorway to enter into each of the *yogasanas*. For example, starting on hands and knees, we exhale as we lift the body into *adho mukha svanasana*, and we lean into *trikonasana* on an exhalation. Though the *yogasanas* are to be entered on the exhalation, the chest should not be allowed to fall toward the pelvis in the process, even in forward bends.

Dead Air

Not all of the air inspired acts to oxygenate blood in the alveoli. Thirty percent of the inhaled air remains in the trachea and upper airway passages as "dead air" and does not make it into the alveoli for gas transfer during the breathing cycle. Assuming that the inspired and expired volumes are the same, the "minute volume" of gas moved is defined as the volume inspired through the nose in one breath (the tidal volume), corrected for the part that is nonfunctional in gas transfer (the dead volume), times the number of breaths taken in a minute. At ten breaths per minute, the minute volume would be $10 \times (1 - 0.3) \times 0.5$ liters = 3.5 liters. As discussed in Box 15.D-1, page 625, the unavoidable reduction in the effective volume of the breath due to the dead volume can be of tremendous importance to undersea divers, to the long-necked dinosaurs and giraffes, and perhaps to *yogasana* students as well, but not to birds.

To recapitulate, when breathing in a restful way, the central tendon of the diaphragm descends 1–2 centimeters (0.04–0.08 inches), and the external intercostal muscles weakly flair the lowest ribs up and to the sides. Exhalation is completely passive, with the diaphragm rising as it relaxes and the ribs falling in at the same time as the external intercostals release. If, however, the breathing is more forceful, then the central tendon of the diaphragm can descend by up to 10 centimeters (four inches) on inspiration, and the rib cage is lifted by the contractions of the external intercostals and the muscles in the neck. The exhalation during heavy breathing also can become a more active process as the antagonist muscles to the external intercostals, the internal intercostals, and the abdominal muscles, come into play, pulling the lowest ribs down and inward.

Though it is widely held that the external costal muscles work to lift the ribs on inspiration and the internal intercostals work to depress the ribs on expiration, this is not agreed to by all. However, if we accept as true that the primary inspiratory muscles are the diaphragm and the external intercostals, then it is then reasonable that the external intercostal muscles in fact are larger and stronger than the internal intercostal muscles.

Valsalva Maneuver

Note the important role the abdominal muscles play in the breathing process. The strength and rigidity of the abdominal muscles give strength and stability to the central tendon. When the central tendon is pulled down, it presses upon the viscera below it; however, the residual contraction of the abdominal muscles at this point supports the viscera, and so acts to stop the downward motion of the diaphragm. When the larynx is open, contraction of the abdominal muscles leads to respiratory exhalation; whereas when the larynx closes by being pulled up against the epiglottis (as when holding the breath) and the abdominal muscles are contracted, the result is urinary and/ or rectal evacuation. If the excretory sphincters too are closed during this pressurization, then the result is the Valsalva maneuver.

Put more simply, when one inhales deeply, then closes the glottis so that no air can escape, and then contracts the thoracic and abdominal muscles, one is performing a forced exhalation against a closed glottis: i.e., the Valsalva maneuver. In this maneuver, the pressure rises substantially in the thoraco-abdominal cavity, thereby transforming it into what is essentially a rigid beam parallel to the anterior spine. Valsalva pressurization is most often used when it is necessary to strain in order to induce a bowel movement, during fetal delivery, or when attempting to lift a heavy weight with the arms. When performing the Valsalva maneuver, the thorax is pumped with air, and so the effective stiffness of the spine is enhanced, much as a balloon is strengthened mechanically by being fully inflated. It is understandable that students might be tempted to employ the Valsalva maneuver in static positions such as *chaturanga dandasana* or in its straight-arm variation, but this holding of the breath is not yogic; it is especially unwelcome in forward-bending *yogasana* postures, where the spine should be in a more relaxed state rather than stiffened. However, it can be useful when lifting a heavy weight while leaning forward, for this maneuver is activated reflexively in support of the pressure that is directly impressed on the lumbar and sacral spine whenever we bend forward to lift a weight with the hands and arms.

When lifting a weight while leaning forward, the Valsalva maneuver reduces the loading on the T12–L1 disc by 50 percent and on the L5–S1 disc by 30 percent, while allowing the erector spinae muscles to relax by more than 50 percent [428]. Were it applied to a student in *sirsasana*, one would guess that the loading on the cervical vertebrae would be assumed in large part by the inflated thorax, and that it also could be used to prevent spinal collapse in *chaturanga dandasana* and *urdhva dhanurasana*.[3] However, though the Valsalva maneuver can be protective of the spinal column when stoop-lifting, such holding of the breath is very non-yogic and can only sustain one for a few tens of seconds at best.

The immediate effect of the Valsalva maneu-ver is to compress the inferior vena cava and there-by decrease the flow of venous blood to the heart and through the lungs. As the filling factor in the right atrium falls, the heart rate increases so as to make up the deficit. At the same time, the aortic pressure rises and then falls as the baroreceptors in the aortic walls respond to the rising aortic pressure. These competing factors lead to an oscillating heart rate having four distinct phases. The Valsalva pressurization is maintained for ten to thirty seconds, and at the start of the maneuver, the momentary systolic pressure in the aorta may exceed 300 millimeters Hg [224]. The cerebrospinal pressure is also elevated during the Valsalva maneuver, suggesting its utility in counteracting the effects of increased blood pressure in the head, as is also the case with *halasana* (Subsection 14.F, page 589).

The twenty-second heart-stopping demonstration of Swami Rama shown in figure 14.A-5b more than likely involves a strong element of Valsalva compression. There is no sign of Valsalva contraction in the practice of *antara kumbhaka* in *pranayama*, though both involve holding of the breath after inhalation [394]. See Section 14.C, page 565, for a further discussion of the danger of employing the Valsalva maneuver when lifting into certain *yogasana* postures.

Explosive Exhalation

Strong action from the diaphragm and abdominal muscles often is called for in acts of expulsion. Thus, when sneezing, coughing, laughing, crying, vomiting, defecating, and giving birth, one may call upon a momentary action of these muscles or invoke the Valsalva maneuver, in which the breath is held after a deep inhalation and the muscles are then used to push for expulsion (see above).

When one coughs or spits, it is the reflexive contraction of the abdominal and internal costal muscles that makes the action possible. Coughing is known to be a rather complex affair neurologically [819], being much more than a simple reflex. When chemical, mechanical, or immunological irritants stimulate receptors in the lungs, afferent signals are sent along types A_δ and C fibers to the

---

3   This would correspond to an internally supported backbend in distinction to the more conventional externally supported backbend discussed in Box 11.D-1, page 453. However, there would be little or no relaxation to be found in such internally supported positions.

brainstem, initiating a deep inhalation followed by a closing of the glottis (figure 15.A-1). When the glottis is rapidly opened, the air in the lungs is released at nearly the speed of sound, and the irritant is forcefully expelled. In the act of coughing, pressure is applied to the heart, and this can be life saving—if the heart stops beating due to a heart attack, consciousness can be preserved if one deliberately coughs strongly once every two seconds, as this can pump sufficient blood through the heart to keep the brain oxygenated for a short time.

It is usually assumed that in the act of vomiting, the stomach contracts and forces its load in the upward direction. In fact, during this act, the abdominal muscles and the diaphragm contract simultaneously and so put external pressure on the stomach to release its contents upward [574].

Should an allergen or a foreign particle of some sort become lodged in the nose, then a reflexive sneeze may be in order to rid the body of this irritant. Irritants in the nasal tract signal their presence to the medulla, which then acts to raise the volume of inspired air to 2–2.5 liters [716]. This is the "aaahhhh" of "aaahhhhchooo." With the lungs filled with air, the glottis closes, and as it does so, the diameter of the trachea collapses. In order to "chooo," the medulla instructs the abdominal muscles and the internal costals to contract so as to compress the air in the lungs, the glottis opens rapidly, and the compressed air is blown through the narrowed trachea at almost the speed of sound (Mach 0.85). During this nasal explosion, the eyes close, to avoid being sprayed with germs (it is said that it is impossible to sneeze with the eyes open), and the muscles of the middle ear contract, so as to lessen the impact of the loud noise on the auditory sensors (see Box 18.A-1, page 694).

Some reflex actions (Section 11.D, page 446) are strictly spinal and so remain active during sleep, whereas those that go as high as the brainstem are turned off during sleep. Sneezing is one of the latter reflexes, and so there is no reflexive sneezing during sleep. We don't sneeze or cough when asleep because much of the central nervous system at this time is inhibited, so that the

reflex arc is incomplete in spite of the stimulus. Strangely, there is a well-known photic sneeze reflex, in which brief exposure to intense light will trigger a sneeze [716], due to the close coupling of the pupilar-eye-dilation reflex and those of the nose. Nasal discomfort, as when one is sneezing with a stuffy, runny, or itchy nose follows the clock, being worst in the morning hours and least from noon to late evening. These hay fever symptoms occur in the early hours when the anti-inflammatory action of cortisol has yet to surge (Subsection 23.B, page 774), but when allergens in the air promote an overabundance of histamine that results in these symptoms.

Hiccups

The hiccup would seem to be a reflex action without a purpose, unlike sneezing, blinking, or coughing, all of which are protective in one way or another. It appears that the hiccup is due to a twitch of the diaphragm when the nerves that drive its contraction are irritated. Thus, when the filled stomach pushes against the diaphragm during an inhalation and the glottis closes momentarily, as when in *sarvangasana* and especially when in *karnapidasana*, the phrenic nerve can become irritated, and the result often is a case of hiccups [716]. With less frequency, the same result may be had when in *sirsasana I*. Irritation of the vagus nerve also can trigger a case of hiccups. Because hiccups are a strongly rhythmic phenomenon involving a central-pattern generator, anything that will break the rhythm can serve as a cure.

The Air We Breathe

When one is at rest, the volume of the inhalation amounts to about 0.5 liters, followed by an exhalation of the same volume. With practice of the control of the breath (Section 15.F, page 637), the volume of air inhaled with each breath can be increased from 0.5 to 6 liters [394]. As the lungs are pressed pneumatically against the rib cage but are separated from it by the well-lubricated pleural membranes (figure 15.A-2a), they are able to move against the ribs without friction.

Changes of Air Composition

It is most interesting to see how the composition of air in regard to its oxygen and carbon dioxide content changes as it is inhaled, circulated through the body, and then exhaled. Air at the moment of inspiration contains 21 percent oxygen and 0.04 percent carbon dioxide (400 parts per million). Once the air has been processed in the alveoli, these concentrations change to 15 percent oxygen and 5.60 percent carbon dioxide. Exhaled air has a composition of 16 percent oxygen and 3.6 percent carbon dioxide; this exhaled air differs from the alveolar air because it is mixed with the unprocessed air in the dead volume of the respiratory tree (Box 15.D-1, page 625). In regard to concentrations of oxygen and carbon dioxide in the body fluids, the concentrations in oxygenated blood are identical to that in alveolar air, but in deoxygenated blood, the figures are 6.1 percent oxygen and 6.9 percent carbon dioxide, while the concentrations in the cells of the body equal those in deoxygenated air. In all of these measurements of gas compositions, there is a constant concentration of nitrogen (79 percent), which generally is inert in the respiratory process. It is seen from these numbers that on exposing air to deoxygenated blood in the alveoli, there is a transfer of oxygen from the air to the blood and a transfer of carbon dioxide from the blood to the air.

When at rest, only about 25 percent of the available oxygen bound to oxyhemoglobin in the oxygenated blood is used by the muscle cells; however, during exercise, this figure increases substantially. Among the many physiological effects attending the vigorous use of the muscles are the rise in temperature of the muscle and the increased acidity of the fluids within the muscle due to the production of lactic acid and the reaction of carbon dioxide with water to form carbonic acid. These two effects of increasing temperature and acidity work to decrease the affinity of oxyhemoglobin for its bound oxygen, and so work to provide more oxygen for the working muscles.

At low exercise levels, the need for more oxygen is accommodated by breathing more deeply; i.e., an increased tidal volume at constant respiration rate. However, at higher levels of exertion, the tidal volume remains more or less fixed, and the extra oxygen then is supplied by raising the respiration rate. Thus one can attain a twenty-fold increase in minute volume (equal to effective tidal volume times the number of breaths per minute) from these two effects. At low levels of exertion, one has considerable latitude in how to dictate to the breath as regards tidal volume and respiration rate; but at higher levels, it becomes more difficult to dictate, as the breathing becomes more automatic and reflexive [827]. Obviously, the ability of the lungs to furnish the necessary oxygen to the working muscles is dependent on the amount of oxygen in the inhaled air. Thus it is that when practicing *yogasanas* at altitudes above 1,500 meters (4,500 feet), where the air is thinner, the hemoglobin in the blood is not fully saturated, and one is easily made breathless.

Cardiorespiratory Arrhythmia

Given that the inspirational breath is energizing and sympathetic, whereas the expirational breath is calming and parasympathetic, it is no surprise that the heart rate is higher during the former than during the latter. Going into somewhat more detail, as the lungs expand on an inspiration, there is a slight pooling of blood in the lungs and a consequent lack of blood entering the heart. In response to this, the parasympathetic excitation in the vagus nerves decreases and the heart rate therefore increases. On the other hand, on expiration, the excess blood is squeezed out of the lungs, the vagal tone increases, and the heart rate slows, as there is sufficient blood to fill the heart's left ventricle [122].

The difference in heart rate during the inspirational and expirational phases of the breathing cycle (figure 15.C-2) is called respiratory sinus arrhythmia, or RSA [119, 576]. Because a nonzero RSA implies a responsive autonomic nervous system, having a large RSA is a general sign of good health, whereas a low or zero RSA suggests many different health problems, including depression and cardiac conditions. A high RSA correlates with a generally high parasympathetic tone to the nervous system and is promoted by deep, slow, rhythmic breathing as per the abdominal and diaphragmatic modes (Section 15.B, page 610). If one emphasizes the exhalation in postures that are meant to be relaxing, then the RSA will lengthen the cardiac-inhibition phase of the breath [143]. In regard to the RSA, Gilmore [275] points out that it is not that the sympathetic excitation is increased on inhalation, but that the governing parasympathetic excitation decreases, and so the sympathetic effect can exert itself more strongly.

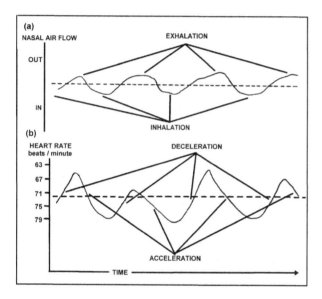

Figure 15.C-2. (a) The relative change of the air flow rates as one inhales and exhales and (b) the acceleration and deceleration of the heart rate as one inhales and exhales.

The results of highly detailed studies of the RSA phenomena, (compare figure 15.C-2**b** with figure 14.A-7) now under the name of "heart rate variability," are quite revealing in regard to the effects of deeply felt emotional states on the RSA and other body functions as well (Subsection 14.A, page 549).

Asthma and the Airways

Should the airways go into bronchospasm (swelling from the inside and constricting from the outside), the airflow is severely restricted, and an asthma attack is underway. During an asthma attack, there is periodic contraction of the bronchi and the bronchioles, making it difficult to inhale and especially difficult to exhale. Because the walls of the bronchioles are almost totally smooth muscle, with no cartilage to hold them open, a bronchospasm can completely cut off the air flow. In general, the bronchospasm is initiated either by a high sensitivity to allergens (such as pollen or cat dander) or by other situations such as breathing cigarette smoke or over-exercising. The excitability of the airways due to vagal stimulation (Subsection 5.D, page 180) can be reversed through a *yogasana* practice that emphasizes the *langhana* aspect of the breath [604], and in cases of mild asthma, *pranayama* also can be an effective cure [794], especially if it has the accent on left-nostril breathing so as to combat the sympathetic stimulation inherent in right-nostril breathing [511]. However, note too the recent report that concludes that "Iyengar yoga conferred no appreciable benefit in mild to moderate asthma" [732].

Hormonal Effects

Our ability to breathe easily depends upon the airways being kept open effortlessly, and this is the case normally when either awake or asleep. However, for those with asthma, the ability of the body to keep the airways open is severely compromised. During the day, the adrenal glands produce epinephrine and cortisol, the effect of the first being to keep the muscles surrounding the airways relaxed and the effect of the second being to reduce any swelling of the airways during the day. Both of these hormones are absent in the evening, and by 4:00 AM, the closing of the airways can be so extreme that one's life is threatened. Asthma attacks in women are often more severe during the menses, and it is thought that changing levels of estrogen and progesterone at that time serve as asthma triggers; progesterone is known to relax the muscles surrounding the airways, but its level in the body falls precipitously just before menstruation (Subsection 21.A, page 737).

The Senses of Smell and Taste

Odor and Emotion

Of all the human senses, the olfactory system is unique in that its sensations are delivered directly to the amygdala, the emotional center within the brain, and to the hippocampus, a memory center within the brain (Subsection 4.C, page 81). The sense of smell also is the only sense in which neural information travels from the limbic (emotional) part of the brain directly to the language areas of the frontal lobe of the cortex. Because the memory of past odors is strongly tied to emotional responses, Freud maintained that once we stood erect and lifted our noses away from the ground, our sense of smell began to degrade, leading to repression and mental illness.

Given the close connection between the nose, olfaction, and the emotions, it comes as no surprise that heavy smokers show significantly higher levels of emotional disturbance than otherwise might be expected [301]. For example, the rate of depression among smokers is double that among nonsmokers, the rate of panic disorder is three times that of nonsmokers, and the rate of generalized anxiety disorder is more than four times that of nonsmokers. It appears that the causative link here is that between breathing disorders and the emotions. On the other hand, some smokers claim that the deep inhalation and exhalation that they practice while smoking is relaxing for them in the same way that deep breathing in *pranayama* is relaxing for the *yogasana* student.

Receptors in the nose appear to be key elements in the attraction between the sexes vis-à-vis human pheromones; this is discussed in Subsection 21.A, page 739.

Receptors

Naked nerve endings of the trigeminal pain nerve (cranial nerve V) are found in the nasal mucous lining, and potent substances can activate them, in addition to those in the olfactory area of the nose. Though the largest number and most obvious of smell receptors are associated with the nose, a few olfactory protein receptors also are found in the brain, the skin, and, of all places, in sperm. It has been shown that when sperm are exposed to a fragrance akin to that of lilies of the valley, Ca^{2+} ion channels are opened in the sperm, their tails wag more rapidly, and they swim toward the source of the fragrance at twice the normal speed![4]

Olfactory Laterality

As the nostrils of the nose are left-right symmetric, one immediately wonders if the sensations of smell are reported to the cerebral hemispheres in a parallel or in a decussated way, as with vision, hearing, touch, etc. It is now known that odors that enter the right nostril are processed in a different way than are odors presented to the left nostril. The olfactory bulb in the left nostril is better at identifying a particular odor, whereas the odors are perceived as more pleasant if sensed by the olfactory bulb in the right nostril. However, the neurons carrying information from the olfactory bulbs to the frontal cortex, amygdala, and limbic cortex do not decussate. Consequently, odors entering the right nostril have a stronger emotional content, because they are sensed in the right cerebral hemisphere [367]. Left-handed people do significantly better at odor discrimination when breathing through the left nostril, and this is reversed in the right-handed. The odor thresholds are equal in the two nostrils [384].

It has been observed that when smelling an unfamiliar smell, the right nostril is superior and that it is the right hemisphere that is dominant in this discrimination; however, if the odor is a familiar one, then there is no asymmetry to the sensitivity [748]. See Section 13.C, page 524, for a brief discussion of how pleasant odors reduce the intensity of pain in women, but not men.

An effect of nasal laterality on the sense of smell itself has been demonstrated [807], wherein it has been shown that odorant perception is dependent upon the rate of nasal air flow and so

---

4   Among the French, the fragrance of lilies of the valley is held to evoke feelings of affection, love, and romance.

Table 15.C-1: Association of the Odor of the Breath to States of Illness

Odor	Illness
Sour	Gingivitis, sinus, chest or tonsil infection, lung disease
Ketonic (nail-polish remover)	Diabetes, anorexia
Fruity, sweet	Oral thrush
Metallic	Ulcers
Ammonia or fishy	Kidney disease
Musty	Severe liver disease

is demonstrably different in the partially blocked and open nostril.

Odor of the Breath

In working with *yogasana* students, teachers have the opportunity to monitor and direct not only the mechanics of the students' breath but to monitor the odor as well. This can be important, because the odor of the breath often can be diagnostic for certain aspects of ill health, as outlined in table 15.C-1. In the absence of burping, breath odors do not originate in the digestive tract, because the throat is normally closed to the stomach; in fact, they are due to noxious substances diffusing into the air within the lungs. Our own bad breath (halitosis) is in part due to a decreased level of salivation; however, breathing through the nose rather than through the mouth helps to keep the mouth well washed by saliva.

Taste/Smell Interaction

In the long history of evolution, the sense of taste is thought to have been among the first developed. Consequently, the gustatory nucleus appears at a site that is far down in the medulla, consonant with its early origin [30]. The tongue itself is capable of tasting only bitter, sweet, salt, sour, and umami (savory); whereas the wonderful tastes of exotic foods come from the combined sensations of the foods' tastes and their smells. When we taste our food, the food odor is exhaled into the nasal tract, and it is the smell of the exhalation that is a measure of our taste pleasure in eating. When the nose is congested with a cold or is simply held closed with the fingers, then food tastes bland at best, as the odor component of the

taste is missing. In general, as we age, the sensitivity of the nose to smells fails, and so the taste of our food becomes impaired.

Since the aromas of foods account for 75 percent of the food-flavor sensation, it is clear that taste in not solely in the mouth. A dry mouth loses its ability to taste food, and high blood pressure also can dull the taste sensation, as does Parkinson's disease. On the other hand, chewing gum promotes salivation and so enhances the flavor of food. Because spicy foods such as hot peppers contain substances that are vasodilators, there is a sensation of a global rush of heat whenever they are eaten. As described in Subsection 3.B, page 47, taste sensations also can be part of synesthesic neural-mode mixing.

Women are thought to use the sense of smell in deciding on the likeability of another person, with the amygdala playing a large role in such decisions. Of course, such reactions to smell are localized deeply within the limbic system and so are reflexive and totally subconscious. Nonetheless, they are subject to review by the conscious centers in the forebrain. See also Subsection 21.A, page 739, concerning the role of the sense of smell in synchronizing the menstrual periods of groups of women living together and of the role of human pheromones in sexual selection.

Section 15.D: *Yogasana* and the Breath

A study comparing the autonomic excitation in a group of trained *yogasana* students versus that in a similar group of untrained students [287] showed that the respiration rate in the steady state of several elementary postures was approximately 50 percent lower in the trained group, while at the same time, the respiration volume was much larger in all postures. Clearly, *yogasana* training can lower the level of sympathetic excitation generated when practicing *yogasana,* as compared to the situation with beginners. On the other hand, Telles et al. [856a] report that "cyclic meditation," in which performance of the *yogasanas* was interspersed with short periods of *savasana,* yielded a deeper relaxation (as measured by oxygen consumption) than did *savasana* by itself when taken at the end of the *yogasana* practice.

It is known that on taking a deep breath, the eyes tend to look up and the cervical and lumbar curves tend to flatten, whereas when exhaling, the opposite tendencies prevail. Experiments show that beginners practicing *uttanasana* more closely approach the floor with their hands when they exhale and look downward as they go into the posture [7].

Spinal-Abdominal Interactions

As determined by electromyography, the abdominal muscles (figure 15.C-1**b**) are only slightly involved in either sitting or standing normally. When standing passively, only the lower parts of the internal abdominal obliques are active; however, in *tadasana,* they become more active and work to pull the linea alba onto the spine as the ribs are lifted and the rectus abdominis relax. Because the abdominals are antagonists to many of the muscles of the back, the abdominals are stretched in backbending but should not be contracted in flexion. All abdominal action is minimal in *savasana,* but if one lifts the head just slightly from the mat, the rectus and then the oblique muscles will contract strongly unless one consciously transfers the work to the psoas instead.

The abdominal muscles can be extremely powerful in driving the expiratory phase of the breath. Ordinarily, the slow relaxation of the inspiratory muscles limits the rate of expiration; however, if one is breathing deeply, so that the

ventilation rate is higher than forty liters per minute, then the intercostals and the abdominal muscles will activate and so play important roles in the expiration [288]. As shown in figure 15.C-1**c**, the muscle tones of the abdominals and the diaphragm are inversely synergistic in a sense, for on inspiration in thoracic breathing, the tone of the abdominals drops and that of the diaphragm increases; whereas in the expiratory phase, the tone of the abdominals increases, while that of the diaphragm decreases [288]. In a sense, the abdominals and the diaphragm may be considered as an agonist/antagonist muscle pair (Subsection 11.A, page 420) [37, 428].

Rationalizing the Effects of the Breath

Neurological

With the above exposition on how the lungs, ribs, diaphragm, and associated muscles work together in order to drive the breath, one can then rationalize the Ayurvedic description of the breath as being either *langhana* or *brmhana* (Subsection 15.A, page 599) in the following way. When breathing in the *langhana* mode, the muscle action on inhalation is largely abdominal, the breathing is shallow, and the effect is stimulating to the parasympathetic nervous system. The exhalation when in *langhana* is rather passive, relying on the elastic energy stored in the muscles and cartilage of the ribs and on alveolar surface tension to return the rib cage to its initial position. The characteristics of *langhana* (table 15.A-1) are most obvious when breathing in the abdominal mode.

In contrast, when breathing in the *brmhana* mode, the diaphragm is pulled down more forcefully, so as to be resisted by the muscle tone in the abdomen, and at the same time, the external intercostal muscles, the sternocleidomastoid, and the scalene muscles contract, so as to lift the ribs upward. This lift of the ribs acts to increase the three dimensions of the thorax, and this volume increase fills the lungs with inspired air. The effect of the muscular action on the nervous system is to stimulate the sympathetic nerves. In the case of *brmhana,* exhalation can be more active, with the contractions of the internal intercostal muscles and those of the abdomen driving the air from the lungs. The thoracic breath is *brmhana.*

Physiological

Physiologically, the effect of abdominal breathing is to drive the level of carbon dioxide in the blood upward, thereby making the body acidic [576]. In response to this mild hyperacidity, there is a decreasing cardiopulmonary stress as the heart rate and blood flow decrease, metabolic activity decreases, as do blood sugar and lactate levels, muscle tone, and skin conductivity. Further, this type of breath promotes oxygenation of the heart and brain, as it promotes blood flow to these areas, and it increases the ease with which hemoglobin can transfer oxygen from the blood to the tissues. In contrast to the above, thoracic breathing promotes the increase of the oxygen level, with physiological results just opposite to those quoted above for abdominal breathing [576].

Psychological

Several psychological effects are reported that also serve to distinguish *langhana* from *brmhana* breathing. Slow, even, deep abdominal breathing increases emotional stability, calmness, and self-confidence while reducing anxiety; whereas thoracic breathing results in the opposite effects [576]. It is also thought that the turbulence of the breath, as it passes through the nasal cavity, is more or less stimulating to sensors in the mucosal linings of the nose that connect to the sympathetic nervous system, and that the neural effects of this turbulence can have profound changes elsewhere in the body (see Subsections 15.E, page 629, and 22.A, page 761), providing one is breathing through the nose rather than the mouth. It is known that the EEG shows demonstrable changes when one switches between nasal and oral breathing (Section 4.H, page 149).

When breathing normally, women tend more toward the thoracic breath, and both men and women will accentuate the thoracic breath during deeper breathing [288]. The emotional profiles of heavy smokers versus those of nonsmokers are presented in Subsection 15.C, page 621, and center on smoke-induced breathing problems.

The Dead Volume

In breathing the way we do, it is unavoidable that in any particular inhalation, a certain part of the air so inhaled is actually stale air from the previous exhalation that was expelled from the lungs but nonetheless was still resident in the airways preceding the lungs. This volume of the airways lying above the lungs is known as the dead volume; its relevance is presented in Box 15.D-1, below.

The Effects of Exercise, Emotion, and Age on Respiration

Short-Term Work

The effects of both long term and short term exercise on the respiration are interesting. Consider first the short-term effects of exercise. The lungs do appreciable work in moving oxygen into the body and carbon dioxide out; when working the muscles at the maximum rate, 10 percent of the total energy is expended in the lungs. In general, systolic blood pressure increases with aerobic exercise, while the diastolic pressure remains constant. However, in isometric exercise such as that found in *yogasana,* both the systolic and diastolic pressures can show large increases.

It is a rising concentration of carbon dioxide that is sensed in the medulla oblongata, which then controls the ventilation of the lungs. If the level of carbon dioxide rises, then the medulla speeds up activation of the intercostals and the diaphragm, increasing the rate and depth of the breathing. Because this response is reflexive on holding the breath, it is impossible to suffocate oneself by consciously holding the breath. The smooth muscle in the walls of the bronchioles is also very sensitive to the level of carbon dioxide in the blood, so that if carbon dioxide concentrations start to rise, the bronchioles dilate so as

Box 15.D-1: Divers, Dinosaurs, Giraffes, and *Yogasana* Students Must Be Aware of the Dead Volume

Dead Volume Defined

In the normal breathing situation, of the 0.5 liters of air inhaled, less than 0.35 liters is truly fresh air, having come from outside the nostrils, with the remaining 0.15 liters being deoxygenated air left within the dead volume of the airways on the previous exhalation; this dead volume is measured from the bronchial bifurcation to the nostrils. Now imagine a diver in her diving suit at the bottom of the ocean, connected to the source of fresh air by a long hose. Ideally, movement of her lungs would be able to expel 0.5 liters of deoxygenated air and to inspire 0.35 liters of oxygenated air to replace it. However, once she is under water, the volume of the hose must then be added to the dead volume. If the dead volume of the system (trachea plus oral cavity plus hose) is larger than 0.5 liters, then the inhalation only succeeds in filling the lungs with the deoxygenated air left in the dead volume by the previous exhalation, and the diver soon suffocates!

Even in the best of situations, the first 0.15 liters of air inspired into the lungs following expiration is stale, useless air left in the airways by the previous expiration; if one is to inhale enough oxygen to survive, the amount of air inspired must be much larger than that of the dead volume. As this was not realized in the early days of diving, many deaths by suffocation occurred, even though the air line to the surface was not blocked. The problem today is solved by having the diver exhale directly into the water through a check valve in the diving helmet, thus reducing the effective dead volume of the apparatus.

In contrast to the sacs of lung tissue that humans must inflate and deflate with each breathing cycle and the inefficiency of the large dead volume inherent in such a structure, birds have an efficient straight-flow-through breathing system that has zero dead volume and never leaves them breathless or sweaty at the end of the day, regardless of how far they have flown!

Dinosaur Breath

The question of the dead volume and breathing also arises for the dinosaurs, some of whom had small heads mounted upon necks up to 12 meters (forty feet) long. It has been suggested that these animals would have suffocated due to the large dead volumes of their trachea if they had lungs such as ours, and that instead, they had unusually large and highly efficient lungs, closely resembling those of birds (to whom they are closely related). As is the case for birds that fly great distances without fatigue, the lungs of dinosaurs are thought not to have been closed subsystems (which must be pumped up and then collapsed in a rhythmic way), but instead to have used a steady stream of fresh air flowing continuously past a set of open-ended tubes, so that there was a continuous flushing of the exhaled air in the windpipe.

Giraffe Breath

Thanks to the long length of the giraffe's neck, the question of the dead volume is again of prime importance. In this case, the dead volume is approximately 8 liters; however, the disadvantage of such a huge dead volume is overcome by an even larger lung volume of 45 liters [61a]!

Emphysema

With nasal breathing, the air is warmed, humidified, and filtered, and almost all of the tidal volume is due to diaphragmatic movement. In deep breathing, for each one-centimeter (0.4-inch) increase of the circumference of the chest, the tidal volume increases by about 0.2 liters [288]. In students with emphysema, the dead volume within the lungs is enlarged and exhalation is a significant problem, and so breathing becomes difficult for them unless their air is supercharged with oxygen. Though a large, rounded barrel chest may be considered normal in heavy people, in those who live at high altitudes or in those who practice *yogasana* and *pranayama,* it also may be a sign of emphysema.

Dead Volume in *Yogasana*

Though no one has died from suffocation in the *yogasanas* (however, see [161]), a similar dead-volume principle applies. In a posture such as *ardha navasana,* the strong contraction of the abdominal muscles reduces the effective tidal volume of the lungs so that it approaches the dead volume of the respiratory system, about 0.15 liters, regardless of circumstances. Were the tidal volume and the dead volume equal, breathing would involve pushing the same air back and forth within the dead volume without it ever being refreshed by oxygenated air from the outside, and one would quickly tire. Similar results are expected in other postures in which the breath's tidal volume is strongly restricted by abdominal contraction, as in *ardha navasana;* by compression of the abdomen, as in postures where one lies belly-down on the floor (*dhanurasana,* for example); or by compression of the chest itself, as in *maricyasana III, virabhadrasana I, urdhva dhanurasana,* etc. In these cases, the tidal volume is diminished but the dead volume remains constant, leading to the situation in which the air being breathed has both a smaller volume and contains a lower percentage of oxygen than when breathing freely. Consequently, breathing in these postures will be rapid but shallow, and the duration of the posture will be shorter than normal. Because deep breathing can raise the tidal volume to as much as six liters, were the dead volume to remain constant at 0.15 liters, deep breathing could be very beneficial in overcoming the dead-volume penalty during *yogasana* practice. However, it appears that the dead volume increases as the tidal volume increases.

to increase the flow of air into and out of the lungs [450].

As the cardiac output (Q̇) increases with work, the arterial blood vessels dilate and so reduce the resistance to the flow of blood to the muscles.

Increased work leads to an increase in the production of lactic acid, and in response to this, the pH of the blood drops from 7.4 to 7.0. Again, all of these changes are those signaling momentary sympathetic excitation (table 5.A-2).

Long-Term Work

The heart rate increases in proportion to the short-term workload (intensity of exercise). With increasing load in standing postures, the stroke volume goes up to a certain point and then levels off, while the cardiac output ($\dot{Q}$ = stroke volume × heart rate) increases from about five liters per minute to about thirty liters per minute at maximum workload. As expected, the venous blood is much poorer in oxygen than is the arterial blood; during work, the concentration of oxygen in the arteries is three to four times larger than that in the veins. As the workload increases, so does $\dot{V}O_2$, up to $\dot{V}O_{2max}$. Following heavy work, there is a remaining oxygen debt. The amount of air breathed per minute is equal to the amount of air breathed in a single inhalation (the tidal volume) times the respiration rate. As the tidal volume is fixed, increased ventilation is due almost totally to an increased respiration rate.

Stroke Volume

When the student goes from lying to standing, the cardiac stroke volume decreases due to the less efficient filling of the right ventricle due to gravity, but the heart rate increases in order to maintain some constancy of $\dot{Q}$, the cardiac output. That is to say, when a *yogasana* is performed with the body in the horizontal plane, the stroke volume is larger and the heart rate smaller than when the same *yogasana* is performed with the body in the vertical plane, all other things being equal.

Respiratory Compliance

How easily the lungs and thoracic wall can be expanded and then collapsed is a measure of their compliance. High compliance results from the presence of elastic fibers in the tissues and from the presence of surfactant molecules on the alveoli, whereas the conditions that promote fibrous character, edema, or a deficiency of surfactant will lead to low compliance. As we age, there is a normal loss of elasticity in the elements of the breathing apparatus; i.e., there is a decrease in compliance, resulting in a decrease in the capacity of the lungs.

Along with this, there is a general decrease in the level of blood oxygenation and of ciliary action in the respiratory tract. Corresponding to this downturn of respiratory functions with increasing age, the elderly are more susceptible to various respiratory disorders [863]. One can only guess as to the positive effects a vigorous *yogasana* practice might have on this otherwise normal rollback of respiratory function in the aged.

Section 15.E: Nasal Laterality

Swara Yogis

For over a thousand years, the *Swara* yogis (*Swara* or *Svara* means "breath") have been aware of a naturally alternating left-right flow of the breath through the nostrils and the subtle psychological and physiological changes that this lateral oscillation promotes [579a]. The process, now called nasal laterality, involves breathing predominantly through one nostril for an extended time (an hour or more) and then slowly shifting to breathe predominantly through the other nostril. A second slow shift to the original nostril completes a "nasal cycle." This lateral oscillation of the breath between the two nostrils can occur without any deliberate effort, as if driven by an internal clock. In the past 100 years, Western science has reaffirmed the observations of the *Swara* yogis and quantitatively expanded on them [36, 38, 118, 123, 215, 258, 259, 373, 374, 579a, 687]. Most recently, Prashant Iyengar has reviewed elements of the original text *Shiva Svarodaya* by the sage Gorakhnath, in which the temporal development of the laterality of the breath is outlined in detail [410].

Connections between nasal laterality, cerebral-hemispheric laterality, and the two branches of the autonomic nervous system are implied in the ancient accounts of the *Swara* yogis, who envisioned the *ida* and *pingala nadis* as dual and opposite in both their respiratory and psychological effects (Section 5.G, page 201). Following

Mohan [579a], air flow through the left nostril is called *ida-swara* and correlates with a mental state that is female, *shakti,* and lunar, whereas air flow through the right nostril is called *pingala-swara* and correlates with a mental state that is male, *shiva,* and solar; the intermediate state, in which air flow is more or less balanced left-to-right is called *sushumna swara* and is characterized as being a state of destruction or affliction and unsuitable for worldly activities. In order to better understand the nasal-laterality phenomenon, we turn first to a discussion of the structure and function of the nose.

Internal Structure of the Nose

Anatomy

For our purposes, we can consider the nose to consist of two chambers side by side, separated by the nasal septum [687]. Two structures known as the "turbinates" or "conchae" (figure 15.A-1), hang down from the roof of the nasal cavity and work to exchange heat and moisture with the incoming and outgoing air. As described below (this page), the turbinates are key factors in directing the breath through either one nostril or the other; veins within the turbinates are served by the external jugular veins on the two sides of the neck.

The innermost tissues of the nose covering the septum and the turbinates exude a continuous layer of mucus, which acts to absorb all airborne particles that otherwise might prove deleterious if allowed into the alveoli of the lungs. This blanket of mucus is actually in motion, the mucus and its embedded particles being transported to the throat, eventually to be swallowed and digested by the acid in the stomach. The nose is innervated by both the sympathetic and parasympathetic branches of the autonomic nervous system (Chapter 5, page 192).

Erectile Tissue

Just below the mucus-secreting tissue covering the bony turbinates of the internal nose lays a much thicker layer of erectile tissue, innervated,

venous, and heavily vascularized [295]. This is erectile tissue that when stimulated, can become so engorged with blood that the nasal passage is totally blocked to the flow of air. Nasal laterality results when the erectile tissue on just one side of the nose is engorged, while that on the opposite side remains flaccid. Air flow is then redirected when the passive tissue expands while the active tissue of the other side shrinks. Interestingly, the nasal erectile tissue responsible for the laterality is closely related to the erectile tissue in the genitals and the nipples of the breasts; sexual stimulation of these latter areas readily causes nasal congestion and difficulty in breathing [36, 687]. This connection led Sigmund Freud to consider the sexual/nasal interplay, and techniques were later developed by him to successfully ease certain PMS symptoms by treating the nerves in the erectile tissue of the nose!

Observing Nasal Laterality

If one is not aware of the disparity of the flow of the breath passing through the two nostrils, it can be made more obvious by holding a small silvered mirror under the nose and noting the differences in the sizes and lifetimes of the two condensation spots on the mirror. Semi-quantitative measurements of the relative fractions of the breath passing through the nostrils can be determined by noting the relative times that the two spots require to evaporate entirely [813]. Sovik also describes a breathing technique called "*sushumna* breathing," which develops this breathing laterality.

Nasal versus Oral Breathing

Because the nose is designed to both filter dirt from inspired air and to warm and humidify it, whereas the mouth is designed instead for eating, we practice *yogasana* only while breathing through the nose, not the mouth. Moreover, there are nerve plexuses in the mucus lining of the nose that are connected to the sympathetic nervous system and which are stimulated when breathing through the nose, but not when breathing through the mouth [385]. Yet another reason for preferring nasal to oral breathing lies in the fact that the brain generates a large amount of heat in the process of metabolizing glucose, and this excess body heat is carried from the brain to the nose by the venous blood. Once the hot blood enters the nose, its heat burden is relieved by heat exchange with the cooler incoming air, but only if the breathing is nasal. Should the brain overheat, the risk of stroke becomes significant.

Relation between Nasal and Cerebral Hemispheric Lateralities

EEG Patterns

The study of nasal laterality has recently taken on a new meaning with the discovery that it is driven in synchronicity with the oscillating dominance of the cerebral hemispheres [259] (Section 4.D, page 105). Furthermore, it is known that each of the cerebral hemispheres is tied closely to one branch or the other of the autonomic nervous system, the left hemisphere being coupled to the sympathetic branch and the right hemisphere to the parasympathetic branch. Experiments show that proficiency at right-hemisphere verbal tasks (table 4.D-1) waxes and wanes within a period of ninety to 100 minutes, while the proficiency for left-hemisphere spatial tasks also oscillates with the same period but is 180° out of phase. That is to say, when the right hemisphere is most active, the left is quiescent, and vice versa. One may also include World Views I and II as given in table 1.A-2 in this group of related but oscillating lateralities.

The suspected connection between the oscillations of the nasal, hemispheric, and autonomic dominances (long ago intuited by the ancient yogis) is strongly supported by the work of Werntz [721], who studied nasal lateralization simultaneously with EEG patterns (Subsection 4.H, page 149). She found that when the left nostril was open, there was increased EEG activity in the right hemisphere, and when the open nostril was switched either naturally or deliberately from left to right, the EEG-active hemisphere switched from right to left. More recently, nasal laterality has been correlated with sweating of the palms

[579a, 852], intraocular pressure [31b], blood glucose levels [31a], and involuntary blink rate [31c], in each case the *ida-swara* breath indicating a smaller contribution of sympathetic activity within the autonomic nervous system and the *pingala-swara* breath indicating a larger contribution of sympathetic activity within the autonomic nervous system.

Werntz hypothesized that both the nasal and the hemispheric oscillations were driven by an oscillation of the relative activities of the sympathetic and parasympathetic branches of the autonomic nervous system (Section 5.E, page 192), via the hypothalamus. Presumably, increased blood flow through the erectile tissue of one nostril is to be associated with increased electrical activity in the contralateral hemisphere of the brain! This suggestion is supported by the observations listed in tables 5.A-2 and 15.E-1, where one sees that all of the effects of having the right nostril open and the left closed are consonant with left-hemisphere sympathetic excitation, whereas those having the left nostril open and the right closed are consonant with right-hemisphere parasympathetic excitation, provided one makes allowance for decussation.[5] However, tests with subjects who were untrained in yogic breathing did not show any such relationship [871b].

Ultradian Rhythms

The phenomena of nasal and cerebral laterality appear related to a number of other "ultradian" phenomena (Subsection 23.B, page 772), which are again under the control of the autonomic nervous system. Experimental work on these ultradian rhythms began in the 1950s, when it was observed that during sleep, there are periodic

---

5   The seemingly strange fact that sensations from, say, the left side of the body are projected onto the cortex of the right cerebral hemisphere is due to decussation, the process in which an ascending fiber enters the medulla oblongata on the left side but, by virtue of a lateral synapse to a secondary relay cell, exits on the right side and travels thence to midbrain, thalamus, and cortex on "the wrong side" [432]. Downward-going neural signals for the activation of skeletal muscles also decussate (figure 4.C-7).

changes of EEG patterns, heart and respiration rates, eye movement, and muscle tone, as well as similar changes for oral behavior, vigilance performance, fantasy content of daydreams, and REM activation during sleep [456].

The periods[6] of these ultradian cycles were found to be three to four hours, and it was hypothesized that the physiological oscillation expresses a phylogenetically old rest/activity cycle that is ever-present but now overlaid by other cycles of different periods. The connection was later made to lateralization of the cerebral hemispheres and an oscillating dominance of one hemisphere over the other.

The alternating effects of left-nostril and right-nostril breathing have been correlated with the two phases of the basic rest/activity cycle, during which left-nostril dominance correlates with the rest period of the basic cycle (parasympathetic dominance); right-nostril dominance correlates with the active phase of the cycle during which the sympathetic nervous system is dominant. Notice, however, that excitations within the sympathetic nervous system are not global in that the excitation of one sympathetic component does not necessarily imply excitation of all components. Thus, for example, as a consequence of right-nostril *pranayama* practice, the rate of oxygen consumption increases as appropriate for increasing sympathetic excitation, whereas the electrical resistance of the skin changes in a way that suggests a lessening of sympathetic activity [852]; this is discussed further in Subsection 5.C, page 174.

Moreover, though one can cite abundant evidence for the four-hour periodic shift of mental and physiologic states in the unperturbed body, higher brain centers may override this underlying rhythm. For example, though the right cerebral

hemisphere controls the facial expression showing emotion, higher centers of consciousness can repress this if the emotion is too strong or too embarrassing. In the calm of *yogasana* practice, the higher centers again may be significant factors in dictating which cerebral hemisphere and which nostril is active at the moment.

Periodicity of Nasal Laterality

Recent studies of nasal laterality show that nostril dominance switches every one to six hours, depending upon the individual; is more regular in the morning than at the end of the day; is often incomplete in some subjects, while being much more complete in others over the course of a day; and can be more complete on one side than the other. In some cases, there seems to be little constancy of the left-right pattern from one day to the next, but averaging the nasal openings, as measured at half-hour intervals over a month, clearly reveals the lateral oscillation and its period (figure 15.E-1). In contrast, the subject in figure 15.E-2 showed nasal lateralization that was constant with respect to the time of day, over a period of three days [215]. In both cases, the period of the oscillations was very nearly five hours.

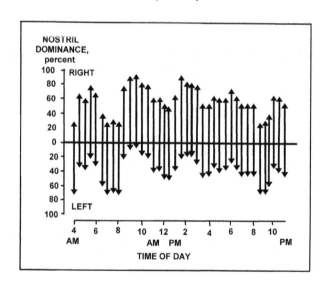

Figure 15.E-1. Oscillation of nostril dominance, as measured every half-hour during the waking hours, averaged over the course of one month, expressed as the percentage of each nostril that is active [258].

---

6   By "period" is meant the time to go from a maximum in the effect in question to the minimum and return to the maximum again. (Some authors define "period" as the time to go from the maximum to the minimum.) Regarding nasal laterality, Gorakhnath [410] has given the time to switch nostrils as "two and a half *ghatikas*." As one *ghatika* equals twenty-four minutes, the period for nasal laterality, as assessed by the ancients, is two hours.

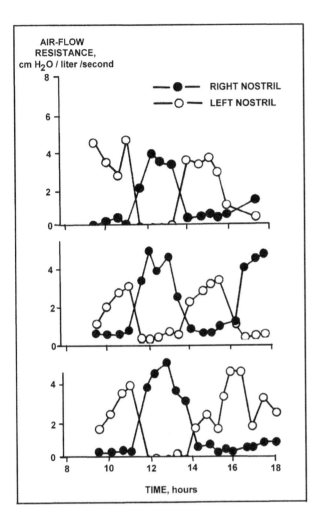

Figure. 15.E-2. Changes in the nasal conductance for air flow through the left nostril (-o-) and through the right nostril (-•-) of a subject for three consecutive days [215].

It is also noted that the nasal oscillation is most obvious in adolescents and fades with age, and it has also been reported in rabbits, rats, and pigs [259]. The periodicity of the nasal laterality is also reflected in the secretory activity of the nasal mucosa. As this is under the control of the parasympathetic nervous system, it is likely that the laterality and mucus production go hand in hand and are controlled by a central hypothalamic center [215].

Physiological Effects of Nasal Laterality

Comparison of tables 15.E-1 and 5.A-2 supports the conclusion that the symptoms attending the oscillating dominance of the nasal breath parallels the shifting dominance of the sympathetic and parasympathetic nervous systems (see Section 5.E, page 193) and the relation of these activities to cerebral location.

Yet other effects of nasal laterality have been mentioned without specifying a left-right correlate: pupil diameter, congestion of the blood vessels of the middle ear, body tone, and higher cortical functions (table 15.E-2). Assuming a one-to-one correspondence between sympathetic and parasympathetic activity on the one hand and right-nostril and left-nostril breathing on the other, one can guess that enlarged pupils, increased resting muscle tone and mental functioning, as sympathetic-system attributes, are promoted by right-nostril breathing, and that the middle ear becoming engorged is promoted by parasympathetic stimulation; i.e., breathing through the left nostril.

The Breath

In an extensive study of the physiological effects of right-nostril breathing when in *surya anuloma viloma pranayama,* Telles et al. [855] report that forty-five minutes of such practice acted to increase oxygen consumption by 17 percent, increase the systolic blood pressure by 9.4 millimeters Hg, decrease the digit pulse volume by 46 percent, and significantly decrease skin resistance. These changes are consistent with stimulation of the sympathetic branch of the autonomic nervous system when practicing *pranayama* exhalation through the right nostril.

The close connection between the dynamics of the breath and the regulation of body functions relates directly to *pranayama.* In fact, it is claimed that the practice of *nadi shodana pranayama* (alternate nostril breathing) not only heightens one's sensitivity to the flow of the breath (Section 15.F, page 637), but when practiced without sound or turbulence, it can promote a more regular rhythm to the normal left-right nasal laterality cycle, thus cleansing the *nadis* [394] and furthering overall good health.

Table 15.E-1: Effects of Nasal Laterality[a]

Left open/right closed	Right open/left closed	References
More quiet, receptive mood, introspective	Outwardly directed	[118, 258]
Passivity	Vigorous activity	[36, 258]
Promotes digestion of liquids (stomach)	Promotes eating and digestion of solids (intestine)	[36, 118, 258, 687]
Reduces body heat in core	Creates body heat in muscles	[118, 687]
Decreases blood pressure	Increases blood pressure	[38]
Induces depression	*Relieves depression*	[38]
Diffuse mental state	Improved mental analysis	[118]
Stronger right-hemisphere EEG activity (alpha waves)	Stronger left-hemisphere EEG activity (beta waves)	[721]
Parasympathetic activation	Sympathetic activation	[118, 721]
Imaginative pursuits	Intellectual pursuits	[373]
Intuitive, holistic thinking	Deductive, rational reasoning	[373]
Subjective decisions	Attention to detail	[373]
Playing music, singing	Hunting and fighting	[373]
Expend energy in a slow, sustained way	Expend energy in a rapid, vigorous way	[373]

a Entries in italics are not reported, but have been interpolated by the author.

Table 15.E-2: Nasal Laterality Effects, Nostril Unspecified

Effect On	Reference
Pupil diameter	[38, 721]
Congestion of blood vessels in middle ear	[38]
Body tone	[259]
Left to right shift on drinking coffee	[118]
Higher cortical functions	[721]

Pranayama

The effects of *pranayama* breathing on the heart rate are interesting. As expressed by the respiratory sinus arrhythmia (Subsection 15.C, page 619), it is known that the low-frequency region (0.05–0.15 hertz) of the heart-rate power spectrum represents the level of sympathetic ac-

tivity in heart action, whereas the higher-frequency region (0.15–0.50 hertz) represents the level of parasympathetic activity (Subsection 14.A, page 549). Studying the ratio of power in the low- and high-frequency regions, Raguraj et al. [680] conclude that when performing *kapalabhati pranayama*, a somewhat less strenuous form of *bhastrika* (see Section 15.F, page 637), the ratio is strongly unbalanced in the direction of sympathetic dominance, whereas following *nadi shodana pranayama,* there is no significant change in this ratio as compared with normal breathing.

Nadis and Chakras

It is amazing how closely the scientific description of the laterality of the breath follows the ancient description of the flow of *prana* through *ida* and *pingala nadis* to terminate at the left and right nostrils (left nostril = *ida* = *chandra*; right nostril = *pingala* = *surya*; see Section 5.G, page 201). If we complete the correspondence, then currents in the *ida* channel correspond to parasympathetic activation, whereas those in the *pingala* channel correspond to sympathetic activation. When the flow of *prana* is balanced through *ida* and *pingala* and is rapid, then *kundalini* rises through *sushumna,* and the mind ascends to higher meditative levels.

General Level of Good Health

Returning to the observations of the *Swara* yogis, prominent oscillation of the nasal cycle was taken by them as a sign of good health, whereas little or no oscillation on a long-term basis presaged illness. This is amply illustrated in figure 5.E-2, showing the strong shift of the responsiveness of the autonomic systems of three subjects, one agitated and anxious, one depressed, and one in mentally healthy balance. Only in the case of the subject who was well balanced is there a significant elasticity in the nasal-laterality response to shifting circumstances. A very compelling story of the negative effects of a frozen nasal laterality on general health and the relief brought about by a simple operation is presented by Johnsen [413]. Flexibility within the autonomic nervous system also is evident in the measurements of heart rate variability (Subsection 14.A, page 549).

A most unexpected consequence of nasal laterality is reported by Shannahoff Khalsa et al. [777], who found that unilateral breathing when deliberately closing off one nostril resulted in different concentrations of the catecholamines in the blood coursing through the two arms! This implies that if one is breathing through one nostril,

one of the adrenal medullas is stimulated more that the other, so that the blood on one side of the body is richer in the adrenal hormones expressed by that medulla.

Nasal muscle tone also shows a shift between the two nasal passages, with a period of one to four hours. This shift of nasal resistance from the left to the right nostril and back was assigned by Eccles as due to a "central rhythm" of nervous activity [216], which we now can interpret as the oscillation of cerebral hemispheric laterality.

Psychological and Emotional Effects of Nasal Laterality

Our interest in nasal laterality stems from the fact that there are distinct psychological and physiological consequences of breathing through either the left nostril or the right. As tabulated in table 15.E-1, breathing through the right nostril is energizing, making a person outwardly directed, somewhat aggressive, and prepared for vigorous physical activity, all the while sharpening mental acuity. In contrast, breathing through the left nostril leaves one more quiet, physically passive, introspective, and tending toward depression. Breathing through the open right nostril promotes digestion of solids while increasing body temperature and blood pressure, whereas breathing through the open left nostril promotes digestion of liquids and lowers the heat of the body. The wide range of physiological rhythms tied more or less strongly to the nasal laterality of the breath is presented in Subsection 23.B, page 774.

Balancing the Laterality

Even when the nasal cycle is in full swing, it is found that both nostrils are simultaneously open about 10 percent of the time [259]. This is the case during orgasm [842], *samadhi,* and sneezing. Though an active oscillation of nasal laterality is a sign of good health and is to be encouraged, more meditative states in yoga can be achieved when the breath is in the intermediate, balanced state [374, 688]. That is to say, one wants a balanced autonomic nervous system, free of any disturbing fluctuations or colorations, in order to achieve higher levels of consciousness. At those times when the left and right nostrils are equally open, it is recommended that one turn away from one's more mundane pursuits and focus instead on spiritual matters, self-study, and meditation [374]. The balanced autonomic state is evident in the heart-rate data of McCraty et al. [550], with balanced subjects being in a state of "internal coherence."

The level of nasal balance necessary to achieve higher levels of consciousness requires diaphragmatic breathing and occurs most naturally in the hours just before sunrise and just after sunset [374]. Note that these times are just those at which the parasympathetic dominance shifts to sympathetic (5:00 AM to 8:00 AM) and the sympathetic shifts to parasympathetic (6:00 PM to 7:00 PM); i.e., when the two states are more or less in balance (Subsection 23.B, page 771).

The Conscious Development and Shift of Nasal Laterality

Making precise and repeatable measurements on nasal laterality is problematic because the laterality seems to vary greatly from one person to the next and can be switched by relatively small events, either internal (thoughts, emotions, etc.) or external (thirst, movement, reading, etc.). On the other hand, this high sensitivity of the nasal dominance to external and internal events means that one can use one's willpower to direct the breath through a specific nostril, provided one is inwardly centered and free from otherwise competing external and internal perturbations. It is reported that deliberate switching of the breathing nostril through willpower can change the location and intensity of a headache or can change a sense of pain into warmth.

Willpower, Savasana, and Coffee

Swara *yogis* deliberately open that nostril appropriate for digestion before eating; when going to sleep, they first turn onto their left sides to warm the body (table 15.E-1) and then onto their right sides in order to relax into sleep. As explained by Ballentine, one can dictate which

nostril will be open by concentrating on which nostril should have the larger flow, or by thinking thoughts that promote either a sympathetic or a parasympathetic dominance, from which the desired nasal laterality follows [38a]. In line with this, getting up from *savasana* by turning onto the right side will leave the student in a more relaxed state than getting up from the left side. As expected for a stimulant, drinking coffee (table 15.E-2) promotes opening of the right nostril and a more active state of mind [118].

Axillary Pressure

It has been found [259, 687] that if you lie on your right side for five minutes or so, the right nostril will close and the left will open, the mechanism seemingly involving preferential swelling of the turbinate on the right side; the opposite is true if one lies on the left side. However, the effect is not one of gravity, as one might at first believe; rather, when the right axilla (armpit) is pressed, there is a reflex reaction closing the right nostril and opening the left. This is suggested by the fact that merely tilting the head does not induce nasal laterality, but walking with a crutch (*danda*) under one armpit does, as one so often sees holy men in India doing for the purpose of switching the nostril dominance [576]. That pressure on the fifth intercostal space leads to an increased sympathetic tone on the opposite side may be related to the effects of axillary pressure.

The Indian crutch-in-the-armpit phenomenon has been investigated by Western physiologists, with the following results. Fifteen minutes on a wooden crutch under one armpit leads to a contralateral decrease and an ipsolateral increase in air-flow resistance in the corresponding nostrils. This is due to reflex changes in the sympathetic tone of the nasal venous erectile tissue [184]. Experiments also were performed using a crutch held for five minutes in one armpit, followed by a thirty-minute rest and then five minutes in the other armpit. It was found that there was a large rise in nasal resistance to air flow on the side of the crutch and a drop in resistance on the other side. The pulse rate and diastolic pressure also rise with axillary pressure (the same on both sides), but the systolic pressure does not rise [895]. The dominance of nasal laterality and axillary sweat production are related, switching sides in concert with one another. In two subjects, the nasal resistance and the sweat rate were in synchronicity and in phase, whereas in five others, they were again in synchronicity but 180° out of phase. These results reflect the actions of the autonomic nervous system in regard to these processes [501].

There is a specific *yogasana* involving axillary pressure, *padadirasana,* that is most effective in switching nasal laterality [774]. In *padadirasana,* one begins by sitting in *vajrasana,* crossing the arms so as to place one of the hands in the opposite armpit, thumb resting on the armpit chest. When the right hand is so placed in the left armpit, then the right nostril will open, and the left will close after a few minutes. The opposite situation is achieved when the left hand is placed in the right armpit, the right hand resting on the thigh. One imagines that performing a posture such as *yogadandasana* in which the hand in the axil is replaced by a foot would have the same effect on nostril dominance, and if so, performance of *yogasanas* such as this on the left and right sides should result in rather different mental states. The use of *yogasana* to direct the laterality of the breath is discussed further in Subsection 4.D, page 106.

Forced Unilateral Breathing

It has been shown repeatedly that if one nostril is blocked with the thumb so that the nasal laterality is forced, the physiological asymmetries will develop if the breathing is continued for about thirty minutes. Under forced nasal laterality, the blood glucose level rises or falls, intraocular pressure falls or rises, eye-blink rate falls or rises, and heart rate decreases or increases, depending on whether it is the right or the left nostril, respectively, that is blocked [775]. Moreover, forced nostril breathing through the left nostril has been found to enhance the performance of spatial tasks (a specialty of the right cerebral hemisphere), whereas forced breathing through the right nostril enhances verbal tasks (a specialty of the left cerebral hemisphere) [412]. In a study of right-nostril forced unilateral breathing, Raghuraj and

Telles [682] report that this mode of breathing recruits more neurons on the right side of the brain and might be useful in treating certain psychiatric disorders involving hemispheric imbalance. The application of this breathing technique to the treatment of obsessive-compulsive disorder is discussed in Section 22.D, page 767.

Emotions

At the level of the emotions, forced breathing through the left nostril correlates with the production of negative emotions in the right cerebral hemisphere, whereas forced breathing through the right nostril correlates with the production of positive emotions in the left cerebral hemisphere [412]. It is but a logical extension of this work to suggest that a simple nose clip designed to close one nostril or the other could shift the autonomic dominance in various *yogasanas,* in support of or in opposition to their natural tendencies. (See Subsection 17.E, page 681, for a related approach to controlling autonomic dominance.)

Possible Mechanisms of Nasal Laterality

Though I can find no explanation for how differential axillary pressure results in differential swelling of the nasal turbinates, one can piece together a tentative explanation. We begin by following Eccles's suggestion that the nasal swelling is due to venous blood pooling, and Gray's comment [295] that the mucus membrane of the nose is thickest and most vascular over the turbinate bones. Note that the subclavian vein on each side of the body drains the blood from the upper body on its side; because it passes over the uppermost rib (T1) at a sharp angle, it is easily compressed and its flow throttled [308]. If the external axillary pressure acts to close off the subclavian blood flow, then the backup pressure of blood within the subclavian vein will tend to swell all parts of the body that otherwise drain into it. Now the part that will swell first and most easily will be the nasal turbinates, for they bring blood very close to the surface of the skin in order to promote the cooling of venous blood, as shown by the ease of nosebleed. This same mechanism may also account for the erection of breast tissue, for this tissue is always susceptible to swelling by circulating blood.

Note too that the flow of lymph in the upper body is strongly asymmetric [308]. Thus, essentially all of the lymph from the lower body flows up the thoracic duct and empties into the venous system, where the left subclavian and left internal jugular veins meet (just above the clavicle on the left side). Lymph draining from the left side of the head, the tissue lining the turbinates of the left nostril, the left arm, and the left chest also uses the thoracic duct just before it empties into the subclavian and internal jugular veins on the left side of the thorax. On the other hand, lymph from the right side of the head, the right nostril, the right arm, and the right side of the thorax enters the right subclavian and internal jugular veins on the right side. Thus, one can argue that axillary pressure on the right side impedes the flow of lymph to the right subclavian vein, so that the lymphatic pressure builds on that side and the turbinates swell in response. From this point of view, axillary pressure leads to the swelling of the nasal turbinates due to the blockage of the flow of both blood and lymph through the turbinates. Perhaps it is also relevant that Kennedy et al. found that the arm in which the catecholamines were higher was on the same side of the body as the nostril that had the higher air flow. That is, both are contralateral to the energized cerebral hemisphere [440].

As mentioned above, nasal laterality also can be induced by appropriate thinking, without any axial pressure being applied. In this case, consider the following. Different portions of the hypothalamus regulate the vascular tone in the two hemispheres of the brain (table 5.B-1) and so control the flow of blood preferentially into one cerebral hemisphere or the other. The dominant, blood-rich hemisphere then dictates to the contralateral side of the body, giving sympathetic (left-hemisphere dominant) or parasympathetic (right-hemisphere dominant) control to all physiological functions that are bilateral, including nasal congestion. Presumably, the initiating mechanism in this case is neural rather

than centered on mechanically restricted blood and lymph flows.

Nasal Laterality's Effects on Asymmetric *Yogasanas*

Given the firm connection of nasal laterality to the laterality of so many other physiological functions, it is likely that nasal laterality is a factor in the performance of lateral (asymmetric) *yogasanas,* and likely as well that they strongly influence one another. I can find only one paper in the literature on what I feel should be one of the more important aspects of intermediate-level *yogasana* practice: taking advantage of the mutual influence of lateral breathing and lateral bending in the *yogasana* postures in order to raise or lower the energy level of the body and mind.

In a highly thought-provoking paper, Sandra Anderson [11] gives detailed guidance as she takes the student through the series *tadasana, trikonasana* right and left, *tadasana, parsvakonasana* right and left, and *tadasana* with the emphasis on keeping the breath calm and stable and on thinking of the breath moving in a unilateral way. I strongly recommend this paper to any student or teacher who wants to connect their *yogasana* practice to the finer aspects of their breath so as to accentuate an aspect of sympathetic/parasympathetic balance. Note that the differences experienced when performing these *asanas* to the two sides will reflect both the nasal laterality at the moment and the inherent laterality/asymmetry of the body (Appendix III, page 845), regardless of nasal laterality.

The practice of nasal laterality while in the *yogasanas* should lead one to the state in which both nostrils are simultaneously open. In this state of nasal balance, the body's energy will flow up the *sushumna,* the mind's awareness will turn inward, and the posture will become meditative.

In addition to the paper of Anderson [11] on developing nasal laterality while in the *yogasana* postures, Sovik [809] gives instructions on how to develop nasal laterality when in a meditative sitting position. There is no strong reason to focus especially on nasal laterality as the key to unleashing other lateralities; it is just that it is the easiest portal through which to go when in search of the other manifestations of laterality in the body and mind.

Section 15.F: *Pranayama*

As several long discourses on the subject of *pranayama* are available to the reader [394, 404, 687] and it is only of tangential interest to our work on *yogasana* for beginning students, only a brief overview will be presented here. In this, we are largely following the discussion of Swami Rama and his coworkers [687, 688, 689, 809] and of B. K. S. Iyengar [394]. Our focus will be on how the practice of *pranayama* affects the autonomic nervous system and bodily functions.

Pranayama is important, because in the eight-step hierarchy of *Ashtanga* yoga, it is the lowest level to explore the direct conscious control of the autonomic nervous system (as viewed from the Western perspective) or (as viewed from the Eastern perspective) to control the fluctuations of the mind by cleansing the energy channels of the body and controlling the flow of the vital force through these energy channels. From either perspective, it is the control of the breath that eventually leads to the desired control of more subtle bodily functions. As such, *pranayama* consists of breathing exercises done with an inner awareness and done in ways that deliberately harness the breath to the autonomic system. Through practiced control of the breath (*pranayama*), one slowly brings all other aspects of the autonomic system under control. *Pranayama* practice demonstrably eases stress when performed correctly [624].

As concentration on the breath is so easily disturbed by external factors, it is important that the body be strong and free of discomfort for the long periods of time during which the breath is being refined. This level of inner strength and quietude is provided by the practice of the *yogasanas*. In what follows, we will briefly discuss a few of the *pranayama* practices that impact di-

rectly on our understanding of the autonomic nervous system.

All agree that there are three basic functions one can perform with the breath: (1) inhalation (*puraka*), (2) exhalation *(rechaka)*, and (3) holding the breath *(kumbhaka)* by closure of the epiglottis (figure 15.A-1) following either 1 or 2. These functions can be exercised rapidly or slowly, using one nostril or both. Simultaneous consideration of these factors in all their permutations and combinations leads to a vast array of possible breathing patterns, the totality of which is called *pranayama;* i.e., control of the life force. Those breathing patterns that stress exhalation over inhalation, with very little holding of the breath, are relaxing; whereas those for which the inhalation and exhalation are equally important, but with holding of the breath after the inhalation, are energizing [662].

In his detailed book on *pranayama* [394], Iyengar ignores the abdominal breath but states that one can breathe into either the lower rib cage, the middle rib cage, or the upper rib cage, and that the breath appropriate to *pranayama* practice involves all three of these. In this breath, the abdominal muscles are quite active, but they are not allowed to press forward on inhalation as they do in the abdominal breath of figure 15.B-1a. In the upper-rib-cage phase of the *pranayama* breath, the lifting of the ribs is aided by the contraction of many accessory muscles in the neck, shoulders, and back. In terms of the diagrams in figure 15.B-1, the Iyengar breath would be closest to the diaphragmatic breath, but with the involvement of the entire chest rather than just the lower few ribs.

There are several lateral-breathing protocols within *pranayama* that promote either *langhana* or *brmhana* in the Ayurvedic sense: in every case, one can rationalize the effect as either heating or cooling (sympathetic or parasympathetic excitation), based upon right-nostril inspiration being very heating, right-nostril expiration being somewhat heating, left-nostril inspiration being somewhat cooling, and left-nostril expiration being very cooling. Taken largely from references [576] and [394], several of these breathing techniques are described briefly below. In these exercises, the fingers are used to close a particular nostril, where appropriate.

Chandra Bhedana: In this technique, one inhales through the left nostril and exhales through the right nostril. This has a calming and cooling effect on the body and so is stimulating to the *langhana* side of our nature; i.e., it is stimulating to the parasympathetic nervous system. Apparently the left-side inhalation has a stronger effect than the right-side exhalation.

Surya Bhedana: This technique, in a sense, is the opposite of that given above, involving inhalation through the right nostril and exhalation through the left nostril. As expected, practice of this technique has a stimulating and energizing effect on the body, and so it is stimulating to the *brmhana* side of our nature; i.e., it is stimulating to the sympathetic nervous system in a way parallel to the practice of *surya namaskar*.

Nadi Shodana: Because this technique uses inhalation and exhalation through both of the nostrils alternately, it is a balanced breathing exercise. In this, one first exhales through the left nostril, inhales through the left nostril, then exhales through the right nostril and finally inhales through the right nostril to complete the cycle. Balance of the body's basic elements (*Vata, Pitta,* and *Kapha*), which is so necessary for good health, is achieved through this practice. *Pranayama* practices such as *viloma* or *nadi shodana* involve the cortical conscious dictating to the subconscious centers in the brainstem that otherwise would control the breathing pattern.

Bhastrika: In this breathing protocol, called the "bellows breath," the shallow breath is driven rapidly in and out by the forceful contraction of the external costal muscles and the forceful contraction of the abdominal muscles, respectively. This forceful action raises the breathing rate into the range of the heart rate (approximately 110 beats per minute), dramatically increases the need for oxygen, and proves to be generally stimulating to the sympathetic nervous system [289, 372]. The practice of *bhastrika* has been shown to decrease both the visual and auditory response times, indicating an improvement in central neu-

ral processing [61]. Hyperventilating, as in *bhastrika,* has the effect of training the body for hard work, so that with such a breathing practice, the sympathetic nervous system is activated and one does not get as tired from strenuous physical labor [25a]. The mechanics of *kapalabhati,* a *pranayama* closely related to *bhastrika* but with the accent on the exhalation [394], is discussed in Subsection 15.E, page 632.

Copeland [156] considers the possibility that the holding of the breath following inhalation (*kumbhaka*) in the course of *pranayama* practice acts to increase the level of carbon dioxide in the blood, which depresses cortical actions and so quiets the mind. Simultaneous with calming the mind, *pranayama* practice has been reported to increase handgrip strength following left, right, or alternate nostril breathing, though with the same increase on the left and right hands; whereas breath awareness and *mudra* practice had no effect on handgrip strength [679]. However, the increase following *pranayama* practice was less than that reported following *yogasana* practice.

Interestingly, the slowing of the respiratory physiology (oxygen consumption, respiratory rate, and volume) attendant to a session of *savasana* was smaller than that following a session in which the practice of various *yogasana* postures was alternated with brief periods of *savasana* [856a].

Hypertension

High levels of stress on the body and mind can result in a general activation of the sympathetic nervous system and a constriction of the arterioles of the vascular system. The smaller diameters of the arterioles then result in a higher, longer-lasting blood pressure. A breathing practice that works to re-establish a balance between sympathetic and parasympathetic stimulation can be effective in reducing this pressure (Section 14.D, page 575), even in beginning *yogasana* students who are otherwise not ready for a sophisticated *pranayama* practice [707]. The technique involves deliberately lowering the breathing rate from a normal fifteen to twenty breaths per minute to ten or fewer per minute, with an accent on switching the breathing mode from thoracic to abdominal and making the exhalation cycle last about six seconds and the inhalation about four seconds. Continue for ten to fifteen minutes in this way, repeating about three or four times a week. On average, after eight weeks, this *pranayama* practice has been shown to lower the systolic pressure by fourteen points and the diastolic by nine points. A deep-breathing program such as this also has the benefit of relieving the discomfort of hot flashes.

Interestingly, it has been shown that the psychological and physiological consequences of vocalizing yoga mantras and rosary prayers when one breathes at a rate of six breaths per minute are very similar, with both promoting a parasympathetic response [58, 511]. Taking this to the extreme, Shannahoff-Khalsa and coworkers [780] report on resetting the cardiopulmonary pacemaker in the brain stem by practicing a one-breath-per-minute *pranayama* in which each cycle consisted of a twenty-second inspiration, a twenty-second holding, and a twenty-second expiration. There appear to be interesting consequences of this technique in regard to preventing heart attacks [579, 780].

Illness and the Immune System   16

Section 16.A: Immunity

It is only relatively recently that scientists have promoted the immune system to the level of one of the body's major regulatory systems, a co-equal with the autonomic and endocrine systems [721]. The human immune system is a wonderfully complex mechanism whereby the body recognizes foreign proteins, microorganisms from viruses to fungi, and parasites, tumors, foreign tissues, and allergens; once having recognized them as foreign, it neutralizes them by killing them. The cells responsible for such actions, the white blood cells, are called leukocytes and are found in the blood, tissue, lymph, and lymphoid structures but are most often manufactured in the bone marrow.

Innate Immunity

In regard to immunity, there are two basic types: innate and acquired. The first of these offers a general nonspecific first line of defense against all foreign cells and toxins and is found, for example, in the antimicrobial action of both the skin and the bones (especially the mandible at the gum line, which is constantly exposed to pathogens in the mouth) and among the digestive enzymes of the stomach. The leukocytes that make up the innate system are cells of large size that function as phages, encountering foreign bodies, enveloping them, digesting them, and then displaying the protein coats of the invaders on their outer surfaces.

Acquired Immunity

The trophy display of the innate immune subsystem then summons a second immune subsystem into action (the acquired immune subsystem); though not as rapidly acting as the first line of defense, the second line has a memory of the particulars of each invader, derived originally from the protein coat of the phagocyte that first encountered it, becoming more potent in defense with each new exposure to the invader. In order to function properly, the acquired-immunity system must distinguish between cells of its own body (Self) and those of any foreign invader (non-Self) by sensing the molecular pattern of proteins on the surface of the cell in question. Because cells of each particular type of invader have a pattern that is characteristic of that invader (much like a fingerprint among humans) but different from that of cells that are of the body, the cell-mediated immune system is species-specific. As this is an acquired immunity, it grows with repetitive exposure to the pathogen; i.e., it is a weak defense on first meeting a particular pathogen but is much stronger should that pathogen be met again.

Foreign Cells

The importance of the recognition and vanquishing of cells with the "wrong" patterns of superficial proteins comes to the fore when one considers the very helpful cells of the foreign bacteria that inhabit the colon (Subsection 19.A, page 709). In regard to bacteria, the womb of the pregnant mother is a sterile place; however, once the infant has been delivered, the infant's gut flora begin to grow; however, secretions from its appendix work to blunt the effects of its immune system in regard to the invading bacteria. The appendix is a very necessary organ in the immune system of the infant but is of little or no use in the adult, except as a spare part available for tissue transplantation without rejection.

Other less-obvious systems are also at work in defense of the body against bacterial invasion. For example, there is a small protein called the endogenous pyrogen, the job of which is to pull iron out of the bloodstream and to deposit it in the liver so that it is not available to invading bacteria [68]. In addition, there are antibacterial enzymes in saliva, and proteins in the blood that kill bacteria in the bloodstream.

Inflammatory Response

Once a foreign invader is detected, an inflammatory response involving redness and swelling at the site of the infection is triggered by the innate immune system [378], followed by fever, body ache, pus, and other flu-like symptoms. This inflammation response of the innate immune system is indiscriminate in regard to the local destruction of foreign cells and cells of the Self, and it is useful only if it does not last beyond a few days. If inflammation persists beyond this time period, then the results are much more negative.

The difference between a useful but short-lived inflammation and a harmful persistent inflammation is that in the former case, neutrophils are brought into the injured area to deal with invaders. Following their attack on the invaders, these neutrophils will commit apoptosis and will then be eaten by resident macrophages. If, instead, the neutrophils die by necrosis and so spill their contents into the adjacent cellular fluid before they can die by apoptosis, the result is an ongoing inflammation, which can become a trigger for other diseases, such as cancers of the colon, liver, and lung. Also possible are autoimmune responses in which the attack is focused upon cells of the body in question, with the result being conditions such as rheumatoid arthritis, heart attacks, Alzheimer's

disease, lupus, multiple sclerosis, asthma, cancer, and allergies [378].

Interaction between the immune system and the nervous system is implicit in the fact that the neurotransmitter acetylcholine, when released by the vagus nerve, binds to macrophages in the gut and thereby prevents an inflammation of the gut normally triggered by the macrophages.

Section 16.B: The Leukocytes

There are three major types of white blood cells (leukocytes) that are found within the immune system: (1) the granulocytes, which engulf and digest pathogens, (2) the monocytes, which become macrophages within the tissues and eat pathogens, and (3) the lymphocytes, which release antibodies. Leukocyte types 2 and 3 also are found in the lymph nodes (Subsection 14.G, page 597). We are especially interested in the type 3 neutrophils and the type 2 monocytes, which are the active components in the innate defense system.

The type 3 neutrophils (45–75 percent of the white blood cell count) attack and destroy foreign cells in the blood, and the type 2 monocytes grow into huge single-cell macrophages capable of enveloping and destroying invaders and dead or dying cells of the host tissue within the body tissue. Because the neutrophils are in circulation, they are able to move to the site of an infection and fight it, so as to keep it from spreading throughout the body. Those leukocytes that die in the service of our bodies appear as pus at the site of the infection. In addition to the lymphocytes, the innate system uses the structural barrier of the skin and various chemical means to defend the body [529].

Among the various types of neutrophil, there is one, the polymorphonuclear neutrophil, that merits special attention, as it is the first to seek out a foreign body and attack it. When this neutrophil is on patrol, it passively rolls along the blood vessel walls, propelled by the current. Once it senses the telltale scent of an invading organism, the neutrophil puts out long legs made of actin (Subsection 11.A, page 382) that are able to pull it rapidly along the vessel wall; the legs also monitor the strength of the invader signal and so propel the neutrophil in its direction. It is the first of the neutrophils to encounter the invader and to engage it in battle [907]. However, there is a limit to the size of a foreign particle that can be excised by the neutrophils, and so, for example, the large dye particles injected into the skin to form a tattoo remain, unless laser irradiation is used to blow the particles into smaller, more digestible fragments.

Because the efficiency of the immune system in defending the body is so dependent upon the patterns of fluid circulation, the work inherent in doing the *yogasanas* has an immediately positive effect on the efficiency of the immune system, since it acts to dramatically increase circulation to all parts of the body.

Lymphocytes

The lymphocytes (15–45 percent of the white cell blood count and one of the five types of leukocytes), which are found largely in the lymph fluid, where they act to destroy invading bacteria, etc., are subclasses of the more general white blood cells so important to the defense of the body against foreign cells. Though the lymphocytes form the backbone of the acquired immune system, they are activated by the actions of the innate system and only then spring into action. There are two general classes of lymphocytes, the B lymphocytes and the T lymphocytes, as discussed below. When the lymphocytes first meet a foreign cell, the response is moderate, but on second and further repetitions of the exposure, the defensive response is far stronger.

The B Lymphocytes

The B lymphocytes (B for bone) are born in the bone marrow, circulate briefly in the blood, and come to collect in the lymph nodes of the body and the spleen [266, 432, 529, 721]. Each of the invading foreign cells is covered in a specific protein or polysaccharide coating that is termed the antigen, and it is by the chemical nature of the cell's antigen that it is recognized by the B cells as Self or non-Self. When a B cell meets a foreign antigen, it engulfs it, digests its protein, and then displays the digested fragments on its surface. Through interaction with the innate immune system via cytokines, each of the mature lymphocytes is thereby encoded to be responsive to a particular type of invading bacterium, fungus, parasite, cancer cell, etc. that may be circulating in the lymphatic fluid. When a B lymphocyte comes into contact with a foreign antigen, its response to it is to generate and release into circulation a particular antibody that is effective in killing the invader and others of its kind once it binds to the antigen. The antibody is a proteinaceous material called an immunoglobulin (Ig), of which there are five general types. Being a mixed blessing, the B lymphocytes not only attack foreign invaders but also are responsible for allergic reactions.

Memory Cells

Not all B cells act as described above. Certain of them, called memory cells, are content to simply record the invader's antigen surface data and then wait for a second invasion of cells bearing that particular antigen. Should that take place within one's lifetime, the memory cells are able to immediately release the relevant antibody in great quantities, thus making a second attack by the foreign cell even less effective. Thus, when we are vaccinated with dead cells of a foreign invader, the memory cells become charged, so that if we were to meet the live organism later on, our antibodies would be primed for maximum defense.

The T Lymphocytes

The T lymphocytes also battle foreign invaders [266, 432] and abnormal but nonforeign cells, such as those within the body that are responsible for tumors and cancer. Like the B cells, the T cells are first born in the bone marrow as stem cells but then migrate to the thymus gland (T for thymus), where they mature into one of three major types of T cell. Like the B cells, the T cells also are activated by the cytokines released by the innate immune system. The helper

T cells identify the intruder cell and signal the killer T cells to attack. In this case, the killer T cells directly bind to the foreign cells and inject toxins that kill the foreign cell. Once the attack of the killer T cells is finished, the suppressor T cells call a halt to the killer T cell activities. The circulating killer T cells are effective in attacking viruses, tumors, cancer cells, parasites, and bacteria [753], while the braking actions between helper and suppressor T cells keeps the immune system in homeostatic balance. The memory T and memory B cells circulate for years, always on the alert for a new invasion. A fourth T-cell type, called Treg, works within the thymus, killing those T cells that are otherwise too aggressive. If the Treg cells allow the super-aggressive T cells to circulate, then the door is open for autoimmune diseases such as multiple sclerosis, rheumatoid arthritis, and lupus.

Though the acquired immune system is relatively slow to come into play, requiring several days for full effectiveness, the B-cell and T-cell arms of the adaptive immune system and the innate immune system are closely coupled to one another and work together to eventually fight off attacks on the body. However, killer T cells also are the active cells responsible for the ravages of autoimmune diseases such as multiple sclerosis. As with the situation in the central nervous system (Section 4.C, page 95), in the immune system, it appears that the largest action is to inhibit the system to keep it from running wild; should this system lack proper inhibition, the results can be disastrous.

Cytokines

Among the great variety of T cells are those with the ability to support or suppress the immune reactions of other types of cells. These T cells are readily influenced by our state of mind [721] and so form the basis of a hypothalamic-immunity axis. Both B and T cells have superficial receptors to specific chemicals called cytokines or immunotransmitters, which allow such cells to turn one another on or off, and to otherwise communicate with one another so as to direct and

influence their behavior in regard to immunity. As such, the cytokines of the immune system are proteins that function like the neurotransmitters of the nervous system and the hormones of the endocrine system [721]. In fact, because the immune system is sensitive to input from the neural and hormonal systems and vice versa [753], it can vary its response with due consideration of factors such as exercise, diet, levels of stress, attitudes, and relationships with others. As an example of this interdependence, note that when a macrophage does battle with a virus, it signals hormonally to the brain to raise the body temperature, as a higher temperature increases the efficiency of the macrophage assault while decreasing the vitality of the virus [186]. Cells infected by a virus are tagged by the viral protein coat and then killed by the T cells before the virus can multiply and spread. As the adaptive immune system becomes more finely tuned and effective, invading bacteria may be met and vanquished so rapidly that symptoms of the invasion do not even appear and one has no sense of a battle having been waged and won on one's behalf.

When two cells of the immune system interact and trade information, they do so through a joint structure that looks very much like the neural synapse shown in figure 3.C-1. Specifically, the structures in both cases are held in an interactive configuration by adhesion proteins and allow communication only between cells that are in physical contact for a few minutes to an hour (Subsection 3.C, page 48). Held in this configuration, the two cells involved in the immune interaction then transfer cytokines across the synapse to waiting receptors. Typically, the two cells are a T cell and a foreign virus that is killed in the interaction of the two; the viral protein coat is then stored in the T cell for use should the cell later encounter further viruses with this protein signature. While in contact, cytokines pass from one cell to the other across the synapse, using an internal network of filaments called the cellular cytoskeletons (Subsection 12.B, page 492) in order to move these proteins within the immune cells [186]. Infections of healthy cells by viruses are thought to involve immune synapses of the sort described here between two cells of the immune system.

Cytokine Effects

Because the cytokines connect the immune system to the brain, a purely somatic medical condition can have an impact on the emotions and moods, as well as on other cognitive brain functions. Thus, when we are sick or stressed, certain cytokine levels are high and remain so, and this often leads to long-lasting depression. This is a recently recognized connection between spirit and body about which *yogasana* scientists have long known.

Strangely, when T cells are activated by the presence of a foreign body, they produce a cytokine that also activates the osteoclasts in the bones (Section 7.C, page 236). Once activated by this cytokine, the osteoclasts work to thin the bones, resulting eventually in osteoporosis; perhaps this takes place because the level of Ca^{2+} in the blood is too low, and so the bone storehouse of Ca^{2+} is called upon for a withdrawal.

Steroids such as cortisol tend to increase the amounts of cytokines in circulation in the body, and when these bind to cell surfaces, they diminish the ability of the cells to fight invading cells. This simple relationship between stress and cortisol and their repressive effect on the immune system is most important. Immunotransmitters such as ACTH (Section 5.E, page 183) allow the immune system to influence the body's other regulatory systems. For example, the inability to cope with stress leads the hypothalamus to promote release of ACTH from the pituitary gland, which in turn forces the adrenal glands to release corticosteroids such as cortisol, which inhibit the immune response. If the release of the corticosteroids is prolonged, the thymus gland, prominent in the armamentarium of the young-adult immune system, shrivels, and eventually the entire organism dies of an irreversible pathology. It also appears that endorphins suppress the immune system, implying that exercise taken to the limit where endorphins (and cortisol, for that matter) become prominent will not be supportive of the immune system.

The B cells and T cells work in tandem during an invasion of foreign cells, and the numbers of such immune cells are readily increased when one thinks positively about an immediate challenge, whereas negative thinking in the same context can reduce their numbers [721]. These changes are likely mediated by cytokines. If, however, the invading virus is HIV, then the helper T cells are killed by the virus, and the body is then laid open to infection by other opportunistic viruses or bacteria, which ultimately can prove fatal. The AIDS virus itself actually hides within the infected T cells and can be detected only indirectly, through the antibody that may be formed in response to its presence.

Section 16.C: The Autonomic Nervous System and Immunity

The autonomic nervous system plays an important role in the functioning of the immune response. In fact, three structures of the immune system, the thymus, the lymph nodes, and the spleen are all innervated by branches of the autonomic nervous system. Thus, when there is a sympathetic activation of the adrenal cortex so as to release cortisol (see above), the immune response is weakened, but at the same time, norepinephrine and epinephrine are released by the adrenal medulla, and these promote the formation of lymphocytes and so strengthen the immune system. Though the adrenal medulla also releases other mineralocorticoids that work to inhibit the suppressive action of the corticosteroids, it now appears that epinephrine and norepinephrine not only stimulate the release of lymphocytes but also promote the growth of disease-producing bacteria in culture [50]! Thus, there are several channels of both suppression and intensification of the immune system, modulated by autonomic factors and working simultaneously to keep the immune system in dynamic balance. Activation of the parasympathetic nervous system also releases acetylcholine, which strengthens the immune system. These hormonal paths are activated by exercise that drives $\dot{V}O_2$ to within 60 percent or more of $\dot{V}O_{2max}$. As appropriate for a physiological function with strong parasympathetic character, the immune system is strongest at about 2:00 AM (table 23.B-1), the time of parasympathetic dominance.

Bird Song

Among songbirds, it is found that the healthiest males immunologically have the largest spleens and the largest repertoire of songs and are the most successful at mating [23]. That the immune system of songbirds could have any relevance to the health of humans in the twenty-first century at first seems far-fetched. However, it recently has become very clear that we humans share a common immune system not just with songbirds but with species as far distant as plants, for it seems that an ancient immune system has been passed down to both plants and animals from a common ancestor [307]. Thus, for example, plants and animals use nearly identical systems to resist common pathogens. This clear link between the immune systems of such seemingly diverse species is less surprising when one reads of the large numbers of genes in bacteria, plants, worms, flies, mice, tree shrews, zebras, and chimpanzees that are found to be functioning in humans [127]. In all of these species, one finds the same set of cytokines at work [634].

Attitudes

Once the links between the autonomic system, the body's hormones, and the immune system are established, it is easy to see how attitudes can affect one's resistance to infection and disease. The more a body resides in the sympathetic mode, the more cortisol is in the blood and the stronger is the inhibition of the immune system. On the other hand, parasympathetic excitation, as when in *savasana,* etc., promotes a strengthening of the immune system [753]. Inasmuch as the autonomic balance is so very much dependent upon psychosocial interactions and events, it is no surprise that moods, attitudes, life's gains

and losses, etc., can have an eventual impact on the immune system and hence on one's health. Tingunait [861] discusses this depression of the immune system from the point of view of depression of the heart *chakra* (*anahata;* Subsection 5.G, page 203), saying that repressing the heart center works to dull the effectiveness of the lymphocytes residing not only in the thymus gland but also in bone marrow, the spleen, and the lymph nodes. See also table 16.E-1, below.

Section 16.D: Malfunctions of the Immune System

It appears that stress is a necessary but not sufficient ingredient in the recipes for many diseases. Thus, for example in peptic ulcer, it is known that there are three essential factors: a high level of pepsinogen in the digestive tract, a dependent personality, and a high level of stress. A person having any two of these will not have such an ulcer, but someone with all three is at very high risk for this condition. In general, the immune system collapses under stress (probably due to chronically high levels of cortisol), whether it is physical stress or mental stress, and this can generate illness when it is coupled to other problems. As another example, consider trench mouth, an infection of the mouth and gums often occurring in college students just before final exams. In this case, there is an ever-present colony of the relevant bacteria living in the mouth but under control of the immunoglobulin IgA in the saliva. At the time of final-exam stress, however, the level of IgA in the saliva drops markedly, and the infection then proceeds at a rapid pace. Similarly, the herpes virus is kept under control by T cells until stress lowers the effectiveness of the T cells, and a herpes episode soon follows.

The immune system can malfunction in three general ways: it can be underactive, it can be overactive, and it can be misdirected [721]. We consider four examples of well-known medical conditions that are now considered to be immune-related.

Cancer

Cancer cells are known to be present at all stages of the growth and development of the human body, but they normally do not grow into recognizable tumors, thanks to the quick and efficient responses of the B and T cells. Cancer as a disease becomes significant to an individual when the immune response is underactive and so does not control the wild proliferation of cancer cells [272].[1] Indeed, it is argued in the cancer community that our cells start shutting themselves down as we go into old age so that they can avoid turning cancerous in a body that is immunologically too weak to defend itself. In this sense, cancer is the price we pay for longevity, and shortevity is the price we pay for staying cancer-free; take your pick!

To date, many of the successful cancer therapies depend upon chemical or radiological poisoning of the tumor, with consequent suppression of the immune system; however, there is increasing evidence that learning how to cope with stress (especially recognizing and dealing with one's emotions) can be an important component of this treatment. The best antidote to cancer is a mechanism called apoptosis, which kills cancerous cells as soon as they go bad (Subsection 16.F, page 653). Still, because cancer is really more than 200 diseases categorized under one name, there is not likely to be a single cure for "cancer."

Experiencing events that lead to the production of corticosteroids (Section 5.C, page 173)—and thence to conditions of anxiety, depression, and low ego strength —all act to further depress the immune system and so interfere with its abilities to fight cancer. Actually, it is not the experiencing of certain events in life that leads to negative consequences as much as it is not being able to cope with them; not everyone reacts negatively to events that may cause depression, etc., in others.

It is a general rule in the oncology field that the risk for cancer is higher the more rapidly a particular tissue divides and reproduces. Thus, the risk for cancer is much higher for bowel, breast, skin, and bone marrow than it is for neural, cardiac, and muscle tissues, which are largely nondividing. That there is little or no cancer of the heart is explained as being due to the fact that cardiac cells have small or zero reproduction rates, and so single-cell mutations do not grow into tumors, in contrast to the situations in breast tissue, the colon, and the skin.

Within a cancerous cell, the energy production is shifted away from the mitochondrion and becomes more global and more glycolytic/anaerobic due to the smothering by the adjacent cells. Production of lactic acid then works to separate adjacent cells and so spreads the cancer. The disruption of the normal mitochondrial functions by cancer deactivates the apoptosis that normally acts to kill infected cells, and so gives the cancer cell "immortality."

Competition for Nutrition

In the environment of the body, the cancer cells compete with normal cells for available nutrition and available space. As the cancer cells multiply and the tumor grows, they overpower the normal cells in their competition for nutrition and eventually drive the normal cells to death through malnutrition. The cancer also expands spatially and so exerts pressure on adjacent tissue, either smothering it or closing off paths of fluid travel, thereby causing an increase of fluid pressure. Moreover, the cancer cells are not as sticky as normal cells, and so they have a tendency to

---

1   Practice of the *yogasanas* is prophylactic in the sense that not only can it cure an illness or condition, but if one does not have a particular illness or condition, then such practice will protect one from contracting that illness or condition. Iyengar [396] rationalizes this by noting that all health problems start with a minor phase of so little consequence that we do not notice it. Only later has it progressed to such a stage that it is noticeable by the person so afflicted. However, if we are innocently doing our practice day by day, then the *yogasanas* work on the nascent health problems without our knowing it, and we seem to stay healthy without having contracted the disease. In truth, we have met and conquered it, though not on the conscious level. According to Iyengar, this is how *yogasana* keeps us healthy [557a].

detach themselves and wander through the tissues of the body (metastasis), spreading their kind through the vascular system to receptive organs distant from the primary tumor [308]. Compared to healthy cells, cancer cells are known to be much more viscoelastic, deforming two to three times as much as normal cells when stressed mechanically, and then not returning to their original shape when the stress is relaxed, in contrast to the behavior of normal cells. This mechanical compliance of the cancer cell may aid in its migration into other organs of the body.

Metastasis

Metastasis of cancer cells from one location to the next is often via the lymphatic channels, and this transfer of cancerous cells can be encouraged by improper *yogasana* practice. Thus, students with active cancer cells should avoid stretching in the affected area so as not to bring increased circulation to that area of concern. The teacher and student should be aware of the direction of lymph flow in the area of concern, because this is a good indicator of the direction in which the cancer cells will move, lodging at a downstream site to begin their uncontrolled growth.

Angiogenesis

In order for an active cancer site to keep growing, it must have a dependable supply of nutrients. To this end, cancer cells form their own capillary network to supply oxygen and nutrients to the rapidly growing cancer cells. This angiogenesis, as it is known, sounds much like the formation of the capillary system encouraged by muscle stretching, but the connection, if any, is obscure.

Lung cancer is the most common cancer and the most common cause of cancer deaths in U.S. males; among women, more die of lung cancer than of breast cancer. Cancers originating in the lungs may be carried in the blood or lymph to other sites in the body; often it is the metastasis of the primary tumor that eventually leads to death. To the extent that *yogasana* practice encourages this type of circulation, students with an active cancer or a local infection must be protected from

unnecessary vascular circulation [450]. The application of *yogasana* practice to cancer patients and survivors is said to yield modest improvement in various body functions, from quality of sleep to cancer-related distress [84].

Menstrual Timing

For pre-menopausal women undergoing surgery or biopsy for possible cancerous growths, there is evidence that the outcome of such a procedure is strongly dependent upon the particular point in her menstrual cycle when the surgery is performed [803]. Similar concerns exist in regard to the best times for radiation therapy and the best time to undergo mammography.

Allergic Reactions and Autoimmunity

Asthma

In contrast to the underactive condition of the immune system, which can be a factor leading to cancer, an overactive or misdirected immune system can lead to asthma and allergies [15, 721]. In the case of allergies, innocuous proteins introduced into the body sensitize it, so that when introduced a second time, there is a meaningless and destructive mobilization of the acquired immune system, and one has an allergic reaction to an otherwise innocuous but foreign protein. Allergic reactions begin with the mast cells of the immune system releasing histamine when stimulated to do so by allergens. The histamine activates receptors in the walls of the blood vessels, causing them to become overly permeable to fluids, protein, and cells from the bloodstream, leaking these into the surrounding tissue. This leads to swelling, itching, and inflammation in the skin; nausea; a runny nose; and asthma (see Subsection 15.C, page 620).

Once again, the hypothalamus has been found to be a prominent player in either softening or exacerbating the effects of allergic reactions, as the sympathetic nervous system promotes the release of histamine, which heightens allergic reactions; whereas parasympathetic stimulation inhibits histamine release.

The basic idea behind the functioning of the immune system is the identification of cells that are a part of the Self and the identification of cells that are foreign. Once this identification is accomplished, the cell in question can be ignored or attacked, depending upon whether it is domestic or foreign. When this identification process breaks down so that the immune system attacks its own cells, then one has an autoimmune condition. This appears to be the case in rheumatoid arthritis (Subsection 7.D, page 249), where the joints of the body slowly become painful, stiff, and swollen in response to the attacks of B and T cells on the synovial cartilage of the joint capsules. Negative emotions are a factor in promoting rheumatoid arthritis through the hypothalamus-pituitary axis. It is possible that though the problem in rheumatoid arthritis would appear to be overly active T killer cells, it may come about instead because the T suppressor cells are underactive and so fail to keep the immune system in balance. Interestingly, as we age and the immune system becomes less effective in doing its job, the severity of autoimmune attacks lessens.

Evidence is accumulating that allergies experienced by older children and adults can be due to "too clean" an environment for small children, who have been denied the early exposure to bacterial and viral infections and whose immune systems as adults are unable to distinguish serious intruders from the incidental casual interloper [310]. Exposure of children to household pets appears to be an important factor in inhibiting later allergic sensitivity as the children become adults.

Interestingly, when the body is infested with parasitic worms, there is an increase of cells called Treg, which control immune response in general. As the number of Treg cells increases, the immune cells responsible for autoimmune diseases such as multiple sclerosis are blunted, so that those persons having such parasitic infections are more resistant to the effects of the immune-system overdrive otherwise aggravating the multiple sclerosis condition.

Chronic Fatigue Syndrome

Symptoms of chronic fatigue syndrome include extreme physical weakness, an inability to think logically, interrupted sleep, and headache, the symptoms being ongoing for years. There has been considerable disagreement as to the reality of the condition, with many medical people claiming that it is all "made up." However, recent studies show that the onset of chronic fatigue syndrome is probably driven by a viral infection of the white blood cells, with consequences in regard to immunity and the genetic expression of various proteins. These proteins play important roles in the function of the mitochondria, the energy sources within our bodies [380]. The point here is that when we must deal with a condition such as chronic fatigue syndrome, we are really dealing basically with a viral infection and its negative consequences on the mitochondrial machinery so important for the production of ATP (Subsection 11.A, page 391).

Fever and Bacterial Infection

Though the quest for cleanliness is laudable, it should be recognized that the human body normally contains and supports well over 100 trillion bacteria and that these, in large part, operate to our advantage. These bacteria help digest our food, are able to synthesize necessary vitamins, do battle with other virulent bacterial strains that threaten to overwhelm the body, and guide aspects of fetal development. Only the liver, gallbladder, brain, thymus, blood, and the lower lungs are free of bacterial colonization in a "clean" and healthy body. On the other hand, there are many secretions of the body, such as those on the skin, that work to keep bacterial populations under control, if not vanquished.

Core Temperature

When there is a superficial local injury to the skin, the body's response is inflammation; i.e., a local swelling and a local rise in temperature (Subsection 13.C, page 519). If, instead, the insult to the body is more global, as with an infection by a pathogenic organism, then the body's core temperature tends to rise. As the monocytes go into action, cytokines are produced, which trigger the release of prostaglandins in the brain. In response to this, the hypothalamus increases the metabolic rate, the core temperature rises yet further, and one has a fever.

By raising the core temperature, the replication rates of the invading bacteria and viruses are slowed, while at the same time, T-cell efficiency increases, as they work best at 38–40° C (100.4–104° F). The heart rate during a fever also increases, so that white blood cells circulate more rapidly through the body. Body temperatures in the range 44.4–45.5° C (112–114° F) are lethal due to the destruction of brain cells at this temperature; body temperatures below 21.2° C (70° F) also can be lethal. When feverish, the body also withdraws the circulating iron in the blood, so that it is not available to the pathogens for reproduction. When infected, the body's response is not only to heat up but also to feel tired and sleepy, with achy joints and a poor appetite, all of which tend to slow one down, thereby speeding recovery. The disabling of foreign invaders and tumors by artificially raising the temperature of the body has been used often in treating syphilis, Lyme disease, and certain cancerous conditions [642].

AIDS

Regarding AIDS, it is not that the immune system is a causative factor in the illness but that the immune system itself is under viral attack. In this case, the human immunodeficiency virus (HIV) infects the CD4 white blood cells (largely within the mucosal tissues of the gut) and disables them so that they are no longer effective in helping to combat other diseases that otherwise are normally overcome. Once the CD4 cells are under attack, they are instructed by the virus to produce more HIV, and having complied, they die; the body is unable to supply new CD4 cells as quickly as the HIV can destroy them. As the CD4 count drops, lymph glands swell, and should they become sufficiently incapacitated, an

AIDS patient becomes vulnerable to certain lung infections and skin cancers. AIDS most often is acquired through contact with infected blood and is not spread by ordinary social contact.

A restorative *yogasana* practice for students infected with AIDS can work to make them more comfortable in living with a condition of overwhelming fatigue [398]. Males infected with HIV also show a 25 percent increase in the stress hormone cortisol in response to the infection. Because HIV has a tendency to attack the basal ganglia (Subsection 4.C, page 83), *yogasana* practice may be very difficult for those so infected.

Because a fragment of the human immunodeficiency virus is adept at disabling T cells, infection with the virus means that certain autoimmune diseases that involve attack of the body by the T cells (such as diabetes, multiple sclerosis, and rheumatoid arthritis) actually can be eased by the infection.

The Brain's Immune System

Thanks to the blood-brain barrier (Subsection 14.B, page 560), the innate immune system of the brain is isolated from that of the rest of the body; it consists primarily of the microglial cells. Much as macrophages function in the rest of the body, the microglial cells of the brain detect faulty cells, kill them with toxins, and then engulf and destroy the remains. Should the microglial cells malfunction and attack healthy brain cells as well, the result is a gradual loss of brain function and a descent into mental illness [420].

Section 16.E: *Yogasana, Immunity, and Illness*

The field of exercise immunology is rapidly changing, with conflicting reports, unsubstantiated findings, and new ideas appearing with great frequency. Our work reports on a few of the more general points in this field, especially as they might relate to the *yogasana* student.

Fatigue

Fatigue, either due to intense manual labor or to intense physical training, has long been known to be a significant factor in the susceptibility to infectious disease [529]. Endurance athletes who train intensely are known to have an increased susceptibility to infectious illness, especially to upper respiratory tract infection. It is doubtful that *yogasana* students work at the level of intensity for this effect to manifest. In fact, there is considerable evidence that moderate exercise of the sort performed in *yogasana* practice infers a small but measurable increase of immunity over that of the inactive person, possibly because the *yogasana* practitioner is adept at optimizing circulation and replenishing the body's energy storehouse on a regular basis through efficient relaxation and through *pranayama*.

Moderate Exercise

The mechanism whereby moderate exercise, such as *yogasana* practice, can stimulate the immune system would appear to be as follows: during exercise, there is a sympathetic release of epinephrine, which promotes an increase in the numbers of circulating neutrophils and lymphocytes, followed by a delayed increase in circulating cortisol, which acts to promote yet higher levels of neutrophils but depresses the lymphocytes. Normal levels of the leukocytes return within twenty-four hours of exercise. The application of *yogasana* practice to the stimulation of the immune system involves many supported-backbend postures so as to open the chest [398]. Though it is often said that these actions serve to stimulate the thymus gland, it should be noted that in the adult, the thymus gland has degenerated to a yellow, fatty blob of questionable function in the health of the immune system (Subsection 6.B, page 216).

Extreme Exercise

According to Nieman [618], exercise done at the extreme level (runners who regularly run for two to three hours nonstop) has the effect of sharply reducing the immune function, for times lasting as long as seventy-two hours. Heavy training, day in and day out, appears linked to a depression of the neutrophil function (to meet bacteria at the site of infection and kill them), whereas more moderate training can increase the strength of the immune system. Thus, in contrast to the immunosuppression found in the dedicated runners mentioned above, those who are over forty years old and walk only forty to forty-five minutes per day cut the incidence of colds by 50 percent, thanks to an increased immune response to this moderate exercise. In regard to the immune system, it appears that moderate physical activity is better than no activity but that too much activity is worse than no activity!

Exercise Timing

The timing of exercise with respect to exposure to an infection is of great importance [529]. Experiments show that moderate exercise done before an intentionally initiated infection can infer resistance to the infection, whereas intense exercise done at the time of infection increases the chance of illness. For example, the severity of paralysis from polio correlates strongly with the exercise pattern of the patient at the time of the appearance of symptoms, with those who exercised moderately before infection showing only mild paralysis and those who exercised with high intensity during and after the symptoms suffering a much more severe paralysis.

Yogasana and Circulation

Yogasana is known to bolster the immune system, as it promotes the formation of both red and white blood cells [753, 755]. Perhaps the largest effect of *yogasana* on the immune system is the effect of such work on the circulation. It is clear that a large part of the immune response is the transport of the infectious agents to the sites of lymphocyte action. If this circulation is brisk, then the maximum immunological response can be expected; however, if the flow of body fluids is

Table 16.E-1: Health Practices and Attitude as Factors in the Strength of the Immune System [753]

Enhances Immune Function	Depresses Immune Function
Health Practices	
Good nutrition	Poor diet (poor quality, improper quantity)
Proper exercise	Lack of exercise
Adequate sleep	Insomnia, somnolence
Relaxation, meditation	Constant stress
Breathing practice	Smoking
Low alcohol consumption	Heavy alcohol consumption
Attitudes	
Active approach to illness	Resigned, helpless approach to illness
Optimistic	Pessimistic
Sees change as challenge	Sees change as threat
Controlled from within	Controlled from without
Inner stability, equanimity	Agitated, volatile
Appropriately self-confident	Self-confidence out of balance
Sense of purpose, commitment	Apathy
Social support system	In isolation
Involvement	Alienation
Warm relationship with parents	Poor communication with parents

sluggish, then so too will be the immune response of the body [753]. Through our practice of the *yogasanas,* we maintain an optimal circulation of the body fluids, thereby ensuring that every last drop of fluid is promptly processed by the elements of the immune system and that all parts of the body are visited regularly by the mobile components of the immune system. A second factor in regard to circulation is the idea that many of the immune factors are stuck to the cell walls in times of poor circulation; however, as your *yogasana* work demands more oxygen and circulation accelerates, the number of your circulating corpuscles increases [15].

Yogasana practice not only speeds the delivery of disease-fighting cells to the sites of infection, but the exercise also works to build high levels of the immune components. Done the correct way, *yogasana* practice will also lead to a more positive parasympathetic response at the expense of the sympathetic response, and this too will bolster the immune system, by reducing cortisol levels. In addition, neutrophils are thought to clear muscle-tissue damage incurred through intense exercise.

Though there is no evidence that *yogasana* practice can either cure or prevent a serious problem such as AIDS, it is clear that it nonetheless can be of use in reducing anxiety and managing stress, and it is a form of exercise that is readily adjusted to the exerciser's limits on strength and energy. Similar statements can be made for other serious diseases [753].

Exercising while Sick

Nieman [618] gives some simple rules for exercising while not feeling well, and these apply to *yogasana* students as well. If your symptoms are above the neck (only nasal), try a simple, undemanding practice. If there are signs of infection, avoid inversions that might encourage it to spread. If the symptoms are below the neck and flu-like (fever, swollen lymph glands, fatigue, sore muscles, aching joints), then the best approach is one of total rest. When the symptoms are below the neck and one insists on working, the door opens wide for much more serious problems.

Schatz [753] presents an interesting table listing common behaviors and attitudes and how they affect the immune system, either bolstering or suppressing immunity. As can be seen in table 16.E-1, the yogic ideals of moderate activity, high spirits, and a calm demeanor all work to keep us healthy.

Psychological Factors

Though psychoimmunology is a very new field, it is already known that older people who are physically and mentally active and healthy have unusually strong immune systems [636], and vice versa. To the extent that our *yogasana* work keeps us physically and mentally healthy, we can expect to be free of the more common diseases of old age. The lack of immunocompetence in the elderly is largely due to inactivity; the positive effects of *yogasana* practice on the immune systems of the young also should work for the elderly, though not so quickly or completely.

Unfortunately, there appears to be a second side to the above argument. As we age and T-cell production and activity begin to wane, the thymus gland degenerates, and the overall strength of the immune system slackens. However, as the immune system weakens, so too does the intensity of allergic reactions.

One of the problems of extended space flight is that the immune system is compromised in a weightless environment [893]. This immediately brings to mind the situation in regard to weightlessness (and bed rest) leading to soft bones and flabby muscles, and this suggests an intimate connection between the immune and the musculoskeletal systems (Subsection 16.B, page 642).

Section 16.F: Apoptosis, Hormesis, and Preconditioning

Apoptosis

When cells die because they have been injured in some way, they swell, leak fluid to the surrounding areas, and cause a local inflammation. In contrast, when cells commit suicide, they shrink instead, and there is no inflammation. This act of suicide, known as apoptosis, can occur as a normal step in the development of the body, as when the fingers and toes form by the apoptosis of the fetal tissues otherwise lying between the digits, when the endometrial tissues in menstruating women slough off, and when the neural circuits in the infant brain are refined by discarding surplus neurons. It is apoptosis that generally is at work when the immune response finishes a battle, and, no longer needing T cells, kills them. Note the significant distinction between necrosis, the disorganized rotting of tissue, and apoptosis, the preprogrammed process of organized cell death, with specific genes and biochemicals guiding the process. However, there appear to be types of cell death that are intermediate between necrosis and apoptosis, depending upon the degree of injury to the cells [849].

Excitotoxins

It must be noted that the sculpting of the brain through experience and learning also involves paring away certain neurons that are otherwise superfluous. One such method to this end is through the use of excitotoxins, neurotransmitting chemicals that kill neighboring neurons by overexciting them. It is known that the excessive release of glutamate ion (a well-known neurotransmitter in the temporal cortex, basal ganglia, cerebellum, and amygdala) can overexcite its neighboring neurons and kill them within twenty-four hours or less. The net effect of these excitotoxic actions is to strengthen certain neural pathways while at the same time destroying others [30]. Excitotoxicity may be a specific form of apoptosis.

Induced Apoptosis

Apoptosis also can occur when cells become seriously infected and become such a threat that the body can be saved only by the suicide of the infected cells. On the other hand, HIV is so effective as a disease because it is able to induce apoptosis in the T cells that normally would fight any infection. Because cancer cells have several mechanisms to avoid apoptosis even though they are unhealthy to the organism, they continue to grow [450]. The continued survival of healthy cells requires that they receive positive signals from other cells and that they adhere to some surface.[2]

Regarding cancer and apoptosis, a relatively small protein known as p53, which is released by healthy cells once they sense the presence of a cancerous cell, serves as a protective agent. The protein p53 induces apoptosis of cancer cells; however, certain viruses related to cancer are now known to disable p53 so that it cannot do its protective job. Strangely, when p53 is at its most active in defending against cancer, it also is accelerating aging. It appears that aging is the price we pay for a cancer-free youth and cancer is the price we pay for longevity! [476].

Protein Misfolding

Chains of amino acids (proteins) are manufactured within cells in accord with instructions from the cell's DNA. In order to be chemically active, the proteins must be folded into very specific spatial configurations, and should the fold-

ing go wrong, the proteins must be destroyed. This is accomplished by covering the misfolded protein with molecules called ubiquitin; the protein within those cells so labeled for destruction are digested by the proteasomes, releasing their basic amino acids. If the protein misfolding, tagging with ubiquitin, and proteasomic digestion process goes awry within the cells of the basal ganglia, the result is Parkinson's disease.

Hormesis

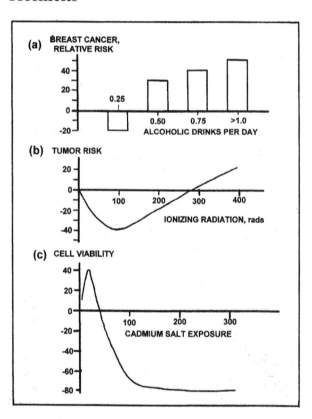

Figure 16.F-1. (a) Variation of the effects of imbibing alcohol on the risk of contracting breast cancer in women. (b) Variation of the incidence of malignant tumors with variation in the dose of gamma rays [701]. (c) Variation of ovarian cell viability with variable exposure to solutions of cadmium salts [701].

Hormesis is generally thought to function through exposure to low doses of a stressor that is harmful at higher doses. For example, figure 16.F-1a shows how the risk for developing breast cancer in women varies with the number of alcoholic drinks imbibed per day [332]. Of course,

---

2   Only those cells that are designed by nature to circulate in the blood are able to avoid death without having to attach themselves to and spread upon some sort of substrate. Experiments [114, 729] show that cells that have been forced to adhere to a solid surface and to spread out on the surface have higher survival and higher proliferation rates than do cells that stick to a surface but remain globular and compact. The conclusion that a mechanically induced elongation of cells controls and promotes their survival and growth may have a direct connection with *yogasana* practice at the cellular level.

there is a nonzero risk even when the number of drinks is zero, due to other cancer-inducing factors. The risk rises above this when 0.5, 1.0, and more than 1.0 drink per day is taken. Note, however, that at a low number of drinks per day, 0.25, the breast-cancer risk is actually 20 percent **less** than when no alcohol is taken! This protective effect of drinking alcohol in low doses is thought to be due to hormesis.

Other Examples

There are many other examples of the beneficial effects of hormesis. Thus, very low doses of gamma rays (25–200 rads) inhibit the formation of tumors more strongly than when there is no such exposure, whereas exposure to 600 rads is strongly stimulating to their formation (figure 16.F-1b). Low doses of radiation, as absorbed by radiologists and by nuclear shipyard workers, have been convincingly shown to extend longevity [500a]. Ovarian-cell viability is strongly increased by exposure to low levels of cadmium as compared to zero-level exposure, but the effects of cadmium become strongly negative at somewhat higher levels (figure 16.F-1c) [701].

Hormesis affects many different body functions. For example, aging is not programmed but is the result of the statistical breakdown of basic biological functions (homeostasis) over time [370]. In this context, it is being argued that the stress of mild exercise (*yogasana,* for example) is just the sort of stressor that exerts a beneficial hormetic effect on longevity [358]. As applied to *yogasana* practice, heavy exercise wreaks havoc with the body, starving some cells of oxygen and glucose while others are flooded with them; the immune system is suppressed and muscle fibers are ripped apart in the process. On the other hand, moderate exercise is a proven benefit to the body. The result is that through hormesis, the body and its immune system are strengthened by moderate exercise, whereas they are truly injured by heavy exercise.

Furthermore, though the aging process may be triggered by free radicals, if the body is mildly stressed by raising the temperature, then heat-stress proteins are synthesized, and these scavenge free radicals, in a hormetic process that acts to extend life. Patients who are heat-stressed before surgery have a higher rate of recovery afterward. For humans, both heat stress and low doses of ionizing radiation decrease the incidence of cancer (figure 16.F-1b) and may increase the life span. Caloric restriction also is a stress that activates various body resistances, and the positive effects of caloric restriction may be due to hormetic effects. Note too that asthma often is due to the lack of stress exposure to foreign substances.

Mechanism

The hormesis phenomenon is observed not only in humans but also in the simplest organisms; apparently many, if not all, organisms have developed the ability to change in beneficial ways on exposure to modest stresses that they encounter in their environments. The hormesis phenomenon appears to be an adaptive response to stress of modest intensity. Hormesis enhances biological function by stimulating the general response to stress (Subsection 5.E, page 182) and strengthening the biological repair mechanisms in the organism. The optimum dose level for hormesis is about 10 percent of the lethal-stress dose. Thus, hormesis acts like a vaccination, priming the body's defense systems [370]. Also, through hormesis, small stresses can be protective of the system, should a large stress of the same sort be met; this is called preconditioning.

Preconditioning

The prevention of horrific events such as stroke or heart attack rests in part on "preconditioning." If one first experiences abbreviated and not too intense deprivations of oxygen, for example, then one can weather a drastic change in the oxygen level much better, should one occur. Those who experience chronic chest pain such as angina, signaling a oxygen deficit within the heart, are much better able to survive a heart attack than those who have not had such oxygen-deprivation preconditioning. Similarly, when a major stroke occurs, those who previously have suffered ministrokes fare better than those who have not. In the same vein, there is much less damage done when a geographic area has many small earthquakes than when there is a long, quiet period preceding a huge quake.

It has been found that the benefits of preconditioning also can be induced by the ingestion of small amounts of poisons such as cyanide, which act to cut the oxygen-carrying capacity of hemoglobin. This leads one back to the effects of hormesis (page 654), wherein small amounts of very poisonous substances have been shown to have beneficial health effects! It appears that what doesn't kill you—as with *yogasana* practice itself!—makes you stronger. This effect of preconditioning is not too far removed from the effects of homeopathic remedies.

How can the healthful effects of preconditioning be introduced into *yogasana* practice? Perhaps performing *sarvangasana, halasana,* or other postures that restrict blood flow to the brain can work to lessen the effects of a stroke, should one occur later. In a similar way, the practice of heavy breathing, as when doing *bhastrika* (Subsection 15.F, page 638), can strengthen us for the hard work we might meet in the future.

Bacterial Priming

Being modern yogis and yoginis and being very health-conscious, we all understand how important it is that foreign organisms be kept out of any open wound. We know that such a wound can be a breeding ground for such foreign organisms and that such contamination can readily lead to a festering sore or worse. Imagine then how surprising it is to learn that this is not true! When foreign organisms infiltrate an open wound, the immune system responds by sending leukocytes to the wound to do battle with the invaders. The result of the battle is the formation of pus and serum, which ooze at the site. And while it is generally held by the public that a sore that oozes pus is a sign of a serious infection, in fact, several medical studies [715] have shown that the oozing pus is a sign that the battle is being won, provided the foreign bacteria are not present in overwhelming amounts. For example, wounds heal better and faster when bathed in non-sterile water than in water that is antiseptic, because the introduction of small amounts of foreign bacteria is stimulating to the immune system, exercising the leukocytes and generating a "laudable pus" in the process, creamy and white, rather than the watery, brown, foul-smelling exudate that signals a systemic infection. This heretical view of the goodness of oozing pus was well known and appreciated by Western medical doctors for centuries until Lister started to apply antibiotics, at which point, oozing pus became a "tomato" from which doctors today do not dare take a bite (see Box 1.A-1, page 5). This situation bears a close relationship to the rapid rise of asthma in children who are brought up in too clean an environment (Subsection 16.D, page 648).

The value of bacterial priming is also shown in regard to drinking water. It has been shown in several cases that in communities in which there is exposure to low levels of bacteria in the drinking water, there is a noticeable resistance to more extreme cases of infection by high levels of these bacteria than is the case in communities where the ambient levels of the bacteria first have been reduced to zero but later rise to high levels. Bacterial priming appears to be a variation of preconditioning.

It is most interesting to think about how the health benefits of *yogasana* practice might be the results of the priming of the body's immune system by processes of hormesis, apoptosis and/or preconditioning as driven by our practice.

Section 17.A: Structure and Function of the Eyes

"Eyes are the windows to the soul," it is said, but that is only half right. Neglected is that not only do others look into the windows of our eyes to see our soul, but we also look out of the windows of the eyes to see the world; fully 80 percent of the information that comes into our brain enters through the eyes! In response to this flood of visual information, between one-third and one-half of the brain's huge capacity is involved with processing visual signals in thirty separate areas dedicated to visual aspects such as form, color, movement, texture, identification of hands, and identification of faces. Needless to say, we would be overwhelmed mentally if all of the visual information received by our eyes were to appear in our consciousness.

Autonomic Control

Inasmuch as the eyes are so much a contributor to our awareness, it hardly seems possible that the eyes are not directly involved with our practice of the *yogasanas* as well. Indeed, being strongly innervated by the autonomic nervous system, the eyes do reflect the levels of physical and emotional tension within the body and so are useful indicators of overall stress when practicing *yogasana*. In periods of stress, the sympathetic nervous system is dominant and the pupils of the eyes dilate, the eyes bulge forward in their sockets, and the blink rate increases, as does the intraocular pressure (table 5.A-2). On the other hand, as pointed out by Ruiz [727], in order to relax the brain and fall asleep, we must close our eyes and so block the otherwise constant stream of visual information (Subsection V.C, page 888). This blocking of the visual pathway allows the parasympathetic nervous system to assert itself, and sleep follows. As many of us are chronically tense visually, the prime consideration of *yogasana* for such students in regard to the eyes is relaxation; whereas for the mentally depressed, it will be important to keep the eyes open and alert. The eyes also can be used to advantage with an active sympathetic nervous system when one is involved in *yogasana* balancing postures, as discussed in Subsection V.C, page 888.

When operating properly, the autonomic nervous system also follows the natural pattern of night and day and adjusts sleep patterns accordingly; however, if it is faulty, then sunrise must be speeded artificially by turning on bright blue lights while it is still dark outside [684a].

External Structure of the Eye

Muscles

The structure of the eye can be divided nicely into two groups: those components within the eyeball itself and those components that are essentially outside the eyeball but still closely related to its function. The six muscles external to the eye that work to position the eyeball in its socket are innervated by cranial nerves (Subsection 2.C, page 24) largely under the control of the autonomic nervous system. Each eyeball is pointed in space

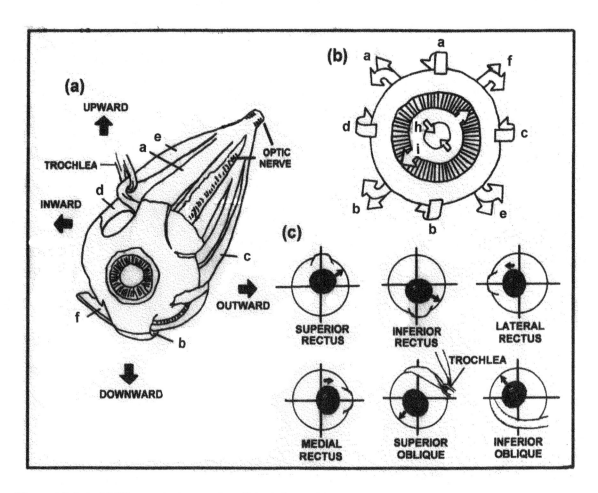

Figure 17.A-1. (**a**) The extrinsic muscles of the left eye, labeled *a* to *f (a* = superior rectus, *b* = inferior rectus, *c* = lateral rectus, *d* = medial rectus, *e* = superior oblique, and *f* = inferior oblique). (**b**) The directions in which the muscles *a* to *f* rotate the left eyeball. The intrinsic muscles surrounding the pupil are labeled *h* (sphincter pupillae) and *i* (dilator pupillae) [431]. (**c**) The extrinsic muscles of the right eye, as seen from the front [613]. Note that the superior oblique muscle, when contracted, is rigged with the trochlea positioned so that contraction will actually pull the eyeball forward and rotate it inward.

using the six muscles shown in figures 17.A-1**a** and 17.A-1**b**. As can be seen there, the four rectus muscles labeled *a*, *b*, *c,* and *d* in figure 17.A-1 are set at the cardinal points so as to give motion in the up, down, left, and right directions, whereas the two oblique muscles labeled *e* and *f* serve to rotate the eyeball around the optic axis. Virtually any movement of the eyeball is complex, in that it involves several or all of the six extrinsic muscles simultaneously [431]. Circumduction of the eye, as when doing the yogic eye exercise in which the eye is moved circularly and slowly past the hours on the face of the clock, can be noticeably jumpy as the various external muscles of the eye are sequentially called into play and then relaxed.

The pattern of two oblique and four rectus muscles positioning each eye is an ancient one, found in almost all vertebrates. The four rectus muscles exert a slightly posterior tension on the eyeballs, whereas the obliques (especially the superior oblique) tend to pull the eyeballs forward; the relative tones of these muscles suspend the eyeball within the bony orbit [288]. Note that the position of the trochlea, which acts as a pulley, is set forward of the position of the ligamentous attachment of the superior oblique to the eyeball (figure 17.A-1**c**), so that when the muscle shortens, the eyeball is pulled forward. In contrast, the ligaments connecting the rectus muscles to the eyeball are placed so that they can act only to pull the eyeball deeper into the eye socket. Because tension in the eyes involves excess contraction of the obliques, the eyes tend to bulge forward when tense, and one must allow the obliques to relax the eyeballs back into the eye sockets.

The medial rectus (*d*) of one eye acts as the antagonist to the medial rectus of the other eye and similarly with the two lateral recti (*c*). Thus, when one eye easily turns in, the other turns out on co-contraction. However, being antagonists, one cannot easily turn both eyes outward simultaneously,[1] though inward turning (co-contraction; see page 422) is easy for focusing in the near field. Motion of the eyeballs is controlled largely by the third, fourth, and sixth cranial nerves (Subsection 2.C, page 24).

Growth

As the volume of the eyeball is only 6.5 cubic centimeters, whereas that of the eye socket is 29 cubic centimeters [68], there is considerable room for movement of the eyeball forward and backward in the socket. However, the eyeball does not rattle around in the spaciousness of the eye socket, because there is a constant tension in the external muscles that keeps the eyeball relatively immobile, though changes in the pattern of tension among the muscles can move the eyeball significantly. Indeed, the position of the front of the eyeball in the eye socket is a reflection of tension in the eyes and facial features, with tension pressing the eyes forward. The tension in the eyes is high if one can see the whites of the eyes as complete circles about the irises.

As we age, the body part that grows the least is the eye; though the adult's body volume is twenty times that of the infant, the volume of the adult eye is only 3.5 times that of the infant's. Nonetheless, it is reported that the eye is capable of relatively rapid growth in the posterior direction in order to bring out-of-focus images back

into focus [129]. On the other hand, too large a growth in the backward direction results in near-sightedness (myopia).

The axis of the bony cavity of the eye socket, or orbit, is offset from the visual axis of each eyeball by approximately 23° outward; that is to say, when at rest, the axis of the eyeball is turned 23° medially with respect to the straight-ahead axis of the eye socket. This inward turning provides large overlap of contents in the left nasal and right nasal fields of view and so makes a stereoscopic synthesis of the scene possible.

Strangely, the extrinsic muscles of the eyes are outfitted with muscle spindles (Section 11.B, page 432) that are capable of monitoring possible overstretching of skeletal muscle, yet these muscles of the eye are never harnessed to an external load and therefore can not be overstretched, nor are they part of any known stretch reflex. It is more likely that they are used as proprioceptive sensors rather than as stretch-limiting safety switches.

Blinking

In addition to aiming the gaze and tracking moving objects, the external muscles of the eyes have two other important mechanical functions: blinking and scanning the visual scene. When our eyes blink, the corneas are being washed down by the upper eyelids in order to keep their surfaces hydrated and free of grime (Section 20.C, page 724). In persons who are twenty years or older, the eyes blink in a reflexive action about twenty-four times per minute. However, the rate is dependent upon one's mood: when we are angry, stressed out, or talking to a stranger, the blink rate increases [297, 716]. Infants, on the other hand, blink less than once per minute. When we blink, the eyes are closed for a significant fraction of a second (400 milliseconds), and in that time, all processing of visual information stops in the brain; however, the brain smooths over these intervals of blackness to present a seamless picture of visual events to the consciousness. What is even more remarkable is that the cessation of visual processing begins about fifty milliseconds **before** the eyelids even begin to move! It is this action of cognitive suppression that is functioning during

---

1   Is it possible that the eyes do not want to look outward simultaneously, since this might present two views to the brain that have no overlapping elements in common and therefore would not allow the brain to form a seamless, stereoscopic picture of the scene?

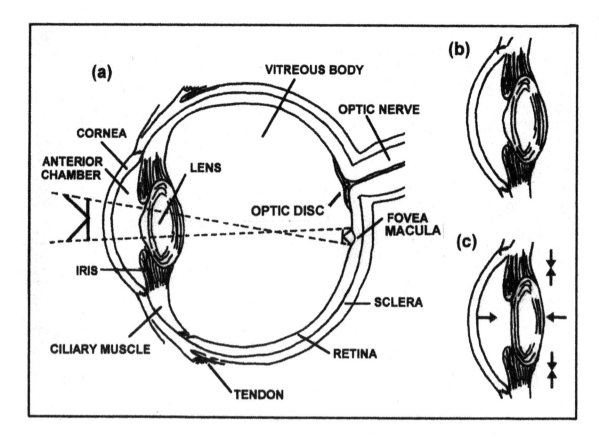

Figure 17.A-2. (a) The inner structure of the eye, as shown in a parasagittal section. Note how the lens works to invert and reverse the image (K) at the retina. (b) High curvature of the lens when the ciliary muscle is relaxed. (c) Reduced lens curvature with the ciliary muscle contracted.

the jumpy saccadic motions of the eyes, and apparently when one tries but fails to tickle oneself but is easily tickled by another (Subsection 13.B, page 511).

The orbicularis oculi surrounds each orbit of the eye and acts as the sphincter of the eye, raising and lowering the eyelids when one is asleep, squinting, or blinking. In these acts, the upper lid moves down considerably and the lower moves up only a relatively small amount. Interestingly, the muscle that lowers the eyelid is innervated by the sympathetic nervous system, thus accounting for the correlation between blink rate and the level of stress [267]. Though the blink rate rises when we are under stress, when concentrating intensely, as when in the *yogasanas,* the blink rate drops significantly, and the corneas tend to dry out. Because the nerves driving the closing of the eyes are reflexively activated whenever we sneeze, it is impossible to sneeze and keep the eyes open.

Internal Structure of the Eye

Optical Parameters

Of the five functions of the eye that are controlled by the autonomic system, three of them involve intrinsic muscle actions that change the eye's optical parameters; i.e., they change the focal length of the lens, open the pupil of the eye, and close the pupil of the eye (figure 17.A-2a).

Light incident on the eye first passes through the transparent cornea, which focuses it; it is then further focused by the lens in a left-to-right (reversed), top-to-bottom (inverted) fashion onto the retina. The final focusing of the image on the retina is accomplished in part by changing the curvature of the lens using the ciliary muscles, as shown in figures 17.A-2b and 17.A-2c. This focusing process is called accommodation. The ciliary smooth muscle attaches to the outer rim of the lens and is normally in a state of contraction, which acts to flatten the lens (figure 17.A-2**c**), thereby increasing its focal length, as appropriate for far-field vision. The ciliary muscle is innervated by cranial nerve III of the parasympathetic system, originating at the oculomotor complex within the hypothalamus. Upon deactivation of cranial nerve III, internal contraction within the lens is released, allowing it to assume a more spherical shape, thereby shortening its focal length, as appropriate for vision in the near field (figure 17.A-2**b**). There are no nerve fibers to the ciliary muscle from the sympathetic nervous system.

In normal use, it is estimated that the internal muscles of the lens contract about 17,000 times a day. Contrary to popular understanding, the lens is not the only structure that determines the effective focal length of the eye, as strong focusing also is obtained at the interface between the cornea and the air outside the eye [297]. In fact, the largest part of the front-to-back focusing of the eye is performed by the cornea, with the lens responsible only for fine tuning [926].

Contents

The anterior chamber of the eye, between the cornea and the lens, is filled with a watery fluid; the second chamber, behind the lens, is filled with a jelly-like material, the vitreous body [450]. The vitreous body is a gelatinous mass supported by a fibrous network of proteoglycan molecules (see Subsection 12.A, page 482). A clear liquid (the aqueous humor) flows continuously in and out of the anterior chamber at the front of the eye, draining at the junction where the iris and the cornea meet. If this liquid does not drain properly, the pressure in this chamber rises, leading to glaucoma.

The Lens

The lens is avascular and is packed with a dense array of proteins called crystallins. Because of the tight packing of the crystallins, there is no light scattering within the lens. Crystallins are the longest-lived proteins in the body; they are present in the embryo and are not replaced once lost. The crystallins in the vertebrate eye are very close-

ly related to heat-shock proteins, which function to help other proteins retain their conformations under heat stress [929]. Should the crystallin proteins begin to denature and clump together, cataracts may form in the lens, and the vision then may become cloudy.

The Cornea and Sclera

The cornea and the sclera (the white part of the eye surrounding the iris) differ in their optical properties. The sclera is filled with loosely packed collagen fibrils (Subsection 12.A, page 483) and so scatters light and appears opaque, whereas the collagen in the cornea is much more tightly packed and does not scatter the incident light and so is transparent. In old age, the collagen bundles in the cornea tend to become less tightly packaged and more like scleral tissue, and light-scattering cataracts are so formed. Because the cornea must be clear, it is avascular and so gets its oxygen by diffusion from the air when the eyes are open, and from the blood vessels on the inner surfaces of the eyelids when the eyes are closed, as when asleep. Contact lenses must be permeable to oxygen or the cornea and lens of the eye will suffer.

Because the cornea has no blood supply and is nourished in part by the aqueous humor (the fluid between the cornea and the lens in the anterior chamber; see figure 17.A-2**a**), it is virtually isolated from the rest of the body. The lens too is free of vascular plumbing. Though the cornea is free of blood vessels, it is richly supplied with nerve endings that signal irritation and pain. If a gritty particle settles on the cornea, a reflex action is activated that leads to blinking and the secretion of tears (Section 20.C, page 723).

The Iris and Pupil

Between the cornea and the lens is the iris, consisting of two circular sets of pigmented, smooth muscles forming an opening (the pupil) to the inner eye. Cranial nerve III innervates one of these, the sphincter pupillae (also called the constrictor pupillae), with muscle fibers running tangentially to the inner rim of the iris (figure 17.A-1**b**). Reflexive excitation of this parasympathetically driven system contracts the muscle fibers so as to decrease the pupil diameter, as when the light incident on the eye is too bright [878]. As agonist to the sphincter pupillae (Subsection 11.A, page 420), there is the second set of muscles, the dilator pupillae, just outside the sphincter pupillae and having their muscle fibers running radially rather than tangentially (figure 17.A-1**b**). Contraction of the dilator pupillae muscle fibers via the sympathetic nerve originating at the uppermost paravertebral ganglion (figure 5.C-1**a**) acts reflexively to increase the diameter of the pupil, as when the light level is too low for clear vision. This response of the dilator pupillae is also present when the adrenal medulla releases catecholamines into the bloodstream, as when under stress.

Returning to the idea that sympathetic stimulation would be in aid of the fight or flight response (Section 5.C, page 170), it can be argued that having a larger pupil diameter increases one's peripheral vision and so adds to the security against peripheral attack, all the while sacrificing spatial resolution. In the battle for dominance of the pupillary diameter, the parasympathetic system generally is the stronger source of excitation.

The diameter of the pupil also controls the amount of light reaching the foveal spot on the retina. In bright light, the pupil diameter reflexively narrows to 2 millimeters (0.08 inches); however, when the sympathetic signal is activated, the diameter of the pupil increases to as much as 8 millimeters (0.31 inches), allowing up to sixteen times as much light to enter. The emotional content of the limbic system also has its effect on the pupil's diameter, as the diameter reflexively tends to increase dramatically whenever we look at someone that we love or admire.

Intraocular Pressure

The intraocular pressure within the vitreous body of the eye serves to keep the eyeball round and the optic image in focus and generally remains constant throughout life, with the rate of intraocular-fluid input into the eyeball being equal to that of its drainage. However, this pressure can become chronically high (up to 70 millimeters Hg) when drainage is impeded. In this case, the added pressure on the retinal artery and on the optic nerve degrades their functions and that of the retina, and the result is a condition known as glaucoma. If the intraocular pressure due to glaucoma is high and persistent, the retina and optic nerve atrophy, and blindness results. Relaxing so that the parasympathetic nervous system becomes dominant is effective in lowering intraocular pressure. Certain inverted *yogasanas,* such as *urdhva dhanurasana, halasana, sarvangasana,* and *sirsasana,* are not recommended for those inclined toward glaucoma, due to the risk they pose for such beginning students. Specifics of these situations as they have been reported in the medical literature are summarized in Appendix II, page 833, and specific cautions also are given for these postures in Iyengar's book [398].

Aging

As we age, the centers of the lenses begin to accumulate dead cells, and the lenses stiffen and become more resistant to changing their shapes. Moreover, with increasing age, the numbers of neural receptors and synapses used in vision decrease, thus impairing sight and ocular reflexes generally [162]. By age forty years, accommodation of the eyes often can be accomplished only with the aid of glasses. Though Western medicine considers the deterioration of one's vision with increasing age and needing glasses to see properly as "natural," it is not true that nothing can be done to impede the course of failing eyesight. Indeed, in many cases, simple yogic eye exercises can be very effective in keeping the eyes in fine condition into old age [262, 288, 581, 686, 862].

Section 17.B: Vision and Neuroanatomy of the Retina

Rods, Cones, and Receptive Fields

Inner Structure

At the point where the optic nerve connects to the retina at the back of the eyeball, the optical

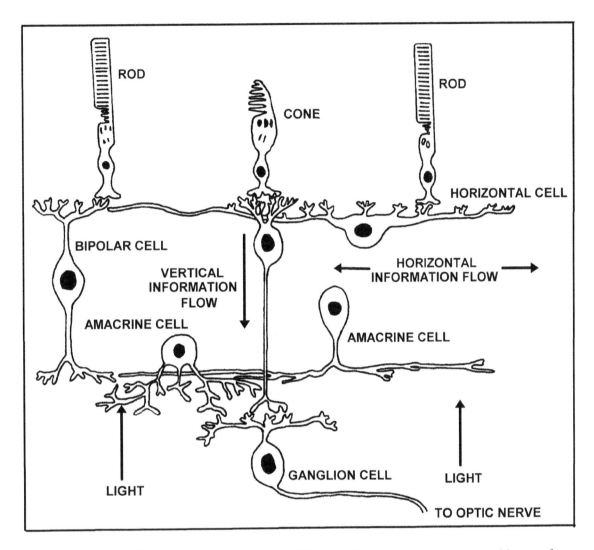

Figure 17.B-1. The cellular structure of the retina. Note that light must penetrate several layers of nerve tissue before reaching the photosensitive rods and cones. The nerve tissue of the retina functions much like brain tissue, in that it too shows a strong neural convergence, with many rods and cones sharing a common ganglion cell.

disc, there are no optical sensor cells, yet the brain smooths over this blank spot in the visual field, regardless of any head motion. The optic nerve tract is myelinated along its length from the brain to the back of the eyeball; however, once inside the eyeball, the optic nerve is not myelinated. Just 3 millimeters (0.1 inches) or so to the lateral side of the optic disc is the broad depression called the macula, and deep within the macula is the fovea (figure 17.A-2a).

Rods

The intrinsic muscles of the eye adjust its optics so that a focused image falls upon the tis-

sue containing the visual receptors, the rods and cones (figure 17.B-1) found in the retina. That the retinas of our eyes contain over 70 percent of the total number of receptors in the human body testifies to the prime importance of these organs in sensing our environment, yet the retina is only 0.5 millimeters (0.02 inches) thick, weighs only 0.5 grams, and consumes just 0.1 Watt of power.

The rods are useful for sensing a black-and-white visual pattern in dim light, whereas the cones operate at higher light levels and are color sensitive, coming in three varieties: red-light sensitive, green-light sensitive, and blue-light sensitive. The rods are most prominent on the periphery of

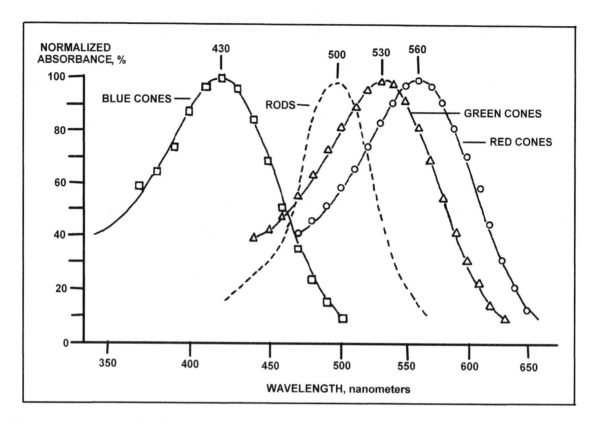

Figure 17.B-2. Normalized absorption spectra of the blue-sensitive, green-sensitive, and red-sensitive cones and the rods within the retina. There is little or no sensitivity at wavelengths below about 380 nanometers, the ultraviolet region, except in persons with very blonde hair and light-blue eye color. On the other hand, overexposure to ultraviolet light acts to desensitize the blue-sensitive cones; interestingly, in many people within cultures in the Earth's equatorial belt, the sensitivity to blue light is so low (presumably due to overexposure to ultraviolet light) that their languages do not even have a word for the color blue, substituting words such as "green" and "dark" instead!

the retina, whereas the cones are tightly clustered about the fovea (figure 17.A-2a). Rods are quite sensitive to motion, as appropriate for detecting a predator moving toward one from the periphery at sunset; whereas the cones offer a high-resolution color scan of a panoramic view in bright light. Signals from the rods often initiate reflexive actions, and rods in the retina are twenty times more numerous than cones.

Cones

Each of the three types of cone in the human eye[2] shows color sensitivity largely in its particular

color band, as displayed in figure 17.B-2, allowing one to sense over two million color hues. The optic signal containing the color-encoded images from the three types of cones travels then from the retina to the occipital lobes, among other places. In contrast, the signals from the rods have no such direct route to the cortex and travel much more slowly into our consciousness, as appropriate for a subconscious process that is essentially reflexive and rapid.

color-sensitive cones. It is thought that our early mammalian ancestors had the full complement of four cones but that they went nocturnal during the Mesozoic period (245 million to sixty-five million years ago), and so two of these cone types (blue and ultraviolet) were lost, with one of them regained by our human ancestors about forty million years ago [282a].

2   In birds, there is a fourth cone present that confers ultraviolet sensitivity, whereas in New World primates, there are only two types of cones: red and green. Only humans and Old World primates have three types of

Visual resolution (the ability to see two nearby features as distinct) is at its highest at the spot on the retina called the fovea, whereas no sensing can be done at the papilla (the optic disc), where the various nerves from the retinal cells and the arteries and veins to these cells coalesce to form the optic-nerve bundle. The fovea is densely packed with cones. One would logically expect that the part of the image at the papilla would be sensed as a black spot within the visual scene, but the brain smooths it over with information borrowed from adjacent areas, so that the blind spot is automatically erased.

Retina as Part of the Brain

The retina and the associated neural net function as a specialized brain center within the eye, performing complex signal processing. In fact, the retina is a part of the brain, growing from the brain in the embryo [450]. Because the neural tissues of the eye are directly traceable to corresponding tissues in the brain, one might rightfully consider the retina to be an extension of the brain. Indeed, it is abundantly clear [383] that the neural layers of the retina are both inhibitory and excitatory in about equal proportions, just as with the brain. Furthermore, in support of this idea, many brain tissues and structures exit the brain and are continued down the optic nerve (channels for cerebrospinal fluid, for example) and even penetrate into the eyeball itself [360]. For example, the white part of the eyeball, the sclera, is just a continuation of the dura mater, the outer covering of the brain; posteriorly, the sclera fuses with the three meninges that surround the optic nerve and the central nervous system itself [251]. In agreement with the idea of the retinas being extensions of the brain, it is observed that animals with very complex eyes have simple brains and vice versa [297]. Vis-à-vis human beings, we have relatively simple eyes and very complex brains.

If the vitreous gel within the posterior chamber of the eye shrinks and pulls away from the retina, it can pull the retina with it, causing a retinal detachment, at which point, vision is lost. This condition may also result if the eye is struck, as with the heel of a student being helped into an inverted position.

Neural Convergence

It is striking that light incident on the rods and cones of mammals must first pass through three layers of nerve cells before reaching the sensory cells of the retina (figure 17.B-1). The outermost layer of the retinal neural cells consists of the retinal ganglia. Within each retina at the fovea, there are three million cones, and though there is a total of 125 million rod and cone receptors in the retina of each eye, there are only one million ganglion-cell axons in the neural net just in front of each of the retinas, and these axons then enter the optic nerve, which contains only about one million fibers. This convergence of the receptor neurons (figure 3.C-2b) onto the neurons of the optic nerve results in a smaller, more flexible optic nerve, which in turn moves more easily when the eyeball moves.

Considerable signal conditioning of the visual signal is done by the neural cells within the retina. This action involves a complex net of excitation, inhibition, and two-way horizontal transfer of signal, eventually to converge upon four types of ganglion cells (figure 17.B-1). These ganglion cells measure local increases and decreases in light intensity and the relative intensities falling upon adjacent cells, allowing them to function as edge detectors.

Receptive Fields

Though every neural fiber originating at a sensory cell (rod or cone receptor) in the retina finds its way to the layer of ganglion cells, there are only 1/125 as many such ganglion cells as there are receptor cells. Thus, there is a strong neural convergence at this point in the visual pathway, with each retinal ganglion being connected to between 100 and 1,000 adjacent receptor cells. Any cluster of receptor rods and cones in the retina having neurons that converge on a common ganglion is called a "receptive field." In the convergence of the visual signals, there is a compression of the signal, so as to finally show a spatial and temporal pattern consisting of receptive-field elements.

Certain receptive fields are configured to show contrast, so as to identify shapes and change of shapes [450]. The smallest receptive fields, and therefore the areas of highest visual acuity, are found in the foveal spot.

Balancing

Studies of the functions of individual receptive fields show that they can be very specific sensors for certain geometric features in the visual pattern. For example, it is known that such a field may be sensitive to sensing straight lines inclined at a specific angle, and that if the angle is turned by 10° or so, then the image no longer activates this receptive field, but activates a different one. Other receptive fields are sensitive to the motions of edges or lines in the visual field, and yet others respond only when the motion is in a specific direction. It is my hypothesis that these motion-sensitive and angle-sensitive receptive fields in the retina are of great use in balancing with the eyes open in the *yogasana* postures, as they can easily sense when a straight line in the field of view begins to rotate as the body starts to fall. On the other hand, trying to balance with the eyes in an environment free of cues as to where the horizon lies or with the eyes closed can be very difficult (Box V.C-1, page 889).

Aging

As we age, our visual acuity decreases. However, the sensitivity of the receptive fields for the movement of a straight edge in the peripheral field actually become more active. As a result, younger people are able to see fine detail in a visual scene but have difficulty with the larger picture, whereas it is the opposite for the older set. It is thought that this difference might relate to the lower levels of the inhibitory neurotransmitter GABA in the brains of older people.

Neural Currents

Even in total darkness, the ganglion cells of the retina are always active, sending a continuous train of action potentials to the brain. The transduction of a visual scene into neural signals is based upon the modulation of this ganglionic dark signal, as described below. There is a significant dark current from the retinal receptors, and on being illuminated, the cells hyperpolarize [383] rather than depolarize, and the amount of released neurotransmitter decreases (Section 3.D, page 53). Thus, the visual signal is measured as a **decreasing** dark current and a lowering of the excitation frequency in the optic nerve! Needless to say, this is completely the reverse of normal nerve action (Subsection 3.B, page 42). When the eyeball is pressed or struck, the increased intraocular pressure on the rods, cones, and optic nerve leads to electrical discharges in the retina and the sensation of bright, flashing lights [798]. This phenomenon can be understood as a consequence of the normal neural action in the optic system, in which pressure on the eyeball presumably throttles the neural current, as with any nerve, but this decreasing dark current then gives rise to optical signals that are interpreted as starbursts, light flashes, etc. Because optical signals are transmitted as decreasing changes in dark current, whereas most neural signals are transmitted as increasing changes in dark current, pressure in the first case leads to enhanced optical sensations, and pressure in the second case leads to weakened sensations.

The two visual systems of the eye, the rods and cones, work together so that the scene that is sensed is seamless. The proportion of rods to cones is larger away from the center of the retina, thus peripheral images appear less colored. But the rods are more sensitive than the cones and so are best used for motion sensing in dim light [347]. Adjacent rods are connected by gap junctions, and several rods may converge on one ganglion, or one rod may connect to several ganglia. If only one rod is excited and it is connected to many ganglia, the brain cannot know where on the retina it is located, and hence, rod vision is not sharp spatially. Nonetheless, the rods are very sensitive to light.

Visual Response Times

Auditory signals require only eight to ten milliseconds to travel from the middle ear to the conscious brain, whereas visual signals require twenty to forty milliseconds to go from the eye to consciousness; the travel time for response to touch is shorter than that for sight but longer than that for sound. In general, the shortest reaction time is obtained when the subject is neither too relaxed nor too tense. Mental fatigue works to lengthen reaction times, but physical fatigue does not; this could be a factor in balancing. Reaction times are shortest when exhaling as compared to the situation when inhaling. Exercise decreases reaction times, especially when the heart rate is 115 beats per minute, as when experiencing a fight or flight situation [462].

Yet another connection exists between the eyes and the passage of time. As we go from normal illumination to dim light and the visual sensors switch from the cones to the rods, the time that it takes the visual signal to travel from the retina to the cortex lengthens appreciably [338, 361]. Because of this slowing of the reaction time in dim light, it is more difficult to balance in the *yogasanas* in dim light (Subsection V.C, page 888) and especially difficult in total darkness (or with the eyes closed).

Chromostereopsis

When white light is obliquely incident on the lens of the eye, there is a refractive bending of the light, with the blue light refracted most toward the center of the eye and the red the least, with green in between. This gives the illusion that the blue object is further away than the red. This color aberration is called chromostereopsis [341] and is discussed further in Subsection 17.E, page 682.

Photopigments

In order to sense light, the cones use a photopigment called retinal (a derivative of vitamin A), whereas the rods use a photopigment called rhodopsin to the same end. In both the cones and the rods, these photopigment prosthetic groups are bound to transmembrane conjugate proteins called opsins. (As with many transmembrane proteins, opsin's alpha helix is woven in and out of the membrane of the retinal cell seven times.) The three cone types, red, green, and blue, have different spectral sensitivities (figure 17.B-2), due to small differences in the molecular structures of the conjugate opsin molecules.

Ion Channels

When light is absorbed by the photopigment in the retina (Section 17.B, page 665), the pigment molecules change their geometry in an act called isomerization. The eventual result of this isomerization is the drastic reduction in the concentration of cyclic guanosine monophosphate (cGMP), a chemical within the retinal cell that effectively holds open the Na^+ channels in the cell's membrane. When the concentration of cGMP drops on exposure of the retina to light, the Na^+ channels close, while at the same time, the K^+ channels remain open to the outward flow of this ion. The net result of the blocking of the inward flow of Na^+ and the unrestricted outward flow of K^+ is the hyperpolarization of the retinal sensor when illuminated.

Hyperpolarization

Remember now that a depolarized excitation wave can propagate for a long distance (over 1 meter; three feet), but hyperpolarization cannot (Section 3.B, page 39). In the retina, the hyperpolarization is able to travel passively for only 2 millimeters (0.08 inches) before it connects to intermediate neurons (bipolar and multipolar) and then to the ganglion cells (figure 17.B-1). It is not yet clear how the hyperpolarization of the retinal cells eventually is transduced into depolarization of the ganglion cells, but the axons of these latter cells are depolarized and send their signals to higher centers in the brain via the optic nerves.

Saccadic and Microsaccadic Motions

Saccades

When the head is held still, rapid external motions of the eyes called "saccadic motions" occur, which successively focus important aspects of the visual scene on the foveal spot, in line with the visual axis (figure 17.A-2a). Saccades are rapid, so as to minimize the amount of time spent in the blurry transitional range, and are synchronized between the left and right eyes. At a normal conversational distance, you will not be able to see both of the eyes of your friend simultaneously, but through the saccadic movement of your eyes you can near-simultaneously see both eyes and the mouth as well. When inspecting a scene with the acuity of the fovea, those areas of the visual image that are important are visited and inspected multiple times in preference to those areas of lesser import. Saccadic motions are very useful, as they are very rapid and allow tracking of irregular motions. Except for the sneeze, the saccadic motions of the eyes are the fastest bodily functions we have. Such saccadic motion is known to be essential for the visual process, as described above in the discussion of the retina (page 667).

Just as with the blink phenomenon discussed above, when the focus of the gaze is shifted through saccadic action, there is a momentary loss of vision during the shift, but the brain smooths this out so that the impression is that of uninterrupted viewing. The density of cones is very high in the 1-square-millimeter area of the fovea, and this is the site of high-resolution vision in the retina at moderate or high light levels. However, the area of the fovea is only a small percentage of the total area of the retina onto which the visual scene is projected. Studies of the saccadic motions show that the attention will be strongest on certain features of the scene—the eyes and mouth of a face, for example—and that the visual process is largely inhibited while the eyeball is in motion, so that the integrated image is not blurred [457]. Those aspects of a scene picked for more intense scrutiny during the saccades are largely out of our conscious control, but the frontal cortex seems to be important in this action. Saccades are an aspect of gaze-holding, of sorts.

Microsaccades

When in that saccadic state in which a small area of the scene is brought to the fovea and held there, microsaccades then take place. Because the pigments in the retina are very rapidly adapting toward zero stimulus (Subsection 13.B, page 506), the image tends to fade quickly (with a lifetime of about one second) if the image is static

on the retina. However, the shifts inherent in the saccades and microsaccades thus act to illuminate and then shield a particular retinal area from light, with the result that the retinal stimulus is constantly refreshed [354]. This is reminiscent of the pose-and-repose action of Iyengar in the *yogasanas* [33], which acts to refresh the mind's proprioceptive picture of the body.

It is said that the eyes move in the same way whether a real scene is being viewed or if one imagines it is being viewed, and that it is difficult to generate a mental image if one's eyes are prevented from moving [76]. The role of saccadic motion in the production of visual stress is discussed above, page 667. It is interesting and perhaps relevant to *yogasana* teaching that there are cultural differences in which aspects of the visual scene are focused on by the saccadic motions. Thus, for example, Americans dwell on the central object of a scene, whereas Chinese focus instead on the background, implying that they are more interested in the context of an object than in the object itself.

Yogasana Teaching

The saccadic motions of the eye are relevant to *yogasana* teaching in the following way. Because processing in the visual cortex is highly competitive, only a small number of all of the distinct features of the teaching scene are given any consideration at all. If the student subconsciously chooses the wrong features of your *yogasana* on which to focus as you demonstrate it, then that student will have missed the point of the demonstration. The lesson here is that you must verbally point out clearly what the student should be focused on visually as you demonstrate, if there is to be any chance of riveting their attention on the relevant aspects of the posture.

The Ocular Reflexes

Connections to the Vestibular Organs

The inner ear contains specialized sensors, the vestibular organs, which contain proprioceptive sensors that are important in static and in dynamic balancing, both upright and inverted (Sections 18.B, page 696, and V.C, page 893). Among these organs are the semicircular canals, which monitor the sense of rotation and speed of rotation of the head, as when falling to the side. Interestingly, there are neural interconnections between the vestibular nuclei serving the semicircular canals and the oculomotor nuclei in the brainstem that direct motion of the eyeballs. These interconnections reflexively integrate the actions of the lateral and medial recti muscles of the eyes with head rotation, so that when the head turns, the eyes rotate oppositely but at a rate so as to keep the fovea fixed on an external point [427]. It is this reflex (known as the ocular-vestibular reflex) that keeps this page static and in focus as you slowly move your head to the left and right. This reflex comes about due to a feedforward response in which the motion of the eyes is fed forward to the brain, which is able to cancel out the sense of motion based on information on the eye orientation [691]. Though the reflex is nominally controlled by centers in the midbrain of the brainstem, it can be overcome by deliberate actions originating at higher centers of consciousness.

The semicircular canals within the vestibular apparatus sense acceleration and deceleration in rotational motion of the head and then couple this to the eyes so as to maintain constancy of the visual field even though the head is turning. However, note that when we stop turning, there is a deceleration and thus a sense of the opposite turning of the head. In this case, the fluid within the canals overshoots and sends a vestibular signal counter to what the eyes may be seeing. The result is a vestibular signal that is in conflict with that of the eyes and nausea that is related to seasickness [346]. Often there is disagreement among the balancing sensations delivered to the brain by the eyes, the vestibular system, and the proprioceptors. When this happens, the brain usually goes along with what the eyes are saying in this regard. Still, such conflicting signals in regard to equilibrium also can generate dizziness and nausea.

Using the Eyes to Balance

The existence of the vestibular-oculomotor reflex leads one to think that balance could be affected by and through the eyes. Indeed, *yogasana* practice shows that the use of the eyes in balancing can be very stabilizing and even can work at a level higher than that of the reflexes (see Box V.C-1, page 889). Thus, it is likely that in moving from *virabhadrasana I* to *virabhadrasana III* and from there to *ardha chandrasana,* for example, the vestibular-oculomotor reflex is of great use in maintaining one's balance during the in-motion phases of the *yogasanas.* As discussed more fully in Subsection V.C, page 888, it is very stabilizing while in stationary balances to fix the eyes on a stationary spot on the wall.

The Heart-Slowing Reflex

The eyes are involved in a second reflex action of great interest to *yogasana* practitioners. Known as the ocular-vagal heart-slowing reflex, this reflex is activated whenever there is external pressure on the orbits of the eyes (figures 4.E-1 and 14.C-2**a**) and results in a slowing of the heartbeat; i.e., it stimulates the parasympathetic nervous system. This is discussed in Subsection 14.D, page 579. An especially interesting visual reflex is described below.

Blindness, Blindsight, and Perceptual Blindness

The First Visual System

The various stages of evolution of brain structure are evident in the morphology and functions of the brain sectors; i.e., the reptilian brainstem evolved so as to first add the limbic system and later to add the cerebral brain, with all three coexisting today in each of us (figure 2.A-1). This developmental path leads to the simultaneous existence and simultaneous functioning of both the conscious arena in the cerebral hemispheres and subconscious neural arenas in the limbic and brainstem areas, and this extends to the visual sensors. Thus, there is considerable evidence for at least two separate visual systems: one slow, conscious, and involving the visual cortex and known as the first system (or the ventral system); and a second being more subconscious, more rapid in response, involving the parietal cortex, and known as the second system (or the dorsal system) [63, 284, 349]. As it is known that the retinal rods are often involved in reflexive acts, perhaps the conscious visual system is tied to the retinal cones and the subconscious visual system is tied to the retinal rods. The dorsal system is the more prominent one in amphibians, reptiles, and birds, whereas the ventral stream is more important in humans and higher mammals. Other visual pathways in humans also exist, such as that which connects the suprachiasmatic nucleus to the retina and which is used for synchronizing various body clocks with the rising and setting of the sun (Subsection 23.B, page 787).

The two visual systems differ in many other respects. The reflexive dorsal stream works in real time and stores visual-motor information for only a matter of a few hundred milliseconds, in contrast to the ventral path, where the visual information may be stored in long-term memory for decades. Further, the dorsal path is essentially involved in an egocentric self-preservation, whereas the ventral path is involved with the wider appreciation of the global scene [284]. The receptive fields operating in the ventral stream are quite complex geometrically (faces, etc.), whereas those operating in the dorsal stream are less complex (straight edges, velocities, etc.) but are activated almost in synchronicity with a variety of motor neurons. It must be said as well that the two visual systems are not totally independent, for the signal from the striate cortex goes in part to the inferior temporal cortex, but a part also goes to the posterior parietal cortex, eventually to be joined there by the dorsal stream coming via the superior colliculus.

The Second Visual System

As compared to the first system, the second (the dorsal system) is of a more ancient age and works much more as a reflexive, intuitive system [30]. That is to say, the first and second visual sys-

tems stand in respect to one another as do the cerebrum and the brainstem of the central nervous system. Indeed, the analogy with the brain is not by chance, for a large part of the visual apparatus is simply a continuation of brain tissue.

As shown in figure 17.D-1, the normal visual signal in the first system passes through the lateral geniculate nucleus and then to the striate cortex. The signal from the striate cortex is then processed in several other brain areas before being presented to the cortex for interpretation. This visual system is used for visual perception of the scene. In contrast, the same signal from the retina also moves to the superior colliculus, upward to the pulvinar area within the thalamus, and then to the posterior parietal lobe of the cortex. Whereas the first system functions in support of the conscious visual system, the second operates in a more reflexive mode, acting with great speed only at the subconscious, intuitive level. As such, it is a visual system for action rather than for perception. For example, when a stone chip is seen as it is sent flying toward the unprotected eye, the second system can activate the eyelid to drop to protect the eyeball in a time far shorter than would be the case were the sight of the chip to be processed by the thinking, conscious brain and then the appropriate muscles activated. To the extent that the second system is concerned with the "responses in relation to orientations in space" [30] it may play a significant role in the visual aid of balancing in the *yogasanas* (Box V.C-1, page 889), especially in the establishment of a visual anchor.

It is no accident that the neural path of the second system has a direct path from the superior colliculus to the lower centers in the brain, to the muscles of the eyes, and to α-motor centers in the spinal cord that control muscle actions in the limbs. In contrast, the connections of the first system to the motor neurons are very indirect and relatively much slower [284].

When the first visual system was momentarily disabled with a transcranial magnetic pulse applied to the visual cortex while the eyes were flashed a momentary colored image, the participants in the experiment were not aware that anything had been seen, but they were able to describe the flashed object, having sensed it subconsciously through the second visual system.

Blindness and Blindsight

If a person is totally lacking in retinal sensitivity, then there is no signal for either the first or the second visual system to process, and the person is blind in every sense of the word. However, it is also possible that a person is blind in the first system because of some neurological malfunction beyond the retina, but that this malfunction does not necessarily incapacitate the second system. In this case, the person is "blind" in regard to the conscious first system, but the ancient second visual system is still operative at the subconscious level and so would allow the person to navigate in three-dimensional space subconsciously! This visual reflex is called blindsight. Those with blindsight report that they have no conscious sense of objects placed in certain parts of their visual fields, but if asked to pick up a specific article among other articles in such a blind area of the field, they can do so easily and correctly. This is the visual equivalent of the proprioceptive sense within the muscular system.

In the context of figure 1.A-1, showing how the conscious and subconscious levels of the mind can become mixed through *yogasana* practice, one must keep the two visual systems in mind, with the thought that they too possibly can be mixed, making the first system more intuitive and automatic and the second system more conscious and deliberate. Those who operate by blindsight have no conscious memory of what they have "seen," but their circadian rhythms are properly entrained with the rising and setting of the sun, which they cannot "see" [835].

Balance

Given that a lightweight stick cannot be balanced on the finger with the eyes closed, experiments on the physics of the eyes-open balancing of a rigid broomstick on the finger support the idea of a second, faster route to "seeing" that is relevant to balancing [99]. The normal route of conscious seeing has a characteristic response time of 70–120 milliseconds on average, whereas

98 percent or more of the corrective motions involved in the eyes-open balancing of the broomstick were found to occur in times of ten to seventy milliseconds! I interpret this as experimental evidence for the rapid, subconscious reflexive action of blindsight in the simple balancing of a broomstick on the finger. Of all the neurons in the optic nerve, about one-third are devoted to carrying the signals of the retinal stream feeding the subconscious dorsal system.

Born Blind

For those who are blind from birth, dreaming is totally auditory but with the auditory cortex shifted considerably into the area normally occupied by the visual cortex; whereas for those who slowly become blind, dreaming slowly shifts from the visual to the auditory mode. In addition to the visual, auditory, and vestibular systems, yet another related phenomenon is the significant difference between a genuine smile, which is a reflexive action, and a forced smile, which is choreographed by the conscious mind and fools no one (Subsection 4.C, page 94). As discussed in Subsection 18.A, page 689, the auditory and vestibular systems not only register higher-level cortical sensations, but they also have older antecedents, which report aural and balance sensations only to the subconscious in a more reflexive manner.

Furthermore, when blind people read Braille with the fingertips of one hand, the sensations appear in the visual cortex of the opposite hemisphere, even though there are no neural signals from the retina to these visual centers! Similarly, when blind people are involved in verbal memory tasks, there is a stimulation of the visual cortex, just as with sighted persons who use the visual cortex to imagine faces, scenes, places, colors, etc., as if they were seeing them directly, just with weaker signals.

Perceptual Blindness

The phenomenon of perceptual blindness in sighted people is the reverse of the blindsight coin and is typified by the following [784a]. A brief video is shown of a three-man team of white-shirted players playing basketball against a threesome of players wearing black shirts. Viewers are asked to count the number of ball passes made by the team wearing white shirts in the first minute of the show. Thirty seconds into the video, a gorilla enters the court, thumps its chest, and only leaves after being on scene for nine seconds. Questioning of the viewers after the game reveals that 50 percent of the viewers did not notice the gorilla, and when watching the video a second time, they felt that a new video had been introduced! Thanks to the perceptual blindness in all of us, much of what we see with our eyes may be invisible to a brain that is focused on something else. This is also called inattentional blindness and is a significant factor in many magicians' acts [690].

In a related study, it has been found that if one is told to look for a specific item in a streaming list, that one is essentially attentionally blind for about a half-second before and after the selected item appears. This failure of awareness is called an "attentional blink" and occurs when we are overloaded in regard to attention.

It appears that "looking" and consciously "seeing" are two very different things. In fact, magicians use verbal suggestion all the time in order to set up their "magic" displays. It is good to remember in our *yogasana* experiences that not only can we fool each other with what we say to others, but we also may be fooling ourselves with what we say to ourselves while practicing. This type of visual blindness relates to the localized focus of the gaze imposed by specific saccadic motions of the eyes (Subsection 17.B, page 667).

Section 17.C: Stress, Vision, and *Yogasana* Practice

The picture painted above assigns the intrinsic muscles of the eye to making accommodations for optimum focusing and light level, whereas the extrinsic muscles are innervated by the cranial nerves and serve to steer the gaze in space. Bates [43], however, finds that imbalance among the six

extrinsic muscles can prevent the intrinsic ones from functioning properly, leading to tension in both the internal and external muscles of the eyes. However, yogic eye exercises [113, 262, 686, 727, 862], which both stretch and release tension in the extrinsic muscles, can indirectly lead to better accommodation by the intrinsic muscles and improved vision.

Stress and Vision

Chronic stress, anxiety, and emotional reactions can lead to refractive changes in the eye and often to blurred vision. Thus, for example, eyes that are 20/20 become nearsighted (myopic) whenever a lie is told [262], and seeing an attractive person tends to dilate the pupils, both signaling tension in the sympathetic nervous system.

Though the visual field spans 200° in an angular sense, the size of the fovea is only 1° [427]. According to Bates [43], the proper function of the eye is to detect details in the small visual field of the fovea (less than 1 square millimeter) and then rapidly switch (at a rate of 70 hertz) to another small field within the overall image. In this way, the visual image is scanned over the fovea (the spot of highest visual acuity), and a high-resolution global image is reconstructed by the brain. That part of the image not scanned by the fovea becomes the peripheral visual field. Bates calls this motion of the eyeball "central fixation and shifting," whereas others call it "saccadic motion" [427]. However, according to Bates, stress, fear, and anxiety trigger sympathetic signals that result in transfer of the optic neural signal away from the striate cortex to the frontal cortex, with dilation of the pupils. It appears that Bates has identified the two visual systems discussed above in Subsection 17.B on blindsight (page 669)! When stressed visually, one has a myopic stare, with the eye attempting to see all areas in sharp detail simultaneously, even though this is not possible, because of the small size of the fovea. Difficulty in focusing the eyes can lead to tonic contraction of several of the muscles of the eyes, and the resulting spasms express themselves as headache.

Muscular Tension

Yogis have found that a general state of high muscle tension in the body can lead to a pull on the eyeballs, pointing them in toward the nose, as is appropriate for sharp focus of nearby objects. Though the muscles of the eyes easily function to force the eyes to cross inward, as when stressed, this is not so for the outward-uncrossing motion, and so the best one can hope for in regard to redirection of the gaze is to allow the eyes to relax toward their straight-ahead orientation. The diminution of the tension pulling the eyes inward probably involves the parasympathetic excitation of cranial nerve III. It is this connection between the extrinsic muscles of the eye (the inferior recti muscles; see figure 17.A-1a and Subsection 11.D, page 446), the parasympathetic nervous system, and the state of body tension that makes this relaxation possible.

Gender Differences

There is an interesting gender difference in the response to being approached by another person and the tension that this can provoke. Because men's vision, in general, is more tightly focused in a narrow, forward tunnel, men feel their personal space is being violated when approached from the front. Because women's vision, in general, is more peripheral and less forward focused, women have the same sense of violation and the need for a defensive posture when approached from the side [554]. With respect to *yogasana* practice, it is the goal visually to transform the student's gaze away from forward and focused (sympathetic, male) toward broadly peripheral and defocused (parasympathetic, female).

Opening and Closing the Eyes

Clearly, when the mind is alert, the eyes are wide open in every sense, and when the mind is relaxed, the eyes close. One can easily observe the extent of sympathetic stimulation in one's students by noting that when there is sympathetic stimulation, the eyelids open so that all 360° of the whites of the eyes (the sclera) are visible, whereas when in the parasympathetic mode, the upper and lower lids move toward one another

and partially block the view of the sclera.[3] Indeed, when light enters the eyes, there is an activation of the reticular formation (Subsection 4.B, page 74) and unavoidable arousal, which would be appropriate in active *yogasanas* such as *trikonasana*, but not in *savasana*.

The standard yogic way of quieting the brain is to quiet the eyes by wrapping them with a soft bandage, thus stilling their motion and blocking the light. At the same time, the bandage acts to initiate the ocular-vagal heart-slowing reflex and a full parasympathetic response. Should the extrinsic muscles of the eyes be overworked and stressed out, they can be profitably exercised using a yogic approach [359, 686, 727]. Practice of the yogic eye exercises leads to an increased ability to relax and to release into sleep, as progressive relaxation of the extrinsic muscles of the eyes leads to reduced mental activity. This will be true for relaxing the mind in *savasana* as well.

EEG

The relaxed watchfulness of *savasana* with the eyes closed generates alpha waves in the EEG (Section 4.H, page 151) of the occipital region, a region of the brain that is dedicated to processing visual information. It has been shown that with training, the alpha-wave pattern can be maintained even though the eyes are opened, if the gaze is defocused [359]. This defocusing of the gaze is important when working to develop the alpha-wave relaxation of *savasana* in all of the more demanding *yogasanas*.

Pressure at the Eyeball

Blood Pressure

If students with high blood pressure are working intensely in the *yogasanas* while slightly hold-

---

3   In the intermediate situation, wherein the whites of the eye are visible on three sides but not on the fourth, one has the condition called *sanpaku*, meaning "three empty areas" in Japanese. The condition is considered to reflect poor health in regard to poor diet and excessive external stresses leading to adrenal stress [631].

ing the breath, they must look down to relax [826], but students with low blood pressure or depression should look up, as long as their eyes do not pull inward toward the bridge of the nose. Though the eyes-up position is a strong indicator of mental activity and is usually inappropriate for *yogasana,* it is appropriate for those who are too strongly directed toward parasympathetic excitation.

Vascular Conditions

Inverted *yogasanas* also can act adversely on the eye by increasing the pressure of the cerebrospinal fluid (Section 4.E, page 107) on the veins of the eyes, leading to papilledema, and by overpressurizing the veins and arteries within the retinal layer, leading to hypertensive retinopathy [360]. Though inversions are contraindicated for glaucoma subjects, they can be done safely by such students with expert instruction [556].

Yogic Relaxation for Visual Stress

The attempt to view a panoramic image (resulting from sympathetic excitation in an effort to form a large pupil diameter) with the high-resolution but very small fovea implies a very high rate of saccadic motion, resulting in eyestrain, pain, frowning, holding of the breath, increased heart rate, tense neck and jaw, shoulders and jaw rotated forward, depressed chest, tension in the mid and lower back, and stiff legs! Moreover, when the stress is habitual, the sympathetic arousal threshold associated with this eye movement is lowered, and the effects last longer. These symptoms correlate with the fear that without special exertion, one cannot hold one's world together, a fear that is said to be common in nearsighted people [520]. As people who are extremely nearsighted are at high risk for retinal detachment [914], *yogasana* students with extreme myopia should avoid extended or challenging inversions or backbends.

Critical Flicker Frequency

When the frequency of a flickering light is slowly raised, a frequency is finally reached

at which the individual light pulses fuse into a steady glow, appearing to be without any flicker. This frequency is called the critical flicker frequency (CFF). Studies of the physiological effects of *yogasana* practice on CFF show that when under stress, there is a decrease in the CFF, but with the relaxation attendant to *yogasana* practice, the CFF increases [680a]. This implies that yoga training has sharpened the temporal aspect of visual perception, as is known for the shortening of visual and auditory reaction times with *yogasana, pranayama,* and meditation practices. It is reasonable to assume that the shorter visual response time that develops with *yogasana* training would be of use when using the eyes in balancing postures (Section V.C, page 888).

Personality

As fine as one's vision may be, it is still the case that what we "see" in our consciousness often is a reflection of our expectations and is strongly colored by our past experiences [251, 339]. Studies show that our vision habits are related to our personalities, and that changing our vision profile can change our personality [520].

Relaxing the Gaze

To avoid tensing the eyes, one must learn to relax the gaze, breathe deeply, maintain elasticity of gaze, and not give in to tunnel vision. One must be more global in one's vision and awareness. If one can do this, the eyes will accommodate in a relaxed way to the large diameter of the pupils and not add yet more stress. As applied to the *yogasana* student, this suggests that our aim should be to keep the gaze broad, soft, and fuzzy, with a global awareness that is the opposite of tunnel vision [359]. To this end, one should work the *yogasanas* in a position where other objects in the surround are not so close that the eyes will be drawn to them and become pulled into a nearsighted condition. As explained above (Section 17.A, page 657), the superior oblique muscles of the eyes also must be relaxed if one is to achieve a globally relaxed state.

Hypnotizability

If it is accepted that the relaxed position for the eyes has them pointing downward and more outward to the sides, then the eyes turned upward and inward must be a position of high stress. Interestingly, it is the ease of attaining this stressful position of the eyes that hypnotists have used to judge the hypnotizability of subjects, with those who can easily turn their eyes in this way making the most easily hypnotized subjects. This position is the gateway into the hypnotic state, as it promotes a strong dissociation of the mind from the body in those who can do it well [507]. While this body-mind dissociation may be appropriate for the more meditative states of *yogasana* practice, it is counter to the aim of the beginning student who is working to reconnect mind and body. Moreover, the connection of eye rolling to hypnotizability has been challenged by Hilgard [368].[4]

Savasana

It is interesting that in *savasana,* there is often considerable random eye movement, reminding one of the REM phase of sleep (Subsection 23.D, page 800). This movement weakens as the relax-

---

4   As mentioned above, looking upward toward the pineal gland (the "third eye," above the brow) by forcefully turning the eyes upward and inward can lead to a mental state in which one senses that the consciousness has left the body; i.e., dissociation. Apparently, this involves interactions within the reticular formation (Subsection 4.B, page 74) and promotes a sympathetic response of the autonomic nervous system. This eye-rolling action could lead to sympathetic excitation if one were to look at the feet while in *sarvangasana* or at the hands while in *urdhva dhanurasana,* and it most certainly results in a very strong sympathetic excitation when in *simhasana II.* Looking upward and inward probably is desirable in very advanced students but could be counterproductive in beginning and intermediate students. On the other hand, looking downward in the *yogasanas* is generally tranquilizing [851] and so would not be recommended if the student is depressed or has low blood pressure. See Box V.C-1, page 889, in regard to how looking up or down affects one's sense of balance.

ing effects of the parasympathetic system take hold. Lacking that, tension in the eyes can be relieved by wrapping the head with a bandage or using an eye bag placed briefly over the eyes when in the supine position; this relief is based upon the ocular-vagal heart-slowing reflex (Subsection 14.D, page 579).

In the act of "seeing," the visual pigments of the retina (retinal and rhodopsin) are temporarily bleached and deactivated, leading to a chemical stress within the eyes that can be released by periodic closing of the eyes, thereby allowing the pigments to return to their active forms [727]. (See also Subsection 17.B, page 667.)

Bright-Light Stimulation

Because bright light entering the eyes is generally a sympathetic stimulant, when doing postures such as *sarvangasana* or *halasana* with a parasympathetic goal in mind, it is best to turn down the intensity of the ceiling lights so as to reinforce the intention of the posture. On the other hand, because one does want a certain nonzero level of sympathetic stimulation in the body when practicing the *yogasanas,* the eyes should not be closed except when performing *savasana* and *viparita karani.* It is the orbicularis oculi (the smile muscles) that surround the eyes and close them.

The Eyes Set the Body's Clocks

The general effect of *yogasana* practice is a slowing of the body's clock, with fast-twitch muscle fibers (types 2 and 3) and their rapidly conducting nerves being converted into slow-twitch fibers (type 1) with slower neural conduction (Subsection 11.A, page 412) and the ascendancy of the body's parasympathetic nervous system. However, it also has been shown that with practice of the *yogasanas* and associated techniques, both the visual and the auditory response times are shortened [532] and visual perceptual accuracy increases [414]. This suggests that though *yogasana* training slows skeletal-muscle action, it can accelerate visual responses.

The Circadian Clock

Many physiological processes in the human body are controlled by an internal twenty-four-hour circadian clock (Subsection 23.B, page 774), including the times of hormonal release each day and the time of the monthly menstrual flow (Subsection 21.A, page 737). The timing of these circadian rhythms is triggered by specific photopigments within cells in the layer of the retinal ganglia having a peak response at a wavelength of 480 nanometers, whereas blue vision involves a set of different photopigments operating in the outer retinal layer [684a, 867], with a peak response at 430 nanometers (figure 17.B-2). This sensory information from the retinal ganglia travels to the suprachiasmatic nucleus within the hypothalamus, where it is processed for eventual response by the autonomic nervous system [360]. The cells responsible for setting the biological clock are a type of retinal ganglion cell which uses melanopsin (melatonin from the pineal gland and its complex with opsin) as photopigment and sends its signal to the brain centers controlling sleep, thereby setting the circadian clock [892]. As light suppresses the production of sleep-producing melatonin by the pineal gland, (with the deep-blue and ultraviolet wavelengths being most effective in this suppression [292]) the complex is destroyed by sunrise, and the suprachiasmatic nuclei are then activated, thereby turning on the internal clocks that regulate the entire endocrine system. If the sun rises later and later as summer turns to winter in your area, then the release of melatonin is set askew and the result can be seasonal affective disorder, or SAD (Subsection 17.E, page 685).

Section 17.D: Vision and Cerebral Laterality

In several of the earlier chapters (especially Chapters 4 and 5), it was explained that many body functions that appear on one side of the body or the other have neural connections that connect the function on that side of the body to the cerebral cortex on the opposite (contralateral) side of the brain. For example, breathing through the left nostril produces a mental state that is characteristic of the excitation of the right cerebral hemisphere (Section 15.E, page 627), and the conscious stiffening of the right arm in *vasisthasana I*, for example, involves excitation originating in the α-motor cortex in the left cerebral hemisphere. Because the sympathetic and parasympathetic aspects of the autonomic nervous system also are strongly lateral, their relative dominance can be shifted by either breathing through one nostril or accenting the muscular action on one side of the body. This neural crossover usually occurs at the level of the spinal cord or brainstem.

Visual Decussation

As discussed below, there are several aspects of vision (anatomic, physiological, and psychological) that lead one to believe that there also are specific neural connections between each of the eyes and the contralateral cerebral hemisphere, and that these hemispheres can be selectively activated through the eyes in order to alter the balance within the autonomic nervous system. One readily can test the visual sense for laterality, as explained in Box 17.D-1, below. Following this, we go on in Subsection 17.E, page 683, to a discussion of how this phenomenon might impact on *yogasana* practice.

Balancing the Dominance

In the box below, a simple test is introduced to expose any visual dominance. However, just as with the *yogasanas,* where we delegate extra work to the side that is the weaker in order to achieve a more balanced situation in the body, so too must we work to lessen the dominance of the stronger eye. If one eye is dominant, one can then wear a patch over the stronger eye for short periods in order to restore visual balance and hence release the tension that comes from imbalance and lack of fusion of the images of the two eyes [285]. The laterality of visual effects also is discussed in Section 4.D, page 103.

Box 17.D-1: Determining Your Lateral Preference for Vision

Visual Dominance

You no doubt have a strong tendency to write with one hand and not the other, to step up onto a step with one foot and not the other, and to hold the telephone to one ear and not the other. All of these lateral preferences reflect a dominance of one cerebral hemisphere over the other. You can check your vision for hemispherical dominance in the following way [337].

With one arm outstretched, extend the thumb toward the ceiling. Adjust the arm position so that with both eyes open, the thumb is seen to be just below some object in the far field. Now close the right eye and notice if the object shifts laterally with respect to the thumb. Starting again with both eyes open, repeat, closing the left eye. Of the people so tested, 54 percent find that the object does not move when the left eye is closed (Coren [159] reports this figure as 70 percent), 4 percent find that it does not move when the right eye is closed, and 41 percent see little or no movement.

If your right eye is the dominant one, then closing the left eye will have no effect on the image, since you are seeing it largely with the right eye, even if both eyes are open, and vice versa for the left eye. That is to say, when you are aiming with your dominant eye, the other eye is essentially nonfunctional. The dominant eye, as found here, is probably the one that you use when looking through a telescope or keep open when you thread a needle. If there is no shift of the image on closing one or the other eye, then you are ambivisual.

Note that according to table 4.D-1, if your right eye is dominant, you show a left-hemispheric preference for vision, suggesting that you preferentially view the world in a logical, analytical way; whereas for those who have the left eye dominant, the right cerebral hemisphere is dominant, and the preferential view is more intuitive and holistic. If you have a strongly dominant eye, then the visual component of your balance in *yogasanas* requiring balance will be more effective with the dominant eye open.

The rivalry between the visions of the right and left eyes can be demonstrated [519]. Look at a scene with the left eye looking through a long paper tube, and place the open right hand about 1 centimeter (0.25 inches) from the right eye, alongside the tube. One will see the image of the right hand and the superposed image of the scene seen through the tube, but in the center of the right hand. The two images are seen simultaneously, but there is no fusion of the images. If the dominance is not too strong, after a short time, the dominance will shift so that the tube image will fade and the hole will fill with the image of the missing part of the right hand. After a short while, it will shift back to the original scene.

Crossover of the Optic Nerve

The phenomenon of stereo-optical images that leads to depth perception requires that the images received by the two eyes be kept separate on their way to higher centers in the brain and then compared for differences. This is performed by having separate neural tracts for the left and right eyes and synaptic neural connections at equivalent sites in the left and right cerebral hemispheres, as shown in figure 17.B-1. But the story is much more interesting than that.

Hemiretinas

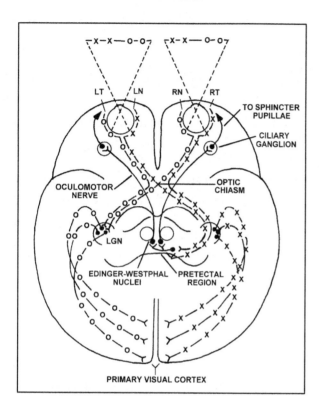

Figure 17.D-1. The neural pathways from the retinal hemifields to the visual cortex, showing the crossing over of the optic nerves at the optic chiasm [360]. Note that the right part of the image (-o-o-) is sensed by the LT and RN hemiretinas and eventually appears as sensation in the left cerebral hemisphere, whereas the left part of the image (-x-x-) is sensed by the LN and RT hemiretinas and appears as sensation in the right cerebral hemisphere. The striate cortex (the primary visual cortex) is not in any way the final picture screen, but rather is just an early stage in the visual processing [382].

The retina in each eye is divided into two hemiretinas, with one half of the retina being closer to the nose and the other closer to the temple. Call those hemiretinas in the right eye RN and RT for right nasal and right temporal hemiretinas, and similarly LN and LT for the hemiretinas of the left eye. Because the lens of the eye inverts and reverses the image on bringing it to a focus on the retina (see figure 17.A-2a), light coming from the right side of the viewer's visual field will illuminate the LT and RN hemiretinas, whereas light coming from the left will illuminate the RT and LN hemiretinas (figure 17.D-1).

Optic Chiasm

As shown in figure 17.D-1, each of the four hemiretinas has its own dedicated neural branch, and as the coding in the figure reveals, the nasal hemiretinal neurons cross over at the optic chiasm, a point just below the suprachiasmatic nucleus within the hypothalamus. Once past the optic chiasm, the nasal hemiretinal neurons continue on to the cerebral hemisphere on the opposite side of the brain, whereas the temporal hemiretinal neurons do not cross to opposite sides. Thus, the LT and RN neural signals come from the left half of the visual field and will synapse in the right cerebral hemisphere, whereas the LN and RT neural signals will come from the right half of the visual field and will synapse in the left cerebral hemisphere. Notice too that each eye nonetheless has direct input to **both** of the cerebral hemispheres. This split-retina-with-crossover has several interesting consequences (see, for example, Box 17.D-1, page 677).

Light falling on the LN and RT hemiretinas generate signals that synapse first at the lateral geniculate nucleus (abbreviated LGN in figure 17.D-1), and then at the parasympathetic center, the Edinger-Westphal nucleus. A reflex arc is completed by stimulation of the ciliary ganglion by neurons from the Edinger-Westphal nucleus in order to drive the sphincter pupillae. The reflex arc is such that with bright light entering either eye, the pupils of both eyes will be reduced in diameter. Because there is no equivalent arc originating at the LT and RN hemiretinas, the pupillary diameter is controlled by the parasympathetic center within the right cerebral hemisphere in the first approximation, but rapid transfer of information between the hemispheres is possible via the corpus callosum (Subsection 4.C, page 97). Also see Box 17.D-1, page 677, for more on the reciprocal effects of mood and visual laterality on one another.

The Higher Visual Centers

It is especially relevant that the center of highest spatial resolution, the cone-rich fovea of each eye, can be in the nasal hemiretina and so is subject to hemispherical crossover of the neural signal, whereas the peripheral rods are more in the temporal hemiretinas and would not cross over. This geometric difference in the neural paths of hemiretina excitation sets the stage for conscious, deliberate visual action on the one hand and subconscious, reflexive visual action on the other (see Subsection 17.B, page 669), as well as separating the signals of the cones in one eye in a lateral sense from those of the rods in that eye.

Once past the chiasm, the contralateral signals from the nasal hemiretinas retain their left-right character and are deposited in the lateral geniculate nuclei (LGN in figure 17.D-1) as alternating slabs of R-L-R-L-L-R information, together with the information from the temporal hemiretinas, but without crossover in this case. Two of the slabs in the LGN contain the information about the shape of the visual image, and four of the slabs contain information about its color.

From the LGN, the visual information is projected backward to the primary visual cortex in the occipital lobes (Brodmann's area 17, figure 4.C-1). The regular deposition of visual information in the primary visual cortex results in a map of the visual receptor fields of the retina projected onto the striate cortex, much like the inputs of the sensory modes and the outputs of the somatic modes are mapped onto the cortex as homunculi (figures 4.C-5 and 4.C-6). Note, however, that the traditional visual pathway from the retina to the primary visual cortex (figure 17.D-1) is generally held to be devoid of any emotional content [786].

Binocular Vision

It is at the level of the striate cortex that complementary cells in the receptor fields of the left and right eyes may interact to form centers of binocular action. These centers in turn may show binocular dominance, with one hemiretina dominating the other. In this way, visual sensa-tions may find their ways preferentially into one cerebral hemisphere or the other. Visual processing occurs at many other centers beyond the striate cortex, as described in the excellent book by Hubel [383], but his text goes far beyond our needs as *yogasana* teachers.

Memory and Visual Laterality

NLP

It is surprising to find that extrinsic eye movements can be correlated with how people store and retrieve information from memory. As studied by those in the neurolinguistic programming (NLP) field, it has been shown that when trying to remember certain sensory events, people tend to use a specific eye movement (figure 17.D-2) to promote easier access to the memory [513]. When first introduced by NLP practitioners, the correlation was presented with more certainty than is presently evident, especially as to what the eye movements might mean. The reader is referred to the NLP website [616] for the current view on this subject.

For a right-handed person with a "normally organized" brain (i.e., sympathetic hemisphere on the left and parasympathetic on the right; see Section 4.D, page 99), and referring to figure 17.D-2, NLP predicts the following:

1. When asked to remember (R) a previous visual image (V), the eyes shift upward and leftward (V^R).
2. When asked to construct (C) a new visual image (V)—for example, imagine Albert Einstein with orange hair in *ardha chandrasana*—the eyes move upward and rightward (V^C).
3. When asked to remember a previous auditory memory (A)—for example, to hum a few bars of one's favorite song—the eyes move laterally to the left (A^R).
4. When the auditory memory involves constructing an auditory scenario, say, the sound of a violin played under water, the eyes move laterally but to the right (A^C).

5. Kinesthetic images (K), including those of taste and smell, are remembered by first looking downward and to the right.

6. When embarrassed, the eyes look downward and to the left (A), as if the emotion is being processed in the right cerebral hemisphere.

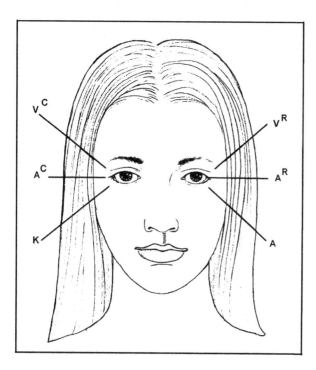

Figure 17.D-2. Directions in which the eyes turn when asked to remember a visual thought (V^R), an auditory thought (A^R) or a kinesthetic thought (K). Alternatively, on being asked to think of a visual construction (V^C) or an auditory construction (A^C), the eyes turn as indicated.

That the directions in which the eyes turn are reversed for people who are left-handed would seem to be evidence for the lateralization of these memory functions in the brain, as handedness and hemispheric laterality are very strongly correlated (Section III.C, page 848).

As might have been expected, searching the brain for visual information involves motion of the eyes upward. In contrast, auditory memory involves only a lateral shift, and kinesthetic feelings will involve motion that is downward and to the right. Deliberate side-to-side motion of the eyes has been used to access traumatic experiences in a subject's life, as have bilateral acoustic tones; the result is an "emotional detoxification" that comes with the surfacing of emotions and their reprocessing.

Mental Eye Movements

The strong connection between mental processes and extrinsic eye movement is easily demonstrated, for it is readily seen that when one is thinking in a logical mode, the eyes tend to shift to the right, as if searching the left hemisphere, whereas when thinking analogically, the eyes tend to shift to the left, as if searching the right hemisphere [721]. On the other hand, when one is asked an emotional question about oneself or is thinking in an emotional, nonlinear way, the eyes look to the left consistently, suggesting that the right cerebral hemisphere plays a special role in emotions [204], as observed (Subsection 4.D, page 102). These observations imply that there is a connection between the extrinsic muscles of the eyes turning them left and right (largely the medial and lateral recti muscles in figure 17.A-1) and the choice of neural branches used for transducing the thoughts.

Studies attempting to test the relationship between the type of memory being recalled and the direction of the associated lateral eye movement have not been uniformly supportive of the sort of ideas expressed above [616]; however, they do agree that the more difficult the memory task, the larger is the amplitude of the lateral eye movement.

The totality of the evidence presented above supports the notion that the unquestioned laterality of brain functions extends to the eyes as well, even though it is not clear just how this comes about. Nonetheless, regardless of the details of the possible mechanism, one can go on to explore the possible relationships between the color of the light entering the eyes, eye/brain laterality, and its effects on the practice of the *yogasanas*, as presented below.

Table 17.E-1: Physiological and Psychological Responses to Color
[1, 267, 435, 473, 761, 824]

Color	Response
Red	Heating, stimulating, promotes circulation and vitality, energizes willpower and nervous system
Orange	Warming, builds sexual energy and high levels of emotional and mental energies; alkaline, relieves congestion
Yellow	Heals, cleanses, purifies digestion; stimulates understanding, intelligence
Green	Balances heart, blood pressure and body temperature; neutral, harmonizing, soothing, cooling, sedative, refreshing, alleviates headaches, lifts depression
Blue	Cool, soothing, contracting, calming, sedating; works mostly on mouth and throat, removes burning sensation
Violet	Sedating, sexual inhibitor, increases mental awareness, lightness in body, opens doors of perception

Section 17.E: Color Therapy and *Yogasana* Practice

The use of color as a therapy appears to have begun more than 5,000 years ago in India with the Ayurvedic physicians. More recently (1933), Ghadiali [513] proposed that there is a color specific to the activation of every organ and another for its deactivation, which immediately brings the sympathetic/parasympathetic dichotomy to mind. As color therapy has changed little through the millennia, we look at the color effects as first put forth by the ancients [435, 473, 513, 824] (table 17.E-1). Indeed, one sees from the table that the colors red and yellow evoke physiological and emotional responses that are understandable in terms of sympathetic arousal, whereas blue and violet act to stimulate parasympathetic responses. Green is held to be a more neutral, balancing color. Though most human eyes do not sense ultraviolet wavelengths below about 380 nanometers, there is considerable evidence showing the role of modest amounts of ultraviolet light in good health [474, 638].

Autonomic Balance

Scientific evidence is available in support of the idea that viewing specific colors can change the balance of sympathetic/parasympathetic activation in the body [786]. In an extended study, Gerard [267] investigated the effects of red and blue light on the physiology of a group of college students. He found that viewing red light raised the respiration rate 2.5 percent but that blue light lowered it by 3 percent. Systolic blood pressure was raised 2.3 percent by red light but was decreased by 1 percent in blue light. Heart rate, palmar conductance, and eye-blink rate were all significantly higher in red light than in blue. On the other hand, viewing red light significantly lowered the percentage of the relaxing alpha waves in the EEG as compared with the percentage when viewing blue light. Also, though red is energizing, viewing pink is sedating, but only for twenty minutes or so, after which it becomes strongly agitating [513, 638]. Extended viewing of lights of specific colors also has been found effective in relieving PMS in some women (Subsection 21.A, page 740).

That the effects of viewing colors can affect the cerebral laterality and thus the balance of the autonomic nervous system would explain some interesting situations. For example, it appears that dyslexia involves a lack of simulation to the left cerebral hemisphere (Subsection 18.B, page 701), so that viewing reading material through properly colored lenses can help those with reading difficulties [513]. This is related to the phenomena discussed in Box 17.E-1, page 684.

Placebo Colors and Sizes

When colored placebo tablets (Subsection 5.F, page 196) were offered to subjects who either are suffering anxiety (and so are in need of sedation) or who are depressed (and so need stimulation), it was found that the placebo-cure effect was strongest when the depressed subjects were given small, yellow sugar tablets and was strongest for patients suffering from anxiety and needing sedation when they were given large blue ones [635]. Similar results as regards sympathetic versus parasympathetic exaltation were obtained when hypnotized subjects were told to visualize the colors and report their feelings and sensations [1].

The Affective Response

Gerard [267] also studied subjective/affective responses and found red light to promote unpleasant thoughts, nervous tension, irritation and annoyance, discomfort, anxiety, heat, and alertness. In contrast, viewing blue light led to responses of comfort, happiness, relaxation, well-being, calm, and pleasant thoughts. The physiological and psychological results of this study are totally in accord with a red-light stimulation of the sympathetic nervous system and a blue-light stimulation of the parasympathetic nervous system. Presumably, these responses to the colored lights originate in the left and right cerebral hemispheres respectively, though there is no mention of any uneven illumination of the retinas. In regard to the above, note that it has been said [761] that one does not really have to look at the colors, because just thinking about them can lead to the same autonomic activation [1, 513, 749]. If this effect is real, it must involve the deliberate activation of higher brain centers to control what otherwise are involuntary responses. The affective response is a key feature of seasonal affective disorder (Subsection 17.E, page 685).

Mechanism

How is it possible that viewing colored lights evenly through the two eyes can change the physiology and psychology of the viewer? Assume first that the two hemispheres of the brain are involved separately in driving either the sympathetic or parasympathetic branches of the autonomic nervous system, with the left hemisphere directing sympathetic action and the right hemisphere directing parasympathetic action (Section 4.D, page 98). It is as if blue light is excitatory to the right cerebral hemisphere and so produces parasympathetic relaxation, whereas red light is excitatory to the left cerebral hemisphere and so produces sympathetic arousal—but how can this be when the illumination is symmetric left to right? For a possible answer, return to figure 17.D-1. When the cornea and the lens work to focus light onto the retina, due to the phenomenon of chromostereopsis (page 667), red light and blue light will be focused to **different** points on the retina. Moreover, those parts of the optic signal that cross over to the contralateral hemisphere (those from the LN and the RN hemiretinas) are stronger than those from the LT and RT hemiretinas.

In this neurological scheme, red light viewed head-on will be found preferentially on the LN and RT hemiretinas, whereas blue light viewed head-on will be found preferentially on the LT and RN hemiretinas. Given this, the red-light signal will appear largely in the primary visual cortex in the right cerebral hemisphere and will stimulate a sympathetic response, and blue-light signals will appear in the primary visual cortex in the left cerebral hemisphere and promote a parasympathetic response (figure 17.D-1).

Alternatively, suppose that the LN and RT hemiretinas are richer in blue-sensitive cones, while the LT and RN hemiretinas are richer in red-sensitive cones. In that case, when both eyes are illuminated with blue light, the LT and RN hemiretinas are excited preferentially, leading to left-hemisphere excitation and the sympathetic response; whereas with red light incident on both eyes, the LN and RT hemiretinas will be preferentially excited, leading to right-hemisphere excitation and the parasympathetic response. The green cones, lying as they do between the responses of the red and blue cones (figure 17.B-2), would be neutral in regard to hemispheric activity, as observed in Section 5.G, page 201.

The explanation given above is based upon the red-sensitive cones being placed in one area of the retina and the blue-sensitive cones being placed in another [70]. If, in fact, these cones prove not to be geometrically segregated, then perhaps something can be made of the fact that the sensation of "red" is known to appear in the consciousness more quickly than the sensation of "blue" [353, 786]; i.e., perhaps the effects of color on the autonomic nervous system involve kinetic rate factors rather than geometric factors.

In any case, there is good reason for thinking that the asymmetric routes of the optic nerves into the cerebral hemispheres (figure 17.D-1) in some way are at the root of the mechanism behind the selective actions of differently colored lights on the autonomic response within the body and mind.[5] Yet other examples of this strange connection between color and physiology are given in Box 17.E-1, page 684.

Yogasana in Colored Lights: A Proposal

Autonomic Response to Color

In the subsection above dealing with the mechanism of color vision, observations were quoted for the physical and emotional effects of colored lights, and possible mechanisms were put forth to explain this. Even if the true mechanism is far from those advanced above, the fact remains that lights of different colors can activate either the sympathetic or parasympathetic responses, shifting the balance between them. As the sym-

pathetic and parasympathetic nervous systems are very active in the changes wrought by *yogasanas* (Chapter 5, page 157), it is immediately interesting to ask if the physiological and psychological effects of *yogasanas* can be modulated by performing them in colored lights. The non-yogic responses of the muscular system to various sensory inputs are discussed at length by Diamond [198].

It is my thesis that energizing *yogasanas* such as *urdhva dhanurasana*, when performed in red light, will be even more energizing, especially when the light is incident on the student's face from the right, so as to excite the left cerebral hemisphere, whereas illumination with blue light from the left will act to stimulate the right hemisphere and so lower the excitation level of the same posture! Similarly, if the *yogasana* is inherently cooling and relaxing, say *sarvangasana*, then the same effects mentioned above still will be expected; i.e., blue-light illumination will be more calming still and red-light illumination will add a component of arousal. Changes of autonomic excitation on changing the frequency of illumination could be measured, using what are by now standard means (blood pressure, heart rate, blink rate, palmar conductance, etc.).

The yogic counterpart to the arm-strength test described in Box 17.E-1 might be performing straight-arm *chaturanga dandasana* or standing in *tadasana* with the arms extended forward or to the side while staring at either a pink or a blue card. In the case of the pink card, one expects a shortening of the duration that the posture can be held comfortably, and the reverse effect when the color of the card is switched to blue.

Optimum Wavelengths

In chromatic *yogasana* experiments such as those described above, one wants minimum overlap of the two test wavelengths but high retinal sensitivity at each; from the data in figure 17.B-2, it is clear that wavelengths of 570 nanometers (red) and 390 nanometers (blue) would do nicely. More interesting yet is the possible effect of blinking the colored lights at the various rhythms of the brain waves (table 4.H-1); i.e., blinking the

---

5   Paradoxically, it was the emotional effects of colors that first piqued my interest in searching the medical literature for an explanation of a phenomenon that I first found in the yoga literature [761], and after ten years of serious searching, I am still uncertain as to the mechanism behind this effect!

Box 17.E-1: The Effects of Colors and Emotions on Muscle Strength

The suggestion that certain colors or emotions can promote a shift of autonomic dominance in regard to muscle strength can be readily shown without any scientific apparatus. In the first case, have a person hold their arms out horizontally and ask someone of approximately the same strength to try pulling their arms down, qualitatively noting the level of resistance to their effort. Then have the person being tested stare at a large square of pink cardboard or construction paper placed about 35 centimeters (fifteen inches) in front of the eyes for about thirty seconds. On testing the arm strength in the same way, it will now be found that the arms are less resistant to being pulled down to the waist! To restore the arm strength, stare at a blue piece of cardboard placed similarly and for a comparable length of time. It is also said that weakness is induced by wearing a wristwatch or wearing clothing made of synthetic blends. Though it is difficult to imagine how this might work, it may be that we will perform the *yogasanas* with more strength if we avoid these energy-sapping objects.

With respect to the arm-strength test described above, Schauss [740] reports that the effect of staring at a pink square of cardboard is evident in less than three seconds, that it works as well with color-blind subjects, and that accomplished athletes and martial-arts practitioners cannot resist the effect, no matter how consciously they try. He invokes the endocrine system in the effect but otherwise offers no explanation.

The color pink has been shown to be quite effective in calming aggressive and potentially violent people, but only if the exposure to the color is of the order of ten to twenty minutes or so, for if the stimulation extends beyond a half-hour, the opposite emotional response results. Thus, the color pink must be used judiciously in the *yogasana* studio, if at all.[1] In distinction to pink, wearing the color red by humans is said to result in a reflexive testosterone surge in the wearer, but a submissive reaction when one sees one's opponent wearing it [530].

The same decrease and restoration of the arm strength can be demonstrated using the emotions, rather than colored cardboard [649]. In this case, it will be found that the arms are more easily pulled down if the person being tested is thinking of something very sad at the time of the test, but that arm strength is restored upon thinking of some very happy situation.

In both of the cases cited above, it would appear that both the color pink (a shade that results from mixing red with white) and sad thoughts stimulate the parasympathetic nervous system, resulting in a relaxation of the muscles and a consequent relative isometric weakness (Subsection 11.A, page 407), whereas happy thoughts and the color blue erase the parasympathetic dominance and restore the isometric strength. These observations are odd, because blue, in general, is a parasympathetic stimulant, and red is a sympathetic stimulant [89], yet in these experiments, the opposite correlation is suggested. However,

---

1   Many prisons in the United States recently have reported that they are painting their community rooms in a shade of pink in order to reduce violence among their populations. Presumably, they have found just that shade of pink that is calming over a period of time longer than twenty minutes.

see page 687 for a discussion on the differing effects of "blue" lights of slightly different wavelength, and the footnote on page 684 for a similar discussion on shades of "pink."

Perhaps the answer to our paradox lies in the visual stimulation involving a left-right neural crossover at the optic chiasm, whereas thinking of positive or negative emotional situations is localized in one hemisphere or the other, but there is no crossover. Moreover, pink is not red, and though blue often may be sedating, it can be relatively energizing with respect to pink. Another possibility is that the effects of the colors are not directly on the muscle strength but on the motivational system within the emotional limbic area of the brain (Section 2.D, page 27), as this controls the tendency to want to use the muscles. Finally—and most likely— it appears that the affective responses to viewing blue and pink objects are very sensitive to small changes in the wavelengths of peak reflectivity of the viewed objects, and this has not been properly controlled for in most experiments yet. (See the footnote on page 687 in support of this point of view.)

red light at 25 hertz in order to promote the alertness of the sympathetic beta-wave state, or the blue light at 6 hertz to stimulate the dreaminess of the parasympathetic theta-wave state (Subsection 4.H, page 153). Additionally, as described in Subsection 15.E, page 629, simply blocking one nostril or the other also is effective in triggering a shift of cerebral dominance and would make an interesting addition to the study of the color effects on *yogasana* practice.

Colored Lights as Props

Though the external manipulation of the autonomic nervous system through the use of blinking colored lights does not sound very yogic, perhaps one can accept it more readily if it is thought of as just another prop, like a bolster or a belt. As such, it can help lead one more quickly to experience the full spectrum of the effects of a particular *yogasana* on the body and mind, but it is to be done with the attitude of eventually working without the prop. Most importantly, the benefits of enhancing the effects of a *yogasana* posture through the use of colored lights could be profound in those cases where yoga is being practiced as therapy for a condition involving imbalance within the autonomic nervous system.

With the regular white lights on in the *yogasana* room, the colors entering the students' eyes will be those of the paint on the walls and the props nearby. These colors should be chosen

with due regard for the physiological and psychological effects desired by the teacher. The color of our clothing when practicing the *yogasanas* also can be a psychological factor, as discussed in Box 17.E-2, page 686.

White-Light Starvation

Seasonal Affective Disorder

In the Arctic Circle, there is near or complete darkness throughout the winter days, twenty-four hours a day. In response to this lack of light in the winter months, the population becomes depressed and the suicide rate soars. In more normal situations, the short days of winter deprive office workers and shut-ins of their optimum dose of natural light, and seasonal affective disorder (SAD) sets in [474]. In the United States, SAD is most prevalent in the states of the northern tier (Washington to Maine), with relatively little occurring in the south; whereas SAD affects only 9 percent of the winter population of Sarasota, Florida, the corresponding figure for the more northern city, Nashua, New Hampshire, is 30 percent.

Women are far more likely to be affected by the lack of natural sunshine in the winter months than are men, especially between the ages of twenty to forty years. It is also the case that the incidences of several cancer types are at their highest in the

---

Box 17.E-2: Hiding behind/within Black Pants

Color is a factor in *yogasana* practice in a rather unexpected way. Three-dimensional shape is perceived by the contrast in shading, shadows, or coloring. Thus, the subtle shadows evident in the seat of your pants when you are wearing white pants is revealing of the true shape of your buttocks. Because such shadows are much less obvious in black pants, your seat clad in black will look much flatter and smaller when viewed by others from the back, but not from the side. This may be why so may *yogasana* students gravitate to black pants when practicing in a group situation. In a similar vein, wearing full-length black pants can make it more difficult for your teacher to see that your legs are somewhat bent in the standing postures. Just as logically, one can change other students' view of your *yogasanas* by wearing vertical stripes when in *vrksasana,* so as to appear more upwardly extended! Actually, one should avoid wearing striped clothing when practicing with a *yogasana* teacher, as the stripes interfere with the teacher's sense of your body position.

---

same northern-tier states that are highest in SAD cases, suggesting that it is the lack of vitamin D as otherwise generated by skin exposure to sunshine in these areas that is responsible for these cancers. This relates to the fact that the vitamin D generated by just a few minutes' exposure to the sun at summer is known to retard the proliferation of colorectal cancers. Of course, excessive exposure to the ultraviolet rays in sunshine raises the risk of contracting skin cancer [62]. Here we see once again how small doses can be beneficial whereas larger doses of the same treatment can be deadly; see Section 16.F, page 654.

Symptoms

SAD is largely an emotional disorder, with symptoms that include strong mood swings, low energy, depression, overeating, low sex drive, social withdrawal, continued sleepiness, and lowered immune function. These symptoms appear with the winter months (December through February are the worst, as with fatal heart attack [803]) and disappear once spring arrives [149, 473]. It is interesting to note that the symptoms of SAD closely match those reported for atypical depression (Section 22.A, page 756). Indeed, just as there is an atypical depression, there is also a summertime SAD, with symptoms opposite to those stated above for wintertime SAD [474] but for which the strongest factor is extreme heat rather than extreme light. SAD resembles depression, except that when depressed, people often lose interest in food, lose weight, and have trouble sleeping, whereas in SAD, all of these symptoms are reversed, especially in regard to the craving for carbohydrates as the days lengthen. People with SAD are parasympathetic dominant; i.e., they show a slowed physiology, as if getting ready to hibernate.

Mechanism

The suprachiasmatic nucleus (SCN), the size of a grain of rice and located in the hypothalamus (figure 5.B-1), is the body's internal clock. As long as there is sufficient light incident on the retinal ganglia, the SCN inhibits the pineal gland from releasing its supply of sleep-inducing melatonin; however, when the sunlight becomes weaker and its time shorter, then the pineal gland is able to release its melatonin into the blood and the drowsy SAD state appears [684a]. Details of the mechanism involving the SCN are given in Subsection 23.B, page 787. In addition to melatonin, serotonin is also implicated in the SAD mechanism, as its level in the blood is very low at midwinter, when SAD is strongest.

Treatment

Patients with SAD are easily treated by exposure to full-spectrum lights with brightness five to ten times larger than that of ordinary room lights. Such exposure drives down the melatonin in the blood (Subsection 6.B, page 215), especially when given early in the morning when the body would normally begin its transition from parasympathetic to sympathetic activities; this treatment can erase all SAD symptoms in a few days [508, 803]. Light therapy for mild to moderate depression associated with SAD is independent of the season. Further research shows that blue-light exposure is more effective than red-light exposure in erasing the symptoms of SAD [684a].[6]

Antidepressant drugs also are effective in reversing SAD; however, this course of treatment usually takes several weeks to become effective. It is possible that the energizing *yogasanas* performed in red light, incident from the left and blinking at 25 hertz, also would be of use in dispelling SAD symptoms, as *yogasanas* are already known to be effective against depression (Section 22.A, page 761). As bright-light therapy is also known to be effective against bulimia and type-D PMS [474], a switch to pulsed colored lights may enhance these therapies as well. A thirty-to-sixty-minute exposure to bright light in the morning is now deemed to be as effective as the use of antidepressant drugs.

---

6   There is a certain amount of confusion in regard to the affective effects of "blue light," but the differences may reflect the fact that some experiments were done with blue light having a strong 430-nanometer component and other experiments were done with a strong 480-nanometer component. In the latter case, there is excitation of ganglion receptors and an elevation of the mood, whereas in the former, it is the retinal blue cones that are excited, and the mood is relaxed. As applied to the yoga studio, it appears that it would be best to use lights that are rich in the 480-nanometer blue wavelengths in the morning, but which then fade toward 430-nanometer wavelength around noon. The lights then should be switched back to 480-nanometer wavelength for afternoon practice to counter afternoon sleepiness among students, and finally switched a second time to 430-nanometer wavelength in the evening to relax them [684a].

Sound, Hearing, and Balance

18

Section 18.A: The Middle Ear

The Mechanics of Hearing

Hearing is another of our sensory organs in which the primary sensor is a hair cell sensitive to the motions of the medium in which it is immersed. The outer ear functions as a funnel, steering sound into the external auditory canal and onto the tympanic membrane of the middle ear (figure 18.A-1). The sound waves, being alternate longitudinal compressions and expansions of the air carrying the acoustic energy, beat upon the tympanic membrane and set it into motion. If the sound is pitched high, the membrane will oscillate at a high frequency, and if the sound is at a low pitch, the frequency of the membrane vibration will be correspondingly low.

Signal Transduction

The inner surface of the tympanic membrane is connected to the first of three small bones in the middle ear (the malleus, the incus, and the stapes, figure 18.A-1), which together function as a mechanical amplifier, increasing the amplitude of the mechanical vibration by a factor of almost twenty [360, 427]. The stapes, in turn, is connected to the oval window that is the thin membrane covering the entrance to the endolymph-filled cochlea. As its name implies, the cochlea is a spirally wound tube resembling a cockle shell; down the center of this tube, there is a basilar membrane

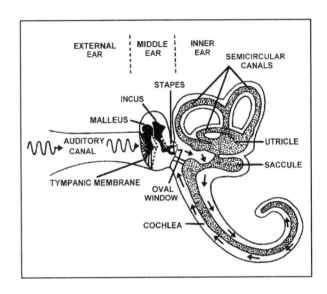

Figure 18.A-1. Structures of the middle and inner ears [360]. The three bones of the middle ear stop growing in infancy and so are the smallest bones in the adult body. Their positions are shown as dashed lines when the tympanic membrane is pushed inward by a sound wave traveling from left to right. In order to more clearly show its internal structure, the cochlea has been drawn partially uncoiled. The arrows show the direction of the sound waves in the cochlea.

of decreasing thickness and decreasing tension, which bears the motion-sensitive hair cells. The middle ear has the smallest number of sensory cells of any sense organ, there being only 3,500 hair cells in the middle ear versus one hundred million photoreceptors in the retina of the eye. Though humans have thirty-eight optic nerve fibers for every auditory nerve, some animals do accentuate sound over sight, and these animals have approximately equal numbers of optic and auditory neurons.

Incoming sound waves that beat upon the oval window set up standing acoustical waves in the cochlea, to be sensed by the motions of the hairs protruding from the sensor cells. The position of largest disturbance along the basilar membrane is dependent upon the frequency of the sound at that moment. High-frequency sound will excite hairs close to the oval window, whereas lower frequencies will produce disturbance further from the window. Whereas intense sound of frequency f can destroy sensitivity at frequency f, it will have a much smaller effect at neighboring frequencies. There are no blood vessels serving the basilar membrane, for if there were, the arterial pulse would be deafening [297].

As seems to be the case with all hair-cell sensors in the body (Subsection 13.B, page 508), those of the cochlea transduce their bending under a mechanical stimulus (sound, in this case) into a modulated electrical wave, the neural frequency of which reflects the intensity of the sound wave at the particular acoustic frequency for which the hair cell is sensitive. Moreover, the neurons that synapse with the hair cells also are strongly frequency-tuned, so that each hair-cell/neuron combination is very frequency-selective and can phase-lock to a pure tone, at least at low frequency. Excitable hair cells use K^+ ions moving outward across the cell membrane rather than Na^+ ions moving inward to depolarize the axonal membrane.

Considering the two ears as antennae, their peak sensitivity will be at an acoustic wavelength equal to the ear-to-ear distance [878]. For humans, this distance corresponds to a frequency of about 2,000 hertz; for the squeaking mouse, it will be at much higher frequency, and for the rumbling elephant, much lower. This law relating the ear-to-ear distance and the frequency of highest sensitivity is obeyed by the ears of all mammals. In young adults, the effective auditory range is 20–20,000 hertz; however, this shrinks to 50–8,000 hertz in the elderly. Interestingly, the

ear can easily detect an acoustic vibration at 5,000 hertz, whereas the maximal neural frequency for mechanical motions is closer to 1,000 hertz. This means that the hair that detects a particular frequency above 1,000 hertz does not do so by necessarily being tuned to that frequency, but is placed within a cochlear structure that shows a frequency dispersion depending upon position [671a].

Hair-Cell Efferents

It is known that there are both efferent and afferent nerve fibers to and from the cochlear hair cells. The former are a puzzle, as other hair-cell sensors in the body are not supplied with efferents (however, see Section 20.E, page 727). On the other hand, other hair cells are not frequency-sensitive as are the hair cells in the middle ear; perhaps the efferent nerve stimulates muscles at the base of the hair cell and in some way helps to fine-tune the stiffness of the hair so as to adjust its frequency response. If so, then its action would be somewhat like that of the contractile γ-motor system at the ends of the muscle spindles (Subsection 11.B, page 430).

The Auditory Nerves

The auditory nerve fibers (cranial nerve VIII, page 25) deliver the acoustic signals to the cochlear nuclei in the temporal lobes, and these signals then ascend to eventually reach the superior temporal gyri in the cortex, where the sound finally makes its impression on the conscious mind. The signals from each of the ears have neural connections to both cerebral hemispheres, but the stronger connection is to the contralateral hemisphere [270, 451], as with two of the hemiretinal signals for vision (figure 17.D-1). There are several sites in the brainstem at which the auditory signal can crossover in order to terminate at the contralateral cerebral hemisphere [621].

Waking Up

Input from the auditory nerve into the reticular formation has a strong effect on the arousal, attention, and wakefulness of the listener, depending upon the quality and intensity of the sound. When we are asleep, the muscles of the middle ear are relaxed, and so the ear has maximum sensitivity to extraneous noises. Moreover, there are collateral neural tracts from the middle ear directly to the reticular formation in the pons (Subsection 4.A, page 74), this being the wakefulness center. If there is a threatening noise while we sleep, the reticular formation will receive the message and immediately awaken both the central nervous system and the muscles, for defensive action.

Psychology

The psychology of our hearing is such that the sound of a waterfall, the sound of tires rolling down the highway, and the sound of raindrops falling on the roof all are soothing and relaxing, being random "white noise" that does not excite the reticular formation. On the other hand, the sound of a dripping faucet is more like the sound of a stalking predator and so has an extremely irritating effect on us as we try to fall asleep. Specific nuclei in the brain receive signals from both ears, compare their timing, and then compute a direction and distance for the sound source, thereby allowing the brain to compose a sound map of the environment.

Competition with Vision

If one focuses all of one's attention on a visual scene, the auditory sensitivity fades toward zero; the *yogasana* teacher should be aware of this in regard to students who may be inclined toward one learning mode or the other, and the teacher should try to maintain a balance between visual and auditory instruction. The opposite situation also seems to hold true: intense concentration on talking on the cell phone while driving, for example, leads to diminished visual awareness and to many auto accidents. It appears that there is a competition between different sensory modes, so that when a person is struggling to hear, there is often a tendency to close the eyes, as if to lessen the visual congestion incident on the auditory path. Similarly, when you remove your glasses, you may strain to "see" and so may lose auditory sensitivity.

There exists an interesting correlation between auditory acuity and blindness that further illustrates the plasticity of the brain (Subsection 4.C, page 80). It is known that people who are born blind are better able to hear than those who can see, and the advantage rests in the processing of the auditory data in the area of the brain normally reserved for visual stimulation! As compared with the seeing, people who are born blind learn to recognize voices at an earlier age, can detect changes in pitch that are undetectable by the seeing, and are better able to pinpoint the sources of sound. In all such situations, it was found that the brain of the blind was recruiting the visual area of the brain, Brodmann area 17 (figure 4.C-1), to help in processing sounds.

Aging

For the general population, the numbers of receptors and synapses in the auditory channel decrease with increasing age, and so the ability to hear degrades with time [162]. However, as inversions such as *sirsasana* and *sarvangasana* bring fresh blood to the head, it may be that for the aging students who do these inverted *yogasanas* regularly, the loss of hearing is slowed.

Second Sound

The above description of the hearing mechanism involves the upward movement of the hearing sensation into the consciousness of the primary auditory cortices within both cerebral hemispheres. However, just as with vision (Subsection 17.B, page 669), there is a second path available for auditory signals involving subcortical centers, resulting in both a reflexive subconscious response and a slower but more conscious response to the sensory signal [30].

Music and the Brain

Auditory Laterality

Inasmuch as the left cerebral hemisphere is more effective at speech processing in right-handed people, the contralateral right ear is more effective at receiving and amplifying speech messages in such people [427], whereas pure musical tones are amplified more strongly in the left ear

[451, 796]; i.e., the left ear is the superior one for the appreciation of music, as it activates the right cerebral hemisphere [204]. Pleasure in hearing music stimulates the same brain centers that respond to eating chocolate, having sex, or taking cocaine.

For beginning students in music, rhythm is sensed in the left hemisphere, in the frontal, parietal, and temporal lobes, and in the cerebellum, but pitch and melody are handled in the right hemisphere. The center for evaluating perfect pitch resides in the upper temporal lobe and must be exercised before age seven years if it is to be effective in the adult.

The experience of mechanical rhythms helps to develop the perception of musical beats. Because our rhythm perception is closely tied to our motor system, if the auditory beat is that of a hot Latin band, we cannot suppress an in-time tapping of the toes. When babies are rocked or bounced to a specific rhythm, they learn to enjoy music with the same rhythms.

Music and Plasticity

As the music student becomes more adept, the active regions of the brain shift, so that these regions are very different for beginners and professional musicians. Moreover, at any given age, the musical-brain structures will be very different for trumpet and violin players [6a]. Though there is an auditory area in the brain, there does not appear to be a specific area in the brain for music, though recognition of rhythm and timbre are strongly localized in one hemisphere or the other. Studies on the effects of music on brain structure yield many examples of brain plasticity:

» When a tone of a particular frequency is coupled with a reward, the area in the brain where the tone of that frequency is sensed increases in size at the expense of neighboring tones.

» Musicians who usually practice certain hand motions for many hours per day for years show hyperdevelopment of certain brain areas. Thus, brain regions that receive sensory signals from the second to fifth fingers of the left hand of violinists are unusually large, whereas those of the same fingers on the bowing hand are no different than those of nonmusicians. (See Subsection 4.C, page 89, for a discussion of the map of the motor cortex.)

» String musicians who began playing before age thirteen years have larger cortical representations of the fingers of their left hands than do those who began to play only after age thirteen years. As with the body, we see that the ability to change one's brain is more difficult the older one is. This extreme plasticity of the brain at an early age no doubt is a factor in the musical genius of children such as Wolfgang Amadeus Mozart [427a].

» The volume of the auditory cortex is 30 percent larger in musicians than in nonmusicians.

» For keyboard players, there is a much stronger coordination of left-hand and right-hand operations, and correspondingly, the anterior commissure connecting the right and left hemispheres is much thicker than normal. In contrast, the inter-cerebral connections within the brains of many autistic "musical geniuses" often are weak or totally missing, thereby assuring that one cerebral hemisphere does not inhibit the functions of the other (Subsection 4.G, page 144).

» The actual sizes of the motor cortex and the cerebellum are both unusually large in musicians as compared with those of nonmusicians.

» The brains of trumpet players react in an intensified manner only to the sounds of the trumpet and not at all to the sounds of the violin [477a].

Yogasana and the Middle Ear

There are several notable facts about the clever mechanical system within the middle ear. First, the two end bones of the middle ear (the malleus and the stapes) are connected to muscles that, when contracted, restrict the motion of the bones and so lower the amplification factor for sound traveling through the middle ear. This is used in the middle-ear reflex [360, 878] wherein the muscles tighten in response to loud sounds and so restrict the motion of the bones whenever the acoustic intensity becomes too high.

The muscles of the middle ear are skeletal muscles, just as the biceps of the arm and quadriceps of the leg are skeletal muscles. However, whereas the latter can be activated when we will them to be so, that is not the case with those of the middle ear, for these muscles can be activated only reflexively, in response to a loud noise or in expectation of a loud noise [268]; however, they can be relaxed voluntarily, as discussed in Box 18.A-1, below. The muscle activating the stapes, the stapedius, is the smallest skeletal muscle in the body, less than 1 millimeter (0.04 inches) long, and its action, when contracted, is to reduce the amplitude of the oval-window vibrations during times of loud noise.

The Autonomic Nervous System

The auditory muscles of the middle ear have a significant muscle tone in the normal, everyday situation, but during relaxation, the parasympathetic branch of the autonomic nervous system is activated—trigeminal nucleus (cranial nerve V) for the malleus and the facial nucleus (cranial nerve VII) for the stapes)—and the muscles of the middle ear relax, thereby greatly increasing the ears' sensitivity. Thus, when in *savasana* with the body very relaxed, the ears become very sensitive, and a modest noise can be very startling [878]. The muscles of the middle ear are very active during the REM phase of sleep (Subsection 23.D, page 800), along with the movement of the eyes in this phase [427]. On the other hand, the three external muscles of the outer ear in earlier times allowed the ears to move without moving the head; they are now no longer of any use to humans, except to amuse children.

Random Noise

Random noise is both physiologically and ethically injurious to us: it leads not only to low birth weight, headache, poor learning, heart disease, high blood pressure, gastrointestinal distress, and fatigue but also makes us less likely to assist strangers in need or to recommend raises for workers; when subject to random noise, we become more willing to administer electrical shocks to strangers [439]. Clearly, the *yogasana* workplace should be as free of extraneous noise as possible.

Students performing *sirsasana I* on the bare floor occasionally report hearing clicking sounds within the head during the first few minutes. Donohue [209] refers to this as a form of tinnitus and attributes this to rapid contractions of the muscles in the middle ear or the palate, whereas von Hippel [878] attributes it instead to electrical stimulation of the middle ear in some unspecified way. That a case of tinnitus recently was cured when the patient's middle-ear musculature relaxed as his collapsed chest and forward-head posture were addressed and corrected suggests that tinnitus could be an encouraging arena for *yogasana* therapy [387a, 790a].

Internally Generated Sounds

Nada Sound

In the human ear, even with no sound incident on the tympanic membrane, there is a 100–300 hertz hum coming from the resting hair cells in the cochlea [443], this being a frequency well within the auditory range. Consequently, when one's meditation is deep and oriented toward hearing the inner sound, the resting signal of the hair cells can be heard loud and clear as *nada*, the sound current [252, 443]. Since the different cilia are tuned to different frequencies, shifting between them can give rise to a variety of sounds, as observed in *nada yoga*. As one ascends the yoga ladder, the *nada* current becomes the inner focus of the practices from *pratyahara* to *samadhi*. From the perspective of kundalini yoga, the *nada* is sensed as the kundalini passes through the *anahata* (heart) *chakra* and is heard in the right ear [841].

Explanations of the *nada* sound run from tinnitus, present in 20 percent of the population, to

Box 18.A-1: Relaxing the Muscles of the Middle Ear

When a bat screeches in order to echolocate flying insects, the muscles in its middle ears become very taut, thereby decreasing the bat's aural sensitivity. This guarantees that the loud screech does not flood the sound sensors; however, immediately afterward, the same muscles relax totally, and the sensitive ears then listen for the telltale echo of the bat's next meal [928]. In humans, something of the same sort happens, for as we sneeze, the stapedius muscles of the middle ears are drawn tight so as to lower the auditory sensitivity to the roar of the nearly supersonic explosion of gas from the lungs through the nose (see Subsection 15.C, page 617). At the same time, the eyes are reflexively closed.

The muscular mechanism protecting the middle ear from acoustic overload is analogous, in a way, to that of the iris of the eye, which contracts under conditions of bright light, thus protecting the retina from sensory overload, but which dilates in dim light to raise the sensory-signal level (Subsection 17.A, page 661).

You can experience directly the effects of relaxing the stapedius muscles of the middle ears in the following way. First, set the volume control of your radio so low that it is barely audible or just inaudible when placed next to your mat. Then lie down in *savasana*; immediately upon relaxing, note how much louder the radio volume becomes as relaxation of the muscles of the middle ears increases the ears' sensitivity. Indeed, people unfortunate enough to have lost control of the α-motor neuron driving the stapedius muscle have uncomfortably acute hearing. Keep this increased aural sensitivity in mind when you speak in order to bring your students out of *savasana*.

The fact that our hearing is the only one of our five cognitive senses that actually becomes more sensitive as we relax suggests that it would be the last such sense to be quieted during the sensory withdrawal sought during meditation [812]. This increased sensitivity of the ear on relaxation may result in the "extrasensory perceptions" sensed during *pratyahara* practice [851].

Relaxing in *Savasana*

The level of relaxation in *savasana* has been measured with and without a guided commentary on how and what to relax, using oxygen consumption and heart rate as indicators of general sympathetic tone. It was found that the relaxation was deeper when the students were guided by such things as being told to relax each part of the body sequentially from toes to head, as compared with the relaxation level reached by students who silently found their own relaxed state [873]. A deeply relaxed state also was achieved while in *savasana* when the teacher instructed the students to sequentially tighten each of the muscles isometrically from toes to head, naming each body part, and then instructing the students to let the body parts successively collapse into the relaxed state [872].

Aural Sensitivity

The contrary response of the ears' sensitivity is also easily experienced. In this case, set the radio volume so that it is just audible, and then lie back over an exercise ball, so as to be in a passive, supported backbend with head below hips. The radio's message will fade within a minute after beginning the backbend, and full auditory sensitivity will be restored immediately (in healthy students) on becoming upright. This loss of hearing on inversion has been reported in the medical literature [668] and has been attributed to high blood pressure in the middle ear, which stretches the ligament attached to the stapes footplate and so stiffens the ear's response. Blood congestion in the middle ear also is reported to be a consequence of nasal laterality (table 15.E-2), which is itself a consequence of unilateral congestion of the nasal passage (Subsection 15.E, page 628). Anoxia also may be a factor in this effect.

This phenomenon of a partial loss of hearing on inversion is much like descending in an airplane and having the pressure outside the ears decrease. In this case too, the level of hearing sensitivity falls. As shown in figure 18.A-1, the middle ear appears to be a closed container, disconnected from the atmosphere outside. However, the nasal-throat cavity within the mouth is joined to the middle ear by the eustachian tube, which connection allows the air pressure within the middle ear to equalize with that within the mouth when we swallow, and the hearing returns.

a spontaneous firing of the neurons that occurs in most mammals whenever there is an absence of sound stimulation; this latter explanation is thought to be due to the brain "listening out."

The Sound of "Om"

It is recently reported that the Earth undergoes free oscillations with a period of between 150 and 500 seconds, as determined from an analysis of seismic data [152, 838]. The most probable force driving this bell-like ringing of the Earth arises from variations in atmospheric pressure alternately pressing inward and outward on the Earth's surface. Note that though we speak of this ringing of the Earth as a "sound," it is at far too low a frequency (2–7 millihertz) to be heard by the middle ear, which has a low-frequency cutoff of 20 hertz. In several experiments, people do report "shivers down their spines" when exposed to sound waves below the 20-hertz cutoff; however, it is not clear that the sensations involve the ears. Is it possible that these two recent scientific discoveries have anything to do with the sound of the universe as reported in the yoga texts as the all-permeating "Om" [253] when in deeply meditative states?

In an independent and totally unrelated study,

it is reported that very small pressure changes of the order of 1/1000 of the total atmospheric pressure, having periods of about fifteen to ninety seconds, are sensed subconsciously by human beings, as witnessed by their clear effects on mental activity and test-taking [881]. Perhaps in the altered consciousness of the meditator, the effects of the low-frequency pressure changes (11–70 millihertz) and the Earth's constant low-frequency hum are brought into the conscious realm and interpreted as sound within the normal acoustic range.

The Earth's hum is now known to rise and fall in intensity, peaking in December-February and again in June-August; one would predict the same for the volume of the "Om" sound if it is really related to the Earth's oscillation! If so, then the "sound" is truly global, if not universal. It is also possible that the Earth's ringing relates in some way to the sense that many animals have of an impending earthquake or tsunami. It is thought that these very low frequency acoustic waves in the Earth's crust are the result of the breaking of wind-driven ocean waves against the sea bottom.

Schumann Waves

Electromagnetic Schumann waves (Subsection 4.H, page 154) have been identified in the Earth's atmosphere at a frequency of 7–10 hertz. Oscillations are also found at this frequency in the brain waves of meditators, clairvoyants, and healers (Subsection 4.H, page 149). The generation of what are said to be Schumann waves in injured bodies helps heal injuries and fractures, the therapy being done with sound speakers and low-frequency gongs at the Schumann frequency. The frequencies of the low-frequency acoustic Schumann waves match the breathing frequency for maximum relaxation in meditation and prayer, and these are invoked to explain a cat's purring when injured. Note, however, that the true Schumann waves are electromagnetic, whereas the therapy described above is acoustic instead, albeit at the Schumann wave frequency. Thus, there is some confusion afoot in this work. Moreover, the frequency of acoustic Schumann waves is below the normal threshold for hearing in humans and so must be sensed by a means other than the middle ear, if at all. Perhaps the mechanism involved in sensing acoustic waves at the Schumann frequency is the same as that used in sensing atmospheric-pressure changes, as explained above for the case of the universal "Om."

The connection of sound to other body/mind processes is well-known. For example, it is known that by playing soft music before surgery, 50–60 percent less anesthetic is required, and that the nausea of chemotherapy also can be reduced by such soft music [103]. In a technique called "toning," singing the vowel "e" is stimulating, bright, and awakening, whereas the same song sung with "ah" resembles the sound of exhalation and brings on the full relaxation response [103]. Yogis will recognize this effect when chanting "Om." The silent chanting of "Om" noticeably reduces the heart rate in experienced meditators, indicating a relaxed state; however, the same meditators also showed an increased peripheral vascular resistance, indicating an increased sympathetic tone acting to constrict the vascular system [854].

Section 18.B: The Vestibular Organs of Balance

Structure and Function of the Inner Ear

In addition to the middle ears so essential for hearing, all vertebrate animals have inner ears (the vestibular organs), which serve as organs of balance [878]. Unlike our other senses, such as vision, taste, and temperature, the sensations of the balancing organs of the vestibule are not at all bright in our consciousness, being more obvious only when we become dizzy or nauseous. The sensory signals from the three types of vestibular organs (called the utricle, the saccule, and the semicircular canals), together with those from the eyes (Subsection 17.B, page 668), pressure sensors in the skin, and the body's proprioceptors (Section 11.C, page 441) work together to maintain posture and balance. The vestibular organs of the inner ear, along with the eyes and the muscles, are key players in the body-righting reflex, the purpose of which is to restore the body to its normal upright position when off-balance. Interruption of the neural signals involved in this reflex can cause nausea and vomiting, in addition to falling.

Sensors for the Static Position of the Head

Utricle and Saccule

The otolith organs forming the vestibular systems within each of the inner ears (figure 18.B-1) are composed of the utricle and the saccule, largely responsible for sensing either the static orientation of the head in the gravitational field (see Appendix IV, page 856) or the direction of linear accelerated or decelerated motion of the head; and the three nearby semicircular canals, which are sensitive to the dynamic forces generated by accelerating or decelerating rotational motions of the head [360, 427, 432, 878]. The vestibular organs on the two sides of the head work together, so that those in one inner ear may reflexively excite extensor muscles on its side of the body, for example, whereas those on the other side inhibit the corresponding extensors on the contralateral side of the body. The utricle and saccule sensors within each ear are sensitive to translation of the body as a whole, all the while keeping the head in the neutral position. Thus, the utricle is activated when moving horizontally as when riding in an automobile, and the saccule is activated when moving vertically, as when in a moving elevator.

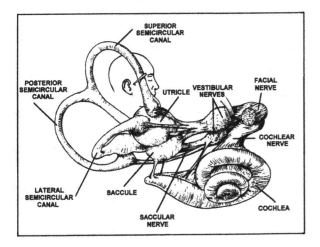

Figure 18.B-1. Details of the vestibular organs and associated nerve bundles within the inner ear, as seen when viewed through the right temple [360].

The entire inner-ear structure is surrounded by a sack of perilymph, which serves to isolate it acoustically from extraneous bone-conducting vibrations and from the sounds of the blood flowing through the skull [878]. The actions of the vestibular organs in maintaining balance in various *yogasanas* are described in Subsection V.C, page 893.

The Kinocilium

The utricle (figure 18.B-1) is a small, closed sac containing both a lymph-like fluid and a gelatinous mass, in which are embedded microcrystals (otoliths) of calcium carbonate. It also contains a horizontal swath of very specialized hair cells, each

of which is in truth a bundle of yet smaller hairs. In this bundle, there is one special hair called the kinocilium, which resides on the outermost surface of the bundle. If, for some reason, the hair bundle were to be bent toward its kinocilium, this would induce a permeability change in the wall of the hair cell, allowing potassium ions (K^+) to flow through the membrane with the development of a transmembrane depolarization voltage. If, on the other hand, the bending were opposite, then the transmembrane voltage across the wall of the hair cell would become hyperpolarized, indicating that the K^+ ions were flowing in the opposite direction. It is the tipping of the head that causes the gelatinous matrix to press obliquely on the hair bundles of the utricle. The mechanism by which the hair cells of the vestibular apparatus sense an external force (gravitational or one of accelerating or decelerating motion) resembles that used by the Pacinian cells (Section 13.B, page 511) to sense pressure on the skin. However, these skin sensors have no directional sense, and they function on the basis of changes in Na^+ permeability rather than K^+.

The kinocilium is always found on the side of its hair bundle, but not on the same side in all bundles. Thus, a force on the plane of bundles, as when tilting the head, will bend some kinocilia in a direction leading to hyperpolarization and others in a direction leading to depolarization. It is this directionality of the hair cells' sensitivity and their ability to both hyperpolarize and depolarize that allow the brain to deduce both the magnitude and the direction of the displacement force. This ability of the vestibular sensors is unique, for most peripheral sensors (such as the Pacinian organs; see Subsection 13.B, page 511) only depolarize or only hyperpolarize (the retinal cells of the eyes, for example; see Subsection 17.B, page 667). Note too that the Ruffini corpuscles (Subsection 11.B, page 440) are sensitive to both pressure applied to the skin and to the direction from which the pressure comes.

Transduction

As with the other mechanoreceptors, the membrane potentials of the hair cells in the inner ear are transduced into frequencies; when the head is held horizontally, the static hair-cell output has a constant frequency of 100–300 hertz, which then is increased or decreased as the hair cells are bent either toward or away from the kinocilium. Strangely, this is the frequency range known for the resting frequency of the middle-ear hair cells, which can be heard when meditating on the inner sound (*nada yoga;* see Subsection 18.A, page 693) [443].

The saccule seems to be much like the utricle, with two exceptions. First, it is exposed to external sound waves, whereas the utricle is not; second, its swath of hair cells is oriented vertically rather than horizontally. It is thought to function in a way parallel to the utricle but sensing tilt away from verticality. The saccule does appear to have an auditory sensitivity in the 50–1,000 hertz acoustical range, and with direct connections to the hypothalamus, it may be responsible for the pleasure derived from chanting and listening to music [540]. Hearing loud bass tones might be pleasurable due to their close relation to the mating calls of lower vertebrates [898].

Sensors for the Dynamic Movement of the Head

Semicircular Canals

The semicircular canals (figure 18.B-1) are composed of three half-circle tubes oriented with their planes mutually perpendicular so as to be sensitive to rotation around any or all of the three axes of the head. Because each of the semicircular canals is open at both ends and terminates at the utricle sac, a set of three complete rings is formed through their common utricle sacs. Semicircular canals operate in the pitch plane (as when nodding the head "yes"), in the yaw plane (as when shaking the head "no"), and in the roll plane (as when tilting the head to the side). The canals are positioned in the head so that when the forehead is tilted 30° downward from its normal position, one of the canals is then truly in the horizontal plane. The two vertical planes within each ear are perpendicular to one another but inclined at 45° to the median plane.

Bent Hairs

Tipping of the head forward stretches the muscles in the back of the neck and so activates static stretch sensors in the capitis muscles (figure V.C-1), which are very important in proprioceptive head orientation and balancing. On the other hand, each semicircular canal has a filling of viscous fluid and a pad of hair cells (with kinocilia that act just as those described above for the utricle and saccule) mounted upon an elastic membrane. In the case of the semicircular canals, it is accelerating or decelerating rotation of the head that stimulates the hair cells, with the canals moving more rapidly than the fluid inside of them due to the inertia of the latter. The inertial drag on the hair cells by the enclosed fluid bends the hair bundles and so alters the rate of firing of the hair cells, with those on one side of the head increasing in rate and those on the opposite side decreasing in rate.

Motion Sickness

The signals output by the semicircular canals travel to the medial and superior vestibular nuclei. The information on the speed and direction of head rotation no doubt complements that from the joint receptors monitoring the kinesthetic stimuli as the limbs move (Section 7.E, page 251). If the head rolls in one or more planes simultaneously, the hyperexcitation of the semicircular canals can lead to motion sickness. This can be cured with anticholinergic drugs [565], but then the vestibular input to the central nervous system is blocked, and one is disoriented and has blurred vision. Random noise in the semicircular canals, as with Meniere's disease, expresses itself as a loss of balance.

The semicircular canals are responsible for the nausea of seasickness and motion sickness. With each lurch to the side, the semicircular canals signal the brain to turn the eyes, to squeeze the internal organs, and to shift weight in order to regain balance. However, just as this is accomplished, the body is tossed in the opposite direction, and a new compensating strategy is set into play. It is this effort to compensate for this back-and-forth motion that sets the signals from the semicircular canals and those from the eyes in conflict, as the eyes readjust more quickly than the semicircular canals, and the result is confusing to both the brain and the digestion.

A strong rap on the head can knock the otoliths of the utricle into the semicircular canals, leading to severe dizziness; should the hair-cell signals of the vestibular apparatus and the visual signals of the horizon then disagree as to the position of the head, then any motion will quickly become sickening [450]. As long as the signal of each particular semicircular canal is the same on the two sides of the head, then the head position is balanced.

Ocular-Vestibular Reflex

The semicircular canals also are important in the reflex action that keeps the eyes turning left, for example, while the head is turning right, thus allowing the eyes to stay focused on a single point in space as the head turns. This reflex involves the neural interaction between the medial and the oculomotor nuclei in the brainstem (Subsection 17.B, page 668). In fact, the association between the eyes and the vestibular system is so intimate that each of the three pairs of external muscles aiming the gaze of the eyeballs lies in one of the planes of the semicircular canals, so that the excitation of one of the canals will excite one of the three pairs of external muscles! This is called the vestibular-ocular reflex, and it works to keep the eyes focused on a point as the head turns. The latency period for the movement of the eyes while engaged in the vestibular-ocular reflex is only seventeen milliseconds, whereas it is seventy milliseconds for a voluntary eye movement. When the vestibular-ocular apparatus is malfunctioning, the result is a visual blurring when the head is in motion. The push-pull contralateral inhibition of the external muscles of the eyes is active in this reflex. Other, more indirect connections between the balancing organs and vision exist, as those *yogasana* students can attest who have tried to balance with their eyes closed (Subsection V.C, page 890).

Vestibular-Spinal Reflex

In addition to the ocular coupling to the vestibular apparatus that works largely to keep the head in an upright orientation, there is a reflexive coupling of the vestibular apparatus to the nerves within the spine, in this case working to activate the legs should one lose one's balance while standing (see Box 18.B-1, below). This vestibular-spinal reflex is much faster-acting than the falling signals generated at the retina by a shift of the horizon (reaction time of about 100 milliseconds) or by the proprioceptors in the muscles of the neck, which also can signal a deviation of the head from verticality (reaction time of about 100 milliseconds).

Innervation of the Vestibular Tract

The afferent nerves from the vestibular balancing organs form a part of cranial nerve VIII, are myelinated, and synapse with the four vestibular nuclei in the lateral parts of the brainstem, just below the fourth ventricle. The vestibular nuclear complex is large, occupying a substantial part of the medulla oblongata. Descending fibers from the medial and inferior nuclei of the vestibular tract go only to the upper part of the spinal cord and are concerned with head and neck movements in response to vestibular excitation. The afferent nerves from the utricle input to the lateral nucleus while the α- and γ-motor neuron efferents from this point are facilitatory for extensor-motor neurons and inhibitory for flexor-motor neurons. Neurons from the cerebellum and spinal-cord proprioceptors also converge on the lateral vestibular nucleus. From its mode of action, it is deduced that the utricle in conjunction with other peripheral sensors can be an important proprioceptor in standing postures.

The cerebellum continuously receives out-of-balance information from the saccule, utricle, and the semicircular canals and then relays corrective information to the motor centers of the cortex in order to regain balance. See the following subsection (page 701) in regard to the possible role of the cerebellum in dyslexia.

Box 18.B-1: Challenges to the Vestibular System

It is simple to demonstrate the action of the vestibular-righting reflex and the conditions under which it is active. Standing with the feet together, fall forward. The vestibulospinal reflex will cause one foot to extend forward in the direction of the fall and the arms to lift so as to protect the upper body from hitting the floor. This reflex is activated by the off-balance vestibular signal, generated when falling. On the other hand, stand again with the feet together and let the head fall forward. In this case, there is no reflexive action so as to break the fall that the vestibular sensors are anticipating on the basis of the head position and motion. Why is this so? The answer lies in the proprioceptive signals that arise from the extensive network of muscle spindles in the back of the neck (table 11.B-1). In matters of balance, it is important to distinguish between a body that is out of balance and falling and a head that is out of balance but not necessarily falling. In the latter case, bending the head forward (or sideward) does unbalance the vestibular sensors; however, the proprioceptive muscle spindles in the stretched muscles at the back of the neck also send a corrective signal to the balance centers in the brainstem, which cancels the vestibular signal when the head is out of balance but the body is not [308]. However, be aware that in the second case, there is no imbalance in the receptors in the soles of the feet, whereas there is in the first case.

It is interesting that tension in just these muscles of the back of the neck that are so rich in muscle spindles is thought to be responsible for many headaches of the tension variety [308].

After rotating and then standing still, the fluid in the inner ear continues to rotate, and so we feel dizzy. The feeling is even worse when the rotation is brought to a sudden stop with the eyes open (as in a rocking boat), for the eyes see no rotation on stopping, but the vestibular organs continue to sense rotation; this sensory mismatch generates a (sea)sick feeling. Because the semicircular canals are dynamic sensors, they are important because they are capable of predicting falling posture, whereas the static detectors only can sense an imbalance after the fact of falling. Thus, the semicircular canals allow one to anticipate and correct posturally the incipient imbalance in a feedforward-like manner (Subsection V.B, page 884) [308].

The utricle and saccule are sensitive to linear accelerations, while the semicircular canals are sensitive to angular accelerations. However, when we fall, it is most likely that the head experiences both types of acceleration, so that both types of sensors are activated. Judging from the imperfect understanding we have of how the vestibular organs work, one can guess that the semicircular canals would still function in inversions such as *sirsasana I*, probably the saccule would also function, but the utricle would not, as the otoliths would not be in contact with the hair cells when inverted.

Neural connections are also made from the four vestibular nuclei to the cerebellum and back again, supposedly for fine tuning of balance reflexes. There is evidence as well that two-way connections also are made between the vestibular nuclei and higher centers, extending up to the cortex. If so, this would allow a conscious sensing of static and dynamic head position in space. Though the signals from the vestibular organs are largely reflexive and thus limited to the subconscious, as they go no higher than the thalamus, there is a slight ascendance to the cortex where one perceives a vague conscious sense of the head's position in space [30].

Yogasana and Dyslexia

A Possible Relation?

There possibly is a most interesting and unexpected connection between the yogic posture *vrksasana,* the vestibular balancing system, and dyslexia, this latter being a condition in which one is able to read, write, and count only with great effort [915, 920]. As mentioned above, the vestibular apparatus feeds its information in regard to balance to the cerebellum, a part of the brain involved in coordinating movement. This is relevant because 90 percent of dyslexic children have problems with vestibular feedback to the cerebellum, whereas non-dyslexic children have few or no problems in this area. Thus, many dyslexics are unable to discern their orientations in space, are forgetful, have poor short-term memories, and often are physically awkward; this disability is three times more prevalent in boys than in girls. There is evidence that dyslexia possibly relates to excess testosterone during pregnancy, which is known to retard the growth and development of the left cerebral hemisphere in boys. It is also true that dyslexic children have great difficulty bringing their finger to their nose with the eyes closed, this being a test of their proprioceptive-sensing system and/or the cerebellum which receives the proprioceptive signals (Section 11.C, page 441).

Types of Dyslexia

There would seem to be two extreme types of dyslexia, one involving the auditory-phonological channel and a second involving the visual-motor channel, with combinations of these two also possible. Given the connection between dyslexia, balance, and cerebellar dysfunction, it is logical then to wonder if practice in balancing might have a positive effect on dyslexic children with problems in the visual-motor channel. In fact, it is reported that practicing *vrksasana* while involved in a second task (such as repeating math tables or tossing a beanbag from hand to hand) for ten minutes a day has profoundly positive effects on dyslexia after a few months' training. Yogic practice of this sort reduced reading difficulties while increasing scores for children in writing, reading, and comprehension tests; conventional treatment for dyslexia without the yogic component is only marginally successful. It remains to be seen how the performance of the other yogic balancing postures (Appendix V, page 865) might measure up against *vrksasana* in the training of the vestibular functions in dyslexic children with visual-motor problems.

Current discussions of dyslexia focus on incomplete brain development with minimal activity in the left cortex of the afflicted [427]. Indeed, in the non-dyslexic, the language area of the brain called the planum temporale is quite large in the left cerebral hemisphere but quite small in the right hemisphere, whereas in the dyslexic, there is little or no size difference of this brain center in the two hemispheres. This difference may relate to an auditory-phonological problem. A second difference lies in the magnocellular cells of the visual system's LGN (Brodmann areas 17, 18, and 19 of the visual cortex, figure 4.C-1), which are specific for the perception of movement and which are noticeably smaller in the dyslexic [909]. In this case, one suspects a problem in the visual-motor channel.

In view of the recognized association of dyslexia with matters of cerebral and possibly cerebellar laterality, the seemingly strange but effective treatments of dyslexics by covering one eye, wearing colored glasses, or playing music into the right ear would seem to make some sense. That each of these treatment modes involves preferential stimulation of one of the hemispheres (see, for example, Box 17.E-1, page 684), is not surprising in hindsight [909].

That covering one eye, listening with one ear, or wearing colored glasses can help certain dyslexic students is consistent with the idea that their dyslexia may involve cerebral and/or cerebellar laterality. In this case, one also can imagine a *yogasana* program (possibly including forced unilateral breathing (Subsection 15.E, page 635) that is preferentially stimulating to one cerebral or cerebellar hemisphere, and not the other, yielding positive results for dyslexic individuals.

The Gastrointestinal Organs and Digestion

19

Section 19.A: Structure and Function

Dimensions

As often has been pointed out, all human beings are hollow. Each of us has an open tube 9 meters (thirty feet) in length, the gastrointestinal tract,[1] running through us from mouth to anus (figure 19.A-1). The inner surface of this tube is just a continuation of the outer surface of our skin; without a seam, the skin of the face becomes the skin of the inside of the mouth, and this continues inward and downward to become the surface of the throat, the stomach, the small and large intestines, the skin of the anus, and the skin of the buttocks (Subsection 13.A, page 501). Though the mucus membrane of the gastrointestinal tract is contiguous with the external skin of the body, it is not protected by keratin from bacterial invasion, as is the case in the latter.

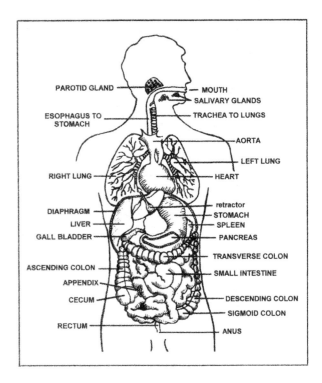

Figure 19.A-1. Enumeration of the organs of the gastrointestinal tract and its accessory organs.

---

1   Actually, the gastrointestinal tract is significantly shorter than this in the living body, due to its ever-present muscle tone; however, it reaches 9 meters (thirty feet) in length in cadavers. The lengths of the gastrointestinal tracts in various animal species depend upon their diets. Vegetarian animals have relatively long tracts, carnivores have relatively short tracts, and omnivores such as humans have tracts of intermediate length.

Closer inspection of the cells and their functions in the various parts of the gastrointestinal tract (also known as the alimentary canal) reveals how very special each of these parts is and the special role each plays. This inner "empty" space as defined by the walls of the gut, expresses our hollowness, and technically is known as the lumen. The exocrine glands deposit their substances into the various lumina of the body—the nasal passages, trachea, lungs, kidney tubules, ducts, bladder, vagina, uterus, etc. [450]—whereas the endocrine glands of the body deposit their hormonal loads into the bloodstream.

Smooth Muscles

In contrast to the situation with skeletal muscles (Chapter 11, page 381), the smooth muscles of the internal organs (the viscera) consist of cylindrical cells of much smaller diameters (10 μ in diameter) and lengths (50-300 μ) than those of skeletal muscle fibers (table 14.A-1). These cells show no cross-striations and no sarcoplasmic reticulum/t-tubule structures (Subsection 11.A, page 384) and are found in the walls of organs having cavities, such as the urinary, reproductive, respiratory, gastrointestinal, and vascular organs. The contractive force of smooth muscle (about forty pounds per square inch) is of the same order as that of skeletal muscle (about fifty pounds per square inch); however, the smooth-muscle contraction times of 500–2,000 milliseconds are much longer than those of skeletal muscle (about fifty milliseconds), and for this reason, there is no need in smooth muscle for a global, highly organized electrical signaling system such as the sarcoplasmic reticulum.

Like the heart, smooth muscles contract largely using gap junctions rather than the traditional neuromuscular junctions; however, where neuromuscular junctions do appear in the gastrointestinal tract, they are very diffuse and spray neurotransmitter over a wide area when energized. Though contraction and relaxation of smooth muscle is slower than is the case for skeletal muscle, one still speaks of "muscle tone" (Subsection 11.B, page 436) for smooth muscle [450].

The job of the smooth muscles is to move material (urine, air, blood, etc.) through the lumina using slow, sustained, rhythmic movements. These smooth-muscle contractions are generally not under voluntary control, but as reflexes, they are responsive to both neural and hormonal stimulation. Smooth muscle, as found in the gastrointestinal tract, can contract for very long periods of time, as compared with most skeletal muscle, which quickly suffers ischemia and fatigue when contracted. Furthermore, smooth muscle can still contract after being stretched 500 percent [432],

and contraction from its resting length can reduce this length by up to 75 percent [308]. That is to say, it has a length/tension curve very different from that of the generic skeletal muscle shown in figure 11.A-11. Unlike skeletal muscle, smooth muscle does not contain muscle spindles and so can be stretched by a very large amount without being reflexively contracted. Yet it can still contract when the need arises, even when extremely extended.

Smooth muscle can be extended over a very wide range with very little resistance to the stretching, and compared to skeletal muscle, smooth muscle requires only 1 percent of the energy to generate the same tension in the tissue. It is known that different tissues have different responses to stimulation. In the case of the gastrointestinal tract, there are no pain sensations if it is manipulated, cut extensively or even burned, but pain is sensed if it is stretched or distended excessively or is in spasm [562].

Smooth versus Skeletal Muscle

Smooth muscle has no striations, but like skeletal muscle, its action is based upon the interactions between actin and myosin myofilaments (Subsection 11.A, page 382). The autonomic nervous system acts to contract smooth muscle using norepinephrine as the neurotransmitter and to relax it using nitric oxide as the neurotransmitter. Smooth muscle also can be activated by paracrine action (histamine in the vicinity) or by hormones (oxytocin in the uterus during childbirth). Neurologically, the central nervous system is able to control muscular action from the mouth to the pyloric sphincter of the stomach and from the colon to the rectum; however, in the intermediate regions of the intestines, it is the enteric nervous system that dictates both the muscular and glandular instructions [268].

In what follows, let us look at the physiological processes that take place sequentially in the gastrointestinal tract (figure 19.A-1) once eating commences [557]. As will be seen, these processes are not without impact on the student practicing *yogasana*.

The Mouth and Esophagus

The Tongue

All of the body's processes require fuel in order to be set in motion. Our fuel is the food that we eat, but as such, it is not directly useable as fuel. It must first be digested in the gastrointestinal tract, and the products of this physical/chemical transformation from large molecules to smaller components are then made available for fueling bodily processes. The mouth is the first station for digestion of food. Mechanically, food is processed into a form suitable for swallowing by the actions (both voluntary and involuntary) of the mouth, lips, teeth, and tongue. As with the eyes (Section 17.A, page 657), the tongue has both extrinsic and intrinsic muscles; the former moves the tongue left and right, using muscles outside the tongue; the latter alter the shape of the tongue, as when speaking or eating. Relaxation of the two types of muscles in the tongue is essential for relaxation in *savasana*.

Salivation

One of the components of the salivary discharge in the oral cavity is the enzyme amylase, the function of which is to digest polysaccharides, reducing them to simple disaccharides, which are further degraded to their constituent monosaccharides in the small intestine; monosaccharides are the only sugars that can be absorbed from the gastrointestinal tract into the bloodstream, and glucose is the most important of the monosaccharides. The enzyme amylase continues to digest the starches in the swallowed bolus but is soon deactivated by the high acidity of the stomach. Simple sugars such as glucose also may be transported directly into the bloodstream within the mouth.

Another of the enzymes released into the mouth during chewing is lysozyme, an antibacterial disinfectant; its presence in saliva is why animals lick their wounds and why people with a persistently dry mouth suffer abnormally high tooth decay [878]. Simultaneously with chewing, the taste buds are activated, as is the olfactory sense

of smell, both using the cranial nerves (Subsection 2.C, page 24). The sensation of "taste" is really a combination of tasting using the taste buds in the tongue and smelling the odor of the food using the receptors in the nose. As the nose's sense of smell is so much more discriminating than the tongue's sense of taste, it is the former that adds so much pleasure to the gourmand's palate (see Subsection 15.C, page 621).

As salivation is a reflex response to stimulation of the parasympathetic nervous system (table 5.A-2), relaxation in *savasana,* for example, often leads to a momentary but noticeable overflow of saliva. When this occurs, it is acceptable to swallow until the overflow subsides.

Swallowing

Proper digestion requires that the food be chewed in the mouth for approximately sixty seconds before it is swallowed. At the same time that glands in the mouth secrete enzymes, lubricants and adhesives are also secreted to further prepare the bolus formed by chewing for transport through the esophagus to the stomach (figures 15.A-1 and 19.A-1). When swallowing food that has been chewed, the larynx lifts, and a cartilaginous flap called the epiglottis folds over its entrance so that food cannot go the "wrong way" down the trachea. At the same time that the epiglottis closes the path to the lungs, the soft palate and the uvula close the path of the food bolus to the nose, leaving the esophagus as the only open path (figure 15.A-1). Because the food or liquid in the swallowed mass is propelled toward the stomach by muscular action and does not depend on gravity alone, we can swallow upward in inverted poses such as *sirsasana* and *sarvangasana;* were it otherwise, as it is with birds, we would have to be sitting or standing upright and tip our heads back in order to swallow. Swallowing is a coordinated reflexive action driven by the medulla oblongata; however, the intervention of the higher cerebral centers can affect this innocent act and so cause a "choking up" for emotional reasons originating in the limbic region.

Breathing Food and Swallowing Air

The esophagus serves only as a passageway between the mouth and the stomach. In the process of swallowing, the epiglottis acts as a lid to close the trachea while leaving the esophagus open during this action. Similarly, during an inhalation, the trachea is open to the outside as far down as the lungs, whereas the esophagus is closed by the uppermost sphincter (the pyloric valve), just above the stomach, so that no air can enter or leave the stomach. Activating the pyloric valve also keeps stomach acid from rising into the esophagus. The passage of solid food from mouth to stomach requires four to eight seconds, but liquids make the trip in about one second.

In the course of eating and swallowing, it in unavoidable that more or less air is swallowed along with our food and drink. Should the upper esophageal sphincter relax after a meal, the result will be the release of the swallowed air as a belch. Anything containing peppermint will encourage the release of this sphincter.

At the two extreme ends of the gastrointestinal tract, conscious and reflexive actions are mixed and present simultaneously, whereas between these points, the action is totally reflexive, involving the parasympathetic and enteric nervous systems.

The Stomach

The stomach is a very muscular organ, these muscles being used to churn the contents so as to intimately mix the chewed food and the digestive juices and to then expel the contents into the small intestine. Thanks to its structure, the stomach is important not only in digestion but is also a holding vessel, capable of expanding greatly to accommodate excessively large meals without an increase in internal pressure. Because there is no excess pressure even when one has eaten excessively, digested food (chyme) is not forced backward from the stomach into the esophagus; however, stretching of the stomach does inhibit food intake [584]. The normal empty volume of the stomach is only 0.05 liter, but it can expand to hold four liters of food before rupturing.

An inner layer of the gastrointestinal tract is strongly muscular but not under voluntary control; it breaks down food mechanically, mixes it with digestive juices, and propels it toward the nether end. This process is known as peristalsis (see below, page 711). The various visceral organs, such as the stomach, are held in place in the abdomen, as they are tacked to the back wall of the abdominal chamber by a ligamentous tissue called the mesentery, which bears many blood vessels, lymph nodes, and nerves.

Digestion

Using digestive enzymes and strong acid produced by the cells lining the gut, the J-shaped stomach is the primary site in the gastrointestinal tract for the digestion of food, though there is very little absorption taking place here. The enzyme pepsin is expressed in the stomach and is used for converting protein into smaller peptide fragments. Inasmuch as all cells have a large protein component, it is strange at first sight that the cells lining the stomach contain protein-digesting enzyme but are not themselves digested by this enzyme. Nature solves this problem by storing the pepsin within the cells in the form of inactive pepsinogen, which then becomes active pepsin only when it is outside of the cell and in the presence of strong hydrochloric acid. This strong acid not only activates pepsinogen but is effective in killing many bacteria. In this regard, see Sections 20.A, page 721, and 20.B, page 722.

Acidity

The gastric glands deliver between 0.4 and 0.8 liter of gastric juice to the stomach at each meal. The concentration of H^+ in the juice is as high as 0.15 molar, corresponding to a pH between 1 and 2. On the other hand, the H^+ concentration within the cells that produce the hydrochloric acid is approximately a million times smaller; i.e., 4×10^{-8} molar in chemical terms. Thus it is seen that the generation of stomach acid involves the active outward transport of huge numbers of hydrogen ions (H^+) through the cell walls and into the lumen in order to raise its acidity. Correspondingly, this transport involves huge expenditures of energy by the local mitochondria [450].[2]

There is practically no absorption of ingested substances taking place in the stomach, except for water, aspirin, and alcohol, which accounts for their fast actions. As regards digestion, the role of the stomach is largely the degradation of proteins into their constituent amino acids. The storage aspect of the stomach also is important, as we eat and swallow food much more rapidly than the small intestine can process it. Were it passed through the small intestine as fast as swallowed, the food would not have time enough to be digested and absorbed.

Neural Signals

There are many signals that precipitate a reflexive release of hydrochloric acid, beginning with signals from the medulla oblongata. In order of increasing effectiveness, thinking about food, smelling food, chewing food, swallowing food, and having food press against the lumen of the stomach all are effective in releasing stomach acid. In the absence of these triggering events, there is no release of pepsinogen or acid. Emotions such as anxiety, fear, and anger can stimulate the sympathetic nerves in the stomach, which will act to slow the release of the digestive juices, which are otherwise under parasympathetic control. Similarly, it is best not to eat before *yogasana* practice, as this practice activates the sympathetic nervous system and thereby stalls digestion. Performing *yogasana* practice upon waking early in the morning seems like the only reasonable alternative, considering the mutually negative effects that *yogasana* practice and digestion can have on one another when practiced simultaneously.

---

2   Within the cells of the gastric glands, an enzyme promotes the reaction of CO_2 and H_2O to produce H^+ and HCO_3^- ions, both of which diffuse out of the cell. At the same time, K^+ is pulled into the gastric cells, and Cl^- leaves the cells for the lumen. In this cycle, carbon dioxide is consumed in a reaction in the gut, unlike the situation in the muscles, where carbon dioxide is generated as a product.

Timing

Even though the stomach dispenses hydrochloric acid whenever something is eaten, its acid output is maximal between 10:00 PM and 2:00 AM, even when fasting. It is thought that this late outpouring of acid not only serves to kill any bacteria that may remain in the stomach after all eating has ceased, but is the cause of both heartburn and peptic-ulcer pain at this time. On the other hand, bleeding of intestinal ulcers occurs most often between 11:00 AM and 1:00 PM.

The residence time of food in the stomach will depend upon just how digestible it is; a heavy meal containing a high proportion of fatty meat may require up to six hours' digestion in the stomach before it is ready to be passed through the pyloric valve to the small intestine, whereas a light meal of carbohydrates may be ready in just two hours, and a meal of lean meat will have an intermediate residence time [774, 878]. Water, on the other hand, is rapidly absorbed from the stomach. See Subsection 19.C, page 716, for the relevance of the residence time to *yogasana* practice.

Generation and Containment of Stomach Acid

Acid Protection

The contents of the stomach when in action are just as easily capable of digesting the cells that line the stomach as they are of digesting beef steak. Though gastric juice will dissolve any other tissue in the body, it will not dissolve the stomach itself. That the cells of the stomach wall are not appreciably attacked is due to an alkaline mucus-gel coating that separates the cell surfaces from the potent brew contained within. In keeping with the rough neighborhood in which the intestinal cells live, they are coated with an alkaline mucus, but even so, they must be replaced every three days [268, 716]. Preventing access of the stomach acid to the other structures in the gastrointestinal tract (the esophagus, for example) that are not so protected is the function of stout valves at the entrance and exit to the stomach, which normally are closed and which open only when absolutely necessary.

Heartburn

The stomach has a special coating that renders it inert to the strong acid involved in digestion. However, should the stomach contents reflux and so enter the esophagus, then the lack of a similar protective coating in the esophagus leads to the sharp, burning sensation of heartburn. Digestive strength can be increased by performing *yogasanas* (spinal twists, supported forward bends, etc.) that increase the blood supply to the digestive system [398, 557].

The cells of the stomach that produce the hydrochloric acid necessary for digestion are called parietal cells; cells that sense the degree of acidity in the stomach and so signal for a greater or lesser release of acid are called G cells. The cell walls of the parietal cells facing the lumen are able to absorb K$^+$ ions from the stomach contents and in return, pump H$^+$ ions into the lumen. It is this H$^+$ that is the acid component of hydrochloric acid (HCl).

Acid production by the parietal cells is triggered chemically by the gastrin released by the G cells, which in turn acts on parietal cells sensitized by their absorption of histamine released by mast cells. This absorption of the sensitizer histamine can be blocked chemically by drugs that compete successfully on the parietal-cell surface for the receptor sites that normally accept histamine molecules. Such "H2 blockers" in this way are able to turn off acid production for many hours at a time. Parietal cells also can be excited to generate hydrochloric acid by both the enteric and central nervous systems. Thus, one needs only to think of food, and the acid will immediately begin to flow into the stomach. This neural activation is much more rapid than the chemically activated one.

Should a parietal cell of the stomach wall die and disintegrate, the door is then open for seepage of strong acid (pH 1) and enzyme into unprotected places, and the possibility of forming an ulcer (self-digestion) in the lining of the stomach. However, this does not happen very often, because when a parietal cell dies, prostaglandins are released in the area, and this stimulates neighboring cells to immediately expand into the opening, thus keeping the parietal layer intact.

The brew of concentrated acid and active pepsin in the stomach is highly effective in dissolving not only the proteins of animal muscle but also the protein of most microbes, parasites, worms, etc. that may be in the food. Any such bacteria that are strong enough to survive the digestive brew in the stomach then go on to colonize the colon (see below). One such bacterium that does survive and in fact prospers in the high acidity of the stomach is *Helicobacter pylori,* the prime culprit in the formation of gastritis and stomach ulcers. In any event, the stomach is a relatively sterile place, there being less than one-billionth the number of bacteria per milliliter in the stomach than are found per milliliter in the colon.

Bacteria in the throat convert nitrate ion (NO$_3^-$) into nitrite ion (NO$_2^-$), which then goes into the stomach, where it reacts further with strong acid to form nitric oxide. This gaseous substance is lethal to bacteria and will kill almost all of the bacteria present in or on our food, including many of those that can survive strong acid alone [450].

Energetics

The absorption of K$^+$ from the lumen and its replacement with H$^+$ on a large scale is a process that is very energy-intensive. The energy needed for this H$^+$ ion pumping is derived from ATP within mitochondria feeding on glucose and oxygen (Section 14.B, page 557). The parietal cells of the stomach are stocked with many large mitochondrial centers; when these are called upon to generate up to a liter and a half of concentrated hydrochloric acid per day, they make a large energy demand on the body, as large as that made by the skeletal muscles. During the digestion of proteins, the oxygen consumption of the body may go up by 25 percent in order to feed the gastric fire that produces hydrochloric acid [197].

The amount of hydrochloric acid required for digestion depends upon what one eats; those who eat large amounts of meat and its associated fat will require much larger amounts of hydrochloric acid, pepsin, oxygen, and energy to digest a meal than will the same person eating a meat-free, carbohydrate-loaded meal [774].

The Small Intestine

Acid Neutralization

The initial step of digestion begun in the stomach is completed in the small intestine. With the aid of the enzymes and alkaline buffering provided by the pancreas, the duodenum of the small intestine is able to handle small aliquots of the highly acidic chyme from the stomach, by neutralizing its acidity (returning it to pH 7–8) and digesting the larger molecular fragments (fats, proteins, and starches) down to their ultimate molecular components. Digestion in the small intestine is aided by the injection of enzymes from the pancreas, the liver, and the gallbladder. The smaller amino acids and monosaccharides that result from this digestive process are then absorbed through the walls of the small intestine directly into the bloodstream. Ninety percent of the nutrients in the food we eat are absorbed in the small intestine, with the other ten percent divided between absorption in the stomach and the colon [632].

The shortest (25 centimeters; ten inches), widest portion of the small intestine is the duodenum, which joins the lower end of the stomach at the pyloric valve; the small intestine then continues downward, surrounded by (but not attached to) the colon in the middle and back part of the lower body, finally to join with the colon at a point just below the navel. The small intestine is about 2.5 centimeters (one inch) in width.

Nutrient Absorption

Absorption of the nutrients in the lumen of the small intestine is efficient because of the huge area of the villi and microvilli covering the inner surfaces of the intestinal walls. These walls of the small intestine are multiply folded, so that the structure has the largest surface area over which nutrients can pass, while occupying the smallest volume. Were the small intestine opened up

lengthwise and stretched taut, it would cover three tennis courts! In this sense, it is not unlike the cerebral cortex in the brain. The combined areas of villi and microvilli in the small intestine amounts to 200 square meters (1,800 square feet), which is about 100 times the external area of the body. The contents of the small intestine are normally sterile as regards bacteria, etc., thanks to the high acidity of the environment in the stomach.

There are two sets of muscles surrounding the small intestine, one to churn the contents without propelling it down the tube, and the second of which sends the contents southward. As described below (Subsection 19.A, page 711), the slurried mass of digested food (chyme) is moved along the 3-meter (ten-foot) length of the small intestine by the reflexive muscular action of peristalsis. Peristalsis in the small intestine is a one-way street, moving the contents only in the mouth-to-anus direction. Peristalsis in the small intestine is very weak compared to that in the stomach and esophagus, and so three to five hours are required to move the fluid chyme through the length of the small intestine. Once the fluid mass has been propelled downward to the end of the small intestine, it is ready for processing by the colon. In the course of processing a typical meal, the small intestine will require nine liters of water and digestive juices, most of which are reabsorbed.

The Colon

Bacterial Content

The lower end of the small intestine is attached to the upper end of the colon (also called the large intestine) but separated from it by the ileocecal valve. The primary function of the colon is to first absorb up to 99 percent of the water and salts in the fluid mass sent to it; if this water is not recovered (two liters per day), the result is diarrhea and a dangerous dehydration of the body. With the water and salts removed, the stool becomes a semisolid mass, consisting largely of the indigestible remains of the earlier meals and of refuse from the liver's purification of the blood. Second, the colon is home to a massive (1.5 kilograms or 3.3 pounds) and wide variety of microbes (approximately 500 different varieties), some beneficial and some not. Every year, one defecates approximately one's body weight in bacterial debris.

The small intestine is essentially a sterile place, whereas the colon is filled with bacteria. The two contrasting environments are kept apart by the ileocecal valve [432], which separates the cecum from the ileum (figure 20.F-2a), thus preventing a reverse flow from the colon into the small intestine. Note, however, that an intense Valsalva maneuver (Subsection 15.C, page 616) can force the ileocecal valve to open and so allow pathogens to pass from the colon into the intestine.

It is estimated that the number of bacteria in the ileum and colon is ten times larger than the number of cells otherwise in the human body, and that the variety of such bacteria in one's body is in part dictated by the mode of infant feeding, depending on whether such feeding was by breast or formula.

The Stool

If our meal contains a sufficient amount of fruit, raw vegetables, and whole grains, then the resultant stool will be high in indigestible cellulosic fibers, will be firm and bulky, and will press strongly against the walls of the colon. The pressure that such a stool generates at the walls is the stimulus for the peristalsis that carries it along from the small intestine to the anus for easy expulsion. Because it requires much more effort to move a solid stool through the colon than to move a fluid slurry through the small intestine, it is understandable that the muscles encircling the colon are larger and stronger than those about the small intestine (figure 19.A-1). Though the colon is less than half the length of the small intestine (but three times as wide), the passage of the solid stool through the former may take up to thirty hours, compared to only three to five hours for the fluid chyme in the latter. The final stage of peristalsis pushes the stool into the rectum. Because this action is reflexive and is stimulated by the presence

of food in the stomach, defecation often can follow immediately after a meal.

If the diet is low in fiber, then the stool in the colon is greasy and small, does not press enough on the walls of the intestine to elicit a strong peristaltic reflex, and is expelled only with great effort and abdominal strain. Many years of a low-fiber diet will result in a colon that is weak and flabby from lack of peristaltic exercise, and quite possibly a very uncomfortable case of hemorrhoids (varicosities of the rectal veins) as well.

If irritated, the colon may discharge its contents before all of the water can be removed; the result is diarrhea. If the colonic contents are retained too long, they become hard and dry, leading to constipation. Society gives us many reasons for deliberately inhibiting the defecation reflex. However, the habitual denial and postponement of the act will eventually lead to a weak defecation reflex and thence to constipation. Having a fixed time of the day during which to defecate—say, in the morning before *yogasana* practice—will pay dividends when you get older, for constipation otherwise can become a problem in old age.

Though very little gas is generated in the small intestine, between seven and ten liters of gas (largely carbon dioxide, hydrogen, and methane) are generated each day in the colon; however, most of this is reabsorbed by the cells lining the intestinal walls [587]. The actions of the bacteria in the colon can generate large amounts of intestinal gas if they are given a high-carbohydrate diet or one rich in certain vegetables. Rice is the only grain that does not produce gas, and eggs, fish, and chicken are also rather innocent in this regard. Several strains of bacteria in the colon are able to synthesize important vitamins that are absorbed by the colon for general use throughout the body, whereas several other strains of bacteria in the colon are pathogenic. In a healthy colon, the populations of the various bacterial strains compete so as to keep one another in check; in the process of fighting an infection, antibiotics or even a change of diet can upset this balance and so lead to other problems. When there is a bacterial imbalance or a new strain of bacteria is introduced into the colon, immune cells in the lining of the intestine may be called upon to reestablish equilibrium.[3]

Pressure in the anus can be varied in both the positive and negative directions through voluntary control by the *yogasana* student, even though the student has done no work otherwise aimed at controlling the anal sphincters [91]. This may be of relevance to the performance of *uddiyana bandha* in the *yogasanas,* or *pavan muktasana.* Negative pressure in the colon is experienced in *ashwini mudra.* The mechanics of defecation are discussed in Subsection 20.F, page 731.

Peristalsis and the Enteric Nervous System

When there is an internal pressure pressing outward against the intestinal wall, a rhythmic action of the intestine is triggered reflexively; it pushes the intestinal contents from the oral toward the anal end, and at the same time, it relaxes the musculature ahead of the contracting wave. This is the peristaltic reflex. Interestingly, if all of the parasympathetic vagal nerves (cranial nerve X) from the medulla oblongata in the brainstem to the intestine are severed in a live animal (including a human), the peristaltic reflex remains active. Like the heartbeat (Subsection 14.A, page 543), peristalsis of the intestine is self-stimulating, yet subject to limited control by the autonomic nervous system. Further, a loop of intestine totally cut out of an animal continues to show this reflex! It is as if the intestine has a nervous system (and brain) of its own and can function without direction from the autonomic or central nervous

systems [268]. This "enteric nervous system" consists of a very dense web of neural tissue wedged between two layers of muscle that encircle the gut. The pacemaker that drives the peristaltic action is contained within cells in the enteric nervous system [17], the peristaltic frequency being three contractions per minute in the stomach and twelve per minute in the small intestine. The enteric system also has its own interoceptive sensors (Subsections 11.C, page 444, and 19.C, page 716), and these too do not synapse with the autonomic or central nervous systems. Whereas this enteric nervous system is able to drive the peristaltic action, the acts of swallowing and defecation do require direction from the autonomic and central nervous systems.

Within the walls of the intestine, there are two layers (three in the stomach) of directionally oriented smooth-muscle fibers of opposing actions. The innermost layer has radially directed fibers that, on contraction, act to pinch off the gut so that its contents cannot move backward if further squeezed. The second outermost layer then squeezes with muscle fibers oriented in the longitudinal direction, so that the digested mass is pushed forward, toward the anus. To be effective, these two muscle actions must be coordinated by the enteric nervous system, as the peristaltic wave moves in one direction only along the gastrointestinal tract [878]. This mechanism of moving fluids by muscle action is reminiscent of the situation in which venous blood and lymph are pumped from the lower body to the heart (Subsection 14.C, page 569). Note too that it is peristalsis that both pushes food down the esophagus into the stomach and pushes urine through the ureters into the urinary bladder. If the swallowed food is in some way defective or toxic, a reverse peristalsis is also possible, in which case the food is vomited in the direction from which it came.

Accessory Organs of Digestion

The Pancreas

There are several organs in the abdominal cavity that are not part of the gastrointestinal

---

3   The foreign bacteria in the colon seem not to set off any sort of an attack by the immune system, even though the bacteria are without question foreign. Normally, foreign bacteria are recognized by their unique coating of sugars on their surfaces; whereas in the colon, the foreign bacteria pass as normal by coating themselves with those sugars normally used by the human cells. However, this mechanism does not function in the newborn, in which case, substances from the appendix act to protect the foreign bacteria from destruction by a temporary blunting of the immune response to foreign species.

tract as such, yet supply important enzymes to it in aid of digestion. Prime among these is the pancreas (Subsection 6.B, page 220), which is able to supply enzymes to the small intestine in wide enough variety as to digest almost anything that can be swallowed, including bacteria, protozoa, and intestinal worms. The pancreas performs two other essential duties: it supplies insulin to the bloodstream, so as to regulate sugar levels in the blood, and it is able to add an alkaline solution of bicarbonate ion to the small intestine to counter the high acidity of the chyme entering the small intestine from the stomach. This latter buffering against acid is essential, as the small intestine is not able otherwise to protect itself against the high acidity of the stomach juices, and because many of the digestive enzymes (such as pancreatic enzyme) that function in the small intestine will not do so at high acidity. The neutralization of acid is keyed to the flow from the stomach; as a small dose of acidic chyme is added to the small intestine via the opening of the pyloric valve, it is neutralized by the bicarbonate solution so as to bring the pH back to 7–8. At this point, another small aliquot of the chyme is moved into the small intestine, and the pancreatic bicarbonate is brought on again for pH neutralization. This step-wise neutralization of the stomach acid continues until the entire contents of the stomach have been moved down and neutralized.

The bulk of the pancreas is an exocrine gland, pumping fluid into the duodenum following a meal. However, within it too are three types of endocrine cells: the beta, alpha, and delta cells. The beta cells secrete insulin when sensors on their surfaces find too high a glucose level in the blood, encourage the liver to convert excess glucose into stored glycogen, promote muscles to convert amino acids into proteins, and promote the synthesis of fatty acids. All of the above work by the beta cells is oriented toward clearing glucose and fat from the blood.

Diabetes

If the beta cells should be killed by an autoimmune reaction, then type 1 diabetes results. Type 2 diabetes occurs when insulin in the extracellular body fluids is present but is unable to gain entrance into the muscle cells. As transport of the insulin across the muscle-cell membrane is aided by vigorous exercise, this condition is more prevalent in the sedentary or overweight [450].

Alpha cells of the pancreas secrete the enzyme glucagon, which promotes the conversion of glycogen to glucose. Glucagon is active when the level of glucose is too low but is inhibited when glucose in the blood is high. The delta cells within the pancreas secrete somatostatin, a factor that inhibits the release of growth hormone. The topic of diabetes is discussed further in Subsection 19.C, page 718, in terms of cell metabolism and *yogasana* practice.

The Liver

The liver is the largest internal organ in the body, weighing approximately 1.3 kilograms (three pounds) in women and 1.8 kilograms (four pounds) in men; its largest part is located just behind the right ribs (figure 19.A-1), and being suspended by two ligaments from the diaphragm, it is massaged during deep breathing. This organ is constructed with a high degree of redundancy; i.e., one can lose 80 percent of the liver and still function without any symptoms. The organ has such a high degree of regeneration that up to 50 percent of a healthy liver can be excised, and it will grow back in a matter of a few months! A liver cell has an average lifetime of 150 days.

Blood Flow

In addition to the hepatic artery, which carries oxygenated blood to the liver (0.35 liters per minute), all of the blood vessels that absorb nutrients from the gastrointestinal tract join to become the portal vein to the liver (1.1 liters per minute). This vein carries the sugars, vitamins, amino acids, drugs, bile salts, and toxins absorbed from the gastrointestinal system to the liver for purification [502]. Not only is the blood supply to the liver quite generous, amounting to as much as 29 percent of the total cardiac output (table 14-A-2), but this expandable venous organ is also an important reservoir for blood storage and supply.

At any one time, the liver holds between 15

and 29 percent of the total blood supply of the body. The capillary beds of most body tissues drain into veins leading directly to the heart. However, the capillary bed from the intestines leads to a second capillary bed in the liver, and these capillaries remove glucose, amino acids, ingested drugs, etc. Thus, the liver is a filter between the intestines and the general circulation, via the hepatic portal system. It monitors the chemical composition of input blood and adjusts it so that the output composition is as much like normal blood as is possible.

Toxins

The liver is known to perform over 500 different functions, including the rendering harmless of numerous substances such as alcohol and nicotine and the storage of toxins such as DDT (see Box 7.B-1, page 234). Though the liver does detoxify alcohol, it can be overwhelmed, in which case, alcohol-damaged liver cells are replaced by scars (alcoholic cirrhosis), which distort the pattern of blood flow in the liver.

Toxins absorbed from the gut are solublized in the liver and then excreted in the feces and urine. It is generally held by yogis that toxins are wrung from the liver and are forced into the body fluids by spinal twists (Box 7.B-1, page 234); however, I can find no scientific evidence either for or against this idea. In this regard, note too that because the rib cage protects the internal organs from outside pressure, one would not expect spinal rotation to offer much mechanical stress to the liver, especially as this organ is highly susceptible to damage by compressive trauma and as it is well served by a very effective blood supply [275]. (See Subsection 8.B, page 294, for more on this subject.)

The liver stores bile and bile salts in the gallbladder between meals, to be excreted just after mealtime when chyme enters the small intestine. The addition of the bile to the chyme occurs only when fat is sensed in the chyme and acts to emulsify any fat so as to make it water soluble. Whereas the digestion products of proteins and carbohydrates are pulled from the small intestine directly into the bloodstream, emulsified fat is pulled instead into the lymph (Section 14.G, page 595),

eventually to be dumped into the venous bloodstream near the neck (figure 14.C-2).

It appears generally true that bodily secretions are driven by the parasympathetic branch of the autonomic nervous system, as opposed to the sympathetic branch, which favors muscle contraction instead. This is also true in the gut, where it is known that gastric secretions are driven by the parasympathetic branch [360] or possibly by the enteric nervous system [268].

In earlier times, when the human diet consisted of more plant material than animal matter, the appendix provided enzymes to aid in the digestion of cellulose. It is still active in the infant in supplying immunological factors but is superfluous in the adult.

The Serous Membrane

All of the visceral organs are covered by a thin, slippery membrane, the serous membrane, and so can be moved over one another without visceral pain when moving, twisting, etc. Pain signals from distressed internal organs often use the same afferent neurons used to signal pain in the skin close to the affected organ. Due to this common neural path, the brain often interprets pain signals from the visceral organs as coming from the associated dermatome or skin area (Section 13.D, page 530). However, in the course of human evolution, the organs and their associated dermatomes have drifted apart geographically, so that real pain in the gallbladder, for example, may be manifest in the brain as a pain in the skin of the right side of the neck (figure 13.D-3).

Surgery in the abdominal area will necessarily sever tissues that otherwise are in contact only through lubrication but that may heal in such a way that the cut fibers of one organ grow onto an adjacent organ. The result is the formation of an internal scar, called an adhesion, at the site of the surgery. Such adhesions following surgery can be painful during *yogasana* practice, as the tissues that were meant to slide over one another as the body moves now pull strongly on one another instead (see also Subsection 11.G, page 480).

Just how many of the internal organs can be excised without becoming a threat to life?

Table 19.B-1: Disorders of the Digestive System

Organ	Disorder
Parotid gland	Cancer
Mouth	Difficulty swallowing (dysphagia)
Esophagus	Dysphagia, spasm, stricture, cancer, achalasia, GERD, hiatal hernia
Stomach	Gastritis, ulcers, gastroparesis, cancer
Liver	Hepatitis, cirrhosis
Gallbladder	Gallstones, cholecystitis
Small intestine	Ulcers, Crohn's disease
Pancreas	Pancreatitis, cancer
Colon	Ulcerative colitis, diarrhea, constipation, diverticulitis, polyps, cancer
Rectum/anus	Hemorrhoids, anal fissure

Apparently, one could live with one-third of a kidney, one-third of the liver, approximately half the brain, less than half a lung, one-tenth of the pancreas, and excision of most of the small intestine. Similarly, one could live with the complete excision of the gallbladder, tonsils, colon, anus, spleen, urinary bladder, external and internal genitalia, and larynx and amputation at the waist. One sees from this how large are the safety factors engineered by nature into the human body.

Section 19.B: Digestive Disorders and the Effects of Stress on the Gastrointestinal Tract

Acidity and Ulcers

If the vagus nerve is intact, then it has a certain neural control over the digestive system, which it shares with the enteric nervous system. It is no surprise that these two entities, through their common location in the gut, can influence one another as well. As the central and the sympathetic nervous systems send their signals to the peripheral effectors in the abdominal area, the enteric system can intercept these and either inhibit them totally or else modulate them in some way [268].

It was long believed that as a result of emotional stress, there was a strong vagal excitation (cranial nerve X) that led to the delivery of excess hydrochloric acid and pepsin to the stomach, and that this excess was able to eat into the lining of the stomach, producing an ulcer. It is now believed that this can happen only under the most extreme stress, and that the normal sort of everyday stress is not a factor here. Instead, many ulcers can be traced to a bacterial infection (*Helicobacter pylori*) of the stomach that is able to promote high acidity [268].

When the body is under stress, the sympathetic nervous system exerts its dominance over the digestive tract. At such times, the blood flow to the small intestine is severely curtailed, as the blood is shunted instead to the large muscles of the body. Consequently, digestion and peristalsis in the small intestine slow and the absorption of nutrients from the small intestine into the intestinal vascular system comes to a halt, while in the upper digestive tract, acidity increases, leading to indigestion and heartburn. If the stress is chronic, one craves complex carbohydrates (pasta, bread, etc.) as these foods trigger the release in the brain of the calming neurotransmitter serotonin. Eventually, through chronic stress, one can become addicted to the calming effect of serotonin release and pay for it with a corresponding increase in weight. As the unfortunate set of gastric circumstances composed of indigestion, hyper-acidity, and heartburn are triggered by stresses that activate the sympathetic nervous system, the symptoms can be countered by *yogasanas* such as *savasana* and supported forward bends, which promote parasympathetic rebalancing.

The digestive system can be the scene of many types of disorder, ranging from the uncomfortable to the fatal. Table 19.B-1 lists the various organs and the more common disorders to which they may fall victim; many of these can be treated with *yogasana* therapy [398] to ease the discomfort or to actually effect a cure. As Prashant Iyengar says, "Yoga can be used to cure what cannot be endured and to endure what cannot be cured."

Section 19.C: Digestion and Metabolism

Yogasana Practice and Digestion

As discussed above, the production of hydro-chloric acid in the amounts and concentrations necessary for digestion requires a great expenditure of energy. Following a meal, the gut demands considerable oxygen, glucose, and ATP in order to drive acid production. Because these materials are also in demand when doing the physical work of the *yogasanas,* it is not a good idea to try to perform *yogasana* and digestion simultaneously. Thus, you should not eat anything requiring a large amount of acid for digestion in the hours preceding your *yogasana* practice; Geeta Iyengar [404] recommends a period of one to four hours between eating and practice, depending upon the size of the meal. If this rule is followed, then one can avoid the unnecessary competition between the gut and the skeletal muscles for energy resources. In regard to delaying the need to eat, it is good to remember that you will sooner die of lack of sleep than of lack of food.

Note too that the digestive juices are set flowing not only by the presence of food in the mouth and the act of swallowing, but the smell of food will kick-start the digestive process, and even just the thought of food is enough to begin acid production! Thus the *yogasana* practice space should be free of the smells of food preparation, and the student should not dwell mentally on the meal to come, hungry though he or she may be. Even drinking water is to be discouraged during *yogasana* practice, as this is known [767] to stimulate the sympathetic nervous system and so increase the resting muscle tone.

Hunger

The sense of hunger originates in the empty stomach with the release of a hormone called ghrelin, which turns on a stimulatory neuron in the arcuate nucleus in the base of the hypothalamus (figure 5.B-1), which then signals the paraventricular nucleus to increase one's appetite for food.[4] Having eaten, a second hormone excreted into the small intestine turns off the appetite signal. Once food is being digested, glycogen is being formed and stored in the liver, and this acts to stiffen the organ in regard to stretching.

In order to appease a demanding appetite, on average, we tend to consume an excess of approximately 15 calories daily, which is equivalent to the caloric content of about half a teaspoon of mayonnaise or half a raw carrot; over the course of a year, this 15-calorie excess leads to a weight gain of approximately 0.7 kilograms (1.5 pounds), and over a span of twenty years, it leads to a weight gain of 14 kilograms (thirty pounds) [67]. To appreciate the effects wrought by an extra half-carrot a day for twenty years, try your *yogasana* practice with two 6.8-kilogram (fifteen-pound) sand bags strapped to your body. Also see pages 444–5 for more on hunger and interoception.

The Sphincters

With the stomach filled with acid during the digestion process, it would seem foolhardy to at-

---

4   Strangely, there are receptors for ghrelin throughout the brain, and even stranger is the fact that stimulation of these receptors with ghrelin appears to stimulate learning!

tempt any sort of inversion, for this would seem to spill corrosive acid into the throat. However, the acid-containing stomach is well sealed off from the upper and lower regions of the gastrointestinal tract connected to it, by the upper and lower sphincter valves that restrict flow out of the stomach in both the upright and inverted positions.

Once having eaten a meal, the digestion process can be accelerated by activating pressure points in the instep of the foot and lower leg [260], as when doing *yogasanas* that press this portion of the anatomy to the floor; e.g., *vajrasana*, or, more ideally, *supta virasana* [404]. Remember too that your stomach empties 50 percent more rapidly after breakfast than after supper, as the body processes food more slowly in the evening. Carbohydrates eaten in the evening are stored in the muscles and liver at night so that they are available the next morning when metabolic energy is needed. We tend to eat more in the evening, in part because our sense of taste is sharper at that time (Subsection 23.B, page 785).

Constipation

At the other end of the gastrointestinal tract, stool in the colon can be expelled only if peristalsis is strong enough to move it into the descending or sigmoid sections of the gut (Subsection 20.F, page 731). This peristalsis is most naturally achieved through the reflex action of the intestinal walls responding to the pressure of the stool on the walls. If this pressure is insufficient, the peristalsis is weak, and the result is constipation.

Note that any pressurization of the wall from the outside toward the inside, as with the wringing actions of *maricyasana III* or *bharadvajasana I* (see figure 8.B-4c), for example, does not activate the stretch receptors in the intestinal wall and so will not promote peristalsis. The yogic approach to overcoming constipation is to perform inversions of long duration, such as *sirsasana I*, *halasana*, *sarvangasana*, and their variations [404]. Perhaps this can be understood in the following way. When in the upright position, moving stool from the ileocecal valve through the ascending colon is uphill with respect to gravity (figure 19.A-1) and

so may prove to be difficult; whereas when inverted, this step is moving with gravity, rather than against it. Moreover, it is the outward pressing of the stool against the intestinal walls that gets it moving; perhaps when inverted, the pressure on the walls is applied to a more sensitive spot, thus stimulating a stronger peristalsis. Variations on *pindasana* in *sarvangasana* or *pindasana* in *sirsasana* are also useful in relieving constipation. In any event, it must be understood that constipation can be a learned response. When the rectum is filled and distended, the internal anal sphincter relaxes, and control then shifts to that conscious center regulating the external anal sphincter. It is important to obey this urge to defecate, for if it is not obeyed, it will go away!

Transit Time

The transit time of food through the digestive system is as follows: from the mouth to the stomach via the esophagus, eight seconds; through the stomach to the small intestine, two hours for carbohydrates, four hours for a high-protein meal, and six hours for high-fat meat; to pass through the small intestine to the colon, three to five hours; and to pass from the colon to the rectum, four to seventy-two hours. The transit time through the colon will depend strongly on the fiber content of the meal. Digestion is best aided by eating slowly and performing *savasana* rather than any other posture immediately after eating, as this will avoid to the maximum any conflict between digestion and any other muscle action. If you have not digested your food within six hours, you have overeaten.

Interoception

As described in Subsection 11.C, page 444, the proprioceptive sense of body and limb position and movement is complemented by a more internal sensing system that monitors the health of the internal visceral organs at a largely subconscious level. This visceral monitoring system is called the interoceptive system in the West [173] and the *antarindriyas* in the East. Interoceptors sense stimuli such as temperature, chemical concentrations, and tissue stretching (as with the vascular walls). Among the interoceptive signals of a more conscious nature are the sense of the heartbeat in the arteries and the senses of hunger and the need to urinate.

Hunger

As an example of the interoceptive system at work, consider the sensation of hunger. Through the hunger center, the hypothalamus is able to sense a low level of glucose in the blood, and in response to this, alerts the cortex to act to find food. Through conscious action, the cortex can ignore the hypothalamic request for about twelve hours before insistent hunger pangs set in. Once our sensors for the sight, smell, or taste of food are activated, the sensations are recorded in the cortex of the brain. From there, cortical messages are sent to the medulla, the upper terminus of the parasympathetic vagus nerve, which in turn has branches innervating the stomach. Activation of the vagus nerve results in the release of hydrochloric acid (more than a liter each day) and other digestive enzymes into the stomach, and the process of digestion is underway.

Other routes to the same digestive end also exist: stretch receptors in the walls of the stomach will be activated as the stomach fills, sending their signals to the medulla oblongata via an afferent branch of the vagus nerve, consequently turning on the digestion process via an efferent branch of the vagus nerve. As the stomach fills, the hunger center is turned off and the satiety center turned on, until the next time the glucose level drops too low and food again must be found. The hunger and satiety centers, both in the hypothalamus, work in opposition to one another, in a sense, with the hunger center always "on" but with more or less input from the satiety center acting essentially to turn it "off," or, at the least, working to diminish it. The level of activity of the satiety center depends upon the levels of glucose and amino acids in the blood, the body temperature, and the physical distension of the stomach.

Local reflexes are also at work, so that digestion can be started or stimulated without any signal going above the spinal cord. Though chewing and swallowing also act to stimulate the flow of the digestive juices, the sensation of hunger persists even in persons having no stomach, for it is the centers in the hypothalamus that control the sensations of hunger and satiety [584]. Note again that the vagal stimulation of the digestive process is driven by the parasympathetic side of the autonomic nervous system; in times of crisis, when the sympathetic nervous system is dominant, blood is pulled away from the viscera, and digestion stops until the crisis is weathered and parasympathetic balance can be asserted again.

Metabolism

In catabolism, large molecules are ingested and degraded into smaller ones (polysaccharides into sugars, proteins into amino acids, fats into fatty acids and glycerol, nucleic acids into nucleotides, etc.). In anabolic metabolism, the reverse takes place, with these smaller fragments being reassembled into macromolecules. The energy released in catabolism is used to make ATP, which in turn is used to drive anabolic processes [450]. The chemical products resulting from the digestion of our food yields high-energy materials that can be used to perform work. However, 80 percent of the calories so derived from our food are used just to maintain a body temperature of 37.0° C (98.6° F). Maintaining this temperature within narrow limits is important, for many of the body's enzymes have been tailored to work best at this temperature. The heat of the body is derived in very large part from the oxidation of the food we ingest, and the rate at which this heat is generated is the metabolic rate. This rate is dependent upon the level of exercise at the moment, the degree of sympathetic excitation in the autonomic system, and the release of certain hormones. As shown in figure 14.A-9, this heating effect due to an elevated metabolic rate is balanced by other factors that work to dissipate the internally generated heat to heat sinks outside the body.

When carbohydrates are used as metabolic fuel, every molecule of oxygen consumed in the reaction yields one molecule of carbon dioxide in the end; however if fats or protein are used instead, then about 70 percent of the oxygen consumed results in the formation of carbon dioxide, and the remainder is used to react with the H atoms in the fat or protein to form water. In the first few hours after a meal, the ratio of oxygen consumed to carbon dioxide released will be close to 1.0, showing that almost all of the food that was metabolized up to that point was carbohydrate (provided the person is not suffering from diabetes mellitus); however, after ten hours, this ratio drops to 0.7, indicating that fats and/or protein have become the sources of metabolic energy.

The endurance of our muscles is largely dependent upon how much glycogen can be stored in it. When on a high-carbohydrate diet, the stored glycogen amounts to thirty-three grams per kilogram of muscle; whereas when on a high-fat diet, this amounts to only six grams per kilogram of muscle; and on a mixed diet, the figure is about seventeen grams per kilogram of muscle. Translated into endurance, the carbohydrate diet allows a marathoner to run for 240 minutes, the high-fat diet allows one to run at the same pace for only eighty-five minutes, and the mixed-diet runner will go for 120 minutes before becoming exhausted.

The basal metabolic rate (BMR) is measured with the body totally at rest and reflects the energy needed to keep the basic physiological processes (neural, cardiac, liver, and kidney function) simmering; it is not the smallest amount of energy necessary to sustain life but is the smallest amount of energy to maintain life, wakefulness, and normal body temperature. The energy expenditure in a normal Iyengar practice for beginning students would be about five times the BMR. The daily oxygen consumption of the various organs while at rest [910] closely follows the blood flow pattern given in table 14.A-2 for light exercise, except for the flow within the muscles, which is considerably higher in light exercise than when at rest.

In the spirit of preconditioning, as described in Subsection 16.F, page 655, it has been shown that restricting the number of calories in the daily diet generates a modest stress in the body, and that in response to this stress, the brain chemistry is altered in such a way that the brain is then more resistant to neurological diseases [98]. As measured by the telomeres of the white blood cells in women, extra poundage reduces our lives by as much as eight years, as does the smoking of a pack of cigarettes a day for forty years (Subsection 24.A, page 813).

Insulin and Diabetes

Using the chemical potential of our ingested and digested food implies that the glucose so formed from our food intake is readily absorbed from the bloodstream into the cells that will eventually do the work based on that chemical potential. In fact, the critical step of absorption from the blood into the cell is dependent upon the presence in the blood of the hormone insulin, produced by the pancreas. When the pancreatic source of the insulin is subject to an autoimmune disease, the body becomes deficient in that hormone, and the result is type 1 diabetes; when the insulin levels are adequate, however, the cell receptors that allow glucose into the cells still may not respond to the insulin. In this case, the result is type 2 diabetes. In both types of diabetes, the blood sugar levels reach very high values (hyperglycemia), but on correction, they may fall to very low levels (hypoglycemia). In either case, these are serious conditions and are potentially fatal. (See Subsection 6.B, page 220, for a further discussion of diabetes and *yogasana*.) The role of insulin in carrying glucose across the cell membranes is not relevant to the brain, heart, or kidneys, for in these tissues, insulin is not required for the transfer of glucose from the blood to the interior of the cells. Insulin also sweeps excess glucose out of the blood and stores it as either glycogen or fat.

The application of *yogasana* practice to the control of type 1 diabetes is described by Cook [151], who found that a vigorous practice combining both sympathetic and parasympathetic stimulations was very effective, provided it was done on a regular daily schedule. Similarly, it is known that type 2 diabetes responds well to moderate exercise; again, *yogasana* practice of about an hour a day is sufficient to reactivate the receptors and allow glucose to flow into the cells.

With respect to the autonomic nervous system, the beta cells of the pancreas that produce the insulin are stimulated by the parasympathetic action of the right vagus nerve (cranial nerve X) and inhibited by sympathetic action [580]. Thus, the cooling postures of *yogasana* would be of help in type 1 diabetes, as they would promote increased insulin production. In addition to the strong effects of insulin, glucose levels in the blood are also strongly affected by other hormones, such as epinephrine, norepinephrine, and cortisol, each of which in turn is more or less susceptible to control through stress reduction using *yogasana* principles (Section 5.E, page 182).

This chapter considers the important exocrine secretions saliva, mucus, tears, sweat, and sebum, together with the nonglandular body wastes, none of which function as hormones. These secretions are transported through ducts to then appear on or at some external surface of the body. Because the hormonal secretions of the ductless endocrine systems are secreted internally, they are considered instead in Chapter 6, page 207. The exocrine secretions considered here are largely under the control of the autonomic nervous system, but, as discussed below, there can be strong conscious components to the secretion processes. As is the case with most subsystems under the control of the autonomic nervous system, release of the secreted substances is often dictated by a circadian rhythm (Subsection 23.B, page 774).

Section 20.A: Saliva

Parasympathetic Excitation

The three pairs of exocrine salivary glands in the mouth are controlled by both the sympathetic and the parasympathetic nervous systems [432]; however, in this case, the parasympathetic system stimulates the production of one type of saliva, and the sympathetic system stimulates the production of a second type. Efferent signals in the salivary branch of the parasympathetic system originate in the salivary nuclei within the brainstem and stimulate the secretion of a thin, watery saliva (saliva in general consists of water, protein, and salts) from the parotid glands via ducts in the mid-cheeks on both sides. The parasympathetically produced saliva is present when food is placed into the mouth or when one simply thinks of food. The parotid secretions are important, as they are bacterial suppressants of tooth decay induced by microbes. Of the 1.5–2 liters of saliva produced each day, by far the larger part is produced by the glands driven by parasympathetic excitation. Rising levels of nasal mucus and the release of tears are driven by the same parasympathetic branch that is responsible for parotid salivation (figure 5.C-1) [427].

Sympathetic Excitation

In contrast to the saliva produced by parasympathetic stimulation, sympathetic stimulation releases a thick, mucoid saliva that is high in amylase (an enzyme important for the digestion of carbohydrates), from glands at the edge of and beneath the tongue. Because the amylase in our saliva turns carbohydrates into the disaccharide sugar maltose, bread tastes sweet as we chew it. The protein in saliva makes it both stickier and a better lubricant for swallowing. Strangely, the same lubricating protein is secreted in the vagina during sexual arousal [68]. As the sympathetic nervous system gains dominance, the activity of the digestive system is blocked, and because salivation is a part of the digestive system, it too becomes sympathetically dominant, and a dry mouth results.

In a situation that is frightening, exciting, or otherwise stressful, as when we have to speak

---

Box 20.A-1: Using the Salivary Glands As Lie Detectors

Salivation is entirely under the control of the autonomic nervous system. The fact that the stress and nervousness that usually accompany lying leads to sympathetic arousal and a dry mouth was used in ancient times as a lie detector. Thus, among the ancient Bedouins of the Arabian peninsula, a suspected liar was made to lick a red-hot poker; if the suspect's tongue burned, that was taken as proof that his or her mouth was dry and that therefore he or she must have been lying. Similarly, the suspect in China was made to chew a mouthful of rice powder and then spit it out. If the powder came out dry, this was considered proof of lying. Among the British, the rice powder was replaced by a large wad of bread and cheese. In spite of the fact that food in the mouth generally promotes salivation, if the suspect could not wet the wad enough to swallow it, this could only be because he or she was a liar. Clearly, these tests were very unforgiving for those with dry mouths due to a fear of test-taking or a distaste of bread and cheese. The modern-day polygraph (lie detector) tries to smooth over these irrelevant responses but can be beat by a yogi in control of his or her autonomic nervous system (see Box 5.E-1, page 192).

---

publicly (see Box 20.A-1, above), the sympathetic dominance of salivation leads to a mouth that feels dry; whereas during a relaxing *savasana,* the parasympathetic system takes over, and the result can be a mouth that is wet to overflowing. Cranial nerves VII and IX are involved in these glandular secretions.

Time Effects

Parasympathetic salivation has its own circadian cycle, being more copious in the morning and least in the afternoon. The quantity of saliva released is also dependent upon posture, being larger when standing up or lying down and less so when sitting [427].

Natural Antibiotics

Saliva plays a major role in the destruction of harmful organisms both in the mouth and in the gut. Compounds called N-nitrosamines are known to be powerful carcinogens in the stomach and are to be avoided at all costs. In order to reduce the chances of forming N-nitrosamines in the gut, large efforts have been made to reduce the amounts of nitrates and nitrites in our food (particularly in cured meats), as it was felt

these compounds could lead to the formation of N-nitrosamines in the digestive tract. However, it is now known that there are common bacteria in saliva that convert nitrate into nitrite before swallowing, and in the absence of sufficient nitrate, the saliva itself will supply the deficit! Once the nitrite in the swallowed saliva reaches the strong acid of the stomach, it is converted into nitric oxide, a gas which is poisonous to salmonella, *E. coli,* and other harmful bacteria. The same gas is found in the sinuses of the forehead, where it acts to prevent the growth of bacteria in these dark, moist cavities, and in the vascular system as well, where it encourages vasodilation.

Section 20.B: Mucus

Despite its lowly status among *yogasana* practitioners, mucus plays several useful roles in the body, unless it is present in excess, as in chronic bronchitis, asthma, and cystic fibrosis. The mucus membranes line the inner surfaces of those body apertures that are open to the outside (the respiratory, digestive, urinary, and reproductive tracts), and along with the skin, the mucus membranes form the body's first line of defense against infection by microorganisms. The mucus membranes also lubricate the tissues lining these tracts.

Particle Filters

Those particles in the air we breathe having sizes larger than 10 μ are trapped in the mucus of the nose and throat. For particles in the range of 4 to10 μ, the inner surfaces of the trachea and bronchi are covered with epithelial cells bearing hairlike appendages, which in turn are covered by a thin mucus film. Any particulate matter (dust or microorganisms) breathed through the nose or mouth is trapped in the turbulent swirl of air in the trachea and bronchi (but not in the alveoli) and is deposited in the mucus film. This film is continuously moving upward at the rate of 1–3 centimeters per hour (0.4–1 inches per hour), eventually to be swallowed when it reaches the level of the esophagus (Subsection 20.B, page 723).

A thin mucus web is also generated within the tissues of the lungs, but it can be very difficult to bring up mucus from the lowest parts of the lungs when standing erect. For this reason, *sirsasana* practice for five or so minutes can be effective in bringing this hidden material in the bronchial tree to a place where it can later be more easily disposed when again erect [112a].

Nasal Sinuses

Mucus is also produced by the linings of the sinus cavities in the regions of the forehead and cheekbones. When the orifices of the cavities are blocked so that mucus cannot flow outward, then one has sinus congestion. Inversions can be of great help in relieving this congestion [398]. The discharge of nasal mucus is increased by parasympathetic excitation and decreased by sympathetic excitation (table 5.A-2). Given that *sarvangasana* is a cooling, relaxing *yogasana,* one concludes that when done in the proper way and for a sufficient duration [388], it leads to parasympathetic dominance. This leads one to expect that the perfor-

mance of *sarvangasana* will bring relief to stuffy, clogged sinuses in spite of the fact that when inverted, the drainage is upward, against the pull of gravity. *Sirsasana* and its variations also will be effective in relieving clogged sinuses [388], if done so that the parasympathetic system remains dominant; however, these postures are contraindicated if one has a sinus infection that might be spread by inverting.

Note that stuffiness of the nasal sinuses can mean either one of two conditions. If neurons in the brainstem stimulate the sinuses to secrete a clear fluid, then there is no sinus infection, and the taking of an antibiotic at this point is unnecessary. Rather than signaling an infection, the secretion of a clear fluid from the sinuses is a sign that one is about to experience a migraine headache. On the other hand, if the secretion is cloudy, then an infection is indicated [586].

Section 20.C: Tears

The lachrymal glands, located in the upper, outer corners of the eyes, exude tears onto the eyeballs through the lachrymal ducts, in order to keep the surfaces of the eyeballs clean and wet. Drainage ducts for the tears are positioned at the lower, inner corners of the eyes and drain the exiting tears into the nose and throat. However, the size of the drainage ducts is often inadequate, and excess tears may spill onto and down the cheeks.

The parasympathetic fibers of cranial nerve VII divide so as to innervate both the lachrymal and salivary glands. Excitations along these fibers produce copious amounts of tears and saliva, respectively. Of course, the lachrymal and salivary responses usually are stronger for emotional stress than for physical stress, but the physical work of *yogasanas* may bring emotional factors to the surface. It is no surprise then that students in *savasana,* a posture with strong parasympathetic action, may need to swallow often and perhaps even cry. Though tears may be squeezed from the exocrine lachrymal glands in part by muscle contraction, this is not the case for endocrine glands (Box 11.D-1, page 453).

Composition

Tears are a complex mixture, containing oil (to lubricate the motion of the lids over the corneas of the eyeballs), salts, sugar proteins that serve as wetting agents, and enzymes that are effective in digesting bacteria [716]. When we blink, the action of the eyelid is to pull tears from the lachrymal glands, sweep the tears across the eyeball, and tunnel them into the drainage ducts. As this process works even when we are inverted, tears still drain into the throat and so do not run down the cheeks when we do long-lasting *sirasanas*. The physiological and psychological effects associated with tears and blinking are discussed in Section 17.A, page 659.

Section 20.D: Sweat Glands

Sweat glands are found all over the body but are at their highest concentrations in the palms of the hands, on the soles of the feet, and in the armpits (axilla). Men sweat at twice the rate of women, and men have more sweat glands on the soles of their feet and in the umbilical region than do women, whereas women have more on the palms, the groin, and the backs of the legs than do men. The mammary glands of women are essentially sweat glands, but they excrete a fluid of a more nutritious sort.

The sweat glands of the skin are found to be of two varieties: the apocrine glands, the exudate of which is warm and smelly, and the exocrine glands, the exudate of which is clear and cool. Both types of sweat glands within the skin perform several useful functions, the two chief of which are discussed below. The sweating reflex originates within the medulla oblongata in the brainstem (Subsections 14.C, page 573, and 20.D, page 725).

As Organs of Purification

Apocrine Glands

The apocrine glands exude a viscous, milky fluid in the areas of the armpits, the outer-ear canal, the nipples of the breasts (when nursing an infant), the external genitalia, and the orifice of the anus. This apocrine fluid is rich in fatty acids and issues from those parts of the skin covered with hair. These glands (approximately 2,000 of them lying beneath hair follicles in the human body) are large, deep glands that become active only after puberty. They release an odorless sweat in the axillae and anal-genital areas, which is rich in body wastes and which is converted into substances of offensive odor by bacteria on the skin.[1] The results of this detoxification is apparent when *yogasana* students sweat, and the action of skin bacteria on this outpouring can be so intense that the air in the yoga room becomes unbreathable after an hour's work. The dirty smell of the air in a closed room after a beginner's *yogasana* class is resolved in time, as their bodies burn their impurities in the course of the regular practice of *yogasana*. The hormonal shifts that result from smelling the apocrine odors of the same and the opposite sex are discussed in Subsection 21.A, page 739. Stress also is said to result in an unpleasant body odor, whereas unstressed people find that bathing without the use of soap is adequate for going in society without offending.

Exocrine Glands

In contrast to the apocrine glands, the exocrine glands secrete a clear fluid of faint odor that appears on skin where there is no hair; it is much more watery and salty than the apocrine excretions. As can be seen in figure 13.A-1, the exocrine sweat duct is a strongly coiled affair; were it uncoiled to full length, it would be about 20 centimeters (eight inches) long, with the total length

---

1 Astronauts are chosen in part based on how dull their sense of smell is, because of the small supply of fresh water in a space capsule, and because a window can not be opened to get fresh air.

of sweat-ductwork in the human body amounting to 1,000 kilometers (600 miles)! The exocrine sweat glands in the skin of the human body outnumber the receptors by a factor of ten to one (there are 65,000 sweat glands in the palm of the hand and five million over the body), though the numbers decrease with age.

Whereas sweat produced by the apocrine glands is a product of stress, anxiety, and fear (i.e., excitation of the sympathetic nervous system), exocrine sweat is activated by heat or exercise. The exocrine sweat glands operate on the basis of acetylcholine as neurotransmitter, whereas in the apocrine glands, the neurotransmitter is epinephrine.

When sweating is copious [360, 431, 432, 582], the electrical resistance of the skin decreases [143]. This is the basis of the lie detector, predicated on the idea that the stress of lying generates a sympathetic response and sweaty palms, which condition is easily detected by measuring the electrical palmar resistance (see Box 5.E-1, page 192).

Though performing the standing *yogasanas* on a hot day can be difficult because of the excessive watery sweat appearing on the soles of the feet via the exocrine sweat glands, more importantly, the exocrine sweat glands are involved in cooling the overheated body through evaporation.

Thermoregulation by Sweat Glands in the Skin

When we are exercised and hot, the skin sweats in order to produce an evaporative cooling, while blood at the surface of the skin radiates heat to the surrounding air (figure 14.A-9). In contrast, when the sympathetic nervous system is aroused, as when fearful, etc., sweating is cold and clammy, and the blood retreats from the surface of the body to better serve the muscles.

Metabolism of fuel within the body continuously generates more or less heat, whereas homeostasis within the body demands that the core temperature of the body (37.0° C or 98.6° F) remain relatively constant. The general problem in regard to body heat is that of transferring more or less of this internal heat to the external

environment, thus keeping the core temperature constant. The importance of temperature regulation is clear once it is realized that if the temperature of the body rises beyond 41.1° C (106.0° F), there is danger of kidney dysfunction, muscle breakdown, loss of brain function, and death. The skin is an active participant in the mechanics of thermal regulation.

The blood vessels of the skin, the body's largest organ, play a central role in the both the nutrition of the skin and the temperature regulation of the body's core, using two mechanisms [432]. Those vessels involved in nutrition and metabolism are the arteries, capillaries, and veins. Less involved in nutrition are subcutaneous plexuses of veins, which carry large amounts of blood and serve to carry hot blood to the skin's surface to be cooled there. Yet another vascular arrangement for heat transfer involves arteriovenous anastomoses, which are direct connections between arterioles and venules and come into play in cold environments. The first cooling mechanism involves the transfer of blood from the core of the body to the skin, there to be warmed or cooled by contact with the ambient air (Subsection 14.C, page 573), and the second involves the evaporative cooling of sweat on the skin.

Evaporation

At temperatures below 37.0° C (98.6° F), water passes from the pores of the skin directly to the vapor phase without really becoming the liquid we know as sweat. However, when one is physically active and the body temperature rises above 37.0° C (98.6° F), as in figure 14.A-9, sweat droplets form on those parts of the skin having an abundance of exocrine sweat glands; only the tip of the penis, the clitoris, and the inner labial lips are totally free of sweat glands. Due to the high heat of evaporation of water (0.6 calories per gram), the evaporation of the aqueous component of exocrine sweat leads to a substantial evaporative cooling[2] of the skin and of any

---

2   At any specific temperature, there is a wide distribution of molecular velocities among the molecules in a liquid, with the kinetic energy of the molecule being

Table 20.D-1: Variation of Skin Temperature over the Body
at Two Different Air Temperatures

Skin of body part	Temperature when air is 21° C (70° F)	Temperature when air is 35° C (95° F)
Hand	28.0° C (82.4° F)	35.0° C (95.0° F)
Head	33.0° C (91.4° F)	35.5° C (95.9° F)
Upper chest	32.5° C (90.8° F)	35.5° C (95.9° F)
Foot	21.0° C (69.8° F)	34.5° C (94.1° F)
Core	36.1° C (97.0° F)	36.5° C (97.7° F)

blood-laden vessels close to the skin. Evaporative cooling normally is called upon to deal with only 15 percent of the body's heat loss, but in a hot, dry climate, this can increase to 90 percent [68]. This evaporative mechanism ceases to be of much utility when the relative humidity is high, as high humidity retards evaporation.

Skin Temperature

The two mechanisms of controlled blood flow to the skin and evaporative cooling are so efficient when working in tandem [187] that the thermal output of the body may be increased twenty-fold by vigorous physical exercise, yet the core temperature rises by less than 1.0° C (1.8° F)! Note too that whereas the core temperature of the body is held at a constant value, the skin temperature will vary over the body and that this variation will depend upon the temperature of the outside air, as seen in table 20.D-1. As might be expected from its location, the foot's temperature most closely follows that of the outside air, whereas the temperature of the head, chest, and body core are the most resistant to such changes of air temperature. If the air temperature is raised to 56.7° C (134° F) , the core temperature of the body increases by

less than 1° C [308], showing the tight regulation that the core of the body can maintain in spite of strong variations of the temperature of the surrounding air. Physical exercise as a way to keep warm is excellent in the short term but quickly leads to exhaustion and thence to dire straits. In very cold weather, the hairs of the body hug the skin, and the skin shivers in order to generate heat at the surface.

Exposure

As with all animals, just how effective the body is in ridding itself of excess internal heat depends upon the extent of its effective surface area with the surrounding air. As this effective area can change with body posture, it will be different in different *yogasanas*. That is to say, cooling of the core can be less efficient in folded but otherwise cooling postures such as *paschimottanasana*, where the upper and lower parts of the body press on one another, as compared with *savasana*, where they do not. *Savasana* in hot, humid weather should be done with the arms well separated from the torso for this reason.

In contrast, when performing the *yogasanas* in a cold room, it is more heat-conserving to work with the body in folded positions such as *adho mukha virasana* than in open positions, all other things being equal. In a parallel way, the sweat pores of the skin automatically close in cold weather and open when it is hot. Note too that long, thin bodies will cool more quickly than short, stout bodies, because their ratio of surface area to volume is larger.

---

dependent on the square of its velocity. As it is the faster-moving molecules that tend to travel from the liquid phase to the gas phase and so evaporate most easily, they leave behind an assemblage of slower-moving, cooler molecules in the liquid phase; thus, the temperature of the liquid drops in the evaporative process.

Emotions

Emotions also have a profound effect on the temperature of the skin. Fear and anxiety lead to a lowering of the skin temperature, pallor, and dryness (the first two of which signal excitation of the sympathetic nervous system), whereas embarrassment and pleasure raise the skin temperature, with obvious blushing. If one is working the *yogasanas* in a vigorous way, then there is a general sympathetic response that acts to move blood from areas devoid of skeletal muscles (such as the gastrointestinal tract, the fingertips, and the toes) to the muscles being used. Consequently, the temperatures in the muscle-free areas of the body will fall when the level of exercise is high.

Yogasana

The effects of a regular *yogasana* practice on thermoregulation have been reported by Bhatnagar et al. [60], who find that the resting core temperature decreases by 1° C after several weeks of beginner's practice, and that the rise of the core temperature following strong exercise is less in those who practice *yogasanas*. These results support the idea that *yogasanas* slow the metabolic processes, and therefore these processes produce less heat in the body per unit of time. A comparison of two groups of trainees, one in "physical training" and one doing *yogasana* instead, showed that the *yogasana*-trained students were more resistant to cold, shivering less and shivering only at a lower temperature, than those taking the physical training [770]. This is in accord with *yogasana* practice raising the level of parasympathetic excitation in the autonomic nervous system, as parasympathetic excitation raises skin temperature and inhibits shivering (table 5.A-2).

The general factors involved in generating and dissipating heat in the body while exercising are summarized in figure 14.A-9. The magnitude of the in-flowing and out-flowing heat will depend upon many factors but will be adjusted automatically so as to keep the core temperature constant.

Section 20.E: Hair and the Sebaceous Glands

In addition to the sweat glands, the skin is host to the exocrine sebaceous glands, which exude a fatty, oily product (sebum). Being most closely related to the hair follicles, they are most numerous on the scalp; it is excessive output from the sebaceous glands that is responsible for oily, greasy hair. Being intimately associated with the hair follicles, the sebaceous glands use the follicle as paths to the corneal layer of the skin. Sebum not only helps to lubricate the skin and keep it pliant, but being acidic, the oil from the sebaceous glands also is bacteriostatic and so helps keep the skin healthy. Many bacteria feed on sweat and sebum and convert these odorless materials into foul-smelling compounds.

Piloerection

In emergency situations where the sympathetic nervous system might be activated, smooth muscles at the base of each of the body hairs of furry animals are activated so that the hairs are brought erect (piloerection), thereby fooling an aggressor into thinking that their bodies are much larger [360, 432]. Clearly, this is no longer a strategy for avoiding conflict in humans, as we have far too little hair, and that hair that we do have serves no serious function in regard to protection. In furry animals, piloerection also works to trap body heat, but this is not a factor for humans, except at the top of the head. In fact, our greatest need in regard to hair is to be hairless in hot weather so that we can reap the largest benefit from the evaporative cooling that follows sweating.

Efferent nerve fibers to the muscles at the base of each hair make it stand on end whenever one is cold or frightened; these are the "goose bumps" we sense in such situations. In practitioners with refined control over the autonomic nervous system, activation of the pilomotor system can be

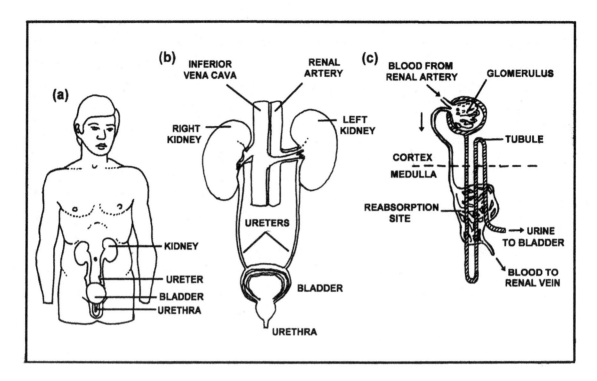

Figure 20.F-1. (a) Location of the kidneys symmetrically around the body's center line, just below the ribs. (b) Details of the organs connected to the kidneys. (c) Detail of the nephron within the kidney, where the filtering action takes place.

brought under conscious control [514]. In such people, conscious stimulation of the sympathetic nervous system not only raises every hair on the body to an upright position but also increases heart rate, respiration rate, and depth of breathing, as well as pupil diameter and sweating; i.e., the general spectrum of sympathetic responses (Section 5.C, page 170).

Section 20.F: Body Wastes

Action of the Kidneys

Specifications

The kidneys are two bean-shaped organs, each situated on its side of the spine at the height of the lowest ribs (figure 20.F-1a). The kidneys are found just forward of the posterior wall of the abdominal cavity, at the level between the T12

and L3 vertebrae; the right kidney is lower than the left in order to accommodate the liver. Each kidney in the average adult is 10–12 centimeters (four to five inches) in height, half that dimension in width, and about 2.5 centimeters (one inch) in thickness. This structure is surrounded by a protective layer of fatty tissue and is anchored to the surrounding tissue and the abdominal wall by connective tissue. The adrenal glands rest upon the upper ends of the kidneys, as shown in figure 5.E-1.

Though the kidneys are only 0.5 percent of the total weight of the body, they directly receive 10 percent of the aortic output during light exercise and perhaps even more when at rest (table 14.A-2). Kidneys are integral parts of the fluid and mineral homeostatic processes, as they filter 180 liters of fluid every twenty-four hours but return 179 liters of this to circulation, with the remaining 1–1.5 liters being excreted as urine. Kidneys in men are about 10 percent larger than those in women, as appropriate for the larger blood volume in men.

Within the kidney, the filtering unit is the nephron, a tube open at one end and closed at the other (figure 20.F-1c). Each kidney contains one to two million nephrons, which remove urea,[3] salts, and other water-soluble wastes. Approximately 1.2 liters of blood (25 percent of the cardiac output; see table 14.A-2) are processed in the kidneys every minute when at rest; however, with heavy exercise, the fraction of the cardiac output sent to the kidneys drops significantly as that to the muscles correspondingly increases. In the course of twenty-four hours, the kidneys reclaim about 650 grams of sodium chloride (NaCl), 400 grams of sodium bicarbonate ($NaHCO_3$), 180 grams of glucose. and about 180 liters of water from the bloodstream! The kidneys are able to maintain electrolyte balance in the body, even when loaded with large amounts of compounds such as the phosphoric acid in cola drinks; however, repeatedly doing such heavy filtration sooner or later takes them to exhaustion. On a short-term basis, the kidneys can handle a 150-fold increase in salt intake or an increase of water intake from pints to gallons without disruption of the electrolyte balance.

Function

In operation, the nephron first filters the blood of its small molecules and ions, stores them temporarily, and then reclaims just enough of these filtered substances to re-form the blood, much as occurs in the liver (Subsection 19.A, page 712). At this stage, the molecules remaining in the filtered fluid are largely the plasma proteins. Surplus or waste molecules and ions not so reclaimed are left to flow out of the kidneys into the urinary bladder [450].

The kidneys are key elements in the water balance in the body, their actions being directed by hormonal release; the most important of these is ADH (antidiuretic hormone or vasopressin; see Subsection 6.B, page 215) from the pituitary gland. The re-uptake of Na^+ is controlled by the concentration of angiotensin II and is closely regulated largely by the action of aldosterone; whereas the reabsorption of water is controlled by ADH. The pH of the urine is also tightly controlled by the absorption and release of the H^+ ion, so as to keep the pH of the blood slightly basic, in the range 7.3–7.4. The four ions K^+, Na^+, Cl^-, and HCO_3^- are key elements in maintaining good health in many cellular processes, and their balance is maintained in large part by the kidneys working with elements of the endocrine system. The kidneys also excrete erythropoietin, a hormone that stimulates the bone marrow to produce red blood cells.

When, in the course of a demanding *yogasana* practice in hot weather, one is perspiring heavily, the release of ADH from the pituitary inhibits the release of water into the urine, but if one drinks too much water so as to dilute the blood, then ADH release is inhibited, and a large volume of watery urine is formed instead. One sees that the kidneys closely regulate the composition of the blood within very narrow limits and so act as one of the body's prime homeostatic mechanisms. The adrenal glands sit atop the kidneys, and their function is discussed in Section 6.B, page 217.

Urination

It is the function of the urinary system to continuously process the bloodstream, to extract from it all toxic materials due either to metabolites or to ingested material, and to homeostatically balance the levels of certain salts in the blood, as well as to adjust the blood volume. A byproduct of this process is the elimination of unwanted materials in the urine. The system working to these ends consists of the kidneys, ureters, the urinary bladder, and the urethra, located within the lower thorax, as shown in figure 20.F-1b. All of the filtering action takes place in the kidneys, the other structures serving as passive conduits and storage vessels for the fluids involved.

---

3   The digestion of amino acids can lead to the production of large amounts of ammonia (NH_3), a very poisonous substance. The body handles this by combining the ammonia with CO_2, to form water and the innocuous compound urea (NH_2CONH_2), which is excreted in the urine.

Blood Flow

Blood from the renal artery first passes into the glomeruli within the nephrons (figure 20.F-1c), where it is stripped not only of the waste products but of many necessary salts as well. Leaving the glomeruli capsules, the depleted blood then passes to a reabsorption site, where the depleted blood is again in contact with the tubules of the glomeruli, wherein the composition of the depleted blood is then fortified so as to have a composition as close to that of fresh blood as possible; this blood exits the kidneys via the renal vein, whereas the unwanted materials are vented to the urinary system via the connection of the tubules to the ureters.

Urine from the kidneys is sent via the ureters to the urinary bladder, a simple organ, being a muscular sac with the ability to hold up to a pint of urine for hours on end if necessary. As the bladder fills, it expands, and when full (0.4 liters of urine), stretch receptors in the bladder walls signal the brain as to the full condition. Sphincters at the two ends of the urethra, the internal and the external sphincters, control the flow of urine, also termed micturition, out of the bladder.

The action of the parasympathetic system during filling and distension of the bladder walls is to reflexively contract the bladder muscles and open the internal sphincter. However, during filling, this parasympathetic tendency toward voiding is momentarily blocked by the action of the sympathetic nervous system on the external sphincter, and no urine passes. Following the sympathetic repression of the micturition reflex, the need to urinate is postponed for up to an hour, only to return more often and more insistently. However, once the bladder distension reaches a high level, the sympathetic inhibition is turned off by supraspinal centers, parasympathetic domination reasserts itself, and urination commences with both sphincters open and the bladder walls contracting. Valves within the ureters are oriented so that on bladder contraction, the voiding is solely through the urethra. In the young, all of the above is just a spinal reflex, but in adults, the control is supraspinal, with conscious control of the external sphincter [427].

Bladder Filling

That urination action usually cannot be begun without releasing the breath is an indication of the parasympathetic nature of this act. When in a tense situation in the presence of others, the external sphincter in men can tighten so that one cannot urinate, even if there is a strong need to do so [68]. When arousal of the sexual apparatus involves the sympathetic nervous system and so inhibits the contraction of the bladder, urination is inhibited. This is a natural reflex.

Because of the large size of the uterus in women, there is correspondingly less volume for the urinary bladder, which can mean frequent trips to the bathroom. When this occurs during a *yogasana* class, one should honor the urge and not try to suppress it, for the bladder should be empty for *yogasana* practice. Inversions and postures that squeeze the abdomen will promote the need to urinate, especially in women. See Box 14.F-3, page 594, for a further discussion of this topic. In the male, because the urethra passes vertically through the prostate gland on its way to the penis, swelling of this gland can lead indirectly to urinary problems.

Urination at Night

At night, the urinary bladder fills so as to stretch to paper-thinness. When in this state, the bladder signals spinal centers to contract the muscles of the bladder and to open the internal sphincter so as to release the pressure. However, when asleep, the external sphincter, controlled by brainstem nuclei, is tightly closed. Only upon awakening does the conscious need to urinate become apparent.

When younger than age seven years, children produce urine at a constant rate throughout the day and night; however, once beyond about seven years, antidiuretic hormone (ADH) is released by the pituitary gland into the bloodstream at night, and so urine production slows at that time by a factor of approximately 70 percent. As one ages, the release of ADH itself slows, and so the pattern of night-time urination reasserts itself, especially when deep sleep is rare.

Inversion

When the water level in the extracellular fluid becomes too low, the hypothalamus stimulates the pituitary gland to release ADH into the bloodstream. This hormone then acts upon the kidneys, encouraging them to retain urine. Somewhat the opposite reaction occurs during inversion. When in an upright stance, there is an insufficiency of blood returning to the heart, and the volume receptors in the atrial chambers (Section 14.E, page 580) report a low blood volume. However, upon inverting, the blood and lymph otherwise pooled in the legs now fill the right atrium, and the volume receptors in this atrium then report an excess of extracellular fluid. Once the extracellular fluid is sensed to be in excess, the body reflexively moves to rid itself of the extra fluid through urination. One understands from this the need to urinate after performing inversions of long duration, or even when thinking about them. This mechanism works only during the day, being nonfunctional at night when the body is horizontal [584]. The volume of urine released also is dependent upon one's emotional state; if one is nervous, so that there is strong sympathetic excitation, leading to an elevated blood pressure, then the excess pressure is relieved by turning blood into urine in the kidneys.

Minerals

The voiding of urine frees the body of excess water and of several salt components, and, as might be expected, the body does this in a regular way by the clock (Chapter 23, page 769). Thus, urination rids the body of Na^+ and K^+ in addition to water, and the amounts lost daily are largest in early afternoon. Similarly, when we lie down at the end of the day and so remove the gravitational stress from the skeleton, the bones begin to demineralize, as with osteoporosis (Section 7.G, page 254), and Ca^{2+} leaves the bones and enters the extracellular fluid, to be released the following afternoon in the urine if not reabsorbed. The acidity of urine is higher at night and less during the day, and the flow of urine through the urethra acts to keep it free of colonization by microbes.

Urine is normally slightly basic; however, this is dependent upon diet, with protein ingestion promoting acidity and vegetarian ingestion promoting alkalinity.

Circadian Cycles

When devoid of twenty-four-hour cues, the body's salt and water excretion become free-running, with periods of either 24.8 or 33.5 hours or both (figure 23.B-2). As shown in the figure, the release of Na^+ and K^+ in the urine conform to the 24.8-hour cycle, with little or no release at 33.5 hours; whereas for Ca^{2+}, there is a prominent 33.5-hour periodicity, with little release at 24.8 hours. The volume of urinary water released during free running peaks significantly at both 24.8 and 33.5 hours, as does the core temperature [584].

Defecation

The processing of food by the gastrointestinal tract up to the point that the digested mass enters the colon is described in Subsection 19.A, page 703. The ascending and transverse sections of the colon function mainly to remove water from the stool and give it solidity, whereas the descending and sigmoid sections (figure 19.A-1) serve largely as storage for the fecal matter prior to the opening of the anal sphincters and defecation. Feces are 75 percent water and 25 percent dry matter, with 50 percent of the dry matter consisting of dead bacterial cells. The weight of the feces depends largely on the amount of undigestible fiber in the diet. If the speed of transit through the colon is fast (i.e., rapid and intense peristalsis), then the stool is dry, and vice versa.

Anal Sphincters

At the colonic end of the gastrointestinal tract, the control of the muscles is again shared by the enteric plexus and by the parasympathetic nervous system, with strong input from higher centers. Peristaltic-like contractions in the descending and sigmoid sections of the bowel compact the fecal matter in the rectum, distending it. Sensed by stretch receptors in the rectum, the distension leads to a reflexive contraction of the rectum, together with the involuntary opening of the internal anal sphincter, just as with the urinary bladder.

The nerve supply to the anus and rectum is largely sympathetic and provides a great many sensors on the anal skin [47]. Because of this, stretching of the anal sphincter accelerates the breathing rate [863]. Perhaps this relates to the anal action in *ashwini mudra*, which lifts and stretches the anal skin and in doing so works to energize the body and mind in whichever *yogasana* posture it accompanies.

Parasympathetic Release

Voluntary release of the external anal sphincter and the act of defecation are triggered by pressure in the terminal part of the colon and are assisted by the parasympathetic nervous system. When this mechanism is active, there is a feeling of relief and relaxation throughout the body. In fact, defecation is medically advised for people suffering from paroxysmal tachycardia in order to bring their heart rate back to normal! If the moment is not right for defecation (as decided by the higher cortical centers), the external sphincter can be kept closed in spite of the involuntary opening of the internal sphincter, and under such conditions, the urge to defecate passes in a few minutes, only to return again in about a half-hour [308]. However, the final release of the external sphincter is under the voluntary control of the parasympathetic pelvic nerves, and so the inhibition of the sympathetic nervous system during defecation makes it generally a very relaxing act, if one does not have to strain to bring it about.

Suppression of the natural defecation reflex by keeping the external anal sphincter closed, using the higher centers in the adult central nervous system, is the unspoken cornerstone of our civilization, for it is only through the intervention of these higher centers that defecation can be postponed to a more socially convenient and private time.

When defecation is difficult, people often turn to the Valsalva maneuver (Subsection 15.C, page 616) to get things started; however, this is a strongly sympathetic activity, and the more natural defecation should be parasympathetically driven.

As mentioned above, the opening and closing of the anal sphincters is under conscious control. Three valves exist in the rectal tissue that allow flatus to pass from the rectum to the anus but that inhibit the simultaneous outflow of feces. Coordination of the rectal valves and the anal sphincters allows one a certain measure of control in regard to passing gas without defecating, as might occur when in *pavan muktasana*, for example.

Constipation

The effects of diet on the stool and on constipation are discussed in Subsection 19.C, page 716. The lack of effective peristalsis that characterizes constipation may be due in part to a sluggish blood supply to the abdominal area [47] and in part to gravitational compression [446]. It is understandable then that the *yogasana* cure for constipation consists of postures that increase abdominal muscle tone (such as straight-arm *chaturanga dandasana*), postures in which the colon is pressed from the outside, and inversions that release the compression due to gravity. In this regard, the most effective cures for constipation will involve one or more of the above factors; i.e., inverted *yogasanas* in which the abdominal muscles are working strongly or the pressure of the heels against the colon massage it and so induce peristaltic movement. Specifically, Mehta et al. [559] recommend either *pindasana* in *sirsasana* or in *sarvangasana* for constipation, postures in which the legs are first put into *padmasana* and the heels are then pressed against the abdomen while inverted. These postures have the advantages of supplying both pressure on the colon and inversion. *Ardha uttanasana* in either *sirsasana* or *sarvangasana* also would be effective.

Readers who follow the Iyengar path are familiar with its method of always performing *yogasanas* that are left-to-right asymmetric, such as *trikonasana*, by first going to the right and then to the left. The intention here is that on going first to the right, the ascending colon is compressed, and then following this with action to the left, the sigmoid colon is compressed, the combination working to move the feces in the direction from the ascending colon to the rectum [646]. Contraction of the abdomen during defecation, as with the Valsalva maneuver (Subsection 15.C, page 616), results in an over-pressure of approximately 100 millimeters Hg in the colon, which may be large enough to force open the ileocecal valve (figure 20.F-2**a**) and so drive feces backward into the small intestine.

Sitting versus Squatting

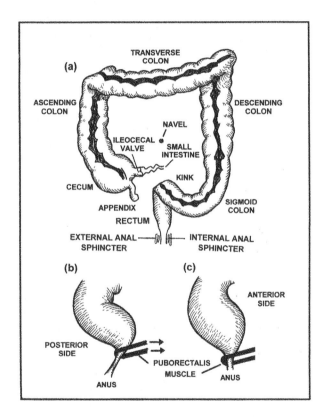

Figure 20.F-2. (**a**) The shape of the colon, connected at one end to the small intestine via the ileocecal valve and to the rectum at the other end. (**b**) Constriction of the lower part of the rectum by the puborectalis muscle when sitting, and (**c**) release of the constriction between rectum and anus by relaxation of the puborectalis muscle, as when in *malasana*.

There are two popular postures for defecation, with decidedly different muscle actions and visceral consequences. In Western cultures, one defecates in the sitting position (*utkatasana*) upon a toilet, often using the Valsalva maneuver to initiate the act. In this, there is an inhalation of the breath by depression of the diaphragm and a simultaneous tightening of the abdominal muscles, the combination of which significantly raises the intra-abdominal pressure (Subsection 15.C, page 616). The consequences of this pressurization are manifold [14, 677, 790, 845, 911] and best discussed using figure 20.F-2, where the colon and its appendages are shown.

We now consider the consequences of defecating in the *utkatasana* position and compare it to defecating while in the *malasana* position.

Utkatasana

When defecation is driven by the Valsalva maneuver while in the *utkatasana* position:

1. The pressure is applied from the top to the bottom of the ascending colon, pressing the contents downward. The effect is to press fecal matter down into the appendix (promoting appendicitis) and backward through the ileocecal valve and into the small intestine (promoting a variety of inflammatory bowel diseases such as colitis, Crohn's ileitis, etc.). Fecal matter will remain in the cecum regardless of the Valsalva strain and will become dry, hard, and cemented to the walls.

2. In order to completely empty the colon, it is necessary to open the kink in the sigmoid colon where it joins the rectum. This kink in the colon acts to prevent incontinence in the long term, taking the pressure off the puborectalis muscle. It is normally is set at an angle of about 90° when in the sitting position and so resists passage of the colonic contents above the kink. Fecal matter trapped in the sigmoid colon can become stagnant, leading to inflammation at that point. The cecum and the sigmoid colon are the top two cancer sites in the colon.

3. Chronic straining at the stool encourages

the development of hemorrhoids and of a type of sigmoid herniation called diverticulosis. It also increases pressure within the thorax and so impedes the venous return to the right atrium of the heart. Consequently, there is a tendency toward fainting (defecation syncope) and even death when strained in this way.

4. In the sitting position, the Valsalva pressure presses the pelvic floor significantly toward the perineum, with appreciable negative consequences in regard to the prostate, bladder, rectum, and uterus. It is a significant problem in women, because the open structure of the vaginal canal is quite vulnerable to the downward pressures on the pelvic floor generated by the sitting posture. It is especially important that pregnant women avoid the Valsalva maneuver when voiding the bowel, and by the same logic, they should avoid Valsalva pressurization in any of the *yogasana* postures. See also the connection of the Valsalva pressurization to childbirth (Section 21.B, page 746). In men at the stool, it is argued that the repeated downward pressure of the daily straining on the pelvic floor stretches the pudendal nerves serving the genital area and thereby isolates the prostate from the central nervous system. This same pressure on the pudendal nerves of women are held to be responsible for the "need" for hysterectomy.

5. In the sitting position, the puborectalis muscle (one of the levator ani muscles; see figure 20.F-2b) is contracted and acts as a noose about the rectum to further impede evacuation in this posture. Its effect can be overcome by maximum straining in the Valsalva position, but this leaves one open to what is essentially a repetitive stress injury.

Malasana

The second posture for defecation is that adopted in so-called less developed cultures. In cultures in which the chair is a luxury available only to very few, defecation is commonly practiced in the squat position; i.e., in *malasana*. This posture is shown in figure 21.B-1 as appropriate for a pregnancy delivery, but it would be quite similar for defecation. In this case, the abdomen is pressurized from the bottom to the top by the pressure of the thighs on the abdomen, so that little or no diaphragmatic pressure is necessary for elimination.

The consequences of this *malasana*-based approach are listed below, for comparison with those of the *utkatasana*-based approach given above:

1. Abdominal pressure is applied by the pressure of the right thigh at the base of the ascending colon from below as the thighs are brought toward the abdomen, with the result that the contents of the cecum (in which there is no peristaltic action) are emptied totally into the ascending colon, where peristalsis then takes over. Any fecal matter trapped in the appendix is emptied upward in the direction of the ascending colon by this pressure of the thigh. Because abdominal pressure in this posture is only moderate at best (only one-third that of the Valsalva maneuver), the ileocecal valve is not forced open, and toxic bacteria do not travel backward into the small intestine.

2. X-ray studies show that in the *malasana* position, the pressure of the left thigh on the sigmoid colon works to support it and open the sigmoid kink from an average angle of 92° when sitting to an average of 132° when in *malasana*, and in some cases, to 180°! With the kink angle opened as it is when in *malasana*, evacuation is complete.

3. As the intra-abdominal pressure is significantly lower when in *malasana*, the risk for diverticulosis or hemorrhoids is low to nonexistent.

4. The various prostate problems of the developed world, such as prostatitis, prostate cancer, and prostate enlargement,

are virtually unknown in the third-world countries and, in fact, were unknown in the Western world before the time of the introduction of the toilet. Using the *malasana* position for defecation is less stressful on the pudendal nerve complex and possibly this relates to the lack of prostate problems in those who use it. Women in squatting cultures have far less urinary incontinence and far fewer hysterectomies than those in sitting cultures.

5. The intra-abdominal pressure necessary for colonic elimination is considerably reduced in *malasana* due to the relaxation of the puborectalis muscle surrounding the rectum.

Gynecology, Pregnancy, and Sexual Function

21

Section 21.A: Ovulation and Menstruation

The Menstrual Cycle

Puberty

The onset of puberty occurs naturally at ages between eight and thirteen years old in girls and a few years later in boys. Puberty is triggered by several nongenetic factors, the most important of which in girls seems to be nutritional status; when the body is well nourished and has stored energy sufficient to support the growth of a fetus, then puberty begins. At this point in both genders, a protein known as kisspeptin is activated in the hypothalamus, which acts to release the gonadotropin-releasing hormone GnRH into the anterior pituitary gland. Following this, the hormones LH (luteinizing hormone) and FSH (follicle stimulating hormone) are released into the blood and stimulate the ovaries to release sex hormones, which initiate the first menstruation, promote the secondary sexual characteristics, and turn off the production of GnRH. When released in boys, the LH and FSH hormones stimulate the testes, again leading to the development of the appropriate sexual characteristics [598a]. The average age at which puberty begins in girls has been falling steadily in Western societies over the past 150 years, from about seventeen to 12.5 years.

Following the full attainment of puberty in girls, every twenty-eight days thereafter, two interlinked gynecological cycles in women, ovarian and menstrual, pass through their respective maximum and minimum phases. Indeed, the words "menstruation," "moon,' and "month" are derived from the Greek word meaning "measurer of time," for a woman's menstrual cycle requires about twenty-eight days, or one lunar cycle. The timing aspect of the menstrual cycle is under the control of the suprachiasmatic nucleus within the hypothalamus (Subsection 23.B, page 787).

Ovarian Phase

During the ovarian phase (also known as the follicular phase), an egg matures under hormonal influence and, under control of a second hormone, is released fourteen days later from an ovary. At this point in the menstrual cycle, there is then a thickening of the endometrium within the uterus, in expectation of the implantation of a fertilized egg, and hormonal levels fluctuate strongly. If the egg is not fertilized, the endometrium disintegrates and menstruation begins. This is described in more detail below.

Menstrual Phase

The menstrual cycle in women consists of the expulsion of blood and tissue every twenty-eight days from the uterus, the flow lasting for three to seven days; let us take day fifteen of the cycle (figure 21.A-1) as the first day of menstrual (luteal) flow. The cycle itself begins approximately fourteen days previous to the time of first menstrual flow, days twenty-six and twenty-seven, when the hypothalamus releases two hormones into the ducts leading to the anterior part of the pituitary

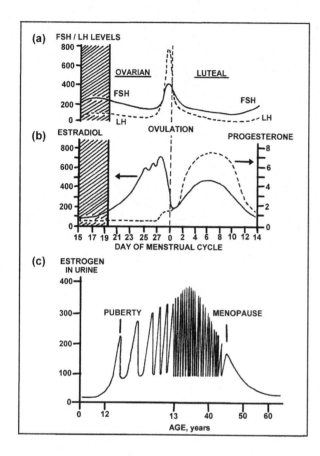

Figure 21.A-1. (a) The ovarian and luteinizing phases of the twenty-eight-day menstrual cycle and the daily variations of LH and FSH. (b) Daily variations of estradiol and progesterone concentrations throughout the cycle. (c) The levels of estrogens in the urine of females from the years preceding puberty to many years beyond the onset of menopause. The monthly rise and fall of the hormonal level within the age range of twelve to forty-five years is obvious.

gland just below it (figure 4.B-1). Called the follicle releasing hormone (FRH) and the luteinizing releasing hormone (LRH), these two substances then promote the release into the bloodstream of the gonadotropic hormones (figure 6.B-3) FSH (follicular stimulating hormone) and LH (luteinizing hormone), both of which peak on the twenty-seventh day (figure 21.A-1a); these hormones have the woman's ovaries as their destination and site of action. In this ovarian phase,

the level of estradiol[1] rises to a peak over the last week, whereas that of progesterone stays relatively low (figure 21.A-1b).

Once in the ovaries, the FSH and LH stimulate one of the follicles in the ovaries to prepare for fertilization, by releasing an egg (ovum) from the follicle into one of the fallopian tubes on the following day (day one). After this ovulation process, there follow fourteen days of relatively low FSH and LH levels, and rising estradiol and progesterone production by the FHS and LH, respectively, eventually turning off the flow of FHS and LH from the pituitary and preparing the lining of the uterus to receive the descending egg.

In this second stage, known as the luteinizing phase, the ovum is called the corpus luteum, and the high estradiol level acts to build up a thick but unstable layer of tissue in the uterus, while the progesterone acts to stabilize this layer and prepare it further for the corpus luteum [814]. The blood flow to the uterine lining (the endometrium) is increased in the luteinizing phase, as is its thickness, and the hypothalamus acts to increase the body temperature by about 0.5° F, so as to provide a more fertile environment for the corpus luteum. By measuring this temperature rise using a basal thermometer, one can estimate the most likely time for fertilization to occur.

If, by the fifteenth day, the corpus luteum has not been fertilized by sperm, the endometrium seedbed of the uterus collapses, tissues disintegrate by apoptosis, and another menstrual flow begins. At the same time, estradiol and progesterone levels have returned to the low values characteristic of day fifteen.

If, instead, the egg is fertilized, then progesterone stays high as estradiol levels fall. As for what happens next, see Section 21.B, page 743. In any case, during the entire twenty-eight-day period, the LH, FSH, estradiol, and progesterone hormones interact and vary in their concentrations, with their relative proportions dictating the events of the cycle as in figures 21.A-1a and 21.A-1b.

---

1   The term "estrogen" refers to a family of closely related chemical compounds, the most important of which, in regard to female reproduction, is estradiol.

Estrogen

The variation of the estrogen levels in the typical woman's body over the years in shown in figure 21.A-1c. One sees that there is a regular rise and fall of the levels on going from age twelve to sixty years and a smooth change of menstrual timing from bimonthly to monthly to yearly in that period. The relative constancy of a regular monthly menstrual cycle in the years between thirteen and forty-three years implies some sort of pacemaker within the body that controls the timing of the process, and it has been postulated that the regulator lies within the pineal gland [814], already known to regulate hormones within a twenty-four-hour sleep/wake cycle (Subsection 23.D, page 794).

Recent studies show that there are changes of the volume of gray matter in the emotional-control centers of the brains of women as they go through their menstrual cycles. In particular, in times of low estrogen, there is a slight increase in the volume of the cingulate cortex, and in times of high estrogen, the volumes of the prefrontal cortex, the left hippocampal gyrus, and the amygdala all increase.

Resetting the Menstrual Clock

Exposure to light can have several important effects on the menstrual period. Thus, those women who live in areas where much time is spent indoors are less fertile than those in sunnier climates; the closer a woman lives to the equator, the more fertile she is. Women with irregular patterns of menstruation can be brought back into the twenty-eight-day pattern by exposure to bright lights (a bare 100-Watt bulb) on nights fourteen through seventeen, as counted from the first day of her last period (days zero through four in figure 21.A-1b). This treatment was effective in shortening the period in women with unusually long periods. Apparently, the light has its effect on either the suprachiasmatic nucleus or the pineal gland, to regularize the period. Note that the suprachiasmatic nucleus is the center within the hypothalamus that responds hormonally to the daily rising and setting of the sun, operating on

the basis of a loosely bound molecular complex formed between a component from the superchiasmatic nucleus and melatonin from the pineal gland (Subsection 17.C, page 675).

Menstrual Timing and Synchronicity

Menstruation occurs only when there is sufficient body fat in the woman's body to support both her needs and that of the fetus, if there is to be one. Thus, menstruation will shut down in the female super-athlete who has too little body fat, and menarche, the time of first menstruation, can be four years later for undernourished young girls in poor countries as compared with that for well-fed girls in the more developed countries [68].

There is an interesting menstrual phenomenon wherein a group of women living together will, in time, synchronize their menstrual cycles so that they occur simultaneously. The entrainment mechanism is thought to involve the pre-ovulation and post-ovulation axillary pheromones of a dominant woman within the group, with the pre-ovulation pheromone inducing ovulation in those other women who have not yet ovulated, and the post-ovulation pheromone inducing delay of ovulation in the others. The result of these two actions sooner or later is to bring the entire group into a state of menstrual synchronicity [904].

Sexual Attraction and the Nose

The timing of a woman's menstrual cycle also is affected by the armpit odors of men, and it has been shown that men prefer the smell of T-shirts worn by ovulating women to those worn by those who are not ovulating. This sensitivity to odor extends to the immune system as well, for a woman will rate the odor of a T-shirt worn by a male as more pleasant, the more different her immune-system genes are from his [905], unless she is on birth-control medication, in which case she will prefer that of males having similar immune-system genes. During menstruation, a woman's face becomes more symmetric left to right, thereby increasing her attractiveness to men (Subsection III.A, page 843) [818].

Given the connection between sexual function in women and the structure of the nose as proposed by Freud (Subsection 15.E, page 628), it is not surprising to find that premenstrual discomfort can be alleviated through the simple inhalation of human pheromones that are mediators of anxiety and hormone-related disorders [924]. Studies show that if there is a high level of stress during a menstrual period, the chance that the next menstrual period will be painful is doubled. For women whose bodies follow this prescription, a relaxing, stress-reducing *yogasana* practice during the menstrual time can make the following month's period significantly less likely to be a painful one.

Sparrowe [814] presents the view that the menstrual flow is purifying and that one should feel that through this process, the body has rid itself of many impurities, both physical and mental. In order for the purification to work, one must not only eat properly but exercise moderately and rest during the first few days in order to give the body every opportunity to do its work.

Hormonal Levels in Males

Detectable levels of both FSH and LH can be found in the male body as well as in the female; however, in the female, there is a strong twenty-eight-day cycle of peak concentrations (figure 21.A-1**a**), whereas in the male, there is no detectable fluctuation of these hormonal levels over the period of a month. The changes in a young girl's body at puberty (i.e., the appearance of breasts, pubic hair, a feminine voice, and broader hips) are all driven by the appearance of estrogen in the body at the time of first menstruation. Sex drive (libido) and the growth of axillary and pubic hair in women also are influenced by the male hormone testosterone, but this gonadocorticoidal hormone in the female is released by the cortex of the adrenal glands. In the male, testosterone is released from the testes, as controlled by LH from the pituitary gland, and if the testosterone level is too high, the amount of LH is reduced, and the testosterone is thereby brought back into line. Thus, it is relatively stable as compared with the hormonal swings in females.

Testosterone in males is used in the manufacture of sperm. However, men with epilepsy frequently have low testosterone levels, as do men at the time of delivery of their pregnant partner. These attentive men also may experience a 20 percent rise in the level of their prolactin during the three weeks before delivery.

Premenstrual Syndromes

The complexities of the menstrual cycle and the delicate balance involved between powerful hormonal forces imply a multitude of ways that the cycle can go wrong. In addition to the specific problems of lack of ovulation, too little or too much bleeding, endometriosis, fibroids, and ovarian cysts, there is a less specific broad class of menstrual-related symptoms collectively called premenstrual syndrome (PMS). It is said that there are at least 150 different symptoms associated with PMS [171], relating primarily to an imbalance of the estrogen and progesterone levels or to a sluggish liver that is unable to handle the efficient removal of toxins generated by the menstrual process. It is most recently accepted that PMS relates to estrogen imbalance [803].

For the sake of specificity, consider the approach taken by Rychner [731] based on an earlier classification scheme of PMS symptoms. She assigned such symptoms to one of four categories: type A (anxiety, irritability, and mood swings), type C (craving, fatigue, and headache), type D (depression, confusion, and memory loss), and type H (water retention, bloating, weight gain, and breast tenderness). Mixed-type symptoms are seen, and the pattern is not necessarily constant from one month to the next. The symptoms, appearing during the days seven through fourteen in figure 21.A-1**b**, are classified into four types below, within a framework of the appropriate *yogasana* postures.

Type A PMS

The *yogasanas* recommended for type A PMS symptoms (anxiety, irritability, and mood swings) are *savasana*, downward-facing *savasana*, and child's posture (*garbhasana*), all of which are consistent with the idea that type A anxiety involves a predominant excitation of the sympathetic nervous system and that parasympathetic balance can be restored by such relaxing postures (Section 22.C, page 766). Note too that the universal antidote for mood swings is regular exercise [171].

Type D PMS

At the other extreme, type D PMS symptoms (depression, confusion, and memory loss) signal the need for more sympathetic energy in the autonomic nervous system, and so it is no surprise that the recommended postures focus on backbending: *urdhva mukha svanasana, setu bandhasana,* and *dhanurasana,* specifically (Section 22.A, page 761). More intense backbending would be appropriate only for those with considerable experience in *yogasana,* as the universal recommendation during menstruation is to take it easy.

Interestingly, the symptoms of seasonal affective disorder (SAD; see Subsection 17.E, page 685) are said to be much like those of PMS, and in some women, phototherapy has been found to be effective in relieving PMS symptoms [539]. As SAD phototherapy involves a rebalancing along the sympathetic-parasympathetic axis, the effects of phototherapy in erasing the SAD-like symptoms of type D PMS are understandable.

Type C PMS

Rychner explains that in type C PMS, the craving for sugar or chocolate is driven by the hyperactivity of the body's insulin at this time and its need for glucose as a substrate (Subsection 19.C, page 718). The cravings are eased by promoting blood flow to the abdominal and pelvic areas, using postures such as *dhanurasana* and *setu bandhasana.* Medically, the craving for sweets relates to a deficiency of serotonin in the brain and is eased by drugs such as Prozac, that work to boost serotonin levels.

Type H PMS

Given that type H PMS symptoms primarily involve water retention and bloating, it is at first logical that the *yogasana* antidotes are relatively passive inversions; i.e., *upavistha konasana* against the wall, wall *padasana,* and *ardha halasana.* Indeed, as mentioned in Box 14.F-3, page

594, inversions do promote urination. However, because full inversions during menstruation are a controversial subject (see the subsection below), even *ardha halasana* just previous to menstruation may cross over the line of permissibility in some teachers' eyes.

Exercise and Estrogen

Many recent studies [618] have focused on the effects of exercise on the menstrual cycle and have found significant effects. Women who exercise regularly and vigorously have two to four times the rates of oligomenorrhea (scanty periods) or amenorrhea (no periods) than do otherwise sedentary women. Moreover, the oligomenorrhea is accompanied by significant bone loss, with estrogen levels depressed and cortisol levels elevated (Sections 5.C, page 176, and 7.G, page 254). Amenorrheic women athletes at age twenty-five years can have the spinal bone mineralization characteristic of women of age fifty-seven years, due to their low estrogen levels. However, oligomenorrhea is rapidly reversible when a young woman returns to a less demanding exercise schedule. For women who are having menstrual difficulties due to intense overtraining in their athletic specialty, the introduction of a *yogasana* practice can be an acceptable mode of restoration and recovery.

In an interesting series of studies, Wojtys et al. [900, 901] have studied the rates of incidence of damage to the anterior cruciate ligament in collegiate female athletes as a function of the phases of their menstrual cycles. They report that there is a statistically significant increased risk for tearing of this ligament during the ovulatory phase (days nineteen through twenty-eight) and the lowest risk during the luteal phase (days zero through fourteen); see figure 21.A-1a. In those athletes using oral contraceptives, increased risk for injury during the ovulatory phase did not appear. As estrogen is high in the ovulatory phase and progesterone is baseline low, it is implied that high levels of estrogen have a weakening effect on the collagen within the ligaments of women, implying in turn that during *yogasana* practice, women may be able to stretch further when their estrogen levels are high, as they are in the ovarian phase, but that they also run a higher risk for injury at that time.

Menstrual Pain

In regard to pain sensations in the two sexes, it is known that for women, there is a much stronger coupling of pain between visceral organs. Thus, women with irritable bowel syndrome often also experience fibromyalgia, headaches, and chronic pelvic pain. The connection between the sex organs and other organs in the female body may explain the odd relief from PMS that can be had by treating other organs. It is reported [844] that the application of gentle pressure to the vaginal area (as when lying upon a bolster, facing downward with the legs spread) can reduce pelvic pain for hours.

Women process pain using parts of the brain concerned with attention and emotion. Thus, distractions away from the pain can bring psychological support and pain relief. For men, the factor most influencing pain is appearing tough in public. Though publicly stoic while in pain, this attitude disappears when in private. See Section 13.C, page 524, for a further discussion of the different reactions to injury and pain shown by the two genders.

During menstruation, there is tissue damage and therefore the release of prostaglandins locally (Section 13.C, page 519) [531]. These hormones not only sensitize the free nerve endings that signal pain to the higher cerebral centers, but they also act to seal off the bleeding area. In doing so, they constrict the arteries so strongly that the arteries can go into spasm, thereby generating the feeling of menstrual cramps. Inasmuch as aspirin works to reduce prostaglandin production, it can be effective in reducing these menstrual symptoms, just as it can help reduce the arterial spasms of a migraine headache. Lower-back pain felt during menstruation is said to be referred pain (Section 13.D, page 532), springing from distress at the uterus [531].

Hormonal Effects on Pain

The sex hormones estrogen and progesterone have a strong effect on pain perception. Just be-

fore a menstrual period, women are less tolerant of pain. It appears that estrogen is excitatory for pain transmission in the central and peripheral nervous systems, and estrogen is at its highest level just a day or two before ovulation (figure 21.A-1**b**). Moreover, estrogen inhibits the production of bradykinin, a potent inflammatory mediator that protects injured tissue. On the other hand, progesterone deadens the nervous system's sensitivity to pain and is at its highest concentration about a week after ovulation; i.e., at the time leading up to the menses. Strangely, the analgesic effect of progesterone is blocked by eating chili peppers [561], whereas progesterone inhibits the action of oxytocin, a hormone closely related to positive feelings about others; a woman will be less trusting of others just after her time of ovulation, when progesterone levels soar.

Inversions at That Time of the Month

Long before the menstruation process was understood scientifically, the ancient yogic texts explained that during menstruation, there is a strong downward flow of *apana* energy and that this natural direction of flow is upset by inversion; however, Lasater [499] states that *apana* energy is increased by inversions. Today, there is general agreement among yoga teachers [404, 405, 531, 750, 758] that full inversions (*sirsasana, sarvangasana, halasana,* all manner of hand balances, and all of their variations) are contraindicated during the menstrual period. *Urdhva dhanurasana* safely may be included in the group of allowed inversions during menstruation [231]. Only MacMullen [531] demurs from outright prohibition of inversions during menstruation, saying that up-to-date (1990) data is not available on this question. Geeta Iyengar holds that inversions can arrest the menstrual flow, as they dry up the uterus. She does open the door somewhat, however, in saying that such a drying action actually may be beneficial if the flow is of an overly long duration or occurs at a time out of synchronicity with the normal flow [406].

Mechanisms

As for the medical reasons why inversions might be forbidden at this time, Schatz first suggested that the ligaments from which the uterus is suspended carry both the thin-walled veins transporting blood out of the uterus and the stout-walled arteries that carry blood into the uterus [750, 758]. Upon inversion, gravitational stresses in the ligaments of the uterus act to stretch them, and so reduce blood flow through the collapsible veins but not through the arteries. As a result, the uterus becomes engorged with blood, leading to increased menstrual flow. According to the drawings of Netter [613], the uterus is suspended from the broad ligament, but inversion would not appear to stress this ligament beyond that stress which is present when upright. Moreover, Schatz's conclusion is opposite to that of Geeta Iyengar, who states that the flow is retarded by inversions. Without further explanation, Lasater [491] argues that inversion blocks the flow of blood to the uterus, thus decreasing or even stopping the flow, but that heavy bleeding then may begin a few hours after the flow has slowed. Clennell [126] points out that inversion at the time of menstruation promotes holding of the unwanted material within the body and then its absorption (rather than its expulsion).

The older ideas that inversions during menstruation act to promote endometriosis or pelvic infection have been convincingly countered by Schatz [757], who shows them to be misconceptions in light of newer data. However, she does recommend strongly that women do not invert at this time, as it would be working against the self-understanding (*svadhyaya* [388]) toward which we strive in *yogasana* practice.

Rolf [714] mentions another point relevant to doing *sirsasana* in or around the menstrual period. She reports that some women experience pain elicited by pressure on a circular area about 2.5 centimeters (one inch) in diameter at the very crown of the head and assigns this to a menstrual disturbance of fascia in the congested region that propagates to fascial tissue at the top of the head. Right or wrong, it is a factor to keep in mind when women want to do *sirsasana* during menstruation.

Section 21.B: Pregnancy

The main focus of the practicing *yogasana* student who becomes pregnant must shift from meeting the challenges of their practice to doing what is most protective of the baby. With this in mind, one does not work so as to become tired or fatigued, and one does not work so hard that one is distressed during pregnancy. That is to say, the pregnant student's *yogasana* practice will have to be ratcheted down a few notches, as she now has something even more important to focus on: the successful outcome of her pregnancy. At this time, she would be wise to continue what she is doing, but at a less vigorous level, and to avoid starting anything new.

First Trimester

During the nine months of pregnancy, the most critical period is the first three months, the time during which the embryo implants in the uterus. Women who have a history of miscarriage or of cervical insufficiency should not start *yogasana* classes during this period, and experienced students who are in this category should do no unsupported standing postures during this time. Yoshikawa [914] recommends no inversions for a pregnant woman in her second and third trimesters; however she allows that this will depend upon the woman's level of *yogasana* experience and condition.

The general effects of pregnancy on the body of interest to *yogasana* students involve changes of numerous hormonal levels, all acting to prepare the body for delivery of a healthy baby and the effects of the growing pressure within the abdomen as the baby and the uterus increase in size. As discussed in Subsection 21.A, page 737, the level of estrogen is low at the time of conception, whereas that of progesterone is high. These factors are discussed below.

The Balance between Estrogen and Progesterone

The condition of the female reproductive apparatus is dictated in part by the relative amounts of circulating estrogen and progesterone, two steroid hormones of closely similar molecular structures but with rather opposite effects; both of these hormones are released by the ovaries. The variations in the relative amounts of these hormones throughout the menstrual cycle are clearly evident in figure 21.A-1**b**. As regards pregnancy, estrogen causes contraction of the uterus and expulsion of the fetus, whereas progesterone works against these tendencies. Early in the pregnancy, progesterone rules the physiology, but with time, estrogen gains the upper hand, and with that, the delivery process (parturition) is set in motion [802].

Delivery

In the early stages of pregnancy, the uterus is a relaxed bag of disconnected smooth-muscle cells, separated by collagenous tissue and closed at its cervical neck by a ring of tough collagen fibers. As delivery draws near and the estrogen from the placenta begins to exert itself by rising in concentration, the uterus synthesizes a protein called connexin that acts to connect the muscle cells electrically, so that when called upon, they can all contract simultaneously, much as the cells in the atrial chambers or in the ventricles of the heart contract in unison (Section 14.A, page 545).

The molecule NO (nitric oxide) inhibits the contractibility of the uterus's smooth muscle walls (as with the smooth muscles within the arterial walls; see Subsection 11.A, page 376). However, as the time for delivery approaches, the nitric oxide concentration diminishes so as to allow contractions. Additionally, under the influence of estrogen, the uterus becomes outfitted with receptors for the brain hormone oxytocin, which increases the force of uterine contractions, induces delivery, and produces prostaglandins, which work to unravel the collagenous ring in the cervix, allowing it to dilate. The hormone oxytocin also acts on the breasts of the new mother, encouraging

the flow of milk, and strengthens the bonds of love between mother and baby and mother and father.

Fetal Hormones

In addition to the hormonal systems of the mother, the hormonal systems of the fetus are active at this time, with the adrenal glands producing cortisol, which acts to eventually inflate the fetal lungs by removing the amniotic fluid that otherwise fills them. As the fetal brain develops, it also begins to release CRF to its pituitary, which in turn releases ACTH in order to promote cortisol release from the fetal adrenal glands. The fetal cortisol in turn stimulates the placenta to produce yet more CRF but on the maternal side. This CRF then acts on the fetal adrenal glands, making them manufacture estrogen! It is the concentration of maternal CRF that controls fetal estrogen production, which then dictates when the delivery process will begin [802].

Third Trimester

Many of the hormones involved in the birthing process are involved as well in the stress-related hormonal shift following excitation of the sympathetic nervous system (Section 5.B, page 165), but in the latter case, there is, of course, no fetal component and no delivery. On the other hand, there is evidence [481] that excessive muscle tension (sympathetic excitation) in the last few weeks of pregnancy can lead to breech presentation upon delivery, but in many cases, purposeful relaxation (parasympathetic excitation) can turn the fetus into the more normal head-first presentation for delivery. *Yogasana* practice directed toward relaxation of the muscles and the breath would thus be of great value where a breech birth and cesarean section otherwise might be the case.

If the birth is by cesarean section, then light stretching around the incised area may start in two weeks following delivery, because the abdominal area is highly vascularized and heals quickly, whereas in the areas of more weakly vascularized tissue following surgery, no stretching should be done for at least three weeks [479]. Light abdominal stretching following a cesarean section avoids the adhesion of the ends of the cut muscles, which would lead to muscle stiffness.

Sensitivity to Pain

The analgesic effects of progesterone are most obvious during pregnancy, when the progesterone levels rise dramatically in the third trimester, in anticipation of labor. The possible consequences of varying sensitivity to pain with respect to the phases of the menstrual and gestational cycles are manifold. Thus, could it be that the freedom of the joints during late pregnancy attributed to relaxin and inhibin hormones in fact involves a decreased sensitivity to pain due to changes in the estrogen/progesterone balance? With progesterone concentrations promoting a lowered sensitivity, does one push further into *yogasana* postures and so suffer more injuries at times when progesterone levels are high?

The ratio of the levels of estrogen and progesterone in the blood varies strongly over the course of a monthly menstrual cycle, being much larger than 1 in the follicular (ovarian) phase and significantly smaller than 1 in the luteal (menstrual) phase (figure 21.A-1**b**). In the first of these, there is high activity in the orbitofrontal cortex and in the amygdala when experiencing reward and/or pleasure. Indeed, other behaviors show a stronger sense of pleasure when the woman is in the follicular phase as compared with the luteal phase. It would be most interesting to see what the emotional swings might be for female students having a standard *yogasana* practice and how they view the pleasure/pain ratios in their practice as they move through their menstrual cycles with strongly varying estrogen/progesterone ratios.

Both estrogen and progesterone have strong effects on cells in the parietal lobes of the brain, these being areas where partial seizures originate, the effect of estrogen being excitatory and that of progesterone inhibitory. Such seizures are far more frequent in premenopausal women around the time of ovulation, when the concentration of estrogen is high and progesterone is low.

Muscles, Joints, Ligaments, and Tendons during Pregnancy

The general structures of joints and their associated substructures are discussed in Section 7.D, page 239. Special mention must be made here of these structures, as they can change considerably when the *yogasana* practitioner becomes pregnant. In preparation for the delivery of the baby, the body produces a hormone called relaxin [479]; as its name implies, relaxin has a relaxing effect on the entire musculoskeletal system, but especially so on the ligaments binding the pubic symphysis together (figure 8.B-7). *Yogasanas*, such as *malasana* (figure 21.B-1), that are done with support and with the feet wide apart also can be used to help open this joint.

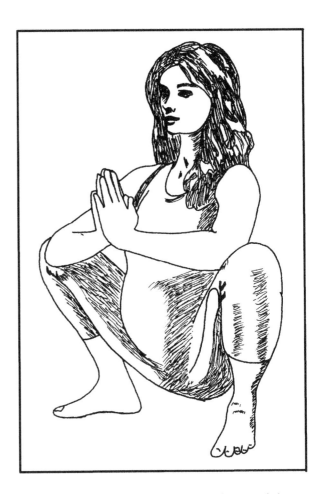

Figure 21.B-1. Squatting in *malasana* while pregnant in order to open the birth canal.

The action of relaxin on the pubic symphysis is easy to understand, for this joint must be able to open considerably in order for the baby to pass to the outside. However, relaxin's similar effect on all the other joints of the body can make problems for the *yogasana* student. As the tension within the ligaments binds the joints together, the pregnant student must be careful not to overstretch, or she runs the risk of destabilizing the joints so opened by overstretching the ligaments. For instance, the medial and lateral arches of the feet are held up in part by spring-like ligaments binding the calcaneus to the navicular bone (figure 10.B-7a), the collagen of which is unraveled by relaxin, with the result that the arches tend to fall and the foot can grow longer by a full shoe size during pregnancy [479].

As pregnancy proceeds, the abdominal muscles are stretched intensely so as to make room for the growing fetus. For this reason, one should do no *yogasana* work that calls for further stretching of these muscles (deep backbends, for example), and on the other hand, any posture that acts to tighten the abdominal muscles *(paripurna navasana,* for example) is also contraindicated, for one can ill afford to have the abdominal muscles contract prematurely. In this regard, there would be a considerable rise in the abdominal pressure when a pregnant woman uses the Valsalva maneuver (holding the breath, closing the throat, and contracting the abdominal muscles; see Section 15.C, page 616) in order to initiate defecation or in the practice of the *yogasanas*. If practical, the much safer way to this end is to assume a squatting posture *(malasana)* while eliminating. The Valsalva maneuver is generally inappropriate for women, as it appears to be a factor in appendicitis, hemorrhoids, endometriosis, dropped uterus, and uterine fibroids [911].

Inversions

In Lasater's recent writing on the subject of *yogasana* and pregnancy [496], she expresses the opinion that though many students perform inversions routinely while pregnant without any apparent problems, there is nonetheless a risk to the fetus involved in this, and so it is better to forgo all risks and just postpone inversions until after the birth. Risks include a breech presentation at delivery and entanglement of the fetus in the placental cord, both brought about by the unnaturalness of the mother's inverted position. On the other hand, an extensive controlled study of the effects of yoga practice (including *yogasanas, pranayama,* and meditation) on the outcome of childbirth involving over 300 pregnant women concluded that the practice resulted in demonstrable improvement in birth weight, decreased pre-term labor, and decreased pregnancy-induced hypertension, without any increased complications [607].

Balancing

The ability of a pregnant woman to balance will be changing rapidly as she adds 16–23 kilograms (thirty-five to fifty pounds) of weight in a very asymmetric way. Standing on one leg for any length of time is especially to be avoided, as this puts too much weight on the leg, especially at the knee joint. On the other hand, during pregnancy, the body can be deficient in calcium, having given so much to the baby, and this can lead to leg cramps, as can the low level of circulation in the legs (see subsection below). In the latter case, wall-supported standing postures are recommended for avoiding such cramps.

Respiratory and Cardiovascular Systems

In response to the growing pressure that the fetus and uterus put on the ribs and diaphragm, the expectant mother's respiration rate increases, and at the same time, the soft tissues of the nose swell and make breathing difficult. At this point, the pregnant *yogasana* student needs to practice relaxing the breath, for this will be basic to all delivery techniques. As the size of the fetus increases, there will be more and more pressure put on the diaphragm, until in the final stage of pregnancy, breathing must involve the intercostal muscles much more, for the range of motion of the diaphragm is severely limited (Section 21.B, this page).

Inferior Vena Cava

The pressure of the baby on the femoral vein (figure 14.C-2) tends to trap blood in the legs and leads to swelling. If one chooses to do inversions at this time, the swelling is best relieved by inversions such as *sirsasana, sarvangasana,* or *viparita karani,* which also serve to reduce the constipation resulting from the pressure of the fetus on the intestines (however, see below). Blood that passes upward through the femoral veins empties eventually into the inferior vena cava, a large vein paralleling the spine and resting just anterior to it on the right side. There is danger during pregnancy that this important vein might be compressed by the weight of the fetus when the mother lies on her back for any length of time, especially after the fifth month. Because closing of the inferior vena cava takes so much blood out of circulation, the student may have a sense of lightheadedness, dizziness, or nausea, as the amount of oxygen reaching the brain is inadequate. Even if no symptoms are evident, it is still a risk, since the baby may be deprived of oxygen, even though the mother feels no symptoms. Thus, the necessary relaxing postures must be done on an inclined plane or while lying on the side. Inasmuch as the inferior vena cava inserts into the right atrium of the heart, it is offset to the right with respect to the spinal cord [613], and so pregnant women are advised to sleep on their left sides rather than on their right in order to avoid pinching off this important blood vessel.

The Nervous and Digestive Systems

Heartburn

As the level of the hormone progesterone increases in the body of the pregnant student, the peristaltic action within the intestines (Subsection 19.A, page 711) decreases while the rising level of relaxin leads to both constipation and indigestion. Furthermore, relaxin loosens the collagen fibers within the sphincter between the esophagus and the stomach, and so allows it to leak stomach acid into the esophagus, leading to massive heartburn. If this is the case, inversions will be inappropriate.

Sciatica

The pressure of the growing fetus tends to press on the sciatic nerve as it passes out of the lumbo-sacral area, thereby generating pain in the mother's buttocks and legs. This, however, can be relieved by the standard *yogasanas* that free the sciatic nerve from pressure by the piriformis muscle (Section II.B, page 837). Carpal tunnel syndrome also can appear during pregnancy and otherwise is very strongly gender-specific, affecting ten times as many women as men.

In terms of the autonomic nervous system, one wants to practice so as to relax the body during pregnancy, which is to say, work the *yogasanas* so as to shift the arousal away from the sympathetic side and toward the parasympathetic (Chapter 5, page 157).

Section 21.C: Menopause

At about forty years of age, nature begins to shut down the production of estrogen by the ovaries, and menstruation becomes scanty and then stops (figure 21.A-1c). This change of hormonal activity, termed menopause, may require two to five years to run its course. Menopause is a natural stage in the life cycle of the female, and when viewed appropriately, it can show her much about who she is and who she is about to become. It certainly is not to be viewed as a disease or a medical crisis of any sort, though there are strong cultural influences directing how women may respond to this event. As compared with the large swings of hormonal levels in the female shown in figure 21.A-1c, the hormonal shifts in the male are much less precipitous over the same span of years.

Decreasing Estrogen

The symptoms of menopause are many and varied, but most, if not all of them, relate to the relatively rapid changes of estrogen levels that characterize menopause. These symptoms include hot flashes (the most infamous symptom), mood swings, depression, night sweats, urinary problems, vaginal dryness, aching joints, reduced libido, and weight gain [491, 836].

When the amount of estrogen from the ovaries starts to decrease, the deficit can be made up by the production of this hormone by the adrenals and kidneys, if they have not been exhausted prematurely by stress [491]. Spinal twists and modest backbending can be used to promote circulation around the adrenals and kidneys at the time of menopause. During the period of low estrogen and progesterone, a more normal level of these materials can be achieved by taking them from external sources; i.e., hormone replacement therapy (HRT). This medical approach decreases the risks of osteoporosis (Section 7.G, page 254) and heart disease, while increasing the risk slightly for breast cancer. If nothing is done to treat menopausal symptoms, a woman's body chemistry will slowly drift toward that of men, with disease patterns and frequencies much like those of older men [836].

Hormonal Effects

Among the many symptoms that accompany the shift of hormonal activity in women at menopause, certain of these relate directly to *yogasana* practice, in that they are either symptoms that affect performance or are antidotal for such symptoms. Several such effects that will especially interest the *yogasana* practitioner are listed below [836].

1. The major component of connective tissue is collagen (Subsection 12.A, page 483), and estrogen receptors have been found on the fibroblasts that manufacture this structural material. As the estrogen concentration in the body drops after menopause, the quantity of collagen made by the fibroblasts decreases, and so connective tissue becomes weaker, as do the bones and skin.

2. Declining levels of estrogen upset the balance between the bone-building cells (the osteoblasts) and the bone-destroying cells (the osteoclasts) in the body, in favor of the latter. The result is weak bones in the wrists, vertebrae, and hips, subject to more frequent fracture than would occur otherwise. Strengthening of the bones during the premenopausal years through consistent *yogasana* practice minimizes the heightened risk of osteoporosis during and after menopause (Section 7.G, page 254).

3. With declining hormonal production, the muscular system loses strength, bulk, and stamina, and the joints may become stiff and painful. Again, *yogasana* practice can prevent or reverse these symptoms. Remember that at this point in life, repair of muscle injuries will be slowed considerably, so that one must be careful not to exceed one's capacity to work physically.

4. Hot flashes appear to be caused by the hormonal imbalance incurred when the ovaries are in the process of shutting down the production of estrogen. This imbalance upsets the hypothalamus, which controls heart rate, sweating, and body temperature. When in this state, the heart rate increases, sweating may be profuse, and heat moves from the core of the body to the skin, resulting in "hot flashes," in which the skin temperature over the face, chest, back, shoulders, and upper arms may increase by up to 4° C (7° F), usually occurring in the late evening. These symptoms suggest a general activation of the sympathetic nervous system (Section 5.C, page 170), and the yogic response to these symptoms would be strongly on the side of those *yogasanas* that activate the parasympathetic nervous system and therefore are cooling. Indeed, the cooling inversions (such as *sarvangasana, niralamba sarvangasana,* and *viparita karani)* are strongly recom-

mended for moderate hot flashes [193, 491], as postures such as these lower heart rate and blood pressure and promote vasodilation, while reducing the hormones that cause retention of water and salt. Inversions stabilize the hormonal systems and so are useful in all hormonal problems, menopausal or not.

5. Sweating is a mechanism whereby the body rids itself of heat through evaporation (Subsection 20.D, page 725); however, the sweat glands do not seem to work as they normally did prior to menopause, for they now sweat profusely during hot flashes, yet there does not seem to be much of a cooling effect. Hot flashes at night also are known as night sweats. In this case, sleep is very disturbed, with decreased REM durations; however, some measure of bodily rest nonetheless can be achieved through relaxing *yogasana* postures such as *savasana*.

6. In the premenopausal female, the heart-healthy ratio of the diameter of the waist to the diameter at the hips is less than 0.8. However, with the onset of menopause, the body's fat distribution will move toward that of men, the ratio in question will go as high as 0.95, and the risk of cardiovascular problems will increase rapidly so as to approach that of men, unless one is involved in an active exercise program. In fact, the waist-to-hip ratio has been shown to be a more accurate predictor of heart attack than is the better-known body mass index (BMI). There are many sites on the surfaces of brain cells that are receptors for estrogen. When menopausal and beyond, the low levels of estrogen can negatively impact the ability to think, to perceive, and to resist anxiety, and they can reduce the mental flexibility needed to accept new ideas. Low estrogen decreases the libido and raises the threshold for sexual arousal.

7. The brain's control of muscles, joints, and movement from within the cerebellum is very strongly dependent upon the levels of circulating estrogen in the body. When estrogen levels are low, tasks requiring fine control over these physical entities will be impaired. As nerve conduction slows with age, balance will be impaired, and memory also will wane.

With a life expectancy of eighty-one years, a woman can look forward to enjoying more than one-third of her life following menopause. Though the time of menopause is one of hormonal imbalance and emotional instability, once past menopause, emotional and hormonal stability set in—increasing one's ability to focus on life goals. It can be a time of peaceful introspection and accomplishment.

Section 21.D: Sexual Function

Gonadotropins

It is fascinating that the same hormones that function in the woman's body to signal the onset of puberty are also working in the man's body to the same end. In the young male, as in the young female, at about age twelve to fourteen years, there is a release of hormones from the hypothalamus to the pituitary gland, leading to the eventual production of the gonadotropins, FSH (follicle stimulating hormone), and LH (luteinizing hormone). In the male body, the FSH promotes sperm production and maturation, whereas LH directs the production of testosterone and the secondary male characteristics: the male pattern of muscle and bone growth, enlargement of the sex organs, growth of coarse body hair, male-pattern baldness, and an enlarged larynx [431, 878]. In the female's body, the generation of the same gonadotropins leads to the appearance of breasts, pubic hair, a feminine voice, and broader hips. The sexual apparatus of the female is totally internal, unlike the structure in males.

Testosterone

In normal development, the increased output of testosterone during the onset of puberty in the male results in the larynx growing larger and the vocal cords growing longer (by up to 60 percent) and becoming covered with an accumulation of collagen. Such changes have the effect of deepening the voice. On the other hand, the castrati of the European opera, by severing the testes from which testosterone otherwise would flow, avoided such changes to the vocal apparatus and so maintained the voices of their childhoods. Thus, they were able to sing with the beautiful voices of the adult woman while maintaining the look of the adult male body. The asexual growth of the body was due to the combined effects of growth hormone and the effect of testosterone deficiency, which allowed the epiphyses on the ends of the long bones (figure 7.A-2a) of the castrati to continue to grow. At the same time, the sternocostal and costovertebral joints within the rib cage (figures 15.A-3c and -3d) remained flexible, so that the castrati grew up to have large, open rib cages with large lung volumes and exquisite breath control [643].[2]

Testosterone in the male body increases the libido (sexual interest), and when it is present at only low levels, the libido is depressed. However, there is no direct link between testosterone and the ability to have an erection [622]. Testosterone levels in men are straightforward barometers of their moods and mindsets; the level surges when men win at games and drops when they lose. It is higher in lawyers and actors than in ministers, and it rises in anticipation of sex but falls if disappointed in that regard. When asleep, testosterone levels in men are at their peaks during the REM phases of sleep. Strangely, testosterone levels in men are at their lowest in the evening, when sexual intercourse is said to be most frequent.

Sperm

On reaching sexual maturity, sperm are manufactured in the testes and stored there. Though the ovaries work best at body temperature (37.0° C or 98.6° F), this is too warm for the sperm in the testes, and so they are stored in the scrotal sac, outside the body, where it is cooler by approximately 1.7°C (3° F). Like the brain, the developing sperm are protected from possible toxins in the blood by a blood-testes barrier. Though the testes prefer a temperature closer to 35° C (95° F), in cold weather or when threatened with a blow, they can be lifted reflexively by the cremaster muscles more or less completely into the body for warmth or safety.

The Penis

A large part of the mass of the penis consists of a spongy tissue carrying a large number of arteries, the smooth muscles of the artery walls being normally contracted due to sympathetic excitation. On sexual excitation, there is a shift to parasympathetic dominance, which releases the muscle tone in the arterial walls of the penis, and it becomes engorged with blood. As with many situations of vasodilation, that in the penis leading to an erection involves the simple molecule nitric oxide, which relaxes the blood vessels in the penis, leading to an erection due to pooled blood in the sinuses of that organ.[3] At the same time, the veins by which the arterial blood would exit the penis are compressed, and so the blood is held in place in the erect penis. Exactly the same mechanism is at work in the female clitoris on excitation and closely resembles the explanation given by Schatz for women not performing inversions during menstruation (Subsection 21.A, page 742).

Circumstances that stimulate the sympathetic nervous system, such as chronic stress, cold, and fear, have a shrinking effect on the penis. In such cases, *yogasanas* performed to ease the level

---

2   There are **no** reports of super-serious *yogasana* students undergoing this operation just to improve the quality of their backbends or their *pranayama* practice!

---

3   This vascular congestion can be generated artificially by taking Viagra.

of stress also will have a beneficial effect on the man's virility. During the recurrent REM phases of sleep (Subsection 23.D, page 800), the sympathetic stress is turned off, and as a consequence, both men and women will experience periods of high sexual excitement between five and six times per night.

Best Times for Sex

In Western societies, the most popular time for sex is 11:00 PM, with the second most popular time being 8:00 AM; Sunday is the most popular day. Within the month, sex is most frequent on the eighth day following the beginning of the menstrual cycle, but in women, sexual desire and fantasies are strongest just before the time of ovulation, in response to the high level of estrogen. Men are most interested in sex in the late fall, when their testosterone level is highest, accounting for the soaring birth rate in late summer.

It is interesting that there are both annual and circadian rhythms to the birthing process in humans. Giving birth at a time of the year that enhances survivability of the baby is achieved by the circadian monitors of the brain, which detect the length of the days and so promote fertility at a time nine months previous to the best delivery date. Furthermore, most deliveries occur between 3:00 and 4:00 AM, just a few hours previous to the daily arousal boost (Section 23.B, page 771).

Redirecting Sexual Energy

The yoga practice of redirecting sexual energy through the practice of celibacy appears to have a basis in physiology. Practice of the *yogasana* postures tends not to stimulate the glands of the gonads but the pineal gland instead, resulting in the production of melatonin. Expression of this hormone decreases the sexual drive [799]. This explanation would seem to follow closely the mechanism for eradicating the effects of summer affective disorder by visually inhibiting the release of melatonin (Subsection 17.E, page 685).

The Hypothalamus

As might have been expected, the hypothalamus plays a significant role in sexual arousal. In males, the preoptic area within the anterior portion of the hypothalamus (figure 5.B-1) is most critical for male sexual behavior. This nucleus is larger in males than in females, contains receptors for testosterone, and is excitatory for the parasympathetic nervous system leading to erection. In females (figure 5.B-1), it is the response to estrogen of the ventromedial nucleus in the central portion of the hypothalamus that controls sexual behavior. This nucleus contains receptors for both estrogen and progesterone and has neural connections to the periaqueductal gray area, which in turn is connected to the spinal cord by way of the reticular formation. Damage to the preoptic area in men or the ventromedial area in women has profound negative effects on sexual behavior. Gay men have a smaller than normal nucleus in the anterior hypothalamus, an area important in determining sex differences generally.

Sexual lust is enhanced by dopamine produced in the hypothalamus, which triggers the release of testosterone. If lust turns to emotional attachment, then oxytocin also is synthesized in the hypothalamus and is released into the bloodstream, surging at orgasm. In the woman, the oxytocin acts to enhance strong pair bonding, whereas in men, it acts to guide them toward smooth social relations when engaged in financial matters.

When there is physical stimulation of the penis, there is a reflexive action, involving inhibitory interneurons, that turns off the sympathetic system and stimulates the erection-generating centers between S3 and T12 in the lower spine [282]. Males in whom the spinal cord has been cut below the hypothalamus can still respond to genital manipulation with erection and ejaculation [204]; however, they cannot be stimulated sexually by thinking sexual thoughts, as can men who have an intact connection between their hypothalamus and their penis. It is likely that a similar mechanism works on the clitoris of women, bringing them to orgasm.

Recent mapping of the sensory cortex of men

has identified that area responding to the soft stroking of the penis; it lies between those of the toes and abdomen in the cortex (figure 4.C-6) and is said to be "very small" [26].

As discussed in Section 5.C, page 170, one of the consequences of sympathetic excitation is that blood is withdrawn from the central body and moved to the skeletal muscles in the arms and legs. Several studies have shown that for males with erectile dysfunction, performing *yogasanas* that promote parasympathetic dominance or *yogasanas* such as *baddha konasana* that bring blood circulation to the pelvic area can be useful in combating this problem [109].

Male Orgasm

At the moment of ejaculation, the autonomic dominance is said to shift from parasympathetic to sympathetic as skeletal muscles are energized to propel the sperm through the penis; however, the EEG at the moment of orgasm in both men and women is strongly centered in the right hemisphere, as appropriate for parasympathetic release of tension [135], leaving one with sympathetic increases of heart rate, blood pressure, and respiration in addition to pleasurable sensations. As with *pranayama, samadhi,* and sneezing, orgasm tends to open both nostrils. Moreover, it has been found that as the female approaches orgasm, blood flow to the amygdala and hippocampus (areas in the brain responsible for alertness and anxiety) are reduced, while that to the cerebellum (an area in the brainstem where movement is coordinated) is increased [505]. However, if the woman is faking orgasm, the blood flow to the amygdala and

hippocampus shows no such decrease. Orgasm in men is apparently accompanied by far less deactivation of the emotional centers in the central nervous system.

Female Orgasm

In a broad study involving both identical and nonidentical female twins aged between nineteen and eighty-three years, it was revealed that only 14 percent of the women always experienced an orgasm during intercourse, but this rose to 34 percent during masturbation. In contrast, 16 percent never experienced an orgasm during intercourse, and this fell to 14 percent during masturbation. It was concluded that 45 percent of the different responses between those females who have orgasm under any condition and those who do not is attributable to genetic variation. On this basis, it is hypothesized that there is little evolutionary pressure driving the female orgasm [379]. During the female orgasm, the pain threshold is said to double, but the effect does not last long enough to serve as a treatment [844].

It recently has been shown that women who have suffered a separation of the spinal cord above T10 nonetheless can be sexually responsive and orgasmic, as the afferent signals are carried by the vagus nerves, which bypass the thoracic vertebrae (Subsection 5.D, page 180) [460].

When in the phase of sexual arousal, there is a release of dopamine in the pleasure centers of the brain in both men and women, and following orgasm, there is a release of prolactin, which serves to induce a sense of satiation in both, and even temporary erectile dysfunction in men.

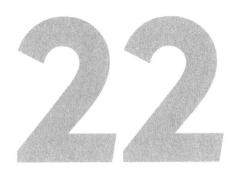

Emotions and Moods

Two categories of emotional state can be differentiated on the basis of time: those states that develop almost instantaneously (in an hour or less) and then recede just as rapidly (sadness, anger, surprise, fear, disgust, contempt, happiness, etc.), and those that develop over much longer periods (weeks) and can become lifelong conditions (depression, anxiety, mania, etc.). The former are called "emotions" and the latter are called "moods." This is not a sharp demarcation, as one can be perpetually angry and only momentarily anxious, but it makes sense in general to distinguish emotions from moods on the basis of duration.

In this section, three generally recognized and related mood disorders—depression, mania, and anxiety—are discussed, along with the impact *yogasana* practice might have on them. That *yogasana* could be in any way prescriptive for these disorders is suggested by the fact that the symptoms for all three appear in part to involve the autonomic nervous system (Chapter 5, page 157), a system susceptible to control and change through *yogasana* practice. Because the emotions and the immune system are under the control of the autonomic nervous system, it is no surprise that the emotions have been shown repeatedly to have an impact on the immune system (Subsection 16.E, page 650). Similarly, it is understandable that mood and respiration have a mutually strong effect on one another [42], and that a particular mood can be strongly associated with one or the other cerebral hemisphere. In regard the latter point, it is known that injection of sodium amital into the right carotid artery and its transport to the right cerebral hemisphere leads to a brief sense of elation, whereas injecting the same substance into the left carotid artery, and its transport to the left cerebral hemisphere, produces a momentary depression [427].

Stress

When we are homeostatically balanced, we are optimally able to function in whatever arena; however, internal or external stresses will act to upset this balance. If the challenge to homeostatic balance is chronically and erroneously perceived to be ever-present, then the individual enters the realm of neurosis, anxiety, and paranoia. It is known that the negative effects of such psychological stress are magnified if there is no outlet for the frustration, no hope for control over the stress, and no hope for a better outcome. If the stress is more or less ongoing, the vigilance necessary to counter the stress becomes constant, even when the stress is no longer a factor, and one has then entered a state of anxiety. Should the stress be constant but with no perceived hope of relief, then the person can easily fall into a state of depression, even if the situation is one that could be overcome in reality. Stress that is unremitting can transform anxiety into depression.

Emotions, Moods, and Facial Expressions

Each of our emotions is written on our face as a particular set of muscular actions [221], and this emotional/muscular system is always turned on and can readily be imitated, even though the true emotion is lacking. It is interesting that if one assumes the facial expression for a particu-

Table 22.A-1: Components of Positive and Negative Attitudes [240]

Positive	Negative
Love	Anger
Trust	Suspicion
Friendship	Alienation
Intimacy	Withdrawal
Sense of community	Me against them / hostility
Responsible for actions	Victim of circumstance
Confidence	Fear
Optimism	Pessimism
Exaltation	Depression
Stimulation	Boredom
Strong goals	No direction

lar emotion, specific physiological changes ensue, and a true emotional feeling appropriate to that face will result. Moreover, being in an emotional state can be mentally paralyzing, in the sense that while we are in such a state, we are closed off to any rational thinking that is inconsistent with the emotion of the moment. This refractory period can be useful if it lasts for just a second or two, for it gives full attention to the emotion, but if it lasts longer than that, then irrational behavior may follow. Regarding the latter, if we come to our *yogasana* practice harboring anger, then our ability to learn the lesson of the moment will be lost on us, unless we are able to discharge the emotion, by chanting, for example. Traffic safety engineers estimate that anger is the equivalent of drinking three beers in regard to crippling one's ability to perform physically.

By consciously assuming a specific facial posture representing a particular emotion, we are able to experience that emotion even though, in a sense, it is forced. Through the action of the mirror neurons (Subsection 4.G, page 142), an observer of our emotion as expressed by our face, also will feel that emotion, showing that our empathy for what others are feeling is a result of the reading and copying of one another's mirror neurons! See also the footnote in Subsection 22.A, page 758.

Emotional Centers

There are two main areas of the brain that are important in exciting emotions and moods. The first is the amygdala in the forebrain, dealing with fear, anxiety, surprise, and anger; the second is the left and right prefrontal lobes (figure 4.B-1), dealing not only with foresight, planning, and self-control, but also with emotions, mood, and temperament. It appears that the amygdala is involved in what are essentially reflexive emotions (those that appear very rapidly and without any prior thought), whereas those that use the prefrontal lobes are more rational and slower to develop but under conscious control [221]. EEG studies show that when one is enjoying good mood and positive emotions, the left prefrontal lobe is very active electrically, and when the mood is strongly negative, it is the right prefrontal lobe that is very active [245]. Buddhist meditators are known to be able to calm the amygdala in addition to activating the proper prefrontal lobe, thereby becoming less angry, less flustered, less shocked, etc. Similar studies on *yogasana* practitioners would be interesting. An excellent review of the literature relating *yogasana* practice to psychotherapy, current to 2001, is given in [799].

A generally positive mental attitude is a fundamental factor in good body health. The thoughts and feelings that form the bases of positive and negative attitudes are presented in table 22.A-1 above.

Role of *Yogasana*

Quantitative measures of the consequences of many of the components of negative attitude given in table 22.A-1 are presented in the work of the Heartmath Research Center [550], citing the connections between mental and emotional attitudes, physiological health, and long-term well-being. In particular:

1. A study of 1,623 survivors of heart attack found that if they became angry during emotional conflicts, their risk of subsequent heart attacks was more than twice that of those who were able to remain calm.

2. Men who complain of high anxiety are up to six times more likely than calmer men to suffer sudden cardiac death.

3. A twenty-year-long study of 1,700 elderly men showed that worry over social conditions, health, or personal finances increase the risks of coronary heart disease.

4. More than half of heart disease cases are not explained by the standard lifestyle factors (high cholesterol, smoking, and sedentary lifestyle).

5. A study of 2,829 people aged fifty-five to eighty-five years old shows that those with the highest levels of "personal mastery" in regard to controlling their lives had a 60 percent lower risk of death in the next year compared to those who felt relatively helpless in the face of life's challenges.

6. In individuals with heart disease, psychological stress was the strongest predictor of future events such as cardiac death, cardiac arrest, and heart attack.

7. In a ten-year study, emotional stress was more predictive of cancer and cardiovascular death than was smoking. Those who could not efficiently manage stress had a 40 percent larger death rate than those who were able to manage their stress.

8. In a study of 5,716 middle-aged people, those with strong self-regulation were more than fifty times more likely to be alive and without any chronic diseases fifteen years later than those who scored lowest in self-regulation.

The positive effects that *yogasana* practice can have in regard to defusing anger and reducing anxiety, worry, feelings of helplessness, emotional stress, and psychological stress while increasing a sense of personal mastery and self-regulation have reached a new high in acceptance by Westerners and should increase many times more in the future. This assures a future for the use of *yogasana* in emotional therapy. Note, however, the caution of Slede and Pomerantz [799], who state that yoga may not be an appropriate treatment for "patients" who do not respond positively after a few months of a daily practice. Moreover, they state that patients with medium IQs do not do as well as those with either higher or lower IQs—those having higher IQs practicing more conscientiously so as to get out of their minds and into their bodies, whereas those of lower IQs possibly using yoga to express themselves when words fail.

Judging from the low rates of cure for mood disorders such as depression, mania, and anxiety and the variable responses to a particular drug, it appears that there are many varieties of each of these mood disorders. Consequently, the effective *yogasana* routines might well be rather different for people suffering from what otherwise appear to be identical disorders. Nonetheless, there are certain broad areas in which *yogasana* can play a positive role. In almost every case, it seems true that the sooner a mood disorder is treated, the more quickly it is overcome. Moreover, almost all of the drug therapies suffer from important side effects, which would be absent in a yogic course of treatment. Because *yogasana* practice can re-balance the autonomic nervous system, it may lead to a diminution of the symptoms of a mood disorder, even if it does not cure it outright. Finally, in regard to psychotherapy, it is said that if the depressed patient and the therapist can form an emotional bond and then work on the common goal of healing, the result can be most beneficial; one might expect the same benefits of such a therapeutic alliance when working with depressed students in the yoga studio [77]. In a recent study, mood was found to be elevated after classes of Feldenkrais, swimming, or yoga activities, but not after aerobic dance or computer lessons [615].

A particularly nice study of the emotional shifts that attend *yogasana* practice is presented by Shapiro and Cline [781], who report that, independent of the postures practiced, there is a general increase in positive moods of the sort listed in table 22.A-1, a decrease of the negative moods (especially frustration, irritation, and pessimism), and a general lifting of energy, the latter lasting for about two hours after the practice. The largest shifts of mood from negative to positive were obtained with backbending, and especially so for those who entered the practice either hostile or depressed.

Mechanisms

It is one of the strong points of *yogasana* therapy that the *yogasanas* are intimately tied to our emotions. Because unexpressed emotions, with their strong connection to the limbic system in the brain (Subsection 4.C, page 82), often are stored as muscular tension in the body (often in the shoulders, stomach, lower back, and jaw [632]), the release of muscular tension through *yogasana* frequently is accompanied by the release of emotional tension. The emotions that can lead to muscle tension include pleasure, pain, anger, rage, fear, sorrow, aggression, and sexual feelings.

Section 22.A: Depression

Symptoms

Postural Reflex

Imagine the self-portrait of Vincent Van Gogh, showing an old man with his head in his hands. This is a graphical depiction of the mental and physical state of depression, and indeed,

Van Gogh died by suicide. The depressed posture is one in which the body is bent forward at the waist, with the chest and the head bent forward, much like a beginner in *paschimottanasana*. The posture resembles the defensive postural reflex described in Subsection 11.D, page 450. Feldenkrais states, "All negative emotion is expressed as flexion." Long before Van Gogh, Hippocrates, in the fifth century BC, used the term "melancholia" to describe the darkness accompanying the depressive state.

In addition to the postural (Subsection 5.F, page 195), other physical symptoms of depression can include losses of appetite, energy, sexual desire, and memory, as well as excessive sadness, restlessness, retardation of thoughts and actions, constipation, decreased salivation, and diurnal variation of the severity of symptoms [427, 609]. Five percent of the world's population suffers from major depressive illness [427], and in the United States, the rate of depression is twice as high among women as among men.[1] Depression is the most common cause of headache [200] (Subsection 4.E, page 114), and there appears to be a connection between depression and excessive dreaming in the REM phase of sleep (Section 23.D, page 800).

The mental and emotional aspects of the symptoms of depression are contained within Hamlet's words: "How weary, stale, flat and unprofitable seem to me all the uses of this world." He spoke of symptoms that include a pervasively unpleasant mood, intense mental pain, inability to experience pleasure, generalized loss of interest in all things, difficulty in concentrating, indecisiveness, feelings of worthlessness and guilt, pessimistic thoughts, and thoughts of dying and suicide [427, 609]. There is a tendency to think of Van Gogh and Hamlet as heroic, and perhaps that depression is even necessary for creating new art; however, it is closer to the truth to say that it

---

1   This 2:1 ratio is very much an upper limit, because studies show that the ratio can be more like 1:1, depending upon the criteria used for defining depression and because the incidence of depression is significantly under-reported for men.

Table 22.A-2: Comparison of the Characteristics of Exogenous and Endogenous Depression [427]

Feature	Exogenous Depression	Endogenous Depression
Onset	Any age, but often below forty years	Over forty years
Recent stress	Yes	No
Familial depression	Absent	Present
Mood variation	Worse late in day	Worse in morning
Sleep pattern	Difficulty in falling asleep, but then stays asleep	Insomnia, middle of night or early morning; short REM phase
Appetite	May increase or decrease	None
Weight change	Little or no loss	Rapid loss; anorexia
Physical ailments	Fewer, less severe	Many, more severe
Mental activity	Mild slowing	Moderate to severe slowing
Attitudes	Self-pity, pessimism	Self-blame, remorse, guilt
Self-esteem	No loss	Complete loss
Interest	Mild/moderate loss	Pervasive loss in everything
Suicidal	Occasional	Common
Psychomotor level	Calm	Agitated
Mental pain	None	Considerable
Response to pleasure	Normal	None (anhedonia)

is constricting, with emotions flat and heavy and having practically nothing in common with the sense of freedom necessary to create.

Types

In the past, the broad category of depression had been divided into exogenous (reactive) and endogenous (physical) subclasses. In the former, there is an external precipitating event of great stress (loss of a loved one, loss of a job, etc.) in which the normal period of grief fails to come to an end, while in the latter, there is no external trigger. In both cases, there are strong genetic tendencies toward the illness. The general symptoms for exogenous and endogenous depression are listed in table 22.A-2, but the dichotomy is not as sharp as implied by this table.

The picture painted up to this point is upset by the 15 percent of depressed patients who show symptoms opposite to those given in table 22.A-2. In cases of atypical depression, patients show overeating and weight gain, extended sleeping periods, and depression worse in the evening hours than in the morning! More will be said of this below.

The American Psychiatric Association more recently has classified levels of depression in terms of symptoms rather than in terms of precipitating causes; in the new description, the two major categories are given as "major depressive disorder" and as "dysthymic disorder." The symptoms of dysthymia (also called dysrhythmia [821]) are the following: relatively mild but chronic depression lasting for two years or more, poor appetite or overeating, insomnia or oversleeping, fatigue or low energy, low self-esteem, poor concentration, and feelings of hopelessness. Dysthymia appears to run in families, though the relative importance of genetics versus environment is not clear.

Dysthymia is closely related to major depressive disorder; however, it is more severe and is episodic rather than chronic. In cases of major depressive disorder, the left prefrontal cortex (a major mood center) is abnormally small and underactive. One possibility is that this underactivity is a response to stress. Because "there is mounting evidence that chronic or acute stress and anxiety play a major role in the disease (depression)," stress management (e.g., *yogasana* practice) could be an important component of therapy [356].

Neurotransmitter Imbalance

To the extent that depression is closely allied with imbalances of the brain's neurotransmitters, descriptions of the conditions may be classified as either "anxiety depression," "anergic depression," or "cholinergic depression." In anxiety depression, there is a predominance of excitatory activity of norepinephrine in the locus ceruleus, of serotonin in the dorsal raphe, and of dopamine in the mid-cortex. If high concentrations of norepinephrine in the brain are maintained for long periods of time through the agency of the fight or flight response, the heart is strained, leading to a strong correlation of high norepinephrine levels and depression with heart failure. The efficacy of electroshock treatment for depression relates to the fact that the shock lowers the output of cells that otherwise oversupply norepinephrine in the brains of the depressed. In contrast, anergic depression follows from the above neurotransmitters acting in an inhibitory way, and cholinergic overdrive results in depression when acetylcholine is overactive in the brain. The correlation of various depressive states with imbalances in those neurotransmitters that otherwise are often met in autonomic imbalance suggests a role for *yogasana* practice in alleviating the symptoms of depression, if they can be caught soon enough.

Opioids

Low opioid levels (Subsection 3.D, page 56) in the brain also have been implicated in depres-

sion. It has recently been reported that the hippocampus, a brain center intimately involved with memory and learning, shrinks with recurrent bouts of depression, and that antidepressants work to reverse the shrinking [333]. In this scenario, excess cortisol produced by various means, including stress, acts to prune the dendrites from the neurons in the hippocampus, eventually killing them. At the same time, the amygdala becomes enlarged. However, it recently has been found that neurons in the hippocampus can be reborn through the process of neurogenesis, which in turn is stimulated by antidepressant medications and by exercise [238].

Medical Treatment for Depression

Stress

The route to the more common exogenous depression starts with the response of the body to stress; in this case, the hypothalamus releases CRF (corticotropin releasing factor) to the pituitary, which in turn releases ACTH (adrenocorticotropic hormone) into the bloodstream (figure 5.E-1). On reaching the kidneys, the ACTH acts on the adrenal cortex (see Section 5.C, page 175), to eventually release, among other things, the powerful chemical cortisol into the bloodstream. Cortisol then promotes physiological changes to support the fight or flight response. The above can be called the hypothalamic-pituitary-adrenal (HPA) axis working under the prod of stress [609].[2]

---

2   It is interesting to note that according to the James-Lange theory, the experience of stress leads to physiological changes that in turn lead to emotional states, rather than the emotional states leading to physiological changes. That physical expression can influence emotional expression has been demonstrated recently [523]. Ekman and co-workers [221] have shown that deliberately assuming a facial expression congruent with a particular emotion leads to the emotion actually appearing in the psyches of the performer and of the observer.

Neurotransmitters

Many of the brain circuits use synapses involving serotonin, dopamine, GABA, or norepinephrine as neurotransmitters, and when there is a loss of activity or hyperactivity in such circuits due to low or high neurotransmitter levels (see Section 3.D, page 53), the result often is depression. Similarly, the neurotransmitter acetylcholine is present in too-high concentrations in the brains of the depressed [266]. Because of the obvious link between the autonomic nervous system, the *yogasanas,* and norepinephrine (Section 5.C, page 170), our discussion will focus on that part of depression involving norepinephrine. It is clear, however, that out-of-range serotonin and dopamine levels also can be important factors in depression, and their involvement, along with norepinephrine, possibly explains why there are so many different symptoms tied to this problem. About 70 percent of depressed patients can be treated effectively with drugs that increase the amounts of either serotonin or of norepinephrine in the synapses of the brain. However, it is now known that a large part of the action of these drugs is to stimulate the growth of neurons in the hippocampus, a center that is involved in depression. Because this process requires time for neural growth, the positive effects of such antidepressants are slow to appear.

Most recently, it has been shown that a brain protein named P11 enhances the effects of serotonin on brain cells and thereby alleviates depressive symptoms, whereas low levels of P11 in the brain correspondingly lead to bouts of mania [133a].

Cortisol

The cortisol produced by the HPA axis prompts the body to shut down all functions not related to self-protection. As cortisol delivers fuel to the muscles and heightens awareness, it also depresses the appetites for food and sex. Indeed, in depressed patients, both the adrenals and the pituitary glands are enlarged, cortisol is hyperexcreted, and CRF levels in the cerebrospinal fluid also are high. It appears, then, that certain types of depression can be the result of a chronic excitation along the HPA axis. Unusually high levels of cortisol also appear to mask the normal circadian rhythm of cortisol production (Section 23.B, page 774) and so lead to the desynchronization of other secondary oscillators in the body that otherwise are entrained with the cortisol rhythm. Austin [31] describes a chronotherapeutic approach (Subsection 23.C, page 789) to depression that involves a major shift of the phases of the circadian rhythms, so as to reset the times of the sleep-wake and rest-activity cycles and with them, the times for peaks and valleys in the concentrations of the relevant neurotransmitters.

Viewed in terms of the sympathetic-parasympathetic balance, the above explanation based upon high cortisol levels and low levels of the catecholamines would lead one to think that depression is a consequence of parasympathetic dominance, as can be seen by comparing table 22.A-2 with table 5.A-2. It is to be noted, however, that there is a negative feedback loop involving cortisol (figure 5.E-1), in which high levels of cortisol inhibit further release of ACTH from the pituitary, thus stabilizing high levels of cortisol in the blood as long as the stress continues. Note too that depression can be the result of either too high a level of norepinephrine or of too low a level of norepinephrine in the brain, and so one must be prepared to find either the sympathetic nervous system or the parasympathetic nervous system to be in overdrive in the depressed student. However, the latter is more likely.

Catecholamines

At the same time that the cortisol level in the depressed is being elevated via the adrenal cortex, the levels of epinephrine and norepinephrine in the brain are being depressed due to inactivity of the adrenal medulla, which otherwise floods the body with these hormones during times of stress by way of the sympathetic nervous system (Subsections 5.E, page 182, and 5.F, page 193). Because it is the symptoms of parasympathetic dominance that are most obvious in depression, any treatment that can raise the concentration of norepinephrine in the brain or increase its effectiveness is likely to have a positive influence on the course of treatment for depression.

Because the cortisol levels in some types of depression are chronically high and the catecholamine levels are depressed at the same time, it appears that the hormonal system under stress can be activated to produce cortisol, while at the same time the sympathetic nervous system is inactive and so produces an insufficiency of the catecholamines. This selective hormonal excitation of the adrenal cortex with respect to the neural excitation of the adrenal medulla relates to our differing responses to situations that are seen as either a threat or a challenge (figure 5.E-1 and Subsection 5.F, page 193).

In line with the diagnosis of anergic depression as involving parasympathetic dominance [626], the standard medical treatment consists of giving drugs that either block the re-uptake of norepinephrine from the brain's synapses or block the enzymes that otherwise clear norepinephrine from the synapses. In either case, the result is a higher, longer-lasting level of norepinephrine in the synapses of the brain and a decrease in the symptoms of depression. Stimulation of the sympathetic branch of the autonomic nervous system [565, 660], leading to the release of the catecholamines, also is effective. To the extent that depression is a response to a depleted level of norepinephrine in the brain, it is thought that an excess of norepinephrine in the brain can lead to mania [609] (Section 22.B, page 764).

Serotonin

As for serotonin, it too seems out of balance in depressed people, and as with norepinephrine, drugs that raise the levels of serotonin in the synapses can be effective in relieving depression. The neural paths that rely on norepinephrine and serotonin as neurotransmitters occur frequently in the limbic area. Therefore, deficiencies in these substances often lead to problems that have to do with emotions, appetite, or thought processing, all features of the limbic brain.

The Hypothalamus

By involving the autonomic nervous system in depression, one implicitly involves the hypo-

thalamus. Indeed, there is substantial evidence for the role that this organ plays in depression [427]. The early morning rise of cortisol levels to abnormal levels in the depressed is known to originate with the release of CRF from the hypothalamus. In turn, the drugs that are effective in reducing the symptoms of depression work on the pathways in the locus ceruleus, a region in the brain that controls hypothalamic activity.

Cerebral Laterality

Brain-excitation studies [705] confirm the cerebrolateral nature of depression, as it is found that in depressed subjects, there is a high level of alpha-wave activity in the frontal lobes of the left cerebral hemisphere and a high level of beta-wave activity in the frontal lobes of the right hemisphere (Brodmann areas 9, 10, and 11; see Section 4.H, page 152) and a correspondingly low level of alpha activity on the right. Recall that because alpha-wave activity is a signal for a relaxed mental state accompanied by significant awareness, the left hemisphere is normally alert and charged with energy. This imbalance in alpha-wave activity is thought to arise from the breakdown of communication between the amygdala (the emotional center) in the limbic system and the relevant prefrontal cortices.

The left prefrontal area that is so alpha-wave active in depressed patients is very alpha-wave inactive in subjects who are deeply in love. Interestingly, people who report high levels of happy feelings have larger and more active left prefrontal cortices than do the depressed [667]. Related evidence for the effects of brain-wave activity on the occurrence of depression is given in Subsection 4.H, page 149).

One wonders how the symptoms of atypical depression might be related to the 70 percent of left-handed people who have their dominant hemisphere for speech on the right side rather than on the left, as do the 96 percent of right-handed people (table 4.D-2). That is to say, perhaps those with atypical depression have atypical stimulation of the "wrong" hemisphere and so show symptoms opposite to those expected. Or perhaps those with atypical depression have the "wrong" imbalance (too high rather than too low a level) of a particular neurotransmitter.

Depressed subjects show abnormally low electrical activity in the left frontal lobes of the cortex [299]. However, using biofeedback, subjects were able to change the left-right ratio of electrical activity, and when this ratio reached the normal value, the depression was largely lifted [817].

Nasal Laterality

As with unilateral muscle contraction, forced unilateral breathing leads to contralateral hemispheric activation [760]. See also the positive effects of forced unilateral breathing in the treatment of obsessive-compulsive disorder (Subsection 22.D, page 767). There is also evidence that some forms of depression relate to left-nostril dominance (Section 15.E, page 633), whereas right-nostril dominance leads to hyperactivity and mania [204]. Indeed, when the breath is forced unilaterally through the left nostril, a more negative emotional state is achieved, with higher anxiety and the telling of stories with a more negative slant. This is in accord with the idea that breathing through the left nostril promoting parasympathetic excitation in the right cerebral hemisphere and breathing through the right nostril promoting sympathetic excitation in the left cerebral hemisphere (Section 15.E, page 627). Electroconvulsive therapy done only to the right cerebral hemisphere is extremely effective in curing certain depressions while leaving the memory intact [266].

Circadian Rhythms

That the autonomic nervous system is tied to the problems of depression (and anxiety; see Section 22.C, page 765) also is suggested by the observation that depressed people can fall asleep easily but awaken at 4:00 to 5:00 AM with a depression headache and cannot return to sleep. Anxiety sufferers, on the other hand, have headaches in the evening and cannot fall asleep. These times of headache onset correspond in a striking way with the shifts of the autonomic nervous system from parasympathetic dominance to sympathetic dominance (between 4:00 to 6:00 AM; see table 23.B-1) and the reverse shift in the time period 5:00 to 8:00 PM, signaling a shift from sympathetic to parasympathetic dominance. Many symptoms of depression can be relieved for a short time by depriving oneself of sleep, for sleep is a very parasympathetic activity.

Efficacy of Cure

If the depression is not too deep, psychotherapy is about as effective as medication in curing the disorder, with placebos (Subsection 5.F, page 196) running not too far behind in effectiveness. Several studies have shown that the use of placebos administered within supportive social conditions (Section 5.F, page 196) are about as effective in reducing the effects of depression as are many antidepressant drugs [602]. However, if the depression is deep, then medication is strongly favored over psychotherapy.

Large and independent studies of the effects of placebos for the treatment of depression agree that the placebos are only insignificantly less effective than are the six most prescribed antidepressants presently on the market [453a], especially in the case of dysthymia. Furthermore, physical exercise has been shown to be as effective as placebos and antidepressants when dealing with dysthymia. Once a person is depressed, the depression exerts its effects on other systems of the body. Severe depression correlates with a reduced functioning of the suppressor T cells of the immune system [635] and to death due to heart-related causes. The latter cause relates strongly to a low variability of the heart rate (Subsection 14.A, page 549).

Yogasana as a Treatment for Mild Depression

Sympathetic Stimulation

Given that many depressions can exhibit parasympathetic, right-hemispheric dominance, it is clear how certain *yogasanas* might work to dispel depression. Meyers [566] and Aldrich [7], for example, have given *yogasana* sequences designed especially for combating mild depression: they feature backbending postures of long duration, both passive and active, along with vigorous hand balancing and finally restful supported-backbending relaxations with the eyes open. Walden [880] presents a softer series of chest openings for relieving depression but also encourages strong inhalations and a mental focus on the body in order to increase the prominence of the sympathetic nervous system [888]. Such chest-opening *yogasanas* are known to be energizing and warming, leading to increased circulation and heart rate, with the blood moving to the surface of the body to cool it [110]; that is to say, they are stimulating to the sympathetic nervous system. A recent study involving the Iyengar point of view in regard to the positive effects of chest lifting and opening on depression used psychological tests, a control group, and measurements of cortisol in order to track the levels of depression in two groups of depressed beginner students. The test group was given two classes per week involving the standard Iyengar beginner's program, as taught by an Iyengar-certified teacher, with jumping, inversion, standing postures, and considerable backbending included. A significant drop in depressive symptoms as measured by both the psychological tests and cortisol measurements was noted in this group, in contrast to the control group, for whom little change was noted [31, 903]. Broad studies of the effects of *yogasana* on depression [566a, 663] conclude that *yogasana* is potentially of benefit to those suffering from anxiety or mild depressive disorders.

As a note of caution, Slede and Pomerantz [799] state clearly that for *yogasana* students with severe psychiatric disorders, *yogasana* practice can lead to depersonalized and dissociated states that can be the doorway to suicide attempts. Moreover, such students often have breathing difficulties that interfere with a true yoga practice, and with some disorders, it is very difficult for students to follow instructions. In these cases, it is advised that one not try to use *yogasana* work as a treatment for a disorder without the assistance of a psychiatric professional.

Immunity

As there is often an immunosuppression of the T cells (Subsection 16.B, page 643) in cases of

severe depression, it is no surprise that the *yogasanas* that are most effective in relieving depression are also the ones that act to revitalize the immune system.[3] If, however, a student showed signs of atypical or anxiety depression, then the *yogasanas* would have to work the other end of the autonomic spectrum, stimulating the parasympathetic response instead.

A possible mechanism connecting backbending, EEG shifts, and depression is put forth in Subsection 22.A, page 761. As depression involves an imbalance of the cerebral hemispheres, *yogasana* therapy for depression would be even more effective if the arousing postures could be done with a strong left-side accent (perhaps the above routine for depression, but with the left nostril blocked, as done by Shannahoff-Khalsa and Beckett in dealing with obsessive-compulsive disorder [776]) in order to energize the right cerebral hemisphere and so decrease its alpha-wave activity and increase its beta-wave activity. Also see Subsection 4.H, page 149, for a way in which postures such as *urdhva dhanurasana* could help ease depression.

Attitudes, Emotions, Fears

Not only could a backbending program work to banish that part of depression involving the autonomic nervous system, but in opening the chest, it may also reveal buried emotions and fears [449], which can leave the student feeling sad at first, but later relieved, if the emotions are dealt with and then set aside. This obvious link between the physiological and the emotional works the other way too, for there may well be hidden fears that keep us from opening the abdominal and solar plexus regions in backbends until those fears are confronted and rationalized (see Section 11.D, page 455). In such cases, the attitude toward backbending may be critical [449].

---

3   There is also a very important time factor in the treatment of depression. Once the depressed attitudes become entrenched, even achieving the appropriate neurotransmitter balance will become an effective cure only a long time thereafter. The symptoms of depression are most easily combated in the early stages of their development [266].

In regard to attitude and the *yogasanas,* note that if the performance of a *yogasana* is seen as a threat and so is laced with an attitude of fear, then excess cortisol will be released by the initial action of the hypothalamus, but release of the catecholamines will be repressed; whereas if the attitude is one of a welcome challenge, then only the catecholamines will be released, and the high cortisol levels characteristic of depression do not appear (figure 5.E-1). These two paths of adrenal excitation differ in that one is driven by a neural excitation and the other is driven by a hormonal excitation of the adrenal glands.

Due to the correlation between stress, high cortisol levels, and depression, it is not surprising to find that among young women who are entering puberty, among mothers who have just delivered, and among older women in perimenopause, there are strong hormonal stresses, great surges of cortisol, and temporary bouts of depression.

Chocolate High

Physiological studies on the effects of hatha yoga exercise have shown that not only can it combat depression temporarily, but it also offers antidotes for anger, tension, sleeplessness, and fatigue [575, 667]. It has been shown that those suffering from mild depression are lacking in the chemical phenyl ethylamine and that either treatment with this chemical or mild exercise can lift the depression for a short time. This chemical is the active pleasure ingredient in chocolate and also may be responsible in part for the emotional high generated by *yogasana* practice [918]. Psychologically, remember: "When we're feeling depressed, we long for genuine connections with others who accept us as we are, and we often can find that in yoga class" [888].

Autonomic Flexibility

Several studies have shown that the occurrence of depression is linked to a lack of variability of the heart rate (Subsection 14.A, page 549), which in turn relates to the ease with which the autonomic nervous system changes its balance between sympathetic and parasympathetic dominance of neural excitation as the heart beats

(Subsection 15.C, page 619). Further, if the depression follows a heart attack and the variability of the heart rate remains low, then the risk of dying immediately following the attack rises. It would follow from this that a *yogasana* practice that stresses an increase in the autonomic flexibility might prove to be an antidepressant.

Colored Lights versus Depression

There is general agreement that regular physical activity is associated with decreases in depression and anxiety for all ages and in both sexes [618], and this includes performing the *yogasanas.* It may be that the euphoria and sense of well-being that follow a *yogasana* practice are manifestations of the alpha waves in the right hemisphere that are known to be generated in the EEG pattern (Section 4.H, page 151) during moderate exercise and that persist long after the exercise is finished.[4] It also is known that exercise can increase norepinephrine and serotonin in the brain.

Notice that the daily depressive low for those suffering from exogenous depression comes at the end of the day, when cortisol levels are lowest (see Subsection 23.B, page 772). This suggests that if done with the proper attitude, backbending at this time of the day might have its largest positive effect (Subsection 23.C, page 789). To further stimulate the sympathetic system (see Subsection 17.E, page 683), one could also introduce red-colored lights, as red is known to stimulate the sympathetic response. Similarly, the relaxed *yogasanas* recommended for the treatment of anxiety and mania could be even more effective if performed with blue lights of the proper wavelength (Subsection 17.E, page 683).

Yet another aspect of depression is that experienced on a yearly basis. When the daylight hours are shorter and the sun is not so bright, the amount of ultraviolet light entering the eyes throughout the day is insufficient, and seasonal

---

4   Note too that the pleasure and satisfaction of exercising also can involve the release of dopamine in specific brain regions, as well as the release of endorphins (Subsection 13.C, page 521).

affective disorder (SAD) results (Subsection 17.E, page 685.) The symptoms of SAD are much like those of depression. However, in this case, there are direct neural connections between the retina of the eyes and the suprachiasmatic nuclei within the hypothalamus, so that direct viewing of supplemental ultraviolet light is effective in lifting the depression (Subsection 17.E, page 685).

Section 22.B: Mania and Bipolar Disorder

Bipolar Symptoms

Recurrent Bouts of Mania

If the catecholamine neurotransmitters in the brain are present at too-high concentrations, then the mood symptoms can be those of mania, and if the concentrations of the neurotransmitters change from too low to too high and back again, then a bipolar disorder is in full swing, carrying one from depression to mania and back to depression.[5]

Approximately 25 percent of those showing major depression symptoms (table 22.A-2) will also show periods of manic (euphoric) mood, with symptoms that are just opposite to those shown in the table. In the manic phase, this alternating pattern of depression and mania, termed bipolar depression, is characterized by symptoms that may include elevated, expansive, or irritable moods; grandiosity; emotional displays; hyperactivity; loquaciousness; increased sexual and physical energy; reckless involvements; and little need for sleep [427]. The symptoms in the depression stage of bipolar disorder remain those for the

unipolar case: excess sadness, apathy, underactivity, loneliness, guilt, and a lowered sense of one's worth (tables 22.A-1 and 22.A-2). It is generally thought that the manic phase of the bipolar disorder is the mind's attempt to keep from sliding into an irreversibly deep depression [74]. Mania without depression is very rare. In some women, mania is experienced close to the time of menstruation.

One may swing between the extreme phases of the bipolar situation in a matter of weeks, or it may require years to go from one phase to the other [74a]. As one swings between these emotional extremes, the time at which the core temperature is maximum is 5:00 PM during the depressed phase of a bipolar disorder but advances to 1:00 PM in the manic phase [584].

Hormonal Imbalances

In the United States, about 1 percent of the population (two to three million) have severe bipolar disorder and about 2 percent have a milder form of the problem. Though there is no biochemical test at present for bipolar disorder, it is known that the level of the neurotransmitter GABA is often low in people afflicted with this condition and that the level of serotonin is low in the depressive phase. The genetic component is a strong one among the risk factors for bipolar disorder [656].

Treatment

Lithium

In bipolar illness, the switch from depression to mania or the reverse can be almost instantaneous or long and drawn out. In the context of the discussion in Section 22.A, page 753, one imagines a rapid or slow shift of the autonomic system between sympathetic and parasympathetic dominance as the cause of the mood swings in bipolar depression. Indeed, the pharmacological treatment for mania is the use of powerful sedatives that inhibit sympathetic dominance.

Lithium (taken as the compound lithium bromide) is often used to treat mania, but it is not

---

5   Though it is good to have a certain emotional flexibility in order to respond appropriately to different emotional stresses, as with the autonomically balanced subject in figure 5.E-2, the bipolar subject overreacts to such stresses and so may be said to be emotionally hyperflexible.

Table 22.C-1: Symptoms that Differentiate Anxiety from Depression [567]

Anxiety	Depression
Hypervigilance	Psychomotor retardation
Severe tension and panic	Severe sadness and anhedonia
Perceived danger	Perceived loss
Doubt and uncertainty	Hopelessness; suicidal thoughts
Insecurity	Self-reproach
Phobic avoidance	Loss of libido
Performance anxiety	Weight change

a cure, and its mechanism of action is not understood. It is known, however, that lithium has the effect of lengthening the period of the X oscillator when it is free-running, so as to lengthen the period of the core-temperature markers (see Section 23.B, page 774) [584]. That mania is more likely in the bright light of summer [721] may be due to the overstimulation of the hypothalamus by the retina. If overstimulation is the case, in a sense, it is a reversed SAD reaction (Subsection 17.E, page 685).

Yogasana

In those cases where the root cause of mania is sympathetic dominance, the *yogasana* approach to dealing with bipolar disorder is to stress the relaxing and restorative postures; i.e., just the opposite prescription given for depression. Consistency and regularity of one's day-to-day routines is a protective factor in combating bipolar disorder, which implies that a daily *yogasana* practice could help in overcoming this condition.

Section 22.C: Anxiety

Symptoms

Emotional Stress

If a stress is a threat not to one's physical being, but instead to one's emotional being, to one's psyche, and at the same time one is afraid to act forcefully against the threat, then the result is anxiety. With anxiety, it is as if one suffers all of the physical symptoms associated with the fight or flight response of the sympathetic nervous system, but in response to a non-physical threat. Anxiety is ever-present in us all but can reach pathological levels during panic attacks, phobia, obsessive-compulsive behaviors, and post-traumatic stress disorder. In normal anxiety, there is a rapid cessation of anxiety symptoms once the stressful event is past, whereas the situation becomes more pathological if the person continues to hold onto the anxiety long after the event. Anxiety is always about fear and the future [95, 810].

Symptoms of anxiety include muscular trembling, sweating, rigid posture, heart palpitations, cold hands, muscle tension, heightened alertness, avoidance behavior, a feeling of dread, fatigue, and fear of losing one's balance [583]. Anxiety headaches appear at or close to bedtime, as the body swings from sympathetic dominance to parasympathetic dominance (table 23.B-4). Just as depression is characterized by a parasympathetic dominance, anxiety is characterized by a sympathetic dominance, which can be countered by taking sedating drugs, such as tranquilizers. The characteristic symptoms of anxiety and depression are compared in table 22.C-1. Note too that a severe case of anxiety is often accompanied by a secondary depression [567] and that anxiety, like depression, is immunosuppressive [635].

Mechanisms

When we experience a frightening situation, the fear is recorded not only in our rational, conscious memory but also is indelibly recorded immediately and directly in a separate location called the emotional memory, within the amygdala. The signal going to the amygdala directly is quite rapid and cannot be edited, unlike that going first to the cortex and then to the amygdala. The direct signal is normally inhibited by large quantities of the neurotransmitter gamma-aminobutyric acid (GABA; see Subsection 3.D, page 55). However, when GABA is lacking, the emotional memory exerts itself, and anxiety ensues. Serotonin also is a factor in anxiety, and so the antidepressants used for depression often are useful in treating anxiety, in spite of the differences listed in table 22.C-1.

Anxiety and *Yogasana*

Parasympathetic Stimuli

As with depression, those who exercise regularly acquire a demonstrable resistance to pathological anxiety [618]. Interestingly, though the same calming, anti-anxiety effect that is promoted by moderate exercise (*yogasana*, for yoga students) also is promoted by meditative rest (*savasana*, for yoga students), the benefits of exercise are longer lasting than those of meditative relaxation.

The γ-motor efferent nervous system is under autonomic control and works to energize the muscles used for posture and balance. Because the γ-system is stimulated by anxiety, this disorder can lead to increased γ discharge and a general tightening of the muscles [157]; i.e., an increased muscle tone. On the other hand, *yogasanas* of the sort that can make us looser in a muscular sense, resulting in muscles of longer resting length (Subsection 11.B, page 436) also can release feelings of anxiety. However, the emotional release often occurring at the end of *yogasana* practice may possibly overwhelm an acutely anxious student, in which case *yogasana* practice may be contraindicated [799].

From the *yogasana* point of view, the anxious or panicked student is in need of postures that are relaxing and promote the parasympathetic response while inhibiting the sympathetic (see [736], for example). A recent study of patients with anxiety has shown significant reduction in anxiety levels when the patients meditated so that thoughts were centered on the body sensations of the moment and not on external, environmental stimuli [575]. It is thought that when one is in a state of relaxation, negative imagery is effectively blocked, thus preventing the right hemisphere from processing any anxiety-producing feelings [479]. Long-term relaxation reduces anxiety.

Pain

Anxiety can be a factor in yet another way for the *yogasana* student. It is known that one's sensitivity to pain is higher when one's level of anxiety is also high, and that if one is both anxious and in pain, the sensitivity to the latter can be appreciably reduced by placebos (Section 5.F, page 196) that reduce the former. It follows from this that a student who is anxious about the discomfort of *urdhva dhanurasana*, for example, will be even more sensitive to the pain, in a self-fulfilling way, so that appropriate anxiety-relieving comments from the teacher could be effective in easing the student's anxiety and heightening the student's performance. It is also known that *yogasana* practice can improve performance on tasks involving learning and memory of non-yogic material, as it reduces anxiety that otherwise interferes with learning and memory [608].

Panic attacks are readily brought on by excess carbon dioxide in the blood, as when hyperventilating by making the inhalation long but the exhalation short. Perhaps improving ventilation through a *pranayama* practice encouraging the shortening of the inhalation and the lengthening of the exhalation, and thereby encouraging a parasympathetic response, could be of help here in dealing with incipient panic attacks, especially when practiced in conjunction with relaxing and restorative *yogasanas* that also promote parasympathetic excitation. Strangely, there appears to be a strong correlation between hyperextension of the joints (Subsection 7.D, page 248) and those with panic disorders or phobias [95].[6]

---

6   Could there possibly be a connection between high flexibility in the musculoskeletal system and high flexibility in the emotional system?

Table 22.D-1: Emotional Distress and the Breathing Modes that Bring Relief [810]

Distress	Breathing Strategy
Anger	As anger builds, divert thoughts to the flow of the breath through the nostrils.
Acute anxiety	Relaxed breath awareness often during the day, perhaps as often as hourly.
Sadness and depression	Breathe in an unbroken flow with breath deep and relaxed, avoiding pauses.
Physical pain	With deep breathing, mentally send the breath to join the pain, rather than fight the pain.

Section 22.D: Other Emotional and Mood Disorders

Obsessive-Compulsive Disorder

Obsessive-compulsive disorder (OCD) is thought to be a variety of anxiety disorder of a very recalcitrant type. Recent experiments show that OCD often involves a lateralized cerebral deficit in the frontal or temporal lobes; realizing the strong lateral effects of unilateral nostril breathing (Section 15.E, page 627), Shannahoff-Khalsa and Beckett [776] have tested this method of treatment on several OCD patients. As the deficit is in the left cerebral hemisphere, gentle, seated exercises were performed while breathing through the right nostril, with the left nostril closed. Working in this way for one year led to significant reduction of OCD symptoms. It is reported that OCD patients are able to scrupulously follow the *yogasana* program and progress more rapidly than others who are less stable and regular in the practice [799].

Schizophrenia

The active symptoms of schizophrenia are delusions, hallucinations, and unusual or disorganized behavior, whereas the passive symptoms are lack of activity, loss of interest, and unresponsiveness. These symptoms of schizophrenia suggest biochemical imbalances and neurotransmitter dysfunctions in the brain. Schizophrenics have very high dopamine levels in the brain, and blockers of dopamine are of help in the return to normal. Glutamate also is involved in schizophrenia, as is the transmission of chemical signals across the lipid bilayers [195]. Persons with mild schizophrenia engage both sides of the brain more evenly than do others, have a thicker corpus callosum, and are unusually creative. On the other hand, the working memory (short-term memory) within the frontal lobes is disorganized and defective in schizophrenics [427a]. Furthermore, schizophrenics show a strong disregulation or lack of circadian cycles with respect to the rising and setting of the sun.

Fear and Anger

Fear is an emotion that usually is not considered to be a disability, but it is something that can hold us back in our quest for a yogic state of body and mind. The physiology of fear is discussed in Subsection 4.F, page 132. As mentioned in Box 11.D-1, page 453, the emotion of fear can be overcome by the practice of backbending [449]. As the emotion of anger is controlled by the hypothalamus, it is no surprise that passive *yogasanas* such as supported *halasana* are effective in defusing anger.

Emotion and the Breath

The intimate connection between our emotional states and the qualities of the breath are obvious and unmistakable. For example, the holding of the breath in a moment of fear or sobbing in happiness is a clear example of the connection between the emotions and the breath. Fortunately, this bridge between the emotions and the breath can be crossed in both directions, so that the conscious use of the breath also can ease emotional pain [42, 810], as indicated in table 22.D-1.

Time and Body Rhythms

23

Section 23.A: The Innate Sense of Elapsed Time

Timing is everything. In our bodies, internal clocks tick out seconds, months, and years [906], and defects in the timing of our biological clocks have been linked to cancer, Parkinson's disease, seasonal affective disorder, and attention-deficit disorder. In general, there are two types of such body clocks: the internal timer that operates essentially as a stopwatch or interval timer on the seconds-to-hours time scale, and the circadian clock that directs bodily processes in ways that depend in a predictable and periodic way upon the time of day, month, year, decade, etc. The first type of clock can be thought of as an interval timer, and the second, being periodic, is known as the circadian clock.[1]

Within each of us, the two types of clocks run at a regular pace, with each independently ticking off time subconsciously. Though many questions still remain, it is now known that the circadian clock rhythmically turns many of our

biological processes on and off at characteristic times that stretch from fractions of a second to as long as decades. Often, the periods of these rhythms are independent of external input and otherwise are only weakly dependent on external circumstances.[2] The internal clock within us senses elapsed time intervals but is neither controlling of any biological process, nor is it periodic in time. This chapter explores the mechanisms by which these clocks operate, the effects of internal-clock time on various body/mind functions, and the relation of such body rhythms to *yogasana* practice.

Interval Timer

In addition to the cyclic, repeating nature of our subconscious time sense, our noncyclical clock is relevant, for as we practice *yogasana*, we become more fulfilled in the moment, and this has the effect of making us more patient in regard to the delayed fulfillment of other needs. With concentration on our practice, small things become less of a distraction, time seems to stretch out ahead of us in a more expansive way [28], and we develop a long-range view of life. In a more practical way, it is the internal interval timer that tells the *yogasana* practitioner that she has spent equal time in *trikonasana*-to-the-right and *triko-*

---

1 It should not come as a surprise to readers of this chapter that the editors of the *Concise Oxford English Dictionary* have determined that the most-often used noun in the English language is "time." In order of their frequency, the top twenty-five nouns are: time, person, year, way, day, thing, man, world, life, hand, part, child, eye, woman, place, work, week, case, point, government, company, number, group, problem, and fact. Almost all of these key words are of fundamental relevance to our *yogasana* practice.

---

2 For cyclic phenomena, the time elapsed between corresponding peaks is known as the period. For example, if body temperature varies rhythmically and is at a maximum at 4:00 AM and again at 4:00 PM and at a minimum at 10:00 AM and 10:00 PM, then the period for this rhythm is twelve hours.

nasana-to-the-left without having to look at her watch.

Location

The interval timers within us all are found within the basal ganglia (figure 4.B-1), in a subdivision known as the striatum [896]. Huge numbers of cortical neurons converge upon the far smaller number of striatal cells, which in turn continuously monitor the signals from the frontal cortex. As discussed in Subsection 4.H, these are the signals that appear in the brain's EEG and that are discharged continuously and apparently chaotically, as the waves run at different frequencies and with random phases. However, it is hypothesized that when an event is first noticed (the change of a traffic light from green to yellow, for example), a brief surge of dopamine in the striatum stops all such oscillatory discharges for a few hundred milliseconds. Following this, the oscillatory behavior then continues in a more orderly way, as all oscillators start their variations at the same time, though the frequencies remain different. The overall voltage patterns that develop in time are complex but will be always the same for a given period after the initial signal. When, in this example, the traffic signal changes a second time from yellow to red, a second burst of dopamine from the substantia nigra to the striatum again freezes the oscillations, and the new pattern of voltages across a given cell in the striatum is then representative of the four-second interval that has elapsed during the yellow phase of the traffic light.[3] This timing information is relayed from the striatum, first to the thalamus and then to the cerebral cortex, for evaluation and direction. Once the variation of the timing pattern in the context of the yellow light has been learned,

the subconscious can then estimate one's speed of travel and calculate whether there is time enough to travel past the yellow light safely, or if too much time has elapsed and one should apply the brakes.

Dopamine

In support of this theory, it is independently known that conditions that lead to low levels of dopamine in the basal ganglia affect the operation of the interval timer. For example, untreated patients with Parkinson's disease have noticeably slower interval clocks; i.e., they underestimate time intervals. Smoking marijuana also has this effect, as does the ingestion of the sedative Valium. On the other hand, schizophrenics have a surplus of dopamine, and their internal clocks run at such an accelerated rate that their circadian rhythms are more or less completely destroyed and their world becomes incomprehensible. Ingesting recreational drugs or stimulants such as caffeine, nicotine, cocaine, or methamphetamines increases the dopamine levels and so speeds the interval timers, making the sense of time pass faster. In states of deep concentration (such as *samadhi*) or of high emotional content, the basal ganglia are flooded with dopamine, with the result that the operation of the interval timer is totally upset and all sense of time is lost. Athletes in this mental state are said to be "in the zone." The interval timers within our basal ganglia are being activated whenever we move muscles in a coordinated way, as when performing any of the *yogasanas*, and especially when we are in motion. They come into play when we kick into *pincha mayurasana* and when we pose and repose in *trikonasana*, moving toward *samadhi*. As we practice, the timing signals of the basal ganglia are refined, and our actions are thereby more coordinated. Activation of the interval timers also can be achieved through motivation; by thinking before we go to sleep that we will awaken at 5:00 AM rather than at 7:30 AM, we awaken at the earlier hour.

---

3   Saying it differently, one can tell elapsed time between start and finish, given a waveform, the amplitude of which varies regularly in time, provided one knows the amplitude at the start and finish times. This applies as well to the situation where many such waves of different frequencies are being monitored but all receive the start and finish signals simultaneously.

Slowing of Time

In contrast to periods of rhythmically-timed events (e.g., temperature change), which change very little as one ages, the periods of elapsed time that are arrhythmic are sensed to lengthen as we age. As described in earlier sections, as we do our *yogasana* practice, our muscle response time lengthens, at least when we are younger. It is possible that this lengthening is related to the apparent slowing of the time sense in older students [19] caused by lower dopamine levels in the brain, for lower levels of dopamine can create a sense that time is passing more slowly than real-clock time. The stretching of real time is most obvious when the aged are busy; for example, subjects aged sixty to sixty-five years who were asked to estimate the passage of three minutes while they worked at a clerical task required almost five minutes to do so [18]. *Yogasana* practitioners during a vigorous practice experience a compression of elapsed time, whereas when in *savasana,* the tendency is for the sense of elapsed time to expand.

When we are sitting quietly in *muktasana,* thirty seconds of real time seems to last for only twenty-six seconds; however, when sitting in Zen meditation, the thirty-second interval seems to last for thirty-seven seconds. These time intervals as perceived by meditators are dependent upon the breathing rate, so that the perceived time is 15 percent longer when breathing rapidly but is 75 percent longer when breathing slowly [30]. Many aspects of the sense of elapsed time, such as clock time, the date, the season, or one's age, also involve the fornix in the limbic system.

The estimation of elapsed time is temperature-dependent, for we tend to overestimate the real time interval when the temperature is high, as at noon. If we are in bed with a fever, everything seems to move at a slower pace, and we tend to become impatient. In the evening, when the temperature drops, we underestimate elapsed time.

Section 23.B: Periodicity of Body Rhythms

Mechanisms of Oscillations

Many cyclical functions in the body apparently are tuned to astronomical phenomena. Some have periods of a day, a month, or a year, corresponding to the Earth's rotational period, the moon's rotational period, or the time it takes the Earth to circle the sun, respectively; while others are of the order of an hour to much less than a second. In the time domain, the time at which a particular function is at an extreme value is called a marker; the peaking of the core body temperature at 8:00 PM every day is an example of a marker. The cyclical appearance in time of a biological marker implies an oscillation in time of some controlling physiological function. One can imagine at least two ways in which such a physiological function could oscillate in time. First, a process would oscillate if it were triggered by some external factor that itself was oscillating in time, as, for example, the sleep-wake-sleep cycle being triggered by the setting, rising, and setting of the sun within a twenty-four-hour period. In fact, many of the body's rhythms have a twenty-four-hour period and are driven by this exogenous celestial oscillator.

For those phenomena that do not have twenty-four-hour periods, another possibility is the following. Suppose that there are sensors in the body that signal when a certain body condition (blood acidity, for example) is too high, whereas other sensors signal when it is too low. On being triggered, each of the sensors promotes the opposite effect. That is to say, if the low-acidity sensor is activated, it triggers a process that sends the acidity up, whereas if the acidity is already too high, the high-acidity sensor will trigger a process that will send the acidity toward a lower value, as shown in figure 23.B-1.

As shown in the figure, with the set points of

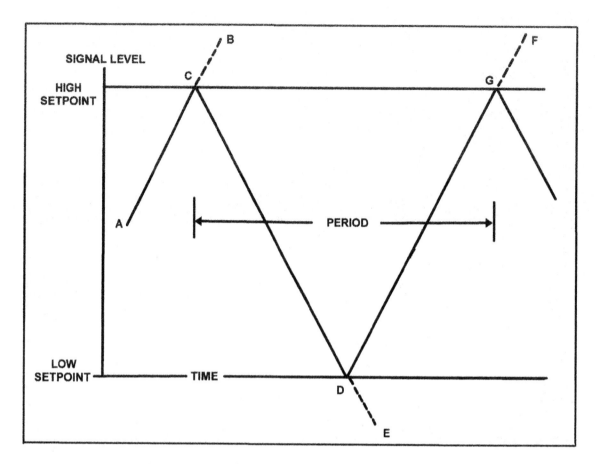

Figure 23.B-1. Producing a signal oscillating in time using a pair of high and low set points. The signal level of some biological condition (acidity, for example) starts at **A** and rises in time toward **B**. However, a high-set-point sensor is triggered at **C** and reverses the rise of acidity, sending the system toward **E** instead. As the acidity approaches **E**, a low-set-point sensor is triggered at **D** and sends the acidity upward toward **F**. On its way to **F**, the system gets no further than **G**, where the high-set-point sensor again intercepts it and sends the acidity downward. The result of this action is an acidity that oscillates between the high and low set points with a period equal to the time interval between points **C** and **G**.

the two sensors placed somewhat apart, the acidity of the blood will rise to the upper set point level and then be sent to the lower level, which in turn will send it upward again to the upper set point. In this way, one sees that the acidity of the blood simply cycles up and down, with a period between high-low-high points that depends upon where the acidity set points have been placed and how rapidly the system can move between them. This is the endogenous mechanism that has been advanced to explain the pulse of the cerebrospinal fluid in the central nervous system (Subsection 4.E, page 109) and would seem to be extendable to other body parameters such as temperature, heart rate, and blood pressure, as

long as they have high and low set points. This is but a variation on the homeostatic control mechanism shown in figure 5.A-1.

Ultradian Rhythms

Body functions that go from peak to valley and return to peak in twenty-two hours or less are termed "ultradian" [585]. Chief among these are the nasal rhythm, in which the nostril used for breathing alternates sides left-to-right-to-left, etc., within a period of about four hours (see Section 15.E, page 630), while the cerebral hemispheric dominance also shifts with approximately the same time period (see Section 4.D, page 104). REM excitation in sleep (Subsection 23.D, page 800), another ultradian process, has a period of ninety minutes; i.e., its onset appears every ninety minutes during sleep. It appears that REM sleep is supported by right-nostril dominance and non-REM sleep by left-nostril dominance. If the ultradian rhythms are to keep their peaks constant in time from one day to the next, then their periods must be submultiples of twenty-four hours; i.e., twelve, eight, six, four, three, or two hours long. The phenomena of nasal alternation, cerebral hemispheric dominance, and REM excitation meet this expectation and so have their peaks at essentially the same times each day, all other factors (such as bedtime) being kept constant.

The Ninety-Minute Period

The periodic release of many hormones in the body shows an ultradian character, with a period of somewhat less than one hour to somewhat more than two hours, and is thought to be related to other autonomic functions of the same periodicity that are governed by the hypothalamus [778]. As we go into puberty, intense spurts of hormones (estrogen for girls, testosterone for boys) are released into the bloodstream at approximately ninety-minute intervals. The same internal clock may be driving the release of insulin and sex hormones in teenagers, as each has a ninety-minute period.

The study of ultradian effects in the human body has been extended significantly by Shannahoff-Khalsa et al. [777], who monitored a select group of subjects for the rhythmic variations of twenty-one different biological functions and found five broad periods within the time interval of forty minutes to six hours. Time variations across all variables revealed ultradian periods of 40–65, 70–100, 115–145, 170–215, and 220–340 minutes, the second of which would fall into the group of those with ninety-minute periods and the last of which falls into the four-hour group. All measurements were taken with subjects at rest in an inclined position. The levels of hormones ACTH, luteinizing hormone, epinephrine, norepinephrine, and dopamine were measured separately in the blood of each arm, along with simultaneous measurements of the air flow through the left and through the right nostrils, cardiac output, heart rate, stroke volume, systolic pressure, diastolic pressure, and mean arterial pressure. While many of these correlated with the nasal flow, the strongest correlation across all of the variables was the correlation of the nasal flow with the stroke volume of the heartbeat, with right-nostril breathing encouraging an increased stroke volume and left-nostril breathing encouraging a decreased stroke volume. Most interestingly, the catecholamines appear alternately in the blood of the left and right arms depending on the phase of the nasal cycle, implying that the hormonal action at the adrenal glands has a laterality that is tied in some way to the laterality of the nasal breath! All of these ultradian rhythms—autonomic, neuroendocrine, cardiovascular, immunological, and behavioral—appear to be under the control of the hypothalamus.

Ancient Rhythms

It has been suggested [456] that the ultradian cycles with approximately four-hour periods are vestiges of a very ancient biological system of activity and rest that has more or less faded in importance in modern man. As such, the effects of the four-hour ultradian cycles can easily be masked by other, stronger influences, but they are still detectable by the alert student of *yogasana*. In any event, it appears that ultradian phenomena with periods much shorter than twenty-four hours are under the control of set-point mechanisms of the sort described in figure 23.B-1.

The One-to-Ten-Second Period

Of course, the breathing cycle (with a period of approximately ten seconds) and the heartbeat (with a period of approximately one second) are two of the body's key ultradian rhythms. A group of neurons having spontaneous rhythmic activity within the nucleus ambiguus of the medulla oblongata may be the respiratory pacemaker [360], whereas the resting heartbeat rate is generated within the heart itself by spontaneous polarization (Section 14.A, page 543) but is subject to strong input from both branches of the autonomic nervous system. Also to be mentioned in this category of ultradian rhythms are the less-obvious pulse of the cerebrospinal-fluid pressure, with a period of around six to ten seconds (Subsection 4.E, page 109), and the period of gastrointestinal peristalsis, also about ten seconds (Subsection 19.A, page 711). See also Subsection 14.A, page 549, concerning an oscillation frequency of 0.12 hertz (period of 8.3 seconds) that can be phase-locked throughout the body when meditating deeply. This wave is closely associated with vascular processes and is known as a Mayer wave.

Ultradian Frequencies Higher Than 1 Hertz

The EEG brain waves (Subsection 4.H, page 149) and the Schumann waves (Subsection 4.H, page 154) are examples of oscillating processes in the body running at values above 1 hertz.

Circadian Rhythms: Physiological Peaks and Valleys in the Twenty-Four-Hour Period

In spite of the tendency toward homeostasis, which is aperiodic (Subsection 5.A, page 158), life-forms from algae to humans also function on a rhythmic basis, which is to say, they display functions that oscillate in time rather than remain static or shift aperiodically; moreover, the shifts are regular and occur at times that easily can be predicted. In those cases where the rhythmic process goes through a maximum, a minimum, and then returns to a maximum once in twenty-four hours, the rhythm is said to be circadian (*circa* = about, *dies* = day). Though the periods of such twenty-four-hour circadian clocks are inborn, the times in the twenty-four-hour cycle at which they reach maximum and minimum values are set by sleep patterns, which in turn are strongly influenced by the light-dark illumination cycle of the rising and setting sun [266]. The details of the mechanism of circadian rhythms are now understood at the molecular level, as discussed briefly in Subsection 23.B, page 787.

Circadian rhythms dictate activity, biochemistry, physiology, and behavior. Though these rhythms persist in the dark, their periods are increased or decreased somewhat with respect to a twenty-four-hour periodicity when free-running in the dark. In many tissues (liver, skeletal muscle, etc.), the endogenous circadian clocks are more or less controlled by the suprachiasmatic nucleus in the hypothalamus. Thus, it is reasonable that the hormonal releases of vasopressin, growth hormone, and cortisol, as controlled from the hypothalamus, show circadian rhythms [450].

General Characteristics

Before going further into the specific details of periodic phenomena in the body, let us consider a few general characteristics of circadian rhythms. Many body processes show a maximum in their rate, their concentration, or their intensity once per day, and always at the same characteristic time of the day for each of the processes. For example, the core temperature of the body is maximal at 8:00 PM every day, the concentration of cortisol in the blood plasma is maximal every day at 9:00 AM, and the urinary excretion of K^+ is maximal every day at 2:00 PM. Minimum values of these functions are observed approximately twelve hours earlier (or later).

Free-Running

It is also known that many of the processes with apparent periods of twenty-four hours in fact show much longer periods when the subjects are shielded from external cues as to the length of the day; i.e., they are kept in constant illumination and constant temperature, take their meals at random times, and have no social contact with the outside world through radio, television, etc. In this free-running state, many processes stretch out in time so as to have periods of up to thirty-four hours or so, whereas others stretch only somewhat to a period of 24.8 hours. All such free-running processes can be brought back into synchronization with the twenty-four-hour clock by exposure to an external trigger having a definite twenty-four-hour period, such as sunrise-sunset or a twenty-four-hour drug regimen. The shift

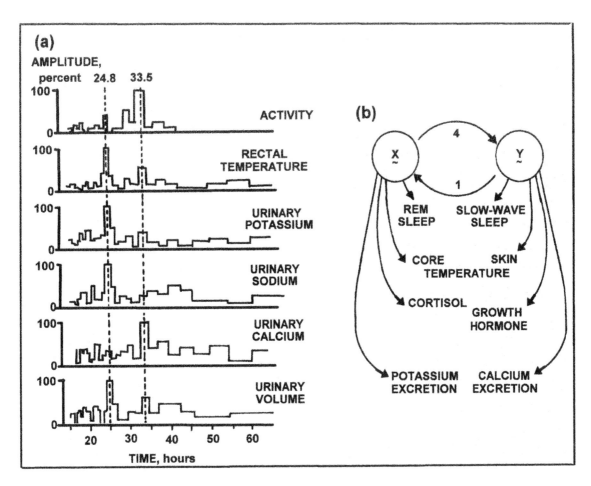

Figure 23.B-2. (a) Temporal display of several biological rhythms in a free-running human subject. Two largely desynchronized rhythms are seen, with core temperature, urinary K⁺, Na⁺, and urinary volume largely following a 24.8-hour rhythm, whereas physical activity and urinary Ca^{2+} have a period of 33.5 hours. Each rhythm shows a small amount of the other. (b) The two rhythms are assigned to oscillator X (24.8 hours) and to oscillator Y (33.5 hours), with oscillator X controlling REM sleep and cortisol production in addition to the processes in (a) having the 24.8-hour period, and oscillator Y controlling slow-wave sleep, skin temperature, and the production of growth hormone in addition to the processes in (a) having the 33.5-hour period. The admixture of X into Y is four times larger than the admixture of Y into X [584].

of the period from the free-running state to that of the twenty-four-hour solar clock is called entrainment. There are many other examples of the entrainment phenomenon. For example, when walking with a friend, we often unconsciously synchronize our walking to be in phase with him, and when the boss at a meeting scratches her nose, everyone else unconsciously repeats the action soon thereafter.

The fact that there are two (or more) circadian clocks keeping time in the free-running human body at two (or more) different rates is apparent

in the free-running data of figure 23.B-2a. Once free-running, one sees clear peaks at 24.8 and 33.5 hours, which Moore-Ede et al. [584], assign to control by two desynchronized oscillators, X and Y, with free-running periods of 24.8 and 33.5 hours respectively (figure 23.B-2b). It is known that oscillator X is the pacemaker for REM sleep, the core temperature, cortisol release, urinary volume, and K⁺ excretion, and it is thought to be located in the hypothalamus (possibly in the ventromedial nucleus). The Y oscillator is the pacemaker for slow-wave sleep, the rest-activity cycle, skin temperature, growth hormone, and Ca^{2+} excretion; it is located in the suprachiasmatic nucleus within the hypothalamus. Entrainment of the above processes by the light-dark cycle of the sun rising and setting results in a resetting of the periods of the free-running pacemakers for both X and Y clocks to twenty-four hours. Note too that there is mixed character to some of the processes in the figure, with both the 24.8-hour and the 33.5-hour periods appearing simultaneously for certain functions.

For most biological processes, a rise in temperature of 10° C results in a doubling of the rate of the process. However, the pacemaker for the circadian rhythm apparently is temperature compensated, for the period of twenty-four hours is independent of body temperature [584], unless the pacemaker is directly entrained to the twenty-four-hour rotational cycle of the Earth.

Rhythm Shifts

As pointed out by Lye [527], the characteristics of an individual's circadian rhythms are not constant throughout his or her life, being present when in utero, reaching peaks during early adulthood, and finally becoming weaker and shifted in phase as the suprachiasmatic nucleus ages and deteriorates. For this reason, humans with a healthy, functioning circadian rhythm urinate during the day but refrain from this during the evening hours. However, with the advance of old age, the circadian rhythm fades, and the necessity of voiding the bladder during the night (called nocturia) becomes more the norm.

What physiological and psychological factors in the body rise and fall over the span of a day, and when during the day are they maximal, and when are they minimal? To answer these questions, all of the physiological peaks and valleys that could be found in the literature are listed in tables 23.B-1, 23.B-2, 23.B-3, and 23.B-4, along with their times of highest and lowest effect [318, 584, 716, 735, 804]. In some cases, there is disagreement among authors as to the times for maximum and minimum effects (by a few hours), but these have been averaged in the tables. For ease of display, the twenty-four-hour clock has been divided into quarters, each covering a six-hour time period. The data shown is that for individuals on a normal sleep schedule (going to bed at about 10:00 PM and arising at about 6:30 AM); abnormal sleep patterns or shifting time zones can shift these patterns [318]. The times of maximum and minimum physiological effects, as listed in the tables, are called circadian markers. Maxima and minima are assigned to lie within one-hour intervals, and where the correlation can be made, the appropriate autonomic dominance as listed in table 5.A-2 is also listed for the marker. Note that the times for the markers for maximum and minimum values in a circadian rhythm are not necessarily separated by twelve hours, as circadian rhythm requires only that the time between successive maximum markers be twenty-four hours and the time between successive minimum markers also be twenty-four hours, but otherwise makes no demands upon the time between successive maximum and minimum markers.

Midnight to 6:00 AM

In the hours between midnight and 2:00 AM (table 23.B-1), the body systems are essentially asleep, and very little would seem to be going on; cortisol levels in the blood are minimal, as are temperature, alertness, blood pressure, and muscle tone in this time interval. However, release of the growth hormone is maximal at this time, as is metabolic activity of the cells lining the digestive tract (so as to release stomach acid) and as is the proliferation of many cells of the immune system.

A low cortisol level is a marker for low physical and mental activity, as appropriate for the late evening hours (a minimum between 9:00 PM and 12:00 AM); however, if this hormone is in disregulation due to chronic stress, then the minimum appears only weakly, if at all. It is during this late-evening resting phase that the immune system (Chapter 16, page 641) strengthens itself, with maximum numbers of T cells, neutrophils, and eosinophils in circulation and maximum activity of the white blood cells and lymphokines. Because asthma can be a symptom of an autoimmune response, the strong activity of the immune

Table 23.B-1: Times for Maxima and Minima of Various Body Functions in the Period between Midnight and 6:00 AM [318, 584, 716, 735, 804]

Time	Extreme Function	Autonomic Dominance
12:00 Midnight	Cortisol secretion min	Parasympathetic
	Growth hormone secretion max	
	T cells max	
	Surgical deaths max	
	Gout pain max	
	Gallbladder attacks max	
	Stomach acidity max	Parasympathetic
	Peptic ulcer pain/heartburn max	
	Liver flow rate max	
1:00 AM	Spontaneous labor begins	
	Surgical deaths max	
	Body temperature min	Parasympathetic
	Alertness min	
	Cholesterol from liver max	Parasympathetic
	Glycogen from liver max	
	Neutrophils max	Parasympathetic
	Eosinophils max	Parasympathetic
	Lymphokine activity max	Parasympathetic
2:00 AM	Sleep deepest	
	Bowel movement min	
	Congestive heart failure max	
	Nosebleed min	
3:00 AM	Skin repair max	
	Blood pressure min	Parasympathetic
	Epinephrine begins drop	
	Histamine begins rise	
	Bone breakdown max	
	SIDS death max	
	Gallbladder symptoms max	
	Hemorrhagic stroke min	
	Variant angina max	
	Muscle tone min	Parasympathetic
	Female alcohol-dehydrogenase activity min	
4:00 AM	Natural childbirth max	
	Skin temperature min	
	Cholesterol production max	
	Lung function min	
	Asthma attacks max	
	Light sensitivity max	

	Cluster/migraine headaches begin	
	Strokes max	
	Pain sensitivity max	
	White-blood-cell activity max	Parasympathetic
5:00 AM	Dreaming most intense	REM
	Airway tension max	
	Endogenous depression max	Parasympathetic
	Heart attack fatality max	
	Auto accidents max	
	Bleeding ulcer min	
	Toothache frequency max	
6:00 AM	Cortisol secretion max	Sympathetic
	Risk of dying of any cause max	
	Insulin secretion max	
	Height max	
	Cold symptoms max	
	Blood pressure/heart rate surge	Sympathetic
	Menstruation begins	
	Platelet clumping max	Sympathetic
	Insulin min	Sympathetic
	Runny nose, salivation, sneezing max	Sympathetic
	Headache discomfort max	
	Bronchial constriction max	Sympathetic
	Melatonin decreases	Sympathetic
	Cortisol begins decrease	Sympathetic

system in the hours around 3:00 to 4:00 AM and the beginning of the release of histamine leads to a preponderance of asthma attacks at this time (80 percent of breathing failures and 68 percent of asthma deaths occur between midnight and 8:00 AM [318]). On the other hand, the occurrence of stroke by hemorrhage in this time period is minimal, as blood pressure is minimal at 3:00 AM, and the epinephrine level starts to drop. Between midnight and 6:00 AM, liver action is at its peak, churning out cholesterol and glycogen. At the same time, alcohol drunk in this early hour of the morning stays in the blood longer and so has an increased effect on one's mental abilities. Length of the spine is maximal at 6:00 AM, thanks to its nightlong rehydration, and menstruation begins at this time, as the blood pressure and heart rate surge.

By comparison with the data of table 5.A-2, each of the circadian markers in tables 23.B-1 through 23.B-4 has been assigned an inferred connection to a branch of the autonomic nervous system, either as sympathetic or parasympathetic. The general pattern of autonomic excitation would seem to be balanced between sympathetic and parasympathetic dominance at midnight but is moving toward clear parasympathetic dominance by 6:00 AM.

7:00 AM to 1:00 PM

Between 5:00 AM and 6:00 AM (i.e., at sunrise), the body-rhythms picture starts to change rapidly. One sees that death by heart attack following coronary arterial blockage or abnormal heart rhythms is three times as likely in the early morning hours between 6:00 to 9:00 AM. The in-

Table 23.B-2: Times for Maxima and Minima of Various Body Functions in the Period between 7:00 AM and 1:00 PM [318, 584, 716, 735, 804]

Time	Extreme Function	Autonomic Dominance
7:00 AM	Testosterone in males max	
	Melatonin secretion min	
	Hay fever symptoms max	
	Rheumatoid arthritis pain max	
	Angina max	Sympathetic
	Blood viscosity max	
	Response to toothache painkillers min	
	Epinephrine increases	Sympathetic
	Helper T cells min	Sympathetic
	Ankylosing spondylitis pain max	
	Newborn medical complications min	
8:00 AM	Bowel movement max	
	Hemorrhagic stroke max	Sympathetic
	Nosebleed frequency max	Sympathetic
	Depression symptoms max	
	Memorization ability max	
	Migraine rate max	
	Bacterial fever max	
	Male alcohol-dehydrogenase activity max	
9:00 AM	Body weight min	
	Migraine frequency max	
	Urinary volume max	
	Cortisol max	Sympathetic
	ACTH max	Sympathetic
	Core temperature min	Sympathetic
	Risk for heart attack max	Sympathetic
	Histamine sensitivity min	
	Stroke max	
	Blood flow, viscera to muscles max	Sympathetic
	Restless leg syndrome min	
	Liver metabolism min	
10:00 AM	Mental alertness/arousal high	
	Heart rate variability min	
11:00 AM		
12:00 noon	Mood elevated	
	Hemoglobin max	Sympathetic
	Digestive strength max	Parasympathetic
	Gallbladder attack min	
	Bleeding stomach ulcer max	
	Time for decision making best	

cidence for stroke also peaks at 9:00 AM. At the same time, hormonal balances begin to shift, and blood pressure and heart rate start to rise, while platelets in the blood clump more easily and tend to form clots at this time. It is in this time period that the various negative complications of heart action appear.

Myocardial infarction is due to several factors: the ability of the blood to coagulate, blood pressure, oxygen requirements, and myocardial susceptibility to ischemia. Each has a twenty-four-hour cycle, and their mutual action places the time of myocardial infarction most often during the morning hours [510]. Strangely, it has been found that an irregular timing between each heartbeat and the next is indicative of good health heart-wise (Subsections 14.A, page 549), but at about 10:00 AM, the time between heartbeats (as driven by the vagus nerve) can become very regular, and this is a signal for heart trouble; this is reflected in the heart attack maximum occurring at 9:00 AM.

In the early morning hours, the nose is runny due to colds and nasal allergies, salivation is maximal [427], and rheumatoid arthritis symptoms peak. Melatonin in the blood decreases with the rise of the sun, as does the insulin level, while the level of epinephrine increases. The hours between 6:00 and 9:00 AM mark the onset of strong sympathetic excitation of the autonomic nervous system, as one can see by comparing the circadian markers of table 23.B-1 with the characteristics of table 5.A-2.

In line with the excitation of the sympathetic branch of the autonomic nervous system in the early morning, the core body temperature (as measured rectally) has fallen to its lowest point by 9:00 AM, as blood is moved from the visceral organs back into the muscles [427]; while ACTH, cortisol, sex-hormone levels (see Chapter 6, page 207), and urinary volume are at their peak values, readying the body for the day's battles. One is at the peak of mental performance in the hours between sunrise and noon, and memorization also is best in the period from 6:00 to 9:00 AM [716].

The fever from a bacterial infection is highest from 5:00 AM to noon, whereas the fever from a viral infection is highest from 2:00 to 10:00 PM [716]. As regards the fever of bacterial infection, its time of maximum temperature does correspond to a low in immune-system response. Babies born in the morning hours are more likely to be healthy; babies born between 2:00 and 4:00 PM are more likely to have medical complications [716]. The level of hemoglobin in the blood is maximal at 12:00 PM, and the digestion is strongest at this time.

1:00 PM to 7:00 PM

There seem to be few extreme values of body functions reached after 9:00 AM and before 3:00 PM, other than the power for digestion, a mental inertness that overcomes the body at about 3:00 PM, and a peak in muscular flexibility that is said to occur at between 2:00 and 5:00 PM. Between 3:00 PM and 5:00 PM, the blood pressure maximizes, as do muscle strength, the ability to learn, lung function, manual skills, and alertness [465]. The velocity of forearm motion is highest during the twenty-four-hour clock at mid-afternoon. Again, all of these responses are driven by sympathetic excitation. We assume that in the intervening hours between 10:00 AM and 2:00 PM, when there are very few extremes of body function, the sympathetic and parasympathetic systems are closer to being in balance.

The steadily rising blood pressure peaks at 3:00 PM, along with peaks in muscular strength and mental powers [465]. The peak blood pressure may be 30 percent higher at 3:00 PM than it is at 3:00 AM. If one takes an hour-long nap beginning at 2:00 PM, then one will have superior performance for visual tasks throughout the afternoon and evening, due to the generation of "slow-wave" sleep. This type of sleep keeps performance from deteriorating.

An hour later (4:00 PM), lung function, skin temperature, and heart rate also reach their peak values; heart rate can vary by up to thirty beats per minute in the span of twenty-four hours [716]. The ability to perform tasks that do not involve memory is greatest when the skin temperature reaches its maximum. Remember that at the temporal antipode (twelve hours later), blood

Table 23.B-3: Times for Maxima and Minima of Various Body Functions in the Period from 1:00 PM to 7:00 PM [318, 584, 716, 735, 804]

Time	Extreme Function	Autonomic Dominance
1:00 PM	Sleep latency min	
	Agitation in dementia max	
	K^+ urinary excretion max	
2:00 PM	Eye-hand coordination max	
	Ankylosing spondylitis pain min	
	Response to toothache painkillers max	
3:00 PM	Power nap deepest	
	Alertness/arousal min	
	Newborn medical complications max	
	Muscle strength max	Sympathetic
	Airway relaxation max	
	Respiration rate max	Sympathetic
	Reflex sensitivity max	
	Mental powers max	
	Salivation min	Sympathetic
	Salt/water excretion max	
	Prednisone for asthma effect max	
4:00 PM	Reaction time fastest	
	Lung function max	Sympathetic
	Core temperature max	Sympathetic
	Heart rate max	Sympathetic
	Blood pressure max	Sympathetic
	Absorption through skin max	
	Tension headaches max	
	Ca^{2+} urinary excretion max	
	Viral fever max	
5:00 PM	Best for sports training	
	Muscle strength/flexibility max	
	Sperm motility max	
	Bleeding intestinal ulcer max	
	Lung/heart efficiency max	
	Exertion for breathing min	
	Toothache frequency min	
	Alertness max	Sympathetic
6:00 PM	Taste most acute	
	Osteoarthritis pain max	

Time	Extreme Function	Autonomic Dominance
	Fibromyalgia pain max	
	Multiple sclerosis fatigue max	
	Multiple sclerosis pain max	
	Endogenous depression max	
	Muscle tone max	Sympathetic
	Insulin secretion min	
	Sneezing, runny nose, salivation min	Parasympathetic
	Cholesterol levels rise	

pressure was lowest at 3:00 AM, as was the risk of stroke, and at that time, the epinephrine concentration in the body dropped and lung function decreased, while at the same time, histamine levels rose, further reducing lung function. It is clear from comparing the maxima of the physiological functions listed in table 23.B-3 with the data of table 5.A-2 that the sympathetic nervous system is in full swing between 3:00 PM and 6:00 PM, in strong contrast to the situation twelve hours earlier; i.e., between 1:00 AM and 4:00 AM, when the autonomic dominance was parasympathetic. Because eating at any time stimulates the release of cortisol, it is good to eat as little as possible in the evening hours.

Osteoarthritis symptoms peak at 6:00 PM, just twelve hours out of phase with the peak in rheumatoid arthritis symptoms (6:00 AM). It is clear that the rheumatoid arthritis symptoms appear when the autonomic balance switches from parasympathetic to sympathetic, whereas the osteoarthritis symptoms appear when the shift is the reverse. Similarly, mood variation is worse for endogenous depression at 5:00 AM and is worse for exogenous depression at 6:00 PM (table 23.B-3). Notice that 5:00 AM marks the time of shift from parasympathetic to sympathetic dominance, while 7:00 PM marks the transition from sympathetic to parasympathetic dominance. Mood swings might be expected to be at their worst at these times of autonomic transition.

7:00 PM to Midnight

By 8:00 to 9:00 PM, the ACTH and cortisol levels are again minimal and core temperature peaks, the incidence of brain hemorrhage rises to its maximum, and blood pressure falls. The brain-hemorrhage rate is maximal at 8:00 PM, just an hour after the time of maximum blood pressure; stroke is more common at 3:00 to 4:00 AM, the time at which the blood pressure is minimum; perhaps death by stroke is related to platelet stickiness (maximum at 6:00 AM) rather than blood pressure. The rate of heart attack is least at 9:00 PM, just the time at which the blood pressure is minimal. Immune and allergic responses are most severe at about 11:00 PM.

Gender Differences

There is an interesting difference in the circadian markers of males and females in regard to enzyme activity: alcohol dehydrogenase works fastest to detoxify the body of ingested alcohol at 8:00 AM in men but is fastest in women at 3:00 AM [716]. Thus, the tendencies of men and women toward inebriation vary differently depending upon the time of day. It is quite possible that the variations of the marker times for various physiological functions (as, for example, the large scatter of the markers for core temperature) reported by investigators are due to inherent but unrecognized gender differences.

Sleep Cycles

Of course, the sleep cycle itself is based upon the circadian rhythm; however, within the sleep cycle, there are several ultradian rhythms as well (see Subsection 23.D, page 794). In regard to circadian markers, we broadly can place sleep in the 8:00 PM to 5:00 AM domain, a time period already

Table 23.B-4: Times for Maxima and Minima of Various Body Functions in the Period from 7:00 PM to Midnight [318, 584, 716, 735, 804]

Time	Extreme Function	Autonomic Dominance
7:00 PM	Body temperature max	
	Blood pressure max	
	Na$^+$/Mg^{2+} urinary excretion max	
	Colic max	
	Handshake strongest	
8:00 PM	Running/swimming abilities max	
	Alcohol tolerance max	
	ACTH min	Parasympathetic
	Core temperature max	Parasympathetic
	Brain hemorrhage max	
	Osteoarthritis pain/indomethacin min	
	Backache pain max	
	Ankylosing spondylitis pain max	
9:00 PM	Melatonin secretion begins	
	Pain threshold min	
	Blood pressure min	Parasympathetic
	Heart attacks min	Parasympathetic
	Cortisol min	Parasympathetic
	Histamine release max	
	Dermatitis max	
	Growing pains max	
10:00 PM	Multiple sclerosis pain/fatigue min	
	Hot flashes rate max	
11:00 PM	Sexual intercourse most frequent	
	Snacking adds most weight	
	Immune response max	Parasympathetic
	Allergic reactivity max	Parasympathetic
	Heart attack risk min	Parasympathetic
	Skin irritability/itching max	
	Restless leg syndrome max	

assigned appropriately to parasympathetic action on the basis of other markers. Interestingly, the normal sleep cycle is thought to involve two intense periods, separated by a less intense period at about midnight [72]. This accords nicely with the generalization that the evening-time period of 6:00 PM to 6:00 AM is home to two parasympathetic periods separated by a more balanced time at about midnight [72]; a similar separation is apparent in the daytime period of 6:00 PM to 6:00 AM.

The Autonomic Cycles

When the times of various maximal and minimal body functions are considered, certain trends become clear regarding the natural times for parasympathetic versus sympathetic stimulation. Looking globally at the twenty-four-hour clock, one sees that the sympathetic stimuli are strongest between 6:00 AM and 9:00 AM, are moderate from 10:00 AM to 2:00 PM, and then appear strongly again between 3:00 and 5:00 PM. This appears to be a baseline fight-or-flight sympathetic response in the body, independent of any specific threat or stress but active during daylight hours and least active around noon. Although Cole [145] argues that mid-afternoon is a poor time for *yogasana* practice, as students tend to fall asleep in *savasana* and otherwise seem to have no energy, this conflicts with the peaks of physical strength, alertness, and mental performance otherwise expected for the period from 3:00 to 5:00 PM (table 23.B-3). The seeming conflict as to the amount of energy and awareness available to students in this period may be age-related, as this time period is more and more transformed from a time of strength and awareness into a time for rest as one ages.

In contrast to the times of sympathetic dominance, the parasympathetic responses cluster in the hours between 8:00 and 10:00 PM and between 2:00 and 4:00 AM, becoming moderate between 10:00 PM and 2:00 AM. It appears that there are four periods of extreme autonomic stimulation, two sympathetic and two parasympathetic, each about three hours long, separated from one another by four periods of relative moderation, each about three hours long, in which it might be supposed that the autonomic system is more in balance. These daily shifts of autonomic dominance are natural body rhythms, driven subconsciously and entrained with the rising and setting of the sun. Because successive maxima markers are separated by twenty-four hours, as are successive minima markers, these markers occur at the same time every day and so are in step with the rising and setting of the sun. It is no accident that the pacemakers for most circadian rhythms are located within the hypothalamus and that the autonomic processes so controlled are largely hypothalamic in nature.

This separation of the times of maximum and minimum effects by other than twelve hours can be an important consideration for the elderly, as they would be more at risk for adverse reactions to medication given at the wrong time (see Section 23.C, page 789). Appropriate timing of medications is especially keen here, as physiological processes are altered by age and chronic illness. One should apply the same reasoning to the importance of timing when doing yoga therapy with older students [595]. As children up to the age of sixteen years are more and more being treated with psychiatric drugs for conditions such as ADHD, OCD, depression, eating disorders, schizophrenia, autism, and bipolar disorder, the medical community is now considering what the best timing is for medication of such conditions; should yoga therapy follow this path, the questions of timing will arise anew.

The clear but simple pattern evident in tables 23.B-1 through 23.B-4 of alternating parasympathetic and sympathetic excitations through the twenty-four-hour clock suggests a possible (but unproved) use for a display of this sort. Thus, for example, it is clear from table 23.B-1 that the parasympathetic nervous system is dominant in the time period 1:00 AM to 3:00 AM, but that not all such processes having maximum or minimum values in this time period have been so identified as being controlled by the parasympathetic nervous system. Nonetheless, it seems a good guess that because the skin repair process and also glycogen production are maximal, and because alertness is minimal in the 1:00 AM to 3:00 AM time period (table 23.B-1), that all three of these processes are being driven by parasympathetic excitation. It remains to be seen whether such interpolations of the times of maximum and minimum effects can be used to infer autonomic dominance.

Morning People versus Evening People

It is generally accepted that there are two kinds of people in the world: those who divide people into two groups and those who do not. The differences between morning people and evening people are no less significant. As shown in table 23.B-5, the characteristics of these two

Table 23.B-5: Extreme Characteristics of the Morning Person and the Evening Person

Characteristic	Morning Person	Evening Person
Age	Over sixty years	Eight to thirty years
Most alert	Noon	6:00 PM
Most active	2:30 PM	5:30 PM
Temperature highest	3:30 PM	8:00 PM
Temperature lowest	3:30 AM	6:00 AM
Mid-sleep time	3:30 AM	6:00 AM
Favorite exercise time	Morning	Evening
Peak heart rate	11:00 AM	6:00 PM
Lowest heart rate	3:00 AM	7:00 AM
Mood shift during day	Declines	Rises
Morning behavior	Chatty	Bearish
Evening behavior	Exhausted	Energized
Favorite meal	Breakfast	Supper
Daily coffee consumption	Cups	Pots
Peak melatonin secretion	3:30 AM	5:30 AM

lifestyles are significant and could play a major role in one's *yogasana* practice if one ignores the tendency. In a normal population, about 10 percent of the people are the extreme morning type, 20 percent are the extreme evening type, and the rest fall in between these two groups. At the extremes, the differences have a genetic component.

The differences in the times of extreme values of the biological processes among individuals displayed in this table (peak heart rate at 11:00 AM versus 6:00 PM and peak temperature at 3:30 PM versus 6:00 AM!), along with any possible gender differences, likely account for the variation in the peak times listed by various investigators in tables 23.B-1, 23.B-2, 23.B-3, and 23.B-4.

From the perspective of the *yogasana* practitioner, one sees from table 23.B-5 that the 20 percent of the average population composed of evening people have physiological and psychological characters that are wildly out of synchronicity with those expected for an early-morning *yogasana* practice. Similarly, that 10 percent of the population composed of morning people will not take well to an evening *yogasana* practice, again for un-

derstandable reasons, both physiological and psychological. People at either end of the extremes of the best-time tendencies as given in table 23.B-5 will not fit the data for more normal lifestyles. It would be very interesting to see if people who are forced to work at times that are out of synchronicity with their natural inclinations in regard to being at their best, either in early morning or later in the evening, eventually suffer adverse mental and/or physical health effects from this artificial and untimely stimulation (See this subsection, page 788, for more on this topic).

Though it is quite reasonable that to exercise in the evening hours might be a poor idea because it may overstimulate the body at a time when it prefers to become quiet as it prepares for sleep, many studies show that light exercise can help one to relax so as to sleep better! An intense backbending practice before retiring would be inconsistent with a sound sleep, but a light stretching practice would be appropriate and even recommended if one otherwise finds it difficult to get to sleep.

Table 23.B-6: Comparison of the Autonomic and Ayurvedic Time Intervals Dividing the Twenty-Four-Hour Day [473]

Time	Autonomic Dominance	Active Dosha	Ayurvedic Characteristics
6:00 AM to 9:00 AM	Sympathetic	*Kapha*	Energetic, fresh, heavy
9:00 AM to 3:00 PM	Balanced	*Pitta*	Eating/digestion, light, hot
3:00 PM to 6:00 PM	Sympathetic	*Vata*	Active, light, supple
6:00 PM to 9:00 PM	Parasympathetic	*Kapha*	Cool, inert, low energy
9:00 PM to 3:00 AM	Parasympathetic	*Pitta*	Digestion
3:00 AM to 6:00 AM	Balanced	*Vata*	Slow, dense, cool

Ayurvedic Rhythms

In Ayurvedic medicine [473], the hours of the day are divided into five periods, with rather close correspondences with the sympathetic and parasympathetic dominances uncovered in tables 23.B-1 through 23.B-4. According to the Ayurvedic point of view, each of the three *doshas* (the active principles determining the biology, psychology, and pathology of the human body, mind, and consciousness [473]) is active in the time periods shown in table 23.B-6. One sees that with a little manipulation, the boundaries of the Ayurvedic and autonomic time periods are amazingly close to one another over the twenty-four-hour period; however, the correlation of autonomic dominance with the phases of the three *doshas* is not as obvious. For example, the period from 6:00 to 10:00 AM is dominated by the sympathetic system and is *kapha* according to the *doshas,* yet in the 8:00 to 10:00 PM time slot, the dominant *dosha* is once again *kapha,* but the autonomic dominance has become parasympathetic. In spite of small problems such as this, the characteristics associated with the four quadrants of the day (table 23.B-6) as assigned by Ayurveda are in general agreement with the circadian trends of sympathetic excitation during the day (energetic, light, hot) and parasympathetic at night (cool, inert, slow, dense).

According to Ayurveda, one should eat the first daily meal at 10:00 AM, with maximum digestion then occurring at noon (table 23.B-2). With an average transit time of eighteen hours

for food to pass through the digestive system, excretion would then occur the following morning at 4:00 AM, this being an appropriate time, since excretion would be driven by the parasympathetic action dominating at that time (Section 20.F, page 732), and would leave one feeling light and unencumbered for *yogasana* practice shortly thereafter.

Yogic Rhythms

The yogic recommendation to commence *pranayama* at 4:00 AM and *yogasana* practice from 6:00 to 8:00 AM is timed perfectly so that the former is done while in a state of parasympathetic relaxation (provided the lights have not been turned on) and the latter takes advantage of the sympathetic energy flowing through the body at the later time. According to table 23.B-3, the next best time for *yogasana* practice seemingly would be late afternoon (3:00 to 5:00 PM), when the sympathetic nervous system again asserts itself, but not necessarily so for the older students. Perhaps this data in respect to *yogasana* practice can be interpreted as showing that a strenuous practice is best done in the early morning hours (7:00 AM to 9:00 AM), and that the early evening hours (7:00 PM to 9 PM) should be reserved for a parasympathetically driven restorative practice.

Giving each phase of the nasal dominance (Subsection 15.E, page 630) a time period of four hours does fill the twenty-four-hour span nicely, but it seems not to have any consistent effect on the twenty-four-hour cycles of the other body functions. So, for example, the right nostril is open for breathing between 5:00 and 7:00 AM, which is consistent with a sympathetic arousal of the body during those hours; however, the same nostril also is active between 9:00 and 11:00 PM, a time when the observed dominance is parasympathetic. That little or no consistent effect is seen for the ultradian nasal cycle on the other circadian cycles is perhaps disappointing, but it is no surprise, since the circadian rhythms represent major physiological surges, whereas the effects of nasal laterality are far more subtle.

It is very interesting that the advice of modern medicine to be especially stress-free in the early morning coincides with the yogi's traditional time for doing *pranayama*. However, since doctors [318] recommend that one do everything one can to reduce stress at this early morning time, as stress can precipitate a heart attack, the more strenuous *yogasana* practice perhaps should be left for the hours between 3:00 and 5:00 PM, when alertness, lung function, blood pressure, muscle strength, and mental performance are all at their maxima. If *yogasana* students' bodies are on the same schedules as those of the myriad subjects whose data led to the average times given in tables 23.B-1 through 23.B-4, then those who practice *yogasana* at about 9:00 AM otherwise seem to be doing their most challenging work about six hours ahead of their peaks in physical and mental abilities. It would appear that the sympathetic dominance is stronger in the first half of the day (around 9:00 AM) than in the second (around 4:00 PM).

On the other hand, for a given level of stress, the largest stress-stimulated release of cortisol occurs at times of lowest ambient cortisol level (10:00 PM; see table 6.A-1) and is least when the level of ambient cortisol is highest (4:00 AM). Accordingly, the amount of cortisol generated by *yogasana* practice will be least for a morning practice and largest for an evening practice. As noted above, morning and evening persons can differ greatly as to the best times for *yogasana* practice (table 23.B-5).

Mechanism of the Circadian Clock and the Suprachiasmatic Nucleus

Some of the most obvious and important aspects of time in our physiological lives involve variations in bodily functions that occur once a day; i.e., those that are tied in some way to the rising and setting of the sun but do not necessarily wax or wane at the times of rising and setting. Furthermore, though such circadian rhythms have twenty-four-hour periods, they continue in their approximately twenty-four-hour rhythm even when kept in total darkness for a week or more, showing that the circadian rhythm is innate rather than simply a momentary response to light and dark.

Circadian Control

In humans, the seat of circadian control rests within the hypothalamus, in a small cluster of cells known as the suprachiasmatic nucleus (SCN; see figure 5.B-1). As one might guess from its name, the suprachiasmatic nucleus is located just above the optic chiasm. The cells within this nucleus have their own circadian rhythm, set in the womb before birth and fully operational at the seventh month of gestation [716]. In the normal, uncontrolled situation, at sunrise, light penetrates the eyelids of the sleeping person, and at the molecular level, stimulates a visual pigment in the ganglion cells of the retina that is different from the ones in the rods and cones responsible for normal vision [867] (see Subsection 17.C, page 675). The response time of this ganglionic system is much longer than that of the rods and cones, and it is triggered only by the relatively slow change of ambient light level as the sun rises and sets.

The "wake up" signal travels from the retina to the SCN over dedicated neural channels within the optic-nerve bundle but does not rise to the cortex. On arrival at the SCN, the signal initiates the splitting of protein complexes within the cells of the nucleus, whereas when the sun sets, the protein complexes are reconstituted during the dark period and are ready then to split at the next burst of light [923]. The smooth changes of the concentrations of the associated and dissociated proteins within the SCN over the course of the day are coupled to hundreds of other aspects of our physiology and behavior, activating and deactivating them once every twenty-four hours [584]. It is this nucleus within the hypothalamus that is the pacemaker for the endocrine system, turning it on and off in synchronicity with the light-dark pattern of ambient light perceived by the eyes. Because HIV attacks the SCN, patients with this virus have a disrupted circadian pattern, especially as regards sleep. Though the SCN is the central pacemaker, circadian-oscillator centers also are found in the peripheral tissues.

Sensitivity to light in regard to setting the circadian rhythm is highest when the body temperature is lowest (4:00 to 5:00 AM); the further one is from one's temperature low point, the less impact light has on setting or resetting the circadian clock. If you must get up at night, use a dim night light so as not to stimulate the SCN. Circadian vision is distinct from normal vision but is different from blindsight (Subsection 17.B, page 669), as shown by the fact that some totally blind people still function on a twenty-four-hour-per-day circadian rhythm [804].

Melatonin

As an example of the visual control of a circadian rhythm, consider that in the dark, the pineal gland releases melatonin, a hormone that promotes sleep. However, at the first light of dawn, the SCN is activated, and as it then indirectly signals the pineal to halt melatonin production, we then become fully awake [162, 878]. Melatonin levels normally start to rise about two hours before bedtime and peak between 2:00 AM and 4:00 AM, before falling again. Because caffeine interferes with the production of melatonin, drinking a cup of caffeinated coffee reduces the melatonin in circulation to only half that normally observed at peak [128] and so can keep us awake at night. Melatonin is intimately involved in the body's physiological response to shifting light levels, as discussed in Subsection 17.C, page 676. However, some people are more sensitive to melatonin than others.

Similarly, the oscillating protein concentrations in the SCN drive changes in the concentrations of vasopressin in the brain, with cyclical consequences in regard to rest and activity [102]. In the brain, vasopressin stimulates learning and memory; its concentration in the cerebrospinal fluid varies over a twenty-four-hour cycle and probably accounts for the circadian oscillation of our ability to learn and memorize throughout the day [721]. In humans, loss of the SCN (a center rich in vasopressin) results in loss of the rhythms of corticosteroid release, feeding, drinking, and locomotor activity [427].

It is clear from the above discussion that melatonin in the blood is highest in the evening and promotes sleep at that time. However, several studies have been carried out on the states of health of those doing consistent day work, consistent night work, and alternating day and night work. It has been found that if the work pattern is consistent and in synchrony with the light-dark pattern, there appears to be no differences in the states of health. However, for those in whom the work/sleep pattern is irregular, the twenty-four-hour circadian rhythm of hormonal release is upset. In women on such alternating work schedules, the rates of breast and colorectal cancers are significantly above those experienced by women who work either consistent day or night jobs, between which there are no differences. Among men, those working on a rotating schedule are three times more likely to develop prostate cancer than among those who consistently work either day or night schedules [312b].

Free-Running Cycles

The chemistry of the visually triggered on-off process that controls circadian phenomena is an ancient one and is innate within us, so that it actually functions with the same characteristic periodicity (twenty-four hours) even when there is no light to drive it [923]! Experiments with human subjects show that when the subjects are shielded from temperature changes and all visual cues as to light and dark, the circadian rhythms continue in some functions (sleep, for example) with periods more like twenty-five to thirty-three hours, and in other functions (rectal temperature in the same subjects, for example), with periods constant at 24.8 hours over many cycles [427]. In the case of sleep in constant darkness, the daily cycle in real time often tends to fall behind by about one hour per day, so that what was a ritual at 7:00 AM on every previous sunlit day will have shifted to 11:00 AM on going from Monday to Friday with a twenty-five-hour period in the dark. Ignoring the twenty-four-hour clock on the weekends and then trying to return to it on Monday is the cause of the "Monday morning blues" during the work week.

At the present point in our evolution, the function of the external light and dark periods is to daily reset the time of the internal clock, but not to change its twenty-four-hour character. That is to say, the times at which the core temperature of the body will be maximal and minimal will depend upon our sleep habits, time zones, jet lag, etc., for example, but still will rise and fall in a periodic way every twenty-four hours in all of us. Through all this, the inherent frequencies of the circadian rhythms are independent of age [923]; however, the differences between sympathetic and parasympathetic dominance fade with age.

Many genes operate on a twenty-four-hour cycle, but not all have the same circadian markers. Thus, it is seen that though the SCN within the brain is important in controlling the timing of many body processes in twenty-four-hour cycles, many other bodily processes on twenty-four-hour cycles are controlled independently by oscillators within the cells themselves (see below). Moreover, the SCN is also the timer controlling the twenty-eight-day menstrual cycle in women.

Unicellular Clocks

As bacteria and other single-celled organisms also show twenty-four-hour cycles in their physiologies but obviously do not have SCNs, one can only conclude that there also must be internal clocks working within a single cell. In fact, circadian rhythms are observed in isolated human cells when cultured. Furthermore, every cell within the human body has within it a circadian clock that directs hormone release, gene activity, and energy production, all with a repeatability of just a few minutes a day!

Section 23.C: *Yogasana* and Chronotherapy

Best Time for Medication

It recently has been realized by doctors that **when** a medicine is taken often can be as important as **what** is in the medicine, because taking a medicine at the "wrong" time of the day can decrease its efficiency while increasing unwanted side effects. To the extent that *yogasana* also is medicine, can it be that the **when** factor also can be important in addition to the **how** and **what** of our *yogasana* practice? The element of **when** enters both yoga and medicine because the body actually is not homeostatic in the short term (Subsection 5.A, page 158); in fact, the productions of most of the physiologically important compounds in the body, such as hormones, enzymes, and neurotransmitters, rise and fall rhythmically over the course of the day. As these compounds are tightly coupled to physiological processes, their variations in time lead to process variations as well; i.e., body rhythms.

The concept in Western medicine called "chronotherapy," in which the times at which drugs are administered are dictated by the peaks and valleys of the relevant circadian rhythms, is new and promising [108, 318, 381, 465, 664, 804]. Considerable evidence has been presented showing that the efficacy of certain drugs can be heightened considerably if their administration is synchronized with the normal circadian swings of body chemistry. For example, it is known that antihistamines, anesthetics, analgesics, aspirin, and steroids work best when given at the appropriate times [149].

Consider, for example, the fact that the heart rate, blood pressure, and blood viscosity rise abruptly at 6:00 AM in most people, as the autonomic nervous system goes strongly sympathetic

Table 23.C-1: The Two-Hour Time Periods for Maximum Activity of the Twelve Organs of Traditional Chinese Medicine When Stimulated by Acupuncture [735]

Time Period	Chinese Character of Time Period	Organ (Condition)
3:00–5:00 AM	Yin	Lungs (immune system, viral attack of respiratory system, asthma, hay fever)
5:00–7:00 AM	Mao	Colon (digestion)
7:00–9:00 AM	Chen	Stomach (heartburn, hyperacidity)
9:00–11:00 AM	Si	Spleen
11:00 AM–1:00 PM	Wu	Heart (angina, cardiac ischemia)
1:00–3:00 PM	Wei	Small intestine
3:00–5:00 PM	Shen	Bladder (urinary flow)
5:00–7:00 PM	You	Kidneys (innate energy level)
7:00–9:00 PM	Xu	Pericardium
9:00–11:00 PM	Hai	Triple warmer
11:00 PM–1:00 AM	Zi	Gallbladder
1:00 AM–3:00 AM	Chou	Liver (flow of substances through body)

at that time (table 23.B-1). In response to this early-morning stress on the cardiovascular system, the incidence of heart attacks and angina discomfort strongly peaks around this hour. Using chronotherapy in Western medicine, drugs are administered to hypertensive patients at a time when the drugs will be most effective in relieving the sympathetic symptoms at the time of greatest cardiovascular risk; i.e., at 6:00 AM. A similar chronotherapeutic approach is now used to treat asthma, a condition with symptoms appearing strongly at about 4:00 AM, for which steroids are best inhaled between 3:00 and 5:30 PM [664]. Circadian variations have been found in arthritis (Section 8.C, page 310), asthma, allergies, peptic ulcer disease, dislipidemia, and cancer, among others [225].

Note too that there are rhythms in the body having periods far longer than twenty-four hours, and these too must be considered when being treated with medication. Thus, the timing is an important but neglected aspect of treating children's psychiatric orders with drugs designed by scientists for use in adults [596].

Multiple Sclerosis

The fatigue associated with multiple sclerosis often is worst in the early morning hours, and so stimulant medications are taken at this time period; the discomfort is especially intense when the temperature rises in the early evening. For those treating their multiple-sclerosis fatigue with *yogasana* practice, it follows that a vigorous early-morning practice between 8:00 and 10:00 AM and/or a more restorative practice between 6:00 and 8:00 PM would be best in regard to keeping the body temperature low. A significant number of women with multiple sclerosis also report symptoms that vary with their monthly rise and fall of estrogen (figure 21.A-1b) and with the onset of menopause [804]. In these cases, a *yogasana* practice with a considerable parasympathetic component at these times could be effective.

Acupuncture

In traditional Chinese medicine, acupuncture is given at specific times of the day, depending upon the illness. The best times for acupuncture for diseases involving the lungs, large intestine, stomach, heart, kidneys, and liver have been listed as per Samuels [735] in table 23.C-1. Though these times for chronotherapy were first enunciated over 2,000 years ago, they agree in large part with those used for modern Western chronotherapy.

In another application of the chronotherapy idea, it has been found that the toxicities of certain chemotherapeutic agents for healthy and cancerous cells vary with the time of day they are taken. Because normal cell processes run on a twenty-four-hour cycle [716], whereas cancer cells run on a twenty-hour cycle, the two cell types can have peak sensitivities to administered toxins at different times of the day; by injecting these drugs at the appropriate times, one can maximize the killing of cancer cells while minimizing the side effects on healthy cells; in effect, chronotherapy has raised the anti-tumor activity of the drug, while its toxicity to normal cells has been lowered. 5-fluorouracil, a potent chemotherapeutic agent in battling colon, breast, and rectal cancers, is best tolerated during the period of mid-sleep, and so is administered at 10:00 PM.

Quite independently of Western medicine and Chinese acupuncture, yogic science has developed specific *yogasana* programs in response to students' health problems. At present, such yoga therapy often is delivered without regard to where students may be at any particular moment in their circadian cycles. Following the lead of Western medical science, one logically can ask, "Given a particular health condition and a prescribed *yogasana* routine as therapy, at what time of the day or night will the *yogasana* practice be most effective physiologically in regard to the condition?" To my knowledge, there is no work in the yoga community as yet on which to base an answer to the above question; however, one can make a guess.

Best Times for *Yogasana*

If the risk of cardiovascular problems is greatest at 6:00 AM and is least at 6:00 PM, then it is most logical that the relaxing *yogasana* routine for such problems should be done just before 6:00 AM or as close to it as possible, and that doing the same routine at 6:00 PM, when cardiovascular risk is low, would be of much less benefit. This timing runs counter to the usual recommendation of doing vigorous *yogasana* practice during the early morning hours and more restful work in the evening (see, for example [800]); however, from the chronotherapy point of view, such a schedule would be best for students who have no medical problems and would be least effective for students with cardiovascular complications.[4] The suggestion that one perform the appropriate therapeutic *yogasana* work at the times of highest risk or discomfort assumes that the beneficial effects of the practice are immediate and not complicated by a chain of cause and effect that would otherwise delay the benefit.

A quick scan of the information on circadian markers in tables 23.B-1 through 23.B-4, and the simple assumption that *yogasana* benefits are immediate, suggest the following times as being the most appropriate for specific *yogasana*-therapy practice:

- » Depression: 5:00 PM
- » Multiple sclerosis: 6:00 AM
- » Anxiety: 6:00 AM
- » Asthma or bronchial constriction: 6:00 AM (or 3:00 to 5:00 PM, if one assumes that the *yogasana* treatment has the same time lag as the steroidal treatment; see page 776)
- » Cardiovascular problems or hypertension: 6:00 AM
- » Rheumatoid arthritis: 6:00 AM

---

4 When the blood pressure surges in the early morning, atherosclerotic plaques which may be in the arteries are encouraged to rupture and the blood also has a hyper-coagulatability, which encourages the formation of thrombi [785a], which can lead to stroke.

» Osteoarthritis: 6:00 PM
» Hot flashes: late evening

The "optimum times" quoted above are average times as appropriate to the average person; one must be careful in this that not everyone will fit into the "average" mold, and so one would profit from having a specific determination of just exactly when the circadian markers occur during the day. That is to say, the therapy should follow "body time" rather than "clock time," and one must be aware that students with central nervous system disturbances or schizophrenia may have altered circadian rhythms (as in table 23.B-5) or even none at all. The sicker someone is, the more likely it is that their markers for circadian rhythm are irregular. If a *yogasana* therapy routine does not seem to be effective when practiced at one time, then consider changing the time of practice.

B. K. S. Iyengar [398] considers disorders of virtually all of the organs listed in table 23.C-1, page 790, and presents detailed suggestions for *yogasana* therapy. It would be most interesting to see if there is a heightened efficacy when the Iyengar *yogasana* programs are combined with the traditional times for acupuncture for the same disorders, and how these times compare with the times thought best according to the precepts of Western chronotherapy. Because the optimal times discussed above for medical chronotherapy include a time interval for the proper chemical activation of the medicine, which would not apply necessarily to the *yogasana* therapy course of treatment, the optimal times for these two modes of treatment might be noticeably different.

The best approach to the question of when is the best time for *yogasana* chronotherapy practice allows for individual variations in order to accommodate the fact that different students will have different but important circadian factors at work, possibly at different times (table 23.B-5, for example). Nonetheless, considering that muscle strength, peak mental performance, and peak lung function are found in the 3:00 to 4:00 PM time slot (table 23.B-3), this would seem to be a good time for a vigorous *yogasana* practice for those younger students who are not "morning persons" and otherwise have no health problems.

Regarding the best time for *yogasana* practice, the question is complicated further by consideration of other new information. For example, if the sleeping hours are unrestricted, it is known that the midpoint of the sleeping period for twenty-year olds will be 5:00 AM, but for sixty-year olds, it will be 3:00 AM. Thus, getting up for 6:00 AM *yogasana* practice will be quite different for these two cases [133], unless there is a restriction on when students go to sleep.

As shown in figure 23.C-1, there is a regular change of sleep pattern as one ages, the extremes being referred to as "larks" (the early risers) and "owls" (the late risers). The points shown in the figure represent the midpoints of the normal sleep cycle as a function of age, and one sees that between ages ten and twenty years, there is a rapid shift from morning-person larks to evening-person owls; then there is a slower reversal of this trend from ages twenty to ninety. Data at the later years appears more random, presumably as the circadian clocks become more erratic with increasing age. It is to be emphasized that tampering with this natural sleep cycle can have ill effects, such as mental and physical disorders, cancer, obesity, and depression, and, least of all, the equivalent of severe jet lag [871a].

Making a teenager go to bed early so as to awake early and refreshed does not work, for their internal circadian clocks will not let them fall asleep at an early hour. When a teenager can only fall asleep after midnight and then must rise to get to school by 7:00 AM, the physiological consequences are significant. As applied to *yogasana* practice, it is clear that students in the age range of twenty to thirty years are largely owls and would not respond willingly to an early-morning practice. Similarly, those over fifty years old are very much larks and so would be more accepting of such an early-morning practice.

Flex Time

A circadian rhythm of sorts also is observed in the flexibility of the body, for many experi-

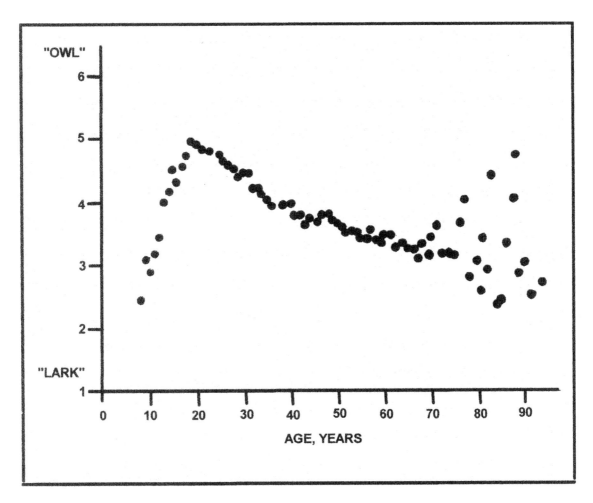

Figure 23.C-1. A plot of the chronotype varying from early-riser larks to late-riser owls, as shown by the hour of the midpoint of their sleep time versus the age of the sleepers. Adapted from [871a].

ments show that the range of motion for shoulder rotation and in *yogasanas* such as *uttanasana, paschimottanasana,* and *trikonasana,* in which the hamstrings are stretched, are least in the early morning and are largest at 10:00 to 11:00 AM and again at 4:00 to 5:00 PM [7]. It would be most interesting to know if this were true for *yogasana* students, who are otherwise advised to practice in the early hours of the morning. Because of early-morning stiffness, there is a greater risk of injury when stretching in the morning (unless one warms up properly; see Subsection 11.E, page 467), and the range of motion will be larger later in the day.[5]

Aged or not, if a posture is more difficult when performed on one side of the body than on the other, the tendency is to spend less time on the more difficult side. Using a timer to balance the time spent on both sides would be wise. Moreover, one actually should spend even longer on the more difficult side, in order to move it toward the level of the easy side (Appendix III, page 845). In fact, in spite of the apparent left-right symmetry in the body, Iyengar prescribes just such a practice to minimize the asymmetry [402].

---

5   The question of timing also appears when one takes protein supplements while trying to increase muscle mass, for those taking the supplements imme-

diately before and after weight training gained twice as much muscle mass as did those who took the same supplements several hours before or after training. It is generally held that amino acids are best metabolized just after exercise.

Table 23.C-2: Medical Conditions Possibly Related to Race through Genetic, Epigenetic, or Social Factors [453]

Condition	Rationale	Race Most Affected
Type 2 diabetes	Mixed genetic and environmental factors	People on Indian subcontinent
Asthma	Major genetic factor	Puerto Rican children
Multiple sclerosis	Genetics most likely; environment least likely	European Americans/rare in Africa
Alcohol	Mutation in gene for aldehyde dehydrogenase	Asians
Cystic fibrosis	Unclear	Caucasians
Schizophrenia	Controversial; possible misdiagnosis	African-Americans
Sickle-cell anemia	Genetics	Africans, people from Caribbean, Asia, Eastern Mediterranean, Middle East
Heart failure	Different causes in white and black Americans	African-Americans
Prostate cancer	Genetics and poor healthcare	African-Americans
Various tumors	Mutation in BRCA genes	Ashkenazi Jews
Hypertension	Unhealthy lifestyles and poor healthcare	African-Americans

Possible Racial and Gender Factors

As discussed above, the daily time factor is a feature of yoga therapy that should be kept in mind by the therapist. Most recently, the idea has appeared in the medical literature that there possibly should be race-specific medical procedures that recognize certain possible race-specific illnesses and conditions. The field is known as pharmacogenomics.

The pharmacogenomic issue is clouded by the confounding of social and political questions with those of genetic diversity. A list of racial differences in regard to various medical conditions are presented in table 23.C-2, with the hope that it may be of value to some yoga teachers and therapists in the future.

It is only a short jump from consideration of pharmacogenomics to questions of the same sort in regard to any differences in treating men and women. Indeed, the more we know about the human body, the more significant differences there appear to be between the anatomies, physiologies, and psychologies of men and women. For example, just look at the gender differences of heart-attack symptoms in men and women (Subsection 14.A, page 556), and you will have good reason to question whether *yogasana* therapy for early-morning heart attack in men will follow the same course for women.

Section 23.D: The Sleep/Wake Cycle and Relaxation

In the average human life, we spend about 30 percent of our time in sleep, yet sleep is so important that a person will die sooner of lack of sleep than of lack of food. During sleep, though the

Table 23.D-1: The Shift of Brain Physiology in Various Sleep Stages Relative to Waking [831]

Physiology Shift	REM Stage 1	NonREM Stage 2	Stages 3 and 4
Synchronous brain wave frequency, hertz	4–6	12–14	0.5–4
Eye movement	↑↑	↓↓	↓↓
Muscle tone	↓↓	↓	↓
External inputs	↓↓	↓	↓
Hippocampus ↔ cortex dialog	cortex → hippocampus	?	hippocampus → cortex
Acetylcholine modulation	↑↑	↓	↓
Norepinephrine modulation	↓↓	↓	↓
Prefrontal cortex activation	↓↓	?	↓
Limbic activation	↑	?	↓
Sensory cortices	↑	?	↓

consciousness appears to have disappeared, the brain is no less active than when awake. Moreover, the more you do not sleep now, the longer and more intensely you will sleep later.

There are two broad subcategories of sleep types, one being rapid-eye-movement (REM) sleep and the other being slow-wave sleep or non-REM sleep. The latter encompasses several subcategories [500, 831]. Because the area of sleep research is very much in flux, not all of those working in the sleep field would agree with the ideas presented here.

Function of Sleep

Though very little is understood about the sleep state, it appears that there are two broad functions of sleep. The first is restoration and recovery of brain energy, sleep being to the brain what rest is to the working muscle. Non-REM sleep appears to be involved in the repair of free-radical damage in the brain, for during this sleep period, genes are switched on that synthesize brain proteins and repair neural-cell membranes. The second function is information processing involving memory.

Little is known about why we need sleep, other than to say that apparently there are centers or neural networks in the brain that require a periodic rest from consciousness. It is known, however, that the transitions from wakefulness to

sleep and from sleep to wakefulness are driven by centers in the brainstem, and that certain aspects of sleep actually show considerable mental activity. EEG studies (Subsection 4.H, page 149) confirm that in certain of the sleep stages, there are close similarities of the brain states with those achieved in both relaxation and meditation [860].

Sleep is induced by the raphe nuclei in the region of the lower pons and the medulla oblongata; this circuitry uses serotonin as the neurotransmitter and sends inhibitory signals to the spinal cord to inhibit pain signals from moving upward into consciousness. There is a possibility that the parasympathetic nervous system has a role in releasing into sleep, for excitations of the parasympathetic cranial nerves IX and X (involved with sucking/nursing and digestion after a large meal, respectively) promote sleep, possibly by triggering the raphe nuclei.

The apparent loss of consciousness on falling asleep is not due to the slowing down of the various nuclei in the brain, but instead is due to the loss of connection between the various nuclei.

Sleep Stages

Once asleep, brain activity does not necessarily become quiet but instead shifts in a cyclic way into other modes. There are five such modes or

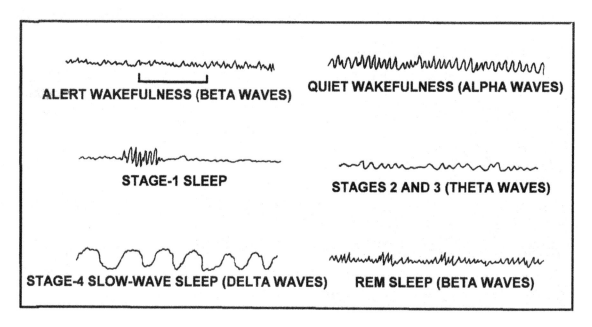

Figure 23.D-1. The basic brainwave patterns that distinguish the various stages of sleep; the horizontal bar in the beta-wave graph represents one second and applies to all of the waves.

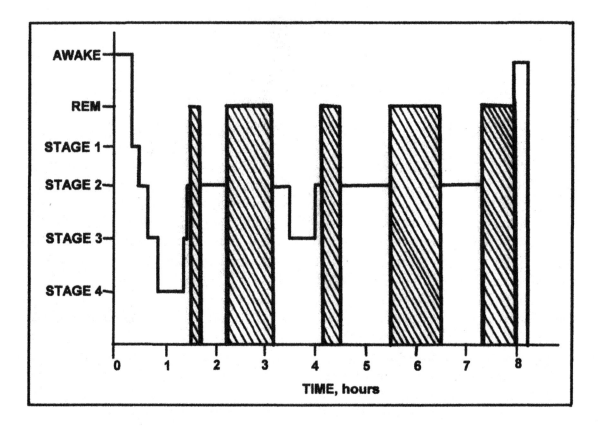

Figure 23.D-2. Shifts of the sleep stages through eight hours of sleep.

stages in the sleep/wake cycle that are recognized, each with its own characteristic EEG brain-wave pattern (Subsection 4.H, page 149), as shown in figure 23.D-1. On entering sleep, one moves from the awake stage, with its attendant beta-wave EEG, and proceeds through sleep stages 1, 2, 3, and 4 (figure 23.D-2). Traversing these sleep stages once in sequential order and then returning in reverse order to stage 1 requires about ninety minutes, and the cycle repeats five or six times during the night. Many hormonal cycles also have the ninety-minute period (Subsection 23.B, page 773). The characteristics of various sleep stages are summarized in table 23.D-1.

Getting to Sleep

When one is having difficulty releasing into sleep, the standard prescription is to "count sheep"; i.e., to imagine a large pen of sheep and count them as they jump over the fence one by one. This can be rationalized in the following way. Mentally imaging the pen full of sheep occupies the right cerebral hemisphere and prevents it from otherwise entertaining any other thoughts of anxiety that might come up. On the other hand, the left cerebral hemisphere is involved in the counting process and so is not allowed to focus on any problematic auditory or verbal thoughts. The counting of sheep thus occupies both cerebral hemispheres and crowds out any other disturbing thoughts that might otherwise keep one awake.

Slow-Wave Sleep

Many sleep scientists hold that stage 3 and stage 4 "slow-wave" sleep is of the greatest importance, and because it appears only in the early part of a normal sleep, one can do well with just three to four hours of sleep at a time. The more sleep-deprived you are, the more quickly you will drop into slow-wave sleep. On the other hand, if you are awakened while in the slow-wave phase, as when asleep for about an hour, you will awaken groggy and require about a half-hour to achieve full consciousness and awareness (this is called "sleep inertia"); whereas if you awake in stages 1

or 2 after a twenty-minute nap, you will become alert more quickly. When a situation will not allow an uninterrupted sleep of six to eight hours, it is better to take several short naps of ten to fifteen minutes' duration as opposed to a one-hour nap. Due to hormone and temperature changes, it is easy to take a catnap at 2:00 PM, whereas at 6:00 AM or 8:00 PM, this will be more difficult, as one is in a more sympathetic autonomic mode at these times. When deprived of their sleep, women tend to slow down in their work but maintain their accuracy, whereas men maintain their speed but work with less accuracy [96].

For early risers, their free-running circadian rhythm period is somewhat shorter than twenty-four hours, and the time of maximum sleepiness comes at about midnight. With evening types, the free-running circadian rhythm is somewhat longer than twenty-four hours, and the time of maximum sleepiness is close to the time of awakening. Those who sleep only a short time do so by decreasing the amount of stage 2 sleep while maintaining the standard amounts of stage 4 and REM-phase sleep.

Coleman [149] presents an interesting chart of circadian variations of physiological functions as they change through the sleep/wake cycle over two days (figure 23.D-3). It is no surprise that alertness drops as we sleep and that we are most alert and awake when our temperature is the highest. Growth hormone, however, behaves oppositely, being almost zero during wakefulness and maximizing during sleep stage 3. Cortisol in the blood peaks in the early morning (table 23.B-1).

It is known that certain chemicals produced in the brain during the waking hours act to induce sleep at night. Interestingly, many of these substances are active immunological agents in the human body. Furthermore, there would appear to be more going on than just repeatedly running through the sleep stages. Thus, there is substantial evidence that the most natural sleep cycle is broken into two equally long sleep phases separated by about one hour of wakefulness [72], the whole requiring nine to eleven hours total. As discussed above, this expectation is born out by the pattern of circadian markers (table 23.B-5).

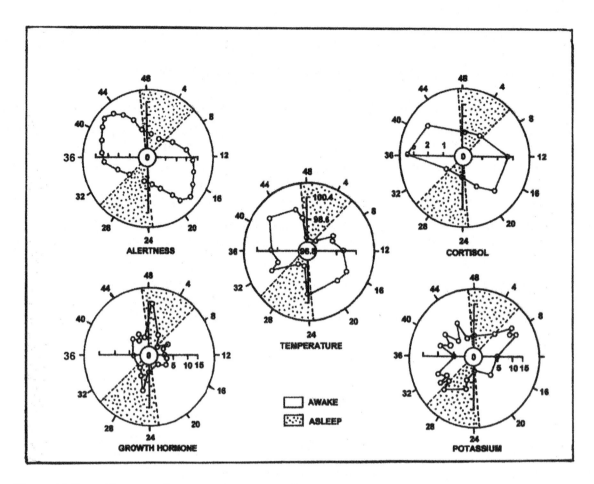

Figure 23.D-3. Changes of various physiological functions according to the phases of the sleep/wake cycle. The figures surrounding the circles are the hours of the clock (6 being morning, 48 being midnight), the time intervals during which the subjects were either asleep or awake are labeled as such, and the amplitude of the function is given as the length of the radius at any particular time during the forty-eight-hour period.

On relaxing in *savasana* after *yogasana* practice, one goes from the beta phase of wakefulness to an alpha brain-wave state and thence to theta relaxation (sleep stages 3–4) [860]. Sleep stages 3–4 are defined as having more than 50 percent theta waves, less than 50 percent alpha waves, and no beta waves. In young adults, the latency period for attaining stage 2 relaxation (the time between feeling sleepy and actually entering sleep stage 2) is about ten minutes [141], possibly passing through a very brief REM period on the way. Consequently, one should allow at least this long with beginners in *savasana* in order to have some hope of achieving a restful theta-wave state. Moreover, because norepinephrine released into the blood by *yogasanas* requires about twenty minutes to clear the bloodstream, a *savasana* of

ten to twenty minutes' duration seems reasonable. Inasmuch as research on circadian cycles shows that even when asleep, the penetration of the closed eyelids by dawn's early light is stimulating to the arousal response within the SCN (see Subsection 23.B, page 787), it would seem prudent to use eye bags during *savasana*, unless the *yogasana* practice room is in total darkness; even when the room is totally dark, one still has the ocular-vagal reflex advantage (Subsection 17.B, page 669) when using the eye bag.

The sleep/wake cycle has a period of twenty-four hours, because this particular body function is entrained with the rising and setting of the sun. If one flies across many time zones in the course of the day, then the sleep/wake cycle and the rising and setting of the sun become momentarily desynchronized, and one has jet lag until entrainment can be reestablished.

Foundation of Memory

It is most interesting to read that recent research strongly implicates the various sleep cycles in the learning and remembering of tasks, such as the mechanics of *yogasana* performance [657]. As discussed further in Subsection 4.F, page 127, the details of material newly learned during the day are transferred from the hippocampus to the cortex during periods of slow-wave sleep and then back again during REM phases (table 23.D-1). This conversation between the two brain areas while asleep results in the memory of the learned process being firmly implanted in the cortex, while the hippocampus memory bank is cleared in order to receive the next day's input. While certain parts of the brain during sleep are profoundly active reviewing what new synapses have been formed during the previous eighteen hours, other parts remain profoundly quiescent.

Quality versus Quantity

The quality of our sleep is more important than the quantity. While asleep, we cycle through ninety-minute periods, as shown in figure 23.D-2. In order to achieve a sense of rest and restoration, one needs to go through at least two full cycles of the sleep phases (three hours) without any interruptions such as might occur during sleep apnea.[6] Sleep fragmented by apnea is devoid of the ninety-minute cycles and so is far from restful. In contrast, relaxation following *yogasana* practice does not rely on any cyclic pattern of mental states and so can be more restful than sleep itself. This is especially so if the sleep is only for an hour or so, since there is not sufficient time in this case to complete even one nine-

ty-minute cycle, whereas a sixty-minute *savasana* can be most refreshing.

Though most people enter their first REM period ninety minutes after falling asleep (figure 23.D-2), depressed people enter REM at sixty minutes or less, and those who have experienced a near-death event enter REM only after 110 minutes.

Normal sleepers are awakened fifteen to thirty-five times a night, but once awake, the body pulls the brain again into sleep. In the extreme case, this can leave one constantly tired and possibly is related to the restorative benefits of yogic relaxation (*savasana*, etc.) which are not involved in this sleep-wake tug of war. To the extent that sleep is a battle between sleep-promoting and wake-inducing neurons, this battle may relate to depression [189]. If one gets about three hours of uninterrupted sleep, so as to have completed two full sleep cycles, then one can awake feeling fine, implying that sleep quality is more important than sleep quantity. In contrast, if one dreams actively and excessively in the REM phases of one's sleep (see below), then one awakes feeling exhausted, unfocused, and unmotivated.

Reticular Formation

Adrenergic excitations in the reticular formation in the upper pons (Subsection 4.B, page 74) are specifically arousing to the mind and the body; however, the threshold for excitation is raised during sleep. When the body is asleep but ready to come awake, a neural signal originates in the reticular formation and moves upward through the thalamus to the cortex, bringing it awake first. Once awake, the cortex sends a descending signal to bring the muscles and reflexes into readiness by increasing the body's muscle tone. As we have seen, as we approach the time of awakening, there also is a release of ACTH from the hypothalamus, leading to the release of cortisol from the adrenal glands and a whole-body energy increase that prepares us for the day ahead. The timing of this process must involve the same internal clock that often awakens us just moments before the alarm clock is set to go

---

6   In sleep apnea, one cycles between deep sleep with no breathing and light sleep with breathing restored. One remains unaware of the non-breathing episodes.

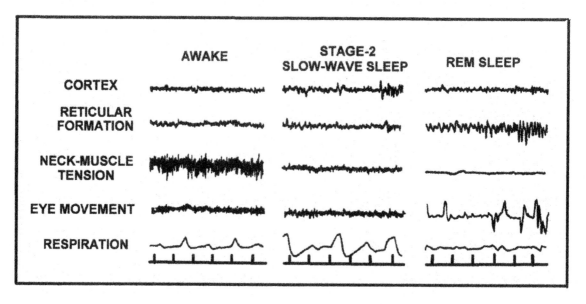

Figure 23.D-4. The variation of several physiological functions when awake and when in the REM and slow-wave sleep stages. Each of the small intervals on the horizontal axes represents one second.

off. What is most surprising is that the release of ACTH can be preprogrammed so as to occur at any convenient hour of the sleep cycle; i.e., if we decide before falling asleep that we should awake at 4:00 AM rather than at 7:00 AM, then ACTH will be released at 3:00 AM, so as to awaken us at the preordained time [908].

REM Sleep

Physiology

The REM (rapid-eye-movement) phase of sleep (stage 1) is most paradoxical. Figure 23.D-4 illustrates how several physiological variables are affected by three sleep stages: awake, REM sleep, and stage 2 sleep. One sees that as the sleeper goes from awake to REM sleep, the reticular formation becomes energized but the neck muscles become slack and passive, as does the respiration. On the other hand, eye movement becomes excessive in the REM phase, seeming to follow the reticular activation. In the REM phase of sleep, the EEG is beta-like; i.e., desynchronized and high-frequency, as appropriate for a level of high alertness. During sleep, the power of the alpha waves in the EEG is minimal in REM periods and maximal during

stage 2 periods. The newest research suggests that the different areas of the brain do not sleep simultaneously and that the global brain waves normally seen in the EEG in fact are very localized but largely uncoordinated globally in both time and space while we sleep [500]. As we drift into REM sleep, the prefrontal cortex (involved in decision making and logic) becomes inactive, and the levels of serotonin and norepinephrine fall, whereas the limbic system is energized, and levels of acetylcholine rise higher than in the waking state.

The heart rate and blood pressure are increased but irregular in the REM phase, respiration is rapid and uneven, and while all gastrointestinal movements cease as we go cold-blooded with little or no temperature regulation, penile and clitoral erections are common [427]. All but the last of these are characteristic of sympathetic nervous activity, whereas erection is a parasympathetic response (table 5.A-2 and Section 21.D, page 749), as are slack neck muscles and passive respiration.

While in the REM phase, autonomic control is nonfunctional and so core temperature, blood pressure, respiration, etc. rise and fall in a random way; when this happens at 6:00 AM (the last REM-sleep period of the night), an extreme blood pressure excursion at this time could lead to a heart attack. Memory consolidation during REM sleep apparently is such a high-energy process that it is given priority over autonomic control.

Periodicity and Extent

In adults, the first REM period occurs about ninety minutes after first falling asleep, and then in each succeeding ninety-minute period, there is less of stages 3 and 4 and more of the stage 1 REM phase. REM sleep amounts to about 50 percent of the total sleep time in infants and 30 percent in children, and it drops to 20 percent in those over eighty years old [4320]. In an eight-hour sleep, one may have between three and five REM episodes, each lasting five to thirty minutes and each lasting longer than the previous one. Normally, an adult spends about 15–25 percent of his or her sleep time in the REM state; however, in women who suffer from PMS, the REM sleep period is reduced to only about 5 percent of the total, and such sufferers are irritable on awakening, even though they have had an eight-hour sleep. When repeatedly awakened during the REM phases of sleep, we awaken finally as anxious and irritable, whereas if we are repeatedly awakened during stage 4 sleep, we awaken finally as physically exhausted. The period and number of REM phases in a night's sleep will be less if there is fatigue present, and even missing entirely when one is bone-tired.

Sleep patterns change as we age, and the need for sleep decreases with age, going from twenty hours in infants to only six hours per day in old age. Also, infants begin sleep with a REM cycle, whereas adults do not. If one takes drugs that reduce the REM time during a night's sleep, and then stops taking the drug, the REM activity will be very high, as if there were a zero-sum game at work.

Strictly speaking, REM sleep, with a period of only ninety minutes, is an ultradian rhythm, not circadian, but it is placed in the latter category since its repeating pattern occurs once per day, at the same time. Note that there are several other physiological processes besides REM sleep that have ninety-minute periodicity (Subsection 23.B, page 773). The ninety-minute period of the REM/non-REM phenomenon in sleep is thought

to be a phylogenetic remnant of an ancient rest/activity cycle in the human constitution [456] and is thought to assert itself during the waking hours as well (Section 15.E, page 627). Though the purpose served by REM sleep is still being debated [427], it is clear that there are aspects of autonomic excitation involved.

Dreaming

Though dreaming is only slightly more common when in the REM phase compared with slow-wave sleep, the latter periods are short and essentially dull and uninteresting,[7] whereas the former are long, vivid, and very exciting. This fact suggests that among other functions, the REM phase is associated in some way with creativity, new ways of looking at things, and bizarre mental associations. REM-phase dreaming is initiated by the release within the brain of acetylcholine, and fifty minutes or so later, other brain cells release norepinephrine and serotonin, both of which counter the effects of acetylcholine and so bring REM dreaming to a halt. During dreaming, both the amygdala and the pons are activated, with the amygdala being the center for emotions and the pons controlling sensory input.

Within the REM-sleep dream phases, the motor neurons in the spinal cord are partially inactivated so that we do not act out our cortical dreams, though we still can move about. The loss of muscle tone (atonia) in the REM phase arises because the actions of spinal motor neurons are inhibited. This atonia prevents us from acting out the active parts of our REM-sleep dreams; specific lesions in the brainstem can block this inhibition and so can lead to a very physical dream life. Emotional memory is processed in the amygdala during REM sleep

---

7   Actually, this is not true for everyone. If one is partially awakened while in the delta-wave stage of sleep, the result may be a sleepwalking episode in which the walker may cook a meal, go for a drive, have sex with a stranger, or even commit murder! In the sleepwalking state, the cerebellum is active, so that motion is possible; however, the higher functions in the frontal and parietal lobes are dormant. In this state, there is no conscious control and no memory of what may have happened while sleepwalking.

whereas spatial memory is processed in the hippocampus during this sleep phase.

Learning during Sleep

It is rather clear that one of the functions of REM sleep is very important in the process whereby the learning of complex tasks, such as how best to perform the *yogasanas,* is implanted into procedural memory and consolidated there (Subsection 4.F, page 127). There is enhanced activity in the hippocampus during REM sleep, signaling the consolidation in the memory of complex actions and procedures learned earlier in the day. This would apply clearly to what has been learned during the day's *yogasana* practice. On the other hand, memories of the personal experience of places and events are consolidated during slow-wave sleep [81].

Learning of certain tasks involves a specific region of the right parietal cortex known as Brodmann area 40 (figure 4.C-1). Studying this area, it was found that if a task was learned in the morning, then retesting in the evening gave no improvement in performance; however, retesting in the morning following sleep showed significant improvement. The busy work of the brain accomplished during the REM phase of sleep stands in direct contrast to the situation during non-REM phases.

Tononi and coworkers [543] recently reported that when the prefrontal cortex was stimulated in awake subjects, using a pulsed magnetic field so as to bypass the reticular formation and the thalamus, a brief stimulation of the prefrontal cortex was localized in that area for fifteen milliseconds and then diffused to adjacent cortical areas in the same hemisphere and via the corpus callosum into the opposite cerebral hemisphere, over the course of the next 300 milliseconds. When the experiment was repeated with the subjects in non-REM sleep stages, the initial excitation was found to be permanently localized in both space and time, showing that when awake, there is significant interaction of the initial stimulus with distant centers in the brain, but when in a non-REM sleep, this delocalizing interaction does not materialize. The corresponding experimental results when in the REM-sleep phase have yet to be reported.

Brain activation during sleep helps sustain body temperature. During sleep, one changes position more than fifty times per night, most often when entering and leaving the REM dream-phases of sleep (figure 23.D-2). The relative phases of the REM/non-REM and left/right hemispheric EEG excitation have been investigated by Shannahoff-Khalsa et al. [779], who report that when in stage 4 sleep (non-REM), greater right-hemisphere parasympathetic dominance was present, whereas when in the REM phase, the EEG dominance (now sympathetic) moves to the left hemisphere for delta and alpha EEG waves.

Energy Consumption

Strangely, the rate of oxygen consumption in the brain during REM sleep is even larger than when one is involved in intense mental exercise but otherwise decreases in the order REM > stage 2 > stage 3 > stage 4 [89]. With all of these aspects taken together, it would appear that there is a paradoxical mixture of sympathetic and parasympathetic features present in the REM state. In this state, dreams are frequent, vivid, and—most importantly—memorable, which is to say, their content has been consolidated (Subsection 4.F, page 127), whereas dreams in the slow-wave stages of sleep are not consolidated and so rarely are remembered. Whereas the brain consumes 20 percent of the fuel spent daily by the body in an adult, the figure is closer to 50 percent in the infant.

Section 23.E: Infradian Rhythms

Bodily processes that require more than twenty-four hours to go through their cycle are termed "infradian." The most obvious is that of the menstrual cycle of women, where there are large swings of progesterone and estrogen hormone levels on a monthly basis (Subsection 21.A, page 737). As with the circadian period, the monthly menstrual period is close to but not quite equal to the natural rhythm of the heavens—in this case, the rotational period of the moon. It is said that the nasal cycle also has a monthly period [123]. The rate of beard

Table 23.E-1: Variation of Body Function Extremes through the Year [804]

Month	Body Function	Extremum
January	SIDS death	Maximum
	Bulimic bingeing	Maximum
	Testicular cancer diagnosis	Maximum
	Cervical cancer diagnosis	Maximum
	Colds and flu	Maximum
February	Heart attacks	Maximum
	Strokes	Maximum
	Male sperm count	Maximum
March	Spring weight loss	Begins
	Hay fever symptoms	Maximum
April	Premenopausal breast cancer diagnosis	Maximum
	Gout flare-ups	Maximum
	Suicides	Maximum
May		
June	Diabetes control	Easiest
July	Multiple sclerosis symptoms	Maximum
	Nail growth	Maximum
August	Birth rate (USA)	Maximum
September	Asthma attack rate	Maximum
	Melanoma skin cancer rate	Maximum
October	Postmenopausal breast cancer diagnosis	Maximum
	Rate of first menstruation	Maximum
	Male testosterone levels	Maximum
	Male sexual activity	Maximum
November	Seasonal affective disorder	Begins
	Childhood diabetes onset	Maximum
December	Perforated ulcer risk	Maximum
	Winter weight gain	Begins
	Blood pressure	Maximum
	Cholesterol levels	Maximum

growth in men is known to go through a maximum once every week [804], and the phenomenon of seasonal affective disorder (Subsection 17.E, page 685) possibly is another infradian rhythm—in this case, the period being one year.

In what appears to be an infradian rhythm, it is known that fatal heart attacks in the northern hemisphere are 33 percent more likely in the months December through February, as compared with the time period June through September. In the southern hemisphere, the peak is reached in July, the middle of winter in that hemisphere. These seasonal differences may be related to the annual cycling of the blood pressure and cholesterol levels and to respiratory infections, holidays, and stress [804]. A more complete listing of the extremes of bodily functions on a month-to-month basis is displayed in table 23.E-1 above.

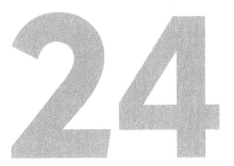

Aging and Longevity

As *yogasana* teachers, it is important that we understand those aspects of aging that are inevitable and those that are avoidable through yogic practices, for this will make our own lives more enjoyable as we age, and it also will allow us to work with and understand aging students in a more effective way. Though not all of our students necessarily will have heart problems, osteoporosis, hypertension, etc., all of them sooner or later will become aged, as will we, and we must understand what that means in terms of abilities, attitudes, etc. Fortunately, it is here that yoga shines, for whereas so many other health and exercise regimes become less appropriate with age, that is not the case with *yogasana*, when practiced with due concern for the natural changes in body processes with age. Moreover, we have many excellent personal examples (B. K. S. Iyengar, for example) of how *yogasana* benefits the aging and aged.

Physiologically, our bodies are constructed from the building blocks of life: DNA, proteins, carbohydrates, and lipids. As we age, there is an unavoidable amount of damage that accumulates in these systems, and by the time one reaches old age, the damage can exceed the body's self-repair capabilities. There then follows the impairment of the cells, tissues, organs, and organ systems, so that they can no longer fight off disease. At the same time, one loses bone and muscle mass, a swift reaction time, visual and auditory acuity, and the elasticity of the skin. Ironically, a significant fraction of the damage originates with the life-sustaining chemical reactions in the mitochondria that drive the production of ATP (Subsection 11.A, page 391). It appears that through the malfunction of the mitochondria,

there is increased apoptosis, and that when this apoptosis impacts the stem cells, aging is in full swing. Actually, those who survive to age sixty-five years are only slightly more likely to enjoy a robust old age than was possible 2,000 years ago. Though our longevity has increased statistically over that time span, the aging seems to continue unabated, regardless of whether we exercise or not. Exercise, diet, lifestyle, changes, etc. can prolong one's life but not retard aging in any significant way. Because the positive effects of exercise fade rapidly once we stop exercising [717], we have good reason to keep the exercise going as best we can, regardless of our immediate condition.

Section 24.A: Aging Symptoms and Statistics

What to Expect

Problems of aging are becoming increasingly more important as the average ages of the populations of the United States and of the world increase. At the moment, the fastest-growing segment of the U.S. population is the elderly, aged over sixty-five years, who will account for 21 percent of the population by the year 2030. Furthermore, today's babies can expect to live to age seventy-five years on average, and if today's adult makes it to sixty-five years, he or she can expect another fifteen years of life for men and nineteen years for women, though not necessarily of the highest quality, for reasons of compromised health. These figures refer to the Caucasian population, with those for American blacks about 10 percent lower. Among the elderly, heart disease takes more than 40 percent, cancer takes 20 percent, and 20 percent of those hardy enough to reach age eighty will suffer from Alzheimer's disease.

At age eighty-five years, the life expectancy is still five years for men and six years for women, and the maximal attainable age for humans is estimated to be 125 years; the oldest documented human being (Jeanne Calment) died in France at age 122. If no particular effort is made to maintain one's body through exercise, one can expect eight to ten years of partial dependency and one year of total dependency before passing on [783]. The suicide rate among white males aged eighty-five years or older in the United States is six times the average rate.

Symptoms of Old Age

Appreciable aging begins in most people at forty to fifty years and is marked by several noticeable but not necessarily rapid changes [181]. Many lists have been compiled to document the symptoms of old age, and three of them will be considered here. Though the three parties involved in generating these lists have divergent professional interests, they are in almost total agreement as to the physical, mental, and emotional effects of aging.

Nieman [618], an exercise physiologist, lists the effects of aging as including:

1. Loss of taste and smell
2. Periodontal bone loss; 50 percent of the U.S. population aged over sixty years has lost **all** teeth
3. Declining gastrointestinal function; less digestive juice, less absorption of nutrients, constipation
4. Loss of visual and auditory functions
5. Decrease in lean body weight, with increasing amount of body fat
6. Osteoporosis; bone weakness with diminished ability to repair fractures

7. Mental impairment; confusion, disorientation
8. Decreasing ability to metabolize drugs
9. Increase in chronic disease; diabetes, cancer, heart disease, high blood pressure, stroke, arthritis
10. Degradation of neuromuscular responses; reaction time, balance, strengths of muscles, tendons, and ligaments all degraded
11. Urinary incontinence
12. Decreased size and function of liver and kidneys
13. Decrease in heart and lung fitness; loss of 8–10 percent per decade of ability of heart and lungs to deliver oxygen

To this list, we would add

14. Decrease in both physical and mental flexibility and range of motion and
15. Lower levels of gonadal hormones

An interesting but qualitative system-by-system description of "normal aging" in women has been presented recently by the Harvard Women's Health Watch [321]:

» **Skin:** Loss of vital cells leads to skin that is thinner, less resilient, and less sensitive to temperature and pressure but is more easily bruised or likely to bleed
» **Brain:** Perceptible loss of short-term memory during the fifth decade; general intelligence decreases in the sixth decade, and capacity for abstract thought lessens in the seventh decade
» **Cardiovascular:** Arteries become less elastic and accommodating as heart walls thicken; contractile force falls off, even if one is in good physical condition
» **Respiratory:** Lung function peaks in early twenties and then falls to about 75 percent by age seventy-five years
» **Musculoskeletal:** At menopause, demineralization rate within bones exceeds bone building as estrogen level starts to fall, all of which can lead to osteoporosis

» **Digestive:** Ages well, with little loss of function

» **Reproductive:** Most eggs are shed or reabsorbed, and estrogen and progesterone production fall off at menopause, leading to hot flashes, etc.

» **Excretory:** Small changes in urinary volume (increase) and timing (less during the day, more at night) with aging

» **Immune:** Thymus gradually degenerates, and T cells decline in number and efficiency, leading to increased susceptibility to infection but possible decrease in allergic reactions as well

» **Endocrine:** While many hormone levels fall, the endorphins increase to reduce sensitivity to pain; thyroid and insulin outputs remain unchanged

» **Sense Organs:** These are most strongly degraded by age; there are losses of sensitivity in hearing, seeing, tasting, and smelling[1]

Not all of the changes listed above are inevitable, and some actually are avoidable in part or reversible; for example, aboriginal peoples not exposed to twentieth-century noise often retain acute hearing into old age [878], and defective vision in old age can be improved through yogic eye exercises [686]. Just how a number of these bodily functions change as one ages are graphed in figure 24.A-1 [618]. It is interesting to note how closely the symptoms of old age resemble those of weightlessness in space [893], physical inactivity [755], and bed rest [618].

---

1   Other aging criteria have been put forward by experts in the gerontology field. As George Burns (who died at age one hundred years) noted: "You'll know when you're old when everything hurts and what doesn't hurt doesn't work; when you get winded playing chess; when you stop to tie your shoelaces and ask yourself, 'What else can I do while I'm down here?' and when everyone goes to your birthday party and stands around the cake just to get warm!"

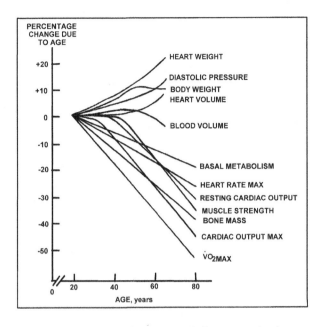

Figure 24.A-1. Physiological changes in body function with increasing age, as compared with the body at age twenty years.

Physical Aging of the Bones, Muscles, and Connective Tissues

Skeletal Height/Bones

The extent of the loss of height on aging due to osteoporosis is a signal that correlates with illness and early death. Thus, for men age 60–74 years, it is found that a height loss of more than 3 centimeters (1.2 inches) on aging correlates with a 64 percent higher risk of death compared with those having a loss of only 1 centimeter (0.4 inches). More specifically, the additional risk for cardiovascular death correlating with loss of height is 39 percent, for respiratory death, 75 percent, and for all other noncancerous deaths, 227 percent.

Loss of Muscle Mass

As we age, there is an unavoidable loss of skeletal muscle mass amounting to approximately 10 percent by age fifty years, 25 percent by age sixty-five years, and 50 percent by age eighty years. On average, up to 30 percent of the motor nerves die by the time we are in our later years. Once a motor nerve dies, then its muscle fiber, lacking innervation, also withers and dies, leading to thinner and weaker muscles. This seems to be especially true for muscles of the legs [621] (see Subsection 11.A, page 381). On the other hand, motor skills of the sort used in *yogasanas* are learned by the aged as quickly as by younger people [702]. In general, as the muscles and nerves age, they atrophy, whereas the connective tissue becomes hypertrophic and increases in stiffness, and the tissues overall become dehydrated. The end results of aging are decreases in neuromuscular efficiency and range of motion, which in turn restrict our mobility [117]. This situation in regard to the aging effects on muscles stands in contradistinction to the situation with heart muscle, which seems to enlarge with time rather than shrink.

Not only do our skeletal muscles weaken with age, but there is a shift of the balance between type 1 slow-twitch muscle fibers and type 3 fast-twitch fibers (Subsection 11.A, page 414), leading eventually to hybrid fibers of intermediate contraction velocity [9].

Muscle-Fiber Changes

Though the loss of strength with aging is due to an atrophy of the muscle fibers, strength gains are still possible beyond age ninety years with proper strength training. With strength training in older people, it is the type 2 fibers that grow the most, whereas these intermediate-type fibers are not even found in younger bodies. In the younger muscle, the fiber types are well mixed, but on aging, fiber grouping by type is observed, this being a symptom of chronic denervation. As we age, muscle fibers are lost, but the fastest fibers (type 3) are lost preferentially (Subsection 11.A, page 412). Even though we exercise into old age, the exercise promotes the effective loss of type 3 fibers, and as the relative proportion of type 1 fibers increases, so too does the muscular endurance. Paradoxically, as we age and lose fast-twitch fibers, our bodies come to be more slow-twitch dominated, and so we are closer to the ideal for *yogasana* practice! Note, however, that though it appears that type 3, fast-twitch fibers and type 2 fibers atrophy faster than the type 1 slow-twitch fibers, not everyone in the field agrees on this point.

Many changes in the motor system accompany aging. For example, muscles become thinner as the muscle bulk falls, the size of the mitochondria decreases, nerve fibers shrink in diameter and become slower in their speeds of conduction, and motor neurons are lost so that less than half of the motor units are still present at age seventy years [549]. Those motor units that still function in old age do so with lengthened reaction times. As we age, the fraction of the muscle dedicated to contractile fibers decreases in favor of fat and connective tissue.

Loss of Strength

Loss of strength commences in earnest after the sixtieth year. For those seventy years old and beyond, the strength of various muscles declines by 35–66 percent as compared with younger bodies. Finally, movements become slower and less precise with age, and circadian rhythms also fade, as discussed in Section 23.B, page 771. Along with the loss of muscle mass on aging, one also can expect to lose height. One will lose 4 centimeters (one and a half inches) in height on reaching age seventy-five years and 8 centimeters (three inches) on reaching eighty-five to ninety-five years.

The rapid fall in the level of strength after about age sixty is due to shifts of the testosterone and growth-hormone levels. As men age, the following functions decline: sexual function, muscle mass, muscle strength, and bone-mineral density. Because these same factors are known to decrease in men having a hypogonadism condition, it raises the question, "Can both be due to a loss of testosterone?" In fact, testosterone treatment does reverse these losses; however, it also seems to open the door to prostate cancer, prostatic hypertrophy, and erythrocytosis. Thus, it is questionable as to whether artificially raising the testosterone levels in older men is really a good idea [805].

On aging, strength decreases due to changes in the muscle fibers and their nerve supplies but not due to changes in motor commands from the brain. The shrinkage of the muscles with age involves men and women equally and involves all muscle groups. In general, there is a 25 percent loss of muscle strength by age sixty-five years as compared with one's peak strength [783]. Neuromuscular end plates also may degenerate and so imperfectly transmit the neural impetus to contract; loss of muscle strength is larger in the legs than in the arms. On the other hand, a few months of resistive exercise such as *yogasana* practice can result in a great improvement in muscle strength. This work is totally beneficial as long as the practitioner avoids the Valsalva maneuver (Subsection 15.C, page 616) during the practice, which might act to raise the blood pressure. *Yogasana* practice has an advantage over Western exercise in view of its accent on keeping the breath moving. One also must be aware that any injury sustained in *yogasana* practice will heal much more slowly as one ages.

Flexibility

Physically, quantitative measures of the change in lumbar flexibility with increasing age have been summarized by Kapandji [428] (tables 8.A-2 and 8.A-3). As can be seen in those tables, the maximum ranges of motion for lumbar extension and lateral bending are achieved in the teen years and then fall to much less than half the maximum values in the sixty-fifth to seventy-seventh years. This loss of spinal flexibility is important, for it will limit severely which physical activities can be enjoyed in the latter years. Loss of spinal flexibility with age is due to the intervertebral discs drying out and shrinking with age, encouraging the vertebrae to move toward one another and then to fuse. Regular practice of backbending, forward bending, *halasana*, spinal twists, and *sarvangasana* can work to slow, if not halt, this tendency.

By age sixty years, the average "sit and reach" distance (*paschimottanasana*) has decreased by 8–10 centimeters (three to four inches). On the other hand, taking the body's aged joints through the full range of motion, as with *yogasana* practice, is held to improve flexibility or, at the very least, to stem the age-driven decrease in flexibility [201a].

Yet another chemical factor in aging and flexibility is due to the cross-linking of the amino acids in adjacent protein chains by bridging glucose molecules, leading to thickening of the arteries,

stiffening of the joints, feeble muscle action, and failure of the organs. Such cross-links accumulate to eventually form hard, inflexible, yellow brown materials that closely resemble the products of the Maillard reaction in which meat is browned and hardened by roasting [560]. As these cross-links between collagen fibrils develop with age within the ligaments, tendons, and joint capsules, there is a natural decrease in flexibility. Free radicals are strongly implicated in this cross-linking reaction.

Reflexes

Elderly persons (especially females) are predisposed to dizziness because of the aging process and so are very susceptible to falling. Physiological changes on aging also include a decline of sensitivity and speed of the proprioceptive (Section 11.C, page 441), visual (Subsection 17.B, page 666), and vestibular reflexes (Section 18.B, page 696). The numbers of receptors and synapses in the visual and auditory channels are reduced, as are the cerebral autoregulation and baroreceptor functions. All of the above lead to a diminished ability to reflexively regulate or compensate for the body's homeostatic needs [162].

Telomeres

A second mechanism leading to aging is popular among those doing research in gerontology at the cellular level. Telomeres are DNA structures that are attached to the ends of chromosomes, much like the tips on the ends of shoelaces, and which function to protect the chromosomes within cells that divide, such as the white blood cells. Each time such a cell divides, the protective telomere is reduced in size at a rate of about twenty DNA base pairs per year, and when the telomere is reduced to a stub, the cell dies rather than dividing again. This much is known to be true for human cells in isolation, and it is hypothesized by many that this is "the beginning of the end" when it happens in the living human body.

Generally, the telomeres are kept in good condition by an enzyme known as telomerase; however, stress has been shown to have a strongly negative effect on this enzyme, so that highly stressed women (mothers giving child care to

Table 24.A-1: Average Ages of Cells in Various Organs and Body Tissues [874a]

Organ or Tissue	Average Age
Cerebral cortex	Calendar age[a]
Visual cortex	Calendar age
Heart	Calendar age
Cerebellum	Two years less than calendar age
Hippocampus	Positive neurogenesis[b]
Intercostal muscle	15.1 years
Gastrointestinal tract (not lining)	15.9 years
Gastrointestinal tract (epithelium)	Five days
Epidermis	Fourteen days
Red blood cells	120 days
Bone	Ten years
Liver	300–500 days

a Your "true" age as measured by the calendar.
b Growth of new neurons observed, but rate is unknown.

chronically ill children, for example) have telomere lengths more indicative of women who are ten years older [97]. Low social status in women, as compared with high status, again results in psychological stress and shortening of the telomeres equivalent to several years of life expectancy. In a study of female twins, one of whom married into a high social class and the other of whom married into a low social class, the latter had telomere lengths that were nine years shorter than those of the former due to increased psychological stress. One infers from this that a relaxing *yogasana* practice that works to reduce one's level of stress will reduce the pressure on one's telomeres and so possibly prolong one's life.

As measured by the lengths of the DNA telomeres, the effect of obesity on longevity is even more negative than that resulting from smoking. In obese smokers, the biological age is ten years less than that of the lean nonsmoker. The decreasing length of the telomeres due to oxidative stress can be halted by lifestyle changes, but this will not bring them back to their original lengths. There is a strong correlation between the length of your telomeres and those of your father, but no correlation with those of your mother.

Aging and the Mitochondria

Using the nuclear methods that have been so successful in dating antiquities, it is now possible to measure the ages of various body tissues, with surprising results (table 24.A-1). One sees immediately from this table that the body parts can have very different ages, with cortical brain and cardiac tissue at any age being just your calendar age at that time; which is to say, as they die off, they are not replaced by new, young cells. In contrast, the hippocampus is now known to grow new cells, but the rate has not been determined; in the cerebellum, new cells are born for the first two years of life, and then they age, as do the cortical tissues. Contrary to earlier reports on muscles in general, it was found that intercostal muscle replaces itself on average every 15.1 years; gastrointestinal muscle replaces itself every 15.9 years, and the full replacement of bone requires about ten years.[2]

---

2   Interpretation of this data on tissue age/replacement is unclear: if the "age" of the tissue is equal to its calendar age, then there is no question. However, when it is less than the calendar age, one asks, is this due to the birth of distinct new cells as in muscle hyperplasia (Subsection 11.A, page 405) or hippocampal

This table immediately raises the vision that the skin should never age, as all of its cells are fully replaced every fourteen days, and similarly, the cells of bones are replaced every ten years. With such ongoing repair mechanisms, why do we age? The answer to this question appears to be essentially that, whereas "new" cells can be manufactured, the mitochondria within these new cells are the old, unreconstructed materials [874a], aged and faulty.

At a deeper level, it is generally accepted that the mitochondria, the energy-generating organelles within the cells, not only control our metabolism but in large part, regulate how long we live (Subsection 11.A, page 375). At the chemical level, much of the blame for aging can be placed at the feet of free radicals produced in the course of ATP production in the mitochondria. Free radicals are molecules with an odd number of electrons, meaning that not all of the molecular electrons can be involved in two-electron chemical bonds, and that the odd electron imparts a very high and nonspecific chemical reactivity to the radical. When we are young, ATP production within the mitochondria is high, and free-radical production is low; but as we age, the ratio shifts, until the ATP supply becomes minimal, and the free-radical production rate becomes maximal in old age [886]. By virtue of their high reactivity, free radicals engage in many deleterious reactions, unless they are mopped up by antioxidants in the diet. It appears that the free radicals produced within the mitochondria attack mitochondrial DNA, leading to mutations that accumulate at faster and faster rates with the years. After 125 years, the lethal dose of mitochondrial mutations finally is reached within "new" cells, and life is no longer possible. If the rate of mitochondrial

degradation can be slowed to match that of DNA degradation, then a significant rise in human longevity will result.

Physical Aging of the Respiratory and Vascular Systems

$\dot{V}O_{2max}$

Of the fourteen physical and mental changes on aging listed above by Nieman, it is the thirteenth that is generally taken by gerontologists as the most direct *quantitative* measure of aging: decrease in heart and lung function; loss of 8–10 percent per decade of ability of the heart and lungs to deliver oxygen to muscles. In particular, it is the quantity $\dot{V}O_{2max}$ that is readily measured and is of the greatest relevance according to Nieman;[3] $\dot{V}O_{2max}$ is a measure of the work capacity of the body, expressed as its ability to deliver oxygen to the muscles as they do their work. As discussed in Subsection 11.A, page 393, the ability of a muscle to do work over an extended time (beyond a few minutes) is dependent upon the delivery of oxygen to the mitochondria within the muscle cells; without sufficient oxygen in the blood, glucose cannot be oxidized, ATP is not produced, and all muscular movement stops. Experiments on men and women show that $\dot{V}O_{2max}$ starts to decline by 8–10 percent per decade after age twenty-five years. It is estimated that half of the decline in this quantity is due to lack of physical exercise, and half is innate and therefore unavoidable.

The avoidable half of the 8–10 percent decline in $\dot{V}O_{2max}$ seems to be more under our control. Experiments show that regular aerobic exercise can lead to the recovery of half of the decline in $\dot{V}O_{2max}$. This recovery holds up to age seventy-five

---

neurogenesis (Subsection 4.C, page 79), or is it due to the slow but ongoing replacement of amino acids in the cellular proteins as described in Subsection 4.F, page 134? The former is based upon the genesis of cells from stem cells, and the latter is based upon the ongoing replacement of components within a static population of cells in a tissue; neither of these situations would apply to tissue having a measured age equal to its calendar age.

3   Note that the factor considered as prime by Nieman is not even mentioned specifically by the Harvard Women's Health Watch. This reflects the fact that $\dot{V}O_{2max}$ is the most quantifiable of the various factors but not necessarily the most important in terms of overall well-being. With this caveat in mind, we focus on this quantity as being of special relevance to *yogasana* students and the athletically inclined, but not so much so to the average person.

years, at which point the decrease of $\dot{V}O_{2max}$ is independent of exercise.

The most recent study of $\dot{V}O_{2max}$ further defines the loss of aerobic capacity as beginning to decline at age forty years, and that the decline accelerates with each succeeding decade, irrespective of one's previous level of exercise or muscle mass. Though the decline in unavoidable, the larger is $\dot{V}O_{2max}$ in the younger years, the larger will it be in the older years, though declining [4, 246]. The largest single factor in forestalling the downward trends of aging is exercise, for this can increase lung capacity, build muscles and bone, and condition the heart and blood vessels. The onset of physical disability in those who do not die accidentally is estimated to be lengthened by up to five years in those who are thin, exercise, and do not smoke [4].

This unavoidable decline in $\dot{V}O_{2max}$ is currently explained by two competing theories: (1) genetic errors accumulate, and the body is unable to correct them, leading to inefficiency and disease; and (2) the body is inherently programmed so that cells divide only a fixed number of times, and then regeneration slows or ceases, leading to disease and degeneration. At another level, natural selection in humans also plays a role in aging, as it has selected against mutations that interfere with our reproductive years, but not against slow-acting mutations that only affect our later years [717].

Cardiovascular System

By age sixty-five years, the mean blood pressure will have increased by 10–40 millimeters Hg, while the maximum heart rate will drop by ten beats per minute per decade, leading to decreased cardiac output; the vital capacity of the lungs will decrease by 50 percent by age seventy years, and the amount of hemoglobin in the blood also will fall. As a consequence of these changes, the aerobic capacity decreases, the cardiovascular risk rises, and both the maximal work capacity and $\dot{V}O_{2max}$ decrease, as does respiratory efficiency. $\dot{V}O_{2max}$ decreases with increasing age, not due to heart factors, but due to the inefficiency of the skeletal muscles [521].

The increase in the size of the heart as we age (figure 24.A-1) is at first sight perplexing, as the size of all other muscles decrease with age. This is explained as the result of the overwork performed by the aging heart in pushing blood through a vascular system that is more and more resistant to the flow of blood. On the other hand, the skeletal muscles of the body become thinner and weaker as the nerves that innervate them die off through lack of use in old age.

Physical Aging of the Neural Systems

In regard to aging mechanisms, neurons (brain cells) and myocytes (muscle cells) cease to divide at all after reaching maturity, and other cell types otherwise reproduce at slowly declining rates. As a result, the general effect of aging is a loss of cells and cell products such as enzymes, hormones, and collagen. Along with the decrease in hormonal levels, it is thought [721] that the numbers of receptors for the hormones on the cell walls decrease with age. Just as the hypothalamus gland initiates hormonal changes via the pituitary gland, signaling puberty, it may also be that it changes the hormonal balance again as one goes into old age, signaling a physiological rollback [721].

Considered at the cellular level, aging is determined almost totally by cell loss and the concomitant loss of cell products. Of those cells that are replaced normally (and many are not), they are replaced at a slower rate as we age, and the products of cell function (hormones, enzymes, collagen, elastin, and neurotransmitters, for example) are produced at slower and slower rates as well [321]. The lowering of the brain's density by the decrease in the numbers of neurons as one ages has been shown to be thwarted by aerobic exercise [706].

As the brain ages and its volume decreases, it necessarily tends to pull away from the rigid structure of the skull. In this process, the veins serving the brain are stretched, and in doing so, they may develop slow leaks of blood into the subdural space between the dura mater and the arachnoid layer. Such leaks, called subdural hematomas, are often seen in the older citizen who has fallen and struck the head on some object or otherwise moved the head so as to subject it to unusual shearing forces. This condition may be further aggravated if the person is also on blood thinners, as is often the case with older people, for the volume of blood leaked will be much larger when the viscosity of the blood is low.

Elderly persons (especially females) are predisposed to dizziness because of the aging process. Physiological changes include a decline in proprioceptive (Section 11.C, page 441), visual (Subsection 17.B, page 666), and vestibular reflexes (Section 18.B, page 696).

Longevity

For 99.9 percent of the time that human beings have populated the Earth, the longevity has been no longer than thirty or forty years. It is only relatively recently that this longevity figure has doubled, thanks to increasing awareness of sanitation, medical techniques, the cultivation of health habits, etc. The influence of health habits on mortality has been nicely set out by Breslow [618], in terms of seven basic rules:

1. Never smoke
2. Moderate alcohol consumption
3. Eat breakfast daily
4. Do not snack
5. Get seven to eight hours' sleep each night
6. Exercise regularly
7. Maintain ideal weight

Figure 24.A-2 shows how ignoring these simple habits become mortality factors. For both men and women, those who practice all seven of the above rules have a 40-percent lower death rate than those who practice only four or five. These seven health habits are clearly compatible with the *yogasana* lifestyle and are even encouraged by it. On the other hand, if one practices only three or fewer of the health habits, the death rate increases by up to 60 percent over that for the median group.

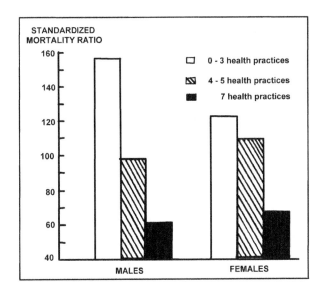

Figure 24.A-2. The relation between the number of good health habits practiced by males and females and the standardized mortality ratio, defined as one hundred times the ratio of the rate of deaths observed to the rate of deaths expected on average.

Note too that although a person with a twenty-pack-per-year smoking history statistically will forfeit three years of life expectancy, there are other indirect factors (stress, for example) affecting longevity other than direct health ones. For example, being a single male also will statistically reduce one's life span by three years, whereas being happily married adds two years [172].

Maintaining one's health into old age can be looked at a second way. In addition to our chronological age, each of us has a biological age as well, the latter depending upon many physical factors such as heart rate, blood pressure, and ability to bend forward. The biological age also can be estimated using a self-reported measure of one's health status. Men and women aged sixty-five to eighty years old who report their health status as "excellent" have a biological age that is five to eight years less than their calendar age, whereas those who report their health as "poor" have a biological age that is five to eight years larger than their calendar age. Reports of "good" or "fair" health status imply near-equality of the biological and calendar ages. Having a lowered biological age strongly im-

Table 24.A-2: Comparison of the Effects of Aging and *Yogasana*

Aging Effects [618]	*Yogasana* Effects [755]
Loss of taste and smell	Heightened senses of taste and smell
Periodontal bone loss	Can reduce TMJ syndrome
Declining GI function	Normalizes bowel function and improves digestion
Loss of visual and auditory sensitivity	Corrects refractive errors in vision, reduces visual headaches, sharpens hearing
Muscle loss/fat gain	Promotes muscle strength, endurance, and flexibility
Decrease of bone strength and density	Bone strength, bone density, and structural integrity of joints increase
Mental impairment	Increased ability to respond positively to stress; increased mental acuity
Decreasing ability to metabolize drugs	Improved sensitivity to insulin; healthy metabolism of lipids and cholesterol
Increase in chronic disease	Increased immune function
Degradation of neuromuscular response	Increase of neuromuscular coordination
Urinary incontinence	Increase of neuromuscular control
Decreasing liver and kidney function	Increase in liver and kidney function
Decrease in heart and lung fitness	Increases in circulation and respiration efficiency; increased tolerance for exercise
Loss of skeletal and mental flexibility and range	Striking increases in flexibility and range of motion
Increasing mental depression	Decreasing mental depression

plies an increased longevity calendar-wise, for it is the biological age that is relevant to longevity. Persons in the sixty-five to eighty year range who maintain themselves in "excellent" health will live ten to sixteen years longer on average than those in the "poor" health group [783].

Today, statistics show that once a person reaches the midnineties, there is a noticeable decrease in the observed death rate as compared to the predicted death rate (i.e., if you are healthy enough to reach ninety-five years, you are healthy enough to live significantly longer than that extrapolated from the data of those who died at earlier ages).

Though it is generally argued that obesity is a factor working against longevity, it appears that if the obese can reach old age, by virtue of their fatness, the obese have a natural reserve of body strength that is a measurable benefit for them, should they be hospitalized. There is a demonstrable protection of obesity in regard to lung cancer.

From the legal perspective, almost everyone dies of the same cause: legal death in most places is now defined as brain death (no brainstem reflexes, no evidence of breathing, and total lack of consciousness). However, this definition is being actively debated among bioethicists, surgeons, and philosophers [296].

Yogasana, Sports, and Aging

Specific data is not available on the effects of aging on the *yogasana* student, but there are

Table 24.A-3: Comparison of the Leading Medical Problems and the Leading Causes of Death in the Age Groups 19–35 Years and Over 65 Years [322]

Age Nineteen to Thirty-Nine Years	Age Over Sixty-Five Years
Leading Medical Problems	
Nose, throat, upper respiratory infections	Nose, throat, upper respiratory conditions
Injuries	Osteoporosis and arthritis
Viral, bacterial, and parasitic infections	Hypertension
Acute urinary-tract infections	Urinary incontinence
Eating disorders	Cardiovascular disease
Violence, rape	Injuries
Substance abuse	Hearing and vision impairment
Leading Causes of Death	
Motor vehicle accidents	Cardiovascular disease
Cardiovascular disease	Cerebrovascular disease
Homicide	Pneumonia and influenza
Coronary artery disease	Chronic obstructive pulmonary disease
AIDS	Colorectal cancer
Breast cancer	Breast cancer
Cerebrovascular disease	Lung cancer
Cervical cancer	Diabetes
Uterine cancer	Accidents other than motor vehicle

Table 24.A-4: Top-Ten Causes of Death in the United States by Gender [791]

	Male	Female
1	Heart disease	Heart disease
2	Cancer	Cancer
3	Accidents	Stroke
4	Stroke	Chronic obstructive lung disease
5	Chronic obstructive lung disease	Diabetes
6	Diabetes	Alzheimer's disease
7	Pneumonia and influenza	Accidents
8	Suicide	Pneumonia and influenza
9	Kidney disease	Kidney disease
10	Liver disease	Blood infection

some generalities for aging athletes that will apply across the board to all athletes. Sports champions can use their speed to secure a competitive advantage in the age range eighteen to twenty-six years, whereas champions in sports requiring coordination can extend their dominance for yet another decade beyond that. Power and endurance are strongest between years thirty and forty, with age being kinder to endurance performers than to power performers. Strength peaks at about twenty-five years but can plateau out to age fifty years, whence it then declines by 20 percent by age sixty-five years and decreases continuously after that. Much of the strength loss is due to the loss of muscle mass and increased body fat. However, in these declining years, resistance training will slow strength loss, as it helps to recruit motor units and promote joint flexibility. In summary, championship-class athletes can expect to first lose their speed, followed by coordination, strength, and endurance.

Yogasana and Aging

It appears to be a different story for those practicing *yogasana* at noncompetitive levels, for Schatz [755] has published a list of how *yogasana* practice can curtail or even reverse the aging process. It is interesting and satisfying to compare her points in regard to anti-aging and those of Nieman in regard to aging (table 24.A-2). Notice that for almost every item listed by Nieman as a negative change on aging, Schatz lists the positive effect *yogasana* practice can have on that factor. This comparison illustrates in a very compelling manner how *yogasana* practice can work to combat the physical and mental decline usually associated with aging. Even more important, yoga done into old age can vastly improve the qualities of our lives and those of our students aside from the possibility of extending life, as it gives the practitioner a focus and commitment to a purpose greater than oneself [755].

It is interesting to see how the profile of leading medical problems and the leading causes of death change between the nineteen- to thirty-nine-year-old age group and the over-sixty-five age group, listed in order of their frequencies in table 24.A-3. One sees there that the medical problems that newly appear once one reaches the older age group (osteoporosis, arthritis, hypertension, cardiovascular disease, and vision impairment) are all addressable through *yogasana* practice. A lifetime of sensible *yogasana* practice will be a prophylactic against many of the items in table 24.A-3, in agreement with the listings in table 24.A-2. The ten leading causes of death in the United States by gender are presented in table 24.A-4.

If we could cure heart disease, then the average life expectancy would rise by three years, and if we could cure all forms of cancer, then the life expectancy would increase by another twelve years.

Following this extra fifteen years of life added by these medical advances, we would then die of stroke or by accidents. At present, women in the United States live five years longer than males. The death rates of males and females are nearly equal in their early years, but once boys start to produce the testosterone that converts them from boys to young men (in the age range fifteen to twenty-four years), their death rate is three times that of girls in the same range. Furthermore, the estrogen produced by women lowers the risks of heart disease and stroke in females, whereas testosterone works in several ways against longevity in men [791].

As long as exercise is pursued diligently, it improves body function; however, it has not been shown to increase long-term survival. Moreover, its effects do not carry very far into the future once one falls back to a more sedentary lifestyle. Note too that anything that would promote the longevity of cells also runs the risk of promoting cancer [717].

Section 24.B: Mental and Emotional Effects of Aging

Brain Shrinkage

Several of the physical factors that decline with aging would seem to have parallels in the mental and emotional sphere. In the latter case, most of the aging changes occur in the cerebral cortex [266], and as with the physical effects of aging, they start at about age forty years. Thus, the cortex of the forty- to sixty-year-old has 15–20 percent fewer cells than that of the twenty-year-old, losing about thirty million cortical cells per year (one per second). By age seventy-five years, the cellular deficit is over 40 percent. With age, brain cells lose dendrites, are less responsive to neurotransmitters, and have atrophied cell parts (Subsection 4.E, page 120). With increasing age, dopamine-producing neurons decrease by 40 percent in certain parts of the brain, and with falling dopamine levels, the sense of the passage of time slows. The locus ceruleus, an area of the brain rich in the norepinephrine needed for arousal, is smaller by 30 percent at age seventy years. By this age, the brain size is smaller by 11 percent, brain weight decreases, and the open volume of the brain ventricles increases [266]. Blood flow to the brain and brain metabolism also decrease with age. In the normal aging brain, the largest fundamental change of size is in the frontal lobes, where 5–10 percent of the tissue can be lost. Unfortunately, this is the brain's center for making plans, organizing one's time, staying focused, and motivating oneself. Without these "executive functions," one loses both a sense of purpose in life (essential to happiness) and the ability to establish and maintain social relations. Once these are lost, it is only a small step to depression.

But there is something to which one can look forward! In a recent functional MRI study, it was found that negative reactions to fearful circumstances are located in the amygdala, whereas positive responses are located in the medial prefrontal cortex. As one ages from twelve to seventy-nine years old, there is a definite shift of the response to a fearful situation that is located progressively less in the amygdala and more in the prefrontal cortex (Subsection 4.F, page 132), in spite of the fact that prefrontal cortical cells die in measurable amounts as we age. It was concluded in this work that older adults are able to successfully transfer potentially fearful thought away from the emotionally negative and subconscious amygdala and to focus instead on the emotionally positive prefrontal cortex [83a] in the conscious sphere.

Neurogenesis

"Facts" regarding brain size have led to the widely held belief that once mature, the number of brain cells decreases uniformly with age, with no replacement of old, dead cells possible. Imagine then the surprise when it was reported that in the human hippocampus, there is strong evidence for the creation of new neurons, even

in the elderly, and that the renewal is spurred by exercise [271]! It remains to be seen if such regeneration of neurons can occur in other areas of the brain. On the positive side, there are experiments that show that a reorganization of neural circuitry is possible as one ages, which compensates for the declining numbers of neurons in the brain (Subsection 4.E, page 120). Yet another factor in the apparent loss of our mental facilities in old age is society's encouragement of the elderly to adopt a sick role and to learn to underachieve. Practice of the *yogasanas* into old age can be a powerful defense against such pressures to prematurely release one's hold on life.

As with the physical side, mental response time increases with age. However, the general level of EEG activity (Section 4.H, page 149) does not decrease until one reaches age eighty years or so. Perhaps this lengthening of response time is related to the apparent slowing of the time sense in the elderly [19], who sense that time is passing much more slowly than does real clock time, possibly due to lower dopamine levels. The stretching of apparent time is most obvious when the aged are busy (Subsection 23.A, page 769).

Diet and exercise are generally held to be of no value in retarding the aging of the brain. This is understandable, because almost all Western forms of exercise are repetitive and require no deliberate mental effort. In contrast, *yogasana* is rich in this mental component, so it can be very different in this regard.

Memory Loss

The largest effect of aging on mental performance is loss of memory as mental resources decline. Most interestingly, there also is, in a sense, a loss of mental flexibility with age, as one is less able to assimilate truly new ideas. "New knowledge" that simply builds upon already accepted ideas is easily incorporated by the aged, but ideas that have no previous foundation are less and less acceptable with increasing age. Resistance to ideas that are too "new" for aged *yogasana* students can be a potent factor in retarding their progress (Section 4.G, page 149). The more closely "new ideas" in *yogasana* practice are related to others already accepted, the more readily they will be accepted. Subjects over sixty years of age who also had high cortisol levels performed poorly in maze tests requiring memory; in animal studies, it is known that high stress levels lead to high cortisol levels, which in turn lead to poor memory retention. The higher your formal level of education, the more your loss of memory with age is compensated; college-educated senior citizens showed considerable activity in the frontal lobes when recalling facts, whereas those who did not go to college had diminished levels of recall and showed intense activity in the temporal lobes under the same circumstances.

Though the older brain does appear to slow down, it also appears to change its tactics in problem solving. In younger brains, problem solving is usually restricted largely to one cerebral hemisphere or the other, whereas in the older brain, there is a more equitable sharing of the thought processes by the two hemispheres.

Maintaining Mental Competence

Four factors have been put forward as key elements in maintaining mental competence into old age [327]:

1. Maintain a high level of mental functioning through an activity that is intellectually engaging. Learn a new skill rather than watching television and talking on the phone all day. Mental exercises keep the brain sharp. Adults who regularly challenge themselves mentally succumb to dementia less often, less severely, and at older ages than do those who do no mental exercise in their later years. Those who are better educated, have high-status occupations, and are more stimulated mentally are somehow protected from mental deterioration as they age. It is as if they have a "mental reserve" that they can draw upon in times of mental stress, or are better able to rewire around minor defects in brain function as they age.

2. Maintain a high level of physical activity. Though the mechanism is not yet understood, it is known that physical exertions that exercise the cardiovascular and muscular systems seem to keep the brain more supple. Though those between seventy and ninety years old who performed little or no exercise over a long period of time showed a far more advanced cognitive decline than those who followed a regular program of moderate exercise, going beyond moderate exercise did not yield any further cognitive benefits. Because the adage "use it or lose it" holds true in both the physical and mental spheres, laws that force high achievers out of their fields of expertise and into retirement have had a strongly negative societal effect.

3. Develop a feeling of self-efficacy so that you feel that you are in control of your life. In order to stay mentally bright, it is important to find mental and physical activities that are challenging, interesting, and enjoyable enough to keep one involved on a daily basis over a long period of time.

4. Do not withdraw from society; it is well substantiated that having a strong social support group and being actively engaged with other people is essential to combating depression. Several studies show that brain function in the elderly is helped as much by social interaction as by physical exercise.

It is difficult to think of anything better suited to these four paths to mental and emotional good health than the daily class practice of the *yogasanas*! It appears that whatever is good for the heart is also good for the brain.

In regard to aging, Nesse and Williams [611] point out that a gene can have multiple effects on the body, some beneficial and some not so beneficial, and that our present situation is a trade-off between longevity and quality of life. For example, the uric acid crystals that are responsible for the pain of gout are also strong antioxidants and can possibly extend our lifespan. In the same vein, Nesse and Williams claim that strong immune defenses protect us from infection, but in the process, they inflict low-level tissue damage. From this point of view, aging is seen not as a disease but rather as a trade-off between lifespan and accumulating tissue damage that eventually works to our disadvantage if we are lucky enough to live to an "old age."

Epilogue

Learning by Rereading

In preparing this revised version of the handbook, I have had the opportunity to reread the earlier version several times over, and each time that I did, I learned something new! But I wrote it, so how could I learn something new by rereading it? The answer is that on rereading, I often found new connections among the plethora of apparent loose ends in that book. In assembling the present version of the handbook, I was keenly aware of how many items have been entered here that may provoke the reader to ask, "Well, what has that got to do with yoga?" My answer is, "I don't know yet, but I am confident that these seemingly out-of-place, irrelevant items sooner or later will be integrated into the larger body of *yogasana* knowledge by some interested reader." I know this is happening because my yoga friends (see Acknowledgments, page *xxi*) who have been proofreading the text keep telling me of the new connections they have been making between seemingly loose ends and the more relevant parts of the text.

Prematurity

In general, most new ideas fit nicely into an existing pattern of understanding and so stand in strong contrast to others which would seem to be premature in their appearance, though they might be no less true [637]. Though the loose ends inserted in this work may well be "prematurities," I think they can be just as true as the full-term ideas, and sooner or later many will find their places in the fabric being woven from yoga and medical threads.

Loose Ends

This particular "open" construction of the handbook was deliberate, done with the hope that it would allow the making of new connections between the old and the new, between the East and the West, between medical science and yoga science, between the conscious and the subconscious, between World View I and World View II (Subsection 1.A, page 3), etc. It has been my aim from the beginning to get readers to view each of the loose ends as an opportunity, sooner or later, to make an otherwise unthought of connection and so advance our thinking. The yoga-medical synthesis we seek should especially encourage large-scale research into the medical powers of *yogasana* practice.

Repeated rereading of the original version of the handbook has confirmed my original intention to place what I felt were interesting loose ends into the text, which others might later integrate into other areas of understanding and so enlarge the cohesiveness of the whole. Well, this is the end, and there are more loose ends than ever (by design) and more connections than ever. When speaking of "loose ends by design," I mean that I deliberately have **not** excluded a loose end just because it was a loose end, but included it with the expectation that some time in the future the loose end would prove to be of some value to the reader in an as-yet-unimagined context.

Divergent Thinking

Go back in this handbook and reread Subsection 4.E, page 124, on convergent and divergent thinking. *A Handbook for Yogasana Teachers* was written within that context, being strongly divergent in nature. The consequence of such an approach is an admitted amount of apparent dead ends and loose ends, but at the same time, the opening of many doors. If I cut out all of the apparent inessentials, this handbook would be far thinner, but it would not be the seed I intend to plant. As it now stands, I don't know what fruit it will bear, but I am optimistic. It is my hope that in reading this handbook, you will have discovered new ideas and come to a greater understanding that illuminates both your practice and your teaching.

Appendix

Yogasana Illustrations

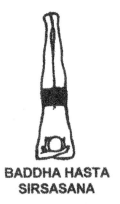

BADDHA HASTA SIRSASANA

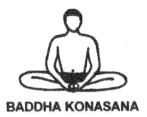

BADDHA KONASANA

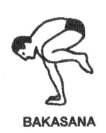

BAKASANA

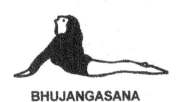

BHUJANGASANA

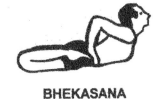

BHEKASANA

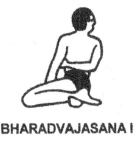

BHARADVAJASANA I

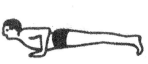
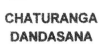

CHATURANGA DANDASANA

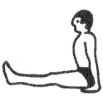

DANDASANA

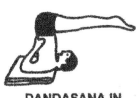

DANDASANA IN SARVANGASANA

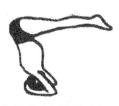

DANDASANA IN SIRSASANA

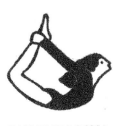

DHANURASANA

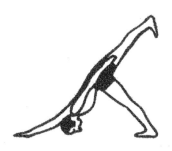

DWIANGA ADHO MUKHA SVANASANA

823

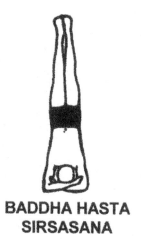

**BADDHA HASTA
SIRSASANA**

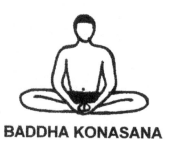

BADDHA KONASANA

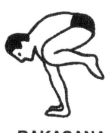

BAKASANA

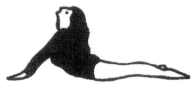
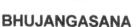

BHUJANGASANA

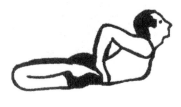

BHEKASANA

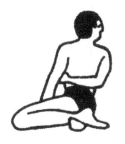

BHARADVAJASANA I

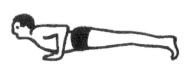

**CHATURANGA
DANDASANA**

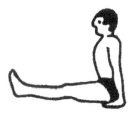

DANDASANA

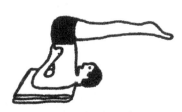

**DANDASANA IN
SARVANGASANA**

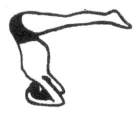

**DANDASANA IN
SIRSASANA**

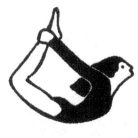

DHANURASANA

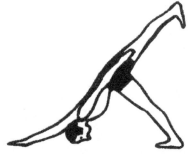

**DWIPADA ADHO MUKHA
SVANASANA**

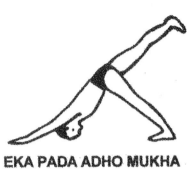

EKA PADA ADHO MUKHA SVANASANA

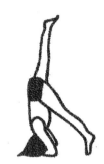

EKA PADA SIRSASANA

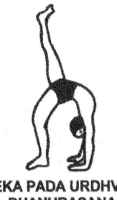

EKA PADA URDHVA DHANURASANA

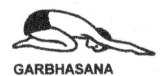

GARBHASANA

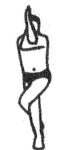

GARUDASANA

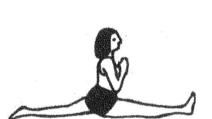

GOMUKHASANA

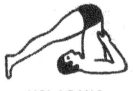

HALASANA

HAMSASANA

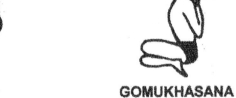

HANUMANASANA

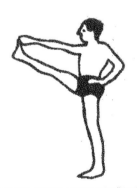

HASTA PADANGUSTHASANA

JANU SIRSASANA

JATARA PARIVARTANASANA

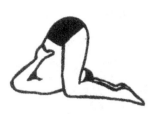

KARNAPIDASANA

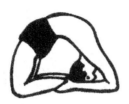

KAPOTASANA

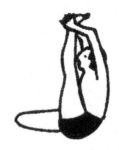

KROUNCHASANA

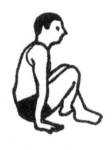

LOLASANA

MALASANA

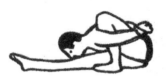

MARICYASANA I

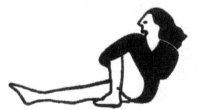

MARICYASANA III

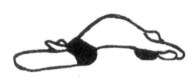

MATSYASANA

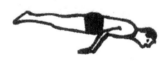

MAYURASANA

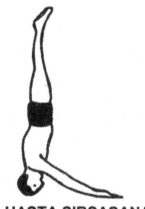

MUKTA HASTA SIRSASANA

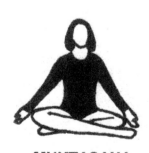

MUKTASANA

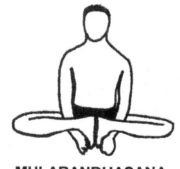

MULABANDHASANA

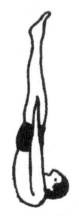

**NIRALAMBA
SARVANGASANA**

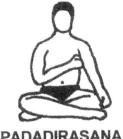

PADADIRASANA

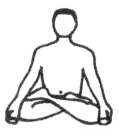

PADMASANA

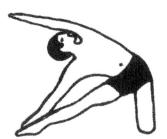

PARIGHASANA

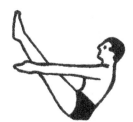

PARIPURNA NAVASANA

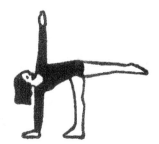

PARIVRTTA ARDHA CHANDRASANA

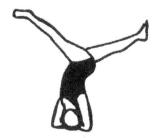

PARIVRTTAIKAPADA SIRSASANA

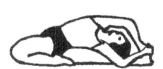

PARIVRTTA JANU SIRSASANA

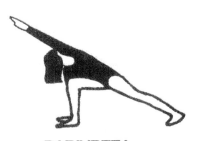

PARIVRTTA PARSVAKONASANA

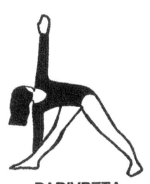

PARIVRTTA TRIKONASANA

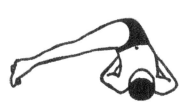

PARSVA HALASANA

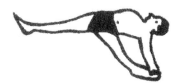

PARSVA HASTA PADANGUSTHASANA

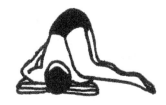

PARSVA KARNAPIDASANA

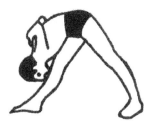

PARSVOTTANASANA

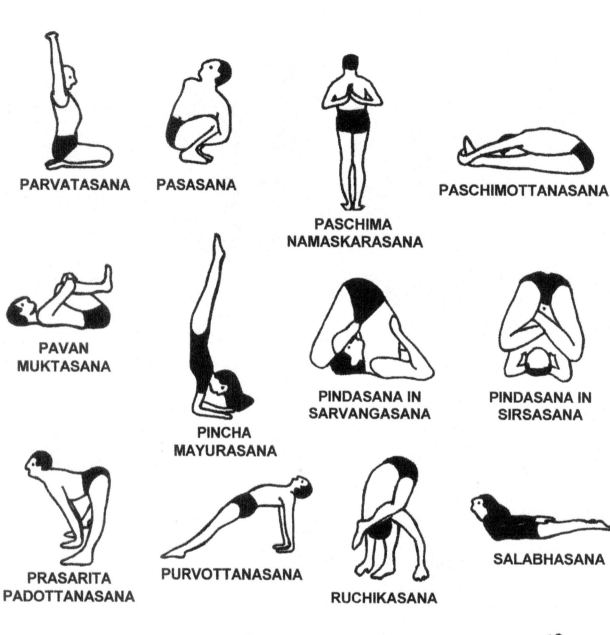

PARVATASANA

PASASANA

PASCHIMA NAMASKARASANA

PASCHIMOTTANASANA

PAVAN MUKTASANA

PINCHA MAYURASANA

PINDASANA IN SARVANGASANA

PINDASANA IN SIRSASANA

PRASARITA PADOTTANASANA

PURVOTTANASANA

RUCHIKASANA

SALABHASANA

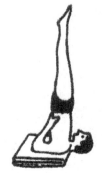

SALAMBA SARVANGASANA

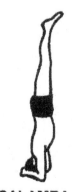

SALAMBA SIRSASANA I

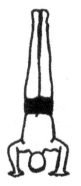

SALAMBA SIRSASANA II

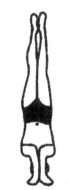

SIRSASANA III

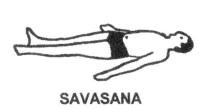

SAVASANA

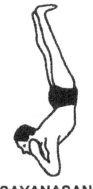

SAYANASANA

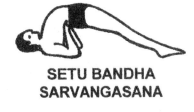

SETU BANDHA SARVANGASANA

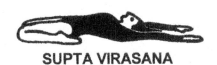

SUPTA VIRASANA

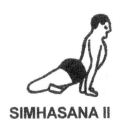

SIMHASANA II

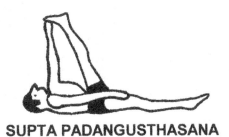

SUPTA PADANGUSTHASANA

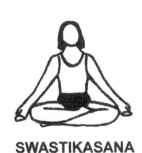

SWASTIKASANA

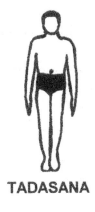

TADASANA

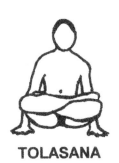

TOLASANA

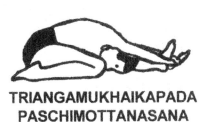

TRIANGAMUKHAIKAPADA PASCHIMOTTANASANA

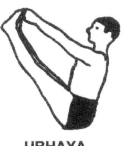

UBHAYA PADANGUSTHASANA

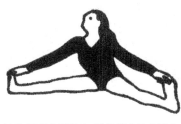

UPAVISTHA KONASANA

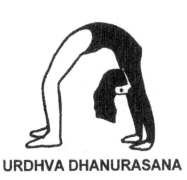

URDHVA DHANURASANA

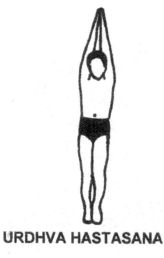

URDHVA HASTASANA

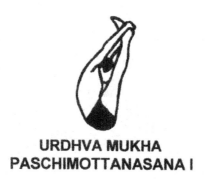

URDHVA MUKHA
PASCHIMOTTANASANA I

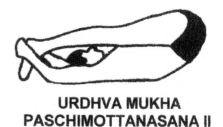

URDHVA MUKHA
PASCHIMOTTANASANA II

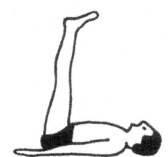

URDHVA PRASARITA
PADASANA

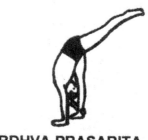

URDHVA PRASARITA
EKAPADASANA

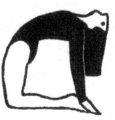

USTRASANA

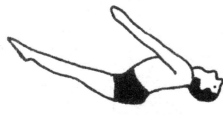

UTTANA PADASANA

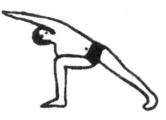

UTTHITA
PARSVAKONASANA

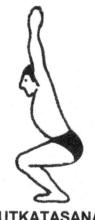

UTKATASANA

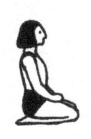

VAJRASANA

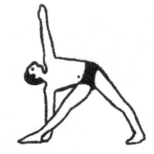

UTTHITA TRIKONASANA

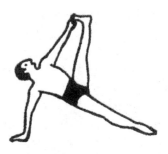

VASISTHASANA

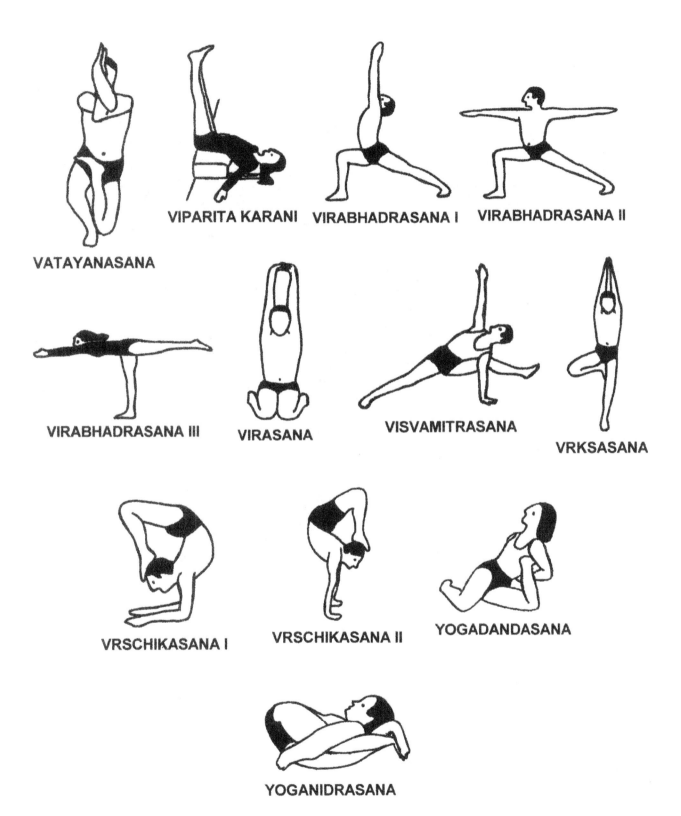

VIPARITA KARANI   VIRABHADRASANA I   VIRABHADRASANA II

VATAYANASANA

VIRABHADRASANA III   VIRASANA   VISVAMITRASANA   VRKSASANA

VRSCHIKASANA I   VRSCHIKASANA II   YOGADANDASANA

YOGANIDRASANA

Appendix 11

Injuries Incurred by Improper Yogasana Practice

Section II.A: Philosophy

Given that the practice of the *yogasanas* can have such a profoundly beneficial effect on a student's physiology, health, personality, philosophy, etc., it is not surprising that *yogasanas* performed improperly can lead to results that actually are harmful. That is to say, *yogasana* practice is a powerful tool, and like a sharp razor, it may do more harm than good in careless or unknowing hands.

"Improper" practice is taken to mean that the postures were done is such a way as to have led to an injury. Ignoring the many, many hearsay stories of injuries incurred in *yogasana* practice, there are nonetheless a significant number of scientific reports in the medical literature concerning such injuries, about which the *yogasana* teacher and practitioner should be aware. These medical reports of serious injury resulting from improper *yogasana* practice form the basis of this appendix.

Unfortunately, the *yogasana* injury reports in question have been written by medical personnel who have no training in yoga, and though the reports are medically complete, they often seem to have omitted vital yogic information, such as the style of yoga being practiced, the possible use of props, their teacher's instructions, or which foot was placed on top of the other thigh. Further, being unschooled in the art of *yogasana,* these medical writers often conclude by condemning *yogasana* practice, without understanding that there is a safe way to do these postures but that the safe way requires an attentive student and a competent teacher [435a]. The situation is not unlike what it would be if a *yogasana* teacher were to pick up a scalpel and attempt surgery with little or no training, and then, looking at the poor results, proclaim surgery to be nothing more than deceitful quackery and a sham!

The following subsections touch briefly upon a few general situations that can lead to injury, as suggested by the specific case histories given in Section II.B, page 835.

Practicing *Yogasanas* from a Book without a Teacher

Because we so easily fool ourselves in regard to our body and what it is doing at any moment, it generally is not a good idea for beginners to practice *yogasanas* using only a book (even a very good book), without input from a teacher (preferably a very good teacher). Those who do so either out of necessity or for philosophical reasons at the very least run the risk of teaching the body the incorrect way to perform the *yogasanas,* and at the worst, they risk injury. The beginning student who has "learned yoga" from a book not only runs a higher risk of being injured unnecessarily but can be a big problem once he or she finds a competent teacher, for considerable erasing of the old technique often has to be done in order to implant the proper technique; indeed, old habits die hard.[1]

---

1   Yes, I am aware of the irony of telling you in this book that you should not try to learn yoga from a book. But I presume that you are not a beginner and that you already know how to take care of yourself.

Being Too Tired Can Lead to Injury

Even with proper technique, the tendency toward misalignment will intrude once one has been in the posture for a substantial time, so that the mood has become more meditative and less concerned with mechanical technique. Related to this is the collapse that often occurs when the student is still in the posture but receives the signal from the teacher to release from the posture. One observes, for example, that many more students lose their balance when coming out of *trikonasana* than when going into it, most likely for reasons of mental and physical fatigue. This premature relaxation of the body's alignment while still in a compromising position can lead to injury (Subsection 11.A, page 400).

Being Too Ambitious Can Lead to Injury

It is natural that when a student is a quick learner, he or she becomes infatuated with *yogasana* practice and wants to try everything in the book as soon as possible. This ambitious attitude can place unwary students in deep water before they are ready for more demanding postures, and so sets the stage for an injury. My own experience in this is that the too-quick student will want to learn "how to stand on my head" and "how to do the lotus position," often before they understand how to do them safely. One must remind the student that *yogasana* practice is intended for a lifetime and that all of the postures do not have to be mastered before age twenty-one! Approaching these postures with caution is not only the safe way, but it also helps the students to control the tendency to go faster in all aspects of their lives. Moreover, as Schatz [758] has pointed out, overly ambitious women who choose to practice demanding postures during their menstrual period may be working with diminished strength and energy and so risk injury. The pros and cons of

doing inversions during the menstrual period are given in Subsection 21.A, page 742.

Yoga Sutras

In regard to *yogasana* and ambition, it is relevant to mention Yoga Sutra II.46:

sthira sukham asanam

In this, the word *sthira* may be translated as "strength, alertness, firmness, or control" and the word *sukham* is translated as "ease, comfort, and openness." Thus:

> *Asana is perfect firmness of body,*
> *steadiness of intelligence,*
> *and benevolence of spirit*
> [401].

I interpret the phrase "benevolence of spirit" to mean without regard to the outcome of the action and performed with a pure heart, free of any ambition or self-aggrandizing goal. If we are overly ambitious or misdirected in our *yogasana* practice, we will fall short of the yogic ideal. Of course, it is difficult at first to be able to perform the *yogasanas* with both strength and firmness, all the while being at ease and comfortable—again the yogic paradox of the simultaneous presence of opposites.

Congenital Weaknesses

Even with an attentive student working with a competent teacher, there is still the possibility of injury due to an unsuspected congenital weakness in the student's body that is uncovered in a particular *yogasana*, even when done correctly. Thus, some students may be injured immediately on performing a particular *yogasana*, and others may do the same *yogasana* in the same way for a lifetime and not experience any problem. The difference here is that in the former case, the student was born with a congenital weakness that was exposed by the *yogasana*, whereas in the latter, the body was strong enough to tolerate the stress of the posture, at least for the short term. This inher-

---

However, I must say as well that even very experienced teachers can hurt themselves in their practice.

ent variability of susceptibility to injury must be kept in mind, and one must realize that even if everything in a posture is in alignment and is otherwise letter-perfect, a congenital weakness can still be present that sooner or later expresses itself as an injury. Further, what is proper for very experienced practitioners will not necessarily be appropriate for beginner and intermediate students, no matter how healthy they might be.

Medically Certified Injuries

One can go too far in condemning *yogasana* practice on the basis of a few medically certified injuries. Thus, Russell [730] has pointed out that, for example, the basilar-artery syndrome (see below) can be precipitated not only by incorrectly performing *yogasanas* such as *sarvangasana* or *bhujangasana,* but also in such innocent situations as tipping one's head back in the dentist's chair, during anesthesia, having a shampoo at the hairdresser's, picking fruit, painting a ceiling, driving a car, swimming the breast stroke, or presiding over a meeting [57, 888]. Certainly none of these are flagged by doctors or by the general public as being too dangerous to consider, and *yogasana* injuries should be given the same benefit of the doubt. Still, not to trivialize the risks in some of the *yogasanas,* students should work on these postures with a knowledgeable teacher and avoid staying too long in static positions (see below).

X-Rated Postures

Alter's book [7], *Science of Flexibility,* has an entire chapter on what he calls "X-rated" exercises, so called because of their risks; all of these X-rated positions are readily recognized as classical *yogasana* positions or their variations. These include *triangamukhaikapada paschimottanasana* (risk to the knee of the bent leg), *supta virasana* (risk to the knees and spine), *malasana* (knees), *uttanasana* (lower back and knees), various backbends from *urdhva mukha svanasana* to *urdhva dhanurasana* (vertebral artery occlusion), gravity inversion as when inverted in the pelvic swing (blood pressure), and *sarvangasana* and *halasana* (vascular and structural cervical problems).

Many of these postures also have been criti-

cized by the medical establishment as dangerous; however, Katz [435a] has exposed the errors behind these warnings issued by medical personnel having no knowledge of *yogasana* practice. Any injuries that may have occurred in these postures underline the need for beginners to work with experienced teachers when first attempting these postures; there are no documented cases of injuries that I know of when these postures were practiced under the guidance of an experienced *yogasana* teacher.

Section II.B: Specific Case Histories

Neurological Damage

Staying Too Long

It is good and proper to encourage students to stay a little longer in the *yogasanas* than they are inclined to do otherwise. In most students, there is a rapid weakening of the nervous system as the posture is held and a rapidly escalating psychological need to come out of the posture. By keeping oneself in the posture just a little beyond the need to come out, one strengthens the neural circuits that drive the muscles holding the posture erect and develops the willpower necessary to progress in the practice. On the other hand, as the medical literature shows (below), one can stay far too long in the postures, to one's detriment. Ideally, one should work with effort but not to the point of struggle, experiencing discomfort but not pain. Done in this way, the postures will show strength and steadiness and at the same time an ease and grace characteristic of the even, focused mind [194]. Resist the temptation to doze in postures that feel very comfortable.

Bone-on-Bone or Bone-on-Floor Contact

In certain postures, one has bone pressing against bone, with muscles and nerves caught between (Section 7.F, page 252), as with the lower legs in *padmasana* or the biceps/triceps pressing the femur in *maricyasana III*; in others, there is a tourniquet effect, and joints close so as to restrict the circulation of blood past the joint, as happens at the knees in *vajrasana,* for example. In such cases, the result is a slowing of the blood flow through the region in question with a consequent decrease in the oxygen being brought to the cells. This slow starvation of the nerves and muscles by compression is of little consequence when the *yogasana* is performed for a short time but can become a serious factor when one feels comfortable in the position and so stays for an extended period. Nerve cells are especially sensitive to this ischemia, for they do not tolerate a lack of oxygen (hypoxia) very well. As discussed below, staying in postures with bone-on-bone or bone-on-floor contact for too long a time creates an ischemic condition, resulting in temporary or even permanent injury to the associated afferent and efferent nerves; i.e., a neuropathy. See for example [882], which describes the bilateral neuropathy of the sciatic nerves in a student who fell asleep in *paschimottanasana* for four hours while under the influence of oral narcotics and an antidepressant. Due to extended compression of the sciatic nerves in the gluteal region, this *yogasana* student lost the use of both of her lower legs (tibial and peroneal fascicles) for at least six months due to a lack of sensory signals below the knee and the weakness of virtually all of the muscles in the lower leg; her doctors question as to whether she will regain full use of the limbs.

In the case of an afferent nerve being injured by compression, the symptoms are a tingling sensation followed by a numbing loss of sensation. If, instead, it is the efferent nerve that is injured, then one has all degrees of loss of muscle control, deliberate and reflexive (Subsection 3.E, page 61). An apparent blockage of the afferent nerves in the upper chest (thoracic outlet syndrome) is reported by Dr. Timothy McCall, who experienced tingling in the arm while staying in *sirsasana* for ten minutes; the tingling sensation receded once he quit *sirsasana* practice [548]. He concludes that not all *yogasana* poses will be suitable for all students.

In addition to ischemia, pressure on the nerves also may result in their demyelination; i.e., a partial or total stripping of the fatty covering of the nerves that is so essential for their neural conductivity (Section 3.B, page 42). When this happens, as in the case of multiple sclerosis, the nerve and the associated sensor or muscle are more or less incapacitated. Yet another possible consequence of external pressure on a nerve is the impediment to the vital flow of internal components within the axon, between the body of the neural cell and its axonal and dendritic tips (Subsection 3.A, page 35).

Consider the case of a meditation student who is reported to have fallen asleep in full *padmasana* for more than three hours [546]. On the next day, the student felt a tingling from the hip to the upper knee on the right side, and after twenty-four hours, the tingling became numbness, with no sensations of pinprick, temperature, or light touch in the area. Apparently the extended time in a position where the afferent sensory nerve on the right upper thigh was so compressed by the left foot that the nerve suffered an ischemia was sufficient to deaden the response of the nerve for more than a month. Not only does the pressure of the ankle on the opposite upper thigh in *padmasana* compress the nerve directly and so interfere with its oxygenation, but it also contributes to a more general ischemia, in that each foot and ankle rests upon the femoral artery of the opposite leg so as to attenuate the overall blood supply to the lower body.

In a somewhat similar case [875], another student of meditation spent two hours sitting with crossed legs, heels under thighs (presumably *muktasana, vajrasana,* or a variation thereof). In this case, the afferent sensory nerves were not damaged; however, the ankle-stretch reflex (foot drop) was affected and was still inactive three weeks after the meditation due to the denervation of the muscles served by the peroneal and tibial components of the sciatic nerve (see below). Apparently, the weight of the body pressing down on the efferent nerves of the lower legs was sufficient to demyelinate the nerves locally, resulting in the loss of the relevant muscle responses [875].

The Sciatic Nerve

Let us consider for a moment the structure and geography of the sciatic nerve, as it is often involved in such neurological injuries. This nerve bundle is composed of five nerves exiting the spine at vertebrae L4, L5, S1, S2, and S3 [295, 483], and it travels diagonally left and right across the back of the pelvis, between the pelvic bones and the piriformis muscles deep within the buttocks (figure 9.B-2c). Each of the bundles then travels down the back of its respective leg, and in the vicinity of the knee, it branches into a smaller division, one part of which stays on the outer surface of the lower leg (the peroneal component), and a larger bundle, which takes a route on the inside of the lower leg (the tibial component). Of the two branches, it is said that the tibial component is the more susceptible to injury by compression [839, 871]. A tributary of the sciatic nerve in the upper leg (the femoral cutaneous branch) innervates the inner, upper thigh [295].

The piriformis muscle runs horizontally, deep in the buttocks, connecting the lower edge of the sacrum to the inner aspect of the greater trochanter (figure 9.B-2c). The sciatic nerve runs vertically and usually passes between the piriformis muscle and the pelvic bone, but in 15 percent of the people, the sciatic nerve actually passes through the piriformis muscle. Piriformis syndrome (sciatica) results when the piriformis muscle is tight and compresses the sciatic nerve, especially in the unlucky 15 percent. Any sport that tightens the hamstrings and buttock muscles can result in piriformis syndrome, and running and cycling are frequently implicated. People who stand habitually with the front thighs rotated externally will promote piriformis tension and thus suffer piriformis syndrome [218]. Should the sciatic nerve penetrate the piriformis muscle, the sciatic discomfort is severe but still treatable through *yogasana* practice. This syndrome is promoted by prolonged sitting, by strenuous spinal twisting, and by falling onto one's buttocks. However, piriformis stretching will relieve sciatica symptoms [328].

In the case mentioned above of the student dozing in *padmasana,* the compressed nerve would appear to be the femoral cutaneous branch of the sciatic nerve, whereas for the student sitting in *muktasana,* the compression was below the knee, more likely where bone presses bone in the crossed-leg position and most likely involving the tibial component of the sciatic nerve in the lower leg.

Yet another meditator commonly sat in *vajrasana* for up to six hours a day, "chanting for world peace" [116, 309]. The result was what is now called "yoga foot drop" in the medical literature, consisting of a loss of muscle strength in the ankles and toes so that the foot cannot be dorsiflexed (toes toward the knee). This outcome was attributed to peroneal neuropathy as a consequence of compression of the relevant efferent sciatic nerves.

Sciatic neuropathies can develop in many seemingly innocent situations. Thus, it is reported that loss of leg strength can occur when the sciatic nerve is compressed for hours on end, as when lying in a coma, when one is bedridden and unable to move to a fresh position, or when having fallen asleep while sitting on the toilet [830, 870, 882]. More bizarre are two independent cases of intense sciatic discomfort brought on by carrying a wallet stuffed with credit cards in the hip pocket of one's trousers [526]! In one of these credit-card cases, the patient earlier had been diagnosed as having a herniated disc and had received chiropractic treatment for his problem.

Ischemia

The effects of compression leading to ischemia of an efferent nerve and paralysis of the relevant muscle are readily demonstrated in two situations familiar to *yogasana* students. First, being in *supta virasana,* for many students, brings on a temporary neuropathy of the nerves in the lower legs due to the heightened pressure at the backs of the folded knees and to the restriction of blood flow below the knees. As a consequence of these effects, after five minutes in *supta virasana,* many students have momentary difficulty standing and walking. A similar momentary paralysis can occur in the arm by sitting cross-legged with the arms in *gomukhasana* and then carefully lying down on the back, thus pinning one arm between the floor and the back body with its hand between the shoulder blades. The weight of the upper body pressing on the nerves of the upper arm for just a minute or two appears to be enough to paralyze the arm for a short time. For those who are susceptible to this type of compression-induced ischemia, it is frightening to think of what the result might be if they were to stay in a position such as this for an extended time.

Vascular Damage

Thrombosis

The inner surfaces of the vascular system are tightly covered with endothelial cells, which keep the platelets that circulate within the system from contact with any of the collagenous material in the outer layers. If the artery or vein is so compressed in a *yogasana* that the integrity of the endothelium is breached, then platelets may gather at the exposed spot, forming a blood clot (a thrombus). The thrombus may grow to cut off circulation in the blood vessel in which it occurs, or it may break loose to form a mobile embolus that may then plug smaller vessels in other parts of the vascular tree. As the tendency to form blood clots is inherited [315], problems of this sort may show up as a congenital weakness in an otherwise strong *yogasana* student.

Note as well that if the blood supply in a limb is cut off for an extended time, as when soaking in a posture, the blood trapped in the limb is then stagnant and easily forms clots when in that state.

The *yogasana*-induced thrombosis/embolism scenarios are most often involved either with the blood vessels of the eyes (often in inverted poses) or with the vertebral arteries of the cervical spine (often with external pressure on the vertebrae or inappropriate turning of the head). It is also advised that inversions be performed only with the help of a qualified teacher if one has glaucoma, detached retina, high blood pressure, heart disease, hiatal hernia, or spinal problems.

It goes without saying that if one has a pre-existing vascular problem, such as varicose veins, one should not spend any length of time in postures that otherwise would further impede venous return from the area in question; i.e., one should not do *padmasana*, for example, if one already has varicosities in the legs.

It is known that pressure on the inside of the upper arm acts to close the axillary vein and that this can lead to thrombosis [619]. Though there are no medical reports on this vis-à-vis *yogasana*, one easily imagines such a situation developing were a student to spend too long a time in either *maricyasana I* or *III*, for in both of these postures, the axillary vein can be pressed tightly against the tibia.

Vertebral Arteries

In traveling up the cervical spine, the vertebral arteries are threaded through openings in the bony transverse processes of vertebrae C6–C1 and then pass through the foramen magnum on their way to the posterior brain (figure 4.E-1). The blood supplies to the medulla oblongata, pons, mesencephalon, and cerebellum are derived from the vertebral basilar-artery system [606]. Serious thrombi or occlusions in the brain can occur when the vertebral arteries are injured, as can happen when flexing the neck or turning the head, especially when the head and neck are bearing weight.

There is a report in the literature [247] of an unfortunate student who performed *sirsasana* without adequate supervision, in her quest for "self-relaxation." In this, a young student is reported to have performed *sirsasana* without a teacher and with only two months' home practice. After five minutes in the position, she felt a sharp pain in the neck, and two months after that, she reported to her doctor that she had only partial feeling and weak muscle control on the right side of the body and a declining level of consciousness. It was concluded that in doing *sirsasana*, she had injured the vertebral arteries in the neck, leading in time to a thrombus in the basilar artery, which is fed by the vertebral arteries. In time, the thrombus was set free in the vascular system, and the embolus so formed found its way into the left hemisphere of the brain, where it interfered eventually with muscle action on the right side of the body. In hindsight, one would guess that the student had placed her head on the floor too close to the hairline, so as to place the neck in extreme extension, and then went inverted without working the arms against the floor; this combination of errors would lead to a shearing action of the cervical vertebrae with respect to the vertebral arteries (Subsection 4.E, page 116). The student returned to near-normal after a year of treatment.

A similarly unfortunate outcome is reported for a *yogasana* student, again working without a teacher or proper instruction [311]. In this case, a young man performed an "inverted standing" (presumably *sarvangasana)* for five minutes every day for eighteen months, without blankets under the shoulders but with his shoulders and head pressed maximally against the bare floor. By the time the student went to the doctor, he was dizzy, was unable to walk, and had bruises over vertebrae C5, C6, and C7; after two months of therapy, he could walk again with a cane. His doctor reports a lesion in the medulla oblongata within the brainstem (Section 4.B, page 72) as the causative factor, most likely induced by the intensity of the posture. The doctor concludes that "inverted standing" on the shoulders and head could be especially dangerous in the elderly, with their underlying vascular and arthritic problems.

Based on this unfortunate event, others have published blanket warnings against doing *halasana* (figure 14.F-2c), without distinguishing between the harm that can come from performing the posture incorrectly and the benefits that it gives when performed carefully, with proper preparation and attention to alignment and the lengthening of the spine [207, 618]. In response to these claims, Lasater has written eloquently, refuting their arguments in every detail [483]. In cases such as the above, the student was not being taught properly, if at all, and furthermore, had blankets been used in the way prescribed for *sarvangasana* and *halasana* [404, 483], the chances for such unfortunate results would have been considerably reduced.

Nagler [606] reports three cases of injury traced to active hyperextension of the cervical spine. In the first, a young student in *adho mukha vrksasana* vigorously pulled his head back as he lost balance backward (overbalance; see figure V.D-2b), inducing an obstruction of the vertebral artery; he was still in a wheelchair eighteen months after the incident. A fifty-five-year-old man performing what appears to have been *salabhasana* forcefully placed his neck in extension in the posture and immediately found that he could not walk or lift his arms. Again, the diagnosis was an occlusion of the vertebral artery and the resulting ischemia. Lastly, a young "yoga enthusiast," while in *urdhva dhanurasana* with her head on the floor, was said to have suffered a cerebellar infarction due to the shutting off of the blood supply in the cervical area. Accidents of this sort are much more likely in those with a congenital disposition toward vertebral occlusion on cervical extension; however, one cannot know one's disposition in this regard until it is tested!

The vertebral artery is most subject to damage at the atlanto-axoid joint between C1 and C2, the point of maximum movement when turning the head to the side. Though no injuries are reported in this regard for *yogasana* students performing spinal twists, the medical literature is rife with reports of people who suffer seriously impeded blood flow to the brain and consequent neurological damage when they turned their heads abruptly but in a seemingly benign manner [784]. For this reason, side-to-side turning of the head would be especially dangerous for a *yogasana* student in postures that are load-bearing on the cervical vertebrae, such as *halasana, sarvangasana,* and their variations.

Rapid movement of the head and/or extreme neck pressure can lead to "arterial dissection," where the formation of a hole in the lining of one of the vertebral arteries leads to a clot forming and thence possibly to a stroke (Subsection 4.E, page 117). This dissection is possible in *sirsasana, parsvakonasana, trikonasana, sarvangasana,* and *halasana*. Extreme neck pressure in the last two mentioned *yogasanas* is minimized by placing padding under the shoulders but not under the head, as shown in figure 14.F-2d. The rate of arterial dissection is only fifteen per million Americans, but it accounts for 2 percent of the strokes and is one of the major causes of stroke in younger people. This sort of vertebral-artery dissection is closely related to the dissection of the aorta when performing a strong muscular action assisted by the Valsalva maneuver (Subsection 15.C, page 616).

Eye Damage

Excessive effort in the *yogasanas* often reveals itself in the eyes. This is possibly due to a fragility of the veins in the eyes and to the fact that at the eyes, the hydrostatic pressure of the blood in inversions is not compensated by that of the cerebrospinal fluid (Section 14.F, page 584).

A *yogasana* teacher with many years' experience was found to have a thrombus in a vein serving one eye; it was concluded in her case that positions such as *sirsasana,* in which the head is below the heart, were a mitigating factor in the development of what was likely a congenital condition [136]. In a similar case, the connection between *yogasana* and thrombosis around the eyes was thought to be much stronger. In this situation [538], the student had performed *sirsasana* for ten minutes, ten times daily for ten years before noticing blue-purple nodules within the conjunctiva of the eyes. It was hypothesized that the thrombi were caused by the increased venous pressure in the eyes, coupled with decreased venous outflow accompanying the inverted position; they were repaired surgically. No mention was made of whether this eager student followed any of his *sirsasana* work with a relaxing *sarvangasana.*

A student who daily performed *sirsasana* and *sarvangasana,* for fifteen to twenty minutes each, allowed his ophthalmologist to measure the intraocular pressures within his eyes as he performed a meditative seated pose, *urdhva dhanurasana, sarvangasana,* and *sirsasana,* recording pressures of 18, 25, 28 and 32 millimeters Hg for these four positions [703]. All pressures returned immediately to the baseline pressure on returning to sitting. It was concluded that inverted postures such as these significantly increased intraocular

pressure and so should be discouraged in those with glaucoma or a tendency toward it. However, it was not mentioned whether the subject of this study was Iyengar-trained or not.

Consider the case described by Fahmy and Fledelius [233], in which a woman who reported episodes of blurred vision following *yogasana* practice was found to have an elevated internal pressure in the fluid of the eyes (momentary glaucoma). Though this increased pressure did not appear after being in *sarvangasana* for one hour, it did appear following one hour in a face-down prone position. Normal pressure returned during the night. Investigation showed that the eyes in this particular case were formed in such a way so as to allow the lens and the iris to collapse upon one another in the face-down position (as in *salabhasana*), thereby pressurizing the internal fluid. This would be a case of a congenital defect in the structure of the eye, combined with an unfortunate choice of *yogasanas* for practice.

The types of eye problems discussed above can be brought about by any extreme effort in which one holds the breath and increases the internal abdominal pressure by tightening the abdominal muscles and closing the throat (the Valsalva maneuver; see Subsection 15.C, page 616). Most healthy people can perform this maneuver without harm, but it is risky for those with cardiovascular conditions. Beginners often resort to this action in an effort to amplify their strength, but this is clearly contraindicated for any but the most advanced *yogasana* practitioners. Perhaps it was this type of action that brought on the problem in the case cited above.

Pranayama

Though many studies have shown the physiological and psychological benefits of *pranayama* practice, adverse side effects can follow when the body is pushed to extremes. There is a tragic story in the literature of a young woman who died of an embolus said to be directly related to her practice of *pranayama* [161]; however, it involved mouth-to-mouth breathing with another student and the heavy use of marijuana. The practice of *kapalabhati pranayama* has been implicated in a case of spontaneous pneumothorax, in which air was found to have accumulated between the two layers of the pleura in the chest cavity, resulting in the partial collapse of the lung [416].

Muscular Damage

Though the favorite topic of conversation among assembled *yogasana* students is their latest muscle pull, spasm, or skeletal pain, I could find no record of such complaints having been taken to a doctor and then finding their way into the medical literature. As discussed in Subsection 11.E, page 467, a proper warm-up should precede any serious attempt at performing a *yogasana* that is challenging. This warm-up will give the muscles a good stretch, lubricate the joints involved, and start the flow of glucose from the liver. Only then is it safe to attempt the more difficult postures.

When doing any of the *yogasanas,* difficult or not, it is important that one does not try to stretch too quickly; if the student will allow himself to ease into the posture slowly and on an exhalation, then there will be no tearing of the muscle fibers as they are stretched (Subsection 11.E, page 467).

When done to excess, eccentric isotonic exercise (Subsection 11.A, page 408) can lead to rhabdomyolysis, a condition in which muscle tissue has been destroyed on a large scale, leading to the appearance of muscle-cell debris in the urine and a fatal blocking of the kidneys by myoglobin leaking from the damaged muscles [177].

Appendix III
Body Symmetry

Section III.A: Symmetry, Beauty, and Health

Sexual Selection

It is clear that animals can be very selective in picking a mate. In this, one wonders just what criteria are used in rejecting one suitor and accepting another. For many animals, it appears that disease or weakness is reflected in a lack of left-right symmetry in the body. Indeed, experiments show that the criterion for selective mating in many animals is high left-right mirror symmetry, for high symmetry is synonymous with fertility, physical and mental health, optimal hormonal function, and sexual prowess. Thus, by the simple assessment of lateral symmetry, animals can assure a strong, healthy mate, free of disease and weakness, and thereby increase the chances of having strong, healthy progeny [665, 878]. This criterion is known to be a factor in mate selection in insects, birds, many other animals, and subconsciously in humans as well [504, 665]. It is also known that insect pollinators are more attracted to symmetric flowers than to asymmetric flowers.

Human Symmetry

It is not unreasonable that humans tend to equate high skeletal symmetry with a strong and healthy mate who can supply strong and healthy progeny, whereas a lack of this left-right mirror symmetry implies physical collapse of some sort and less than perfect health. In humans, there appears to be a link between left-right asymmetry in the body and aggression, for people with the largest side-to-side differences in the sizes of their ears, big toes, or hands are those most easily provoked into aggressive responses.

Beauty

Among humans, symmetry also is a factor in beauty in all cultures, and beauty is very important in choosing a mate. Tests of perceived facial beauty for both men and women consistently show that those who are thought to be "most beautiful" have the highest left-right facial symmetry [665].[1]

Our faces reveal our emotions, health, fertility, and general suitability for perpetuating the species. Women's features become even more symmetric as they approach the most fertile point in their menstrual cycles, thereby increasing their attractiveness to men [818].

Positive emotions such as joy, warmth, and affection are processed primarily in the left cerebral hemisphere, whereas negative emotions such as anger, fear, and disgust are processed primarily by the right cerebral hemisphere. However, due to decussation, the positive emotions of the left cerebral hemisphere distort the face more strongly on the right side, whereas the negative emotions of the right cerebral hemisphere distort the face more strongly on the left side of the face [348].

---

1   However, do not confuse "most beautiful" with "most interesting."

Thus, when smiles are asymmetric right to left, it is the right side of the smile that is accented. That infants in the womb prefer to turn their heads to the right (as do people who are kissing) and fetuses most often suck their right thumbs in utero shows clearly that left-right hemispheric discrimination is functioning in utero.

There are also molecular forces at work in human mate selection [134]. It has been found that a woman prefers a man's face that is most like her own, which can be translated as showing that the eyes of women prefer a mate with a face displaying a group of immune-system genes (the major histocompatibility complex) similar to that of her own. In contrast, the noses of women prefer a mate with a somewhat different major histocompatibility complex, as determined from the smell of sweat.

The natural conjunction of the concepts "beauty" and "symmetry" is a well-known facet of the most profound theories of the mathematical physicists. That is to say, the most profound theories of the nature of matter and the universe often share elements of high mathematical symmetry, which bring those who understand them to say that they are absolutely "beautiful" [569]. This developing union of science and art within physics is already flowering in the world of Iyengar Yoga, where it is held that "The whole body should be symmetrical. Yoga is symmetry. That is why yoga is a basic art [393]."

Asymmetry

Organisms having bilateral (left-right) symmetry can be found in species having lived as far back as 550 million years ago. The flip side of the relation between symmetry and beauty is that we all show a reluctance and unease in having to look at asymmetric deformities in others. This may relate to the unavoidable empathy that we show for others through the actions of the mirror neurons (Subsection 4.G, page 142).

Luckily, we have few opportunities for looking into one another's bodies, for in spite of the superficial high symmetry of the body as seen from the outside, the inside of the body is quite

asymmetrical. This is odd, for the adult human body, as seen from the front, appears to be highly symmetric across the midsagittal plane dividing left from right. There are two equally placed cerebral hemispheres, two eyes, two nostrils, two arms and two legs, etc., and with only one mouth and one nose, even these are placed symmetrically on the midsagittal plane. Even the external symmetry is more apparent than real, since each of the pairs mentioned above has one partner of the pair that is functionally dominant, often in a way that depends upon what the task is at the moment.

In the early stages of human embryonic development, the embryo is perfectly symmetric until the heart starts to form. However, from that point on, the asymmetries begin to accumulate. It is known that in the embryo, the placement of the heart and liver are dictated by gene expression, so that if the genes are active on the right side, the liver is formed there, whereas the heart forms on the left, where the genes do not operate [541]. Looking within (figure 19.A-1), other asymmetries abound. There are two lungs, but the left one is divided into only two lobes because of space constraints, whereas the right lobe is divided into three. Also, the left and right bronchi are tilted at different angles so that if an object is inhaled into the lungs, it always will be found lodged in the right lung. Note also that according to Ayurvedic thinking, the long-term lack of symmetry when breathing alternately through the nostrils (Section 15.E, page 633) is a strong signal for incipient disease or an unhealthy condition [473].

There is only one heart, but it is not placed symmetrically in the chest, nor is it right-left symmetric. The left side of the heart is larger and stronger than the right, as it pumps blood through the entire body, whereas the right side only pumps it through the lungs [5]. Kimball [450] points out that the drainage of the lymph from the upper portions of the body is very different on the left and right sides of the torso. This is used to rationalize the effects of asymmetric pressure on the armpits to direct nasal laterality (Section 15.E, page 634).

The other internal organs are even more asymmetric: the liver, gallbladder, spleen, stomach, and colon are placed in the abdominal cavity on the basis of packing efficiency, without regard for symmetry.[2] Furthermore, though the vagus nerve (cranial nerve X) branches to both the left and the right, the left branch reaches only to the upper stomach, whereas the right branch continues on to innervate almost all of the abdominal organs, being far more extensive and important than the left branch [626]. The internal asymmetry of the human body may be responsible for much or all of the asymmetric weight distribution observed for students in *tadasana* (Section IV.D, page 861).

Coren [159] points out that in gymnasts who are both right-handed and right-eyed, the center of gravity is moved noticeably to the right in their bodies, and this tends to introduce a twisting motion to their performance. If true, the same effect would be present in the *yogasana* student having a simultaneous preference for the right hand and the right eye; i.e., clockwise and counterclockwise twisting postures may feel very different on the two sides of the body. Right-handed *yogasana* students most often twist their front bodies more easily to the left, bringing the right arm across the front body and the left arm behind. This parallels the fact that such students also find *gomukhasana* easier with the right arm overhead and the left behind, rather than the reverse.

Yogasana

Could the connection between geometry and health be related in some way to our striving for high left-right symmetry in the *yogasanas* when performed in the Iyengar way (*trikonasana*, for example), regardless of the overall inherent asymmetry of the posture? In fact, one of the basic principles of the Iyengar style of *yogasana* teaching is the attempt to recover the high symmetry

---

2   One in every 25,000 babies is born with all of the internal organs transposed to the "wrong side" [51]. This can be a serious threat to health and longevity, for those born with two "right sides" rarely live past the first year, whereas those with two "left sides" have a normal life span.

of *tadasana*, even in the most asymmetric postures. As discussed in Subsection VI.H, page 946, Iyengar [403a] advises that there should be "no contortions in any asana."

Section III.B: Symmetry, Asymmetry, and *Yogasana*

Tadasana Standard

Continuing along this line of thinking, consider *tadasana* to be the standard of high left-right symmetry and thus, indirectly, the standard of optimal strength and health. In going from *tadasana* to one of the less symmetric standing postures (*trikonasana*, for example), is it not reasonable that we nonetheless perform the posture in such a way as to promote strength and health; i.e., we perform the posture with maximal left-right symmetry? But how does one do an inherently asymmetric posture with maximal symmetry? The answer to this is to perform these globally asymmetric postures in a way that the **local** symmetry is as high as it can be, given the nature of the posture. Referring to *trikonasana*, we attempt to perform as many of the relevant *tadasana*-like actions as we can in *trikonasana*, trying to keep the **local** left-right mirror symmetry as high as possible and avoiding collapse in all parts of the body; see Subsection 9.B, page 320, and Box III.B-1, below, for more detailed examples of what is meant here.

Top-to-Bottom Symmetry

Going beyond left-right mirror symmetry, there is a second element of symmetry to be considered occasionally when discussing *yogasanas*: many inverted postures have their complements in the standing postures, and the proper top-to-bottom symmetry and actions of the inverted posture is just that appropriate to the complementary standing posture. Thus, virtually all of the actions appropriate to *adho mukha vrksasana*

Box III.B-1: Preserving the Symmetry of *Tadasana* in *Trikonasana*

Tadasana is as symmetric as one can get with respect to the left-right mirror plane of the body. Let us first list all of the local symmetry elements present in *tadasana*:

1. Back body (back of head, scapula, buttocks, little fingers, calves, and heels) in a vertical plane
2. Legs active and straight with foot, ankle, and knee of each leg in alignment
3. The axes of the spine (vertical) and of the pelvis (horizontal) are mutually perpendicular, whereas the axes of the shoulder girdle and of the pelvis are parallel
4. The distance from the right iliac crest to the lowest right rib is equal to that from the left iliac crest to the corresponding rib on the left
5. Normal spinal curvatures, with cervical vertebrae in line with those of the thoracic spine left to right
6. Lifting the energy from the pit of the abdomen into the chest, with scapula dropped away from the ears and tipped into the rib cage to open and lift it while lengthening the spine and spreading the collarbones

As compared with *tadasana* symmetry-wise, *trikonasana* has lost the left-right mirror symmetry totally, yet the proper action in *trikonasana* is such as to restore the local symmetry as outlined by the six points above, though of course, one can not restore the global symmetry and still be in the posture. Consider the six points given above, but as applied to *trikonasana*-to-the-right:

1. Rotate legs and ribs so that the back body parts (back of head, scapula, buttocks, backs of the hands, calves, and heels) as much as possible lie on a vertical plane
2. Legs active and straight with the foot, ankle, and knee of each leg in alignment
3. Tip the pelvis so that the axis of the pelvis remains perpendicular to the axis of the spine and parallel to the axis of the shoulders
4. Press the right sitting bone toward the left ankle and lift the right ribs away from the iliac crest on the right, so as to make the two sides of the upper body equally long from pelvis to lowest ribs
5. Maintain normal curvature in the spine, especially in the lumbar, and lift the head so as to keep the cervical vertebrae of the neck in line with the rest of the spine
6. Lift the energy from the pit of the abdomen into the chest, with scapulae dropped away from the ears and tipped into the rib cage to open and lift it while lengthening the spine and spreading the collarbones

When compared in this way, one sees immediately that at a certain low level, the work of *trikonasana* is largely that of trying to restore or preserve the local symmetry around certain key areas of the body while forfeiting the global symmetry. How many of the symmetry-preserving elements of *tadasana* can you find working in *parivrtta trikonasana*?

(figure V.G-1**a**) are found as well in *urdhva has-tasana* (except the neck extension; see Subsection V.D, page 907), its foot-standing complement. In a similar vein, lordosis in *sirsasana I* or kyphosis in *sarvangasana* are no more appropriate in these postures than they would be in *tadasana*, and the actions appropriate for upright *ardha uttanasana* are those appropriate for the inversions *halasana* and *dandasana* in *sirsasana* as well.

Though not as obvious as handedness (Section III.B, below), our bodies also have preferred sides for many other asymmetric motor tasks, such as which foot first steps onto the lowest step when climbing stairs, which eye opens first when slowly opening the eyes, which foot turns out more in *urdhva dhanurasana*, and which index finger crosses over the other when interlacing the fingers. We are similarly bound reflexively when we turn our heads to kiss; it is always in the same direction, usually to the right.

In terms of left-right symmetry, the muscle on the side of neuromuscular dominance is known to be slightly quicker in its action and more easily fatigued, and it contracts to a larger extent than the corresponding muscle on the less-dominant side [822]. The result of such unavoidable muscular imbalance is an asymmetry in movement and even in stance.

Handedness

In addition to the unavoidable asymmetry imposed upon us by the placement of our organs, the preferential handedness in humans also affects our *yogasanas* in a purely mechanical way. For example, it is almost always more difficult for *yogasana* students to place the right hand behind the back in *gomukhasana* than it is to place the left. This is due to habit, for right-handed people "live" in the forward-right quadrant of space, so the backward-right quadrant is foreign to their right hand and thus a difficult place to visit. The same factor would come into play in *ardha baddha padma paschimottanasana*. Interestingly, the right-arm-behind-the-back problem for right-handed students doing *gomukhasana* does not appear as often for left-handed students when placing their left hands behind their backs, again showing that they are less committed to their dominant hand than are the right-handed students. This subject is treated further in Subsection III.C, page 848.

Brain Asymmetry

Though the brain at first sight appears to be left-right symmetric, the inner body's asymmetry penetrates into that region as well. As discussed in more detail in Section 4.D, page 98, the gross symmetry is deceptive, for the corresponding parts in the two hemispheres can have different sizes, and the hemispheres themselves each have their special functions. In 95 percent of the population, the language functions are restricted to the left hemisphere, which is also dominant for manual motor skills in right-handed people. On the other hand, the right hemisphere is dominant for spatial ability, music, and emotional behavior (table 4.D-1). It appears that our brains are about as symmetric as our bodies, which is to say to about the same degree as males and females are alike in their symmetries, functions, and constructions.

To the extent that our lack of left-right symmetry of the cerebral hemispheres may be a factor in the performance of the *yogasanas*, it is interesting to note that the proprioceptive sense of alignment is more accurate on the left side of the body, thanks to the specialization of the right cerebral hemisphere to synthesize global pictures. In the general population, greater strength, coordination, and balance are observed on the side of the dominant hand [7]. However, with the accent in *yogasana* practice on working both the dominant and less dominant sides, one would expect the lateral imbalances to be lessened (see Section 4.D, page 106).

Maintaining Symmetry

That we think of each of the muscles as a distinct entity with a characteristic name is a useful approximation, but nonetheless it is only an approximation, for in truth, the two most widely separated muscles are intimately connected by the web of fascia and connective tissue that surrounds all muscles down to the level of the nuclei within each cell; moreover, this web incorporates the connective tissues that surround the bones and support the internal organs (Section 12.A, page 481). Rolf [714] points out that if we could somehow extract all of the myofibrils from the body of a friend, leaving only the connective tissues, the result would still look recognizably like that person as we ordinarily know him or her.

Given that the internal organs are very asymmetrically placed left and right within the body and that they are held in place by webs of connective tissue (which are themselves just a part of the larger web holding all of the body in its shape), it seems inescapable that the pull of these asymmetric organs on all the muscles of the body must in some small way make the muscle actions similarly asymmetric, as implied by figure 12.B-1. This line of thinking brings us to a seemingly odd impasse: when doing the asymmetric *yogasanas*, one must work to retain as much local symmetry as possible; yet even in the most symmetric posture, *tadasana*, one should sense a great local asymmetry, for that is the nature of our inner construction. See also Box V.F-2, page 920, for an example of how the body's neural crossover can affect our sense of left-right balance. *Trikonasana* done to the left and to the right with sufficient inner awareness must feel different to some degree, in spite of the efforts to make it otherwise; and even *tadasana*, the standard of high symmetry, must be asymmetric to some extent, due to the basic asymmetry of the human body plan. Iyengar has addressed this inherently asymmetric situation from the point of view of the *yogasanas*, recommending that one must acknowledge the basic asymmetries of the body but work to minimize their effects, rather than ignore them and have them become even more pronounced [402]. Thus, for example, one should perform the lateral postures for a longer time on the weaker side to strengthen it and thereby maintain balance between the two sides as much as possible.

A second aspect of asymmetry in the postures is presented by Mehta [557a], who points out that in performing *trikonasana*-to-the-right,

for example, one's consciousness moves strongly to the right, so that the left side of the body is bereft of awareness unless a special effort is made to keep that side of the body alert and alive.

Section III.C: Handedness

Handedness is of interest to students of *yogasana*, because its dominance can be so strong as to force a one-sided dominance on other functions that are otherwise unrelated to handedness. For example, 70–97 percent of humans show left-hemisphere dominance for language specialization and vocalization [432], whereas 90 percent of the population is right-handed, thanks to decussation of the efferent nerves in the spinal cord (Section 4.A, page 69). As shown in table 4.D-2, the dominant hemisphere for speech is the left one for not only right-handed people but for many of the left-handed, as well as the ambidextrous; however, this tendency is much stronger in the right-handed than in the others. In general, left-handed people are more symmetrical than are the right-handed, which is to say, they are less committed to their handedness. The lack of mirror symmetry between the hemispheres for both language specialization and handedness is clouded further by the fact that many people are right-handed for some tasks and left-handed for others. Nonetheless, Corballis [158] has proposed that our right-handedness developed early in the course of human development, at a time when speaking (controlled by the left hemisphere) involved considerable right-hand gesturing (again controlled by the left hemisphere).

If one defines the cerebral hemisphere that controls verbal expression as the dominant hemisphere, then 96–99 percent of right-handed people have a dominant left hemisphere. More specifically, the dominant center resides in the left frontal lobe. For people who are left-handed, 60–70 percent have a dominant left hemisphere; in those cases where the cerebral dominance is on the right side, the center in question is the right frontal lobe [427]. People with a strong excitation in the right prefrontal cortex tend to be more nervous and pessimistic, whereas when the left prefrontal cortex is strongly excited preferentially, the patients show depression.

Cerebral Lobe Asymmetry

The parietal lobe of the dominant hemisphere plays a significant role in calculation, writing, and the reading of words. As the temporal lobes of the brain are closely associated with hearing, injury to the temporal lobe on the dominant side leads to an inability to understand spoken words [621]. Cerebral laterality also seems to have its effect on sexual orientation, for the proportion of left-handed lesbians among left-handed women in the general population is double that of right-handed lesbians among right-handed women in the general population. The more left-handed you are, the larger is the corpus callosum, that

nerve bundle that serves as the main communication highway between the right and left cerebral hemispheres [590]. This would follow from the idea that left-handers are more left-right symmetric than are right-handers (Subsection III.C, page 848). It is well known among neuropsychiatrists that slight damage to the brain in the fetal state can turn a significant number of infants from right-handed into left-handed [733].

Dominance

A number of simple experiments show that though there is a dominance for a particular hand performing a particular task, the nondominant hand substantially aids the action, but at the subconscious level. For example, right-handed people will write 20 percent more rapidly when they hold the paper with their left hands than when holding the left hand in their laps [351].

Appendix IV

Gravity

Note: A shorter version of this work has appeared in [712a].

Section IV.A: The Gravitational Attraction between You and the Earth

You Have No Choice

Newton's Law

Gravity affects us as *yogasana* students in several important ways, the most obvious being in regard to maintaining balance and resisting gravitational collapse. In order to understand how gravity affects us and how we might respond to this, let us first look at the inviolable Law of Universal Gravitation first deduced by Sir Isaac Newton. Given two objects of mass m_1 and m_2 separated by a distance d, the gravitational force F attracting each of the objects to the other is given by Newton as:

$$F = Gm_1m_2/d^2 \text{ (equation IV.A-1)}$$

where G is a fixed number called the gravitational constant. When we practice standing *yogasanas* on the floor at the surface of the Earth, then F is the gravitational force with which our feet press the floor, m_1 is our mass, m_2 is the mass of the Earth and d is the Earth's radius. The magnitude of this force, F, can be measured directly by anyone, scientist or not, by simply standing on a bathroom scale and reading the dial. As G, m_2 and d are fixed quantities, the only way we can change the force with which our feet press into the floor or the scale when in *tadasana* is to change our mass m_1; i.e., eat a cheesecake, slim down, or hold a sandbag. Note that in regard to the gravitational force F with which the soles of our feet press the floor, there is no room in the above equation for personal choice, willpower, the number of trips you have taken to Pune, or your years of yogic practice.

It follows from Newton's Law that, contrary to what is said by many teachers in *yogasana* classes, you cannot simply:

1. "Press your feet into the floor," as teachers often instruct students in the standing postures. If you could press your feet into the floor on command, then you could change your weight as measured on the bathroom scale at will, instantaneously. In fact, your feet press into the floor in *tadasana* whether you want them to or not, and how hard they press into the floor cannot be changed as long as you stay in *tadasana* and neither gain nor lose weight.

2. "Come up by pressing your feet into the floor" in *trikonasana*. Actually, your feet unavoidably are pressing into the floor as you start the posture, remain pressing while you are in the posture, and press the floor as you come out of the posture; this pressure of your feet on the floor does not change unless your weight changes. The only way to increase your weight on the floor on coming up from *trikonasana* is to start eating more and exercising less.

3. "Press your forearms into the floor" in *pincha mayurasana*. Just as when standing with your weight on your feet, your weight on the floor in *pincha mayurasana* will not respond to your teacher's advice to press the floor harder or heavier in this posture, because Newton's Law got there first. Similarly, you can not "press your right palm down" when attempting to lift the hips in *vasisthasana*. However, as explained below, you **can** press your forearms into the floor to good effect when in *sirasana I*.

One has the illusion that the soles of the feet can be pressed into the floor in *tadasana* because we are generally not aware of the pressure on the soles of the feet resulting from the Earth's gravitational pull on our mass. However, when the teacher says "Press the feet," we become quickly aware of the pressure and so think that the teacher's instruction immediately made the pressure increase. Actually, the pressure has stayed constant, but the **awareness** of the pressure increased when the teacher gave her command.

Though you cannot change the weight that presses your feet onto the floor in *tadasana*,[1] what

you can change is the *distribution* of your weight among the various parts of the foot touching the floor. That is to say, in *tadasana*, you can be heavier on your heels by being lighter on the balls of your feet, you can move the weight from the inner edges of the feet to the outer edges, and you can shift the weight from one foot to the other. You can press your feet more strongly into the floor in *adho mukha svanasana* by shifting your weight away from your hands and toward your feet. When coming up from *trikonasana*, though one shifts the weight between the left foot and the right and also between different parts of each foot, simply "pressing the feet into the floor" has no meaning. And though you simply cannot "press your forearms into the floor" in *pincha mayurasana*, you can lift your upper arms away from your forearms to achieve the same end, or you can be heavier on the hands and lighter on the elbows, and you can press the forearms into the floor in *sirsasana I* so as to be heavier on the forearms and lighter on the head. The question of differentially pressing your weight into the floor is discussed from an experimental point of view in Section IV.B, page 853, and in Subsection IV.D, page 858.

Actually, there is a yogic way of pressing your feet into the floor in *tadasana*: if, in this posture, you press your arms upward against the ceiling with a force of Y pounds, then the weight on the soles of your feet will increase by Y pounds. If you are standing on your partner's thighs while doing this, he will feel the extra push. Strangely, you *can* very slightly increase or decrease the force of your feet on the floor when in *tadasana* by either coming into *malasana* or *urdhva hastasana*, respectively, as explained in the subsection below. One also can reduce the weight of the feet on the scale, in principle, by flapping one's wings in the air; birds do this all the time and can reduce their weight on the scale to negative values; i.e., they can fly

---

1   This is not strictly true, actually. The rotation of the Earth produces a centrifugal force that tends to push the body **away** from the center of the Earth. This antigravity force is stronger at the equator and weaker at the poles, so that a person weighs about 0.25 kilograms (half a pound) less at the equator than at the north pole; if the Earth spun so rapidly that a full day required only seventy-five minutes, the outwardly directed centrifugal force at the equator would then equal the inwardly directed gravitational force, and your weight on the floor would be zero in *tadasana*. As the Earth requires twenty-four hours per rotation, one must be satisfied with the thought that the body in *chaturanga dandasana* is nonetheless 0.25 kilograms lighter at the equator than at the poles! Furthermore, you will weigh more when lying down than when you are standing up, because the distance (d) in equation IV.A-1 (given above) is smaller by about three feet when you lie down. Because the distance (d) from your center of gravity to that of the Earth is 120 million feet, the measured change in weight (F) when going from standing to lying will be

totally negligible, yet this very small difference in gravitational potential energies when standing and lying is enough to pull us down onto the Earth if we relax. If circumstances demand it, the strength of the body is such that it can resist the gravitational pull for hours on end without surrender.

by lifting their weight off the ground and pressing their weight onto the air instead. Humans do something of the same sort when they walk on the tightwire while holding an open umbrella. Pulling down on the umbrella traps air in the bell of the device and acts to momentarily lift that side of the body. *Yogasana* students may want to try a difficult balancing with an open umbrella in hand as an aid.

Section IV.B: Significance of the Center of Gravity

When standing in *tadasana,* the different body parts are at different distances (d) from the center of the Earth, and so each body part experiences a very slightly different gravitational force; i.e., it has a very slightly different weight from that which it would have in *savasana,* where every part of the body is equidistant from the center of the Earth. The single force (weight) that you register on the bathroom scale when in *tadasana* is equivalent to what you would experience if all of your mass were concentrated at one particular point in space, a point called the center of gravity.[2] In the human body when in *tadasana,* the center of gravity is a few inches below the navel (at about the height of the S2 vertebra) and halfway back along the line from front to back, (figure IV.B-1).

_____

2   Technically, every atom of the student's body interacts gravitationally with every atom of the Earth, as per equation IV.A-1. However, this impossibly complex interaction is simplified once it is realized that it is equivalent to reducing each of the two objects (the student's body and the Earth, each with its complex spatial distribution of matter) to two points in space, each carrying all of the mass of each of the distributed objects. The two points in space that allow this simplification are called the centers of gravity of the two objects, body and Earth in our example. If any object is suspended by a string from its center of gravity in the gravitational field, it will hang without any turning; i.e., it is that point around which there are no gravitational torques.

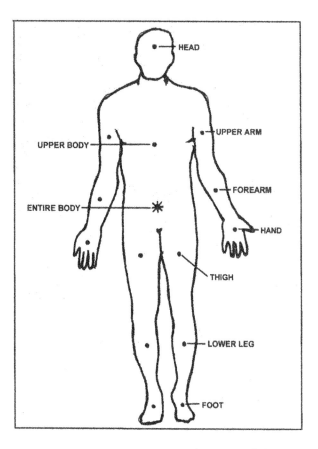

Figure IV.B-1. The centers of gravity of various body parts and of the entire body.

For a spherical object such as the Earth, the center of gravity is the geometric center of the object. However, the center of gravity of an object need not be within the object; i.e., the center of gravity of a doughnut is within the doughnut hole rather than within the doughnut itself, and that of half a doughnut (*urdhva dhanurasana*) is about halfway up from the floor, toward the lumbar spine.

When in *tadasana* and then lifting the arms overhead so as to be in *urdhva hastasana,* the center of gravity moves upward and similarly, when the legs are bent so as to go from *tadasana* to *malasana,* the center of gravity moves downward. For a given placement of the body parts, the position of the center of gravity is fixed with respect to the posture regardless of the body orientation in space; i.e., the position of the center of gravity with respect to the body is the same in *urdhva hastasana,* in *supta urdhva hastasana,* and in *adho mukha vrksasana*, and when in *savasana*, it is in the same place in the body as when in *tadasana*. The **direction** of the gravitational force between the body of a yoga student and the Earth is coincident with the line between their centers of gravity as in figure V.D-1.

Pressing the Floor

Often what is sought by "pressing the feet into the floor" is a lengthening of the distance between two points in the body, one of which is constrained to the floor. The lengthening does not press the hands, feet, or forearms more into the floor, but it does lift the center of gravity. Thus, to be more accurate, we should be saying to students in *tadasana*, "Lift your center of gravity by lengthening the distance between your feet and your pelvis" rather than "Press your feet into the floor so as to straighten your legs." The work involved in doing the *yogasanas* is largely the work of lifting the center of gravity of the body away from the center of gravity of the Earth, and correspondingly, the body is most relaxed when its center of gravity is closest to the center of the Earth; i.e., in *savasana*. Experimental proof for this point of view comes from measuring the forces on the hands and feet in postures where the corresponding arms or legs are either bent or are "pressed into the floor" in order to straighten them (Section IV.D, page 856). Thus, moving from *parsvakonasana* to *trikonasana* by straightening the front leg does not increase the pressure of the foot of the front leg on the floor, nor does moving from *chaturanga dandasana* to straight-arm *chaturanga dandasana* increase the pressure of the hands on the floor, though one has the illusion that the feet or hands are being pressed to the floor.

Falling and Balance

The concept of the center of gravity is most useful to *yogasana* students in another context. In order to avoid falling in balancing poses, the line between the Earth's center of gravity and the center of gravity of the body must pass through the area of the base of the body that is in contact with the Earth (Section V.A, page 867). One can remain balanced in a posture only as long as the line between the centers of gravity of the body and the Earth falls within the area of the base of the posture on the floor and the student is strong enough to keep from collapsing along the line of centers.

Section IV.C: Gravitational Effects on Anatomy and Physiology

---

Retrograde Processes in Zero Gravity

For the *yogasana* student, the physiological effects of a lack of gravity are manifold. In the zero gravity of outer space (or to a lesser extent when confined either to bed rest or to old age), the body's processes tend to go retrograde. Nausea can develop as the vestibular signals conflict with the visual signals in regard to just what is "upright," blood and lymph pool instead in the chest rather than in the feet and legs, the heart weakens as its load decreases, muscles become feeble, and bone demineralizes at a rate greater than 10 percent per year. In zero gravity, muscles not only atrophy, but in some postural muscles, the slow-twitch fibers so necessary for long-term muscle strength and for *yogasana* practice are converted into fast-twitch fibers, which act more quickly but which rapidly fatigue. As the bones demineralize and become brittle, this demineralization raises levels of Ca^{2+} to dangerous levels in the serum. The immune system seems also to be adversely affected by weightlessness, as is sleep quality and motor coordination. Unfortunately, many of the symptoms of living gravity-free appear in a reduced form when we are bedridden for any length of time or make the mistake of becoming old. On the other hand, these symptoms are minimized when we are physically active.

Retrograde Processes in Nonzero Gravity

Many scientists hold that on evolving from a quadrupedal to an upright bipedal stance, the human body has suffered greatly as the downward gravitational pull on our upright bodies has moved us toward flat feet, slipped intervertebral discs, hernias, various prolapsed organs, and a slumped posture, much of which must be counteracted through use of the postural, antigravity muscles. These consequences induced by a lack of gravitational stress can be minimized by an active physical *yogasana* practice that enhances both the antigravity muscles and our postural awareness.

Gravity and Body Fluids

Though the skeleton and the antigravity muscles can support the body against the pull of gravity, it is not as effective in shielding the body fluids from this downward pull. In the gravitational field, these fluids tend to pool in that part of the body closest to the floor: i.e., when standing upright, in the legs; when sleeping, on the side of the body closer to the floor; when inverted, in the head and neck. In regard to *yogasanas* performed in the supine position, there is a more efficient filling of the right atrium when horizontal, and in consequence of this, the volume receptors in the atrium report a high value to the hypothalamus, which in turn decreases the heart rate as compared to the situation where the posture is performed in a standing position. It is this aspect of assuming the supine position that generally leads to a global relaxation of the body and mind (*savasana*, for example). However, even in the standing position, there are indirect ways of using the bones and muscles to elevate fluid (see Subsection 14.C, page 569, and Section 14.G, page 597), thereby keeping the fluid distribution more or less uniform.

In contrast, without gravity, fluids move more to the head when standing and so cause stuffiness and congestion. The senses of taste and smell degrade, and in zero gravity, each leg loses about one liter of fluid, with overall plasma volume decreasing by 20 percent. Once plasma volume decreases, red blood cell production shuts down, and anemia sets in.

Because the brain has a somewhat lower density than does cerebrospinal fluid, the brain floats in the skull, at the top of the cranium when standing upright and against the roof of the mouth when inverted (Subsection 4.E, page 107).

Bed Rest

With the advent of space travel, bed-rest studies were instigated in order to simulate the physiology of extended stays in a gravity-free and exercise-free environment. After twenty-one days of enforced bed rest, it was found that the male subjects had suffered a 28 percent loss of $\dot{V}O_{2max}$ (equivalent to more than thirty years of aging!) and a 25 percent loss of their cardiac stroke volume. Moreover, their heart volume had shrunk by 11 percent. Publication of these results in 1968 led to an immediate shift of hospital practice, shifting heart patients from bed rest to exercise. Following the study, it was found that the cardiac deficits of bed rest were erased by placing the subjects onto their feet, the cardiac recovery time being much shorter than is required for atrophied skeletal muscles to respond to weightlifting [522].

Old Age

The effects of weightlessness due to a lack of gravitational pull on the body are of interest to us, not only because they point out several important factors here on Earth that we have come to ignore due their constancy, but also because the effects of weightlessness seem to mimic closely those of bed rest and of old age (Chapter 24, page 805) [893]. Thus, space travelers suffer from poor balance when they return to Earth's gravitational field, and mental deterioration sets in: they suffer from motion sickness, vomiting, headache, poor concentration, and loss of appetite. All of the above observations parallel many of the body changes observed in the aging process following prolonged bed rest. Clearly a regular *yogasana* practice works against all of the negative effects of too little gravitational pull on the body, by keeping us out of the sickbed and by giving us opportunities for actively responding to gravity's pull.

Section IV.D: Gravitational Effects on *Yogasana* Postures

We are dealing with the effects of gravity whenever we are in any posture in which balance is a factor. In outer space, where there is little or no gravity, balancing has no meaning, since all orientations of the body are equally energetic, and thus there is no force that can lead to a fall. Said differently, in outer space, one can not "fall down," as the direction "down" is defined as the direction of the gravitational force, and this force does not exist in outer space. It is for this reason that people on the southern hemisphere do not fall off the Earth, but instead are pulled toward the center of the Earth, just as are those in the northern hemisphere. On the other hand, balancing on the surface of a planet such as Jupiter also would be impossible, as the strength of gravity is 317 times larger than that on Earth, and one's body would be crushed before it could be balanced. Only here on Earth have gravity and balancing reached a *sattvic* state, for gravity is neither too low nor too high, and balance is possible (and necessary) for the *yogasana* practitioner.

The body's reaction to the pull of gravity begins once we are born, for from that moment on, the pull of gravity is a mechanical stress to which the body must react. As discussed by Myers [603], the body's web of connective tissue is responsive to gravitational stress, either thickening the tissue in places where the stress is intense and continuous, or going beyond this to form bone where only cartilage and a vascular net existed before, all in mechanical support of the body against the pull of gravity. In fact, each of us is born with approximately three hundred bones, many of which are adjacent but disconnected at birth; however, once these bones are used in ways such that they experience gravitational stress, the independent bones may be knit into more solid structures, leading to only 206 distinct bones in the adult body. As

vertebral life has come to inhabit Earth, certain muscles in humans have evolved in the legs, back, and neck with the main purpose of holding the skeleton erect; i.e., they are the antigravity muscles (Subsection 11.A, page 414).

Origins and Insertions: What Moves?

When a joint opens within a body that is free-floating in space, the two articulating bones both move, and the amplitudes of the two motions are inversely proportional to their masses. That is, the bone with the lighter mass moves more, and the bone with the heavier mass moves less. In this case, the end of the muscle attached to the more massive body part is called the origin, and that connected to the lighter body part is called the insertion (Subsection 9.B, page 320). Rephrased, the bone attached to the origin moves less, and the bone attached to the insertion moves more. In contrast, when we work the *yogasanas,* one side or the other of the two bones often is connected to the Earth and thus, in effect, has infinite mass. This means that because it is connected to the Earth's mass, its motion is blocked and so does not move, regardless of how low its true mass might be. As an example, stand in *urdhva hastasana* with the upper arms vertical but with the elbows flexed. Then open the angles at the elbows by contraction of the triceps, and observe that the forearms move but the upper arms/body/earth do not. Next, "stand" on your forearms in *pincha mayurasana* with the arms flexed again at the elbows. Again open the angles at the elbows through contraction of the triceps and note that with the forearms attached to the Earth, they do not move, but it is the upper arms and the rest of the body that move instead. In summary, the part of the body that moves when activating a particular action around a joint depends on which part of the joint is connected to the Earth/floor/wall; that part connected to the Earth/floor/wall essentially has infinite mass and so will not move at all (and so becomes the origin), whereas the part that is free of the Earth/floor/wall moves maximally (and so becomes the insertion). Thus, it is seen that due to gravitational effects, the definitions of "origin" and of "insertion" in regard to a muscle spanning a particular joint will depend totally on which of the two bones is in contact with the wall or floor.

Resting Muscle Tone

The reticular formation within the brainstem (Subsection 4.B, page 74) plays an important role in our anatomic battle with gravity. The general effect of gravity is to pull us flat onto the floor, whereas the general anatomic goal of our *yogasana* practice is to lift the body parts upward, as far from the floor as possible. Even when not thinking of the proper *yogasana* actions in our daily lives, the reticular formation is busy behind the scenes, subconsciously arranging contractions of the "postural" or "antigravity" muscles in the neck, back, and legs so that the body is held in extension and is supported against gravity's tendency to pull us into a flexional posture.

When standing, there is a continuous transmission of neural impulses from the reticular formation (Subsection 4.B, page 74) to the antigravity extensor muscles in order to support the body against the force of gravity. The reticular formation performs these actions following its receipt of sensory signals from our four types of balance sensors (Section V.C, page 893), contracting and relaxing muscles appropriately so as to maintain both balance and support [308]. These subconscious balancing and supporting actions will be active whether we are intensely working our *yogasana* practice or just conversing with a friend as we walk to the coffee shop. They are part of our resting muscle tone (Subsection 11.B, page 436).

In regard to balance and support of the body, we continuously monitor subconsciously where our limbs are in space by integrating visual cues with information from our eyes (Box V.C-1, page 889); from the vestibular system (Section 18.B, page 696); from proprioceptors on bones, muscles, and joints (Subsection 11.C, page 441); and from mechanoreceptors on our skin (Subsection 13.B, page 506). Of these balance sensors, all but the visual cues depend partly or completely on our body's response to gravity.

The gravitational force that keeps us fixed to the Earth also works to pull us flat onto the floor, however, thanks to the rigidity of our bony skeleton, we remain more or less upright. The endless work of the *yogasanas* to "lift up" against gravitational collapse (Subsection V.B, page 884) is done in response to this downward pull, and we work against the downward pull of gravity when we work to raise our center of gravity.

Balancing

All of the *yogasanas* except for *savasana* can be considered as balancing postures if one is sufficiently unsteady. When falling out of balance in the Earth's gravitational field, there are two distinct modes. In the first, there is an induced rotation (torque) of the body as one falls forward, backward, left, or right. In the second case, one yields to gravity along the line of centers (Subsection V.B, page 884), and so there is no rotational torque, but instead, one has a postural collapse, most often a sinking of the chest and a dropping of the body's center of gravity. It is the tendency toward this postural collapse that we work so hard to negate in Iyengar yoga. This lifting is highest and most sustainable when the bones of the body are positioned so as to bear the most weight (gravitational stress) and the muscles are used only to keep the bones in alignment and the joints open (*tadasana*, for example). Of course, purposely nonaligned positions are also possible (*utkatasana*, for example), but here, a larger part of the gravitational stress falls on the muscles, and so the posture cannot be held as long. Bones fatigue in the course of years, muscles in the course of minutes. Nonetheless, both bones and muscles are strengthened by resisting the pull of gravity, and both wither in a gravity-free environment or in an environment where there is gravity but no effort is expended to resist its pull, as when lying in bed.

Muscle Actions

As discussed in Subsection 11.A, page 407, muscle actions in the gravitational field can be divided into four categories: isometric, concentric isotonic, eccentric isotonic, and passive stretching. In the absence of a gravitational field, the difference between concentric and eccentric isotonic actions becomes moot; however, the difference between isotonic and isometric can be maintained either by external forces (being pulled forward by one's teacher into *paschimottanasana*, for example) or by internal forces (pulling on one's own ankles with the hands in *uttanasana*, for example).

The gravitational pull of the body toward the Earth's center gives us a proprioceptive handle on our orientation in space (see Appendix V, page 886), which is so valuable for balancing. Note, however, that the body's sensors cannot distinguish between the gravitational force and any other external force that is unavoidably present when the body is in accelerating or decelerating motion, other than that the gravitational force is always toward the center of the Earth and the non-gravitational forces can be in any direction.

Certain of the *yogasanas* are relatively unaffected by the pull of gravity, as, for example, *supta padangusthasana*, whereas others are strongly affected, *chaturanga dandasana*, for example. With respect to the latter, in the presence of gravity, lowering from the plank position to *chaturanga dandasana* involves an eccentric isotonic extension of the triceps, whereas the same motion in the absence of gravity would involve a gripping of the floor and a concentric isotonic contraction of the biceps (Subsection 11.A, page 407). To experience what *yogasana* practice would be like in the zero gravity of outer space, try the postures while submerged in your swimming pool.

Postural Goals

It is gravity's intention to pull us flat onto the floor, bringing our center of gravity as close to the center of the Earth as possible (Box V.A-1, page 868). Even when we are able to resist this action of the Earth's gravitational field, our resistance is not total, and so we tend to collapse our chest over time, especially as we grow older or become tired. This collapsed posture is not only unattractive, but it is very inefficient physiologically, as it inhibits the return of venous blood to the heart and often becomes the origin of negative emotions or a reflection of them; it is one of the postural goals of *yogasana* practice to correct the spinal collapse initiated by the downward pull of gravity. The mechanics of this adjustment in regard to the spine are discussed in Subsection 10.A, pages 331 and 337.

Measuring Weight Distributions in the *Yogasanas*

One cannot say that a subject is "understood" as a science until it has been measured quantitatively. As such, measurements of the weight distributions in the *yogasanas* would be one of the first steps in this direction. To this end, measurements of the distribution of the body weight on the floor while in the *yogasanas* are discussed here. These measurements were performed by placing bathroom scales (electronic and spring balance) under the various body parts otherwise in contact with the floor when in a particular *yogasana* and reading the proportion of the body weight born by each such contact. For example, one such scale was placed under each foot with the student in *trikonasana*-to-the-right (figure IV.D-1), and on average, it was found that the front foot carries 63 percent of the total body weight and the back foot carries 40 percent of the total body weight for the intermediate practitioner. As described below, the numbers are noticeably different with beginners.

Five intermediate-level students (with an average of six years' experience) participated in this study along with three beginner-level students (with less than two years' experience), with body weights of 50–80 kilograms (110–176 pounds); average values attained by the two groups are reported here. Interpreting the weight-distribution data is aided by Gorman's illustration of the local centers of gravity [288], as shown in figure IV.B-1. Though we found that the sum of the scale readings in almost all postures was equal to or very close to the total weight of the student while in *tadasana*, in some cases, this was not so, and so the calculated percentages in some instances do not quite add to 100 percent.

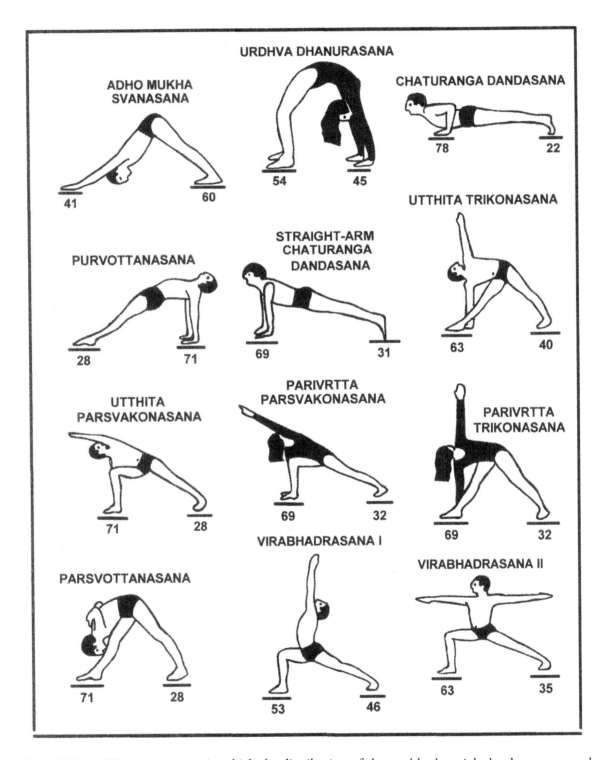

Figure IV.D-1. Various *yogasanas* in which the distribution of the total body weight has been measured between the hands and the feet or between the two feet, all on the floor, as appropriate to the posture. The percentage values given for each limb contacting the floor are averages of the values found for a group of five intermediate-level Iyengar students.

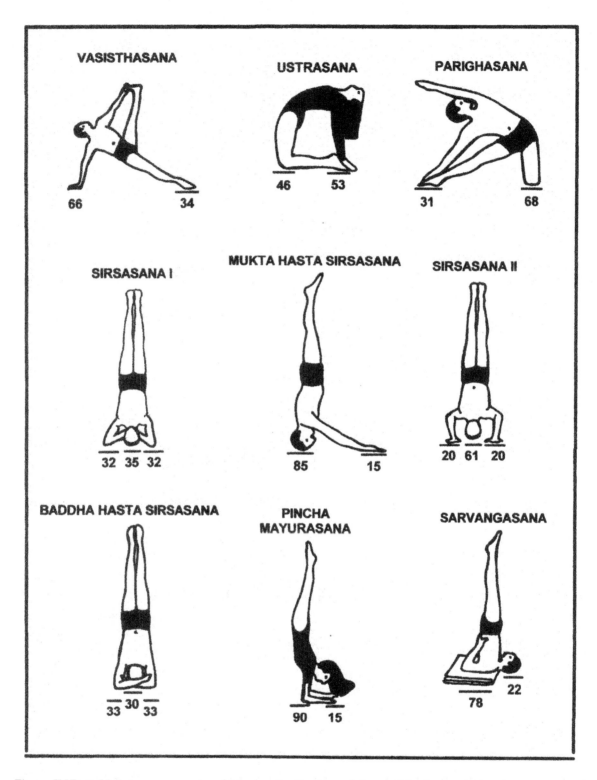

Figure IV.D-2. Various *yogasanas* in which the distribution of the total body weight has been measured between some combination of the hand, the foot, the elbow, and the knee on the floor, as appropriate to the posture. The percentage values given for each limb contacting the floor are averages of the values found for a group of five intermediate-level Iyengar students.

Adho Mukha Svanasana and Variations

With the beginner in *adho mukha svanasana,* the hands-to-feet weight ratio is close to 50 percent hands and 50 percent feet, but the more experienced students could effectively move 10 percent of their total body weight from hands to feet, achieving weight ratios more like 41 percent hands and 60 percent feet. This shift is a consequence of the experienced students being able to work the posture so as to move the pelvis upward and backward, thereby making the legs more vertical and lengthening the spine. If, instead, the student moves the pelvis forward to plank position (straight-arm *chaturanga dandasana*) from *adho mukha svanasana,* the weight becomes much more imbalanced, favoring the hands, of course (69 percent hands and 31 percent feet); this imbalance increases yet further (78 percent hands and 22 percent feet) on moving to *chaturanga dandasana,* where the center of gravity is shifted yet more toward the head as the arms are bent. Plank posture done facing upward (*purvottanasana*) has the same hand-to-foot weight ratio (71 percent hands and 28 percent feet) as straight-arm *chaturanga dandasana* itself, and nearly that of *vasisthasana* (66 percent hand and 34 percent foot; see figure IV.D-2).

Note too that on attempting to move from *chaturanga dandasana* to straight-arm *chaturanga dandasana,* the teacher might reasonably ask the students to "press their hands into the floor in order to lift the chest up," as discussed in Subsection IV.A, page 851. However, if "pressing the floor" were the way to lift the chest (or any other part of the body), then the percentage of the weight on the hands would **increase** significantly, whereas it is observed that the weight percentage actually **decreases**, going from 78 percent to 69 percent (figure IV.D-1)! One can take this as experimental proof that encouraging students to "press the floor" in order to lift a part of the body farther from the floor can be poor advice.

Backbending

Thinking of *urdhva dhanurasana* as the result of turning *adho mukha svanasana* inside-out, it is not surprising that the weight distribution for *urdhva dhanurasana* (45 percent hands and 54 percent feet) is much like that of *adho mukha svanasana* (41 percent hands and 60 percent feet); this is also evident from the locations of the centers of gravity being very much the same (figure IV.D-1). *Ustrasana* performed with the hands lying flat on the soles of the feet results in a weight ratio of 46 percent knees and 53 percent feet, a ratio rather close to that of *urdhva dhanurasana,* showing that in both postures, the centers of gravity lie left-to-right about halfway between the arms and those parts of the legs that are off the floor.

Standing Postures

In the symmetric postures *tadasana* and *adho mukha vrksasana,* scales were placed under each of the feet (*tadasana*) or under each hand (*adho mukha vrksasana*), with the expectation of equality of the weights on the left and right sides. Though the postures appeared to observers to be well balanced left-to-right, the scales showed significant imbalances, often amounting to side-to-side differences of 9 kilograms (twenty pounds), implying that the architecture of the internal body is significantly less symmetric than that of the external body!

With the body bent strongly to the right side, it is no surprise that the weight ratio in *trikonasana* is found to be 63 percent right foot and 40 percent left foot. These figures shift measurably (to 69 percent right foot and 32 percent left foot) when *trikonasana*-to-the-right is rotated into *parivrtta trikonasana.* If the difference is significant, this suggests that among the intermediate students, spinal elongation to the right is not as large in the rotated variation, or that spinal twisting results in an unavoidable shortening of the spine. On taking *parsvakonasana*-to-the-right, the center of gravity is further drawn to the right as compared to that in *trikonasana,* and the weight ratio becomes 71 percent right foot and 28 percent left foot, independent of whether the posture is *parivrtta*-rotated or not. The measured weight ratio for *parsvottanasana* is exactly that observed for *parsvakonasana,* as one might expect.

Not unexpectedly, all of the standing postures

done on one straight leg and one leg bent strongly to the right (*parsvakonasana, parivrtta parsvakonasana,* and *virabhadrasana II*) have similar weight ratios on the right and left feet; however, the right foot is noticeably lighter in *virabhadrasana II* as the upper body in this posture remains erect. It is at first sight surprising that the left-right weight distribution in *virabhadrasana I* (53 percent right foot and 46 percent left foot) is as close to even as it appears to be, given the imbalance observed in *virabhadrasana II* (63 percent right foot and 35 percent left foot); see figure IV.D-1.[3]

The weight ratio on the two feet is more even in *virabhdrasana II*-to-the-right (63 percent right foot and 35 percent left foot) than in *parsvakonasana* to-the-right (71 percent right foot and 28 percent left foot), as it holds the upper body more vertically erect and so has its center of gravity moved to the left.

Bending the left leg in *trikonasana* and dropping the knee to the floor brings one to *parighasana*-to-the-right. Being on the left knee in this posture, the center of gravity can be seen to have moved far to the left, and so the weight ratio becomes 31 percent right foot and 68 percent left knee.

Inverted Postures

With beginners in *sirsasana I,* an average weight ratio of approximately 50 percent head and 50 percent forearms was measured; however, they were very unsteady in this posture, and so for each of them, the weight was constantly shifting between wide limits. Because the intermediate students are more able to lift their shoulders up and away from their elbows, taking the additional weight on their forearms, they are able to generate a ratio of 32 percent head and 64 percent fore-

arms (figure IV.D-2). Actually, the intermediate students easily were able to lift their heads totally off the floor in *sirsasana I,* achieving a ratio of 0 percent head and 100 percent forearms; however, they were asked to perform the posture as they would for a ten-minute practice of the posture. When placed in *sirsasana II,* the pressure of the hands on the floor is no longer transmitted efficiently to the shoulders, and consequently the weight ratio rises to 61 percent head and 40 percent hands for the intermediate students versus 32 percent head and 64 percent forearms in *sirsasana I.*

That the percentage of the total weight on the head when in *sirsasana II* (61 percent) is significantly larger than that on the head when in *sirsasana I* (33 percent) suggests why the former posture is usually performed for only two minutes or so by students who are easily able to perform the latter posture for ten to fifteen minutes. Note that the percent-head-to-percent-hand ratio increases yet again when the arms straighten and the backs of the hands are placed on the floor, as when in *mukta hasta sirsasana* (85 percent head and 15 percent hands). In these *sirsasanas,* one of the roles of the hands or forearms is to work the floor so as to shift the weight off the head and onto the hands or arms.[4] Comparing the percentage of the total weight on the head in *sirsasana I* (33 percent), *sirsasana II* (61 percent), and *mukta hasta sirsasana* (85 percent), one sees how important it is to keep those parts of the anatomy (hands or forearms) that work to keep the weight off the head, as close as one can to the head, balance permitting.

When in *pincha mayurasana,* the intermediate students again lift the shoulders away from the hands, leading to a weight distribution of only 15 percent hands and 90 percent elbows as appropriate for having the vertical line of the body over the elbows in this posture. In contrast, in the beginner, the shoulders will be more over the hands than over the elbows, and the hand-to-elbow

---

3   It appears that in *virabhadrasana II*-to-the-right, the lateral bending of the upper body to the left is inhibited by the bone-on-bone contact in the left hip joint (Subsection 7.F, page 252), and consequently results in a lesser weight on the left foot. On the other hand, in *virabhadrasana I,* the backbending toward the back leg is relatively easy and so the front-to-back weight distribution is more evenly divided.

---

4   Yes, it is correct to "press the floor" in these postures, for that is how we shift the weight off of the head and onto the arms and shoulders.

weight ratio will be much larger than that for intermediate students.

In this preliminary study, it was found that in vertical *sarvangasana* with blankets under the elbows and shoulders, the elbows and shoulders carry 78 percent of the total weight, and only 22 percent of the weight rests on the back of the head. As with the *sirsasanas* discussed above, the importance in *sarvangasana* of keeping the point of contact with the floor close to the centerline of the posture, *i.e.*, keeping the arms under the posture so as to exert the maximum sustainable lift, is apparent.

This preliminary and admittedly crude study involves the awkward placement of large scales between the floor and certain large body parts. However, with very little effort or expense, the measurements could be made using very small and inexpensive strain gauges; with these simple sensors and a cheap meter, one could sense the pressure differences between the first and fifth metacarpals (the thumb and little finger) with the hand on the floor as in *adho mukha svanasana* and/or between the first and fifth metatarsals (big toe and little toe) or between inner ankle and outer ankle with the foot on the floor as in *urdhva dhanurasana*, etc. Once this small step in regard to instrumentation is taken, it should be relatively simple to make quantitative measurements of relative pressure in both static postures and balancing postures. Such simple experiments will allow comparison of the relative weight distributions in a set of common postures as performed by beginners, intermediate-level students, and senior-level performers. In this way, a doorway to a fresh understanding of the anatomy of Iyengar *yogasana* practice will open for whoever chooses to walk through it.

Appendix V
Balancing

Balancing (*tola* in Sanskrit) is especially important to the *yogasana* student, because it is a significant part of every *yogasana* more elevated than *savasana*. If one loses balance before the *yogasana* is brought to completion, then fully one-third or more of the going-into-the-posture/remaining-in-the-posture/coming-out-of-the-posture three-part cycle has been lost. Maintaining balance can be especially difficult when the posture requires: (i) being inverted on the head, as in *sirsasana*; (ii) balancing on the hands, either inverted as in *adho mukha vrksasana* or nominally upright as in *bakasana*; (iii) standing on one leg, as in *vrksasana*; (iv) moving from one balanced position to another, as when going from *ardha chandrasana* to *virabhadrasana III*; (v) balancing on the ischial tuberosities (sitting bones; see figure 8.B-7) of the pelvis, as in *paripurna navasana*; (vi) balancing in a posture in which the left and right sides of the body are reversed in their positions as compared with their normal positions, as when in *parivrtta trikonasana* (bending to the right but with the left ear below that of the right); (vii) rotating in a balanced position so that the left and right sides of the upper body are reversed with respect to the lower parts, as when moving from *trikonasana* to *parivrtta trikonasana*; and (viii) balancing on two feet but in an unusual position, as when in *virabhadrasana I*. Some postures combine aspects of the points listed here, as, for example, *vasisthasana*, an inclined balancing posture involving support on one arm and one leg. Maintaining balance is also critical when coming out of a posture in a state of fatigue (Subsection II.A, page 834). It is nonetheless common to find beginning students for whom balancing in more mundane postures such as *sarvangasana* or even *trikonasana* is chal-

lenging and for whom the special cases mentioned above are more or less completely out of reach. Finally, it must be said here that as defined in this appendix, virtually all *yogasanas* (save *savasana*) are balancing postures.

Fear of Falling

In addition to the frustration of struggling to maintain balance in the *yogasana* postures, fear of falling is natural and can inhibit our attempts at being totally present in the posture. Fear of falling can be an inhibiting factor even in a standing posture such as *trikonasana*, in which students are reluctant to place the plane of the upper body in the plane of the legs. Even when we are just walking, we are only 0.3–0.5 second from falling forward onto our faces, for it is imbalance that propels us forward; this has special meaning as we age and our reaction times tend to lengthen.

Falling and Aging

Approximately 20 percent of Americans suffer difficulties in balancing. These difficulties can be triggered not only by aging but also by viral infections of the inner ear, head injuries, multiple sclerosis, Parkinson's disease, Meniere's disease, poor blood circulation, stroke, and diabetes [675], or even by the taking of some antibiotics. Among the elderly, falls are the leading cause of fracture and disability and account for more than $20 billion per year in hospital bills.

It is widely acknowledged that both the frequency and the severity of falls increase as we age. Once past age seventy-five years, the death rate due to falls is more than three times larger than for any previous decade, and it is known that falls among elderly nursing-home residents correlate more strongly with insomnia than with sleep-inducing medication; a lack of sleep for twenty-four hours puts one in a mental fog equivalent to that when the blood-alcohol level reaches the limit of intoxication as defined legally. It is clear that regardless of cause, a loss of balance can be a significant factor in the premature deaths of older people.

In addition to the risk of the serious consequences of falling and breaking bones, there is also the risk to the brain of developing a hematoma in the older person, in whom the veins are stretched by the normal shrinkage of the brain with age (Subsection 24.A, page 812).

Fear of falling among the elderly is also known to be a significant factor in keeping them housebound and reluctant to venture outside to become participants in life. In fact, once having fallen, many seniors are so fearful of falling again that they cannot walk without trembling or losing their balance and soon find themselves walking with canes or sitting in wheelchairs. Fortunately, the balancing senses can be sharpened by *yogasana* practice, thereby lessening the risks of a bad fall and its consequences.

Though our focus is on balancing the body, it will be useful to first discuss two preliminary situations, that regarding the static mechanical stability (support) of a rigid block (Subsection V.A, below) and that regarding how the body balances a rigid block using a dynamic approach (Subsection V.A, page 872).

Section V.A: Balancing a Rigid Block

Aspects of Mechanical Stability

Falling Sideways

Let us consider the factors involved in balancing a solid, inanimate block of unspecified shape resting on the floor. Qualitatively, a block that is mechanically "stable" is in a configuration in which it is absolutely still for very long periods of time in spite of small external perturbations (i.e., it does not fall even when rocked modestly from side to side). Because there can be more than one stable state of the block, there is a spectrum of relative stability, with one particular orientation being most stable and the others being only relatively stable with respect to the position of greatest stability.

There are situations in which a block is stable in theory, but in fact, such a block resting on the table will fall, because its base is so small that small external perturbations will rock it to the side and it cannot resist falling. This situation in which a block is theoretically stable but in reality is unstable (imagine a pencil balanced on its sharpened point) is called "metastable." Moreover, even when in a relatively stable position, there may be different degrees of stability with respect to falling in different directions. A sheet of cardboard set on edge can be very stable with respect to falling in the left-to-right direction but very unstable with respect to falling in the front-to-back direction.[1] This directional variability of stability is termed "specific metastability." The most stable state will not show metastability of any type, but the relatively stable states may or may not show aspects of metastability.

In opposition to the most stable state of a system, positions or orientations of the block that lead in both theory and practice to immediate falling, either down or to the side, are called "es-

---

1   In the realm of *yogasana*, this example of metastability arises when in *prasarita padottanasana* with the hands and the head on the line between the feet, for the stability in the left-right direction in this *yogasana* is very high, whereas the stability in the front-to-back direction can be relatively very low, as witnessed by the large proportion of students who somersault forward the first time they come into this position. It is of great value in *yogasana* balancing to understand the directions of stability and metastability when in the various postures and to understand how to reduce the risk of falling in the direction of metastability, if there is one.

sentially unstable," in distinction to those that are only unstable in a practical sense.

When left to themselves and given enough time, it is a law of thermodynamics (called the Second Law; see Box V.A-1, page 868) that a rigid, inanimate object (such as our block), with very little prompting, will move from essentially unstable, metastable, and relatively stable configurations to the most stable state, the one of maximum attractive gravitational force F (equation IV.A-1), but not the reverse (i.e., inanimate objects can fall down but cannot fall up). You can experimentally test the truth of this statement as described in Box V.A-1, below.

A Balancing Rule

Understanding mechanical stability, relative stability, metastability, and essential instability (as illustrated by the block toss in the box below) is aided considerably by the concept of the center of gravity of the object being balanced; it is strongly recommended that you read or review Section IV.B, page 853, on this point. The center-of-gravity concept is discussed further in Section V.B, page 874. For a rigid body, a simple balancing rule governs whether a particular orientation of the block on a surface in the Earth's gravitational field is mechanically stable, relatively stable, metastable, or essentially unstable, depending in part upon just where the center of gravity lies with respect to the supporting surface on which the object lies:

> Given a particular flat surface of a rigid block in contact with the floor, the block will be mechanically stable, relatively stable, or metastable in this orientation only if the line between the center of gravity of the block and the center of gravity of the Earth lies within the area common to the block and the floor. The line between centers is coincident with a plumb line hanging from the object's center of gravity and perpendicular to the floor. If the line between centers falls outside the common surface area of the block and the floor, then the block is essentially unsta-

ble and will fall sideways to achieve one of its more stable, higher-gravitational-force orientations. For a nonrigid block, mechanical stability also may be lost by internal collapse, wherein the object falls toward the floor along the line between centers, without rotation. Among those states that are stable, the most stable state is that one of smallest separation of its center of gravity with that of the Earth. The higher is the center of gravity of a relatively stable state above that of the most stable state, the higher is its relative instability (i.e., the easier is the object tumbled as it is pulled closer to the center of the Earth).

Referring to figure V.A-2 (page 869), one can readily see how the above rule of balance comes to be. Imagine an oval object firmly attached to a rectangular base, resting on the floor as in figure V.A-2**a**. In this case, the gravitational force on the object (F) is coincident with the line between centers and so acts only to pull the object more forcefully onto the floor; in your mind, imagine the line between centers to be a string to be pulled, and pull it. Should the internal strength of the oval be low, the object may collapse along the line of centers without a loss of balance (figure V.A-2**b**). If the object instead is off balance as in figure V.A-2**c**, the force (F) still passes through the base and will generate a rotational torque about the point marked ∗, which tends to rotate the object clockwise (pull on the string again to see this). However, if the initial rotation is so large (figure V.A-2**d**) that the force (F) falls to the left of the point marked ∗, then the sense of the rotational torque will be counterclockwise, and the object will continue to fall to the left (as you pull the string).

Examples of Stability

Consider the three-dimensional rigid object shown in figure V.A-3 (page 870). By the balancing rule stated above, it is seen that configuration "a" has its line between centers within the base (A) and is most stable on the basis of the nearness of

Box V.A-1: The Second Law of Thermodynamics and Rigid Blocks

Everyone in your class takes a **foam** block, for which we will consider five possible orientations on the floor: *savasana* (largest surface on the floor, figure V.A-1**a**), *anantasana* (block on edge, intermediate area on the floor, figure V.A-1**b**), *tadasana* (block on end, smallest area on the floor, figure V.A-1**c**), *vrksasana* on one toe (block with only a corner touching the floor, figure V.A-1**d**), and *ardha chandrasana* (block with one edge on the floor, figure V.A-1**e**). On a signal from the teacher, everyone throws their block high into the air, and a qualitative tally is made of which orientations are preferred by the blocks once they come to rest on the floor. One might assume beforehand that all positions of the block would be equally likely; however, in practice, *savasana* wins by a landslide, because it is mechanically the most stable orientation for an inanimate block, with *tadasana and anantasana* in the minority, as they are only relatively stable with respect to *savasana*, and *ardha chandrasana* and *vrksasana* being totally absent, as the first of these is only metastable and the second is essentially unstable (as shown in the figure). *Savasana* is the overwhelming winner because its position experiences the largest attractive gravitational force, having the smallest value of d in equation IV.A-1 (i.e., its center of gravity is closest to the center of the Earth, and the posture is inherently stable).

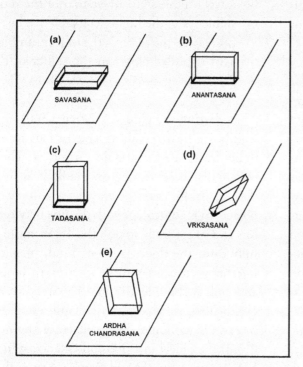

Figure V.A-1. (**a**) Block in the *savasana* position, with the largest surface on the floor shown by heavy lines; (**b**) block in the *anantasana* position, intermediate surface on the floor shown by heavy lines; (**c**) block in the *tadasana* position, with the smallest surface on the floor shown by heavy lines; (**d**) block in *vrksasana* position, standing on one corner, shown by heavy lines; (**e**) block in *ardha chandrasana* position, with one edge (the heavy line) in contact with the floor.

In regard to body postures rather than block stabilities, it is also the case that the *yogasana* position of absolute largest attractive gravitational force is that of *savasana* and that this will be the most relaxing posture possible, because all other postures experience a smaller attractive gravitational force (equation IV.A-1) than it, and so must be supported or maintained in some way against the downward pull of gravity, by some expenditure of energy.

its center of gravity to that of the Earth; "b" and "c" are relatively stable, because in these cases, the line between centers again passes through the bases B and D, respectively. However, the same object when placed in configuration "d" does not have its line between centers within the area of surface C and so is essentially unstable and will fall, turning around the point marked ∗, to place

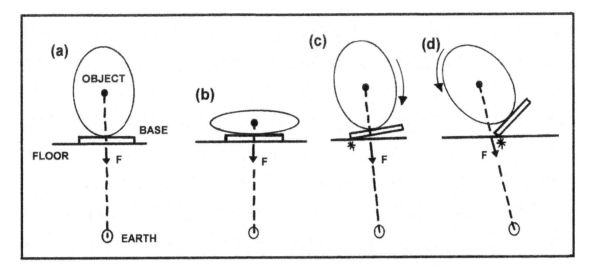

Figure V.A-2. (a) An oval object and its rectangular base are pulled downward by the gravitational force (F) onto the floor. (b) In response to the force (F), the object could collapse along the line between centers without falling to the side. (c) The object falls to the left about the point marked ∗; however, the line between centers remains to the right of this point, and so the force (F) rotates the object clockwise. (d) The object has fallen so far to the left that the force (F) lies to the left of the point marked ∗ and the gravitational force acts to rotate the object counterclockwise (i.e., it falls to the left).

stable surface D on the floor. However, if the falling end of the block when in configuration "d" is supported by a wall, as shown in configuration "e," the block is again stable. In this case, the balancing rule still applies, for the "block" is now mechanically defined as including the wall, so that the effective area of the base relevant to balancing in figure V.A-3e extends from the left-hand edge of the block all the way to the outer surface of the wall.

Were the block in figure V.A-3d jointed as in figure V.A-3f, it would still be unstable unless the block were folded so that the joint were closed as in figure V.A-3g, in which case the line between centers is once again within the base, as the center of gravity has moved to the left by moving mass to the left.

If the object in question is a spherical ball rather than a wedge, then its line between centers is just within the area of the base when it is resting motionless on the floor. Given just the slightest push to the right, the ball's center of gravity then falls outside the area of its base (as defined by the point in contact with the floor) and so the ball begins to "fall" to the right. In this case, the center

of gravity of the ball is always just to the right of the point of contact of the ball with the floor but is never just over it as when stationary; this rolling of a spherical object is a case of continuous falling and is in every way analogous to the gravitational force that keeps a satellite or the moon in continuous orbit around the Earth.

Specific Metastability

If the line between centers lies within the area of the base but very close to an edge of the area, as for object 1 in figure V.A-4, then only a very small angle of sway toward the left or the right is allowed before the line between centers falls outside of the base and so topples the object. Object 1 theoretically is stable, for it is in accord with the balancing rule; however, in a practical situation, it immediately will fall in response to small but unavoidable oscillations of air pressure or vibrations of the table and so is here classified as metastable. The stability of object 2 is increased considerably compared to that of object 1 (figure V.A-4), because it has three widely separated points of contact on the floor, and the effective area for stability includes the stippled area be-

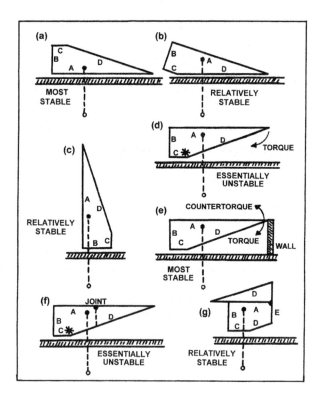

Figure V.A-3. A chisel-shaped block of wood in the four orientations (**a**), (**b**), (**c**), or (**d**), having the respective bounding surfaces **A**, **B**, **C**, or **D** placed on the floor; the dashed lines represent the lines between the centers of gravity of the Earth (○ - -) and the block (- - ●). In the unstable configuration (**d**), relatively stability can be achieved by placing the block against the wall as in (**e**). Now introduce a joint in the block as in (**f**), but leave it open. Again the block is essentially unstable when resting on surface **C**, but if the joint is flexed as in (**g**), the center of gravity is shifted to the left, and the block then becomes relatively stable when resting on surface **C**, as its line between centers now passes through the area of the base.

tween these points. Object 2, in a practical sense, may be taken as relatively stable, rather than unstable. Object 1 might be a mechanical model for a person trying to balance on one leg (*vrksasana*) on the deck of a rolling ship, whereas Object 2 is a model for a person standing on the deck of a rolling ship with legs separated and both feet and both hands planted solidly on the deck in *adho mukha svanasana*.

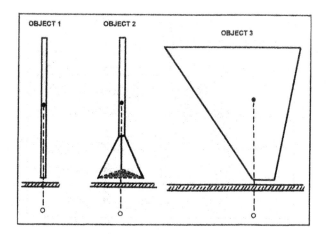

Figure V.A-4. In object 1, the dashed line between its center of gravity (- - ●) and the center of the Earth (○ - -) is just barely within the effective area of the base; for this reason, object 1 will be unstable with respect to small oscillations that carry its line between centers outside the area of its base. In contrast, object 2 is constructed so that the base is the stippled area between the feet of the tripod legs and so will be far more stable than object 1; it is relatively stable, as it is not in the state of lowest energy. Object 3 is specifically metastable, as it can easily fall to the left but is relatively stable in regard to falling to the right.

Notice that if the very stable, two-dimensional block in figure V.A-3**a** were of the size shown but as thin as paper in the third dimension, it would be very stable toward tipping in the left-to-right direction but very susceptible to tipping in the front-to-back direction. In such cases, we speak of specific instability (i.e., a situation in which stability is very high in one direction but very low in a second, usually perpendicular direction). Object 3 in figure V.A-4 shows a specific metastability, as it is strongly resistant to falling to the right but is easily toppled by any small external perturbation that would push it to the left. Object 2 is relatively more stable toward external perturbations than is either object 1 or object 3. Object 1 in figure V.A-4, being unstable in all directions perpendicular to its long axis, can be said to be unequivocally metastable. Several examples of specific metastability in *yogasana* practice are presented in Subsection V.D, page 897.

Collapse along the Line between Centers

Imagine a leaking ball that slowly loses its inflation and so is pulled more and more toward the center of the Earth as it slowly deflates, yet the line between centers does not fall outside the base of the ball on the floor. In contrast to such a deflating ball, the blocks in figures V.A-1, V.A-2, and V.A-3 are assumed to be rigid, so that the possible collapse of the block toward the center of the Earth, all the while keeping the line between centers within the area of the base of the object, is moot.[2]

---

2   In the earlier parts of this section, a number of aspects of relative mechanical stability were defined and illustrated. For the sake of easy comprehension and ready availability, they are summarized here.

» **Stable:** The orientation and geometry of an object showing the strongest gravitational attraction to the Earth according to equation IV.A-1 (i.e., the one having the closest approach of the object's center of gravity to that of the Earth). In *yogasana* practice, the stable orientation/geometry is attained in *savasana*. In a mechanical sense, the lower is your center of gravity, the more you are "grounded."

» **Relatively Stable:** Orientations and geometries of an object that are stable in time toward small external fluctuations but that experience a lower gravitational force than in the stable posture due a larger value of the distance between centers. In *yogasana* practice, most of the postures displayed in Appendix I are relatively stable with respect to *savasana,* the stable posture of the body. Relatively stable states will revert to the state of highest gravitational attractive force if given enough time.

» **Metastable:** Refers to orientations and geometries that on paper are clearly relatively stable, but that are not so in practice. For most of us, the full arm balance performed on one arm theoretically is a posture of only relative stability with respect to *savasana*; however, in practice, it falls immediately (as with object 1 in figure V.A-4) and so is given the label "metastable."

» **Specifically Metastable:** Refers to orientation and geometries that in theory and in practice

Intelligent Balancing of a Block

Though the rigid blocks are stable with respect to collapse along the lines between centers, should any of the blocks in figures V.A-1, V.A-2, or V.A-3 fail to satisfy the rule regarding the relation of base area to line between centers for balancing, the fall cannot be halted, because the blocks are lacking in all aspects of sensing imbalance and reacting to resist it. Though the possibilities of either vertical collapse or of resistance to sideways falling are moot in wooden blocks in stable or relatively stable states, they can be real problems for *yogasana* students in balancing postures. These differences aside, both the student and the wooden block are required to obey the dicta that an object will rest on the floor without falling only if (1) the line between its center of gravity and the center of the Earth passes through the surface common to the object and to the floor and (2) it is strong enough to resist collapse along the line between centers.

In regard to Newton's equation IV.A-1, the **magnitude** of the gravitational force (F) is relevant to falling down along the line between centers, whereas the **direction** of F (coincident with the line between centers), as we shall see, is the

---

are very stable toward falling in certain directions but are very unstable toward falling in one or more other directions. For example, object 3 in figure V.A-4 is stable with respect to falling to the right but is specifically metastable with respect to falling to the left. In *yogasana* practice, *trikonasana* is relatively stable in the left-to-right and forward directions but is specifically metastable in respect to falling backward. Similarly, one might be both front-to-back and left-to-right stable in *tadasana* but still be specifically metastable with respect to collapse along the line of centers. One might just as well speak of specific metastability as "differential stability."

» **Essentially Unstable:** Any orientation or geometry in which the balancing rule is not obeyed and falling is inevitable and immediate, as with *tadasana* attempted with the body at 45° to the vertical.

key factor of interest in trying to avoid falling to the side in balancing postures. The direction of the force (F) is always along the line between centers.

Torque and Countertorque

Actually, the unstable block in figure V.A-3**d** does not simply "fall" to the right, but more precisely, in falling, it rotates around the point marked * clockwise (as viewed by the reader). When the line between centers falls outside the area of the base as in configuration "d," a rotational force called torque is developed. Torque, unopposed, leads to rotation and falling. One way to keep such a block from falling on the floor is to lean it against the wall instead; i.e., have it fall onto the wall instead of onto the floor (Section V.D, page 901). In this case, the wall supplies a countertorque (figure V.A-1**e**) that resists the falling torque, so that further falling is avoided. When the object is in balance, the sum of the torques acting on it is zero; i.e., there is no net rotational force acting on it when stable.

The configuration depicted in figure V.A-3**e** is a two-dimensional model of the body in *vasisthasana I*, with the tug of the Earth on the body's center of gravity pulling the hips to the floor. Mechanical stability implies that there is no net torque on the object in question, and in this handbook, the phrase is synonymous with "balanced" when used in reference to inanimate objects that could fall but do not; the terms are not synonymous when referring to the human body in the *yogasanas*.

The Articulated Block

Imagine now that the unstable block in figure V.A-3**d** not only is articulated (i.e., has a single joint, as in figure V.A-3**f**), but also has a motor to flex the joint, a torque sensor, and a computer. In that case, it would be possible for this intelligent block to balance without leaning on the wall. To do this, it would sense the clockwise "falling" torque, and with the aid of the computer and motor, flex its joint to generate a counterclockwise torque that would just counterbalance the falling torque. In regard to the block in figure V.A-3, the

countertorque involved in going from figure V.A-3**f** to figure V.A-3**g** is equivalent to a shift of the center of gravity of the block to the left, so that the line between centers now falls within the area of surface C, and mechanical stability is attained. The proper countertorque can be thought of as either countering the falling torque or, equivalently, as that shift of the center of gravity of the block required to ensure the intersection of the line between centers and the base of the block.

Balancing a Broomstick

A more instructive model of balancing in the *yogasanas* is that of a human being, complete with balance sensors (Section V.C, page 886), moveable limbs, muscles to move the limbs, and a nervous system, all coupled mechanically to a rigid block (e.g., a human being balancing a broomstick on the end of one finger). In this scenario, there is a single joint, in effect, where the broomstick rests on the finger. Were the broomstick to rotate clockwise in falling in the gravitational field, the eyes would sense the resultant change of position due to the unbalanced torque, and with the aid of the brain and the muscles of the wrist and upper arm, the hand supporting the broomstick could be swung in a counterclockwise way to generate a countertorque and so cancel the falling torque and preserve the balance. However, if the countertorque is too large, it brings the broomstick past vertical and starts a falling rotation counterclockwise. In response to this, the eye again alerts the brain, and the hand then is sent in a clockwise arc so that the broomstick rotates clockwise. Feedforward (Subsection V.F, page 917) is important here in anticipating the overcorrection.

Dynamic Balance

When a block is balanced (as in figures V.A-3**a**, **b**, and **c**), it is static in every sense of the word and will never fall due to gravitational forces, whereas in the case of the balanced broomstick, the broomstick is in dynamic balance in the gravitational field and is always falling. In this metronomic *pas de deux*, it is as if there are two swinging pendulums (the broomstick and the hand), the motions of which are synchronized to keep the net torque on the vertical broomstick averaged to zero over time. The motions of the two pendulums are essentially out of phase (i.e., when the wrist swings to the left, it sends the broomstick to the right, and vice versa). Yet another way to interpret this balancing act is that once the eyes sense an imbalance, the base (where the broomstick rests on the fingertip) is moved to intercept the moving line between the centers of gravity. This constant **dynamic** interplay of falling torque and countertorque is the key to balancing the body in the *yogasanas* and stands in contrast to the static situation, in which an inanimate block is mechanically stable or relatively stable while resting on the floor. The dynamic aspect of maintaining the broomstick in balance is especially relevant to the application of our understanding of *yogasana* practice and distinguishes "balancing" (Section V.B, page 875) from simple "support or mechanical stability" (Section V.A, page 866).

Furthermore, if the end of the broomstick is sharpened to a point, the area of "the base" can be made as close to zero as one would ever want, yet the balancing of the broomstick is no more difficult, as long as the appropriate swaying motions of arm and broomstick are maintained! One could say that the effective base for balance of the broomstick is the arc covered by the swinging of the point of contact of stick and finger.

If a *yogasana* posture were being performed by an acrobat on the slack wire, then the point of contact of the foot and the wire would be exceedingly small, but it could be smoothly moved left and right to maintain the base under the line of centers, in exact analogy with the finger and broomstick exercise above. Note, however, that when balancing in a *yogasana* on the floor, one cannot readily move the base of the posture (call this option "i") to keep it always under the center of gravity, as we did with the broomstick or our image of the acrobat on the slack wire. When losing one's balance on the floor, though, it can be recovered by awkwardly hopping on the foot to re-establish the base beneath the center of gravity; however, this is more like replacing balance with support. Balance can be better maintained instead by moving the center of gravity of the body

using countertorques, so that the line of centers is always within the area of the base; it is this approach (call this option "ii") that we use in the floor-based *yogasanas*.

As mentioned elsewhere, the act of maintaining balance by generating countertorques in response to the sensations of falling torques can be phrased in an equivalent way: When falling is sensed, one moves one or more body parts in a way that shifts the body's center of gravity to reposition the line between centers over the base of the body. These two equivalent modes of thinking about balancing the body in the *yogasanas* are used interchangeably in the following sections.

In the broomstick illustration above, the object being balanced (the balancee) is unintelligent and inanimate, whereas the eyes/finger/arm/brain ensemble organizing the balancing (the balancer) is essentially playing the role of the floor. In order to balance the body intelligently, what we want is to make the floor solid and inanimate so that the body becomes both the balancee and the balancer. Still, there are many aspects of the broomstick experiment that are relevant to balancing in the *yogasanas*.

Section V.B: Balancing the Body

Resisting Gravity

We now turn to balancing the body in the *yogasanas*. Translating the above theoretical discussion of balancing an inanimate block into the practical world of balancing the student in a *yogasana*, it is gravity's intention in every posture to pull the student toward the center of the Earth and flatten him onto the floor, either by tumbling to the side to lower his center of gravity or by falling straight down, again lowering his center of gravity. This falling brings his center of gravity as close as is possible to that of the Earth. Our work in *yogasana* practice is to resist the effects of this natural attraction of our body to the floor in all of the postures, except for *savasana*, where the body is in the lowest possible energy state (gravitationally speaking) and there otherwise is no resistance to gravity; in this case, the effects of gravity work to support relaxation. Because any muscular tension in the body when in *savasana* raises the body's center of gravity off the floor, a truly relaxed *savasana* allows every part of the body to come as close to the floor as possible.

The Body's Center of Gravity

For a person of normal weight and proportions standing in *tadasana,* the center of gravity of the body lies just below the navel and about halfway back toward the sacral spine (Section IV.B, page 853). In this posture, the body is in balance as long as the line between this point within the body and the center of the Earth falls within the area delineated by the placement of the heels and toes on the floor. However, as described in Section IV.B, though the center of gravity of the body lies within the body when in *tadasana,* it is not necessarily the case that the center of gravity of the body will lie within the body in all of the *yogasana* postures.

In *urdhva dhanurasana,* for example, the body's center of gravity rises more toward the solar plexus (because the arms are lifted overhead) and is positioned in the empty space behind the dorsal spine (because the spine is lifted well above the line connecting the heels and the wrists); as with *adho mukha svanasana,* the effective area of the base for *urdhva dhanurasana* is that delineated by the placement of the hands and feet on the floor. When hanging from a horizontal bar by one's hands, the center of gravity is below the point of support, and no falling is possible other than straight down, without the generation of any torque.

The Base

In *yogasana* practice, the concept of the base is a critical component and has complications that go beyond that of blocks with flat surfaces. There is no confusion as to what "the base" is when the student stands with feet together in *tadasana.* If one then opens the stance by separating the feet

laterally, as when setting the feet for *prasarita padottanasana,* then the effective area of the base becomes the area of a rectangle having the heel and toes of one foot at two of the corners and the heel and toes of the other at the other two corners, just as with the stippled area in object 2 in figure V.A-4. This expansion of the base of *prasarita padottanasana* makes the posture more stable, but only in the left-to-right direction, not in the front-to-back direction, which retains its original dimensions. Because the posture in *prasarita padottanasana* is less stable in the front-to-back direction than it is side to side, it is specifically metastable.

Similarly, with two hands and two feet on the ground in *adho mukha svanasana,* the effective base for balancing is that defined by the positions of the two hands and two feet at the corners of the rectangle. If one hand and the foot on the same side are lifted from the floor while in *adho mukha svanasana,* the base becomes very narrow, as defined by the remaining hand and foot on the floor, and balance is precarious in the front-to-back direction. However, if one instead lifts one hand and the opposite foot (*dwianga adho mukha svanasana*), stability can be maintained in both the front-to-back and the left-to-right directions, the more so the more the balancing hand and foot are separated front to back and left to right. This subject of the effective size of the base is discussed further in Subsection V.D, page 899.

Static Support versus Dynamic Balance

If one is to avoid a loss of balance through a collapse along the line between centers, it is necessary to be strong and supportive but essentially static and subconscious. In contrast, the solution to the problem of balancing to avoid falling to the side will be dynamic and more than a little involved with the conscious sense of the falling torques.

Going beyond the balancing rule given above regarding mechanical stability, balancing in the *yogasanas* amounts to having a continuous sense of the falling torques and continuously developing countertorques within the body that bring it back into balance (i.e., movements that dynamically maintain the line between centers within the effective base of the posture). Notice how similar this prescription for balancing in the *yogasanas* is to the general situation in *yogasana* practice, where the postures are not static but are constantly being refined by returning to each of their elements and extending their actions so as to go deeper into the posture (i.e., we pose and repose) [33]). In speaking of conscious action, William James appropriately describes it as "the marksman ends by thinking only of the exact position of the goal, the singer only of the perfect sound, the balancer only of the point of the pole whose oscillations he must counteract [229]."

Though it is possible to recover from a loss of balance using the great strength of the supporting limb in contact with the floor, the student will find this tiring and from there will come to see that the long-term use of strength to maintain balance is secondary to remaining constantly aware of the balanced position and not letting the body move too far toward falling. The use of strength to maintain balance also is at odds with the yogic dictum to perform the *yogasanas* with grace and ease (Subsection II.A, page 834). However, see also Subsection V.B, page 874, where the strength aspect of maintaining a balance is discussed.

Proper balancing of the body involves transforming it mechanically into a broomstick and then balancing that broomstick dynamically using the generation of countertorques. The ideal position of the body when balancing will be the position of minimum effort in order to conserve energy and prolong the duration of the posture. Deviations from this ideal position will be expensive in terms of energy and the time for which the position can be held in balance. Resistance against gravitational collapse is a matter of inner strength; given this resistance to collapse, the resistance against imbalance is a matter of sensitivity, awareness, and swift and appropriate (but momentary) response.

Distinguishing Support from Balance

If it is accepted that balancing involves the sensing of a falling torque and the activation of an appropriate mechanism by the falling object

to generate a countertorque having the correct timing, strength, and direction, it follows that because inanimate objects have none of these abilities, none of the stable objects (blocks) in figures V.A-1, V.A-2, V.A-3, or V.A-4 really are balancing; instead, **they are supported**. This distinction between balance and support applies to *yogasana* postures as well, even though we are all supplied with a full complement of sensors and balancing strategies. For example, *sirsasana I* can be performed as either a support (performed against the wall) or a balance (performed in the middle of the room), and *sirsasana II* is essentially a supported posture (weight of the body leaning upon the bent arms) rather than a balanced posture, as one can see from the weight distribution shown in figure IV.D-2.

The key elements of support in regard to the body are an internal rigidity, a large element of strength, little or no mental involvement, no sense of falling torque, and a motionless body. For example, stand 30 centimeters (one foot) away from the wall, lean your right shoulder on the wall, and, using your strength to keep the body stiff, place the left leg in *vrksasana,* and "support" this position with the mind empty and the body motionless. In contrast, stand in the middle of the room, lift one leg into *vrksasana,* and "balance" in this position by responding to the body's balance sensors, having a deep inner awareness of what is needed to achieve your goal but using little or no strength to this end, except for that needed to keep the secondary joints as close to their limiting ranges of motion as is possible while focusing on the primary balancing joint (Subsection V.B, page 877).

The main difference between "support" and "balance" of a body is that in the former, there is a rigidity sufficient to resist further falling while the body is motionless, and there are no falling torques to be counterbalanced, as with a block supported on the floor; in the latter state, the body is in motion side to side and/or front to back, and motion sensors activate muscular contractions that resist the falling. When "balancing" in the *yogasanas,* you will never be motionless, yet you must work appropriately to maintain the line of centers within the base of the posture with a minimum of swaying.

As with most things, the reality of most of our *yogasana* balancing postures will be a mixture of support and balance, but it will be important to know just how much of each we are depending upon to keep from falling. For example, the two aspects of support and balance are evident when performing *tadasana*. True alignment of the skeleton in *tadasana* involves being heavy on the heels and light on the toes, as this puts the maximum stress on the skeleton for maintaining the posture, and the least on the muscles. On the other hand, this alignment places the line between centers very close to the heels, so that the balance (such as that for object 3 in figure V.A-4) can be precarious. If the balance is difficult in this position, it is a reasonable compromise to slightly move the weight of the posture onto the toes, taking the skeleton slightly out of full balance and truly vertical alignment and putting the body more into the muscular-support mode by slightly leaning forward onto the toes. Specific metastability can be maintained in several ways: through static support, through dynamic balance, or through some combination of the two.

As will be shown below, in some cases, we use an appendage on the floor for mechanical support against collapse, and at other times, as an aid to balance. Sometimes we do both, and sometimes these two aspects of support and balance stand in opposition to one another.

Interestingly, it is the extreme flexibility of the body as compared with a block of wood that makes balancing the body so much more difficult, and at the same time, it is the extreme flexibility of the body and mind that allows one to maintain the balance of the body!

On Becoming a Broomstick

The description given in the previous section for balancing a broomstick on the end of the finger holds the essence of what must be done to balance the body in the *yogasanas*. In order to balance, one must keep certain parts of the body as immobile as a broomstick, while at the same time, one must maintain a mobile joint close to the floor, which joint is given 100 percent of the responsibility for keeping the whole structure in balance. It does this by sensing the falling torques and generating countertorques.

Because object 1 in figure V.A-4 essentially is a broomstick, it is mechanically stable as long as there are no external or internal disturbances; however, even a slight tipping to the side will take the line between centers beyond the minuscule base, initiating a fall that cannot be negated by a countertorque. In contrast, the broomstick placed on the end of the finger poses no problem, as long as the joint formed where the finger contacts the broomstick works with the eyes to apply the appropriate countertorques to the falling torque.

Now imagine that the broomstick has been cut horizontally into ten pieces and that a thin elastic band has been placed between each pair of adjacent pieces. As will be seen below, this is a more realistic model of a beginning student attempting to balance, for example, in a standing posture. In this case, the broomstick has become eleven individual but strongly interacting pendulums by the introduction of ten joints along its length, with each pendulum in the altered broomstick now representing the motion around a particular collapsed but all-too-mobile joint in the student's body.

Eye-Hand Coordination

In theory, the eye and the hand of the supporting arm could work together in a complicated way in order to keep all the relative torques of the eleven individual broomstick pendulums sufficiently compensated to maintain balance, at least for a short time. However, all too quickly, the complexity of keeping the torques of eleven independent pendulums in balance becomes overwhelming, with the result that the center of gravity of the broomstick soon falls outside the base of its support, and irreversible falling begins. How much easier and more sensible it is to replace the elastic bands with stout metal sleeves, making the broomstick integral again, with only the one joint between finger and broomstick mobile and totally responsible for balancing.

Correspondingly, the best plan for balancing on one leg in a standing posture, for example, is to focus all of the attention on the ankle joint of the standing leg and keep all of the other joints in the body immobile by opening them to the limits of their ranges of motion. In all upright standing postures, it is the proprioceptive feedback from the ankles (the primary joint for balancing in this type of posture) and from the Pacinian corpuscles in the soles of the feet that are crucial for the control and maintenance of the balance [427]. The involvement of the other, higher joints unnecessarily complicates the picture if they too are allowed to participate in the balance.

There is yet another benefit of the broomstick approach to balancing. It is known that the afferent neural channels that carry information about being out of balance can be easily overloaded to the extent that even a strong signal becomes lost in the noise (Subsection 13.C, page 523). This implies that if many parts of the body are active in trying to maintain balance, the changing signals in the proprioceptive afferents in the ankle may be swamped by those coming from other joints; whereas if only the ankle is active in balancing, then its proprioceptive signal should be read loud and clear by the central nervous system, if one can keep the mind focused on it.

Extraneous Motion at Secondary Joints

Lasater [486] points out that in *sirsasana*, beginners tend to go up into the inverted position using the strength of their arms and then balance with their legs, whereas one should do the reverse. As Farhi says with respect to balancing in *adho mukha vrksasana*, one should instead keep a neutral position of the legs with respect to the pelvis [234] (i.e., do not swing the legs back and forth to maintain balance). I agree with this totally and feel the same reasoning applies in the other inverted balances.

In *sirsasana,* if one extends the body straight up to take all of the looseness out of the joints (the body is taut), then the balancing action is in the hand and wrist, as it should be. If the body is loose instead, then balancing action reverts to points far above the point of contact with the floor, and complex body oscillation ensues. Not only is the balance impaired by this upper-body motion, but maintaining the motion is very energy-draining. Finally, only in *sirsasana I* and *savasana* are we unable to see any part of the body; all of the alignment then must be via the proprioceptive system of the body [485].

Unfortunately, when beginners have to balance in *yogasana* practice, they instinctively take the opposite route by flailing their arms and legs, swinging their hips, and otherwise fully expressing their multi-jointedness. Students who do not use the broomstick-countertorque technique put forward here can balance momentarily by generating countertorques through such motions around joints higher in the body (for example, by swinging the legs and hips to generate a countertorque in *adho mukha vrksasana*). However, these have a way of transforming into complex movements and premature falling; such flailing around the secondary joints in the arms, hips, and/or legs is often seen in gymnasts just a few seconds before they fall off the balance beam.

How then does one inhibit motion around the secondary joints, when balancing on the foot, to localize the balancing action in the foot? The extraneous motion around joints other than the ankle can be minimized by energetically opening each of these joints in the body maximally, making each of the joints taut (Iyengar says "poker stiff") and the body thereby unitary and monolithic. The stabilization of the secondary joints follows naturally from the yogic elongation of the body normally performed in the posture when bringing it into alignment and sending the energy to the extremities. Nothing more is needed than to realize that the effort to extend the secondary joints (your "broomstickiness") also serves the sense of balance; mentally placing this deliberate extension on second attention stabilizes the secondary joints so that one can give undivided attention to the primary joint working the floor. With practice, one works to minimize the amplitudes of the oscillations in the primary balancing joint to make the balance-conserving motions imperceptibly small and thereby energy-conserving as well.

One can gain an appreciation for the increased

level of complexity involved when going from one balancing joint active in *vrksasana* (the ankle) to two independent joints. Come to balance in *vrksasana* with a broomstick in one hand, and then balance this broomstick on the finger while supporting the body on one leg. The simultaneous balancing of the body by the ankle and the broomstick by the hand can be challenging, especially if the hand and foot are on the same side of the body and so are using the same cerebral hemisphere for the reception of falling sensations and their corrections. If there is no difference when one goes from ipsilateral to contralateral hand/foot balancing, there must be a rapid side-to-side transfer of balancing information going on between the cerebral hemispheres in the latter case.

When the secondary joints are wide open, they become silent, as their proprioceptive signals become constant and so are blocked by the reticular formation (Subsection 4.B, page 74), whereas the ever-changing signal from the primary joint is easily heard by the balancing mechanism.

Generating a Countertorque When Falling

Given that one has learned how to transform the body into a broomstick for the purposes of balancing, how then does one achieve the second action necessary for balance: the generation of a torque countering that of falling? The answer to this is illustrated by the exercise described in Box V.B-1, below.

Because nature has placed the ankle over the heel and far from the toes, a strong countertorque can be generated when leaning forward on the foot but not backward. If the ankle were centered between the toes and the heel of the foot, then one could balance forward and backward by generating clockwise and counterclockwise torques, but this is not the case. The awareness of the action of the toes, foot, and ankle on the floor in this exercise should be uppermost in the minds of the students as they practice balancing in the standing *yogasanas*. This also applies to balancing on the side body, as in *anantasana* (see below), and to hand balancing, where there are fingers

on one side of the palm, but not on the opposite side.

Useless Knee and Elbow

In contrast to the hand and the foot, the knee and the elbow have no appendages on any parts of their peripheries with which a countertorque can be generated against the floor. Consequently, balancing on the knee (as in *vatayanasana*) or on the elbows (as in *sayanasana*) is exceptionally difficult, as is *anantasana* for those with feet held in plantar flexion rather than in dorsiflexion. However, the forearms can act like fingers for the elbow when in *pincha mayurasana* (i.e., they can be used to generate a countertorque if one is falling backward, and so the balance is relatively easy, compared to that in *sayanasana*). However, this is the case when in *pincha mayurasana* only if the center of gravity of the body is over the forearms; if it is forward of the elbows, then the posture is lost, for the line between centers is outside the base, and one simply falls forward onto the toes, as there is no way to apply a countertorque in this situation.

If balancing in *vasisthasana I* is trivial for you, try the variation with one hand on the floor and the lower leg bent so that its foot rests on the thigh of the upper leg and its knee rests on the floor; having a chair in front of one is a great help in getting into this posture. Once there, release the chair and balance on one hand and one knee. Because the knee is of no use in balancing in this posture, all of the work falls to the one hand on the floor, and this elevates the posture to the level of difficulty that one finds in doing a one-arm hand-balance! Similarly, sit in *vajrasana* placing a belt so as to bind ankles to thighs. Holding on to a chair, come on to the knees, feet off the floor, heels to buttocks. Release the chair and balance on your knees. You will see how useless the knees are in balancing, because they do not have any primary joint that can be used to develop a countertorque from the floor. If, on the other hand, the feet are lowered onto the floor so that the shins can work the floor, as in *ustrasana,* then the balance is so stable that one really should call it "support," as with a block.

Box V.B-1: Using the Floor When Balancing

Repeating the lesson of Section IV.A, page 851, you cannot consciously press your feet further into the floor in *tadasana,* because you press the floor with whatever your weight is, and you cannot change that pressure unless you change your weight. What can be changed is how you transfer weight from one part of your foot to another (e.g., from the medial edge of your foot to the lateral edge, from one foot to the other, or from heel to toe). The shift of the pressure among the various parts of a limb on the floor can generate a rotational torque.

In order to discover the counter-rotating force so useful in balancing, come to stand with your right side about two feet from the wall, and then come into *vrksasana* on the right leg. Purposely lean to the right and break your fall by pressing the wall with your right hand. This pressure against the unmoving wall provides the countertorque needed to restore balance.[1] When the wall is not there, a similar action of foot on the floor serves the same purpose. Next, stand with your feet 45 centimeters (eighteen inches) from the wall, lean your seat onto the wall, and fold forward into *uttanasana.* Using your hands, gently push off the wall to be in classical *uttanasana,* legs vertical and weight somewhat on the balls of the feet (the metatarsal heads) and heavily on the heels. Now further tip your weight forward to generate a momentary forward-falling torque and notice how pressing the toes and their metatarsals (especially those of the big toes; see Box V.F-1, page 916) into the floor generates the countertorque that keeps one from falling any further. That is to say, by pressing

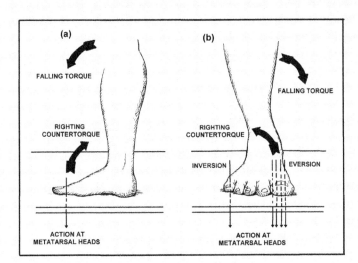

Figure V.B-1. (a) As one falls forward in *uttanasana,* generating a falling torque, the toes and their metatarsal heads are pressed into the floor to generate a countertorque, restoring balance. (b) Schematic of the right leg and foot as they stand on the floor in *vrksasana.* If the leg/torso falls to generate a clockwise falling torque (upper arrow), then the reflexive action is for the big-toe side of the foot to press the floor, generating a counterclockwise torque (lower arrow) that acts to align the body vertically and restore balance.

---

1   The need for a strong, immobile surface against which one can generate a countertorque is obvious if one will just imagine how ineffective the counterbalancing action would be if the wall were made of Jell-O rather than of wood and plaster. With that in mind, think of the disadvantage of trying to balance when standing on a soft yoga mat. This need for a strong, immobile anchor against which one can work in order to maintain balance is closely related to the use of anchors when stretching (Subsection 11.F, page 468).

the forward parts of the feet into the floor, using the gastrocnemius and peroneus longus muscles of the lower legs (Subsection 10.B, page 356), one generates a torque counter to that appropriate to falling forward (figure V.B-1**a**) and so returns to the upright position, provided the countertorque is of the proper magnitude and comes at the proper time.

Similarly, if standing on the right foot and falling to the left (figure V.B-1**b**), one generates the countertorque by pressing the base of the big toe and inner edge of the foot into the floor. In *vrksasana,* maintain a high level of "broomstickiness" from the shins up to the crown of the head, but from the shins down to the sole of the foot, be a well-oiled machine, operating as described in figure V.B-1. This clearly shows how one works the floor in order to generate countertorques that maintain balance. However, this assumes that one is able to raise and lower the medial arch of the foot (arch 1–3 in figure 10.B-8). If this arch has fallen and cannot be activated, then the broomstick-countertorque technique will not work as well to maintain balance in the standing postures.

The extent of the countertorque that can be generated by either the hand or the foot is quite limited. For this reason, one must enter balancing postures gently and use the hand or foot to maintain balance rather than to establish balance.

Asymmetric Hand and Foot

The effects of the asymmetry of the hand and foot on hand balancing and foot balancing become evident on considering the factors determining the magnitude of the countertorque being developed while balancing. Consider figure V.B-2**a**, in which the line between centers is forward of the base of the standing foot and so results in a counterclockwise-falling torque of magnitude -FR, where F is the gravitational force (equation IV.A-1) and R is the distance from the line between centers to the vertical line passing through the base of the toes.

The magnitude of the countertorque is given by the product of the size of the force being exerted and the length of the lever arm over which the force is exerted (i.e., by the product of the counterbalancing force and the distance from the point of application of the force to the line of centers). As applied to foot balance (figure V. B-2**a**), the countertorque for falling forward will involve the product of the force (Q) exerted on the floor by the toes times the distance (r) from the toes to the line between centers, the latter being essentially through the ankle and just slightly forward of point 3 in figure 10.B-6**b**. Balance is preserved in figure V.B-2**a** if the clockwise countertorque is

slightly larger than the counterclockwise falling torque.

The rotational torque when falling backward equals the product of the gravitational force F times the distance -R′ from point 3 on the heel to the line between centers. In turn, the countertorque for falling backward is the product of the force Q′ with which the heel can press into the floor times the distance -r′ from point 3 on the foot to the mid heel. Because this distance factor in the case of falling backward is so small, falling backward in a foot balance is very difficult to counteract, and the best strategy for maintaining balance is to keep the weight somewhat forward on the toes and away from the heels. Maximum ease is developed in foot balance by having a long foot, leading to both a large base for the posture, a large lever arm (r) for generating a countertorque, and high toes-to-the-floor strength. Students with short, weak feet are at a distinct disadvantage in all three regards when foot balancing.

If falling sideways when foot balancing (figure V.B-1**b**), the distance factor (r) in regard to the countertorque is essentially the same when falling to the left or to the right; however, the force (Q) that can be applied by the big toe is substantially larger than that which can be applied by the

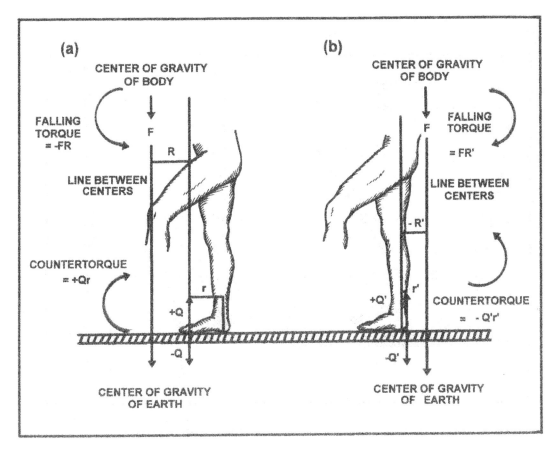

Figure V.B-2. (a) Diagram of forces and torques acting at the foot when falling forward on the right leg. The falling torque is to be countered by the torque generated by pressing the forward part of the foot into the floor with force Q, which expresses itself as a torque (T) when multiplied by the length of the lever arm (r), this being the distance from the point on the foot for the application of the force on the floor to the point on the foot about which the countertorque rotates (i.e., point 3 in figure 10.B-8c); T = Qr. (b) Diagram of forces and torques acting at the foot when falling backward on the right leg. Note the much smaller value of r′, the length of the lever arm, and hence the smaller value of T′, the generated countertorque when falling backward as compared with falling forward.

little toe; thus, it will be advantageous to keep the weight more on the big-toe side of the foot than on the little-toe side.

The difference in the countertorques when falling forward or backward is accentuated even more when hand balancing (figure V.D-3a), because the lever arm through which the countertorque acts will be the length of the hand for overbalancing but essentially zero for underbalancing. For one-arm balances such as *vasisthasana I*, the force developed by thumb pressure on the floor will be much stronger than that for the little finger, and so the weight should be kept more toward the thumb side.

Finally, the countertorques at our disposal are at their extremes in the *sirsasana* variations. In *sirsasana I*, it is abundantly clear from figure V.D-2 that the balance-conserving lever arm for underbalancing (length of forearms) is far larger than that for overbalancing. Thus, the very strong tendency in *sirsasana I* to be heavy on the elbows (underbalanced) is seen to be a psychological defense against falling backward into the unknown, against which there is very little resistance. The opposite situation is met in *pincha mayurasana*.

In contrast, now allow the weight to fall backward when in free-standing *uttanasana* at the wall; because there are no toes at the back of the foot to press onto the floor, a countertorque cannot be generated at the ankle, and one ends up falling backward into the wall. The simple lesson illustrated by the above applies to any standing posture, on one leg or two, regardless of the position of the upper body; keep the weight slightly forward toward the toes in order to avoid falling backward over the heels.

Falling too far forward is avoided by pressing the base of the toes **gently** into the floor, so that the forward lean does not become excessive, and so that the toes do not try to grip the floor.[3] Leaning backward is to be avoided, because one cannot generate a countertorque in this case, and falling is certain. Consequently, we attempt subconsciously to have the countertorque be just short of that necessary to bring the body into perfect balance, thereby avoiding the chance of losing balance by falling backward over the heels.

As another example of generating a countertorque on the floor, sit in *vajrasana* with buttocks on heels, and then start to fall backward; pressing the insteps of the feet heavily into the floor generates a countertorque which lifts the hips upward and forward to regain balance.

In *vatayanasana*, the balance is on one foot and the opposite knee and is very difficult unless one can get the complete foot on the floor, as the knee is of no use, and having only the toes of the other foot on the floor is not enough to generate strong countertorques. However, *adho mukha*

svanasana done with both the knees and the elbows on the floor is perfectly stable, because we can shift weight between these anatomic parts on the floor even if each by itself is unable to generate a countertorque!

Try standing up but with feet replaced by knees, i.e., sit in *virasana* with ankles belted to thighs and then "stand up" on the knees, using a chair for momentary support. Balance can be maintained if at all, only by wildly swinging the arms about, which is very unyogic. However, the extreme sensitivity of the fingertip as sensor (Subsection V.D, page 901) can be exploited here, for just a gentle touch of one fingertip to the chair is all that is needed to maintain this balance.

In general, the idea that the hand and foot are strong enough to generate torques large enough to shift the body's center of gravity seems unlikely. However, as Myers points out [603], the body contains "anatomy trains," in which small muscles at the extremities are integrally linked to larger and even larger muscles in the fashion of a train, and in which contraction of the small muscles at one end of the train results in the near-simultaneous contraction of the larger muscles at the other end of the train. This would offer a simple mechanism by which pressure on a certain part of the hand when balancing results in the distance activation of large muscles in the back, which pull the center of gravity to a more favorable position, much as the action of the thumbs on the floor results in the scapulae of the back being pressed onto the rib cage (Subsection 10.A, pages 328 and 331).

Gripping the Floor

When on the feet, as in *tadasana* (or on the hands, as in *adho mukha vrksasana*), the toes (or fingers) rest on the floor, stretching forward from the ankles (wrists). Neither the toes nor the fingertips should grip the floor in these postures. However, when one comes to balance on one foot (or the hands), it is then advantageous to move the weight somewhat forward onto the toes (or fingertips) in order to generate the necessary countertorque for balancing. That is to say, add a little more support to the support/balance mix if maintaining balance requires it.

---

3   Ideally, for either the hands or the feet on the floor, the phalanges should extend forward and rest gently on the floor, whereas the heads of the metacarpals and metatarsals are pressed more or less strongly into the floor to generate the torques required for maintaining balance. When learning to balance, it is more excusable to also grip the floor with the tips of the fingers and toes, especially in *adho mukha vrksasana* and *bakasana*, where bending the fingers and pressing the fingertips into the floor gives one a great advantage in retaining balance, provided one avoids leaning the body weight backward into the heels of the hands in these postures. The use of the tip of the little finger as a balance sensor rather than as a generator of countertorque is described in Subsection V.D, page 902.

The leg is stronger than the arm, and the foot is stronger than the hand. In postures such as *dwianga adho mukha svanasana,* where both a hand and a foot are on the floor for balance, if the sole of the foot can be placed fully on the floor, then it will be the stronger contributor to balance, and the head should be tipped to look at the foot. If, on the other hand, one can only get the toes on the floor in this posture, then the hand is the stronger balancing element, and one should look at the balancing hand instead (Subsection V.C, page 892).

Size of the Base

The student will readily appreciate the advantage of having a base of large dimensions when balancing, by comparing the increasing difficulty of balancing after tipping into *uttanasana* first with the feet hip width apart, then with the feet successively together, with one leg in *ardha padmasana,* and finally when standing on just the toes of one foot. Similarly, compare the ease of balance in *sarvangasana* with that in *niralamba sarvangasana,* a posture with a much smaller base. See Subsection V.D, page 899, for more on this subject. In addition to concern about the area of the base, when balancing on the hands or other parts of the anatomy, the principles of "broomstick and countertorque" to keep the line of centers within the base still must be enforced.

The general instruction to "broaden the base of the hand (foot) from left to right, stretching the fingers (toes) forward" is appropriate for *adho mukha svanasana,* even though there is no balancing involved; but when in *dwianga adho mukha svanasana,* these actions also broaden the bases of the hands (feet) used for maintaining balance in the posture and so become doubly important. In all balancing postures on hands and/or feet, the skin placed on the floor should be as broad as possible in all directions. This stretching of the skin also may function to bring the Ruffini corpuscles of the skin (Subsection 11.B, page 440) into the sensor picture as aids to balancing. However, this stretching action also brings one to the limit of range of motion and so weakens any muscle action needed to maintain balance; see Box 11.A-2, page 401, in regard to the minimum strength of muscles when at the limits of their ranges of motion.

The Order of Muscle Recruitment

When the body in standing position is momentarily tipped off balance, as in the *uttanasana* described in Box V.B-1, page 879, and figure V.B-1a, it has been shown [427] that the first reaction is for the balls of the feet to be pressed into the floor by contraction of the type 3 (fast-twitch; see Subsection 11.A, page 414) gastrocnemius (calf) muscles, in order to generate a countertorque. This is then followed by further countertorques, generated by contraction of the hamstrings and erector spinae muscles. These successive reflex actions are set in motion by the simultaneous activation of the four receptor modes mentioned in Section V.C, page 886: cutaneous, vestibular, proprioceptive, and (possibly) ocular. The sequence of muscle actions in this balancing is that the muscle closest to the base is activated first, while those more distant are activated at later times; this may be taken as a general rule when using countertorques in balancing. In regard to the actions of muscles of different types, it is most likely that type 3, fast-twitch muscles are more involved in the balancing act at the primary balancing joint and that type 1 postural muscles are more active in keeping the secondary joints fully taut and open.

Response Times

Conscious action in regard to balancing requires time to receive the off-balance signal, evaluate it, compute a new course of action, transmit the action plan, and finally execute it. When time is too short for this, the body takes the reflex route to quick action, bypassing the higher brain centers (see Section 11.D, page 446). Postural response time is shortest when the imbalance is sensed proprioceptively by the muscle spindles (seventy to one hundred milliseconds), whereas response times are perhaps twice as long when the off-balance signal is vestibular or ocular [427]. When the balancing task is slow, simple, and undemanding, the proprioceptive joint inputs are used more than the vestibular sensors; however, when the task is more complex or more rapid, then the latter can increase in importance.

The joint sensors are relatively inactive when standing on a soft surface, in which case, the slower vestibular apparatus takes over [782]. If there is no need for haste, then the conscious mind can intercede in the decision making, though the elapsed time for action will be longer than when reacting reflexively [277].

There is a unique aspect of the balancing reflex that should be encouraging to the *yogasana* student. Whereas the patellar knee-jerk reflex (see Section 11.D, page 448), for example, remains always the same, the balancing reflex becomes both quicker and more refined with practice. That is to say, one eventually can balance on one's hands by practicing, as the balance reflex can maintain balance for a longer and longer time with less and less effort through practice [427]. This is possible because our bodies are capable not only of responsive feedback (a reaction to an imbalance already in motion) but also of responsive feedforward, a process in which the imbalance is anticipated and adjustments made in preparation for it. So, for example, in the case of falling forward in *sirsasana I*, the reflexive action in the elbows may be too strong at first, and the body then starts to fall backward. With practice, one can reflexively anticipate the over-reaction and moderate the first response while being prepared to counter it with the second by anticipating it. In this way, practice sharpens the balancing ability and makes progress possible.

Conscious versus Subconscious Actions

That the subconscious mind can contribute to our mechanical balance is evident from the fact that we are largely unaware of our balance when walking or bending over to pick up a yoga belt, yet we rarely fall when so involved. In these cases, it is the slow-twitch, antigravity type 1 muscles, together with the four types of balance sensors, that are involved in the balancing act at levels below consciousness. When intermediate-level students come to balance in the *yogasanas*, there is a strong element of deliberate, conscious effort.

Though the subconscious effort certainly is evident in beginners learning to balance, with practice, they too will come to balance with a higher consciousness.

Falling Straight Down: Gravitational Collapse

Intelligent Use of the Bones

In the context of a rigid block, the possibility of its falling straight down along the line between centers is moot if it is assumed that the block is truly rigid; however, the issue of collapse along the line between centers of body and Earth while balancing is a real one, because the human body is not necessarily a rigid block. Though not a factor for a rigid body such as a wooden block, gravitational collapse along the line between centers is a real possibility for the *yogasana* student, who otherwise must keep the following in mind: Even in a *yogasana* in which balance is not a factor, as with *adho mukha svanasana*, for example, the intent of gravity to pull the body onto the floor must be dealt with. The strongest steel-link chain in the world will collapse gravitationally if you try to balance it on end, for the strength of the chain is in tension, whereas resisting gravitational collapse involves strength in compression. Because each of our bodies is a tensegrity structure [387] involving a balance between the soft tissues in tension and the bones supporting compression, it is the compressive strength of our bones and the proper placement of them by the muscles that resists gravitational collapse.

The best defense against collapse along the line between centers involves placing the bones of the body in such a position to best support the posture for a meaningful period of time. If the body is in *vasisthasana I*, supported on one arm, that arm must be kept straight (but not necessarily vertical), with the bones of the upper and lower arm in alignment. Though this position can be held with the arm bent, it cannot be held very long. Similarly, in *utthita hasta padangusthasana*, the standing leg must be straight if one is to stay up for any length of time, as the bent leg is effectively in a one-legged crouch. When the leg is bent, this can be sustained for only a short time using the strength of the leg muscles, but it can be sustained indefinitely by the strength of the leg bones when the leg is straight.

Muscles versus Bones

On those occasions when the geometry of the posture requires that the skeleton be arranged in a way that muscle support is not optional, then you have no choice but to employ a larger strength factor than is usual in *yogasana* practice. For example, this is the situation in both *chaturanga dandasana* and in *utkatasana,* in which the bent arms and the bent legs (Subsection 11.A, page 428) must do hard work in order to support the body weight. The importance of using the skeleton to support the body rather than the muscles in *yogasana* postures will be evident to your students if half the class is put into plank position (straight-arm *chaturanga dandasana*) and the other half simultaneously is put into conventional bent-arm *chaturanga dandasana*. Which half stays in position longer: those supported by the bones (straight-arm *chaturanga*) or those supported by the muscles (bent-arm *chaturanga*)? A similar comparison of endurance with the two halves of the class performing either bone-supported *tadasana* or muscle-supported *utkatasana* teaches the same lesson.

Bone Placement

Regarding gravitational collapse, a wooden block is very strong, a soufflé is very weak, and your body is in between—strong if you act intelligently regarding how to use it, but not so strong if you are careless about how to use its parts to resist gravity.

Given that straight-arm *chaturanga dandasana* position is more strongly supported by the skeleton than is bent-arm *chaturanga dandasana,* go into the straight-arm position and then incrementally move your hands apart laterally with the arms kept straight. The added difficulty of opening the arms to the side while in straight-arm *chaturanga dandasana* demonstrates the importance of keeping the arms directly beneath the body in order to support it against gravitational collapse. This simple requirement is often ignored by beginners in postures such as *sirsasana, bakasana,* and *sarvangasana,* when they allow the elbows to be placed far from the center line of the body. Even with the arms bent in *chaturanga dandasana,* beginners still should keep the elbows close to the sides of the body for support, as letting them out to the sides only increases the possibility of gravitational collapse.

As another example of the importance of keeping the bones in alignment, consider inverted *sarvangasana*: stand with back to wall with arms in the *sarvangasana* position, elbows as close to one another as possible. Lean back to bring the elbows, the upper arms, and the head onto the wall, and note the pressure on the wrists as hands press into the kidneys and rib cage in support of the body weight. Now just let the elbows slide out to the side (as with *sarvangasana* in the beginner), and see how the pressure at the wrists disappears and the arms are no longer in position to support anything. It is for this reason that the elbows must be kept close to the center line of the body in *sarvangasana,* and the same reasoning applies to *sirsasanas I* and *II* as well.

Thus, in a balancing posture such as *adho mukha vrksasana,* the effect of gravity becomes doubly disadvantageous, for it requires that the body be kept in balance in spite of gravity, and at the same time, it must be elongated upward, again in spite of gravity. However, as discussed above, the act of yogic elongation against gravity actually makes balancing easier in almost all cases, as it damps the motions in the secondary joints, thereby making the balance more sustainable.

Belt Support

In an arm-supported hand balances such as *lolasana, tolasana,* or *dandasana* with the legs held off the ground, the center of gravity of the body lies between the shoulders and the floor, and the act of support can be so challenging in regard to falling straight down that one hardly has a chance to test the balancing aspects of the postures. In that case, the legs can be supported by a belt looped around the chest from the back and under the ankles or feet, thus allowing one to focus solely on the balance. In a similar way, if the student's arms will not support the body weight in *adho mukha vrksasana,* a belt placed just above the elbows will keep the bones of the arms in alignment and thereby prevent gravitational collapse while allowing one to focus more intently on working toward balance.

Section V.C: The Four Balance Sensors

There are four distinct sensory systems in the body that are relevant to the act of balancing in the *yogasanas.* Just how effective the four sensors are in sensing a falling torque around a specific axis of the body and reporting the falling in a timely fashion are key elements in balancing. Furthermore, different sensors may be brought into play depending upon the posture in question, and which sensor is activated will depend upon which part of the anatomy is in contact with the floor when in the posture.

The four sensors used for balance in the human body are:

1. Proprioceptors in the muscles, joints, and skin that sense the positions and rates of motion of the various body parts with respect to one another, using the muscle spindles (see Section 11.B, page 429), the joint capsules (see Section 11.B, page 440), and the stretch receptors in the skin (see Subsection 11.B, page 440)

2. The eyes, which play a key role in determining if the head or body is being held in an upright position or is falling front to back or side to side (Subsection 17.B, page 666)

3. Vestibular organs in each of the inner ears, which sense both the static head positions and any dynamic forces on the head, as when one falls (Subsection 18.B, page 696)

4. Large numbers of pressure sensors located at several locations in the skin (soles of the feet, for example; see figure 13.B-2), which indicate any shift of weight that occurs when one is falling while in a standing, sitting, or inverted posture

Specific Insensitivity

In addition to instability in regard to specific directions in a posture due to the shape of its base (Subsection V.A, page 869), one also must consider the possible specific insensitivities of the balance sensors. The pressure sensors (figure 13.B-2) are not of much help when trying to balance on a part of the anatomy devoid of pressure sensors, as is the case with the upper back body in *niralamba sarvangasana.* Because retinal streaming of the eyes (Box V.C-1, page 889) is more effective when it detects sideways falling as compared with front-back falling, the eyes are of little or no use when balancing in *sirsasana I.* Probably because they are used more in the upright position, the semicircular canals (Subsection 18.B, page 698) are more effective when upright than when inverted, so it seems that all upright variations of a balancing posture are easier than the corresponding inverted postures, at least for beginners.

The Subconscious

The highest spinal levels generally reached by signals from these four types of receptors are the medulla oblongata, the mesencephalon, and the vestibular part of the cerebellum (i.e., the oldest part of the brain phylogenetically, figure 4.B-1 and Section 4.A, page 72). Thus, the balancing motions under the control of these receptors initially are largely (or totally) in the subconscious unless they can be deliberately brought to higher levels.

Proprioception

As discussed in Section 11.C, page 441, although proprioceptive signals are relatively little understood and their role in balancing is not at all clear, their actions can be readily demonstrated. It is the proprioceptive sense that unerringly guides the fork into the mouth without error, and it is the same sense that keeps the fork from moving so far back in the mouth that it stabs the throat. Watching an infant's first attempts at eating with a spoon convinces one that proprioceptive skills are learned by practice. In *yogasana* practice, the proprioceptive sense comes to the fore when we perform *eka pada adho mukha svanasana,* for example, with the lifted leg in alignment with the spinal column, even though we are not able to see it.

In regard to balancing, proprioceptive information is generated especially in the talus joint of the ankle, the hip joints, the spine, and the suboccipital muscles of the neck [168]. Information from these joints and muscles goes to the brainstem and cerebellum for processing [782], and a map of the body in space is then constructed by the subconscious brain.

Neck-Spindle Sensors

Proprioceptive sensations of muscle tension are transmitted to the brain from the muscle spindles within the rectus capitis posterior minor muscles in the back of the neck. These muscles, left and right, run parallel to the spine, with origin at the posterior tubercle of C1 and insertion on the dura mater at the skull's occiput (figure V.C-1). The extraordinarily high density of muscle spindles in such a small muscle as the capitis (table 11.B-1, page 431) suggests that its value to the cervical spine rests more in its function as a proprioceptive monitor of head position than as a muscle for support against gravity [111, 112]. As one moves toward old age, the capitis sensors become the major sensors used to monitor balance of the head and therefore of the body.

Differences in the muscle-spindle signals from these tiny muscles are used proprioceptively to determine the left-to-right orientation of the head. Subconscious comparison of the muscle-spindle tension in the left and right capitis muscles offers a simple measure of the left-to-right tendency of

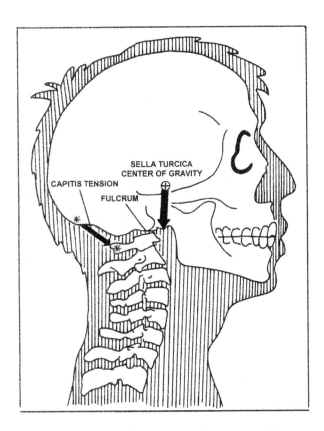

Figure V.C-1. The center of gravity of the head lies at the sella turcica, just forward of the atlas, which is the fulcrum upon which the head rests. Muscle tension in the capitis muscles of the neck serves as a countertorque to the falling torque of the head, and so keeps it erect. The origin at C1 and insertion of the capitis muscles at the dura mater covering the occiput of the skull are indicated by *s.

the head or the body to lean to one side or the other. Note, however, there is little or no tension in the capitis muscle sensors if the head is held in extension, as when looking upward in *vrksasana,* for example, and therefore, this position of the head lessens the amount of postural information available to the brain.

Though the capitis muscles are slack when the neck is in extension and there is no significant proprioceptive signal from these sensors, still the rise and fall of the muscle-spindle signals as the head moves between flexion and extension while retaining left-right symmetry does provide some information about front-to-back falling.

Because the rectus capitis are bound to the dura mater surrounding the brain, faulty action of the rectus capitis can lead to the instability known as "cervical vertigo." Yet if these sensors are functioning properly and optimally, one can stand in *vrksasana* for thirty seconds with eyes closed and arms crossed over the chest.

The Eyes

As more than one-third of the neurons in the brain are involved in some way in the visual process, it is no surprise that the eyes are strongly involved in balancing. Readers can readily test for themselves the truth of this statement by performing the simple exercises described in Box V.C-1, below.

Candlepower

Muscular actions in response to visual cues are slowest in dim light and fastest in bright light [338, 361]. This means that balancing in *yogasanas* will be easiest with bright illumination, because the responsiveness to imbalance is quicker; conversely, balancing will be more difficult in very dim light. It is conceivable that poor vision could interfere with using the eyes to advantage in balancing. Try *vrksasana* with and without your glasses on, to see if this is the case.

Falling with Closed Eyes

The extent of the involvement of the eyes in a particular balancing posture can be determined easily by performing the posture with the eyes open and then closing them; if you fall immediately on closing the eyes, then streaming retinal visual cues are clearly involved strongly in your balancing. Try this with a number of balancing positions in order to see for yourself that the extent of involvement of the eyes can be variable, being perhaps large in *vrksasana* but minimal in *paripurna navasana* and in *sirsasana*. Apparently there is no loss of sensitivity with time due to adaptation of retinal streaming (Subsection 13.B, page 506).

When balancing a broomstick, first watch the upper tip of the broomstick and see how easy it is to balance. Then, keeping the eyes open, watch the lower tip of the broomstick instead. In this case, falling is immediate! In order to balance the body, not only does the balancing sensor have to be switched on, but it has to be coupled directly or indirectly to some part of the anatomy that is falling. In *sirsasana I*, one can close the eyes without falling because (1) the eyes are not able to focus on a falling part of the body and so are irrelevant and (2) the head is not falling in *sirsasana I*, as it is the feet that fall.

If you find that you are unable to balance for a reasonable time in *vrksasana* with the eyes closed, then you must drive with great care. Police in certain locales now use the time for which one can stand on one leg with the eyes closed as a standard field sobriety test. Being able to balance for ten seconds on one leg with the eyes closed can mean the difference between avoiding a serious ticket and not!

It is of great interest to our discussion to note that whereas a light stick cannot be balanced with the eyes closed, the balancing of a heavy stick can be so balanced [99]! Apparently, when the stick is light, there is too little stimulation of either the pressure sensors or the proprioceptive sensors, and so visual cues predominate, whereas if the stick is sufficiently heavy, these balance sensors are functional and the visual route can be turned off.

Visual Grasp

The concept of visual concentration (visual grasp) while balancing in the *yogasanas* perhaps can be logically related to the meditative practice of *dristi*, which involves the use of the eyes to concentrate the mind. Because the eyes are so important to concentration and balancing, one assumes that there must be an optimal way of using them to stabilize a standing posture. Indeed, the eyes can be used to best advantage when balancing in the following way. Having first come into position in a standing posture, pick a stationary object on the far wall, and work the countertorques to keep the object attentively in the center of your field of view. As long as the image of the object is stable on the retina, the retinal streaming signals from the receptive fields will not change, and this will serve to keep you balanced. In effect, one has a visual grasp on a stable anchor in the visual field. Of

---

Box V.C-1: Using Your Eyes to Balance

Retinal Streaming

The rods and cones in the peripheral region of the retina are wired to each other in small groups called receptive fields, the purpose of which is to identify any movement of the external world with respect to the retina (Subsection 17.B, page 665). In particular, the receptive fields are composed of individual cells wired together in such a way that each group is sensitive to motion of a specific image shape at a specific angle. Some of the receptive fields are sensitive to left-to-right motion of the straight edge of a bar, and others to the opposite motion; some are sensitive to longer bars, and others to shorter bars; and some are sensitive to the motion of curved lines of specific curvature and orientation. The receptive fields within the retina present a steady stream of information in regard to the motions of objects in the visual field. Twenty percent of the fibers in the optic nerve are dedicated to carrying the messages of retinal streaming to balancing centers in the brain. In part, this is why there are so many more fibers for the optical nerve than for the auditory nerve, as the latter is not used for balancing.

The motions within the peripheral visual field to which the receptive fields respond may be either due to the relative motion of an external object moving with respect to the immobile retina, or due to the relative motion of the retina when off balance with respect to immobile visual anchors. There is an ongoing stream of receptive-field data being sent to the brain, a part of which refers directly to the state of the head's orientation with respect to vertical. These streams of data change with every step we take; however, in walking or bending over, we have learned what to expect in regard to retinal-stream changes, and no alarms are sounded. Only when the retinal streams change in a way that is inconsistent with non-falling behavior does the body respond to preserve balance.

Notice that if one is falling either to the left or right with the eyes open, changes in the retinal streaming signal will be generated as the visual field sweeps across the retina. However, when falling to the front or the back, there is little or no perceived motion of the visual field, and so retinal streaming in this case is much less effective in signaling a fall. For example, because *trikonasana* shows a front-to-back specific metastability, as do *bakasana* and *adho mukha vrksasana*, the tendency toward losing one's balance in the forward-backward directions is primary, whereas the retinal streaming signals are relatively small or lacking totally for falling in this direction. In contrast, in *virabhadrasana I*, the specific instability is in the left-to-right direction, and retinal streaming will be very important in signaling a fall in progress. Retinal streaming is not a factor when in *adho mukha svanasana* but is a left-to-right factor when balancing in *dwianga adho mukha svanasana*.

As discussed in more detail in Subsection 17.B, page 669, there are two major retinal streams from each retina with very different properties; one stream (the ventral stream) is essentially in the conscious sphere, has a long response time, and is long remembered; whereas the other (the dorsal stream) is essentially subconscious, requires a rapid muscular response, and is instantaneously forgotten. It is the second of these that is active reflexively in those cases where one is using the eyes to balance.

There will be a strong contribution of the eyes' receptive-field sensors to the act of balance as long as the eyes are open and as long as the falling is in a direction that changes the position of a distinctive marker in the visual field that can leave a trace on the edge sensors of the retina as the head falls. As a corollary to this, if one is trying to balance, motions of external objects in the field of view can easily be confused with the sensation of falling and so can misdirect the balancing efforts [708]. This optokinetic effect is discussed below.

Closing the Eyes

More than one might think, we use our eyes to sense the visual markers in the environment (e.g., we all use retinal streaming in order to adjust our verticality). The general truth of this statement for the student of *yogasana* is easily shown. Perform *vrksasana* as you normally do, and then close your eyes and see how much more challenging the balancing becomes. The key factor here in using the eyes to balance is the presence in the eye of receptive fields, many of which are sensitive to the angular alignment of straight lines in the visual field. As one starts to fall, the changing angle of these straight lines, as sensed by the eyes, serves to initiate corrective actions to preserve balance, provided the eyes are open.[1] The use of the eyes as a visual anchor is like a visual mantra, in that it acts as an aid to maintaining mental focus and therefore balance. In fact, due to the existence of vestibular-ocular reflexes, both postural stability and gaze stability (*dristi*) are affected when the vestibular system is dysfunctional. Such vestibular dysfunction can be assessed using the Romberg test for balance, in which one stands in *tadasana* with the eyes closed for thirty seconds and tries not to fall.

In addition to the obvious implication of the eyes in balancing, there is a more general damping down of all of the body's motor systems when the eyes close. Thus, being blindfolded for two minutes results in a slowing of the firing of all of the motor units, regardless of the task at hand, and all reflexes slow when the eyes are shielded from light [30]. Though this must be a significant factor in the relaxation occurring in *savasana* with the eyes closed (or when in any *yogasana* with the eyes bandaged), closed eyes, darkness, or just squinting the eyes are impediments to balancing in the *yogasanas*. That the balance is not affected in *vrksasana* by closing only one eye shows that the visual effect on balancing does not involve stereoscopic vision. As the practice of *bhastrika pranayama* has been shown to decrease the reaction times for both visual and auditory sensing [61], it is possible that the visual (and auditory) components of balancing in the *yogasanas* could be helped by practicing this *pranayama*.

---

1   Children raised in tepees where the lines of construction are oriented at angles other than 90° or 180° see the real world in a way measurably different from that of children raised in rooms having lines oriented at 90° or 180°.

course, if you have other students in your field of view who are wobbly or falling, this visual grasp of external objects can work to upset your balance too! For a similar reason, the teacher should not be walking aimlessly around the room while students are working in the balancing postures. Only with intense mental concentration can the balance be kept if the visual field is either unmarked or is in motion.

Not all changes in the retinal stream elicit a

quick reflexive readjustment. Bending over rapidly to pick up a belt changes the visual scene at the retina, but there is no reflex akin to the closing of the eyes as a stone chip flies toward the eye. Apparently the ventral streaming system is selective in what it reacts to and what it ignores.

Note that the left-to-right placement of the eyes in the face means that the eyes are more useful in balancing when the falling sensation is in a sideways direction than when it is in a front-to-back direction. Thus, the eyes are more useful in balancing in *virabhadrasana III*, where the falling is more likely to be sideways, than in *trikonasana*, where the falling is more likely to be front-to-back.

Breaking the Habit

The other side of the visual-fixation coin is that one can become habituated to this mode of balancing, always using the same objects on which to focus. When this becomes the case, trying to balance in a different environment can be very destabilizing. Moreover, using the eyes in a visual grasp promotes a certain tension in the visual system (Section 17.C, page 672), which can be counterproductive in the long term. As you become more adept at balancing in the *yogasanas*, you will rely less consciously on the grasp of the eyes to hold you up, and you will be able to relax the tension in the eyes.

The Ganzfeld Effect

Use of the eyes in balancing is predicated upon a visual field with stationary markers that can serve as visual anchors. In fact, if the visual field is lacking in any pattern or feature, the movement of which can be sensed by retinal streaming, the result can be a feeling of blindness or disorientation and a loss of balance, just as when experiencing a whiteout in a snowstorm. Called the Ganzfeld effect, the difficulties it can cause are readily apparent in balancing *yogasanas*, as when one tries to balance with the face only a few inches from a solid-colored or patternless wall, unless of course the student is adept at balancing without visual cues. (You can know this by closing the eyes in *vrksasana* and seeing how large

an effect it has on your balance. If you fall readily when you close your eyes, then you will also suffer a strong Ganzfeld effect when trying to balance too close to a patternless wall.) Even when facing a wall in *trikonasana*, the Ganzfeld effect can create a sense of imbalance that is normally not present in the posture when it is performed in the middle of the room. Note that Iyengar is careful not to place beginning students in the standing postures too close to a facing wall (see Appendix VI, page 946). Similarly, the eyes may well suffer a Ganzfeld effect when looking at the floor in *adho mukha vrksasana* or *pincha mayurasana*, and so the balance may be aided by placing a coin between the hands on the floor. Balancing postures attempted on a mountaintop on a clear day with nothing visible but the clear sky also will suffer from the Ganzfeld effect.

The Optokinetic Effect

The optokinetic effect comes into play when the head is held still but the background is in motion, as when trying to balance while others around you are falling or walking through your field of view. Most familiar is the optokinetic situation when we are sitting still in an automobile and the car next to us starts to pull forward, in which case our retinal streaming subconsciously tells us that we are rolling backward, and we respond by consciously pressing frantically on the brake! This is a result of an illusion within the optokinetic apparatus of the brain. However, we quickly learn to release the brake so that a second car pulling forward does not elicit the same response from us [782]. As applied to the situation when in a balancing posture while the background is in motion, the tendency is to move opposite to what is being observed and then to fall.

Eye Action When in Motion

In situations in which one is moving but not rotating while balancing, as when going from *virabhadrasana I* into *virabhadrasana III*, for example, fixing the eyes upon a distant point for balance is impractical. In this case, imagine instead a black line painted on the floor and running through the forward foot while in *virabhadrasana*

I. Keep this imaginary runway beneath the standing foot well lit and centered in your visual field as you lean forward, lifting the back leg for takeoff and lowering it to land. The visual instructions for moving into *virabhadrasana III* from *tadasana* via *virabhadrasana I* might be thought of as a virtual construct designed to overcome the Ganzfeld effect, as the anchoring line is imagined, not real; however, the line does not waver in the imagination, because it must run beneath the foot, unlike an imagined spot on the wall for *vrksasana,* for example.

An oculomotor reflex comes into play when one starts in *ardha chandrasana* and then slowly rotates into *parivrtta ardha chandrasana,* keeping the arms outstretched laterally throughout. The balancing difficulty arises in the transition between the postures, where the arms are horizontal so that neither hand is on the floor. In cases such as this, pick a point on the floor on which to focus the gaze. As the head and body turn, the vestibular-oculomotor reflex (Section 17.B, page 668) automatically will turn the eyes at the same rate, but in the opposite direction as the head, to keep the chosen object centered in the field of view, even though the head is in motion. This action will not cover the full 180° range of motion of the head but can be done in a few angular increments, advancing the point of visual fixation with each increment. Again, putting a coin or two on the floor as visual markers can be of great help in such balances.

Blindsight

The function of the eyes in balancing takes place in the subconscious sphere, coming into consciousness only as we fall irreversibly. As described in Subsection 17.B, page 669, we have two visual systems: one supplying visual images to the conscious brain, and one operating reflexively at the lower level of the superior colliculus of the midbrain. This second visual system is strongly involved with the innate tendency to gaze at an object, the "visual grasp reflex." It seems likely that our use of the eyes to hold on to visual anchors when balancing involves the reflexive visual system, as it responds much more quickly than

does the conscious visual system and so places balancing more in the realm of reflex than mentation. In particular, experiments on the balancing of a broomstick on the fingertip show that corrective actions to maintain balance occur significantly faster than the normal visual reaction time, the implication being that even when a sighted person balances a broomstick on the finger, the rapid response of blindsight is a significant factor in the balancing act.

Sutra I.2

In regard to using the eyes to balance, there is a strong reflexive, automatic, subconscious component to "seeing," and that subconscious part is much faster acting than the conscious part. This subconscious visual signal works to uphold balance, provided that one's concentration on balance is not contaminated by superfluous thoughts. Sutra I.2, "Yoga practice acts to still the fluctuations of the mind," is very much to the point for the student learning to balance (i.e., if the student's mind wanders from the task of staying in balance, falling ensues immediately). In a similar vein, Iyengar speaks of using *yogasana* practice to "harness the wild horses of the mind"; these wild horses will tip you over if you are trying to balance in the *yogasanas,* however, they can be tamed by cultivating an inward awareness of the body as it balances.

Visual Focus on the Primary Joint

A second and very practical use of the eyes involves focusing their attention on the joint of highest priority. Most of the balances are considerably easier if one focuses the eyes on the joint at the floor. If the balance is on the foot, then looking down at the foot (flexion of the neck) helps to concentrate the mind on the job at hand, which is balancing; if the balancing is inverted, as when in *pincha mayurasana,* then use extension of the neck to keep the hands and fingers in view. See, however, Subsection V.D, page 909, for instruction on what to do when both a hand and a foot are on the floor for balancing.

Mobility of the Head

Simple testing in different balancing *yogasanas* shows that the eyes can aid balance in both upright and inverted positions through the agency of retinal streaming, but only if the head is free to move. That is to say, they are of great value when balancing in *adho mukha vrksasana*, in *vrksasana*, and in *vasisthasana*, yet they are of no value when balancing in *anantasana*, *sirsasana*, or *niralamba sarvangasana!* The difference here is that in the first class of balancing postures, the head and eyes fall when the body falls, whereas in the second class of postures, the head and eyes are more or less immobilized when the body falls (because they are already so close to the ground even when in balance), and so visual signals are of little use in maintaining balance. In people who have lost both the vestibular apparatus and the proprioceptive functions, vision is still useful for maintaining balance as long as the eyes remain open, the posture is such that the head falls when the body falls, and the required corrective balancing measures are not too rapid [308].

The Vestibular Organs

Two types of vestibular sensors deep within the inner ears (figure 18.B-1) monitor the static positions of the head relative to the downward pull of gravity, as well as the rotational motion of the head (see Section 18.B, page 698). The vestibular organs are quite small, being less than the size of a dime, and consist of two static and three dynamic sensors deep in each ear. The latter (the semicircular canals) are stimulated only when there is an acceleration or deceleration of the head; motion of the head at constant speed will not excite these sensors.

Static Sensors

Within each of the two ears, there are two vestibular organs called the utricle and the saccule, each of which contains small calcium carbonate stones (otoliths), the movements of which are sensed by the bending of hairs within the organs when the head is tilted. The utricle senses forward, backward, and sideways static displacements of the head, and the saccule senses up and down static alignment. The head-righting reflex involves the otolith organs' response to the pull of gravity and works to keep the head looking straight ahead, whether the eyes are open or not [782].

It is said [98a] that the practice of *yogasana* inversions results in the specific increase of extensional muscle tone in the postural muscles paralleling the spine, whereas slow, rhythmic movement relaxes one's muscle tone. The increased muscle tone of spine and chest when inverted is thought to be the source of the enhanced mood when one is otherwise suffering from grief or depression.

Dynamic Sensors

Each of the three semicircular canals of the vestibular system is filled with a viscous fluid, the endolymph, surrounding position-sensitive hairs, and in turn, each semicircular canal is surrounded by a second fluid, the perilymph. The three canals within each ear monitor the head motions in three mutually perpendicular planes and are insensitive to the static position of the head. Should there be an acceleration or deceleration of the head, as when falling, the semicircular canals respond to the force associated with the change of speed. This response involves the bending of the hairs within the canals due to the viscous drag between the rapidly moving canals and slowly responding viscous fluid within them. The imbalance signal strength and direction of the force is then derived subconsciously from the extent and direction of hair bending, as recorded in the six semicircular canals within the skull. Because the semicircular apparatus within each ear consists of three mutually perpendicular sensors, they are equally sensitive to falling in any direction.

Innervation

Because the afferent signals from the vestibular apparatus go to the brainstem via the vestibular branch of the acoustic nerve (cranial nerve VIII) and the returning efferent nerves from the brainstem activate the muscles in the head and upper back, it is an interesting question then as to whether such upper-body sensors are of any value when balancing on the feet. In fact, the brainstem nuclei involved in vestibular balancing do have tracts to the cerebellum (Subsection 18.B, page 699), and from this point, there are efferent neural tracts to muscles in the leg, foot, and ankle that control the balance when standing.

The various sensors recording imbalance send their afferents to the brainstem, where the signals are integrated. From there, the signals travel to the cerebellum, where corrective muscle actions can be activated if they have been learned by previous experience. If, instead, the imbalance is a product of an unfamiliar occurrence (seeing the whirling of the trees when one does a cartwheel on the lawn, for example), then part of the integrated message moves as high as the cerebral cortex, which learns to accommodate whirling trees, and which by habituation comes to recognize such motion as nonthreatening.

As discussed in Section 18.B, page 699, there is a very interesting coupling of the balancing signals from the inner ears and the proprioceptive signals from muscle spindles in the back of the neck that work to distinguish a full-body fall from a simple tilting of the head. Of equal importance to balancing when upright are the proprioceptive sensors in the ankles.

Vestibular Dysfunction

There is a wide variety of vestibular dysfunction that can be operating in a student, most of which is beyond a yoga teacher's level of understanding. One that is within our reach, however, is the question of diet. The endolymph and perilymph within and outside the semicircular canals are different fluids, each with a precise composition. Should these compositions be upset by dehydration, excess salt, simple sugars, caffeine, alcohol, nicotine, or aspirin in the diet, the result can be a vestibular dysfunction having a negative impact on the balance. There also is evidence for a cause-and-effect relation between vestibular dysfunction and scoliosis [676].

When stressed, tense, or fatigued, the brainstem nuclei responsible for integrating balance

information function less efficiently, and loss of balance becomes more likely in this case.

Pressure Sensors

Deep-Pressure Sensors

Deep-pressure sensors in the skin (see Section 13.B, page 511) detect the pattern of pressure within the skin as it presses the floor. This shifting pattern of pressure is readily translated into a sense of balancing or falling. Thanks to the bilateral symmetry of the cortex, an afferent signal from a pressure sensor in the right hand, for example, will go to the left cerebral hemisphere, and the responding efferent motor neuron will travel from that hemisphere back to the right hand. Afferent signals from the left hand similarly terminate in the right cerebral hemisphere. The contribution of the pressure sensors to balancing becomes apparent if one tries to balance with the left hand on the right side of the body and the right hand on the left, thereby confusing the hemispheres. For example, perform the one-legged table posture with hands crossed at the wrists, palms on the floor, as described in Box V.F-2, page 920. The difficulty experienced when the hands are in this configuration suggests that the balance involves considerable input from pressure sensors in the hands.

Of the four balancing senses, the pressure sensors in the skin use signals that are felt consciously in real time as we balance, but the other senses are more or less confined to subconscious reflexes in most of us. Note that the pressure sensors used for balancing show a rapid adaptation toward zero signal (i.e., given a constant pressure, the afferent signal falls rapidly toward zero; the pressure signal is largest at the moment the pressure is applied and falls thereafter). This rapid loss of sensitivity is curtailed when balancing by the dynamic nature of the balancing action, which rapidly moves the pressure from one part of the body surface on the floor to the another part, thereby resulting in a pressure signal that is constantly refreshed and so is available for a relatively long time.

Some workers in the balancing field consider

the pressure sensors to be part of the proprioceptive sensor system, but I take them as separate. Proprioceptively touching the end of the nose with the fingertip with the eyes closed clearly requires a different mechanism than sensing the differences in pressure on the bottom of the foot when balancing in *vrksasana,* for example.

Judging from the low density of pressure sensors on the upper back body (figure 13.B-2), one would expect that balancing in *niralamba sarvangasana* would have a very small contribution from these sensors. Neither the vestibular apparatus nor the eyes would be of any value here, since the head does not move in this posture should the feet begin to fall. Consequently, it would appear that balancing in *niralamba sarvangasana* is largely in the realm of the proprioceptive sensors.

Aging, Random Noise, and Swaying

It appears that the deep-pressure sensors in the feet of senior citizens lose their sensitivity, so that they sway through much larger angles before sensing the imbalance, thereby increasing the risks of a fall [734]. Recent research in improving the standing balance of older citizens has focused on increasing the sensitivity of the pressure sensors in the soles of the feet and thereby decreasing the sway angle [674, 675].

It is generally held that random noise in the sensory channel connected with balance is an interference in that activity; however, it is now known that through stochastic resonance (Subsection 3.F, page 66), noise may contribute in such a way as to **increase** the sensitivity of the sensory signal. It is suggested that balance may be poor because the signals from pressure sensors are so weak that they do not reach the threshold necessary for neural transmission, whereas the addition of a random-noise component lifts the signal above threshold. Thus, balance would be improved if one were to wear insoles in shoes that would vibrate in a random way and so raise the sensitivity of the pressure sensors in the soles of the feet. In the same way, standing on a vibrating plate would add just enough noise to pressure receptors in the feet to lift their signals above threshold.

Studying the effects of random noise on balance, Collins et al. [673] placed each of sixteen senior citizens (average age: seventy-two years) on a vibrating stage, with vibrations that were so slight that they could not be sensed consciously. Measuring the subjects' degree of displacement from vertical when standing barefoot on the platform with eyes closed and arms at their sides, they performed as well as did the age-twenty-three group standing on solid ground! On the other hand, when they could sense the vibrations in the soles of their feet, there was no measurable increase in their performance over that when simply standing on solid ground. The benefits of subconscious stochastic resonance to balancing were even larger when the senior citizens wore vibrating gel insoles in their shoes, their stability being even higher than when on the vibrating platform. Perhaps the benefits of balancing on vibrating gel at subconscious amplitudes can be gained by balancing on a soft surface, such as a rolled-up yoga mat.[4] Similarly, older adults who practice walking on uneven cobblestones have been shown to have improved balance, as this type of walking stimulates the pressure sensors in the soles of the feet.

The muscular responses necessary to maintain balance when standing on a vibrating plate are effective stressors on the associated bones and so result in increased bone mass and density (Subsection 7.A, page 233). *Yogasana* students who practice the standing postures and the foot-

---

4 It is paradoxical that we recommend that one **not** practice balancing on a soft mat; however, the possibility exists that this could be good exercise for sharpening the balancing sense, perhaps working like preconditioning (Subsection 16.F, page 655). Though standing on a soft mat does not necessarily provide the vibrations necessary for stochastic resonance, a soft-mat practice still may be useful for exercising an injured but recuperating ankle. On the other hand, the act of resistive balancing (as discussed in Subsection V.D, page 909) is not unlike the macroscopic resistance that is so useful when muscle stretching (Subsection 11.F, page 468) in which it is clear that the object offering the resistance must be solid and unmoving. As this applies to balancing as well, it is equally clear that soft-mat balancing will have its disadvantages in regard to falling.

balancing ones also should benefit from working in this way, both in regard to balancing and to increased bone density.

Comparison of Sensors

Of the various balancing systems, the proprioceptive is the most rapidly responding, with the visual and vestibular apparatus being significantly slower [427]. Moreover, the relative importance of the different balancing sensors may vary from one person to the next and from one *yogasana* to the next. As we age, the first balancing mechanism to fail is that of the vestibular apparatus, likely due to a lessening of blood flow through the semicircular canals. Balancing in the older student is especially difficult if it is coupled to other aspects of the posture (high intensity of hamstring stretch, for example) that act to pull the student's attention away from the work of balancing.

Because loss of balance can lead to falls and injuries in the older student, it is most relevant that as we age, the composition of the muscles changes from fast-twitch, type 3 fibers toward more slow-twitch, type 1 fibers. This means that as we age, we are less able to apply a balance-saving countertorque in a timely manner to prevent a fall. An active *yogasana* practice with a prominent balancing component will be of great help to such people.

Sensor Interactions

In discussing the mechanism of balancing in the body, note must be made of the cerebellum and the basal ganglia of the brain (see Subsection 4.C, page 83), for these two centers are intimately involved in the act of balancing. The proprioceptive sensors (Section 11.C, page 441) relay their information in a constant stream to the hemispheres of the cerebellum, where this detailed information is transformed into a total-body map indicating where the various muscles and limbs of the body are located, which limbs are moving, how fast they are moving, and in which directions. At the same time, signals from the vestibular apparatus in the inner ears (Section 18.B, page 696) also converge upon the cerebellum, indicating the

alignment of the head in the gravitational field and its angular motion, if any. Ocular information is also of great importance here, but the information does not go to the cerebellum; rather, it travels directly to the occipital lobe, from whence it spreads toward many other areas of the brain.

With the proprioceptive, visual, deep-pressure, and vestibular information in hand, the cerebellum and basal ganglia then work together to devise a muscular strategy, so that balance is maintained with smooth but corrective movements. If the movement in question involves a conscious act of balance, then the plan devised by the cerebellum and basal ganglia is sent upward to the motor cortex of the cerebrum and from there, downward to the relevant muscles. If, on the other hand, the balancing is more postural or reflexive, then the cerebellar plan does not involve the cortex, but instead is loaded directly into the medulla oblongata for transmission downward to the muscles.

When Sensors Disagree

All four of these sensor modes working more or less simultaneously and in harmony to keep the body in mechanical balance during *yogasana* practice. If, on the other hand, the signals from the various balancing modes do not agree as to what is needed, then the result is some combination of cold sweats, drowsiness, dizziness, vertigo, pallor, nausea, vomiting, and falling.

Motion sickness results when the outputs of the various motion and position sensors disagree. Thus, when one decides to read a book while riding in a car, the eyes tell the brain that everything is still as they scan the page of the book, yet the vestibular apparatus signals the brain that we are moving and bouncing about. The result of this discordance between the visual and vestibular sensors is motion sickness. On the other hand, though the vestibular system of the driver also senses the bouncing motion of the car, his eyes are on the road and so sense a scene that also is unsteady, but in a way that is consistent with that sensed by the vestibular apparatus. Consequently, the driver's visual and vestibular sensors are concordant, and no motion sickness follows. Similarly, when you are staring at the back of the unmoving seat in front of you and the airplane hits rough weather and drops 200 feet in a second, the effect is a feeling of butterflies in the stomach, as visual and pressure-sensor signals no longer agree.

It is also true that the relative prominence of the various sensor modes may depend upon external factors. Thus, when walking on a smooth solid surface, the sense of balance is 70 percent proprioceptive/pressure sensors, 20 percent vestibular, and 10 percent visual whereas the same person when walking on cobblestone would have a distribution that is 60 percent vestibular, 30 percent visual, and 10 percent proprioceptive/pressure sensors.

Section V.D: Other Aids to Balance

One can do several things in aid of balancing in the *yogasanas,* in preparation for eventually using the broomstick-and-countertorque model in the middle of the room. In order to balance in *yogasanas,* the student must be sensitive to changes in one or more of the sensory receptor modes (whether the body is upright, inclined, horizontal, or inverted) and must be able to activate the proper response. Until that higher level of performance is reached, several aids to balancing can be instituted when the student's balancing organs are not yet up to the demands of the posture. These aids to balancing are discussed here, as adjuncts to the discussion in Section V.B, page 873. Note that the information and advice given in this Section will aid balancing for the beginning student, but as mentioned below, it may tend to promote habits that eventually must be broken if one is to progress in *yogasana* study. Several of these aids to balance have been discussed by Cole in his introduction to balancing in the *yogasanas* [147a].

Shifting the Body's Center of Gravity

Sway: Dynamic Shifting

As discussed in Section IV.B, page 853, the center of gravity of the body when standing in *tadasana* is just below the navel and halfway back toward the spine; the posture is balanced mechanically when the line from this center to that of the center of the Earth passes through the footprint of the feet on the floor. Consider also that in the real-world situation, the body while in balance will not be static, but will instead be undergoing oscillations in space and time as it constantly reads the balance sensors and makes the appropriate postural adjustments. This is the dynamic aspect of balancing in the *yogasanas,* which can be quantified by the sway angle θ. When in *tadasana,* for example, the body may sway through an angle θ without falling; however, should this angle exceed a critical value θ^*, then falling commences, as the line between centers no longer falls within the footprint (figure V.D-1a). If, instead, the center of gravity of the performer is raised, as when coming from *tadasana* into *urdhva hastasana* (figure V.D-1b), then the critical sway angle θ^* becomes correspondingly smaller (i.e., the posture is less stable because falling occurs at a smaller sway angle θ). Correspondingly, if the center of gravity of *tadasana* is lowered by moving the body into *malasana,* then the critical sway angle θ^* within which one is constrained becomes larger than that in *tadasana* (figure V.D-1c), and the posture becomes more stable with respect to swaying and falling.[5] Similarly, the balance in *hasta padangust-*

---

5   The same reasoning holds for sports cars. If the center of gravity is kept low, then the **angular** displacement that is allowed before the car rolls over is much larger than when the center of gravity is higher, as in sport utility vehicles. One can take corners at high speed in the low-slung sports car, but not in the top-heavy SUV. A moment's reflection on figure V.D-1 convinces one that any adjustment while in a *yogasana* that redistributes its weight to **lower** its center of gravity while maintaining the area of the base will make it more stable with respect to falling.

On the other hand, doing *vrksasana* while stand-

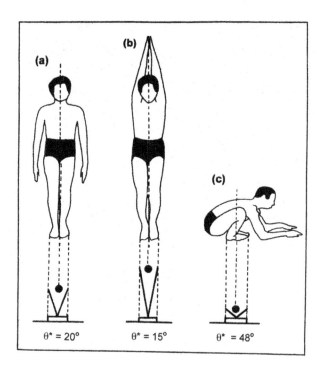

Figure V.D-1. (a) The posture *tadasana* and the corresponding mechanical diagram showing the relation between the body's center of gravity, the area of the footprint of the feet on the floor, and the critical sway angle, θ*, beyond which the performer loses balance and falls. (b) The raising of the center of gravity on going from *tadasana* to *urdhva hastasana* and the corresponding diminution of the critical sway angle θ*. (c) The lowering of the center of gravity on going from *tadasana* to *malasana,* and the corresponding enlargement of the critical sway angle θ*.

ing on a wooden block raises the distance of the body's center of gravity with respect to the center of the Earth; however, the balance is not affected (except for the fear factor), for the surface of the block has become the new "floor." In a similar way, there is no benefit to be gained by lowering the center of gravity by trying to balance in the basement of your studio, as compared with balancing on the roof! The important factor here is the height from the center of gravity of the body to whatever surface the body is being balanced upon, regardless of the height of this surface from any underlying support structure. In this regard, see footnote on page 901, where the situation when balancing in a human pyramid is discussed.

hasana performed on a straight leg is far less stable than the same posture performed with the supporting leg fully bent so that the buttock rests on or close to the heel of the supporting leg.

However, there is a compensating feature of the arms-over-head position in *urdhva hastasana* that make it the preferred manner of performing this *yogasana*: it promotes a tautness in the secondary joints that eradicates unnecessary wobbles that otherwise contribute to enlarging the sway angle θ (Subsection V.C, page 895). Thus, the more elongated posture that we always seek in our practice is not necessarily the most stable one in terms of the relation of the height of our center of gravity above the floor; however, it does lead to smaller sway angles, θ, in other ways.

Static Shifting

The student can experience the consequences of the static shifting of the effective center of gravity in balancing postures in the following ways. First, come into *vrksasana* by standing with your right shoulder to the wall, feet together, and right foot as close to the wall as you can get without falling. In this posture, the line of centers between the Earth and the body passes through the base area of the soles of the feet. Now, keeping the right shoulder touching but not being supported by the wall, slowly lift the left foot off the floor. Falling (instability) to the left is inevitable here, because with the left foot off the floor, one cannot move the center of gravity of the body enough toward the right to force the line of centers to pass through the footprint of the right foot, the base of the posture when the left foot is lifted. On the other hand, when at the wall with the right shoulder touching, stability can be maintained easily while lifting the right foot; this is accomplished by shifting the hips rightward and the torso far to the left, thereby keeping the line between centers passing through the footprint of the left foot on the floor. This static shifting in *vrksasana* performed free of the wall is unavoidable but should be done as little as possible to keep the standing leg and the spinal column as close to vertical as possible.

Next, come to *vrksasana* in the middle of the

room with arms overhead, and note the level of inner awareness necessary to keep the posture in balance. Then repeat, but with each of the hands holding a sandbag at the level of the knees. The inner awareness and effort necessary to keep the posture in balance will be far less when holding the sandbags, because the effective center of gravity of the body is substantially lower when holding the bags at the knees. Similarly, one has a more difficult time balancing in *vrksasana* if the sandbags are raised overhead while balancing on one leg, as lifting the bags overhead makes θ^* smaller.

To experience the effect of shifting the center of gravity when inverted, first come to *sirsasana I*, either in the center of the room or positioned about one foot from a wall. Then have a friend gently place a sandbag on the soles of the feet, thereby raising the center of gravity of the posture. In this case, the elevated center of gravity means that the performer is constrained to a much smaller critical sway angle θ^* (i.e., she must maintain a much sharper awareness of body position to avoid falling) Because of the heavy sandbag placed on the soles of the feet in *sirsasana I*, the body must not be allowed to assume the feet-forward, heavy-on-the-elbows, more support/less balance attitude so common in beginners' headstands, because holding this heavy weight in the out-of-balance position can severely strain the muscles of the lower back. Conversely, having beginning students balance with sandbags on the soles of the feet ensures a more erect, centered, balancing posture in *sirsasana I*, provided they are strong enough to resist falling straight down along the line between centers.

In *sirsasana I*, the posture with hips directly over head is more stable if bent somewhat at the hips and the legs bent to place the heels on the buttocks; it is the posture used by beginners when first coming off the floor and heading toward the fully extended position, and it is used by more experienced students when moving between *sirsasana* and *bakasana*. Because this folded posture has a much lower center of gravity but the same base as the fully vertical posture, it is more stable mechanically and is the easiest posture to control if one is not too competent when inverted. In the same vein, if you perform *niralamba sarvangasana*

bent at the waist to be in a V shape, balance is easier than being in the classical I shape for this posture, because the center of gravity is lower when bent at the hips.

Increase the Size of the Base to Increase Stability

It follows from the balancing rule stated in Subsection V.A, page 867, and from the consideration of the sway angle θ given above that increasing the size of the base of a *yogasana* will make θ^* larger, thereby making the balancing easier in general, provided that opening the base does not significantly reduce the support given the posture against gravitational collapse. Because the line between centers connecting the student's body and the Earth must intersect the area of the base of a posture if a student is to be balanced, any action that increases the area of this base aids in the balance. The benefits of increasing the size of the base when balancing are expanded upon below, using several *yogasana* examples.

Ardha Chandrasana

If either the hand or foot is on the floor in a balancing posture, it will be stabilized by an opening of the hand or foot to increase its area on the floor.[6] This understanding can be refined.

---

6   A possible increased stability from stretching and opening a hand or foot on the floor involves a competition between at least three competing effects. First, opening the hand or foot increases the area of the base on which one is attempting to balance and so increases the critical sway angle, θ^*. It also increases the lever arm (R) involved in generating the countertorque (figure V.B-2), and so increases the strength of the countertorque. On the other hand, the countertorque that one can generate by pressing a body part onto the floor will be minimized by an elongation that takes the involved muscle to the outer limit of its range of motion (Subsection 11.A, page 400). That is, working at the limit of the range of motion reduces the force (Q) otherwise used to maintain balance. On balance, it appears that the "Q" and "R" factors work against one another, leaving the larger area as the governing factor when spreading the hand or foot while balancing.

When in *ardha chandrasana,* the challenge to balance is not in the left-to-right direction but in the front-to-back direction, especially if the standing foot is truly aligned left to right (i.e., *ardha chandrasana* shows an element of specific metastability, Subsection V.A, page 869). Thus, when placing the hand on the floor, it should be placed under the shoulder and to the little-toe side of the standing foot, so that the effective front-to-back dimension of the posture is enlarged. Because *ardha chandrasana* is specifically metastable, placing the hand in line with the standing foot is a very difficult balancing position, as it increases the effective area of the base in the direction (left-to-right) in which the student is not likely to fall, while offering no help in the critical front-to-back direction! In contrast, the balancing problem in *bakasana* (another specifically metastable posture) is front-to-back, and so setting the hands further apart left-to-right will not increase front-to-back stability.

Balancing in *ardha chandrasana* is aided by removing all unnecessary motions in the body other than that at the supporting ankle (Subsection V.B, page 877). This means that one must pin the hips by pressing the inner thighs outward and the outer thighs inward on both legs in order to avoid any pelvic motion in the balancing scenario. A variation of *ardha chandrasana* that is more challenging to the balancing senses is described in Subsection V.D, page 905.

Eka Pada Urdhva Dhanurasana

The close relation between *adho mukha svanasana* and *urdhva dhanurasana* was mentioned in Subsection IV.D (page 861), and this applies as well to the variation done with only one hand and one foot kept on the floor. B. K. S. Iyengar performs this amazing variation of *urdhva dhanurasana* using the hand and foot on the floor on the same side of the body (the right side), [388, plate 502]; however, they are clearly offset left to right with respect to one another to offer a reasonable base area for balancing.

Gomukhasana

Gomukhasana done in the classical manner has one sitting upon the folded legs with the shins

touching side-by-side (Appendix I, page 825). Balance here is difficult, not only because of the left-to-right neural crossover of the pressure sensors in the lower legs (Box V.F-2, page 920), but also because the base is so narrow left to right, and because the mind is distracted from balancing by the discomfort of bone-on-bone contact in the lower legs. If one has a balancing problem with this aspect of the posture, then keep the knees in contact with one another, but increase the area of the base by separating the ankles and sitting between the ankles rather than on top of them. This action increases the size of the base, lowers the center of gravity, and removes the problem of bone-on-bone discomfort.

Parivrtta Trikonasana

A specifically metastable balancing problem similar to that in *ardha chandrasana* arises when *parivrtta trikonasana* is performed with the feet parallel and essentially in line with one another, for this again offers very little stability in the front-to-back direction when the upper body is rotated. As with *ardha chandrasana,* the balance in *parivrtta trikonasana* is aided by placing the hand on the floor far off the line of the feet, and also by separating the feet in their left-to-right direction. In all of the balancing postures with one hand and one foot on the floor (i.e., *ardha chandrasana, parivrtta ardha chandrasana, dwianga adho mukha svanasana, visvamitrasana,* and *ardha baddha padmottanasana*), the hand and the foot can be placed with wide front-to-back and/or left-to-right separations as aids to balancing for the beginner.

Sirsasana

Balancing in *sirsasana I* is a special case, in that it would seem to make sense, from what has been said to this point, that there is something to be gained by opening the elbows wide in order to increase the area of the base. Note that this will only stabilize the posture in the left-to-right direction, whereas the balancing problem and specific metastability in *sirsasana I* is largely in the front-to-back direction. Furthermore, if the elbows are widely separated left to right, then the base shrinks in the front-to-back direction, and there will be a reduced ability to balance in that direction; even more importantly, separation of the elbows in *sirsasana I* violates the dictum that one should work with the bones under the posture (Subsection V.B, page 885) to give it maximum support. In conclusion, there are good reasons (both for balance and for resisting gravitational collapse) for keeping the elbows no wider than shoulder width in *sirsasana I*.

Just as in *sirsasana I*, the elbows in *sirsasana II* must not be allowed to separate any farther than shoulder width for reasons of gravitational collapse. If the base of *sirsasana II* is narrowed by working with the forearms touching and the hands supinated (*sirsasana III*; see Appendix I, page 828) balance in the posture becomes exceedingly difficult. In contrast to the small base of *sirsasana III*, that of *mukta hasta sirsasana* (figure IV.D-2) is huge by comparison, and maintaining balance here is trivial, provided the neck is strong enough to support 85 percent of the full body weight (figure IV.D-2). One often can see multi-jointed pendulums in the circus, stabilized using several of the balancing principles given in this chapter.[7]

---

7   For example, the human-tower circus stunt begins with acrobat 2 standing on the shoulders of acrobat 1. Acrobat 3 then climbs up to stand on the shoulders of acrobat 2, making a three-high tower. Should the lights go out at this point, the tower will fall immediately, for keeping this construction in the air requires many visual cues, especially because there are so many flexible joints in the construction. The fact that the tower's center of gravity also is very high contributes to the instability as well. If the circus is a good one, they will then attempt to stand acrobat 4 on the top of the three-high tower, making a four-high tower. Because the weight on the shoulders of acrobat 1 is becoming appreciable, acrobat 4 will be a young child, who is often flung to the top of the tower. Balancing such a tower is a mighty feat, even with the lights on, as there is independent movement at the "joints" of the tower formed by the feet of acrobat 1 on the floor, by the feet of acrobat 2 on the shoulders of acrobat 1, and so on up the tower. Balance can be maintained for only a few seconds before the tower falls (always forward) and acrobat 4 is caught by acrobat bystanders. The balancing of an equally long and heavy pole

Using an External Wall

In regard to balancing postures, use of the wall for support of the body weight can be very useful to beginning students, as it allows them to work on developing strength and on the postural details of the *yogasana* without having to worry about balancing. Once these preliminary aspects are satisfied, just a light touch on the wall can be used advantageously to sharpen the sense of balance. However, when learning to balance in the *yogasanas,* use of the wall can be both a great teacher and an impediment to growth. The wall can help the beginner to approach a difficult position, but in doing so, the student runs the risk of becoming wed to the prop, unable to function without it. Once we are comfortable working against the wall, we must take the next step of cutting the umbilical cord connecting us to the wall, and work to take our place in the larger world without props. The same philosophy applies to using the eyes to balance (Box V.C-1, page 889); they are useful props, but the intent of our practice eventually is to cut ourselves free of these aids.

Moving from Support to Balance

If one stands with the side of the body parallel to the wall, one can support the body in *vrksasana* position with one hand heavy on the wall; howev-

---

is trivial compared to the problems of balancing four pendulums moving independently, as when stacking four acrobats.

Much more stable constructions (pyramids) can be built of acrobats if several of them are positioned close to one another in a bottom layer. The acrobats of the second layer then place their feet on one shoulder each of the adjacent acrobats in the first layer, and the tower is built layer by layer. This approach illustrates how interlacing acrobats can minimize the allowed motions of the whole by lowering the center of gravity, and especially how broadening the base makes the structure much more stable. The stability of the many-person tower is increased again if each of the layers has the people side-by-side in a circle rather than side-by-side in a straight line, for reasons of front-to-back stability. We try to use both of these approaches when balancing in the *yogasanas.*

er, if the aim is to balance in *vrksasana,* it is sufficient to use just the fingertip of one finger lightly
on the wall to sense the imbalance. Thanks to the
many pressure sensors in the little finger (figure
13.B-2), it is possible to balance more easily using
the tip of the little finger pressing lightly on the
wall as balance sensor than by using all of the sole
of the foot on the floor! Close your eyes and see
how effective the gentle pressure of your fingertip
on the wall can be in maintaining balance in *vrksasana,* especially when compared with the balance when the fingertip is removed from the wall
with the eyes still closed. Because the fingertip is
of little or no help in regard to support, using the
fingertip on the wall contributes solely to the refinement of the balancing action; notice how the
oscillations of the balance become smaller once
the fingertip placed lightly on the wall enters the
balancing-versus-support equation.

As discussed in Subsection 4.C, page 95, the
cerebellum is the site where muscular actions are
controlled and one's intensions are compared to
the proprioceptive signals showing body posture.
Discrepancies between intention and performance are corrected in real time in the cerebellum; adjustments are made to correct imbalances,
for example. Because the proprioceptive and pressure signals are especially strong and sensitive
from the fingertips, it is not surprising in hindsight that the balance in foot-balancing postures
such as *vrksasana* and *ardha chandrasana* is aided
by fingertip contact with the wall or floor.

The aid of the fingertip to the wall in *vrksasana* changes substantially if one aligns the shoulders
parallel to the wall, extends the arm forward, and
then touches the wall with a fingertip. The hoped-
for advantage when the balancing finger and the
supporting foot are in parallel alignment is especially absent if one then closes the eyes. Can you
rationalize this difference? The answer is below.[8]

Now repeat this exercise with *ardha chandrasana* in the middle of the room, first using one hand
on the floor to both support and balance the posture, as in Subsection V.D (page 899), and then
using just one fingertip on this hand to balance
but not support the posture. Of course, in many
cases, such as *dwianga adho mukha svanasana,* the
foot or the hand on the floor can be critical for
both support and balance in equal measure.

Sirsasana

In regard to the distinction between support
versus balance (Section V.B, page 885), notice
that *sirsasana I* is a balancing posture when the
body line is truly vertical; however, beginners
will keep the body line leaning onto the elbows
so that the posture becomes more supported than
balanced.[9] This forward imbalance develops in
order to avoid the possibility of falling backward
into the unknown, the possibility being greatly
increased by the fact that resistance toward falling backward in *sirsasana I* is much less due to
the smaller length of the lever arm ("r" in figure V.B-2), the distance from the point of the
application of the force to the balancing point.
Sirsasana I, when vertical, is a true balancing
situation, with the hand placement alternately
allowing gentle front-to-back and back-to-front
adjustments of the body's center of gravity, with
65 percent or more of the body weight borne by
the upper arms and shoulders (figure IV.D-2).
The two sets of muscles (agonist and antagonist)
used when balancing in *sirsasana I* are alternately
contracted and relaxed out of phase, as balanc-

---

8   Mary Dalziel [179] answers this by pointing out
that because side-to-side balance is more difficult in
vrksasana than is front-to-back balance, the sideways
help of the little finger against the wall will be much
more useful in maintaining balance than when using
the same finger in the front-to-back mode.

9   This tendency to let the weight fall onto the elbows in *sirsasana I* is most apparent when the student
tries to move from *sirsasana I* to *sirsasana II* while inverted. In this case, when the student tries to move the
hands from behind the head to forward of the head,
being heavy on the elbows immediately results in a
drop to the feet; the transition from *sirsasana I* to *sirsasana II* can be accomplished only if the *sirsasana I* position is **fully** vertical, with substantial weight on the
head and lightness at the elbows. This kind of thinking leads one to understand readily why the transition
from *sirsasana II* to *sirsasana I* is even more frightening
than going in the opposite direction.

ing swings the center of gravity alternately from front to back and then from back to front, so that each of the relevant muscles has a duty cycle of only 50 percent.

On the other hand, *sirsasana II* and all other variations in which there are no hands behind the head are never done with a truly vertical line from the crown of the head to the soles of the feet, and the line always is inclined so that the weight is heavy on the hands. In *sirsasana II*, the hand placement only allows the body to assume an inclined body line with a significant fraction of the body weight (40 percent) supported on bent arms, and rarely is it done with leg or torso variations. Though the weight distributions in *sirsasana I* and *II* are surprisingly alike (figure IV.D-2), in *sirsasana II*, the body is perpetually underbalanced, with the weight significantly forward on the hands and the upper arm and shoulder muscles perpetually tensed (100 percent duty cycle) to keep the posture metastable (i.e., it is a support rather than a balance). For most of us, *sirsasana II* is so taxing in the muscular sense that it can be supported for only a few minutes, unlike *sirsasana I*.

Advantages

With the above caveat in the minds of the students and their teachers in regard to balance versus support, the students can then use the wall to great advantage in the following ways:

1. Use the wall to steady the posture, so that the student can feel more comfortable in the position, without fear of falling. *Ardha chandrasana* is a good example of a posture that beginners struggle with in the middle of the room but take special delight in doing with the support of a wall at the back and a block under the hand.

2. Once supported by the wall, the student can devote full attention to the elongation and alignment of the posture without worrying about falling. In this case, the wall not only ensures mechanical stability but is a reference plane onto which one works to place key points of the back body (i.e.,

the back of the head, the shoulder blades, the backs of the hands, the buttocks, and the heel of the elevated leg). Again, *ardha chandrasana* performed with support of the wall is a good example of working on elongation and alignment while postponing the issue of balance.

3. When using the wall for support, the student should work sufficiently close so that the wall can be reached without distorting the body's alignment in the process. For example, if the feet and supporting hand are placed 30 centimeters (twelve inches) from the wall in *ardha chandrasana,* and the student then uses the wall for balance by placing the back of the hand of the upward arm and the heel of the elevated leg on the wall, then the arms and spine will not be in the ideal alignment that otherwise is enforced when the posture is set closer to the wall from the beginning.

4. In standing postures such as *vrksasana, utthita hasta padangusthasana,* and *parivrtta trikonasana,* and in seated postures such as *paripurna navasana,* where balance is a significant factor, have the students lean slightly backward (or forward or sideward) onto the wall for support and alignment. As they progress, then shift their weight slightly off the wall to attempt the freestanding balance.

Converting Strength to Balance

Balancing in *ardha chandrasana* illustrates another useful point: Balance is aided considerably by the proper placement of all five fingers on the floor and letting the body weight fall onto this five-finger support. Intuitively, when on the fingertips, we tend to place less weight on them and more on the supporting leg. In fact, with practice, it is only necessary to gently rest the tip of the index finger on the floor to maintain balance in *ardha chandrasana.* A fingertip in gentle contact with the wall or floor is all one needs in order to sense a strong element of proprioceptive and pressure-sensitive signaling in aid of balance. When the hand or finger on the floor or wall is used gently for balance in *ardha chandrasana,* then the supporting leg and the pelvis must work harder to maintain support against collapse along the line between centers. Finally, remove the single finger from the floor, and balance using only proprioception and actions in the ankle of the supporting leg, with the body doing its best imitation of a broomstick while the mind is intently focused on maintaining balance.

As discussed in Subsection 11.E, page 461, time is on your side when stretching: go deeper into the posture by incremental amounts, with long pauses between movements, and continue to maximum elongation. Time is also on your side when balancing. Move slowly and incrementally with minimum disturbance, raising as little dust as possible as you work toward trading support of the posture for balance of the posture. This is best illustrated by taking *ardha chandrasana* in the support mode (five fingers on the floor) and then slowly releasing each of the fingers from the floor in turn to slowly, gradually come into a one-leg foot balance with hands free of the floor.

Making an Internal Wall for Support

The advantages and disadvantages of constructing an internal wall in regard to balancing are presented below using several illustrative *yogasanas.*

Sarvangasana

For those students with less than perfect balance who nonetheless are ready to wean themselves away from the wall and work in the middle of the room, the internally generated wall can be of great value. Consider the balancing posture *salamba sarvangasana.* As described by Iyengar [388], *salamba* means "supported" or "propped up," as the bent arms support the torso. In a sense, then, one has created an "internal wall" with the arms in *salamba sarvangasana,* against which one can lean the rest of the body for support. In this case, one attains mechanical stability by internal bracing or support; however, there is little or no balancing in this posture in the broomstick-countertorque sense. In contrast, with practice, one can

move from pure support in *salamba sarvangasana* to pure balancing in *niralamba sarvangasana* by releasing the support of the back body by the wall otherwise formed by the arms and shoulders.

Note, however, that using an internal wall for support is much like leaning sideways onto an external wall for support: the wall must be mechanically strong enough to support the weight pressed onto it and must offer resistance to falling when the body is pressed into it. Consider *vrksasana,* with right shoulder toward the wall, and stabilized by placing the right hand on the wall. Where then should the hand be placed for most efficient support: opposite the shoulder, far forward of the shoulder, or far behind the shoulder? Clearly, the hand should be placed just opposite the shoulder because it is the shoulder that falls to the wall and this configuration offers the maximum direct support of the falling body. In a similar way, when in *sarvangasana* or *sirsasana I,* the elbows are placed on the floor so as to offer maximum support to the upper body, i.e., the elbows are placed at just shoulder width for maximum efficiency in working the floor.

Anantasana

Though other postures are not identified by the word *salamba,* they too can use the internal wall for mechanical stability. By way of example, consider *anantasana.* With one arm supporting the head and the other connected to the toe of the upward-extended leg, the balance on the side of the body can be precarious if all of the body parts are appropriately in line. However, if the ankle of the leg on the floor is dorsiflexed so that the toes point toward the knee, then the little toe (fifth metatarsal) is forward of the line of the body on the floor, and tipping the body forward onto the little toe provides an internal wall onto which one can lean as effectively as when one leans backward on a brick wall. Practice *anantasana* with the toes of the lower leg pointed first away from the knee in plantar flexion, and then dorsiflexed toward the knee, all the while keeping the body weight rolled slightly forward in order to see the advantage of the latter position in regard to balance. Note also that once the weight is allowed to roll backward in *anantasana*, it makes no difference what the toes are doing; the battle is lost, and one rolls out of the posture and onto one's back.

Ardha Chandrasana and Visvamitrasana

The balancing situation for beginners is exactly the same in *ardha chandrasana* as in *anantasana*, in that if the fingers of the arm touching the ground are placed in line with the foot on the ground, the effective base of the posture is much smaller than if one places the fingers instead to the little-toe (fifth-metatarsal) side of the standing foot and then leans back on the arm. That is to say, placing the fingers off the line of the foot in *ardha chandrasana* provides an internal wall onto which beginners can lean to stabilize the posture.[10] With practice, the fingers can be brought more and more onto the line of the standing foot and more and more lightly on the ground, leading to a truly foot-balanced posture, just as the case where, with practice, one can move from mechanical stability in *salamba sarvangasana* to balancing in *niralamba sarvangasana*.

Visvamitrasana is a balancing posture related to *ardha chandrasana*, in that both involve balancing with one hand and one foot on the ground. As with *ardha chandrasana*, balance in the front-to-back direction is difficult while in *visvamitrasana* if the hand and foot are placed in the same line; however, it is much easier if the hand of the supporting arm is set on the floor so that it is somewhat behind the foot on the floor and is bent so that it supports the other leg in the air. When done in this way, the posture has the advantage of both a larger base and an internal wall for support.

Adho Mukha Vrksasana

For *adho mukha vrksasana*, stay slightly overbalanced, leaning slightly on the wall offered by the pressure of the fingertips on the floor, and avoid rolling over the wrists, as when underbal-

---

10   As mentioned in Subsection V.D, page 899, the placement of the fingers off the line of the feet in *ardha chandrasana* aids balance by increasing the effective size of the base under the posture.

anced. In this case, the wall formed by the fingers is strengthened if the fingers are somewhat curled so that the fingertips grip the floor more tightly. However, the hand position on the floor is reversed in *mayurasana*, so one must again keep the weight heavy on the fingertips, but this time by staying slightly underbalanced. The hand position in *hamsasana* is reversed again with respect to that in *mayurasana*, and so in this case it is appropriate again to be slightly overbalanced, as in *adho mukha vrksasana*.

Many other balancing *yogasanas*, such as *parivrtta trikonasana, parivrtta ardha chandrasana,* and *pincha mayurasana*, are performed by constructing such an internal wall and then leaning against it. In fact, each time we press the floor in order to generate a countertorque, in essence, we are leaning momentarily on a self-constructed wall. The generation of a countertorque in aid of balancing is described in more detail for *vrksasana* in Subsection V.F, page 914. The point here is that in many balancing positions, the lessons of Box V.B-1, page 879, regarding the asymmetric nature of hands and feet apply. Thus, when on the foot, it is best to lean somewhat forward, taking advantage of the internal wall that exists forward of the heel, not backward, and which is stronger in the forward direction than it is side to side. In a similar way, when on the hand, keep the weight somewhat forward on the wall formed by the pressure of the fingertips on the floor (slightly overbalanced) and away from the wrist side of the palm (underbalanced). In this way, one can generate a swaying interaction of torque and countertorque without the risk of falling off the heel of the wrist. As discussed in Subsection V.B, page 878, you can depend on the knees and elbows for support, but not for maintaining balance.

Redistributing the Mass: The Balancing-Pole Effect

Visualize the circus acrobat balancing on the high wire, carrying her long pole held crosswise to the wire. Though this pole does not in any way increase the area of the performer's base (sole of the foot on the wire), it does aid greatly in stabilizing the left-right balance. The mechanical stability of airplanes, rockets, and bombs is aided by their outstretched lateral appendages (their wings and fins), which keep them from tumbling through the air.

In the standing *yogasanas,* you too can be helped by this balancing-pole action if the synchronization of falling-body torque and foot countertorque cannot be realized. Rather than working to extend the arms upward, as in many standing postures, extend them outward to the sides instead and feel the mechanical stability that comes from lowering the center of gravity and from this redistribution of mass, which generates a useful counterbalancing torque.[11]

_____

11   This leads to the temptation to balance on the arms by swinging the legs and vice versa. Try to minimize this aspect of mass redistribution. Actually, there is a competition between balancing by generating a countertorque against the floor using the feet and balancing by the movement of large body parts in order to reposition the center of gravity. In the latter case, there may be gross and unwelcome distortions of the posture, whereas in the former, the countertorque may be too small to counter the falling. As with most things, the truth lies somewhere between the two extreme cases: it is best to use the countertorque generated by working the primary joint against the floor as best you can when balancing, while using the "un-broomstick-like" gyrations if necessary. With time, maximize the former and minimize the latter.

The competitive nature of these two balancing modes is shown in *uttanasana,* done at the wall. The competition between balancing by the gross movement of large parts of the body versus that obtained by working the floor to generate a countertorque is illustrated in the following *uttanasana* exercise. Start with *uttanasana* at the wall, setting the feet at a comfortable distance from the wall and adjusting the position of your pelvis over your feet so that your weight rests only lightly on the toes. From here, in steps, sequentially halve the distance of the heels from the wall, and note how as your heels are set closer and closer to the wall, the wall more and more inhibits shifting the pelvis backward, and as a consequence, the toes (and fingertips!) are more and more called upon to press the floor in order to avoid falling forward. Practicing *uttanasana* with the heels at the wall, minimal fingertip pressure on the floor, and strong foot action to press

Application to Yogasana

Students having trouble balancing in *vrksasana,* *virabhadrasana III,* or even *virabhadrasana I* for example, profit from redistributing their mass by extending their arms to the sides to form balancing poles in these specifically metastable postures. If you can balance easily in these postures but fall when you close your eyes, try them again with your eyes closed but with your arms held outward at the sides to increase your stability. In the same vein, any left-right falling while in *paripurna navasana, ubhaya padangusthasana,* or *urdhva mukha paschimottanasana I* can be stabilized by left-right spreading of the legs, as in *upavistha konasana.* Similarly, the balance in *ubhaya padangusthasana* is easier in the forward-backward direction than is that in *urdhva mukha paschimottanasana I* because of the larger angle at the hips in the former as compared to the latter. Balancing in these seated postures with the angles of the legs opened is easier than when the legs are together or pulled closer to the chest, because the hamstring stretch is not as intense in the legs-opened positions (Subsection 10.B, page 345), and so gives one more psychological space in which to maneuver. It is very difficult to balance when we are constrained by the limits of our range of motion!

When in *parsva hasta padangusthasana,* the balance in the left-right direction can be precarious with one leg outstretched to the side. If finding stability in this posture is difficult, try extending the opposite arm to form a left-to-right balancing-pole combination with the oppositely extended leg. Though raising the opposite arm does raise the center of gravity of the posture, this disadvantage is more than offset by the advantage of having formed a balancing pole in this posture.

Holding an open umbrella in the free hand not only adds a theatrical touch to your balancing but may prove to be just what you need to stay up. In this case, the motion of the umbrella displaces a certain volume of air in its motion, and a

_____

the buttocks to the wall strengthens the action necessary for foot balancing.

useful torque then develops from the momentum generated by the displacement.

The above deals with weight redistributed about the line between centers of body and Earth. A strong effect on balance also is observed and expected when the center of gravity is moved upward or downward on the line of centers. This is considered in Subsection V.D, page 897.

The Importance of Head and Eye Positions

Several aspects of the various roles of vision in balancing are discussed in Subsection V.C, page 888. In this subsection, we discuss the relationships between head position, eye orientation, and ease of balancing. The positions of the head and eyes in general are coordinated in the following ways. Tipping the head backward (extension) or forward (flexion) tends to turn the eyes either toward the upper eyelids or the lower eyelids, respectively. The ocular-vestibular reflex (Subsection 17.B, page 668) operates when the head is rotated around the axis of the cervical spine so that the eyes reflexively turn left to right when the head is turned right to left, thus allowing the line of sight to remain stationary, though the head is turning. These reflexive tendencies are easily nullified if the practitioner chooses to do so.

Autonomic Nervous Excitation

Note that the two head positions, chin to chest and chin away from the chest, are respectively calming (*jalandhara bandha,* figure 11.D-2) and arousing to the body and mind (*urdhva dhanurasana,* Box 11.D-1, page 453) and so may be competing factors in achieving the calm mental state required to balance. With the head down (flexion) in a standing position, there is a parasympathetic stimulation and a calmness that enhances mental concentration during the balancing efforts. Neck flexion also is a right-hemisphere function, which is the hemisphere for better proprioceptive sensing. On the other hand, with the neck in extension, as in *simhasana II,* there is an excitation of the sympathetic branch of the autonomic nervous system, which may interfere with the mental con-

centration necessary for balancing. Note too that balancing in *vrksasana* with the neck in flexion but with the eyes looking downward is easier compared with keeping the neck in flexion but with the eyes looking upward.

When inverted and balancing, the effects of head and eye position are also inverted, with the eyes-toward-the-upper-eyelid position being the more relaxed and more stable one, all other things being equal [851]. Presumably, in the case of inversion, the parasympathetic relaxation allows a more undisturbed concentration on maintaining balance. It is an open question as to how important the head position is in balancing when the eyes are closed, if at all.

The Neck Muscles

There are important groups of muscle-spindle stretch sensors in the capitis muscles on the left and right sides of the cervical spine (figure V.C-1), which are activated when the chin drops toward the chest or toward one shoulder. These sensors are used proprioceptively to monitor the deviation of the head from the erect posture by comparing the tension in the muscle spindles on the two sides.

It is understandable, in part, that keeping the neck in flexion should be advantageous when balancing in the upright position, because in this situation, the muscles at the back of the neck are in tension. In this case, the muscle-spindle proprioceptors within the neck muscles are activated and so can act as left-to-right balance sensors, whereas there is no such activation when the neck is in extension and thus there are no out-of balance signals to be sensed. I can find no information on the possible role of the joint-capsule proprioceptors between the cervical vertebrae on maintaining balance, so one can only assume that they also play some role in regard to the attitude of the head. On the other hand, the utricle of the vestibular system (Subsection 18.B, page 696) would seem not to be activated in the inverted position with the head in flexion, but it is so when in extreme extension.

Yoga experience shows that in standing balances with the eyes open, the visual support of balance is greatest when the eyes look down, is less so when looking straight ahead, and is least when the head is turned to look upward. The truth of this statement is easily tested by doing *vrksasana* with each of the three head positions. These differences probably involve the extent of stretching of the capitis muscles, the use of different parts of the vestibular apparatus when balancing in the different head positions, and also the fact that we are more habituated to looking downward (when walking, etc.) than we are to looking upward, and so the visual-balancing mechanism is simply more effective in the head-down position. When looking up at the ceiling, across the room, or down at the floor, having a point of visual focus will be mechanically stabilizing in the balancing postures. Note, however, that when the eyes are closed in *vrksasana* and the balance maintained by use of the little finger on the adjacent wall (Subsection V.D, page 902), the balance is unaffected by the position of the head; apparently, the sensors of the little finger are more important than tension in the capitis muscles in this case.

Head/Eye Positions and Swaying

Though the situation is somewhat muddled, there is substantial evidence [782] that there is at least some interaction in regard to balancing between the vestibular apparatus and the proprioceptors in the neck, which monitor both muscle tension by the muscle spindles and also send proprioceptive signals from the joint capsules in the cervical vertebrae. Guyton [308] describes this interaction in terms of falling and head bending. In a number of situations, balance is strongly affected by head position:

1. In *vrksasana*, the balancing is easiest when the eyes are looking down and most difficult when looking up. A similar statement holds for *trikonasana, ardha chandrasana,* and *virabhadrasana III*. Note that in *trikonasana*, the head position is looking over one shoulder rather than in extension or flexion. Neck proprioceptors can still be of use here, as they report left-right imbalance. There is further evidence con-

necting these muscle spindles of the neck with eye motion in [603].

2. In *adho mukha vrksasana* (full arm balance), the balance is easiest when the back of the head is lifted (neck in extension) than when the neck is held in flexion. This is opposite to 1, but the posture is inverted with respect to 1.

3. Head position doesn't seem to be as large a factor when balancing in *pincha mayurasana*.

4. There is little or no effect of head position when balancing in *anantasana*.

5. In *sarvangasana*, do not look at the ceiling, as this is an eyes-up position and thus serves to activate the intellect in a posture that does not require it. Similarly, do not look at the solar plexus, as this tends to pull the eyes in toward the nose, thus creating visual tension. Looking at the knees in *sarvangasana* is a good neutral position for the eyes in this posture. Regarding body position, keep the weight slightly overbalanced in *sarvangasana*, so that the weight is somewhat shifted off the neck and more on the elbows. Inasmuch as one can see only oneself in *sarvangasana*, it is an ideal posture for self-examination [477]. In contrast, in the counterposture, *sirsasana I*, one can see everything except oneself. In this way, one can rationalize the fact that *sirsasana* is energizing and heating whereas *sarvangasana* is meditative and cooling.

One is tempted to generalize, from the above cases, that head position is more of a factor in balancing the further the head is from the floor. This makes sense, as it implies that the closer the head is to the floor, the less it is moved during a fall, and the less it is therefore responsible for sensing the fall.

Balancing with the Head in Motion

There is evidence that lifting the gaze makes the sway angle θ larger and therefore leads to a more challenging balance. Tipping the head backward to look upward may not cause dizziness but still results in increasing the extent of sway. With the gaze held level, young adults sway by about 2.5 centimeters (one inch) when in *tadasana*; however, senior citizens sway by 50 percent more, and the sway increases even more when looking up at 45°; this angle of sway may readily exceed θ*, the critical angle for falling. On the other hand, the ocular-vestibular reflex (Subsection V.C, page 890) can work to keep the eyes stationary, even though the head is in rotary motion.

Head Rolling

Yet another aspect of head position involves balance and head rolling. One is easily convinced that the head must be kept still while balancing in the *yogasanas* by coming into *vrksasana,* for example, and then rolling the head to randomly excite the semicircular canals (Subsection 18.B, page 698). The effect will be an immediate falling over when in foot, forearm, or hand balances, but again the effect is not as strong when in seat balances. Apparently the seated balances largely involve the pressure sensors of the anatomy in contact with the floor and rely only weakly on coherent excitations within the vestibular apparatus.

Keeping the Eyes on the Prize

Experience shows that balance in general is most easily maintained when the eyes are open and focused on the balancing joint placed on the floor, and least easily maintained when looking away from this joint. Also, when head down in an upright position and head up in an inverted position, one is always in a position to view the hands or feet on the floor. Thus, difficulty in a particular balance possibly can be relieved by changing the head position.

When in foot-balancing postures such as *ardha chandrasana, virabhadrasana III,* and *utthita hasta padangusthasana,* it is most stabilizing to hold the neck in flexion. In contrast to this, balancing in *urdhva prasarita eka padasana* is easier with the head tipped upward (neck in extension); however, the neck can be held in flexion as in *ardha baddha padmottanasana* when the hands are on the ground. Similarly, balancing in *pincha*

mayurasana, bakasana, and *adho mukha vrksasana* is far easier with the neck in extension than in flexion. Have a partner help with the balance in *adho mukha vrksasana* by bracing the front of the thighs with a thumb and index finger of one hand and bracing the back of the calves with a thumb and index finger of the other hand. In this position, moments of balance can be readily achieved if the balancer holds her neck in extension. In contrast, if the head is held in flexion, the moments of maintained balance are much fewer and farther between.

It seems to be that balance is most easily maintained with the neck in flexion when upright but in extension when inverted. What, then, is best in a balancing posture such as downward-facing dog performed with opposite-side hand and leg lifted (*dwianga adho mukha svanasana*)? The answer, I believe, depends upon what the foot is doing in this posture; if the foot is in the straight-ahead position with heel lifted, then more balance control comes from the hand, and one should keep the neck in extension to focus on the hand; however, if the foot is fully on the floor, even though angled, it is stronger than the hand and should be given the responsibility for maintaining balance, i.e., keep the neck in flexion. In seat-balancing postures such as *paripurna navasana* and its variations, neither head position nor lack of vision seem to play a role. However, see Subsection V.D, page 906.

As for why turning the eyes to look at the joint on the floor that is responsible for the balance is so effective, perhaps it relates to the idea that balancing is a very mental activity and that distractions that interrupt one's concentration on what is going on in the primary joint(s) can only lead to premature falling. Looking at the primary joint while in a balance aids the depth of concentration supporting that balance.

Resistive Balancing

Imagine our beginning student trying unsuccessfully to balance away from the wall in *sirsasana I*. For many such students, the proper muscle actions for balancing in *sirsasana I* seem

Box V.D-1: Resistive Balancing

For practice in resistive balancing when working with a student in an inverted posture, first hold the student in the balanced position, and then slowly push him or her out of balance, either to underbalance (feet too far forward) or overbalance (feet too far backward), but maintain the support in the unbalanced position. The support by the teacher or helper in the off-balance position is minimal; usually just placing the tips of the thumb and index finger of one hand on the upper thighs (front or back) is enough. From the position of supported imbalance, the student then works to generate a countertorque (as exemplified in figure V.D-2) that overcomes the imbalance, and, using feedforward as well, brings the off-balance position back to stability. By working in this way, the student has the time to sort out the proprioceptive and vestibular signals and to try various righting strategies. Over time, this practice results in the training of the various neuromuscular groups necessary for activating the complex balancing patterns. Note too that even when not falling in *sirsasana I*, the net effect of working to open the angles at the wrists and at the elbows while balancing results in a beneficial net relocation of the shoulders, both away from the floor and away from the hands. The technique of resistive balancing can also be used in standing postures such as *ardha chandrasana* and *parivrtta trikonasana*.

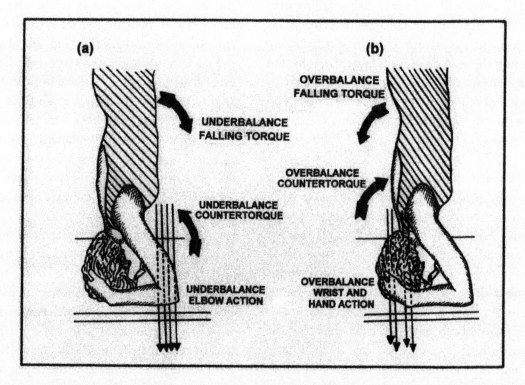

Figure V.D-2. (a) Schematic representation of the forearm and wrist in *sirsasana*, with the torso underbalanced and rotating clockwise. In this case, the counterbalancing torque is generated by pressing the elbows into the floor. (b) If the torso is overbalanced so that it would fall in a counterclockwise sense, then application of the wrists to the floor will generate the necessary countertorque and so restore balance.

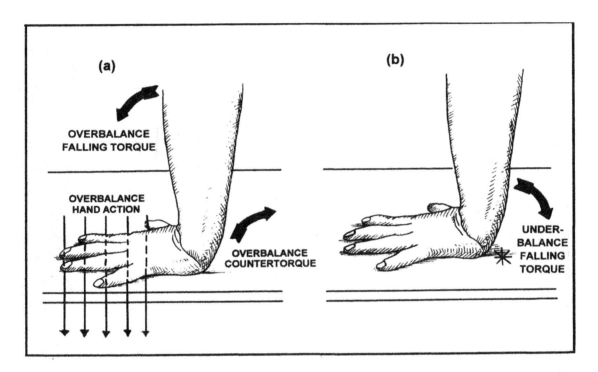

Figure V.D-3. (a) Resistive action of the fingers and metacarpals when overbalancing in *adho mukha vrksasana* or other hand-balancing postures, and (b) the situation when in the same posture but underbalanced. In this latter case, no resistance is possible, and one simply rolls about the point marked * and drops the feet to the floor.

not to be accessible when inverted, or the falling is so rapid that they cannot be brought into play quickly enough to save the falling posture. One way around these problems, for some, is to practice the technique of resistive balancing [181] described in Box V.D-1, above.

If the student is unable to generate enough countertorque to compensate for the falling torque when overbalanced, the magnitude of the countertorque can be increased by pulling the wrists closer to one another. This will move the fingers further from the head and so increase the length of the lever arm (r) over which the restoring force is working (figure V.B-2).

Using the support given in resistive balancing also can be very useful in implanting in the student's mind the consequences of letting a balance become too far underbalanced. For example, support a student in *adho mukha vrksasana* in the overbalanced position (figure V.D-3a), and the student will be able to work the hands against the floor to recover the balance point. However, if the same student is supported in the underbalanced position (figure V.D-3b), he or she will quickly discover that recovery is not possible while keeping the arms straight and so learns to avoid that situation in the future.

Once a resistive-balancing exercise on the hands is finished, have the fully inverted student return to the beginning position (feet on the floor) slowly, with as little outside help as possible. This latter is a resistive strengthening exercise involving eccentric isotonic work (Subsection 11.A, page 408), and will quickly build the strength needed to go into the inverted *yogasana* without jumping or kicking, as well as enhance the student's ability to increase the duration of the inverted posture.

Visualization Practice

It has been shown in several non-yogic studies that the neuromuscular skills of the sort that we work to perfect in *yogasana* practice are in fact enhanced by confident thinking, conversations with oneself, and passive visualization of the activity prior to practice [602a]. The last of these is an interesting idea well worth exploring in its applicability to *yogasana* practice in general and to balancing postures in particular. Presumably, exercising the thought processes involved in the activity without actually activating the requisite muscles is of value, thanks to the strengthening effect it has on the neural patterning that eventually will drive the muscles (Subsection 4.G, page 135). In a similar vein, practicing an exercise on only one side actually works to improve the performance on the second side through a lateral transfer of the neuromuscular pattern learned and refined on the first side.

It is becoming increasingly recognized that optimizing athletic performance does involve a certain amount of neurological practice and neurological warm-up. Applying this idea to balancing, just prior to attempting a balancing *yogasana* that is difficult for you, meditate first on the actions you will take as you come into the posture, visualize the actions in the joint that will keep you stable as you stretch into the "broomstick" state, and sense the stability as you remain in the posture. Finally, imagine the completion of the action and the successful outcome of your attempt as you release from the balanced position without falling. The effect of such warm-up imagery is to program the neurological system to perform optimally. Perhaps something like this is at work when students are asked to be still and just watch the teacher demonstrate a new *yogasana*. In this way, their neurological systems (actually, the mirror neurons, Subsection 4.G, page 142) are primed to do the work asked of them. Not only do such mirror neurons help us learn the postures from our teachers, but they also prompt us to look more and more like them!

All of the general points described in the discussion above in regard to foot balancing will apply generally as well to the inverted *yogasanas* (Section V.G, page 922). In order to illustrate the basic facts of balance, the balancing aspects of several specific *yogasanas* (standing balances, hand balances, and a few others) that are well known to all who practice this discipline are discussed below. In this, we integrate the information in the previous sections 17.A, page 657, 18.B, page 696, and V.A, page 866.

Section V.E: Coming into the Balancing Position

This and the following sections are devoted to somewhat more detailed discussions of the balancing actions in illustrative upright and inverted postures. As beginners, we are generally better able to balance in the upright versions of the *yogasanas* than in the corresponding inverted postures, probably for reasons of familiarity. When first practicing an inversion, it is recommended that you move into it as slowly as your strength will allow.

The strength to move into the inversion with muscular control can be attained by practicing coming down from the inverted posture with as much muscular control as you can manage.

The slow approach to balance not only exercises the powers of balance without overwhelming them but lessens the necessity of a large correction of the balance that cannot be anticipated or counterbalanced. If one enters a posture without the proper control, there is little chance that the mistake can be corrected while fully in the task of balancing in it; it is much more profitable to enter balancing postures slowly and with maximum control, but not so slowly that getting into the posture leaves one exhausted. In the same vein, it is good to think beforehand of what actions you will perform in the balancing posture but to do this while you are still on your feet and not when you are in whatever posture is the doorway into the balance. That is, run through the actions you will take to get into and remain in *adho mukha vrksasana* while still on your feet rather than when you are ready to kick up from *adho mukha svanasana* with one foot up in the air.

Vrksasana

Often with the *yogasana* beginner, falling is so rapid that one has no time in which to organize a muscular rebuttal before one is irrevocably out of the posture. In this case, placing the posture against the wall will prove to be of value, for it removes the time element while still allowing the student to practice coming back into balance once he or she is ready to lean away from the wall (Subsection V.D, page 901). As discussed in Subsection V.D, a light touch of the finger on the wall is all that is needed to balance in *vrksasana*.

With the feet placed properly in *vrksasana*, the posture resembles the broomstick labeled "object 2" in figure V.A-4, and like object 2, it is easily tipped out of balance. To balance on the right leg in *vrksasana*, start first in *tadasana*, either next to the wall or in the middle of the room. With both feet still on the floor, first imperceptibly shift the weight from the left leg onto the right leg. If you try lifting the left leg without first shifting, you will fall immediately. It is better then to move the weight slowly off the leg to be lifted and transfer it onto the standing leg; in general, it is most effective to try to achieve a balanced position as you are entering the posture, rather than trying to find it in the confusion of being in an off-balance position. If you balance on one leg and fall before you can raise your arms, try raising the arms to vertical before lifting the leg. Balance is easier still if the arms are just lifted in the plane of the body to horizontal to take advantage of the balancing-pole effect (Subsection V.D, page 905).

As you bring weight onto the standing leg, select a stationary object across the room as a visual anchor, and keep its image centered in your field of view. With practice, you will be able to release your visual hold on the anchor and allow your gaze to become broad and soft. Extending the fingertips to the ceiling will then serve to open all of the secondary joints fully, keeping them taut and immobile.

Sirsasana I and Bent Legs

A fully inverted posture such as *sirsasana I* can be approached in steps, each of which will require an increased prowess in balancing. When attempting *sirsasana I* in the middle of the room, the easiest balancing position is that with the legs bent, knees pulled into the chest but pelvis directly over the head. This posture takes advantage of stability that follows from the low center of gravity of the folded position. Once the balance is mastered in this position, keep the legs bent at the knees, but lift the knees over the axis of the head and pelvis to raise the center of gravity significantly. The final position, with the legs straight and the body truly vertical, is only slightly more challenging than the intermediate position with legs folded at the knees.

Sirsasana I and Straight Legs

The basic balancing principle of Section V.A, page 867, in regard to keeping the line between centers within the base is relevant not only to maintaining balance in *sirsasana I* but also is the key to lifting straight legs from the floor to the inverted position. With the head and arms on the floor appropriate to *sirsasana I*, straighten the legs. If, when in this starting position, the line of centers between the body and the Earth (see figure V.A-2d) is outside the triangle of the lower arms and head on the floor, you are in the falling position, the feet will be heavy on the floor, and it will be difficult (if not impossible) to get the legs moving upward. The secret to coming into *sirsasana I* with straight legs is to get the line between centers of the body and the Earth within the balancing triangle of the arms on the floor while the feet are down. To do this, (i) with hands and head in *sirsasana I*, walk the feet toward the head as far as they will go; (ii) separate the legs as in *prasarita padottanasana*, and walk them yet further toward the line defined by the elbows; (iii) bend at the hips to bring the buttocks as much overhead as possible—this is more easily achieved by the beginner with the legs separated than together for the same reason that *upavistha konasana* for the beginner is easier than *paschimottanasana* (Subsection 10.B, page 345); (iv) come up on the toes; (v) once the pelvis is as much as possible over the head, roll **slightly** back on the head to bring the cervical vertebrae closer to vertical, and simultaneously lift the legs so that the weight on the toes becomes negligible; (vi) mentally prepare the wrists to counter rolling too far backward as the legs literally lift themselves upward; (vii) once the spine and the legs are in the vertical plane but with the legs separated, bring the legs together vertically over the vertical spine. If you are not able to get the posture to move in this way, it is likely that the bottleneck involves a lack of hamstring flexibility, which first must be addressed through the appropriate practice. A strategy similar to that given above will also work for jumping or pressing into *adho mukha vrksasana* with straight legs; i.e., at first work with the legs widely separated, and concentrate on getting the buttocks over the wrists before working on getting the legs together and vertical.

Dwianga Adho Mukha Svanasana

One can approach this balancing posture by making it progressively more inverted at each step. First, set the hands at the wall at hip height, and walk the feet under the hips to be in the *adho mukha svanasana* posture with feet on the floor but hands on the wall (*ardha uttanasana*). Lift the opposite arm and leg to come into the *dwianga* posture. Balancing here is easy, because all of the weight is over the standing leg, and its foot is strong enough to keep the posture in balance with minimal help from the hand on the wall. Repeat, placing the hands on a chair seat instead, and progress from there to hands on two and then one block on the floor. As the balancing hand approaches the floor, it carries more of the weight, and as it is weaker than the foot for balancing, the difficulty increases. In this way, walk the balancing hand of *dwianga adho mukha svanasana* stepwise down the ladder until it is on the floor. See Subsection V.D, page 907, in regard to how best to hold the head in this posture.

One has the option as well of entering *dwianga adho mukha svanasana* from *adho mukha svanasana* by first lifting the leg and then the arm or the reverse; I find the balance is easier if I lift the arm first, then the leg.

Section V.F: Maintaining Balance in the Standing *Yogasanas*

Localizing the Balancing Action in *Vrksasana*

Consider that one starts to fall while in *vrksasana*. As shown schematically in figure V.B-1b, if the right leg tends to fall clockwise (as seen from the front), then pressure applied by the big-toe (first metatarsal) side of the right foot to the floor will generate a counterclockwise torque within the foot, ankle, and leg; the foot and ankle in *vrksasana* play the roles of the hand and wrist in the broomstick balance. This action in *vrksasana* essentially is one in which the foot pendulum creates a countertorque to balance the falling torque of the upper-body pendulum.

Balance is restored and maintained by pressing first one side of the foot to the floor and then the other to always (in time and space) counterbalance (countertorque) with the foot and ankle the falling imbalance (torque) of the upper body. Because the first metatarsal is so much stronger than the fifth, one can stay up in *vrksasana* longer if the weight on the standing foot is deliberately kept slightly on the side of the first metatarsal.

When in *vrksasana*, the front-to-back foot action required to retain balance is largely plantar flexion and so is driven by the peroneus longus muscle (Subsection 10.B, page 356), whereas the left-to-right balancing action in this posture is a matter of inversion and eversion of the ankle (figure V.B-1b). In this, the inversion of the foot involves pressing the lateral edge of the foot to the floor via the extensor hallucis longus, and eversion involves pressing the medial edge of the foot to the floor via the peroneus longus and peroneus brevis muscles. In these actions around the ankle, inversion is said to be stronger than eversion, and plantar flexion is stronger than dorsiflexion [101]. See Box V.F-1 (below) for a further discussion of the innervation of the first metatarsal.

In support of the line of reasoning given in Box V.F-1, below, Myers [603] points out that the foot is naturally divisible longitudinally into that part involving the first three metatarsals and the talus, and a second part consisting of the two outer lateral toes and the cuboid bone (figure 10.B-7c). The two parts of the foot, so apportioned, have distinctly different innervations [613]. The first of these is the major weight-bearing portion of the foot, as emphasized by Iyengar, and should be the part most involved in a foot balance. This is especially true considering that it is the talus that is so rich in balancing mechanoreceptors.

With the arms over head in *vrksasana,* the upward lift of the body in the course of opening the joints leads to the sensation of hanging by your fingertips from the ceiling rather than standing with your foot on the floor. While balancing in *vrksasana,* the mind focuses totally on the countertorquing motions of the ankle joint but ignores the other joints of the body, because they are fully elongated and thus immobilized.

Having reduced the act of balancing in *vrksasana* to localizing the action in the foot and ankle of the standing leg, we now consider how anatomically and neurologically the ankle keeps the body balanced in the pose. With the cervical vertebrae in line with those below it, the balanced position in *vrksasana* is aided by the utricles of the inner ears, by the appropriate receptive fields in the retinas of the eyes engaged in retinal streaming, by the proprioceptive sensors throughout the body, and especially by the pressure-sensitive Pacinian receptors on the bottom of the foot. Apparently, the relative amounts of these different balancing sensors used while in *vrksasana* varies among students.

The beds of mechanoreceptors at the level of the joint capsules surrounding the talus in each ankle are significant factors when balancing on the feet. Should these sense an imbalance, they will report the off-balance condition upward to both the higher centers of the brain and to the muscles of the body in reflex arcs that automatically right the body.

Note, however, that because of the flexibility of the cervical spine, the head may be truly balanced according to the vestibular organs, while the rest of the body is not. Thus, verticality of the entire body along the length of its axis must involve the participation of proprioceptors other than the vestibular organs if the head, torso, and legs are to be in the proper aligned relationship [885] (see Section 11.B, page 431, regarding the role of the mechanoreceptors in the back of the neck). If, while in *vrksasana,* one turns the head in small circles at a modest speed, all balance will be lost as the confusing signals from the vestibular apparatus swamp those from the Pacinian sensors in the sole of the foot and the joint-capsule sensors in the ankle. Keep the head still, and let the sensors in the foot and the visual cues control the balance.

When standing, there is a synergism between two sets of balancing organs. On the one hand, the elements of the vestibular apparatus work to alert the body to a fall, under the questionable assumption that if the head is falling, then the body must be falling. On the other hand, the proprioceptors in the muscles spindles of the neck muscles and in the joint receptors of the neck report on the relative muscular tension at the back of the neck. These two balancing signals work against one another in the following way. If the vestibular apparatus reports falling and the neck proprioceptors do the same, then the signals cancel one another, as appropriate for a simple tipping of the head without loss of balance. However, if the vestibular apparatus reports a forward fall but the back of the neck does not report a corresponding stretch, then there is no counterbalancing of the signals, and a real fall is signaled as imminent. This may be relevant to the relative difficulties of balancing in *vrksasana* with the head looking down, straight ahead, and upward, as different neck signals are generated in the three cases. When the head is flexed downward, the vestibular reflex tends to extend the arms in anticipation of a fall, whereas relaxation of the neck receptors tends to relax the arms [308]. This should be relevant to all postures in which the head is placed into *jalandhara bandha* or tipped backward.

Box V.F-1: You Have More Sensitivity in Your Big Toe than You Ever Imagined

Figure 13.B-2 shows a plot of the measured mean separation between surface pressure receptors in various parts of the body. The larger this mean separation is, the fewer the number of sensors in this area and the lower the resolution of the touch (i.e., the coarser the sense of touch). Accordingly, the very large areas of the cerebral cortex devoted to the areas of the lips, tongue, fingers, and thumbs (figures 4.C-5 and 4.C-6) have the finest resolution for touch and movement. The exacting command over the movements in these areas makes speech and tool-making possible for human beings, as well as balancing with just the tip of the finger on the wall for sensing the balance. Notice, however, that the resolution of the touch sensors of the big toe (hallux) is finer than those of the palm of the hand, the sole of the foot, the calf, thigh, belly, back, forehead, shoulder, upper arm, or forearm!

What can it possibly mean that the big toe has such a high resolution for pressure on its underside? I interpret this as showing that in our evolution to bipedalism, we have developed extraordinary strength and sensitivity in the area of the big toe in order to balance on two feet, using the pressure sensors in and around the big toe as the prime sensors and prime movers. From the point of view of the *yogasana* student, this interpretation should seem logical in hindsight, for in the *yogasanas,* we often depend strongly on the actions of the big toe against the floor to maintain both alignment and balance.

In making this argument, I have used the fact that the distribution of light-pressure sensors appropriate to figure 13.B-2, which are active in sensing the weight distribution on the big toe when standing, is mirrored by that of the deep-pressure sensors used in sensing any falling torque. The idea proposed here receives support from the sensory cortex, which shows about as much cortical area devoted to foot and toe sensors as to hand and finger sensors [427]. When balancing in *vrksasana,* trust your big toe, and keep the body's primary intelligence in the toes, foot, and ankle of the balancing leg.

Once in the classical position, maintain balance by connecting the conscious mind to the balancing joint, being aware of the mechanical actions being performed by the joint, assessing them mentally to keep them within bounds, and then lessening their amplitudes so that the balancing actions become more subtle and refined.

If *vrksasana* is wobbly, stability can be gained by broadening and lengthening the standing foot and by spreading the arms laterally. For students seeking more challenge, coming up on the toes of the foot of the straight leg in *vrksasana* makes the base yet smaller and hence the posture even more challenging.

Though the body is left-right symmetric while we stand in *urdhva hastasana,* this is no longer the case in *vrksasana,* for if we balance on the left leg, the lumbar spine tends to move to the right, the thorax to the left, and the cervical spine to the right again [428]. However, these lateral curvatures of the spine are very much reduced if the body is extended upward, as recommended for better balancing, for this elongation acts to straighten the spine in both the front-to-back and left-to-right directions. When standing on one leg as in *vrksasana,* the pelvis on the unsupported side tends to drop from lack of support, but the gluteus medius muscle (figure 11.A-2) on that side then contracts to hold the pelvis stable and in position.

In the case of the muscles, too rapid a stretching of the muscle spindles leads to a reflexive contraction of the stretched muscle (Section 11.B, page 432). Just as happens with the spindles in the muscles, if the head is moved impulsively (as might occur when rotating it in a circular motion in the discussion above), there is a strong torque within the semicircular canal sensors, prompting an immediate reflexive righting action to occur, which often is destabilizing in the long run. However, if we move the head slowly from head down to head up in *vrksasana*, for example, then vestibular response is slow, smooth, and under conscious control, just as for slow, conscious stretching of the muscle (Subsection 11.B, page 433), and there is no reflexive countermotion.

As with feedback, there is also a control loop in a feedforward response, but with parameters to be adjusted to achieve a goal in the future. For example, in attempting to perform *vrksasana* on the right leg from *tadasana*, feedforward circuits adjust the positions and motions of the limbs in anticipation of raising the left leg. Similarly, if one moves from *tadasana* to *virabhadrasana III*, feedforward actions originating in the basal ganglia anticipate the swinging action around the standing leg and bring it to a halt when the body reaches the horizontal position. These examples of feedforward reflexes are brought into the conscious realm with practice.

The Ill and the Elderly

It is said that the elderly are unable to balance while standing on one leg [266]. Thus, the average balancing time on the dominant leg has been reported to vary with age in the following way: age forty to forty-nine years (15.5–7.2 seconds), age fifty to fifty-nine years (8.7–3.7 seconds), age sixty to sixty-nine years (4.5–2.5 seconds), and age seventy to seventy-nine years (2.6–1.5 seconds) [317]. This rapid falling off of the balancing time (about 50 percent every decade) is thought to be the result of incidental damage to the afferent sciatic nerve running from the foot to the base of the spine, the longest in the body, for it is considered unlikely that such a long single

neuron could remain intact and functioning over a lifetime. Because elderly *yogasana* students daily are able to do *vrksasana* for minutes rather than seconds shows that this idea is in error.

In addition to the risks of falling for the elderly, there are risks for those who are not elderly but who might be suffering from neuropathy associated with diabetes, poor vision, vestibular disorders, weak muscles or weak bones, spinal injuries, or stroke. Priplata et al. [675] have made a special study of balancing in diabetics and those with stroke, and they compared the parameters of their balance performance with a subgroup of healthy but elderly subjects. It was found that the use of noise-enhanced vibrating insoles (Subsection V.C, page 894), significantly improved balance in all three groups.

Healing

Once a sprained ankle is in its healing mode and can bear weight without pain, the promotion of circulation into and out of the sprained area can be very healing. This circulation is promoted by balancing on the affected ankle in *vrksasana*, for early mobilization of the ankle speeds recovery and lessens the pain of injury. Also, see Subsection 18.B, page 701, for a discussion of the helpful effects of *vrksasana* practice on dyslexia in children.

Balancing in the Other Upright and Horizontal *Yogasanas*

Considerable attention has been given to the balancing aspect of *vrksasana*, the archetypical balancing posture in the standing postures. With these points now out in the open, much less needs to be said about the other standing postures, for the balancing points are essentially the same.

Anantasana and Vasisthasana

In both *anantasana* and *vasisthasana*, the balancing problem is front to back, whereas the ocular support, being generally from left to right, is of reduced value in these postures. Balancing will be easier in *vasisthasana* than in *anantasana* because of the high torque that can be generated by the hand on the floor in the former posture, and because with the hand on the floor, the countertorque can be either clockwise or counterclockwise. The hand on the floor for *vasisthasana* should be as broad as possible, to allow one to generate the maximum countertorque and to provide the largest base for balancing.

Utkatasana and Malasana

We are stable when standing in *tadasana* because the line between centers connecting the body and the Earth falls within the area defined by the feet on the floor. On coming into *utkatasana*, bending the legs moves the knees forward and the pelvis backward in an effort to maintain balance. However, there is still a backward overbalance present in this movement, which also requires the torso to lean forward, with front ribs dropping toward the thighs, knees together. When compensated in this way (chest forward and pelvis backward), the posture is in balance but the spine is far from vertical. The work in *utkatasana* is then to make the spine as close to vertical as possible while maintaining balance.

If the knees are maximally flexed to place one in *malasana*, then front-to-back balancing with the feet fully on the floor requires that the knees open laterally so that the torso can be placed fully forward and between the knees, with the spine as close as possible to the horizontal position.

Trikonasana

Consider the student bending to the right, coming into *trikonasana*. Because the feet are widely separated left to right in *trikonasana*, there is no problem with wobbling or falling in the left-to-right direction, whereas in the front-to-back direction there is no less stability in *trikonasana* than in feet-together *tadasana*.[12] Leaning

___
12   As pointed out to me by Carol Wipf, beginning students actually are more stable in *trikonasana* when they are bent at the waist, with the chest far forward of the triangle of the legs and the buttocks pushed backward. This can be understood as a front-to-back balance enhanced by the mass redistribution (Subsection V.D, page 905) in the front-to-back direction result-

to the right in *trikonasana* will activate that semicircular canal having its axis parallel to that of the rotational axis (pubis to coccyx). According to the physiologists, this action will not stimulate the vestibular oculomotor reflex (see above), since this reflex is only activated for the canal in each ear having its axis parallel to the body's long axis; however, the utricle in each inner ear does sense the deviation of the head from verticality. Nonetheless, if you go into *trikonasana* with your eyes closed, you will tend somewhat more to fall forward or backward, showing again the utility of consciously using the eyes for balancing in *trikonasana*, as you did in *vrksasana*. Note too that the student needs static balance when balancing in *trikonasana*, which is essentially a supported position, but dynamic balance when going in both directions between *tadasana* and *trikonasana*. To the extent that the vestibular apparatus of the inner ears is involved in moving in and out of *trikonasana*, congestion and stuffiness in this area can upset one's balance. If *trikonasana*-to-the-right is further embellished by turning the head to look at the upraised left hand, then the vestibular oculomotor reflex will come into play, as the rotation of the head is around the proper internal body axis.

Parivrtta Trikonasana

Balancing signals from the left vestibular and ocular organs are processed in the right cerebral hemisphere, which in turn activates muscles on the left side of the body. Similar decussations (lateral crossings) occur for signals originating on the right side. If, as we lean to the right for *trikonasana*, we instead place the left hand down and rotate the spine to look backward (*parivrtta trikonasana*), the eyes still can be of great use in balancing. However, note that on leaning to the right in *trikonasana*, we are accustomed to having the right ear and the right eye closer to the ground than are those organs on the left, whereas in *parivrtta trikonasana*, it is the left ear and the left eye that are closer to the ground, even though the tilt of

___
ing from pressing the chest forward and the buttocks backward.

the upper body is to the right! Furthermore, with respect to the face in *trikonasana,* the directions of "front" and "back" also have been reversed in *parivrtta trikonasana.* This means that the inputs from the left and right vestibular sensors, from the left and right eyes, and possibly from the right and left edges of the soles of the feet must be reversed left to right at some point in the neural arc if the balance is to be maintained. This mental adjustment can be slow to develop at first, and so *parivrtta trikonasana* is often much more wobbly than is *trikonasana.*

Pulling the outer thighs toward one another and the inner thighs away from one another in *parivrtta trikonasana* pins the hip joints and so stabilizes the legs and pelvis in this posture by removing any possible oscillation in this area, thereby returning full control to the feet and ankles. However, the pressing of the thighs in *parivrtta trikonasana* is an action, not a movement (Chapter 11, page 405) and so the thighs actually do not move toward one another, as this would collapse the groin. See Box V.F-2, below, for further discussion of the effects of physical crossover on balancing.

Virabhadrasana III

The general rules elaborated above for *vrksasana* would apply to balancing in *virabhadrasana III.* Start in *urdhva hastasana,* with all of the secondary joints elongated and stabilized, and, keeping the ankle balance in one's consciousness, pivot slowly over the standing leg. The joints of the body other than the standing ankle are fully opened and thus too taut to wobble, and the gaze is focused on a line on the floor, real or imagined, which runs from the sole of the foot to the forward wall (Subsection V.C, page 888). Like landing lights on an airport runway, this line will guide you and hold you steady if you keep it centered in your field of view as you slowly and with intense consciousness move in and out of *virabhadrasana III,* all the while working the sole of the standing foot against the floor to generate the countertorques needed to balance. Additional stability of balance in *virabhadrasana III* comes from keeping the palms facing one

another (thumbs rolling inward) while rotating the biceps of the upper arms outward [276] to keep the upper body taut (Subsection 10.A, page 328).

The balancing-pole effect is already working for you in *virabhadrasana III,* as the torso and one leg are stretched forward and backward, respectively, to aid balance along this line. In order to gain the same balancing-pole advantage along the left-to-right line in *virabhadrasana III,* extend the arms sideways rather than forward. In this position, you are now fully the airplane landing and taking off from the runway on the floor.

As one moves from the vertical to the horizontal head position coming into *virabhadrasana III,* the saccules will become active as the balancing organs in the face-down position. Of course, the proprioceptors will be active in all body orientations, and especially the pressure-sensitive receptors on the sole of the foot of the supporting leg contribute to the balance, as do the eyes and joint capsules. As in *vrksasana,* balance in *virabhadrasana III* is more readily accomplished if the weight on the standing foot is kept somewhat to the big-toe side and the arches of the foot are kept broad.

Note than when pinning the hips in *virabhadrasana III,* etc., the hip joint is being closed rather than opened when the outer thighs press inward (i.e., the femoral heads are being driven directly into the acetabulae of the hip joints). Moreover, the contraction of the peroneus longus of the lower leg (Subsection 10.B, page 356), as when pressing the bases of the big toes (the first metatarsals) away from the knees and those of the little toes (the fifth metatarsals) toward the knees, also works strongly to pin the hips. Finally, one should minimize the contraction of the gluteus muscles.

Other aids to balancing are available to the student practicing balancing in the upright position (see, for example, Box V.F-1, page 916, Subsection V.F, page 917, and Section V.G, page 928).

Box V.F-2: Physical Crossover Requires Neural Repatterning

As we repeatedly practice the balance in a particular *yogasana,* we develop a deeply ingrained neural pattern of muscular responses in order to maintain that balance (i.e., we learn how to balance in that posture). This patterning is useful up to a point; however, as with *yogasana* practice in general, we can get so strongly patterned in one way that we can no longer react appropriately to new balancing situations (see Juhan's comments in regard to the dangers of ingrained neural patterning, Section 1.B, page 8). Perform the following simple *yogasana* work to see the unbalancing effect that results from taking a part of the body normally on the right and placing it on the left.

A. First stand in *tadasana* with the medial edges of the feet touching. Then repeatedly gyrate the hips in a circular way, pressing them forward, to the right, backward, and to the left in a continuous circular movement, increasing the speed with each rotation. Note any difficulty in maintaining balance on the feet.

B. Now stand in *tadasana,* but with the lateral edges of the feet touching and the legs crossed at the ankles. Again gyrate the hips as in A above, with increasing speed on each rotation. Note now how much more difficult is to maintain balance with the positions of the feet reversed from that normally used in *tadasana.* Difficulties arise in balancing with the ankles crossed, because we are not accustomed to working the left ankle when leaning to the right, and vice versa for leaning to the left. With practice, the balance can be maintained equally for the two foot positions. A more difficult crossed-limb balance is presented below.

C. Assume the Table position on hands and knees, with the hands under the shoulders and separated by shoulder width, and the knees set under the hips and feet placed hip-width apart. Now straighten the right leg and hold it parallel to the floor. Balancing in this position is trivial because of the large area of the base formed by the two hands and the knee (and foot) of the bent leg. Repeat, lifting the left leg instead.

D. Assume the Table position, but with the knees together and the hands as close to one another as possible, adjacent fingers of each hand touching one another, thumbs touching, knees touching, and big toes touching. Perform the right-leg lift again, noting how much more difficult the left-to-right balancing is with the left-to-right dimension of the base so much smaller. Notice also how the inner and outer edges of the hands sense the imbalance and work against the floor in order to generate the appropriate countertorques for maintaining balance. For example, as you sense a fall to the right, you instinctively press the little-finger edge of the right hand on the floor to generate a countertorque, and vice versa for a fall to the left. Repeat, lifting the left leg instead.

E. Set up as in D above, hands touching and knees and feet touching, but now cross the right arm over the left, so that the arms are crossed at the wrists and the little fingers of the two hands are touching rather than the thumbs. With the right leg lifted, the balancing action of the hands on the floor now must be deliberately reversed left to right in the nervous system in order to keep from falling. That is, to maintain balance while falling to the right, for example, one must now press the thumb side of the left hand to the floor in order to generate the same countertorque as was generated in D above by pressing the little-finger side of the right hand to the floor. Note the increasing levels of concentration necessary to keep from falling as one goes from position C to D to E.

In this crossed-over orientation, the hands feel as if they are on the "wrong" sides of the body; maintaining balance would appear to require that the balancing reflex signals received by the higher centers in the "wrong" side of the central nervous system transfer the signals to the corresponding part of the "correct" side of the central nervous system and correspondingly reroute the efferent signals to the muscles to the opposite side of the balancing organ.

One might guess that this left-right transfer of neural signals is achieved via the corpus callosum, a large bundle of nerves connecting the left and right cerebral hemispheres of the brain. However, there is specific evidence that neither the hands nor the feet are associated via the corpus callosum, and so a different mechanism must be at work; presumably it is the anterior commissure that is involved in the hemispheric transfer. If, instead, the pressure sensors in the palms of the hand are being used as sensors, then we simply have to respond to their pressure signals and disregard the fact that the hands are not in their "correct" places as regards the sides of the body. Either way, if we are to hand-balance in the crossed-arm position, we need to learn a new neural pattern that essentially transposes the muscular responses of the inner and outer edges of each hand in response to the falling torques sensed in either the vestibular organs or the pressure sensors. The neural transposition is aided by looking at the hands while balancing.

Similar static crossover balancing problems arise in *gomukhasana*, *parivrtta trikonasana*, and when doing *adho mukha svanasana* with arms crossed at the wrists and one leg lifted. The balancing problem in *gomukhasana* is twofold. First, when done in the classical way with the shins touching, though the center of gravity is quite low, the base is very small. Second, with the legs crossed at the knees, the right shin monitors pressure on the left side of the body, and the right shin monitors pressure on the left side of the body. This then is another case of neural crossover, which is best overcome through practice. In *parivrtta trikonasana*, one of the hands is crossed over to rest on the floor on the outside of the opposite leg. This means that the right hand, for example, is placed on the floor to the left of the left foot, so that when one presses the right hand to the floor, it creates a countertorque that shifts the center of gravity backward, whereas normally in *trikonasana*, the right hand is outside the right foot and pressing the hand to the floor creates a countertorque that shifts the center of gravity of the body forward. In this case, one must use considerable feedforward control of the countertorques to keep from overcompensating and falling.

Practicing these and similar postures in the crossover positions promotes a keener sense of balance overall and is excellent exercise for reconnecting the mind to the body. (See also Subsection 4.D, page 98, for further discussion of the topic of neural crossover.)

Balancing deficits in patients with cerebral hemispheric lesions have been observed in patients balancing on two feet with the eyes closed [652]. Interestingly, it has been found that the larger balancing deficits occur in those for whom the cerebral lesion is carried in the left cerebral hemisphere [713]. That the task of balancing on two feet is cerebrally asymmetric for these people implies that, as with handwriting, etc., they are naturally right-footed.

Section V.G: Balancing in the Inverted *Yogasanas*

Until one is very well exercised in balancing in inversions, it is generally true that the inverted position is more difficult to maintain than the equivalent upright position. Thus, *tadasana* is easier to maintain than is *sirsasana I*, *urdhva hastasana* is easier to maintain than *adho mukha vrksasana*, and *utthita hasta padangusthasana* is easier to maintain than is *urdhva prasarita eka padasana*. Actually, the base is larger in *sirsasana I* than it is in *tadasana*, and there is less wobble when in *sirsasana I* than in *tadasana*, though admittedly it can require more energy to stay in the former than in the latter, because the arms are not as strong as the legs!

Aids to Balancing in the Inverted *Yogasanas*

The inverted postures are defined as those in which the heart is below the head; *uttanasana* and *adho mukha svanasana* are inverted postures, but *tadasana* and *urdhva mukha svanasana* are not. The neural confusion that is inherent when balancing in the left-to-right crossover position discussed above is likely to be exacerbated when the student is top-to-bottom inverted. Expect beginning students to be totally disoriented and out of touch with their muscle control when they are inverted for the first few times. Though many of the points made in the discussion of upright balancing on the feet (Section V.E, page 912, and Section V.F, page 914), apply as well to inverted balancing on the hands and on the head, there are

several useful points not mentioned in the earlier sections as they apply most readily to the inverted positions. We consider a representative set of examples to highlight the relevant aids.

Adho Mukha Vrksasana

Balancing in *adho mukha vrksasana* (full-arm balance) is best learned by first using the wall for support. The ideal body alignment in this posture is that of *urdhva hastasana*; however, if the student places the hands 30 centimeters (twelve inches) or more from the wall and then uses the wall to hold the heels steady, then the body is necessarily in a banana shape: belly forward and lumbar spine collapsed. Because this posture has the heels too far overhead, encouraging compression in the lumbar spine, it is called overbalancing, whereas underbalancing refers to the heels being too far in front of the face, encouraging bending at the hips when inverted. As beginners become more accomplished in this *yogasana*, they should be encouraged to move the hands ever closer to the wall in order to bring the arms, spine, and ribs into *urdhva hastasana* vertical alignment (however, see below).

Once proper alignment and elongation are achieved at the wall, the student next should be encouraged to work away from the wall in order to develop independence. With this latter point in mind, set the balancing point on the floor at a distance from the wall equal to the heel-to-shin length of the legs. Kick up into the inverted position, bending both legs and bringing the toes to the wall, belt around elbows if necessary. Lift one leg to vertical, and then lean slightly into the room to drag the second foot slightly off the wall and straighten the second leg as well. If the student then overbalances from here, bending one leg will bring the toes to the wall without bending the rest of the body out of position [276]. Hand balancing also can be practiced by kicking up into the position with the hands placed far from the wall. If one leg is then brought forward while the other stays back, one then has a front-to-back balancing-pole advantage, and one can from that point gently lift the back leg off the wall by slightly tipping the pelvis in the appropriate direction and by working the fingertips against the floor. Balance is then achieved free of the wall but with the legs separated front to back.

With beginning students, inverted balancing postures should be performed either close to the wall, a shin's length removed from the wall, or very far from the wall. Do not let students practice the balance at a distance of, say, one meter (three feet) from the wall, for if they start to fall backward from there, the wall is too far away to support their balance, and they otherwise will fall heavily into the wall and possibly be injured.

Fear of falling backward is a strong emotion for students in inverted postures [765] and may lead to a permanent relationship with the wall. In order to overcome this, it is useful to eventually set students in the center of the room, away from the wall, and practice deliberately falling backward from inverted positions. Use helpers to lower the performing student's body onto the heels and back body as they slowly fall backward, with a helper's support, into the unknown. Once this fear of falling backward is conquered, then the student can practice the balance unassisted in the center of the room.

Assuming that the students are using the one-legged kick to come into *adho mukha vrksasana* in the middle of the room, it is wise to coach them into pulling the armpits forward as they go up (that is, in the direction appropriate to *adho mukha svanasana*), as the opposite action at the shoulders is apt to drop the student onto his head or back following the kick. There are many excellent articles describing why students should be doing *adho mukha vrksasana* and how to get into the inverted position [234, 388, 484, 766, 800], however, there is precious little on how to stay there without leaning against the wall. Similar expositions are readily available for wall-supported

sirsasana [388, 486, 800] and *pincha mayurasana* [388, 800]. At this point, we discuss how to stay up, once in these inverted postures.

To practice the balancing action of *adho mukha vrksasana,* begin at the wall, and, as discussed in the previous subsections:

1. Work with the hands at shoulder width and with palm and fingers spread to maximize the area of the base of the posture
2. Use nothing soft under the hands
3. With the eyes open, fix the gaze on a point on the floor just forward of the fingertips [234], tilting the head to lift the chin away from the sternum; gazing at a coin placed forward of the fingertips can be very stabilizing
4. Begin the *yogasana* in full *adho mukha svanasana* extension and alignment, step one of the feet halfway toward the hands, and then kick the body into the inverted position, retaining the hand and shoulder actions of *adho mukha svanasana*. In the transitional phase between *adho mukha svanasana* and *adho mukha vrksasana,* the pelvis should arrive at the wall before the shoulders or the back of the head.[13]

---

13   When learning to kick into *adho mukha vrksasana,* it is helpful to consider the line between the left and right shoulders as a horizontal axis around which the body must rotate in order to become inverted. If this axis is bent (as when the shoulders approach the ears), then the rotation will be difficult, but if the axis is straight (as when in *adho mukha svanasana*) then the rotation is smooth and effortless. Thus, to kick up into either *adho mukha vrksasana* or *pincha mayurasana,* start with the shoulders lifted away from the ears as for *adho mukha svanasana,* and keep them lifted as you come to verticality. As explained in figure 11.A-14, the resistance of the fingers on the floor will be strongest when the wrist is in the neutral position and weakest when the wrist is in extension. Consequently, the resistance of the fingers and metacarpal heads to falling backward will be stronger in *pincha mayurasana* than in *adho mukha vrksasana.*

In Box 11.A-5, page 424, a chain reaction of sorts is described, in which the specific action beginning at the bases of the thumbs and index fingers on

5. Kick gently and with deliberation into the final position, so that the momentum of the kick does not lead to excessive overbalance. A slow ascent also allows the vestibular-organ signals to change smoothly as you come into the inverted position. You will want to kick into a position of approximate balance and then use the feedforward reflex (Subsection V.F, page 917) to pull the body in a controlled way into the final position. If you do not learn how to kick into the inverted position without either overbalancing or underbalancing, you will never learn how to get into the posture in the middle of the room.

6. In the inverted posture, keep all of the secondary joints open and taut as you extend the body upward from above the wrists to the heels. In *vrksasana,* this is done by stretching the arms up and pulling the rib cage away from the pelvis. In *adho mukha vrksasana,* this is done by lifting the heels and the bases of the big toes toward the ceiling to pull the pelvis away from the rib cage. Give full attention to the actions of the hands and wrists on the floor. Balance is aided by keeping the lock of the shoulder blades onto the rib cage (Subsection V.F, page 919) that is so useful when balancing in *virabhadrasana III.*

7. Once in the position, do not move the head, as this will only create extraneous noise within the vestibular organs, which already have enough to do without this added burden. The outward look of full arm balance is very much like that of *urdhva hastasana,* except that in the former, the head is decidedly thrown back more than is proper for the latter [388]. This head-back position, in fact, is absolutely necessary for all hand-balancing *yogasanas* which in general are very difficult with the head turned down, chin to sternum. Note that this head position for inversions is opposite to that recommended for erect positions (Section V.D, page 907), even with the eyes open. Because the chin-to-chest flexional position encourages rolling backward more or less in a "front somersault" when inverted, it is best in inverted postures to keep the neck in extension, chin away from chest.

8. Slowly lift the buttocks off the wall, but keep the weight somewhat heavy on the fingertips. Just as the leg is stronger than the arm, so are the foot and ankle stronger than the hand and wrist. This means that one can afford to lean far forward in *vrksasana,* and the strength of the ankle can supply enough countertorque to keep the body from falling further, whereas the wrist and hand, being much weaker, will tolerate only a much smaller overbalance in full-arm balance before being overcome.

9. With the body off the wall but leaning slightly backward, heels lightly on the wall, press the fingers against the floor so that the body is torqued slightly in the falling-forward direction. This counterbalancing action of the fingers on the floor compensates for the overbalancing action of falling backward and keeps the posture stable mechanically. This torque is stronger yet if the fingers are bent so that only the tips and lowest knuckles of the fingers press the floor, in addition to the metacarpal heads, of course. On the other hand, if the falling torque is clockwise (underbalancing), as shown in figure V.F-2b, there is little or no countertorque that can be generated, because the bones of the wrist are at the very heel of the hand, and the balance is lost by rotating around the spot marked ✳. That is to say, if you want to stay balanced with the arms

---

the floor in *adho mukha svanasana* results in specific movements of the collar bones, rib cage, and shoulder blades. The action of the thumb and index finger in *adho mukha vrksasana* coincides with that of the same appendages in *adho mukha svanasana.* Progress from the one-legged kick to jumping up (or pressing up) with the legs together, big toes touching.

straight in this posture (and in *bakasana*), you must actually stay a little overbalanced, with the weight of the body always heavier on the fingers and base of the knuckles than on the heels of the hands. A similar statement holds for keeping the center of gravity of the posture somewhat away from the elbows when balancing in *pincha mayurasana*.

10. As a variation, start with the hands well away from the wall. When in the inverted position, extend one leg forward while the other is extended backward (as in beginning *parivrtta ikapada sirsasana*) to gain a balancing-pole advantage in the front-to-back direction. Once in this position, gently tip the back leg off the wall, but remain slightly overbalanced; do not swing the legs excessively, but work more from the wrists.

11. As a second variation, when in the fully extended position at the wall, try sliding the heels down the wall to come into the full arm balance but with the heels resting on the buttocks, knees toward the chest and buttocks still on the wall. This position significantly lowers the center of gravity and so makes balancing easier when the buttocks are gently lifted from the wall.

The yogic full arm balance, figure V.G-1a, is very different from that often seen in the circus. For circus performers, the principal concern is keeping balance rather than gaining yogic elongation. To that end, the circus full arm balance is often done with an extreme backbend in the lumbar region, with the abdomen and chest very forward of the arms and the heels far behind the head (figure V.G-1b). This posture works for them because the trunk of the body itself serves as a front-to-back balancing pole, rather like the situation with beginners in *trikonasana* (Section V.F, page 914), and the extreme spinal extension (backbending) lowers the center of gravity. When the equilibrist shifts to balance on one arm (figure V.G-1c), the legs are then separated left to right,

thus acting as an additional balancing pole for imbalance in that direction. Needless to say, the "banana" or "circus handstand" is a totally inappropriate posture for *yogasana* work for beginners or intermediate students, and any tendency in this direction is to be discouraged [234, 484]. In the same vein, compare the posture for *pincha mayurasana* done circus-style in figure 8.B-5c with the yogic posture depicted in Appendix I, page 823. On the other hand, one does see *yogasana* postures (performed by more advanced students) that closely resemble circus postures, as, for example in *vrschikasana II*, compared in figure V.G-1d (circus style) and in Appendix I, page 831 (with *yogasana* alignment).

Getting a Kick out of Inversions

One final point should be made with respect to the safety of the teacher when teaching inversions. The time will come when some of your students will have to be hoisted into the inverted positions because they do not kick hard enough to reach the wall on their own and/or need shoulder support from behind. In this situation, your face will be in the direct line of fire of their heels unless your students understand **when** they are to kick and you then turn your head away from the action at the appropriate moment. If you neglect to turn away, sooner or later you will get kicked in the face [484].

Sirsasanas I and II

Most interestingly, the very strong feedback that one gets from the eyes in the other inverted postures is not a factor at all in *sirsasana I*! Not only is *sirsasana I* stable with the eyes closed (try it), but it can be even more stable than *tadasana* with the eyes open if one monitors the degree of sway in each. Why is this so?

To answer this question, note first that *sirsasana I* can be more stable than *tadasana* both because the area of the base is larger and because the center of gravity of the body in *sirsasana I* is much more over the center of the base, whereas in *tadasana*, the center of gravity is more toward the heels and so is less tolerant of any backward motion. As for closing the eyes having no impact

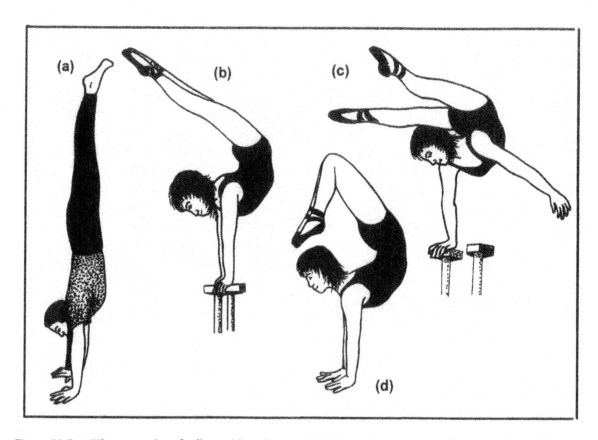

Figure V.G-1. The two styles of *adho mukha vrksasana*. (a) The yogic position, with maximal spinal lengthening and verticality (Theresa Rowland), and (b) the circus posture, with extreme spinal extension to gain the balancing-pole advantage in the front-to-back direction. (c) In the one-arm hand balance, circus style, the legs also separate left to right so that the performer now has both front-to-back and left-to-right balancing-pole advantages. Notice that the body is positioned so that the center of gravity is progressively lower on going from **a** to **b** to **c**, thereby increasing the stability of the posture. (d) The *yogasana* posture *vrschikasana II* does embody elements of the circus posture (**b**), with extreme curvature of the spine as well as the upper body and legs counterbalancing one another in the front-to-back direction.

on balancing in *sirsasana I*, this is at first quite a surprise, since it is very important in *vrksasana* and *adho mukha vrksasana*, for example. Notice, however, that the contribution of the eyes to balancing comes from their sense of the visual field shifting as the head moves. But in *sirsasana I*, the head is pinned to the floor, and because it does not move, neither the retinal streaming signal nor the vestibular system is of any value in determining the balancing response! Presumably, the situation would be different in *sirsasana I* if we had eyes or vestibular sensors on the ends of our toes. As regards the semicircular canals (see Section 18.B, page 698), they too are unresponsive in *sirsasana I*, since they only respond to accelerating rotations of the head. Similarly, the utricle and

saccule of the inner ear and the muscle spindles at the back of the neck (Section 18.B, page 696) could help balance the body if the head position reflected the body position, but with the head firmly on the floor, these sensors will give constant signals independent of the body position.[14] Hence, balancing in *sirsasana I* is largely a matter of proprioceptive sensing and adjustment, with significant input from the pressure sensors

---

14   Actually, the mat of sensor cells in the utricle lies in a horizontal plane with the gelatinous mass above it when standing upright. When inverted, it is possible that the gelatinous mass pulls away from the sensor hairs, and thus the hairs are not bent in response to an imbalance.

in the lower arms. As is the case with *sirsasana I* (Section V.E, page 913), working in *adho mukha vrksasana* with the legs folded into the chest lowers the center of gravity of the posture and so makes balancing easier.

The Balancing Point

The center of gravity of the head is at a point called the sella turcica (figure V.C-1), and as can be seen in the figure, this point (the seat of the pituitary gland) is anterior to the occipital condyles. Because the center of gravity of the head is forward of the occipital condyles, when standing erect but at rest, the head tips forward, chin on chest, so that the upright erect position of the head is maintained by a constant muscle tone at the back of the neck. The proprioceptive signals from such postural muscles and the joint receptors in the cervical vertebrae, working in the reflexive mode, help keep the head on an even keel when standing in *tadasana,* without any conscious action on our part. On the other hand, the sella turcica is just below the crown of the head when standing erect, suggesting that the crown of the head is an ideal spot on which to balance in *sirsasana* (as recommended by Iyengar [388] but not necessarily by Coulter [167]), provided the postural muscles at the back of the neck remain active and the cervical curve is normal (see Subsection 8.A, page 264, for a discussion of body weight versus risk to the neck in *sirsasana*). Assuming that when in a balanced position in *sirsasana I,* the crown of the head is just over the sella turcica, the situation in many beginners is to place the balancing point of the head closer to the hairline and then lean the body's weight more onto the elbows. This tendency toward strength and away from balance in *sirsasana I* will be even stronger in *sirsasana II.* See Subsection IV.D, page 862, for a discussion of the position of the center of gravity when switching between *sirsasana I* and *sirsasana II.*

Another function of the posterior neck-muscle spindles is as proprioceptive sensors, keeping the head erect except when asleep and therefore relaxed. These proprioceptors would not be very active in *sirsasana,* as the head and neck are largely immobile in this posture, with the fulcrum of the

broomstick action being at the shoulders, moving through the actions of the hands and elbows on the floor.

Yet another useful approach to balancing while inverted is to gradually alter the angle of inversion when this is possible. Thus, for example, starting in *adho mukha svanasana* with the hands on a chair seat, lift the left hand and the right leg, balancing on the right hand and the left leg in *dwianga adho mukha svanasana.* This will be relatively easy. From here, lower the right hand onto ever lower blocks until the right hand and the left foot are both at floor level. This is more difficult but is attainable if approached incrementally. At a higher level, start in *vrksasana* and then move the practice to *ardha uttanasana* while in *vrksasana.* Once balancing in this position is mastered, bend more deeply, finally to take full *urdhva prasarita eka padasana* once the sense of balance has been refined. In all of these inverted balances, the neck should be kept in extension and the eyes focused on the foot and ankle for the easiest balance.

Other Inversions

Much of what has been outlined above for balancing in *adho mukha vrksasana* can be carried over in toto for balancing in postures such as *bakasana* and *pincha mayurasana.* In these postures, lean to develop a slight overbalance torque, and then compensate this with a countertorque generated by pressing the fingers or parts of the forearms (Appendix V.B, page 879), against the floor appropriately. If, in any of these *yogasanas,* the posture becomes underbalanced, there is no way to regain balance (unless one can bend the arms), and one must start over, remembering to keep the weight somewhat heavy in the overbalanced direction. In all of these postures, coming down slowly with control will help build the shoulder, chest, and back strengths needed for performing the postures without the support of the wall.

In the context of what has been said above in regard to balancing in inversions, *sirsasana I* is especially interesting from several points of view. First, unlike *adho mukha vrksasana,* balancing in *sirsasana I* is much easier: its base area is larger, the center of gravity is lower, there are fewer joints above the floor that can go into motion, and the placement of the hands on the floor (figure V.D-3) allows both clockwise and counterclockwise compensating torques to be applied for balance. This last point does not apply to those variations of *sirsasana* in which both the hands and elbows are forward of the head (Appendix I, page 828). In these cases, one must stay slightly underbalanced in order to not overbalance and roll backward.

Blood Pressure in the Head

In preparation for going up in *sirsasana I*, take *adho mukha virasana,* with the weight of the head pressing the brow onto the floor for several minutes. Pressure at this point in the head promotes the ocular-vagal heart-slowing response (Subsection 14.D, page 579), and so lowers the blood pressure before inverting. This could be useful for all inversions where increased blood pressure upon inversion is a problem. See Subsection 8.A, page 265, for more information as to the loading on the cervical vertebrae while in *sirsasana I.*

Gender and Age

There is evidence [185] that at the time of menopause, women lose their muscle strength and their reflexes slow down, making them more prone to losses of balance and broken bones. Presumably, *yogasana* practice would be of preventative value here. Mortality among post-menopausal women who fall and break their hips is frighteningly high at 30 percent. Elderly students, especially women, are predisposed to dizziness as a consequence of the aging process, as aging implies a physiological decline in proprioceptive, visual, and vestibular reflexes, all of which serve normally to keep us in balance. The performance of older yoga students who have practiced *yogasanas* for a long time suggests that this decline in the balancing senses does not necessarily have to occur or can be slowed significantly by *yogasana* work. Balancing questions aside, one must use care and good judgment when bringing new students into the inverted positions, especially the elderly, as discussed in Appendix II, page 833.

Section V.H: General Points on Keeping Your Balance

Many of the specific points raised in the sections above can be generalized to apply to any and all balancing positions in yoga, whether upright or inverted, inclined or horizontal. These generalities regarding the balancing aspects of the *yogasanas* are gathered together in this place.

1. It is very difficult to balance on one or more appendages when said appendages are barely strong enough to support the posture. Any work that strengthens these appendages in general will consequently make the balancing easier.

2. Make the area of the base of the posture large, so that the line between the center of gravity of the student and the center of the Earth is well within the area of the base. This does not mean that practicing *adho mukha vrksasana* with the hands as far apart as possible will help the balancing, because the balancing problem in this *yogasana* is forward-backward, and separating the hands only would aid in the left-right direction. On the other hand, putting the hand on the floor in *ardha chandrasana* so that it is behind the standing foot rather than in line with it does aid the balance tremendously. Spread the hand so that the span of the knuckles is maximal; spread the foot so that the span of the base of the metatarsals is maximal.

3. Enlarge the area of the base to avoid wobble. Balance means not only not falling over, but a steadiness in the position that denotes complete neuromuscular control of the body.

4. The closer the student's center of gravity is to the floor, the easier the balance, in part because the time available for response is longer if the student starts to fall, and also

because the critical sway angle beyond which one falls is larger.

5. The surface supporting the posture must be solid and unyielding. Try balancing in *vrksasana* while standing on a soft foam block or on a multiply-folded sticky mat to see how important it is that the support be firm and resistive.

6. Keep all of the joints of the body (except the lowest) fully extended to avoid unnecessary wobble at these joints. Assuming that the balancing is being done on the floor, use the joints that rest on or close to the floor to do the balancing, keeping all others fully open but immobile. The big toe will be very important in standing postures, both for reasons of strength and balance. A similar statement applies to the thumb in many one-hand balancing postures.

7. When balancing on the hands (feet), let the weight of the body fall lightly on the fingers and metacarpal heads (toes and metatarsal heads), and with the body's secondary joints fully extended, work the floor with the fingers and metacarpals (toes and metatarsals) to generate compensating countertorques to the falling-body torques.

8. Appendages held out to the side or front to back will stabilize balance in the plane of the appendages. This is the balancing-pole effect often used in the circus and by small children walking on top of narrow walls with arms extended sideways.

9. Once in the posture, keep the head still. When the head moves, the motion sensors in the inner ear will activate reflex arcs that may conflict with the balancing efforts of the joints on the floor.

10. When balancing on the feet with eyes open, keep the head in the neutral position so that the cervical vertebrae are in alignment with the remainder of the spine, if possible. If not, it will be easiest then to balance when the neck is flexed into the *jalandhara bandha* position and

most difficult when the neck is in extension. This will not be true when in the inverted *yogasanas* where the head-up, neck-in-extension position is more appropriate.

11. Keep the eyes open when balancing; fix the gaze on an immobile object in the far visual field, and keep the object centered in the visual field. In those cases where balance is involved in moving into the *yogasana,* imagine a line painted on the floor; keeping the line centered in the visual field while moving is very stabilizing. Avoid trying to balance when the visual background is in motion, and avoid having to look at a blank wall having no distinguishable features (Subsection V.C, page 891). If the posture is an inverted one, keep the neck in extension and look at a small object placed between the hands. Balancing in the open with no walls for visual support can be an added burden [276]. Try wearing glasses in order to see if poor vision could be a factor in your balancing.

12. Balancing will be easier if the same background is present as when the *yogasana* was first learned. Face the same wall each time, so that the same visual anchors are present during the practice. Once these visual tricks are mastered, then work to disengage from the anchors, so that the posture can be done facing in any direction, in any room, or open space. At this point, the eyes can be kept with the gaze broad and defocused to relax the muscles of the eyes.

13. Move slowly and with awareness into the final position of balance, starting in a balanced position and adjusting the balance as you go, so that there is a minimum of readjusting to be done once in the posture. Moving slowly also promotes the mental steadiness that is required for physical steadiness. Your steadiness in a balance at a particular moment will reflect your emotional stability at that time; do not be

surprised if a balance that was easy on one day appears difficult on the next.

14. One comes most smoothly into the balanced position by leaning the posture first on a wall and then gently moving the weight off the wall to balance freely.

15. When kicking into an inverted position, do not try to kick into exact balance; instead, either over-kick or under-kick slightly, and using the feedforward reflex (Subsection V.B, page 884), capture control of the posture and then either push or pull it into position in a controlled way.

16. Practice; the balancing reflexes are refined by practice, practice, practice in a deliberate and conscious manner.

Conclusions

Balance and the Subconscious

Balancing is generally a subconscious action, but our goal in *yogasana* work is to make it maximally conscious, by deliberately making the body taut, and by focusing the consciousness on that part of the anatomy in contact with the floor.

How then does one maintain balance? One can look in vain in all of the books on *yogasana* and not find a word in answer to this question. It seems that one balances by not falling over! Actually, there is a certain amount of truth in this flip reply, for we seem to balance using a reflexive strategy, with all of the neural and muscular actions occurring largely in the subconscious, rather than in the conscious sphere. However, if the balancing act remains reflexive, there will be no improvement with practice; without deliberation in the act, there is no pivotal experience that seeds the brain as worth "learning" and which then is engraved on the brain as a resource for future attempts at balancing. More so than with other reflexive actions, the balancing system is adaptive, allowing one to balance in new situations, and most importantly, learning follows from repeated conscious attempts to balance (i.e., from *yogasana* practice) [782]. Once the balancing act becomes deliberate and effective, its further practice makes

the proper actions again somewhat reflexive in the more advanced student.

As our nervous system matures, we are able to bring the subconscious to the surface (figure 1.B-1), where we can act consciously to adjust the actions to suit our needs, just as we learn how to consciously manipulate subconscious actions such as the breath, the heart rate, and the finger temperature through *yogasana* practice. It is the goal of this discussion to stress how to make aspects of the balancing act more conscious and less reflexive.

Balance Requires Mental Concentration

The balancing *yogasanas* set themselves apart from the others in the *yogasana* lexicon by the degree of concentration one must exert in order to do them even modestly well. Though it may not be apparent to others that while you are in *adho mukha svanasana*, you are thinking about what you had for breakfast that morning, the same train of thought while in a balancing posture such as *dwianga adho mukha svanasana* will lead to an immediate fall to the floor! As balancing requires constant attention and a steady mind, external sensory inputs and the variety of internal thoughts are reduced when concentrating on balancing (see Subsections 1.A, page 12, and 4.C, page 78). The intense look of concentration on the face of the balancing student is most evident in the eyes and testifies to the degree of inward attention to the body that the beginner exerts in the balancing postures (see also the footnote on page 81 quoting William James). Indeed, Austin [30] says clearly that the state of inward attention is a mental state in which all eye movements stop. Such high levels of inner concentration place the balancing postures closer to the higher meditative levels of *Ashtanga* yoga, such as *pratyahara*.

From the neuroscientific point of view, there is a brain-wave state that is characteristic of intense concentration and inward awareness: the gamma-wave state. Found in the EEGs of meditating adepts in the 40–90 hertz range with almost global synchronization (Subsection 4.H, page 149), one expects that these gamma waves will be most prominent in the EEGs of *yogasana* practitioners when in the balancing postures.

Balance and the Emotions

We must distinguish between two aspects of lack of balance. In the context of *yogasana* practice, we might run up against beginners who are not able to balance because the postures are new and they have not had sufficient practice in their performance; the solution to their balance problem is obvious. We may also find students whose balancing problems have real organic roots, such as blindness, Meniere's disease of the vestibular organs, cardiovascular or neurological problems, hormonal fluctuations (as with low thyroid function), hypertension, hypotension, etc. In these cases, the lack of balance may be commingled with fears of falling, various phobias (claustrophobia, for example), depression and anxiety, frustration, and high stress levels. Difficulty in balancing may raise stress and consequently lead to high blood pressure; it also may lead to a less active life, fear of leaving the house, feelings of missing out on life, and frustration that no one seems able to help. Such balancing problems associated with conditions such as these are hard to describe, hard to diagnose, and hard to treat, even for professionals, and they are best left to professionals for treatment.

The Neural Connection

All sensory inputs involving movement, touch, and body awareness are effective in stimulating the parietal cortex (Subsection 4.C, page 92), and one might reasonably expect that neural processing in this area is a significant element in the balancing act. Consider, then, that experiments on the interpretation of a visual scene (the differences between two faces, for example), when challenged by extraneous input such as a flickering light or counting mentally, show that the interference leads to the loss of the sense of difference between the two scenes; in the visual sphere this is called change blindness [46]. Transcranial magnetic stimulation (Subsection 4.D, page 105) when aimed at the right parietal lobe to disable it clearly demonstrates that this region is intimately

involved in the change blindness phenomenon, whereas the left parietal lobe is not so involved. Note that proprioceptive signals are integrated into a whole in the right hemisphere (Subsection 11.C, page 441). It appears that inattention, as when lacking in a strong focus on a task, leads to confusion in the right parietal lobe, which lessens its ability to discriminate in regard to differing sensory signals. This may be the neurological connection to the observed necessity of being totally focused on the balancing signals when trying to balance in the *yogasanas*. It is my hypothesis that this focused concentration is intimately involved with the firing of a specific subset of place cells in the hippocampus, and with the possible discontinuities of such firing patterns when in strange environments or in environments without any distinctive markings (Subsection 4.G, page 140).[15]

Bringing conscious awareness to a balancing-joint action seems to focus the fast subconscious actions on this joint as well, to the advantage of more sensitive balancing. In contrast, while in *vrksasana,* try counting backward from 679 by increments of 17 in order to see the impact of mental actions that disturb the mind's focus on the balancing process.

At first thought, the two facts of balancing appear contradictory, with the speed of action and reaction being available only to subconscious reflexes, whereas at the same time, balance requires a conscious focus on the balancing act. This seeming contradiction may be resolved by the conscious focus on balancing being the motivator or catalyst for the subconscious balancing function to operate. Or, perhaps more likely, the balancing act is subconscious because reflexive responses are

---

15   The method of forming a spatial map in the hippocampus is known to be gender specific [427a], for women form the map by focusing on landmark features and use the right parietal and right prefrontal cortices to form the map, whereas men form an internalized geometric map using the left hippocampus. If such spatial maps are relevant to the use of the eyes when balancing in the *yogasanas,* as I suspect, then men and women may be balancing in the *yogasanas* by two different mechanisms!

so fast, and the role of conscious action is to keep the neural channels clear of extraneous neural traffic, which it does by concentrating the mind on the balancing action. Returning to the suggestion of Section 1.B, page 9, that subconscious and conscious sensations differ only in the magnitude of their neural currents, the raising of the subtle balancing sensation into the conscious sphere can become a reality if all competing strong signals from other sources are minimized. That is to say, if one is very quiet mentally and devotes full attention to the signals from the balancing sensors, they will be sensed in the conscious realm and so can be controlled consciously to maintain balance. Once the concentration on balancing is broken by extraneous thoughts, the door is open to falling.

This concentration required for balance is maintained by restricting the afferent and efferent balancing signals to only the primary joint in the balance, by placing the mind's attention solely in the primary joint, and by then working consciously to reduce the sway angle θ at the primary joint to as small a value as possible.

It is interesting that Iyengar differentiates between concentration and meditation [391]. When one is in a state of concentration, one is inwardly focused on a single aspect of the body (remaining balanced, for example); whereas when meditating, the focus is on everything simultaneously. From this point of view, *yogasana* balancing for beginners is strictly a matter of mental concentration, as with *pratyahara* or *dharana,* but not one of meditation. Being in either a state of *pratyahara* or *dharana,* balancing in the *yogasanas* is nonetheless strongly concerned with stilling the fluctuations of the mind.

In synopsis, one can imagine the following scenario for balancing. When we assume the broomstick position for balancing, we flood the brain with proprioceptive signals from all of the muscles, joints, pressure sensors, and joint capsules in the body. Amongst the flood of signals is that of the primary balancing joint, with its information in regard to falling/not falling. Just as when the body is in pain, the stimulation of surrounding sensors can drown out the primary sensation of pain, so too is the proprioceptive balancing signal blunted by the plethora of irrelevant stretching and bending signals being sent upward to the brain. However, through the conscious effort to focus on the primary balancing signal and to sense it free of extraneous interference, one comes to balance subconsciously while consciously focused on the one signal that must be sensed in order to maintain balance. It is the focus on the proprioceptive signals coming from just one joint of the body, while holding the other proprioceptive signals at second attention and blocking those random thoughts that can appear in a mind that wanders, that differentiates the balancing *yogasanas* from the others.

Hemispheric Interference

See for yourself the consequences of conflicts that arise within and between your cerebral hemispheres when trying to balance. First, engage the left hemisphere by counting backward from 1,043 by increments of seventeen, and time the length of time you can balance (a) while standing on the left foot and balancing a broomstick on the left index finger, (b) while standing on the right foot and balancing the broomstick on the right index finger, (c) while standing on the left foot but balancing the broomstick on the right index finger, and (d) while standing on the right foot but balancing the broomstick on the left index finger. Compare these values with those when the mind is not engaged in mental arithmetic [337].

Appendix VI

Iyengar Yoga and Western Medicine

It is interesting to compare the aphorisms of B. K. S. Iyengar with the medical understanding of the body as currently put forth by the Western medical establishment; as shown below, there is an overall broad agreement that is very satisfying. That is to say, there is no apparent disagreement in the comparison that would lead one to think that one side or the other is in error, Additionally, because many of the aphorisms of Iyengar extend far beyond the body and into more ethical and philosophical realms, there is no comparison to be made with Western medical ideas in such cases. Most of the aphorisms used here are taken from the book *Iyengar: His life and Work,* [390] and from references [391, 394, 851].[1]

It goes without saying to readers of this handbook that the Iyengar family has developed an approach to yoga that is totally unique and almost completely independent of Western ideas of the body and mind. This approach is largely subjective and personal, based upon a penetrating awareness of the feelings within and sensitivity to the outward effects of various postures. As Iyengar yoga is a self-contained science that clearly stands on its own, it is not in need of any support from Western ideas. In fact, much of what the Iyengars say is, at present, beyond what Western science can comment on, for the Western approach to the body and mind is largely objective and imperson-

al, based on experiments, instrumental readings, and theoretical analysis.

The two approaches, Western and Eastern, are largely independent in their developments but not unrelated; it is of interest, especially to us Westerners, to compare several concepts expressed by the Iyengar family over the past fifty years with modern concepts taken from Western science and medicine. In assembling this comparison, I have relied on the many written works and spoken words of this family and on my own study of the connection between *yogasana* practice and Western medicine. That we should attempt to reconcile Western medicine with Iyengar yoga rather than with other yoga programs is most reasonable in view of the many statements from the Iyengar family regarding their support of the scientific approach to *yogasana* practice.

Of course, because very little Western medical research is directed at studying the neuroscience, physiology, or anatomy of *yogasana* practice, we must allow some latitude in applying medical principles to *yogasana*. What follows below is the best that I can do in this regard. Listed below are my personal interpretations of the connections between certain aspects of Iyengar *yogasana* practice and the relevant Western medical ideas. In this, the Iyengar ideas have been synopsized and presented in italics, with the Western interpretation given immediately below each such concept. The Western descriptions purposely are kept brief, but references to more complete discussions in specific chapters are included for readers who wish to go somewhat deeper.

Like Patanjali's sutras, the aphorisms of the Iyengar family are brief and can be interpreted in

---

1   This appendix first appeared in an abbreviated form [711] as an article written in honor of Guruji in celebration of Guru Purnima, 2003. It is a pleasure to acknowledge the contributions of Carol Wipf to the expansion and the refinement of this material following the original publication.

different ways. The interpretation given here is that within the context of Western neuroscience, physiology, and anatomy, though other interpretations also are possible. In several cases, two or more closely related aphorisms have been combined into one.

This chapter is based totally on the assumption that I have correctly understood the meaning of Guruji's sayings. I must point out that if this is in error, then the explanations put forward to explain them in Western medical terms are meaningless.

Section VI.A: The Postures

There are two I's in us. One of the I's is intuitive and the other I is conscious. And the conscious I is the one that is the enemy, which puts up the screen for you not to see the hidden guru of that conscious I—the intuitive I. Now you're all doing the asana, *but you do not know if you are doing it with the conscious I or the intuitive I. You are all doing it with only the conscious I. But I do it with the intuitive I. For me, the conscious I is subordinate; for you, predominant.*

I would interpret this in terms of the conscious/subconscious mixing discussed in Subsection 1.B, page 12, where it is proposed that without *yogasana,* the conscious Self and the subconscious Self are sharply divided and unmixed, with the former being very evident and directing the actions of the posture, whereas the latter is hidden from view. However, with concentrated practice, the barrier between the conscious Self and the subconscious Self begins to melt away, so that more and more of the subconscious neural sensations achieve sufficient neural current to reach the thalamic or cortical regions and so become more or less evident to us. With extended practice and concentration, the sensations of the subconscious come to be more important to the practitioner than those of the conscious realm. However, it is the reverse, I feel, when in the balancing postures (Subsection V.H, page 929).

One must also mention the relevance of the autonomic nervous system to the performance of the *yogasanas* and the fact that this neural system is most active in the intuitive, subconscious realm but can be brought into the realm of conscious sensation through *yogasana* practice.

In trikonasana, *the brain of the pose is in the big toe and the thumb that is touching the ground.*

Differentially pressing the mound of the big toe (the head of the first metatarsal) on the floor in *trikonasana* brings the entire forward leg into a proper orientation and also offers the inward-turning resistance against which the upper portion of the forward leg rotates outward (Subsection 11.F, page 468). By pinning the leg to the floor via pressure on the big toe, outward rotation of the anterior thigh presses the groin of that leg forward, thereby opening the pelvis (Subsection 10.A, page 337). In a totally similar way, the pressure of the thumb on the floor (as in *adho mukha svanasana*) turns the lower arm inward and, working against this, the anterior upper arm rotates outward and so activates the shoulder blade on its side; as a consequence of this disrotatory action, the rib cage is lifted and pressed forward (Subsection 10.A, page 331).

It was the mention of the thumb action in *trikonasana* that appears in Telang's book [851] that encouraged me to think further about the role of the thumbs in *yogasana* practice (Subsection 10.A, page 331). Note also that the thumb and big toe have unusually high densities of pressure sensors (figure 13.B-2a), and so also are well suited for roles as balance sensors.

Precision in action comes when the challenge by one side of the body is met by an equal counter-challenge of the other. This ignites the light of knowledge.

This is a broader statement than that given above in regard to the opposable thumb, and it refers to the use of anchors (also called macroscopic resistance) in the *yogasanas* (Subsection 7.A, page

232). The point here is that in order to stretch a particular muscle, it is necessary to anchor one end so as to resist the pull of the other end. This macroscopic resistance of one muscle in support of the stretching of another is discussed specifically in Subsection 11.F, page 468, and otherwise throughout the text.

In sirsasana, *balance on the crown of the head.* Sirsasana *is done posteriorly;* sarvangasana *is done anteriorly.*

One is truly balanced on the head when the line between the point of contact of the scalp on the floor and the center of the Earth passes through the center of gravity of the head. This center of gravity in the human head, called the sella turcica, lies just below the hypothalamus (figure V.C-1), and placing the sella turcica in the *sirsasana* balancing position requires that the crown of the head be placed on the floor. This stands in contrast to the bregma positioning [167] of the head in *sirsasana*. *Sirsasana* is done with an accent on elongation of the back body, whereas in *sarvangasana*, the accent is on elongation of the front body.

Allow not only the body but the brain to relax in savasana. *If the mind is to be made still, the eyes must be still. The eyes control the brain. Tenseness of the eyes affects the brain. If the eyes are still, the brain is still.*

The brain operates on the basis of electrical voltages that drive electrical currents through electrical resistances. Vestiges of the low-voltage brain waves, of the order of microvolts, signaling brain activity can be sensed on the scalp, as when one records the electroencephalogram (EEG; see Section 4.H, page 149). Specific brain states are characterized by specific voltage patterns over time. When one is outwardly directed, fully conscious and alert to outside events, then the EEG pattern consists of electrical waves rising and falling in time, with wave peaks separated by one-thirtieth of a second; i.e., oscillating at a frequency of 30 hertz. This frequency character-

izes the beta-wave mental state, as when one is working intensely under the teacher's guidance to stretch the body in *parsvakonasana,* for example. As the beginner goes from the fully alert, outwardly engaged beta state of *parsvakonasana* to the inward mental exploration of the body as occurs when one relaxes the body in *savasana,* the EEG frequency drops from 30 hertz to 7–8 hertz. This lower-frequency mental state is called the alpha state, characteristic of mental and physical relaxation and inward turning. Thus, the body and brain have distinct states corresponding to being either energized or relaxed. For the beginner in *parsvakonasana,* the body is dominated by the sympathetic nervous system (Subsection 5.C, page 170), and the brain is in the beta-wave state; whereas in *savasana,* the body is dominated by the parasympathetic nervous system (Subsection 5.D, page 178), and the brain is in the alpha-wave state.

The eye is a strongly innervated structure, much like the brain. In fact, many of its most important parts are constructed largely of brain tissue, unlike any other sensor in the body. Thus, it is no surprise that motion of the eyes and stimulation of the brain are concurrent (see Subsection 23.D, page 794). If the eye motions are depressed, as with an eye bag in *savasana,* then the corresponding brain activity also is depressed.

Jalandhara bandha *acts to keep the pressure from rising in the head.*

The vascular system, consisting of arteries and veins, contains sensors (called baroreceptors) at specific sites, the purpose of which is to monitor the blood pressure at each of the sites. If the blood pressure moves outside of a specific range (called homeostasis), afferent signals are sent from the baroreceptors to the brainstem, and via efferent signals sent along the appropriate branch of the autonomic nervous system, the characteristics of the heart action are modified so as to return the blood pressure to a state of homeostasis (Section 14.E, page 581). If the baroreceptor records too low a blood pressure, the heart action will accelerate and intensify, whereas if the pressure is sensed by the baroreceptors as being too high, the heart action will slow and decrease in intensity. Baroreceptors acting in this way are found in the internal carotid arteries in the neck, which otherwise carry blood from the heart to the brain.

When the head is held in the *jalandhara bandha* position (figure 11.D-2), as when in either sitting *pranayama* or in *sarvangasana, halasana,* or *savasana,* the carotid arteries are compressed, resulting in a **local** excess pressurization of the carotid baroreceptors. If the baroreceptors have been well exercised, the out-of-range baroreceptor signals immediately impact on the medulla oblongata in the brainstem, which then uses the vagus nerve (cranial nerve X) to signal the heart to reduce both the heart rate and the force of the cardiac contraction. Working in this way, the blood pressure is kept within an acceptably low range when the head is held in a *jalandhara-bandha* position, even when the body may be inverted. Due to the general heart-slowing action of *jalandhara bandha,* this head position is relaxing in all postures in which it is prescribed.

To bring the whole body into correct alignment, you have to work each and every part of the body. When performing asanas, *no part of the body should be kept idle.*

The muscular anatomy of the body is arranged in linear arrays of closely linked individual muscles. Each array is known as an "anatomy train" [603]. Through the activation of an anatomy train, the actions of the fingers in *adho mukha svanasana,* for example, can direct the actions of a particular chain of muscles up the full length of the arm, through the shoulder, and down the back so as to impress the scapulae on the rib cage (Subsection 11.A, pages 423, and 424), pressing it forward and up! Activation of anatomy trains helps to involve the maximum number of parts of the body in the performance of any one *yogasana* and also allows an apparent action at a distance, with the action at the thumbs dictating the movement of the scapulae, for example,

or the action of the big toes instigating movements in the pelvis and hip joints. In addition to the anatomy trains, there also are the agonist/antagonist muscle pairs and muscle synergists to be activated, in relative proportions as suits the particular posture.

The effect of appropriate yogasana *practice on depressed students can be healing. If you open the armpits, the brain becomes light. You cannot brood or become depressed. If the lungs collapse, the brain becomes dull and morose.*

Because *yogasana* practice reveals how the body, the mind and the emotions are bound to one another, it is no surprise to *yogasana* students that negative feelings of depression, guilt, sorrow, apathy, fear, etc. correlate with a spinal posture that is strongly flexional (collapsed forward), whereas the spinal posture appropriate to positive feelings is strongly extensional (backward bending); see Subsection 22.A, page 756. This latter posture emphasizes lifting the rib cage upward and forward and is an ever-present component of Iyengar *yogasana* practice. The use of the arms and scapulae to open both the armpits and the rib cage in order to elevate both the mood and the chest is discussed in Subsection 10.A, page 328.

In addition to our central nervous system, we have the autonomic nervous system, consisting of the sympathetic and parasympathetic branches (Subsection 5.A, page 157). When first put forward, this system was termed "autonomic," because it was believed at the time that all homeostatic actions of this system were automatic and that they could not be activated or deactivated by direct will of the subject. It is now known that energizing the sympathetic branch by external means leads to a mental and physical state of atypically high energy, alertness, positive feelings, etc., whereas the function of the parasympathetic branch is to calm the body, returning the system to its baseline resting state. It would appear that in the depressed, there often is too strong a parasympathetic action in the frontal lobes of the left cerebral hemisphere, and that this can be relieved by lifting the EEG into the beta level; i.e., by performing energizing, uplifting *asanas* such as *urdhva dhanurasana* and *sirsasana*. When in these postures, the adrenal glands are stimulated to raise the levels of epinephrine and norepinephrine in the blood, and these hormones then activate the sympathetic branch of the autonomic nervous system (table 5.C-1). Thus, we see that depression is countered by the physiological effects of opening and lifting the chest and by the effects this opening has on the activation of the sympathetic nervous system. A key factor in this hormonal and anatomic action is the lateral rotation of the upper arm, which presses the upper, inner armpit forward.

The intellectual person thinks that he is only in his head and nowhere else: his intelligence cannot spread beyond the brain to inhabit the rest of the body. But the yogi says, "Diffuse that energy from the brain to the other parts of the body, so that the body and the brain work in concord and the energy be evenly balanced between the two." Extend the intelligence from the head to the extremities; as we move away from the brain, our control of muscles and sensitivity of sensations decrease.

During the first year after birth, physical development of the infant is cranial to caudal (head toward foot), from proximal to distal (near toward far) in the limbs, and motor control is refined from coarse to fine in the proximal to distal direction (Subsection 3.A, page 33).

Our nervous system undergoes strong modifications as we mature, casting away neurons that are not used, and developing nerves that are fully covered with a fatty substance called myelin by the time of sexual maturity. Neural conduction is about 100 times more rapid in such myelinated nerves than in those that are not so covered. At birth, there is little or no myelination of the nervous system, but with time, the myelination proceeds from the central body to the appendages. As a consequence of this, a baby first learns how to wave his arms, then later learns how to bend the arms at the elbows, and finally how to perform delicate tasks with the hand and fingers. At the same time, the infant first is able only to wave its legs from the hips, followed by using the legs for locomotion (as when crawling), and finally develops the use of the more distal parts of the legs, as when walking. In this way, our neural dexterity is seen to move from the central axis to the extremities; to the extent that we are less than fully developed neurologically as adults, we will need to be reminded by our *yogasana* teachers that we must continue to extend our intelligence and awareness from the head to the extremities.

As discussed in Box 8.A-1, page 270, as we go from fetus to an adult, the body goes through a series of changes that mirror the evolutionary changes we have gone through as a species. In this, we again progress from a wiggly fish to an upright, bipedal human.

There is a second neurological aspect to be considered in regard to extending the intelligence throughout the body and mind. For many years, it was known that certain brain processes involved specific neuropeptides functioning as neurotransmitters. What is so surprising and so unavoidably clear is that these same neuropeptides found originally in the brain are actually active with respect to receptors found throughout the body [654]! From the neurological point of view, it is now clear that the neurotransmitters that are so active in the intelligence of the brain in fact extend their activities throughout the body; i.e., our intelligence can be body-wide when fully developed. Moreover, this communication is reciprocal, for it is now known, for example, that the hormone grehlin which triggers signals of hunger in the gut has a large number of receptor sites in and on the hypothalamus just above the brainstem (figure 4.B-1). The global nature of the body's intelligence is further demonstrated by the strong interactions between the neural, immune, and endocrine systems.

Finally, the proprioceptive map of body limb orientation and velocity of movement generated proprioceptively in the subconscious is of great value to us if we can use the body's global intelligence to bring our yogic intentions into congruence with the body's actions.

Section VI.B: Sensations

Opening the eyes wide releases pain and stops dullness of the brain.

There are two aspects of the eyes that lead to a stimulation of the sympathetic branch of the autonomic nervous system; it is known that sympathetic excitation erases pain and stimulates mental alertness. First, when the eyes are closed, there is no light impinging upon the retina, and a restful state ensues. In contrast, when the eyes are opened wide, there is a strong retinal stimulation of the sympathetic nervous system. Moreover, if the eyelids are lifted subconsciously so high that the most or all of the sclera is visible, this too is a sign of strong sympathetic involvement. In addition to erasing pain, sympathetic excitation pulls the eyeballs forward, giving the impression that the eyes are bulging (Subsections 11.A, page 406, and 17.C, page 672).

In the yogasanas, *one must read the messages of the skin. Self-knowledge starts from the skin on the soles of the feet when standing. Because you cannot see the back, it is forgotten. The back must be activated in all the poses. Everything cannot be observed by our two eyes. Each pore of the skin should act like an eye. Your skin is a most sensitive guide. All knowledge comes only from the skin. The skin is the intellect—a sense organ; flesh is physical.*

The soles of the feet are studded with a high density of pressure sensors (Pacinian corpuscles, etc.; see Subsection 13.B, page 511), the signals of which can be used intelligently to discern the distribution of the weight on each foot. This is essential knowledge in regard to building a proper foundation for every standing posture. In contrast to the situation on the bottoms of the feet, the density of the pressure sensors is very low on the back body. Moreover, the muscles of the back are largely antigravity muscles and are in states of mild contraction for long periods of time while one is upright. As their contractions are largely reflexive and subconscious, it can be very difficult to establish conscious control of the muscles of the back.

Pressure receptors in the skin, such as the Pacinian corpuscles, also are activated by the pull of the underlying muscles and connective tissue on the overlying skin. Because the skin is tightly bonded to the muscles beneath it, the skin experiences the tensile stresses that are present in the underlying muscles. Interestingly, the skin also contains mechanoreceptors called the Ruffini corpuscles, which subconsciously report not only the tension in the skin due to the underlying muscle stretch but also the direction of the stretch! Apparently, with enough *yogasana* training, one can bring the Ruffini signals into the realm of consciousness, thereby making the Ruffini corpuscle information not only a part of the proprioceptive map, but also a part of our consciousness.

Another message borne by the skin depends upon its translucency, for one can assess the condition of the blood supply to the underlying muscle by the color and temperature of the skin above it. So, for example, if the muscle is taut and there is no blood in the muscle due to vascular constriction, then the color of the skin is ashen white; if the skin is cold with a sluggish flow of deoxygenated blood, then the skin has a bluish cast, whereas if the muscle is hot and flushed with blood, then the skin will appear red (Subsection 13.A, page 503).

The eyes are the windows of the soul; the ears are the windows of the mind. You see the external world with the eyes, the internal world with the ears. To understand the outer world, open your eyes. To understand your own inner world, close your eyes and open your ears. The ears control the mind.

This simple statement has intrigued and puzzled me for years, with the first part concerning the eyes being so obvious and the second part concerning the ears being so obscure. Perhaps it is relevant that all tactile sensory signals are processed in the temporal lobes (Subsection 4.C, page 93) of the cortex, in a small spot just behind each ear. Perhaps Iyengar once again has conscious access to the signals within the temporal lobes coming from the pressure on the skin and from the stretching of the skin by the underlying muscles, sensing signals that otherwise are subconscious in most of us. In reference [403a], he mentions the "vibrations" from the back body to be sensed "through the ears." These may well be proprioceptive, signaling the tensile stress in the skin over contracted muscles.

We must be constantly aware in the yogasanas *that we do not allow the poses to become routine, for we must always search for the new feeling, the new awareness.*

As we practice our *yogasanas,* neural patterns are first reinforced in the subconscious regions of the central nervous system. Starting in the subconscious, these patterns then move into the conscious realm. However, if practiced in this way without any shift of awareness, the neural pattern then relocates in the subconscious. Only if we can make the posture (or our awareness of it) novel in some way will it remain in the conscious realm (Subsection 4.B, page 77).

Section VI.C: Breathing

As leaves move in the wind, your mind moves with your breath.

An autonomic excitation of the sympathetic nervous system occurs with each inhalation we take, and a parasympathetic relaxation follows with each exhalation. As a consequence, the heart beats faster and with more force on the in-

halation and correspondingly slows and weakens with each exhalation. As is normal with sympathetic excitation, there is also a rise in blood pressure along with decreasing arterial diameters and increasing bronchial diameters and muscle tone. When exhaling, these autonomic changes are reversed. On the mental-psychological plane, the inhalation is arousing and energizing, and the exhalation is restful and relaxing. As we inhale and exhale during the breathing cycle, the body and mind cycle through alternating dominance of the sympathetic and parasympathetic nervous systems, each with its own unique somatic and psychological characteristics (Subsection 15.C, page 619).

During exhalation the intellectual center is completely purged—this is renunciation.

According to Iyengar [394], the intellectual center is served by the *vijnana nadi,* which carries *prana* to this center in the form of peripheral receptor signals. This center would appear to be the sensory cortex or a lower, subconscious center just below the cortex, such as the thalamus. In contrast, the *karma nadi* has two afferent branches from the intellectual center, the *ida* and the *pingala,* relating to breathing through the left and right nostrils respectively. From the physiological point of view, traffic through the *vijnana nadi* would involve sympathetic stimulation of the intellect (a left-hemisphere function; see table 4.D-1, page 99) when there is an inhalation, and it follows then that on an exhalation, stimulation of the intellect (a left-hemisphere function) is relaxed, i.e., purged.

Going beyond pranayama *and to* pratyahara, *let go of the external senses and go within.*

Subconscious signals from the external body (muscles, joints, skin, etc.) are sensed by the proprioceptive system, whereas one subconsciously senses signals from the internal, more visceral organs of the body using the interoceptive system (Subsection 11.C, page 444). In order to "let go of the external senses and go within," one must switch from proprioceptive (external) to interoceptive (internal) sensing.

Section VI.D: Physiology

Make intelligent contact with each cell of the body, sensing the tension in each cell.

We are familiar with the afferent nervous system that carries sensations such as vision, hearing, touch, stretch, and taste to the brain, and of the efferent nervous system that carries instructions from the brain and spinal cord to the muscles, glands, and visceral organs of the body. What is new and interesting in medical experimentation today is the study of yet another nervous system within the body, the "perineural nervous system" (Section 2.C, page 26, and Subsection 12.B, page 492).

Each muscle fiber of the body is surrounded by a layer of connective tissue, and this connective tissue in turn is connected to that of adjacent cells, forming a macroscopic web that runs through the body from head to toe. Though it has long been thought that a cell in the body structurally was little more than a bag of fluid, modern work with the electron microscope reveals that each cell has an internal structure called the cytoskeleton. The cytoskeleton is itself very highly structured; it tends to fill the cell volume and is rather rigid mechanically. In fact, the connective tissues surrounding all cells penetrate the cell walls and then form structures within each cell that mechanically link the various cell components, such as the cytoskeleton, the nucleus, and the mitochondria, to one another. The body-wide system of connective tissue connecting the largest tissues surrounding muscles to the submicroscopic cytoskeletons within each cell in the body is called the perineural nervous system. It is becoming clear to researchers that there is a direct, unavoidable connection between the stretching of connective tissue as in *yogasana* practice and stretching forces that are readily transmitted from the muscles and

bones to the most elemental components of each of the cells in the body.

How then are the electrical signals developed and read in the perineural system? Virtually all of the connective tissues in the body, at all levels of magnification, possess the property of piezoelectricity; i.e., they develop electric charges on their surfaces in proportion to how large the mechanical stress is at each of those points. Whenever we stretch a muscle, all of the elements of the relevant connective-tissue perineural system, from the tendons and myofascial sheaths down to the membrane surrounding the nuclei within every cell, will become more or less charged electrically due to the stresses felt there; these charged areas can then stimulate chemical reactions of the most profound kind. For example, when the nuclei of the muscle cells are electrically charged in this way by stretching, the genetic machinery of the nuclei is set in motion and generates proteins relevant to muscle growth and remodeling of the connective tissue!

Within the context of the perineural model, the sensation one experiences as a "blockage of the flow of energy" while stretching relates to snags in the connective tissue that do not allow the tensile stress to propagate unimpeded throughout the perineural system. When Guruji encourages us to extend the energy of the body beyond the points of blockage, he is asking us to extend our sensations of the tensile stress within the perineural nervous system to the furthest reaches of the body. It is the genius of our Guruji that such subtle but well-founded signals at the subcellular levels have been revealed to him at the conscious, cortical level.

When stretching, the muscles and tendons should be wet and juicy.

The Iyengar family often mentions that in order to stretch fully, the muscles and joints of the body must feel "wet and juicy." Technically, this may be interpreted as meaning that the muscles must be well hydrated with water, and this can be understood in the following way.

Many of the body's elements have a semirigid

structure but float in a more fluid soup called the ground substance (Subsection 12.A, page 485). The ground substance is an integral part of the connective-tissue system, functioning as a lubricant (among other things) whenever one body part moves against another. If the ground substance is dehydrated and therefore viscous, then movement is impeded, whereas if the ground substance is kept well hydrated, the muscles and joints will be wet and juicy and will move with the least resistance. Guruji reports that as we age, the sternocostal joints of the rib cage are the first to become dry and inflexible.

Water enters the question of stretching in a second way: a significant fraction of the resistance to muscle stretching involves, in part, the lengthening of the collagenous connective tissue of the tendons, which is interwoven with the contractive parts of the muscle. That stretching is aided by the presence of water in the connective tissues [143] implies that the hydration of the collagen helices in the connective tissue reduces the hydrogen bonding between the helices while increasing it between each collagen strand and water, and so allows stretching to occur with less effort.

In the postures, squeeze the muscles so as to drive the blood out, and then relax and let fresh blood flow into the muscle.

During contraction of a muscle, an internal pressure is developed, which acts to collapse the venous system and so stymies the flow of blood. This then results in the accumulation of vasodilators and metabolic products such as lactic acid within the contracted muscle. Once the contraction is relaxed, the metabolic products in the muscle then speed the flow of blood through the muscle. The net result of this relaxation is a rapid flushing of stagnant blood from the muscle and its replacement with fresh blood. In turn, this increased circulation can lead to the formation of new capillaries in the affected muscle, especially in the young. This process of accelerated blood flow following a period of blockage of the flow, called reactive hyperemia, will require a

time period approximately as long as that given to the blockage; i.e., if the blockage was for thirty minutes, then the reactive hyperemia will last for about thirty minutes (Subsection 14.C, page 561).

One easily sees the effects of stagnant metabolites on blood flow when coming out of a long session in *sirsasana*. In this posture, the blood supply to the feet is sparse due to the effect of gravitational pull, and the color of the feet is ashen as metabolites accumulate. However, on standing up from there, the metabolites encourage the feet to be engorged with fresh blood and assume a deep red color.

Precision in action comes when the challenge by one side of the body is met by an equal counter-challenge of the other.

The muscles of the body are paired together as agonist and antagonist, so that any action of agonist contraction is undone by the contraction of its antagonist. For example, the biceps and triceps of the upper arm form such an agonist/antagonist pair; contraction of the biceps flexes the elbow, whereas contraction of the triceps puts the arm in extension. Precise control of the angle at the elbow is attained by a proper balance of the simultaneous contractive strengths of the biceps and triceps muscles.

Iyengar's statement can be viewed from a second perspective. In stretching some body part in the +x direction, the maximum stretch is obtained if some other body part or parts resist by moving in the -x direction (Subsection 11.F, page 468). By challenging the movement in one part of the body by moving another part in opposition, one generates the maximum stretching of any tissue positioned between the two body parts moving in opposition. Extensive examples of the efficacy of macroscopic resistance in *yogasana* practice are given in Section 11.F, page 468.

Each of the postures described in Light on Yoga *is to be held for at least thirty seconds or longer.*

The first step in stretching a muscle is to overcome the natural contraction of the muscle in its resting state. The resting-state muscle tone (Subsection 11.B, page 436) is due to a certain nonzero contraction of the muscle driven by the corresponding γ-motor neuron. However, in an effect known as autogenic inhibition (Subsection 11.B, page 439), if the muscle is gently stretched for twenty to thirty seconds, the Golgi tendon organ associated with the muscle in question sends a signal to the spinal cord, which leads to the inhibition of the γ-motor neuron and so releases any resting-state contraction of the muscle. By maintaining the stretching beyond thirty seconds, the resting muscle tone is released by the autogenic inhibition, and further stretching is then possible with lower resistance.

Section VI.E: Neurology

As there is space between thoughts, there is a space between action and thought.

In one of the classic experiments of neuroscience, Lisbet [516a] found that when we consciously decide to contract a muscle, there is an activation of the muscle-contracting neurons that occurs about 300 milliseconds **before** the conscious awareness of the decision to contract! This 300-millisecond space between action and thought is interpreted as allowing other inhibiting neural centers in the brain to come to the fore and either inhibit the proposed action or allow it (Subsection 4.C, page 94).

Perfect understanding between the nerves of action and the nerves of knowledge working together in concord is yoga. Thus, analysis in action is required in yoga. Fusion of the energies in the ida *and* pingala *nadis makes energy available throughout the body through the* sushumna nadi.

The "nerves of action," the *karma nadi,* correspond anatomically to the efferent nerves that connect the central nervous system (brain and spinal cord) to the muscles, organs, and glands, whereas the "nerves of knowledge/analysis," the *jnana nadi,* correspond anatomically to the afferent nerves that connect the sense organs to the central nervous system. If the two nervous systems work together in concord during *yogasana* practice, then the muscular actions of the body are integrated with the sensations and knowledge of the body; i.e., our yogic actions are integrated with our yogic intentions (Subsection 5.G, page 201).

Furthermore, the *karma nadi* can be dissected into those nerves that energize the body and those that relax the body. Iyengar identifies these two subsystems as the *ida* and *pingala nadis,* intertwined around the *sushumna nadi* of the spine. Correspondingly, the *pingala* and *ida nadis* can be interpreted as the sympathetic and parasympathetic nervous systems, which are known to have their neurological plexuses aligned within or alongside the spine. The first of these *karma nadis* is activated automatically when we are in a fight or flight situation and the second when we are in a rest and digest situation. On the other hand, the *sushumna nadi* corresponds to the central nervous system. When the sympathetic and parasympathetic nervous systems are in balance with respect to one another, then *kundalini* energy rises, and we are healthy, neither too tense nor too relaxed.

Section VI.F: The Brain

Self-correction comes with perception.

One of the functions of the cerebellum is to perceive the body's position in space and to then compare it with our intention for the body. If the perceived performance does not match the intention, then the cerebellum introduces small adjustments so as to bring action and intention into concordance. Through this specific action of the cerebellum, "self-correction comes with perception."

When in a yogasana, *recycle the awareness continuously so that all parts of the body are kept alert and involved, but all the while keep the body relaxed; i.e., pose and repose. In each posture, there should be repose.*

The muscles and joints of the body are home to many types of mechanoreceptors, the purposes of which are to report to the brainstem the extent of the tensile stress in all of the muscle fibers and their tendons and the angles at all of the joints (Subsection 11.B, page 428). From this type of information, the brain synthesizes an instantaneous picture of the body geometry. This ability to sense the body's posture is called the proprioceptive sense and is what we as children first used to guide the spoon into our mouths without looking and then to stop its travel before it pokes the back of our throats. As yoga students, thanks to the operation of our proprioceptive senses, we lift the legs and arms to exactly 45° in *uttana padasana,* even though we cannot see either the arms or the legs in this posture.

Within the brainstem, an area called the reticular formation stands guard over the pathway to the conscious brain, and it is wired so as to allow into the conscious sphere only signals that are changing rapidly in time; were it otherwise, the system would be swamped with huge amounts of irrelevant, static information. It also happens that any such proprioceptive signal of the body map fades rapidly with time, even if the pressure stimulating the signal remains constant. This effect of the fading of a sensory signal with time is called receptor adaptation (Subsection 13.B, page 506).

Were we to be truly static in a *yogasana,* the proprioceptive picture would quickly fade from our consciousness, because there is no change in the proprioceptive signals, and because the signals otherwise adapt rapidly to zero response. For example, notice how aware one is of the pressure of the floor on first lying down in *savasana,* but after a few minutes, there is no longer any sense of the back body pressing the floor. This fading of the sense of pressure on the back body is due to both the unmoving nature of the body posi-

tion and the adaptation of the pressure sensors on the back body. However, in a *yogasana* other than *savasana,* one can update and refresh the proprioceptive picture by continuously making small adjustments to the posture by contracting and relaxing various muscles; i.e., to pose and repose. It would appear that these adjustments not only make the posture dynamic in time, but are necessary if one is to maintain that proprioceptive connection between the brain and the body that constantly refreshes the picture of the posture in one's mind! Because the pose-and-repose mechanism also repeatedly activates and deactivates the muscles, it also encourages venous blood and lymph flow back to the heart (Subsection 14.C, page 569).

A play on words is also contained within this aphorism, for "repose" in this context means not only to reposition the parts of the body, but also to attain a state of relaxed mental serenity in the posture, as per Yoga Sutra II.46 of Patanjali (*sthira sukham asanam*) [401].

The visual signals from the eyes bifurcate so that copies go both to the conscious (cortical) brain and to subconscious (subcortical) brain centers. At the same time, the eyes perform a rapid jitter motion (at about 70 hertz) called saccadic motion, which in effect sweeps the visual image repeatedly over the fovea, the point of highest visual acuity on the retina. As this saccadic action is "visual pose-and-repose" in a sense, it may serve to continuously refresh both the visual pigments and the subconscious visual field. This visual but subconscious afferent signal could be a significant factor in balancing, where the eyes are very important sensors (Subsection V.C, page 888).

In the beginning, the brain moves faster than the body; later, the body moves faster than the brain. The movement of the body and the intelligence of the brain should synchronize and keep pace with each other.

It is known that there are two major paths for muscle action: the reflexive path, which is subconscious (subcortical/spinal) and operates very rapidly (tens of milliseconds); and the voluntary, deliberate path (cortical/supraspinal), which is conscious and operates much more slowly (hundreds of milliseconds). In the beginning, these two paths are separate and noninteracting, but with *yogasana* practice, their unique characters become mixed and synchronized (Subsection 1.B, page 12). This dual-path structure of response is found not only in the muscles, but also in the visual and auditory systems and in the emotional and decision-making systems within the central nervous system.

Bring the unknown into the sphere of the known. Go to the unknown more and more.

In our bodies, the highest brain functions involve conscious thinking within the brain's cortical area, and beginning there, the conscious activation of skeletal muscles through the action of the central nervous system. For example, the deliberate response to specific instructions of Iyengar yoga such as "keep the quadriceps toned in order to keep the leg straight" is an action that the thinking brain initiates and so takes place in the conscious sphere (Subsection 1.B, pages 12 and 15). In contrast, many of the body's housekeeping functions, such as regulation of the breath, regulation of the blood pressure, regulation of the acidity of certain body fluids, and the temperature of fingertips, are handled by lower brain centers that operate subconsciously, at levels below our awareness. These latter functions are handled by the autonomic nervous system (Chapter 6, page 207). In the normal person, there is a sharp demarcation between the conscious and subconscious spheres of influence.

With diligent *yogasana* practice, the conscious sphere can become more aware of what lies in the subconscious; as a result, formally subconscious functions (say, the breath and the blood pressure) can then be controlled by willpower and conscious action. Conversely, certain actions that can be activated only by deliberate thought (say, the toning of the quadriceps), now become, through *yogasana* practice, more automatic and intuitive; i.e.,

subconscious. This mixing of the subconscious (unknown) events with the conscious (known) events through yoga practice truly "brings the unknown into the sphere of the known" and at the same time, brings the conscious, deliberate acts of the "known" more into the realm of the intuitive, subconscious "unknown." Through extensive practice, we come to a place where we intuitively keep the quadriceps toned and at the same time, use our intellect in a deliberate way to regulate the breath and the blood pressure. In essence, *yogasana* practice has made the barrier between the known and the unknown, between the conscious and the subconscious, between the physical and the mental, more easily traversed from either direction (figures 1.B-1 and 1.B-2).

Section VI.G: Teaching and Learning

Memory is necessary to see whether we are regressing or progressing. Memory is a friend when used for progress.

Guruji emphasizes the importance of capturing the student's total attention, for without this, there is often no comprehension of the instructions. In order to learn something, we must store it in long-term memory and be able to access it when called upon to do so (Section 4.F, page 127). Information from our sensory organs first goes into immediate memory, and after a few seconds, is either transferred to short-term memory or is forgotten. If embedded in short-term memory, information can remain there for a matter of tens of hours before it is either forgotten or transferred to long-term memory. Retention of memories in long-term storage has long been held to be permanent, on the scale of a lifetime; however, it is now known that when a long-term memory is recalled, it is then subject to editing, embellishment, etc., so that it can be brought into line with more recent learning experiences. This mechanism allows the possibility to unlearn certain postural behaviors and to replace them with more appropriate ones, given a good teacher.

It is generally held that only 1 percent of the information gathered by the senses actually makes it into the long-term memory bank. With odds one hundred to one against, one must speak forcefully and make the *yogasana* lesson indelible if it is to make it into the top 1 percent of long-term sensations to be remembered and learned by the student that day.

The important transfer of *yogasana* instruction from the momentary short-term memory into long-term memory is aided considerably by a period of rest following the lesson. Thus, *savasana* is an important part of the overall *yogasana* lesson, in that it aids considerably in the retention of the lesson for recall during later classes; i.e., the lesson has been learned (Section 4.G, page 135).

Give a hint, nothing happens. Give a hit and see what happens! To love is to be merciless. To make the pupil sattvic, *the teacher has to be* rajasic.

We are flooded constantly with external information, all of which competes for our attention and a permanent resting place in the brain. It is known that how well an external event is recorded in the brain (i.e., remembered) depends upon its novelty or the emotional content of the information. Should one receive a hit from the teacher because one refuses to learn the lesson, the shock of it is so strong that the lesson will never be forgotten from that time on. This approach has a name outside of *yogasana* practice; it is called "superlearning."

When teaching a new posture, have the students just watch as you silently demonstrate the pose. First observe, then use the intelligence.

When we decide to move the body, the neural impulses that will drive the muscles originate in the motor cortices of the cerebral hemispheres. However, just prior to the activation of the motor cortices, a "warm-up" of the neurons takes place in an area of the brain called the premotor cortex. This excitation of the premotor cortex is a necessary preamble to movement. Most interestingly, when students watch a movement being made, their premotor cortex is being activated in synchrony with the movement being observed. As a result, when they then perform the movement, they have, in essence, already learned through watching, thanks to the warm-up (and subconscious memory) of their premotor cortical neurons! The premotor neurons are called "mirror neurons," reflecting the mirror relationship of the premotor neuron patterns of the teacher and the students (Subsection 4.G, page 142). For students who are able to learn through the visual channel, the phenomenon of mirror neurons can be very helpful.

In yogasana practice, the first side teaches the second.

The two cerebral hemispheres of the brain appear superficially alike but in fact have very different functions and paths of action (Subsection 4.D, page 98). They are, however, connected by two cords of neural tissue, the corpus callosum and a smaller one, the anterior commissure, which shuttle neural information back and forth from one hemisphere to the other. This initial functional independence of the cerebral hemispheres was shown in medical surgeries in which the corpus callosum was severed; as a consequence, the patients behaved as if they had two distinctly independent brains! For example, if a picture of a ball is projected only to the left visual field of such a split-brain subject, the image of it appears in the right cerebral hemisphere due to the neural crossover that occurs in all of us. When asked to describe the shape of the object in the image, the subject is unable to respond, because the image is locked in the right hemisphere, whereas language ability operates in the left hemisphere, and the hemispheres are disconnected. Though the shape of the object cannot be described verbally, the subject can readily point to the correct shape, as shape recognition is a right-hemisphere function. If, instead, the image of the ball is presented to the right visual field of the subject, there is an immediate verbal response to the question as to the shape. The distinct functions of the two cerebral hemispheres are listed in table 4.D-1.

It is known also that the nerves that connect muscles on the left side of the body to the brain switch sides in the spine so as to be connected to the right hemisphere, and vice versa for the nerves serving the muscles on the right side (Section 4.A, page 69). This left-to-right neural crossing is called decussation. When one performs *ardha chandrasana* to the right, the muscular actions of the right leg originate in the left hemisphere, and those of the left arm originate in the right hemisphere. It is reasonable to assume that the same neuromuscular messages then go via the corpus callosum and/or the anterior commissure to the relevant opposite hemisphere when this posture is performed to the left side. Due to this ready transfer of information between the cerebral hemispheres through the corpus callosum and anterior commissure, it is understandable that one side of the body and its associated cerebral hemisphere can "teach" the other side of the body and its cerebral hemisphere, provided the interhemispheric nerve bundles are not severed or otherwise faulty. If, on the other hand, a *yogasana* student has a transmission problem between the cerebral hemispheres, then one side will not be able to teach the other.

Section VI.H: Balance

Balance is the state of the present—the here and now. If you balance in the present, you are living in eternity. Balance is a gift of the creator. The median line is god! As a goldsmith weighs gold, you have to adjust your body so that it is perfectly balanced in the median plane. Mind must remain in the same state of the present.

The median line in *tadasana* and in all other postures connects the center of the Earth with the center of gravity of the body (Subsection IV.B,

page 851, and Section V.B, page 874). As long as the median line falls within the base of the posture, the posture is stable and will not fall. However, once it goes outside the area of the base, the body, posture, and state of mind are upset as the posture falls to the side; i.e., there is a loss of physical, mental, and emotional equilibria once we lose control of the median line (Appendix V.A, page 866). The act of balancing demands high levels of mental concentration, as any wandering of the mind, either forward or backward in time, leads to a fall.

Beginners should never do the standing postures facing a nearby wall.

Whenever one is facing a wall that is too close, the eyes lose the sense of the true horizontal and vertical directions. In this case, one is essentially snow-blind, with all directions equally likely as "vertical," and as a result, one's sense of balance is strongly impaired. The lack of balance that follows from a lack of markers in the visual field is known in neuropsychology as the Ganzfeld effect (Subsection V.C, page 891).

An asana *performed with total awareness is as good as a mantra or as meditation. In meditation, the mind is still but razor-sharp, silent but vibrant with energy.*

When adepts meditate, their EEGs are dominated by gamma waves of very high frequency (40 hertz), high intensity, and global synchronization (Subsection 4.H, page 153). This unique EEG is held to be a physical manifestation of their deep awareness when in the meditative state. Presumably this is the well-documented mental state (as characterized by the global 40-hertz waves in the EEG) Iyengar refers to when he speaks of "an *asana* performed with total awareness."

Your whole being should be symmetrical. Yoga is symmetry. That is why yoga is a basic art. There should be no contortions in any asana.

This is a very intriguing comment, given the apparent conflict between it and the demonstrated physical, temporal, and functional left-right asymmetries of the two hemispheres of the brain; the asymmetry of the heart, lungs, and viscera in the thorax; the asymmetry of the normal breathing pattern; the asymmetry of the muscle strength of the limbs; etc. Given these unavoidable asymmetries of the human body, it is at first difficult to see how our whole being could be symmetrical. Iyengar's dictum here is that in spite of these inherent asymmetries, we must work the body so as to lessen the extent of the felt asymmetry [402] (Section III.B, page 845).

Of course, all of the above asymmetries may express themselves only in very sensitive individuals; however, one would think that in highly accomplished yoga practitioners, an asymmetric posture such as *trikonasana* would feel inherently different when done to the two sides, or when done at two different times of day, or when performed when different neural systems are ascendant, etc. The only thing I can find in the literature, Western or Eastern, is the fascinating article by Sandra Anderson [11] relating the standing postures done to the left and right and the nostril through which one is breathing at the time.

The alignments and actions in the various *asanas*, regardless of how asymmetrical they may appear, are oriented toward retaining as much of the alignment and actions that operate in the standard position of highest symmetry, *tadasana* (Subsection III.B, page 845). At the postural/geometric level, this is a key difference between yoga and contortionism.

Section VI.I: Metabolism

Depending upon what has been eaten, wait between one and four hours before attempting yogasana *practice.*

To digest food, the stomach requires huge amounts of oxygen, ATP, and glucose in order to generate sufficient acid in the stomach (Subsection 19.C, page 715). As this energy-intensive process of digestion competes with the energy-intensive processes that fuel the muscles needed for *yogasana* work, it is unwise to perform the *yogasanas* while the stomach is still in the process of generating acid for digestion. The time for digestion will depend upon what has been eaten, being four hours and beyond for a greasy meal having a large amount of meat, and as short as one hour for a light meal of vegetables.

Section VI.J: Aging

Aging lessens one's strength; however, by constant practice, one can continue to increase one's efficiency and so maintain one's performance.

The muscular strength of our body is dependent not only on the size of our muscles, but just as importantly on the efficiency of the nerves that activate these muscles. In fact, in athletic young students, the muscles hardly increase in size, while their apparent "strength" grows greatly with daily practice. This gain in apparent strength is due to a refining of the neural patterns driving the relevant muscles, encouraging the muscles to work more efficiently rather than to increase in size. A related phenomenon, referred to as "muscle memory," operates when we try for the first time in twenty-five years to ride a bicycle again and find that nothing has been lost (Subsection 4.G page 140).

The refinement of the neural patterns used in *yogasana* and their implantation in the memory can be achieved not only by physical practice but also by imagining or thinking deeply about the sequences of movements involved in the practice without doing them. Thus, it appears that one can increase shoulder strength by sitting and thinking of moving in and out of *chaturanga dandasana*, in effect mentally exercising the neural patterns

Table VI.K-1: Aphorisms of Albert Einstein

"The most beautiful thing we can experience is the mysterious.
It is the source of art and science."

"Imagination is more important than knowledge."

"God is subtle, but He is not malicious."

"We should take care not to make the intellect our God; it has, of course,
powerful muscles, but no personality."

"Everything should be made as simple as possible, but not simpler."

"Science without religion is lame, religion without science is blind."

"Whoever is careless with the truth in small matters cannot be trusted with important matters."

"Art is the expression of the profoundest thoughts in the simplest way."

needed for performing this action rather than exercising the muscles themselves. This shows in a most dramatic way the cooperative interaction between mind and body.

The above is but an abbreviated list demonstrating the high congruency between the Iyengar and Western approaches to the physiology of the body in the *yogasanas*. This close matching hopefully will prove to be an advantage to both. More interestingly, there are discrepancies as well, and so there is still work to be done and there are lessons to be learned in rationalizing these two approaches.

Section VI.K: Iyengar and Einstein

In preparing this appendix, I have been struck by how closely the public thoughts of that genius of Western thinking, Albert Einstein, often parallel those of the Iyengar family, the geniuses of Eastern thinking. I list above (table VI.K-1), without further comment, a few of the aphorisms of Einstein and leave it for the reader to place them in concordance with those of the Iyengars.

Glossary

Many but not all of the technical terms used in this handbook are adequately defined in the text and can be found using the index. However, this glossary also can be used for finding succinct definitions of many of the technical terms used in the text. The definitions given in the glossary are not the widest possible, but are suited to the level of technical discussion used in this handbook.

Å: See **angstrom**

abductors: Muscles that lift the limbs away from the center line of the body

accommodation: The change of the curvature of the lens in response to a change in the viewing distance

acetabulum: The socket of the hip's ball-and-socket joint within the pelvis

acetylcholine: One of several neurotransmitters released into the neuromuscular synaptic gap in the course of the neural activation of muscle, and between neurons as well

ACh: The neurotransmitter acetylcholine

ACTH: Adrenocorticotropic hormone

actin: The thinner of the two protein strands in skeletal muscle (the other is myosin) responsible for its contraction

action potential: The voltage that propels the neural signal down the axon and toward the waiting synapse. This voltage is generated by the selective motions of various ions through channels in the cell membrane

acute: A biological process that is brief and intense but not chronic

adaptation: The loss of a receptor's sensitivity over a period of time in spite of continuous stimulation

adductors: Muscles that pull the limbs toward the center line of the body

adenosine diphosphate (ADP): The chemical product formed from the energy-producing reaction of ATP with water

adenosine triphosphate (ATP): The key biological chemical used to produce energy in the body

ADH or antidiuretic hormone (vasopressin): A mineralocorticoid released by the adrenal cortex to inhibit urination

adhesion: Following an injury to tissue, the binding together of the injured tissue and the subsequent loss of its elasticity

adrenal gland: An endocrine gland resting on top of the kidney, composed of the cortex (secreting corticosteroids such as cortisol) and the medulla (secreting epinephrine and norepinephrine)

adrenergic: Said of synapses in the body, such as the postganglionic sympathetic fibers of the autonomic system, that involve norepinephrine as neurotransmitter

adrenocorticotrophic hormone (ACTH): A pituitary hormone that stimulates the adrenal cortex to release cortisol. Production of ACTH is initiated by hormonal release of corticotropin-releasing factor (CRF) from the hypothalamus

aerobic oxidation: Pertaining to oxidation processes within the body that require oxygen pulled from the air and dissolved in the blood

affective sense: Relating to an emotional feeling such as happy, depressed, or lightheaded

afferent fiber: A nerve fiber that conducts

impulses from a sensory receptor to the central nervous system or from lower to higher levels in the sensory projection systems within the central nervous system

agonist: One half of a pair of muscles, each of which moves a body part in a direction opposite to that moved by the other; see **antagonist**

AIDS: A viral infection leading to impairment of the T cells of the immune system

aldosterone: A hormone, released by the adrenal cortex, that promotes water retention

allergen: A substance that produces an allergic reaction; the response to an allergen is called an allergy

alpha brain waves: Electrical voltage waves sensed in the scalp at a rate of 8–13 hertz, indicating relaxed wakefulness, early stages of meditation, sleep, and receptivity to ESP; a creative state of mind

alpha-motor neuron: An efferent neuron originating in the ventral horn of the spinal cord and terminating on a muscle fiber, controlling the innervation and contraction of skeletal muscle

alpha receptors: Generally responsive to norepinephrine, causing a constriction of the smooth muscles in the organs of the gastrointestinal tract

alveoli: The smallest branches of the bronchial tree, being the sites at which gas exchange of oxygen and carbon dioxide between blood and breath take place

amenhorreic: Lacking in menstrual periods

amino acid: A molecule bearing both an amino group ($-NH_2$) and a carboxylic acid group ($-COOH$). Amino acids combine chemically to form proteins

amphetamines: Stimulants to the central nervous system, increasing blood pressure

amygdala: The region of the limbic brain dealing largely with emotions such as fear

amylase: An enzyme in saliva converting starch into maltose

anaerobic oxidation: Pertaining to oxidation processes within the body that obtain their oxygen from sources other than air

analgesia: The loss of sensitivity to pain without loss of consciousness or the other sensory qualities

analgesic: A drug that relieves pain

anatomic position: *Tadasana* with the forearms supinated

androgen: A male hormone responsible for the development of male characteristics

aneurysm: A swelling in the wall of a blood vessel

angiotensin II: A neuropeptide promoting the drinking of water

angstrom (Å): A unit of length measurement on the atomic scale, equal to one hundred millionth (10^{-8}) centimeter; the diameter of the hydrogen atom is 1.2 angstroms

anoxia: The condition in which tissue is deprived of oxygen

antagonist: A muscle that produces a result opposite to that produced by the contraction of its agonist muscle; if the biceps is considered to be the agonist, then its antagonist is the triceps

antecubital: The anterior elbow

anterior: The front part of the body

anterior hypothalamus: That forward part of the hypothalamus controlling the excitation of the parasympathetic nervous system

antibody: A protein, also called an immunoglobulin, that binds to the surface antigen of a particular infectious organism and either neutralizes, inhibits, or kills it

anticholinergic: A substance that blocks the action of the neurotransmitter acetylcholine

antidepressant: A drug or *yogasana* that is mood-elevating

antidiuretic hormone: See **ADH**

antigen: A foreign protein that triggers the formation of antibodies by the immune system

aorta: The large artery leaving the left ventricle of the heart and supplying oxygenated blood to the entire body

apocrine glands: Located mainly in the armpits and surrounding the genitals, they release a smelly fluid when the body is under emotional or physical stress

aponeurosis: A broad band of tendon, connecting bone to bone or muscle to muscle

apoptosis: Process by which cells kill themselves

aqueous humor: The fluid filling the space between the cornea and the lens of the eye

arterioles: Small arteries positioned between the larger arterial branches and the capillaries, controlling the rate of flow of blood from the heart and hence the blood pressure

articular cartilage: The smooth tissue covering the ends of bones within joints

articular processes: The small protruding wings on each side of the vertebral bodies, each of which is used in forming a vertebral facet joint in the spinal column

articulation: The formation of a joint by bringing two bones together

Ashtanga: The eight limbs of the yoga tree, the third and fourth limbs being *yogasana* and *pranayama*, respectively.

astrocyte: A type of neuroglia that forms sheaths around the capillaries in the brain

atherosclerosis: A plaque composed of fatty substances that can coat the inner walls of the large arteries in response to stress and thereby reduce blood flow

atlanto-occipital joint: The cervical joint between the atlas of the skull and C1 of the vertebral column

atlas: The first cervical vertebra

atmosphere (atm): atmospheric pressure; 1 atm = 14.7 pounds per square inch or 760 millimeters Hg

atrium/atria: The right and left upper chambers of the heart, which collect blood from the body (right atrium) and the lungs (left atrium) and then pump it to their respective ventricles

autoimmune: Pertaining to the attack of the body's immune system on one of its own cell types

autonomic ganglia: Nerve plexuses serving the autonomic nervous system

autonomic nervous system: Referring to that part of the nervous system that operates without conscious control, as with the nerves that innervate the internal organs, the smooth muscles, and the glands

autoregulating: Self-regulating (as for organs)

avascular: Tissue (such as cartilage) that lacks blood vessels

AV node: The point in the ventricles of the heart that triggers ventricular contraction

axial spinal appendages: The skull and pelvis

axon: The output part of a nerve cell that conducts the neural signal away from the cell body and forms a synapse to another cell, be it neuron, muscle fiber, or gland

axon hillock: The point on the cell body that is the origin for the axon and the point at which the many incident receptor potentials are summed

axon terminal: The distal tip of the axon, filled with neurotransmitter and forming a synapse with other nerve or muscle cells

ballistic stretching: A very rapid stretching, limited by the protective response of the muscle spindles that promote muscle contraction; the opposite of *yogasana* stretching

baroreceptor: A sensor within the body that is sensitive to pressure, transducing it into a neural signal

basal ganglia: Brain structures deep within the cerebral hemispheres controlling motor activity, learning and memory

basilar artery: An artery at the base of the brain, connecting the carotid and vertebral arteries

B cells: Lymphocytes that originate in the bone marrow and that produce antibodies; they are responsible for antibody memory

beta blocker: A medication that decreases the heart's activity and prevents blood vessels from dilating (among other effects) by binding to the beta receptors and preventing their stimulation by epinephrine and norepinephrine

beta brain waves: Asynchronous brain waves in the 13–30 hertz range, signaling a state of arousal and energy

beta receptors: Found in the heart and responding to epinephrine, the effect being to increase the heart rate and strength of contraction and to dilate the vascular system of the skeletal and cardiac muscles

bifurcating: The branching of a single vessel into two

bilateral: Having distinct left and right sides

bioelectrochemistry: Processes in the body simultaneously involving elements of biology, electricity, and chemistry; said of the process of neural conduction

biofeedback: A technique in which instruments detect the level of body function and display this to the conscious awareness of the subject, who then responds physiologically and mentally so as to change or maintain the level

biogenic amines: Organic compounds within the body bearing the amino group NH_2, as with the catecholamines

biorhythms: The regular variation in time of the body's basic functions, with repeat periods that stretch from seconds to years

bipolar disorder: A psychosis in which periods of depression alternate with periods of mania

blindsight: A reflexive visual system bypassing the visual cortex, often operating in people who are otherwise found to be "blind" due to defects in the more common visual-cortical pathway

blood-brain barrier: A membrane surrounding the brain that allows only small molecules (such as glucose) to pass from the blood into the brain

bolus: The wad of material formed in the mouth by chewing food wet with saliva, just prior to swallowing

bone marrow: Soft tissue filling the porous cavity of the bone shaft; may be red and produce red blood cells or yellow and fatty depending upon age

bone spurs: Sharp, bony projections that grow to eventually press painfully upon nerves

bow legs: Legs in which the knees fall outside of the straight lines between the hips and the ankle joints on the respective sides

brain: That part of the central nervous system above the spinal cord and within the cranium, controlling all mental functions and behavior

brainstem: That part of the brain between the cortex and the spinal cord, including the medulla oblongata, the pons, and the midbrain but excluding the cerebellum

brain waves: Electrical signals on the scalp detected with an electroencephalograph, indicating the state of cortical activity

breathing centers: Those neurological nuclei within the brainstem controlling the timing of inhalation and exhalation of the breath

Broca's area: A posterior part of the left frontal cortex involved with expression of language; see also **Wernicke's area**

bronchiole: A small airway in the respiratory system; a subdivision of the bronchial tree lying in size between the bronchi and the alveoli

bursa: A small, fluid-filled sac serving as lubrication or cushioning between bone and muscle or between muscle and tendon

bursitis: Painful inflammation and swelling of a bursa

C1, C2, etc.: The first, second, etc. cervical vertebrae

Ca^{2+}: The positively charged ion of the calcium atom; essential to the release of neurotransmitters in all neural processes and the formation of bone

cancellous bone: Porous bone of light weight but high strength; also called trabecular bone

capillary: A short blood vessel of very thin walls, standing between the arterial and venous systems, allowing the passage of nutrients and waste products between the fluids inside and outside the capillary wall

carbon dioxide (CO_2): A product of the reaction of sugar (fuel) and oxygen (oxidant), carried by the blood to the lungs and expelled on exhalation

cardiac muscle: The contractive muscle within the heart

cardiac output, $\dot{Q}$: The rate at which blood is pumped through the heart, milliliters per minute

cardiopulmonary system: Pertaining to the heart and lungs

cardiovascular system: Pertaining to the heart and associated arteries and veins

carotid arteries: Arteries within the neck that carry blood to the forward part of the skull and brain

carotid sinus: An expanded portion of the carotid artery containing the baroreceptor sensor, which measures the blood pressure at that point and then reports this to the central nervous system

cartilage: A form of collagenous tissue, avascular, dense and often weight-bearing, as found in the larynx, trachea, and nose, and within and surrounding joints

catecholamines: The neurotransmitters epinephrine, norepinephrine, and dopamine

caudal: Away from the head and toward the tail

celestial oscillators: The sun as it rises and falls daily; the moon as it waxes and wanes monthly

center of gravity: That point, inside or outside of the body, around which the body would not rotate were it supported at that point when in the gravitational field. In *tadasana,* the center of gravity is just below the navel and halfway back from the front body.

central nervous system (CNS): The brain and spinal cord lying within the skull and the spinal column, respectively

central-pattern generator: A neural plexus in the spine capable of driving a repeating muscular pattern (such as walking) when triggered by higher centers

cephalic: Toward the head

cerebellum: The coordination center within the brain for posture and equilibrium, situated above the pons and medulla and involved in both learning and performance

cerebral cortex: The convoluted outer layer of the gray matter covering the cerebral hemispheres, divided into frontal, parietal, temporal, and occipital lobes

cerebral hemispheres: The left and right halves of the brain, composed of the cortex and the deeper-lying limbic nuclei but lying above the thalamus

cerebrospinal fluid: A fluid resembling blood plasma in which the brain and spinal cord float

cervical: Pertaining to the neck; for example, the cervical vertebrae

CFF: Critical flicker frequency

chakras: The points along the center line of the body that are the common intersections of the *sushumna,* the *ida,* and the *pingala nadis;* several *chakras* correspond to nerve plexuses

CH_3COO^-: The negatively charged acetate molecular ion

chelation: The binding of metallic ions to organic molecules having a claw shape

chemical synapse: A synapse operating on the basis of a chemical release from one neuron and its reception by an adjacent neuron

cholinergic: Said of synapses in the body, such as those in the postganglionic parasympathetic system, that involve acetylcholine as the neurotransmitter

chronic: A biological process that has a long onset and is long-lasting; not acute

chronotherapy: A therapeutic program in which consideration is given to the time at which the therapy is applied in order to increase its effectiveness

chyme: The partially digested semisolid that passes from the stomach into the small intestine

ciliary muscles: Controlling muscles that alter the shape of the lens of the eye and so adjust its ability to focus

circadian marker: The point in time during the day when a particular biological process is either at a maximum or a minimum

circadian rhythm: A rhythmic process within the body that is maximal and minimal once per day, always at the same time each day; i.e., it has a twenty-four-hour period

circumduction: The path of circular motion of a limb or organ

Cl^-: The negatively charged ion of the chlorine atom

claudication: A cramping muscle pain, caused by an inadequate blood flow

centimeter: Approximately 0.4 inch

CO_2: Carbon dioxide

coccygeal: Pertaining to the four fused vertebrae at the base of the spine

cochlea: The spiral organ within the middle ear that transduces sound waves into auditory nerve signals

co-contraction: The simultaneous contraction of the two components of an agonist/antagonist muscle pair

collagen: A fibrous protein of which many body parts, from soft tissue to bones, are constructed; it is a principal component of connective tissue

color therapy: The exposure of the eyes to various colors as a therapeutic mode for non-visual problems

commissural fibers: Tracts of nerve fibers that connect opposite sides (left and right) of the brain or spinal cord

compliance: The ease of distortion of a substance by an external force

compressive stress: The mechanical stress imposed on an object when its ends are pressed toward one another

concave: Curved away from the viewer when viewed posteriorly, e.g., the cervical spinal section

concentric isotonic action: The contraction of a muscle as it works isotonically to move a load

conchae: Shell-shaped structures projecting from the lateral walls of the nasal cavities

condyle: The surface of the enlarged, rounded end of a bone, such as that at the lower end of the femur

cones: The light-sensitive elements in the retinas of the eyes, used for daylight vision, with sensitivity to red, green, and blue light

conrotatory: A spinal twist in which the rib cage and the pelvis rotate in the same sense; also applicable to the relative rotations of the opposite ends of arms and of legs

consolidation: The process whereby memories are moved from fleeting short-term memory to permanent long-term memory

contralateral: Said of two structures on the opposite sides of the body

convex: Curved toward the viewer when viewed posteriorly, e.g. the thoracic spinal section

core temperature: The temperature of the interior of the body, usually measured rectally

cornea: The transparent outer coating of the eye

corpus callosum: A thick bundle of nerve fibers connecting the left and right cerebral cortices of the brain

cortex: The outer covering of an organ, such as the cortex of the brain or the cortex of the adrenal glands. In the brain, the cortex is the site of consciousness and the initiator of deliberate action

cortical bone: The dense form of bone

cortisol: An adrenal hormone released when the body is under stress (as when the sympathetic nervous system is activated), in order to stabilize blood glucose levels

cranial nerves: A set of twelve nerves exiting the skull at the base of the brain, serving the region of the head and neck without passing through the spinal column

crepitation: Production of noise through movement of muscles or bones

CRF: Corticotropin releasing factor

cross bridge: The molecular fragment between the actin and myosin filaments of the muscle fiber that is responsible for their relative motion when the muscle contracts

cross-bridge heads: Molecular knobs at the ends of the cross bridges; responsible for the attachment and detachment of the myosin cross bridges to the actin chains within muscle

cross-link: A short molecular bridge joining two longer molecular polymer chains

CSF: Cerebrospinal fluid

cutaneous: Pertaining to the skin

cytokine: A molecule that is able to transfer information within the immune system, acting much like a neurotransmitter in the neural system

cytoplasm: The totality of the contents of a cell, except for the nucleus

cytoskeleton: The rigid inner elements of the cell that dictate its shape and resistance to changes of shape

d: The Earth's radius

declarative learning: The conscious acquisition of information about people, places, and things

declarative memory: The storage of information about people, places, and things, requiring conscious action for recall

decussation: A crossing of a neuron from one side of the body to the other

defibrillator: An electrical device used to shock the heart's four chambers into beating rhythmically at appropriate rates

° C: Temperature, degrees Centigrade

° F: Temperature, degrees Fahrenheit

delta brain waves: Synchronous electrical waves in the brain of very low frequency (1–4 hertz) appearing during sleep

demyelination: The stripping of the myelin sheath from around a myelinated nerve fiber, as occurs in multiple sclerosis

dendrite: An extension of the neural body that receives messages from other neurons via synapses and transmits them toward the neural-cell body

dephosphorylation: A chemical process in which a phosphate group (PO_4) is split from a larger molecule such as ATP

depolarized: The condition of a neuron that has received an electrical signal from a nearby neuron and, as a result, has a potential of -65 millivolts or less, as compared with -70 millivolts when in the resting state

dermatome: The area of skin innervated by a single sensory root of the spinal cord

detraining: To stop a physical-training program

diaphragm: A thin, domed muscle spanning the bottom of the rib cage, the contraction and relaxation of which helps fill and empty the lungs of air

diaphysis: The shaft of a long bone such as the femur, bounded on the ends by the epiphyses

diastole: The phase of the cardiac cycle during which the atria fill with blood while the ventricles rest

diencephalon: The middle brain, consisting of the thalamus and hypothalamus

diffusion: The tendency of molecules to move from a region of high concentration to one of low concentration

disc prolapse: See **herniation**

dislocation: The movement of a bone from its normal position in a joint

disrotatory: A twisting of the two ends of a long bone, a limb, or the spinal column in which the ends are rotated in opposite senses

dissociation: An abnormal mental state in which it is felt that one is leaving the body

distal: The furthest point on the arms or legs from the center of the body; the fingertips are the distal end of the arm

DNA: Desoxyribose nucleic acid

DOMS: Delayed onset of muscle soreness

dopamine: A neurotransmitter responsible for control of attention, voluntary movement, learning, pleasure, and reward

dorsal: Toward the back of the spine (posterior) in four-footed animals

dorsiflexion: The bending onto itself of the back body; for example, the bending backward of the head at the neck (also called extension) or pulling the toes toward the knees

dowager's hump: See **kyphosis**

eccentric isotonic action: The elongation of a muscle as it works isotonically to resist the movement of a load

eccrine/exocrine gland: A gland that releases its secretions into a duct; a sweat gland used for cooling the body

edema: A swelling of the body tissue with excess fluid

EEG: Electroencephalogram

effector organ: The target site for an efferent neuron

efferent fiber: Nerve fiber that carries impulses away from the central nervous system to muscles, viscera, or glands, or from higher to lower centers in the central nervous system

elastic: The mechanical behavior or property of a stressed material to return to its original dimensions when the stress is relieved

electrical synapse: See **gap junction**

electrocardiogram (ECG): A graph of the heart's

electrical activity in time

electroencephalogram (EEG): A recording of the electrical activity of the brain's cortex, usually through electrodes placed on the scalp

embolus: Matter, such as a blood clot (thrombus), that travels in the vascular system to eventually occlude (block) an artery; if within the brain, an embolus can cause a stroke

endocrine glands: Ductless organs that secrete hormones directly into the blood

endogenous: Originating or produced internally

endoneurium: The innermost layer of collagenous tissue surrounding an axon

endorphins: Natural, morphine-like substances produced in the body

endosteum: The inner lining of a hollow bone

endothelium: The cells forming the capillary wall, allowing the transfer of gases and nutrients across the wall; also the inner lining of vascular elements separating the collagen in the vessel walls from the blood within

end plate: The plate-like ending of an efferent axon, forming the neuromuscular synaptic junction to a muscle fiber

enteric nervous system: The totally independent nervous system within the gastrointestinal system

entrainment: Said of biorhythms that are synchronized with the twenty-four-hour period of the rising and setting sun

enzyme: A chemical that accelerates a chemical reaction without itself being consumed

epicondyle: The thick, rounded section of bone just adjacent to the condyle of a long bone

epidermis: The outer layer of the three layers of the skin, consisting largely of dead cells

epigenetic: A genetic trait that can be turned on or off by nongenetic factors such as lifestyle

epimysium: The connective tissue sheath binding a bundle of muscle fascicles

epineurium: The outermost collagenous sheath surrounding a nerve and bearing the vascular supply for the nerve

epiphyses: The knobs on the ends of the long bones, separated by the bone shaft

epithelium: The innermost lining of hollow tubes in the body such as blood vessels

erectile tissue: Tissue that becomes engorged with blood when stimulated to do so

erector spinae: Muscles paralleling the spine, used to keep the spine erect and in alignment

essential instability: The condition in which an object falls either because of internal collapse or because the line of centers between the object and the Earth falls outside the area of the object's base

estrogen: A family of sex hormones responsible for maturation and maintenance of the female genitalia

eversion: Shift of the weight on the ankle toward the big-toe (medial) side of the foot

excitotoxicity: The death of neurons by excessive excitation, usually involving the glutamate ion as neurotransmitter; a form of apoptosis

exocrine: A gland delivering its secretion to a surface through a duct, as with tears

exogenous: Originating or produced externally

explicit learning: See **declarative learning**

explicit memory: See **declarative memory**

extension: Movement of the bones tending to open the joints; to extend a part of the body; backbending is a front-body extension

extracellular fluid: Any fluid that is not contained within the cells but lies outside of them

extrafusal muscle fiber: Muscle fiber that is not part of the muscle spindle

F: The force and direction of gravitational attraction

facet: A solid plane or shallow depression

fascia: Fibrous connective tissue

facilitation: The strengthening of the synaptic connection between adjacent neurons

fasciculus: A bundle of muscle fibers, usually with a common function

fast-twitch muscle fibers: Muscle fibers that are able to contract rapidly and with great force, but only for a short time; also known as type 3 fibers

FC: The force of cardiac contraction, as measured in Newtons (N)

feedback: The return of sensory information to

its source, resulting in a change of activity of the source

fibrils: Small bundles of fibrous molecules

fibrocartilage: Dense connective tissue found between the vertebrae and in joint capsules and related ligaments

fight or flight syndrome: The active response of the sympathetic nervous system to a perceived threat

flexion: Movement of the bones tending to close the joints

flexor: A muscle that bends the body by closing one or more joint angles

fMRI: Functional magnetic resonance imaging of the changes of blood flow and oxygen consumption in the brain nuclei during various mental tasks and emotional episodes

foramen/foramina: An opening between two larger vessels in the body

foramen ovale: the opening in the interventricular septum of the heart at birth

forced unilateral breathing: Breathing through one nostril only due to the forceful closing of the other by mechanical means

fovea: The spot on the retina having the highest resolution and having only the color-sensitive cones as receptors

free nerve endings: Sensors found in the skin that are sensitive to tissue damage; they function as pain receptors when connected to nociceptive neurons

FRF: Follicle-stimulating hormone releasing factor

frontal lobe: The most forward lobe of each of the cerebral hemispheres

FSH: Follicle-stimulating hormone

G: The gravitational constant

GABA: Gamma-aminobutyric acid, the primary inhibiting neurotransmitter in brain function

gamma-motor neuron: A motor neuron with cell body in the ventral horn of the spine and terminating at the intrafusal fibers of the muscle spindle; intimately involved with the tension in and stretching of the skeletal muscles

ganglion: An aggregate of unipolar nerve-cell bodies, usually outside the central nervous system and traveling through the ganglion without synapsing

gap junction: A variety of fast-acting synapse, not using a neurotransmitter but transmitting ionic current directly across the synaptic junction, as in the heart

GAS: General adaptation syndrome

gastrointestinal tract: The digestive tract from the mouth to the anus

genu valgum: Knock-knees

genu varum: Bowed legs

GHRH: Growth-hormone releasing hormone

gland: An organ specialized for secretion, usually of a hormone or of body waste

glenohumeral joint: The shoulder joint

glenoid fossa: The socket of the shoulder joint, formed by the union of the scapula and the clavicle, into which the humerus fits so as to form the glenohumeral joint

glia: Cells within the nervous system that support the nerves mechanically and perform many housekeeping chores in the vicinity

glucagon: A liver enzyme that promotes the conversion of glycogen to glucose

glucose: A simple sugar used by the body as a source of fuel for oxidation by oxygen, etc.

glutamate: The major excitatory neurotransmitter within the brain

glycogen: A polysaccharide broken down by glucagon into glucose

Golgi tendon organ: A stretch-sensitive receptor in the muscle tendon

gray matter: Slowly conducting, unmyelinated nerves in the nervous system

gram: A unit of weight; a penny (US) weighs approximately 2.2 grams

GRH: Gonadotropin-releasing hormone

growth hormone: A stimulant for the growth of the body prior to sexual maturation

H+: The positively charged ion of the hydrogen atom

habituation: The process in which the response to an innocuous stimulus decreases the more it is experienced

hallux: Referring to the big toe

HCO$_3$-: The negatively charged bicarbonate

molecular ion

H_2CO_3: Carbonic acid

heat-loss centers: Nuclei in the anterior hypothalamus that promote cooling of the body

hematocrit: The percentage of red blood cells in whole blood

hemiretina: That half of the retina viewing either the nasal or the temporal halves of the visual field

hemorrhage: Heavy bleeding from a damaged blood vessel

herniation: A rupture of the annulus of an intervertebral disc, allowing the nucleus pulposus to leak out; also known as disc prolapse

hertz: A measure of frequency; the number of times an event occurs in a second. An EEG wave that rises and falls twenty-three times in a second has a frequency of 23 hertz; 1 hertz = 1 cycle per second

Hg: The element mercury, used in manometers to measure blood pressure

hillock: See **axon hillock**

hip joint: The ball-and-socket joint formed by the juncture of the head of the femur and the acetabulum of the pelvis

hippocampus: Repository for the storage of declarative memory deep within the temporal lobes

histamine: A chemical released when tissue is injured; responsible for the pain sensation when its presence is sensed by free nerve endings

HIV: Human immunodeficiency virus, responsible for AIDS

H_2O: Water

homeostasis: Refers to the many processes through which the body maintains a state of internal equilibrium, as reflected in (for instance) temperature, heart rate, blood pressure, and the chemistry of tissues and body fluids regardless of changes in external or internal environments

hormone: A chemical substance liberated by an endocrine gland into the bloodstream, which then circulates throughout the body,

activating other organs

HPA: The hypothalamus-pituitary-adrenal axis

HR: Heart rate; beats per minute

HRT: Hormone replacement therapy following menopause

hydrolysis: A chemical reaction involving the splitting of H_2O into H and OH radicals, and the reactions of these radicals with a second, different molecule

hydroxyapatite: The hard, mineral component of bone and teeth, containing a form of calcium phosphate

hyperemia: The accelerated blood flow following the release of a blockage to the flow

hyperflexibility: The ability to stretch easily into positions that are so far beyond proper alignment that they risk damage to the ligaments

hyperpolarization: The change of the transmembrane potential of a neuron wherein this potential becomes more negative and, as a consequence, the neuron is inhibited from propagating a neural current

hypertension: Persistently high blood pressure, systolic and diastolic, usually taken as a reading above 140/90 millimeters Hg

hypertrophy: Increasing in size, as of an exercised muscle

hyperventilation: Breathing at a rate of more than fourteen breaths per minute, with the exhalation shorter than the inhalation

hypotension: Persistently low blood pressure, usually taken as below 100/60 millimeters Hg, systolic/diastolic

hypothalamus: A part of the diencephalon, beneath the thalamus; an important brain center controlling the autonomic nervous system and endocrine and visceral functions

hypoxia: A state in which there is a deficiency of oxygen

iatrogenic: Pain or other medical problems arising as a result of medical treatment

ida: The *nadi* originating at the right side of the coccyx and terminating at the left nostril after crossing the *sushumna* several times

idiopathic: Of unknown cause, seemingly

appearing spontaneously, as with an illness

immune system: The system with which the body identifies foreign proteins and destroys them

immunoglobulin: The antibody synthesized by a lymphocyte in response to an antigen

immunotransmitter: A molecule allowing communication between different parts of the immune system; also called a cytokine

impingement: Encroachment

implicit learning: The subconscious learning of neuromuscular processes, as by habit; also called procedural learning

implicit memory: The subconscious recall of neuromuscular processes learned by habit

incus: One of three bones of the middle ear; also called the anvil

infarction: A portion of tissue that is occluded by an embolus and is dying from this cause

inferior vena cava: The major vein returning blood to the heart from the legs and trunk

inhibition: A neural blockage of the response to a stimulus

innervation: Nerves serving tissue or organs; not all tissues or organs are innervated

insertion: In an articular joint, the end of the muscle tendon attached to the bone that moves when the joint is opened or closed

insulin: An important pancreatic hormone that controls blood glucose levels by converting glucose into glycogen when glucose levels are too high and by facilitating the transfer of glucose through cell membranes

interneuron: A type of neuron that always acts to hyperpolarize its synaptic neighbor, thereby inhibiting neural conduction

interoceptive: Subconscious sense of the conditions within the visceral organs

interossei: Muscles joining two adjacent but parallel bones, as between the adjacent fingers of the hand or between the adjacent toes of the foot

interosseus tissue: Nonmuscular tissue binding together two parallel bones otherwise not forming a common joint

interstitial: Space between cells within a tissue

interventricular septum: Tissue separating the left and right ventricles of the heart

intervertebral discs: Soft pads of tissue separating neighboring vertebrae

intraocular: Within the eyeball

inversion: Shift of the weight on the ankle toward the little-toe (lateral) side of the foot; to turn the body upside down

ion: An electrically charged atom or molecule, called a "cation" if the charge is positive or an "anion" if the charge is negative

ion channel: A pore within a membrane that allows certain ions to pass through it

ipsilateral: Said of two structures on the same side of the body

iris: Muscles surrounding the pupil of the eye, controlling the pupillary size

ischemia: A condition in which an area of the body is momentarily or constantly underserved by the vascular system, as in muscles rarely used, flesh under external pressure, etc.

isokinetic: The action of a muscle against a resistive load, moving it at a constant velocity

isomerization: A change of molecular geometry while retaining the molecular constitution. Ethyl alcohol and dimethyl ether have the same chemical formula (C_2H_6O) but different spatial geometries and so are geometric isomers

isometric: A static muscle contraction in which tension is generated in the muscle but there is no change in muscle length

isotonic: The action of a muscle in moving a load offering a constant resistance

K^+: The positively charged ion of the potassium atom

keratin: A tough protein forming the outer layer of hair and nails

kilogram: One thousand grams, equal in weight to 2.2 pounds

kilometer: One thousand meters; one kilometer equals 0.6 miles

kinesthesia: The sense of the positions of the body's parts and their rates of movement, using muscle-tendon-joint sensors

knock knees: Legs in which the knees fall to the inside of the lines joining the hips to the ankles

kyphosis: A condition of the spine in which the thoracic vertebrae are excessively rounded convexly (bowed toward the observer) when viewed from the back

lacrymal: Referring to tears and the tear ducts

lactate ion/lactic acid: Chemicals produced by the muscles through their incomplete oxidation of glycogen

lateral: Outward; to the side; opposite of medial

lateral flexion: Bending to the side, as in *trikonasana*

left brain: The left cerebral hemisphere, responsible for excitation of the sympathetic nervous system

leukocyte: An important element of the immune system in fighting foreign cells within the body

LGN: Lateral geniculate nucleus within the brain

LH: Luteinizing hormone

ligament: Connective tissue that joins two bones within a joint

limbic system: A group of nuclei within the brain responsible for emotions, etc.

lipid bilayer: The outer cell membrane formed by a double layer of end-to-end phospholipid molecules

lipolysis: The reaction of fatty substances (such as lipids) with water, usually accomplished by the fat-splitting enzyme lipase

liter: Unit of volume, approximately equal to one quart

LN: Left nasal hemiretina

LT: Left temporal hemiretina

load/loading: The stress imposed on an object; for example, the weight of the body stressing the bones of the legs when standing

long-term memory: Memory that is stable for a very long time, formed by consolidation of events stored first in short-term memory

lordosis: A condition of the spine in which the lumbar vertebrae are excessively pressed forward (concavely) as viewed from the back

lower hinge: The hip joints, as opposed to the upper hinge formed by the sacroiliac joints and the intervertebral joints within the

lumbar spine

LRF: Luteinizing hormone-releasing factor

lumbago: Lower-back pain, often attributed to a herniated intervertebral disc in the lumbar region

lumbar: The part of the back body and sides between the lowest ribs and the top of the pelvis

lumen: The empty spaces within the organs of the digestive tract and other hollow organs

lymphocyte: A white blood cell of the immune system having only one nucleus and residing mostly in the lymph; lymphocytes produce antibodies, fight tumors, and respond to viral infections

lymphokine: An immunotransmitter in the immune system

m_1: The mass of one's body

m_2: The mass of the Earth

macrophage: A large cell residing in tissue; it attacks invading cells recognized as other than Self

malleus: The "hammer," one of the three bones of the middle ear

mania: Period of unusually elevated mood, interest, and engagement, in contrast to depression

masseters: The muscles connecting the lower jaw to the skull, used in mastication (chewing)

master gland: The pituitary gland

max: Maximum

Mayer waves: Physiological waves in the body having a frequency of approximately 0.15 hertz

mechanoreceptor: A sensor within or upon the body that is sensitive to mechanical pressure

medial: Referring to the inner aspect of the body, closer to the center line; the opposite of lateral

medulla: The central part of an organ, surrounded by the cortex

Meissner's corpuscle: An encapsulated organ of the skin, sensitive to touch

melatonin: A hormone produced by the pineal gland, involved with the light/dark and sleep cycles

membrane: A thin structure composed mainly of

lipid molecules surrounding each cell of the body

meninges: The three-layer covering of the brain and spinal cord

metabolism: The sum of all energy-changing chemical processes that take place in an organism

metalloprotein: A protein containing one or more metal atoms; hemoglobin, containing four iron atoms per molecule, is a metalloprotein

meter: A length equal to 30.5 inches, approximately one yard

microglia: One of the prevalent cell types in the brain, different from the neurons but used both for signaling and housekeeping

micron (μ): A metric unit of length equal to one millionth of a meter; 0.00004 inch or one-thousandth of a millimeter; a human hair has a diameter of 75 μ

microtubule: The system within a neuron connecting the cell body to the axonal tip and transporting materials between these points

microvilli: Microscopic fingers lining certain cell membranes, thereby increasing their area and absorptive powers

midbrain: The brainstem between the pons and the thalamus

middle ear: The chamber between the eardrum and the inner ear, containing the three bones (the malleus, the incus, and the stapes)

milligram: One-thousandth of a gram

milliliter: Approximately one-thousandth of a quart

millimeter: One-thousandth of a meter; one millimeter equals 0.04 inches

millimeters of mercury: Pressure expressed as the height of a mercury (Hg) column; 760 millimeters Hg equals 1 atmosphere (14.7 pounds per square inch)

millisecond: One-thousandth of a second

millivolt: One-thousandth of a volt

min: Minimum

mineralization: The process whereby soft organic tissue is reinforced by crystals of the mineral hydroxyapatite, turning the tissue to bone

mineralocorticoid: Corticosteroid hormone from the adrenal cortex (such as ADH) that maintains Na$^+$ and K$^+$ levels in body fluids

mirror neurons: Neurons in the premotor cortex that are activated when a physical action is viewed

mitochondrion: An organelle within cells responsible for the generation of ATP for the cell's energy needs

mitotic: Descriptive of a cell within the body that is capable of division

monocytes: Cells that clean up debris after neutrophils within the immune system kill invading bacteria

motivational system: A function within the limbic system that dictates the level of effort to be applied toward performing a certain task

motor cortex: That part of the cortex containing the neural machinery that stimulates the skeletal muscles using motor neurons

motor end plate: That part of an efferent neuron that synapses to a muscle fiber and energizes it

motor unit: A motor nerve, its branches, and the assembly of contractive muscle fibers connected to it

mucopolysaccharides: See **proteoglycans**

muscle memory: The subconscious memory of how to use the muscles to perform a learned task (for example, how to work the legs in *dandasana*); also called reflexive memory

muscle spindle: A receptor structure within a muscle giving feedback information for adjusting and controlling the extent and speed of muscle elongation

musculoskeletal: Pertaining to the muscles and the skeleton

mu waves: A variety of alpha wave in the EEG (9–11 hertz), closely related to the mirror-neuron phenomenon

myalgia: Pain in a muscle

myelin: The fatty material surrounding certain nerves, making them rapid conductors of nerve impulses; myelin consists of a wrapping of Schwann cells in the peripheral nervous system and of oligodendrocytes in the central nervous system

myofibril: A subunit of the muscle fiber running the length of the fiber

myoglobin: The oxygen-carrying metalloprotein serving slow-twitch muscle fibers

myofascia: The connective tissue surrounding muscles and binding the muscle fibers to one another

myosin: One of the two proteins within muscle fibers responsible for its contractile properties

myotatic stretch reflex: The reflexive recoil of the body from a situation in which certain muscles are being overstretched or are in pain

N: The Newton, a unit of force

Na+: The positively charged ion of the sodium atom

negative feedback: A biological process in which an effect is produced but which effect acts to retard further advance of the process

nerve: A bundle of afferent and/or efferent neural axons outside the central nervous system but connecting the central nervous system to peripheral body parts, including connective tissue, blood vessels, and even some white blood cells

neural: Relating to the nervous system

neural crossover: The neural shift from left to right that accompanies the physical shift that occurs when a part of the right side of the body is placed on the left, and vice versa

neuralgia: A sharp pain usually associated with a pathology within the nerve itself

neuroendocrine: The chemical-electrical interaction between elements of the neural and hormonal subsystems

neurogenesis: The formation and growth of nerves to replace those that have died

neuroglia: Cells within the central nervous system dedicated largely to housekeeping

neurohormone: A hormone released into the bloodstream to be bound by neural receptors, thereby initiating receptor potentials in far-distant places

neuromodulator: A molecule that works to increase the long-term strength of the neural

signal at a synapse; see **second messenger**

neuromuscular junction: The synapse between the axon of a stimulating efferent neuron and the receptor site on the muscle fiber to be energized

neuron: A nerve cell consisting of a bulbous cell body, trees of signal-detecting dendrites, and a long axon extending from the cell body and carrying neural signals to other cells; the basic unit of any nervous system

neuropathy: A malfunction or affliction of the nerve

neuropeptide: A short peptide capable of acting as a neurotransmitter

neurotransmitter: A molecule that carries neural information across the synaptic gap, from one neuron to the next

neutrophil: A white blood cell that forms the first line of defense against foreign substances, bacteria, etc.

NLP: Neurolinguistic programming

nanometer: Equal to 10^{-9} meter, used in reference to the wavelengths of visible light

nocebo: The placebo effect working toward a negative response, in contrast to the placebo itself, which elicits a positive response

nociceptor: A receptor especially sensitive to noxious stimuli (those capable of producing tissue damage); the afferent neurons that carry pain signals to the brain

noise: Random fluctuations of current or voltage within the neural circuitry, present even when there is no significant signal from the receptors

nonsteroidal anti-inflammatory drugs (NSAIDS): Aspirin-like agents (ibuprofen and indomethacin) that reduce swelling and reduce pain

noradrenaline: See **norepinephrine**

norepinephrine: A neurotransmitter hormone released by the adrenal medulla into the blood, activating the sympathetic nervous system and also neuroactive in the brain

nucleus: In neuroanatomical terms, a collection of a few hundred to a few million adjacent nerve-cell bodies, functioning together with a common purpose; also that component of all cells in which the genetic material is contained

nucleus pulposus: The soft central component of the intervertebral disc

O$_2$: The oxygen molecule

occipital: At the back of the head

occiput: The posterior base of the skull

occlusion: An embolus that is born in the bloodstream and becomes lodged in a too-small blood vessel; also a shrinking of the diameter of a vessel by outside pressure

ocular-vagal heart-slowing reflex: The reflexive slowing of the heart rate when the orbits of the eyes are pressed

ocular-vestibular reflex: When the head turns, this reflex rotates the eyes in the opposite direction at the same rate as the head turning, so that the field of view appears not to move, though the head is in motion

oligodendrocyte: One of the neuroglia within the brain, and the myelin-forming cell in the central nervous system

ontogeny: A history of the development of an individual

opsin: A transmembrane protein within the cell membrane of the retinal cone cells that binds to the photopigment retinal; the different color sensitivities of the cones are due to slightly different opsin configurations

optic chiasm: The point within the skull where the optic nerves from the inner (nasal) retinas cross left to right

optic disc: On the retina, the point of exit of the optic nerve, this being a blind spot with no visual receptors

organelles: The discrete organs within a cell, such as the mitochondria and the nucleus

origin: In an articular joint, the end of the muscle attached to the bone that does not move when the joint is activated

ossification: The transformation turning cartilage into bone, driven by the presence of a local vascular system

otolith: A small stone of calcium carbonate within the balance sensors of the inner ear

overbalance: To fall backward when in an inverted balance posture

overdrive: Hyper-excitation of a physiological process

oxidation: The chemical reaction of a fuel such as glucose with oxygen to yield the energy necessary to sustain biological processes

oxidative phosphorylation: The oxidation process whereby ADP is converted into ATP

oxytocin: A hormone released by the posterior pituitary that acts to contract smooth muscle, as in the uterus during childbirth; also responsible for the feelings of love in women

pain: A protective mechanism signaling the brain that there is something wrong in the body that requires attention

palmar conductance (or resistance): The electrical conductance or resistance of the skin of the palm due to stress-induced sweating

palpate: To touch from outside the body

palpitations: Usually of the heart; regular or irregular rapid beating of the heart

paracrine: Descriptive of cells that secrete hormones locally for use by adjacent cells only

parallel processing: The ability to perform different mental tasks simultaneously, as in the right cerebral hemisphere

parasagittal: A vertical plane not passing through the midline of the body

parasympathetic nervous system: A major branch of the autonomic nervous system, responsible for the relaxation response following the activation of the sympathetic nervous system; it stimulates vegetative functions using the cranial and sacral nerves

paravertebral: Along side the vertebral column

patency: The time between stimulus and response

pathogen: A virus, bacterium, or parasite that invades the body and produces disease

Pb^{2+}: The positively-charged ion of the lead atom

pennate: Type of muscle having fascicles arranged obliquely to a long central tendon, or about a common central point

perimysium: A connective-tissue sheath

surrounding a bundle of muscle fascicles

perineurium: The connective tissue surrounding a bundle of nerve fibers (neural fascicles)

periosteum: The outer covering of bone, interwoven with the attached tendons and ligaments

peripheral nervous system: Those bundles of nerve fibers that connect sensory or motor organs to the central nervous system; the cranial and spinal nerves and the peripheral ganglia lying outside the central nervous system

peristalsis: A progressive muscular movement down the gastrointestinal tract, designed to move its contents in the mouth-to-anus direction

permeability: The ability of a membrane to allow certain chemicals to pass through it

pH: An inverse logarithmic measure of acidity in aqueous solutions; high acidity is reflected by low pH, and vice versa

phasic reflex: An instantaneous and short-lived muscular response to a stimulus, as when stepping on a sharp object with a bare foot

phospholipid: A highly polar molecule based upon a glycerol backbone, fatty side chains, and a charged phosphate group; cell membranes are formed by a double layer of phospholipid molecules

phosphorylation: A chemical reaction in which a phosphate group (PO_4) is joined to another chemical group, often a protein

phylogeny: A history of the development of a species

physical crossover: To displace a body part from the right-hand side of the body to the left and vice versa, as in *parivrtta trikonasana,* for example

piezoelectric effect: Appears when certain materials are stressed and develop intense electric fields on their surfaces; bone and cartilage are piezoelectric materials

pilomotor response: The lifting of a hair by contraction of smooth muscles at its base

pingala: The *nadi* originating at the left side of the coccyx and terminating at the right nostril after crossing the *sushumna* several times

pituitary: The master gland, located just below the hypothalamus, that directs many other hormonal processes, the forward portion of which is itself under the neural control of the hypothalamus; also known as the hypophysis

place cells: A subset of hippocampal cells that are excited only when in a specific location within the environment, thereby forming a map of the environment as one moves from place to place

placebo: A Latin word meaning "I will please"; often an inert pill or solution of salt or sugar given in place of an analgesic agent

plantar flexion: Attitude of the foot having the heel pulled upward toward the back of the knee and the toes pointed away from the knee

plasma: The fluid portion of blood when freed of suspended cells

platelet: A disc-like cellular component of blood that is responsible for clot formation at the site of vascular damage

plexus: A local network of neurons, veins, or lymphatic vessels

PMS: Premenstrual syndrome

PNF: Proprioceptive neuromuscular facilitation, a non-yogic stretching procedure

$PO_4{}^{3-}$: The negatively charged phosphate ion

polymer: A very large organic molecule formed by the joining together of many smaller molecules, either all of the same kind or of related types. For example, collagen is a polymer of the amino acids glycine and proline, and cellulose is a polymer of glucose molecules

polymodal: Said of nerve endings that are sensitive to more than one type of stimulus (temperature, pressure, pain, etc.)

positive feedback: A biological process in which a compound is formed and its formation promotes its further production

posterior hypothalamus: The rear part of the hypothalamus, controlling the excitation of the sympathetic nervous system

postganglionic neuron: A part of the autonomic nervous system originating in an outlying ganglion and terminating at an effector organ

postural muscles: Those muscles having an ongoing muscle tone of a relatively low level but which hold the body in an upright posture for long periods of time when in the gravitational field

power stroke: That phase in the cardiac cycle where the left ventricle contracts in order to pump oxygenated blood through the aorta. Also used to describe the action of the cross bridge in the sliding filament theory of muscle action

Pranayama: The fourth level of the *Ashtanga* yoga system, focusing on the breath

prefrontal cortex: The most forward parts of the frontal lobes

prime mover: That single muscle most responsible for a particular muscle action, often assisted by adjacent muscle synergists

preganglionic neuron: A part of the autonomic nervous system originating in the central nervous system and terminating in an outlying ganglion

progesterone: A hormone produced by the ovaries and significant in both menstruation and pregnancy

prolapse: To fall out of place, as said of an organ

prophylaxis: Steps taken to prevent a disease or harmful condition

proprioception: A subconscious sense of where the various body parts are in space and in what direction and how fast they are moving; the sensors reside in the muscles, tendons, joints, and vestibular organs

prostaglandins: Cellular compounds that are released when cells are injured, causing swelling and inflammation

proteasome: An organelle within a cell where misfolded proteins are decomposed into their constituent amino acids

protein: Large networks of amino acids joined to one another

proteoglycan: A huge molecular complex containing proteins, sugar molecules, and variable amounts of water; when combined with collagen, the result is cartilage.

proximal: The closer point on the arms or legs to the center of the body; the shoulder is the proximal end of the arm.

PS: The parasympathetic nervous system

pulmonary circulation: The movement of blood from the heart to the lungs and the return of the blood to the heart

pyrogen: A substance in the body that promotes a high fever

Q̇: Blood flow rate through the heart, milliliters per minute

radiating pain: Pain sensations that move away from the spine toward the extremities with time

rate of change of length: How rapidly a muscle's length is changing on being stretched or contracted

rebound headache: The headache that may follow once a particular treatment modality for headache is withheld

recall: The retrieval of information from its storage sites in the short-term or long-term memory

receptive field: A group of sensor cells in the retina that work together to detect a particular geometric or kinetic aspect within the visual field, such as a horizontal straight line or a slanted line moving from left to right

receptor: A cell specialized for sensitivity to a particular physiologic variable such as light, touch, temperature, or acetylcholine concentration

recruitment: The employment of specific motor units depending upon the task to be performed

reflex: The simple, innate response of a system to a particular stimulus; it is unlearned and involuntary

reflex arc: The direct link between the receptor and the effector organ via the central nervous system

refractory period: The brief period during or following a neural impulse during which no second impulse is possible

relaxation: Not contracted; a state of restful alertness; the aspect of alertness differentiates relaxation from sleep

REM sleep: A phase of sleep characterized by rapid eye movement, dreaming, muscular paralysis, and a desynchronized EEG; occurs about every ninety minutes during a night's sleep

renin: An enzyme released by the kidney in times of low blood volume, which acts ultimately to restrict urination

respiratory sinus arrhythmia (RSA): The difference between the heart rate when inhaling and exhaling

resting muscle tone: The degree of muscle contraction (tonus) when in a restful state

reticular activating system: See **reticular formation**

reticular formation: The center in the brainstem from the lower medulla to the diencephalon, involved with arousal, alertness, and control of neural traffic ascending and descending the central nervous system

retina: The light-sensitive cells and the associated neural networks at the back of the eyeball

retinal: The photopigment in the cones of the retina

rhodopsin: The photopigment in the rods of the retina

right brain: The right cerebral hemisphere, promoting excitation of the parasympathetic nervous system

right vagus nerve: The right branch of the vagus nerve (cranial nerve X), extending from the hypothalamus to the lower regions of the digestive system

RN: Right nasal retinal hemifield

rods: The light receptor cells in the retina functioning only in dim light and without color sensitivity

rotator cuff: The four muscles holding the humeral head in the shoulder socket and responsible for glenohumeral movement

RT: Right temporal retinal hemifield

S: The sulfur atom; also the sympathetic nervous system

S1, S2, etc.: The first, second, etc. sacral vertebrae

saccule: A vestibular receptor in the inner ear, for sensing lateral head tilt

sacral: Referring to the fused vertebrae (the sacrum) at the base of the spinal column

sacroiliac joint: The joint at the base of the spinal column joining the sacrum of the spine and the ilium of the pelvis

SAD: Seasonal affective disorder

sagittal: The vertical axis of the body or a plane containing the vertical axis

sarcolemma: The connective-tissue sheath surrounding a bundle of myofibrils within a muscle

sarcomere: The bundle of interleaved myosin and actin myofibrils between adjacent Z discs in a myofibril; when the muscle contracts, the actin fibers are pulled along the myosin fibers and the Z discs move toward one another

scapulae: The shoulder blades

Schwann cell: A fatty cell that is wrapped about an axon in the peripheral nervous system, thereby myelinating it and significantly increasing its conduction velocity

sciatica: Discomfort in the buttocks and legs arising from impingement on the sciatic nerve

SCN: The suprachiasmatic nucleus

scoliosis: A deviation of the spine in the lateral direction

second messenger: A chemical within a cell that responds to a molecule outside the cell and so initiates a chemical/physical reaction; often increases the conduction across a synapse, thereby increasing the strength of long-term learning

selective permeability: The property of a membrane allowing the passage of certain particles from one side to the other, but not others

semicircular canal: One of three perpendicular semicircular organs within the inner ear sensing the rate, sense, and axial direction of head rotation

sensitization: An increasing sensitivity to pleasurable sensations with time

sensorimotor integration: The interaction of the sensory and motor systems of the body to accomplish a specific task

serotonin: A pituitary hormone and neurotransmitter found throughout the body, implicated in depression and having other functions in the body in regard to regulation of anxiety, food intake, and impulsively violent action

serous membrane: Any membrane secreting serum into the large body cavities

serum: A thin, watery fluid secreted by serous membranes

set points: The upper and lower limits of a physiological variable (temperature, pH, etc.) between which a regulatory mechanism operates; the body adjusts automatically so as to keep the variable at a value between the set points

short-term memory: The storage area for briefly storing memories before they are either erased or moved to long-term memory

signal: The change or propagation of transmembrane potential following activation by a sensory receptor or by another neuron

sinus node (SN): Heart muscle fibers within the atria of the heart, triggering their contraction

skeletal muscle: Striated muscles used to open and close joints

skin tension: The tension detected by sensors in the skin due to tension in the muscles underlying the skin

slow-twitch fibers: Type 1 muscle fibers that contract relatively slowly but that are capable of contraction for a long time

slow-wave sleep: Stages of deep sleep in which the EEG displays synchronous waves of low frequency

smooth muscles: Non-striated muscles, usually under autonomic control, as those within the intestines, blood vessels, etc.

soft tissue: Any tissue other than bone

somatic: Referring to the muscles and skin of the body

spasm: An involuntary muscle contraction

specific metastability: The situation in which an object is stable toward falling in specific directions but is unstable toward falling in

one or more other directions

sphincter: A ring of smooth muscle that opens or closes an orifice of the body

spinal appendages: Primarily the skull and pelvis, but indirectly, the arms and legs as well

spinal flexion: Forward bending

spinal root: A spinal nerve bundle consisting of afferent fibers from the dorsal spine and efferent fibers from the ventral spine

spinal stenosis: A narrowing of the spinal canal, possibly placing pressure on the spinal cord

spinous process: The posterior aspect of each of the spinal vertebrae, forming the chain of bumps that can be felt as the spinal column from the outside

spontaneous polarization: The spontaneous development of an action potential in a muscle cell leading to contraction without any initial stimulation by an efferent nerve, as with cardiac muscle

sprain: A sudden or violent twist or wrench of a joint that injures the ligaments at that joint

stable: The mechanical state of an object in which the line between its center of gravity and that of the Earth falls within the area of the base of the object

stapes: One of the bones of the middle ear, shaped somewhat like a stirrup

stasis: The inhibition of the normal flow of a fluid; stagnation

stem cells: The basic cells that give rise to each of the types of tissue, such as brain, lung, and muscle

stenosis: The narrowing of an opening in the body, as with the spinal canal, for example

sternal notch: The depression at the point where the clavicle meets the manubrium in the front upper thorax

stochastic resonance: The enhancement of a neural signal by random noise within the neuron

strain: A muscle or its tendon injured or weakened by maximal extension, most often by overuse, misuse, or excessive pressure; also the fractional change in length of a substance following an applied stress

stress: Mechanical or emotional pressure applied to the body or mind

stress fracture: A microfracture of bone that grows into a full-blown fracture due to ongoing applied stress

stressor: An emotional or physical factor that leads to emotional or physical stress in the body

stroke volume: The volume of blood pumped by one cycle of the heartbeat

subcortical: Referring to centers in the brain at a level lower than that of the cortex; the thalamus, for example

subluxation: A momentary decrease in the normal area of contact between bones in a synovial joint

sudomotor: Referring to sweat production in the palms of the hands, as controlled by the autonomic nervous system

superior vena cava: The large vein draining blood from the head, arms, and chest into the right atrium of the heart

suprachiasmatic nucleus (SCN): A nucleus within the brain resting just above the optic chiasm; responsible for many of the body's circadian rhythms

supraspinal: Involving brain centers higher than those in the spinal cord and more likely to add a conscious component to the spinal reflex mode

SV: Cardiac stroke volume, milliliters per beat

sympathetic nervous system: A major branch of the autonomic nervous system; responsible for the fight-or-flight response to a threatening situation

symphysis: A fibrocartilaginous joint

synapse: The very narrow space between the ends of adjacent neurons, the synapse being the relay junction between them

synchronicity: The timing of brain waves of a particular frequency in the EEG such that they reach their peak voltages at the same time in different areas of the scalp

synergist muscle: A muscle that participates in a muscular action, but only in a supporting role in regard to the action of the prime mover

systole: The period of the heart action during which the ventricles contract and blood pressure rises to a maximum

T cells: A part of the immune system identifying foreign cells in the body in order to attack and destroy them

tactile: Pertaining to touch

temporal antipod: The halfway point in a biorhythm cycle, which often is the time of minimum activity of the function

TMJ: The temporomandibular joint connecting the mandible to the temporal portion of the skull

tendinitis: Inflammation of a tendon, resulting in limited motion of the attached muscle

tensegrity: A stable geometric structure involving the interplay between elastic and compressive elements

tensile stress: The mechanical stress imposed on an object when the ends are pulled away from one another, as when stretching a muscle, bone, or nerve

terminal: See **axon terminal**

testosterone: The most important male sexual hormone (androgen) generated in the testes

thalamus: A nucleus serving as a major relay point in the brain, evaluating sensory and muscle-activation information before sending it to or receiving it from the cortex

thermoregulation: The process whereby an organ or body controls its temperature over a narrow range

thoracic: Pertaining to the chest

thrombus: An immobile blood clot formed within a blood vessel

tonic reflex: A muscular reflex of low intensity and long duration, as with the resting muscle tone

trabeculae: Spongy bone consisting of thin bony plates in an irregular lattice

tract: A bundle of nerves all beginning and ending at common points within the central nervous system

traction: Putting a bone or muscle under tensile stress in order to lengthen, immobilize, or align it

transduction: The conversion of a sensory stimulus (light, pressure, etc.) into an electrical signal in the associated afferent neuron

transmembrane potential: The voltage appearing across a membrane due to the differing numbers of charged particles (ions) on its two sides

TRH: Thyrotropin-releasing hormone

triglyceride: A compound formed by the union of one molecule of glycerol with three molecules of a fatty acid

tripartite brain: The division of the brain into the forebrain, the midbrain, and the hindbrain, the latter being the oldest and most primitive part

t-tubule: Transverse structures within muscle fibers that carry signals from the sarcolemma to the myofibrils within

tumor: A benign or malignant tissue having an abnormally high growth rate

ultradian: Biorhythms with periods shorter than twenty-four hours; for example, the heartbeat

umbilicus: The navel

underbalance: To have the weight falling forward when in an inverted posture

unilateral breathing: Breathing through one nostril only for a prolonged time, either naturally or forced by mechanical closure of the opposite nostril

unipolar depression: Periods of depression that do not alternate with periods of mania

upper hinge: Bending of the body in the area of the sacroiliac joint and the lumbar vertebrae, as distinct from bending at the lower hinge (the hip joints)

utricle: A vestibular organ for sensing forward/backward tilt of the head

vagal: Referring to the vagus nerve (cranial nerve X) and responsible for much of the parasympathetic control of the heart, stomach, and intestines

Valsalva maneuver: Squeezing the abdominal muscles while holding the breath, allowing one to generate momentary strength in the thorax and maximum pressure at the ends of the gastrointestinal tract

varicosity: A swelling of a vessel or organ

vascular headache: A headache brought on by tension in the smooth muscles of the vascular system in the brain

vascularity: The extent of the development of the vascular system in a particular location

vasoconstrictors: The nerves or substances that cause the diameters of blood vessels to narrow, causing a slowing of the blood flow

vasodilators: Nerves or substances that cause the diameters of blood vessels to increase, causing a relaxation of the vessel walls and an accelerated blood flow

velocity: An object's speed, centimeters per second

ventral: Referring to the front side of the body

ventricles: The lower chambers of the heart that pump blood through the arteries of the body; also, empty spaces within the brain, filled with cerebrospinal fluid

ventricular node (VN): The point within the ventricles of the heart at which electrical excitation and contraction originate

venule: A small vein, lying in size between the capillaries and the veins

vertebrae: The twenty-three or so block-like bones that form the spinal column, found in the cervical, thoracic, lumbar, sacral, and coccygeal regions

vertebral arteries: Arteries that are threaded through foramina in the cervical vertebrae and serve the rear portion of the brain

vertebral wedging: Having wedge-shaped vertebrae and/or discs, leading to an excessive curvature of the spine

vertigo: A vestibular disorder leading to the hallucination of movement

vesicle: A small vessel filled with a particular compound or mixture that can release its contents into the body fluids by rupturing the vessel's walls; prominent in neural transmission across the synaptic cleft and the release of hormones into the body fluids

vestibular apparatus: Organs within the inner ear, responsible for many aspects of balance and equilibrium, sensing the orientation in the gravitational field and rates of angular motion

villi: The projections of the intestinal lining

functioning in the absorption of food

viscera: The internal organs of the abdomen

viscoelastic: Describes a solid (such as muscle) showing both viscous and elastic mechanical properties; when stressed briefly it appears to be elastic, but when stressed for an extended time, it appears to be viscous and flows in the direction of stress

viscous: Describes a very thick fluid or solid that moves only slowly when stressed mechanically and does not return to its original shape when the stress is removed

visual crossover: The crossing over of a branch of the optic nerve of an eye on one side of the head to the cerebral hemisphere on the other side, the crossing occurring at the optic chiasm

vitreous body: The viscous fluid filling the chamber between the lens and retina of the eye

$\dot{V}O_2$: The rate of delivery of oxygen to the muscles, liters of oxygen per minute, while working at a constant rate

$\dot{V}O_{2max}$: The maximum rate of delivery of oxygen to the muscles, liters of oxygen per minute, while working at the maximum rate

water balance: Control of the salt concentrations in the body by intake and voiding of water

Wernicke's area: Area within the left parietal lobe involved with language comprehension and production

white matter: The rapidly conducting neurons of the central nervous system, which are myelinated, i.e., covered by oligodendrocytes

working memory: Short-term memory located largely in the prefrontal cortex

xiphoid process: The small bone attached to the lower end of the sternum

Yogasana: The third level of the *Ashtanga* yoga system, focusing on the traditional Indian postures

Z discs: Terminal structures at the ends of the sarcomeres that are pulled toward one another when the muscle fiber contracts

References

In order to make this handbook as current as possible, references to the newest work in the literature have been cited in the text and in the reference list, while the main text was in preparation for publication. As the *ex post facto* addition of each of the approximately fifty new citations to the reference list would require the renumbering of all other references in the entire text and in the reference list, these new additions instead have been inserted alphabetically in their appropriate places but with the reference numbers appended with letters a, b, c, etc.

[1] Aaronson, B. S. "Color Perception and Affect." *American Journal of Clinical Hypnosis* 14 (1971): 38.

[2] Abraham, I. "Prolotherapy for Chronic Headache." *Headache* 37 (1997): 256.

[3] Abrams, M. "Can You See with Your Tongue?" *Discover* (June 2003): 53.

[4] Ades, P. A., and M. J. Toth. "Accelerated Decline of Aerobic Fitness with Healthy Aging: What is the Good News?" *Circulation* 112 (2005): 624.

[4a] Adler, J. "B. K. S. Iyengar Sheds Light on Life." *Yoga Samachar* 10 (Spring/Summer 2006): 7.

[4b] Adler, J. "B. K. S. Iyengar Sheds Light on Life." *Yoga Samachar* 10 (2007): 9.

[5] Ainsworth, C. "Left, Right and Wrong." *New Scientist* (June 17, 2000): 40.

[5a] Alden, T. "The Anatomy of Choice." *International Journal of Yoga Therapy* 13 (2003): 35.

[5b] Aldrich, V. "Yoga and Depression." *Yoga Samachar* 10 (2007): 7.

[6] Alexander, R. M. *Bones: The Unity of Form and Function.* New York: MacMillan (1994).

[6a] Altenmuller, E. O. "Music in Your Head." *Scientific American Mind* 14 (2004): 24.

[7] Alter, M. J. *Science of Flexibility* (2nd ed.). Champaign, Illinois: Human Kinetics (1996).

[8] Ananthaswamy, A. "Injury Puzzle Solved." *New Scientist* (April 5 2003): 21.

[9] Andersen, J. L., P. Schjerling, and B. Saltin. "Muscles, Genes and Athletic Performance." *Scientific American* (September 2000): 48.

[9a] Anderson, A., and L. Middleton. "What Is this Thing Called Love?" *New Scientist* (April 29, 2006): 32.

[10] Anderson, S. "The Supple Spine." *Yoga International* (Jul/Aug 1994): 14.

[11] ———. "A Play of Opposites." *Yoga International* (Jun/Jul 2000): 17.

[12] Angus, C. "Don't Let Osteoarthritis Get the Best of You." *Yoga International* (Feb/Mar 1998).

[13] Anon. *Nature* 46 (1892): 451.

[14] ———. "Cardiovascular Events at Defecation: Are They Unavoidable?" *Medical Hypotheses* 32 (1990): 231.

[15] ———. "Exercise May Toughen Immune System." *Yoga Journal* (May/Jun 1990): 14.

[16] ———. "The Color of Stress." *Discover* (May 1997).

[17] ———. "Making Waves." *Discover* (October 1998): 24.

[18] ———. "Why Does Time Seem to Speed Up as I Get Older?" *Health* (Jul/Aug 1998): 128.

[19] ———. "Housecalls." *Health* (Jul/Aug 1998): 128.

[20] ———. "Pricking for Endorphins." *Scientific American* (August 1999).

[21] ———. "The 1998 Nobel Prizes in Science." *Scientific American* (January 1999): 16.

[22] ———. "Neural Ties That Bind Perception." *Science News* 155 (1999): 122.

[23] ———. "Healthy Serenades." *New Scientist* (February 5, 2000): 25.

[24] ———. "The Rhythm of Mind." *Discover*

(January 2000): 24.

[25] ———. "No Way Out." *New Scientist* (January 26, 2002): 34.

[25a] ———. "Breathe Deep." *New Scientist* (November 23, 2002): 26.

[26] ———. "Brain Scans Find the Penis at Last." *New Scientist* (June 25, 2005): 22.

[26a] Arpita. "Physiological and Psychological Effects of Hatha Yoga: A Review of the Literature." *Journal of the International Association of Yoga Therapists* 1 (1990): 1.

[27] Arria, S. A., and C. I. Staley. "The Dangers of Sitting." *Muscle and Fitness* (September 1994): 244.

[28] Atmarupananda, S. "What Can We Expect from a Life of Vedanta?" *Yoga International* (Jun/Jul 1999): 24.

[29] Aum, L. "Feldenkrais Bends." *Yoga Journal* (Jan/Feb 1998): 30.

[30] Austin, J. A. *Zen and the Brain*. Cambridge: MIT Press (1999).

[31] Austin, J. "A Yoga Intervention for Young Adults with Elevated Symptoms of Depression." *Yoga Rahasya* 12 (2005): 34.

[31a] Backon, J. "Changes in Blood Glucose Levels Induced by Differential Forced Unilateral Nostril Breathing, A Technique which Affects Both Brain Hemisphericity and Autonomic Activity." *Medical Science Research* 16 (1988) 1197.

[31b] Backon, J., N. Matamaros, and U. Ticho. "Changes in Intraocular Pressure Induced by Differential Forced Breathing, A Technique that Affects Both Brain Hemisphericity and Autonomic Activity." *Graefe's Archive for Clinical and Experimental Ophthalmology* 227 (1989): 575.

[31c] Backon, J., and S. Kullock. "Effect of Forced Unilateral Nostril Breathing on Blink Rates: a Relevance to Hemispheric Lateralization of Dopamine." *International Journal of Neuroscience* 46 (1989): 53.

[32] Badeer, H. S. "Does Gravitational Pressure of Blood Hinder Flow to the Brain of the Giraffe?" *Comparative Biochemistry and Physiology A* 83 (1986): 207.

[33] Baier, K. "What Is an Asana?" *Yoga Rahasya* 2 (1995): 89.

[34] Bailey, J. "Balancing Act." *Yoga Journal* (Sep/Oct 2003): 87.

[35] Balasubramanian B., and M. S. Pansare. "Effect of Yoga on Aerobic and Anerobic Power of Muscles," *Indian Journal of Physiology and Pharmacology* 35 (1991): 28.

[36] Ballentine, Jr., R. M. "Nasal Functioning." *Research Bulletin of the Himalayan International Institute* (Winter 1980): 11.

[37] Ballentine, R. "Breathing: The Chest Cavity, Part I." *Research Bulletin of the Himalayan International Institute* 2 (1980): 8.

[38] ———. "Clinical Significance of the Nasal Cycle." *Research Bulletin of the Himalayan International Institute* 2 (1980): 9.

[38a] ———. "Nostril To Nostril: Balancing the Breath." *Yoga International* (Feb/Mar 2003): 40.

[38b] Bandler, R., and J. Grinder. *Reframing: Neuro-Linguistic Programming and the Transformation of Meaning*. Real People Pub. (1981).

[39] Barrett, J. "Heart to Heart." *Yoga Journal* (December 2002): 100.

[40] ———. "The Trouble with Touch." *Yoga Journal* (Mar/Apr 2003): 102.

[41] Barsky, A. J., R. Saintford, M. P. Rogers, and J. F. Borus, "Nonspecific Medication Side Effects and the Nocebo Phenomenon." *Journal of the American Medical Association* 287 (2002): 622.

[42] Bass, C., and W. Gardner, "Emotional Influences on Breathing and Breathlessness." *Journal of Psychosomatic Research* 29 (1985): 599.

[43] Bates, W. H. *The Bates Method for Better Eyesight Without Glasses*. New York: Holt, Rinehart and Winston (1968).

[44] Baumgart, T. "Brain Rejuvenation." *Yoga Journal* (Nov/Dec 1998): 20.

[44a] Bauman, A. "Sinusitis Survival." *Yoga Journal* (Jan/Feb 2003): 34.

[45] Beardsley, T. "Truth or Consequences." *Scientific American* (October 1999): 21.

[46] Beck, D. M., N. Muggleton, V. Walsh, and N. Lavie. "Right Parietal Cortex Plays a Critical Role in Change Blindness." *Cerebral Cortex* (May 2006): 712.

[47] Behanan, K. *Yoga, A Scientific Evaluation*. New York: Dover, (1937).

[48] Beilock S. L., and T. H. Carr. "On the Fragility of Skilled Performance: What Governs Choking under Pressure?" *Journal of Experimental Psychology; General* 130 (2001): 701.

[49] Bekoff, M. "Beastly Passions." *New Scientist* (April 29, 2000): 32.

[50] Belay, T. "Stress Express." *New Scientist* (May 27, 2000): 21.

[51] Belmonte, J. C. I. "How the Body Tells Left

from Right." *Scientific American* (June 1999): 46.

[52] Benjamin, B. E. *Listen to Your Pain*. New York: Penguin (1984).

[53] Bennett, D. "Don't Tickle My Funny Bone." *Muscles and Fitness* (May 1998): 212.

[54] Benson, H. *The Relaxation Response*. New York: Morrow (1976).

[55] Bera, T. K., M. M. Gore, and J. P. Oak. "Recovery from Stress in Two Different Postures and in Savasana: A Yogic Relaxation Posture." *Indian Journal of Physiology and Pharmacology* 42 (1998): 473.

[56] Berg, M., and M. Basta Boubion. "Zapping Postexercise Pain." *Muscle and Fitness* (May 2000): 106.

[57] Beringer, G. B., and G. S. Golden. "Beauty Parlor Stroke: When a Beautician Becomes a Physician." *Journal of the American Medical Association* 270 (1993): 1198.

[58] Bernardi, L., P. Sleight, G. Bandinelli, S. Cencetti, L. Fattorini, J. Wdowczyc-Szulc, and A. Lagi. "Effect of Rosary Prayer and Yoga Mantras on Autonomic Cardiovascular Rhythms: Comparative Study." *British Medical Journal* 323 (2001): 1446.

[59] Berridge, M. J. "The Molecular Basis of Communication within the Cell." *Scientific American* (October 1985): 142.

[60] Bhatnagar, O. P., A. K. Ganguly, and V. Anantharaman. "Influence of Yoga Training on Thermoregulation." *Indian Journal of Medical Research* 67 (1978): 844.

[61] Bhavanani, A. B., Madanmoham, and K. Udupa. "Acute Effect of *Mukh Bhastrika* on Reaction Time." *Indian Journal of Physiology and Pharmacology*. 47 (2003): 297.

[61a] Biel, A. *Trail Guide to the Body*, Boulder, CO. Books of Discovery (2005).

[62] Biever, C. "Bring Me Sunshine." *New Scientist* (August 9, 2003): 30.

[63] Blackmore, S. "The Grand Illusion." *New Scientist* (June 22, 2002): 26.

[64] Blackwelder, R. B. *Alternative Medicine* (monograph, edition 219, Home Study Self-Assessment Program). Kansas City, Missouri: American Academy of Family Physicians (August 1997).

[65] Blanchard, E. B., and L. D. Young. "Self-Control of Cardiac Functioning: A Promise As Yet Unfulfilled." *Psychological Bulletin* 79 (1973): 145.

[66] Bloom, H. "Reality Is a Shared Hallucination" in *Global Brain: The Evolution of Mass Mind from the Big Bang to the 21ˢᵗ Century*. New York: Wiley (2000).

[67] Bloom, S. "The Fat Controller." *New Scientist* (August 9, 2003): 38.

[68] Bodanis, D. *The Body Book*. Boston: Little Brown (1984).

[69] Bonnick, S. *The Osteoporosis Handbook*. Dallas: Taylor (1994).

[70] Borish, I. M. *Clinical Refraction* (3rd ed.). Chicago: The Professional Press (1970): 568.

[71] Bowe, C. "Body Briefing: The Endocrine Glands." *Lear's Magazine* (Jan/Feb 1989): 69.

[72] Bower, B. "Slumber's Unexpected Landscape." *Science News* 156 (1999): 205.

[73] ———. "Schizophrenia May Involve Bad Timing." *Science News* 156 (1999): 309.

[74] ———. "Pushing the Mood Swings." *Science News* 157 (2000): 232.

[75] ———. "Forgetting to Remember." *Science News* 164 (2003): 293.

[76] ———. "Whiffs of Perception." *Science News* 164 (2003): 308.

[77] ———. "Allies in Therapy." *Science News* 164 (2003): 357.

[78] ———. "Juggling Takes Stage as Brain Modifier." *Science News* 165 (2004): 78.

[79] ———. "The Brain's Word Act," *Science News* 165 (2004): 83.

[80] ———. "Neural Aging Walks Tall," *Science News* 165 (2004): 115.

[80a] ———. "Female Brains Know How to Fold 'em." *Science News* 166 (2004): 46.

[81] ———. "Wayfaring Sleepers." *Science News* 166 (2004): 294.

[81a] ———. "Synchronized Thinking." *Science News* 166 (2004): 310.

[82] ———. "Brains Disconnect as People Sleep." *Science News* 168 (2005): 23.

[82a] ———. "Mirror Cells' Fading Spark." *Science News* 168 (2005): 373.

[83] ———. "Smart Shoppers Use Unconscious Tactics." *Science News* 169 (2006): 124.

[83a] ———. "Older but Mellower." *Science News* 169 (2006): 389.

[84] Bower, J. E., A. Woolery, B. Sternlieb, and D. Garet. "Yoga for Cancer Patients and Survivors." *Cancer Control* 12 (2005): 165.

[85] Bower, J. M., and L. M. Parsons. "Rethinking the Lesser Brain." *Scientific American* (August

2003): 51.

[86] Bowman, A. J., R. H. Clayton, A. Murray, J. W. Reed, M. M. Subhan, and G. A. Ford. "Effects of Aerobic Exercise Training and Yoga on the Baroreflex in Healthy Elderly Persons." *European Journal of Clinical Investigation* 27 (1997): 443.

[87] Boyle, C. A., S. P. Sayers, B. E. Jensen, S. A. Healey, and T. M. Manos. "The Effects of Yoga Training and a Single Bout of Yoga on Delayed Onset of Muscle Soreness in the Lower Extremity." *Journal of Strength and Conditioning Research* 18 (2004): 23.

[88] Brainard, G., V. Pratap, C. Reed, B. Levitt, and J. Hanifin. "Plasma Cortisol Reduction in Healthy Volunteers Following a Single Session of Yoga Practice." *Yoga Research Society Newsletter; Philadelphia* (Apr/Sep 1997): 1.

[89] Brebbia, D. R., and K. Z. Altshuler. "Oxygen Consumption Rate and Electroencephalographic Stage of Sleep." *Science* 150 (1965): 1621.

[90] Brechue, W. F., and M. D. Beekley. "What Does the Body/Muscle Remember?" *Women's Health Digest* 2 (1996): 221.

[91] Broden, G., A. Dolk, C. Frostell, B. Nilsson, and B Holmstrom. "Voluntary Relaxation of the External Anal Sphincter." *Diseases of the Colon and Rectum* 32 (1989): 376.

[93] Brooks, M. "13 Things That Don't Make Sense." *New Scientist* (March 19, 2005): 30.

[94] Brown, B. B. *New Mind, New Body.* New York: Harper and Row (1974).

[95] Brown, P. "In the Shadow of Fear." *New Scientist* (September 6, 2003): 30.

[96] ———. "Sleep: Who Needs It?" *New Scientist* (November 6, 2004): 37.

[97] Brownlee, C. "Tug of War." *Science News* 167 (2005): 197.

[98] ———. "Eat Smart." *Science News* 169 (2006): 136.

[98a] Brownstone, A. "Therapeutic Mechanisms of Yoga Asana." *International Journal of Yoga Therapy* 11 (2001): 11.

[99] Cabrera, J. L., and J. G. Milton. "On-Off Intermittency in a Human Balancing Task." *Physical Review Letters* 89 (2002): 158702.

[100] Cahill, L. "His Brain, Her Brain." *Scientific American* (May 2005): 40.

[101] Calais-Germain, B. *Anatomy of Movement.* Seattle: Eastland Press (1993).

[102] Caldwell, M. "Mind Over Time." *Discover* (July 1999): 52.

[103] Campbell, D. "The Mozart Effect and More." *New Visions* (September 1998): 6.

[104] Cannon, W. B. "Voodoo Death." *American Journal of Public Health* 92 (2002): 1593.

[105] Carbonnel, J. www.positivehealth.com/permit/ Articles /Regular/joel46.htm

[106] Cardoso, S. "It's No Laughing Matter." *New Scientist* (May 18, 2002): 48.

[107] Carlson, N. R. *Physiology of Behavior* (3rd ed.). Boston: Allyn and Bacon (1986).

[108] Carter, B. L. "Optimizing Delivery Systems to Tailor Pharmacotherapy to Cardiovascular Circadian Events." *American Journal of Health-System Pharmacy* 55 (1998): S17.

[108a] Carter, R. "Tune In, Turn Off," *New Scientist* (October 1999): 30.

[109] Castleman, M. "Alternative to Viagra." *Yoga Journal* (Jul/Aug 2002): 36.

[110] Cavanaugh, C. "Urdhva Mukha Svanasana." *Yoga Journal* (May/Jun 1991): 34.

[111] Chaitow,L. www.positivehealth.com/permit/ Articles/Regular/chaito38.htm

[112] ———. "Fibromyalgia Update 2000." www. Healingpeople.com

[112a] Chandra, F. J. "Medical and Physiological Aspects of Headstand." *Journal of the International Association of Yoga Therapists* 1 (1990): 29.

[113] Chaney, E. *The Eyes Have It.* York Beach, Maine: S. Weiser (1987).

[113a] Cheikin, M. "Yoga Hatha Medica: An Integrated Medical Yoga Curriculum," *International Journal of Yoga Therapy* 13 (2003): 15.

[114] Chen, C. S., M. Mrksich, S. Huang, G. M. Whitesides, and D. E. Ingber. "Geometric Control of Cell Life and Death." *Science* 276 (1997): 1425.

[115] Chohan, I. S., H. S. Nayar, P. Thomas, and N. S. Geetha. "Influence of Yoga on Blood Coagulation." *Thrombosis and Haemostasis.* 51 (1984): 196.

[116] Chusid, J. "Yoga Foot Drop." *Journal of the American Medical Association* 217 (1971): 827.

[117] Clark, M. A. *Integrated Flexibility Training.* Thousand Oaks, California: National Academy of Sports Medicine (2001).

[118] Clarke, J. "The Nasal Cycle, Part II." *Research Bulletin of the Himalayan International Institute.* 2 (1980): 3.

[119] ———. "Respiration, Heart Rate and the

Autonomic Nervous System." *Research Bulletin of the Himalayan International Institute* 3 (1981): 4.

[120] ———. "Resting Breath Pattern." *Research Bulletin Himalayan International Institute* 3 (1981): 15.

[121] ———. "Asana and Aerobics." *Yoga International* (Jan/Feb 1994): 31.

[122] ———. "Slowing Down: The Practice of 2-to-1 Breathing." *Yoga International* (Nov/Dec 1994): 56.

[123] ———. "The Nasal Cycle: Ancient and Modern Studies of Body-Mind Balancing." *Yoga International* (reprint series, 1995): 13.

[124] Clay, C. C., L. K. Lloyd, J. L. Walker, K. R. Sharp, and R. B. Pankey. "The Metabolic Cost of Hatha Yoga." *Journal of Strength and Conditioning Research* 19 (2005): 604.

[125] Clayton, J. "Caught Napping." *New Scientist* (February 26, 2000): 43.

[126] Clennel, B. "A Woman's Yoga Practice." *Iyengar Yoga Association of Greater New York Newsletter* (Summer/Fall 1999): 7.

[127] Coghlan, A. "Beg, Steal or Borrow." *New Scientist* (May 20, 2000): 17.

[128] ———. "Late-Night Drinking." *New Scientist* (April 20, 2002): 18.

[129] Coghlan, A., and M. Le Page. "The Fix That Fails Kids' Eyes." *New Scientist* (November 23, 2002): 6.

[130] Coghlan, A. "Deadly Poisons Reveal Their Friendly Side." *New Scientist* (February 15, 2003): 10.

[131] ———. "How Sensitivity to Pain Is Really All in the Mind." *New Scientist* (June 28, 2003): 17.

[132] ———. "Elite Athletes Are Born to Run." *New Scientist* (August 30, 2003): 4.

[133] ———. "Does Youth End When You Go to Bed." *New Scientist* (January 8, 2005): 13.

[133a] ———. "Found: a Dimmer Switch for Depression." *New Scientist* (June 14, 2005): 13.

[134] ———. "Love's a Fight between the Eyes and the Nose." *New Scientist* (July 23, 2005): 12.

[135] Cohen, H. D., R. C. Rosen, and L. Goldstein. "Electroencephalographic Laterality Changes During Human Sexual Orgasm." *Archives of Sexual Behavior* 5 (1976): 189.

[136] Cohen, J., D. H. Char, and D. Norman. "Bilateral Orbital Varices Associated with Habitual Bending." *Archives of Ophthalmology.* 113 (1995): 1360.

[137] Cohen, P. "Forget Me Not." *New Scientist* (July 1, 2000): 12.

[138] ———. "Mental Gymnastics Increase Biceps Strength." *New Scientist* (November 1, 2001).

[139] Coker, K. H. "Meditation and Prostate Cancer: Integrating a Mind/Body Intervention with Traditional Therapies." *Seminars on Urology and Oncology* 17 (1999): 111.

[140] Cole, R. "Physiology of Yoga" in *Newsletter, B. K. S. Iyengar Yoga Institute of South Africa* (December 1988): 26.

[141] Cole, R. J. "Postural Baroreflex Stimuli May Affect EEG Arousal and Sleep in Humans." *Journal of Applied Physiology* 67 (1989): 2369.

[142] Cole, R. "Science Studies Yoga," as reported by A. Cushman in *Yoga Journal* (Jul/Aug 1994): 43.

[143] ———. "Relaxation Physiology and Practice" (unpublished notes, 1994).

[144] ———. "Physiology of Inversions," (unpublished notes, July 1997).

[145] ———. Personal communication (1999–2000).

[146] ———. "Hips and Knees: Anatomy and Asana" (unpublished notes, October 2001).

[147] ———. "Losing Strength from Yoga?" *Yoga Journal* (Sep/Oct 2002): 42.

[147a] ———. "Plumb Perfect." *Yoga Journal* (May/June 2004): 98.

[148] Coleman, M., and K. Bendall. "Keeping Your Nerves," *New Scientist* (August 27, 2005): 31.

[149] Coleman, R. M. *Wide Awake at 3:00 AM: By Choice or by Chance?* New York: Freeman (1986).

[150] Collins, C. "Yoga: Intuition, Preventative Medicine and Treatment." *Journal of Obstetrics, Gynocology and Neonatal Nursing* 27 (1998): 563.

[151] Cook, B. "Controlling Diabetes." *Yoga International* (Feb/Mar 1998): 51.

[152] Coontz, R. "The Planet That Hums." *New Scientist* (September 1999): 30.

[153] Cooper, R. S., C. N. Rotimi, and R. Ward. "The Puzzle of Hypertension in African-Americans." *Scientific American* (February 1999):56.

[154] Copeland, P. "Yoga, the Heart and the Breath." *Yoga Journal* (May 1975): 6.

[155] ———. "Yoga and the Endocrine System." *Yoga Journal* (Jul/Aug 1975): 9.

[156] ———. "Pranayama and Physiology." *Yoga Journal* (Nov/Dec 1975): 9.

[157] ———. "Yoga, Mind and Muscle." *Yoga Journal* (Mar/Apr 1976): 27.

[158] Corballis, M. C. "From Mouth to Hand:

Gesture, Speech and the Evolution of Right-Handedness." *The Behavioral and Brain Sciences* 26 (2003): 199.

[159] Coren, S. *The Left-Hander Syndrome.* New York: Free Press (1992).

[160] Cornelius, W. L., and K. Craft-Hamm. "Proprioceptive Neuromuscular Facilitation Flexibility Techniques: Acute Effects on Arterial Blood Pressure." *The Physician and Sports Medicine* 16 (1988): 152.

[161] Corrigan, G. E. "Fatal Air Embolism after Yoga Breathing Exercises." *Journal of the American Medical Association* 210 (1969): 1923.

[162] Corrigan, M. V., and C. V. Tyler, Jr. *Common Problems in Elderly Persons* (monograph, ed. no. 223, Home Study Self-Assessment Program) Kansas City, Missouri: American Academy of Family Physicians (December 1997).

[163] Couch, J. "In Defense of Stretching." *Yoga Journal* (Jul/Aug 1983): 11.

[164] Coulter, D. "Self-Preservation." *Yoga International* (Nov/Dec 1994): 67.

[165] ———. "Moving Gracefully: The Role of the Knee-Jerk Reflex." *Yoga International* (Jul/Aug 1994): 55.

[166] ———. "For Clarity of Mind: the Diaphragmatic Breath." *Yoga International* (reprint series, 1999): 9.

[167] Coulter, H. D. *Anatomy of Hatha Yoga: A Manual for Students, Teachers and Practitioners.* Honesdale, PA: Body and Breath, Inc. (2001).

[168] Coulter-Parker, N. "Brain Training." *Yoga Journal* (Sep/Oct 2002): 79.

[169] Councilman, J. E. *The Science of Swimming.* Englewood Cliffs, NJ: Prentice Hall (1968).

[170] Cousins, N. *Anatomy of an Illness.* New York: Norton (1979).

[171] Couzens, G. "PMS Workout." *Self* (October 1991): 150.

[172] Cowley, G. "How to Live to 100." *Newsweek* (June 30, 1997): 54.

[173] Craig, A. D. "How Do You Feel? Interoception: The Sense of the Physiological Condition of the Body." *Nature Reviews, Neuroscience* 3 (2002): 655.

[174] Crawford, A. M. "Hormones Demystified." *Yoga Journal* (May/Jun 1997): 34.

[175] Criswell, E. *How Yoga Works: An Introduction to Somatic Yoga.* Novato, CA: Freeperson Press (1987).

[176] Curtis, V. "The Art of Persuasion." *New Scientist* (December 18, 2004): 21.

[177] Dajer, T. "Deadly Knee Bends." *Discover* (May 1999): 38.

[178] Dalal, A. S., and T. X. Barber. "Yoga, Yogic Feats and Hypnosis in the Light of Empirical Research." *American Journal of Clinical Hypnotism* 11 (1969): 155.

[179] Dalziel, Mary. Personal communication (2005).

[180] Damasio, A. R. "How the Brain Creates the Mind." *Scientific American* (December 1999): 112.

[181] Darling, R. C. "Physiology of Exercise and Fatigue" in *Therapeutic Exercise*, S. Licht, ed. Baltimore: Waverly Press (1958): 21.

[182] Das, J. P. "Yoga and Hypnosis." *International Journal of Clinical Hypnosis* 11 (1963): 31.

[183] Datey, K. K., S. N. Deshmukh, C. P. Dalvi, and S. L. Vinekar. "Shavasan: A Yogic Exercise in the Management of Hypertension." *Angiology* 20 (1969): 395.

[184] Davies, A. M., and R. Eccles. "Reciprocal Changes in Nasal Resistance to Airflow Caused by Pressure Applied to the Axilla." *Acta Otolaryngologica* 99 (1985): 154.

[185] Davies, J. "Menopausal Falls." *New Scientist* (November 16, 2002): 24.

[186] Davis, D. M. "Intrigue at the Immune Synapse." *Scientific American* (February 2006): 48.

[186a] Davis, K. "How to Lose Weight without Even Trying." *New Scientist* (September 15, 2004): 7.

[187] Davson, H. *A Textbook of General Physiology.* Boston: Little, Brown (1959).

[188] Day, S. "Pain Memories." *New Scientist* (March 2, 2002): 29.

[189] Dayton, L. "Snooze Control." *New Scientist* (February 23, 2002): 38.

[191] Demers, C. "Chaos or Calm: Rewiring the Stress Response." *Yoga International* (Feb/Mar 2004): 76.

[192] Dennett, D. C. *Consciousness Explained.* Boston: Little, Brown (1991).

[193] Derrick, J. M. "A Routine for Menopause." *Iyengar Yoga Association of Greater New York Newsletter* (Summer/Fall, 1999): 4.

[194] Desikachar, T. K. V. *The Heart of Yoga.* Rochester: Inner Traditions International (1995).

[195] Deth, R. C. "What Happens to the Body and Brain of Individuals with Schizophrenia?" *(SciAm Asks the Experts, no date)*

[196] Devereux, G. "Hatha Yoga and the Five Energies of Nature." *Yoga International* (Aug/Sep 1999): 30.

[197] Diamond, J. "Dining with the Snakes." *Discover* 15 (1994): 48.

[198] Diamond, J. A. *Your Body Doesn't Lie*. New York: Warner (1979).

[199] Diamond, M. C., A. B. Scheibel, and L. M. Elson. *The Human Brain Coloring Book*. New York: Harper Perennial (1985).

[200] Diamond, S. *Hope For Your Headache Problem* (second ed.). Madison, Conn.: Intern. Univ. Press (1988).

[201] ———. *The Hormone Headache*. New York: Macmillan (1995).

[202] DiCarlo, L. J., P. B. Sparling, B. T. Hinson, T. K. Snow, and L. B. Rosskopf. "Cardiovascular, Metabolic and Perceptual Responses to Hatha Yoga Standing Poses." *Medicine, Exercise and Nutritional Health* 4 (1995): 107.

[204] Dimond, S. *Introducing Neuropsychology*. Springfield, Ill.: C. S. Thomas (1978).

[205] Dobbs, D. "Zen Gamma." *Scientific American Mind* 16 (2005): 9.

[206] Dodes, J. E., and M. J. Schissel. Letter to the editor. *Discover* (October 1999): 16.

[207] Dominguez, R. H., and R. Cajda. *Total Body Training*. New York: Scribner's (1982).

[208] Donelson, R., G. Silva, and K. Murphy. "Centralization Phenomenon: Its Usefulness in Evaluating and Treating Referred Pain." *Spine* 15 (1990): 211.

[209] Donohue, P. G. "Ear-Muscle Contraction Renders Clicking Noise." *Newark Star Ledger* (October 2, 1998): 70.

[210] Douglas, K., A. George, B. Holmes, G. Lawton, J. McCrone, A. Motluk, and H. Phillips, "Eleven Steps to a Better Brain." *New Scientist* (May 2005): 28.

[210a] Douglas, K. "It's in Your Hands." *New Scientist* (August 19, 2006): 33.

[211] Douillard, J. *Body, Mind and Sport*. New York: Harmony (1994).

[212] Draper, D. O., J. L. Castro, B. Feland, S. Schulthies, and D. Eggett. "Shortwave Diathermy and Prolonged Stretching Increase Hamstring Flexibility More than Prolonged Stretching Alone." *Journal of Orthopaedic and Sports Physical Therapy* 34 (2004): 13.

[213] Dunavan, C. P. "Blindsided by Tetanus." *Discover* (January 2000): 39.

[214] Dunn, S. "How Yoga Saved My Life." *Yoga Journal* (August 2000): 78.

[215] Eccles, R. "The Central Rhythm of the Nasal Cycle." *Acta Otolaryngologica* 86 (1978): 464.

[216] ———. "Sympathetic Control of Nasal Erectile Tissue." *European Journal of Respiratory Disease, Supplement*. 128, pt. 1 (1983): 150.

[217] Eckberg, D. L., F. M. Abboud, and A. L. Mark. "Modulation of Carotid Baroreflex Responsiveness in Man: Effects of Posture and Propranolol." *Journal of Applied Physiology*. 41 (1976): 383.

[218] Editors, *Yoga Journal*, quoting Mary Schatz.

[219] Edmonds, K. www.IUS.ed

[220] Ekkekakis, P. "Pleasure and Displeasure from the Body: Perspectives from Exercise." *Cognition and Emotion*. 17 (2003).

[221] Ekman, P. *Emotions Revealed*. New York: Times Books (2003).

[222] Eliade, M. *Yoga, Immortality and Freedom*. Princeton: Princeton U. Press (1969).

[223] Elefteriades, J. A., I. Hatzaras, M. A. Tranquili, A. J. Elefteriades, R. Stout, R. K. Shaw, D. Silverman, and P. Barash. "Weight Lifting and Rupture of Silent Aortic Aneurysms." *Journal of the American Medical Association* 290 (2003): 2803.

[224] Elefteraides, J. A. "Beating a Sudden Killer." *Scientific American* (August 2005): 64.

[225] Elliott, W. J. "Timing Treatment to the Rhythm of Disease: A Short Course in Chronotherapeutics." *Journal of Postgraduate Medicine* 110 (2001): 119.

[226] Englert, H. "Sussing Out Stress." *Scientific American Mind* 14 (2004): 56.

[226a] Erickson, S. "How to Understand Tissue Memory and its Implications." *Massage Therapy Journal* 42 (2003): 70.

[227] Etaugh, C., and P. Ptasnik. "Effects of Studying to Music and Post-Study Relaxation on Reading Comprehension." *Perceptual and Motor Skills* (August 1982): 141.

[228] Evans, P. R. "Referred Itch (Mitempfindungen)." *British Medical Journal* 2 (1976): 839.

[229] Evarts, E. V. "Brain Mechanisms of Movement." *Scientific American* (September 1979): 164.

[230] Ezraty, M. "Asana." *Yoga Journal* (Mar/Apr 2002): 138.

[231] ———. "Dropping Back into Urdhva

Dhanurasana." *Yoga Journal* (December 2002): 128.

[232] Faber, W. J., and M. Walker. *Pain, Pain, Go Away*. Mountain View, Cal.: Ishi Press (1990).

[233] Fahmy, J. A., and H. Fledelius. "Yoga-Induced Attacks of Acute Glaucoma." *Acta Ophthalmologica* 51 (1973): 80.

[234] Farhi, D. "Asana: Handstand." *Yoga Journal* (Jan/Feb 1993): 35.

[235] ———. "Karnapidasana: Pain in the Ear Pose." *Yoga Journal* (Nov/Dec 1993): 40.

[236] ———. "Holding Your Breath." *Yoga Journal* (Mar/Apr 1996): 75.

[237] ———. "Padmasana." *Yoga Journal* (Nov/Dec 1999): 84.

[238] Farley, P. "The Anatomy of Despair." *New Scientist* (May 1, 2004): 43.

[239] Feinstein, A. *Training the Body to Cure Itself*. Emmaus, PA: Rodale (1992).

[240] Feltman, J. (ed.). *Prevention's Giant Book of Health Facts*. Emmaus, PA: Rodale (1991).

[241] Fetler, L., and S. Amigorena. "Brain Under Surveillance: The Microglial Patrol." *Science* 309 (2005): 392.

[242] Fields, R. D. "The Other Half of the Brain." *Scientific American* (April 2004): 55.

[242a] ———. "Making Memories Stick." *Scientific American* (February 2005): 75.

[243] Fischman, J. "Conquering Pain." *U.S. News and World Report* (June 12, 2000): 59.

[244] Fitzgerald, L., and R. Monro. "Follow-up Survey on Yoga and Diabetes." *Yoga Biomedical Bulletin* 1 (1986): 61.

[245] Flanagan, O. "The Colour of Happiness." *New Scientist* (May 24, 2003): 44.

[246] Fleg, J. L., C. H. Morrell, A. G. Bos, L. J. Brant, L. A. Talbot, J. G. Wright, and E. G. Lakatta. "Accelerated Longitudinal Decline of Aerobic Capacity in Healthy Older Adults." *Circulation* 112 (2005): 674.

[247] Fong, K. Y., R. T. Cheung, Y. L. Yu, C. W. Tai, and C. M. Chang. "Basilar Artery Occlusion Following Yoga Exercise: A Case Report." *Journal of Clinical Neuroscience* 30 (1993): 104.

[248] Fox, C. "The Speed of Life." *New Scientist* (November 1, 2003): 42.

[249] Fox, D. "Breathless." *New Scientist* (March 8, 2003): 46.

[250] Francina, S. "The Fountain of Youth." *Yoga Journal* (May/Jun 1997): 87.

[251] Francis, C. C. *Introduction to Human Anatomy* (4th ed.). St. Louis: C. V. Mosby (1964).

[252] Frawley, D. "Yoga and Sound." *Unity in Yoga News* 2 (Winter 1990): 1.

[253] ———. "Mantra and the Energetics of Sound." *Clarion Call* 3 (1990): 35.

[254] ———. "The Chakras and Modern Science." *Yoga International* (Sep/Oct 1993): 5.

[255] Freedman, J. Personal communication (1990).

[256] Funderburk, J. *Science Studies Yoga*. Honesdale, PA: Himalayan Press (1977).

[257] Funk, D., A. M. Swank, K. J. Adams, and D. Treolo. "Efficacy of Moist Heat Pack Application over Static Stretching on Hamstring Flexibility." *Journal of Strength and Conditioning Research* 15 (2001): 123.

[258] Funk, E., and J. Clarke. "The Nasal Cycle: Observations over Prolonged Periods of Time." *Research Bulletin of the Himalayan International Institute* (Winter 1980): 1.

[259] Funk, E. "Biorhythms and the Breath: The Nasal Cycle." *Research Bulletin of the Himalayan International Institute* (Winter 1980): 5.

[260] Gach, M. R. *Accu-Yoga*. Tokyo: Japan Publications (1981).

[260a] Galle, S. "The Awareness/Energy Connection through Hypnosis, Yoga, and Neurofeedback." *International Journal of Yoga Therapy* 11 (2001): 77.

[261] Gallese, V., and A. Goldman. "Mirror Neurons and the Simulation Theory of Mind-Reading." *Trends in Cognitive Science* 2 (1998): 493.

[262] Gallup, C. "A Yoga for the Eyes." *Yoga Journal* (Nov/Dec 1986): 19.

[263] Gardner, J. *Color and Crystals: A Journey Through the Chakras*. Freedom, CA: The Crossing Press (1988).

[264] Garfinkel, M. S., A. Singhal, W. A. Katz, D. A. Allen, R. Reshetar, and H. R. Schumaker, Jr. "Yoga Intervention for Carpal Tunnel Syndrome: A Randomized Trial." *Journal of the American Medical Association* 280 (1998): 1601.

[265] Gavin, J. "Understanding Psychoanatomy." *IDEA Health and Fitness Source* (May 2000): 61.

[266] Gazzaniga, M. S. *Mind Matters: How Mind and Brain Interact to Create Our Conscious Lives*. Boston: Houghton-Mifflin (1988).

[267] Gerard, R. M. *Differential Effects of Colored Lights on Psychophysiological Functions* (PhD dissertation). Los Angeles: University of California (1958).

[268] Gershon, M. D. *The Second Brain*. New York:

HarperCollins (1998).

[269] Geschwind, N., and W. Levitsky. "The Human Brain: Left-Right Asymmetries in the Temporal Speech Region." *Science* 161 (1968): 186.

[270] Geschwind, N. "Specializations of the Human Brain." *Scientific American* 241 (1979): 180.

[271] Gibbs, W. W. "Dogma Overturned." *Scientific American* (November 1998): 19.

[272] ———. "Untangling the Roots of Cancer." *Scientific American Special* 14 (2004): 60.

[273] Gillespie, P. R. "Beyond Relaxation." *Yoga Journal* (Jul/Aug 1988): 37.

[274] Gillespie, S. "Taking Yoga to Heart." *Yoga International* (Mar/Apr 1995): 19.

[275] Gilmore, R. Personal communication (2004).

[275a] Gilmore, R. St. C. "The Effects of Yoga Asanas on Blood Pressure." *International Journal of Yoga Therapy* 12 (2002): 45.

[276] Giubilaro, G. Personal communication.

[277] Gladwell, M. *Blink. The Power of Thinking without Thinking*. New York: Little, Brown, (2005).

[278] Glausiusz, J. "Brain, Heal Thyself." *Women's Health Digest* 2 (1996): 224.

[279] ———. "Wired for a Touch." *Discover*. (December 2002): 13.

[280] Glazier, W. H. "The Task of Medicine." *Scientific American* 228 (1973): 13.

[281] Goleman, D. "Too Much Rest Prolongs Muscle Pain." *The New York Times* (May 19, 1988).

[282] Goldstein, I. "Male Sexual Circuitry." *Scientific American* (August 2000): 70.

[282a] Goldsmith, T. H. "What Birds See." *Scientific American* (July 2006): 68.

[283] Gonzalez-Alonso, J., and J. A. L. Calbet. "Reductions in Systemic and Skeletal Muscle Blood Flow and Oxygen Delivery Limit Maximal Aerobic Capacity in Humans." *Circulation* 107 (2003): 824.

[284] Goodale, M., and D. Milner. *Sight Unseen*. UK: Oxford Press (2004).

[285] Goodrich, J. "Freeing the Inner Eye." *East West* (April 1990): 54.

[286] Gopal, K. S., and S. Lakshmanam. "Some Observations on Hatha Yoga: The Bandhas." *Indian Journal of Medical Science* 26 (1972): 564.

[287] Gopal, K. S., V. Anantharaman, S. D. Nisith, and O. P. Batnagar. "The Effect of Yogasanas on Muscular Tone and Cardio-Respiratory Adjustments," *Indian Journal of Medical Science*

28 (1974): 438.

[288] Gorman, D. *The Body Moveable*. Guelph, Ontario: Ampersand Press (1981).

[289] Grady, M. "Tempering the Mettle: The Practice of Bellows Breathing." *Yoga International* (Jan/Feb 1994): 56.

[290] Graham-Rowe, D. "Teen Angst Rooted in Busy Brain." *New Scientist* (October 19, 2002): 16.

[291] ———. "When a Low-Fat, Salty Taste Strikes a Chord" *New Scientist* (March 15, 2005): 8.

[292] Graves, A. "Wakey, Wakey," *New Scientist* (September 1, 2001): 11.

[293] Gravitz, L. "Why We Crack Under Pressure." *Discover* (May 2000): 15.

[294] ———. "Rain Man's Brain Explained," *Discover* (May 2006): 17.

[295] Gray, H. *Anatomy, Descriptive and Surgical*. Philadelphia: Running Press (1974).

[296] Greenberg, G. "As Good As Dead" in *The Best American Science and Nature Writing, 2002*, N. Angier (ed.). Boston: Houghton Mifflin (2002).

[297] Gregory, R. L. *Eye and Brain* (5th ed.) Princeton University Press (1997).

[298] Grilley, P. "Anatomy for Yoga" (video). Pranamaya (2004).

[299] Griffiths, J., and A. V. Ravindran. "Disrhythmia." *(Sciam* Asks the Experts, no date)

[300] Grillner, S. "Neural Networks for Vertebrate Locomotion." *Scientific American* (January 1996): 64.

[301] Grimes, K. "Hunted!" *New Scientist* (April 13, 2002): 34.

[302] Gudmestad, J. "Take a Stand." *Yoga Journal* (May/Jun 2002): 137.

[303] ———. "Backbends and Headaches," *Yoga Journal* (Jul/Aug 2002): 18.

[304] ———. "The Gripping Truth," *Yoga Journal* (Sep/Oct 2002): 137.

[305] ———. "Anatomy of a Yogi," *Yoga Journal* (November 2002): 127.

[306] ———. "Spread Your Wings," *Yoga Journal* (December 2002):145.

[307] Gura, T. "Roots of Immunity." *New Scientist* (February 19, 2000): 24.

[308] Guyton, A. C. *Textbook of Medical Physiology* (7th ed.). Philadelphia: Saunders (1986).

[309] Haga, E. "Yoga." *Journal of the American Medical Association* 218 (1971): 98.

[310] Hamilton, G. "Filthy Friends." *New Scientist*

(April 16, 2005): 34.

[311] Hanus, S. H., T. D. Homer, and D. H. Harter. "Vertebral Artery Occlusion Complicating Yoga Exercises." *Archives of Neurology* 34 (1977): 574.

[312] Harder, B. "Up and Down Make Different Workouts." *Science News* 166 (2004): 380.

[313] Harden, N. "Sciam Asks the Experts: "What is a Headache?" (no date).

[314] Harman, W. "Science and Yoga, Friends at Last?" *Yoga International* (Jul/Aug 1991): 21.

[315] *Harvard Medical School Family Health Guide*, A. L. Komaroff (ed.). New York: Simon and Schuster (1999).

[316] Harvard Medical School. In *Neuron* (Summer 2002).

[317] *Harvard Women's Health Watch*. "Exercise." (Vol. III, January 1996): 5.

[318] ———. "Chronotherapy." (Vol. III, April 1996): 2.

[319] ———. "High Blood Pressure." (Vol. III, July 1996): 2.

[320] ———. (Vol. IV, No. 9, May 1997): 4.

[321] ———. "What Is Normal Aging?" (Vol. IV, June 1997): 3.

[322] ———. "Prevention." (Vol. IV, 1997): 2.

[323] ———. "Sciatica." (Vol. V, September 1997): 2.

[324] ———. "Excess Hair." (Vol. V, September 1997): 4.

[325] ———. "By the Way, Doctor." (Vol. V, September 1997): 8.

[326] *Harvard Women's Health Letter*. "A Special Report on Headache" (revised). Boston: Harvard Medical School, Health Pub. Grp. (1999).

[327] *Harvard Women's Health Watch*. "Aging, Memory and the Brain." (Vol. VII, No. 11, July 2000): 1.

[328] ———. "Piriformis Syndrome." (Vol. VIII, No. 7, March 2001): 8.

[329] ———. (Vol. IX, No. 6, February 2002): 7.

[330] ———. "Syncope: What Is It and Why Does It Happen?" (Vol. IX, July 2002): 2.

[331] ———. "Soft-Tissue Knee Injuries in Women." (Vol. IX, July 2002): 4.

[332] ———. "Alcohol and Breast Cancer." (Vol. X, May 2003): 8.

[333] ———. "Antidepressants Protect Brain from Depression-Related Shrinkage." (Vol. XI, No. 2, October 2003): 3.

[334] ———. "Uphill or Down: The Health Benefits of Hiking Depend on Where You're Going." Vol. XII, July 2005): 3.

[335] ———. "Small Vibrations Can Improve Bone, Increase Muscle Mass." Vol. XIII, No. 6, October 2005): 6.

[336] Harvey, J. "Patterns of Response to Stressful Tasks: the Biofeedback Stress Profile." *Research Bulletin of the Himalayan International Institute* 2 (1980): 4.

[337] Haseltine, E. "Your Better Half: How to Tell Which Side of Your Brain Is Controlling Your Life." *Discover* (June 1999): 112.

[338] ———. "Slow Pain Coming."' *Discover* (August 1999): 88.

[339] ———. "Gre-t Exp-ct-ti-ns:- What You See Is Rarely What You Get." *Discover* (September 1999): 107.

[340] ———. "How Your Brain Sees You." *Discover* (September 2000). 104.

[341] ———. "Bending the Truth." *Neuroquest, Discover* (November 2000): 112.

[342] ———. "The Long and Short of Memory." *Neuroquest* (no date).

[343] ———. "Anthropology of the Brain." *Neuroquest* (no date).

[344] ———. "Poltergeists Are Real." *Neuroquest* (no date).

[345] ———. "What Kind of Meat Are You?" *Neuroquest* (no date).

[346] ———. "Your Built-In Steadicam." *Neuroquest* (no date).

[347] ———. "Double Vision." *Discover* (August 2000): 96.

[348] ———. "Face Facts." *Discover* (April 2001): 92.

[349] ———. "Blindsight." *Discover* (July 2002): 92.

[350] ———. "Say Cheese." *Discover* (August 2002): 88.

[351] ———. "One Head, Two Hands." *Discover* (December 2002): 96.

[352] ———. "Seeing Double." *Discover* (February 2003): 88.

[353] ———. "Black and White in Color." *Discover* (April 2003): 88.

[354] ———. "The Joy of Jitters." *Discover* (June 2003): 88.

[355] ———. "Forecast: A Chilly Scorcher." *Discover* (December 2003): 100.

[356] ———. "Depression: Is Stress a Contributing Factor?" *Neuroquest* (no date).

[357] Haslock, I., R. Monro, R. Nagarathna, H. R.

Nagendra, and N. V. Raghuram. "Measuring the Effects of Yoga in Rheumatoid Arthritis." *British Journal of Rheumatology* 33 (1994): 788.

[358] Hechtel, S. "Cruel to Be Kind." *New Scientist* (March 17, 2001): 43.

[359] Hedstrom, J. "A Note on Eye Movements and Relaxation." *Journal of Behavioral Therapy and Experimental Psychiatry* 22 (1991): 37.

[360] Heimer, L. *The Human Brain and Spinal Cord* (2nd. ed.). New York: Springer-Verlag (1995).

[361] Helmuth, L. "Slow Motion Sets in When the Lights Dim." *Science News* 155 (1999): 228.

[362] ———. "Neural Teamwork May Compensate for Aging" *Science News* 155 (1999): 247.

[364] Herbert, R. "Spirited Stuff." *New Scientist* (February 1, 2003): 45.

[365] Hermann, N. "Sciam Asks the Experts: Is it True that Creativity Resides in the Right Hemisphere of the Brain?" (no date).

[366] ———. "Sciam Asks the Experts: What is the Function of the Various Brainwaves?" (no date).

[367] Herz, R. S., C. McCall, and L. Cahill. "Hemispheric Lateralization in the Processing of Odor Pleasantness versus Odor Names." *Chemical Senses* 24 (1999): 691.

[368] Hilgard, E. R. "Illusion That the Eye-Roll Sign Is Related to Hypnotizability." *Archives of General Psychiatry* 39 (1982): 963.

[369] Hilgetag, C. C. "Learning from Switched-off Brains." *Scientific American Mind* 14 (2004): 8.

[370] Hively, W. "Is Radiation Good for You?" *Discover* (December 2002): 74; and www.belleonline.com.

[371] Hoenig, J. "Medical Research on Yoga." *Confinia Psychiatrica* 11 (1968): 69.

[372] Hoffman, K., and J. Clarke. "A Comparative Study of the Cardiac Response to Bhastrika." *Research Bulletin of the Himalayan International Institute* 4 (1982): 7; *Journal of the International Association of Yoga Therapists* 7 (1997): 35.

[373] Hoffman, K. "Moving with the Current: Observations on Nostril Dominance." *Yoga International* (Sep/Oct 1993): 10.

[374] ———. "Nostril Dominance: Experiencing Subtle Energy." *Yoga International* (reprint series, 1995): 10.

[375] Hogan, J. "Eye Can See Better When It's Noisy." *New Scientist* (June 7, 2003): 20.

[376] ———. "Is This the Way to Keep Skin Young and Beautiful?" *New Scientist* (March 26, 2005): 15.

[377] Holloway, M. "The Mutable Brain." *Scientific American* (September 2003): 79.

[378] Holmes, B. "Fanning the Flames." *New Scientist* (May 22, 2004): 41.

[379] Hooper, R. "Satisfaction Not Guaranteed." *New Scientist* (June 2005): 6.

[380] ———. "Chronic Fatigue Is Not All in the Mind." *New Scientist* (July 23, 2005): 9.

[381] Hrushesky, W. J. "Cancer Chronotherapy: Is There a Right Time in the Day to Treat?" *Journal of Infusional Chemotherapy* 5 (1995): 38.

[382] Hubel, D. H., and T. N. Weisel. "Brain Mechanisms of Vision." *Scientific American* (September 1979): 150.

[383] Hubel, D. H. *Eye, Brain and Vision*. New York: Sci. Am. Lib. (1995).

[384] Hummel, T., P. Mohammadian, and G. Kobal. "Handedness Is a Determining Factor in Lateralized Olfactory Discrimination." *Chemical Senses* 23 (1998): 541.

[385] Hymes, A., and P. Nuernberger. "Breathing Patterns Found in Heart Attack Patients." *Research Bulletin of the Himalayan International Institute* 2 (1980): 1.

[386] Imms, F. J., F. Russo, V. I. Iyawe VI, and M. B. Segal. "Cerebral Blood Flow Velocity During and After Sustained Isometric Skeletal Muscle Contractions in Man." *Clinical Science (London)* (April 1994): 353.

[387] Ingber, D. E. "The Architecture of Life." *Scientific American* (January 1998): 48.

[387a] Ireland, T. "Noise Control." *Yoga Journal* (Mar/Apr 2002): 36.

[388] Iyengar, B. K. S. *Light on Yoga*. New York: Schocken (1966).

[389] ———. *Body the Shrine, Yoga Thy Light*. B. I. Taraporewala (1978).

[390] ———. In *Iyengar, His Life and Work*, M. Manos (ed.). Porthill, Ida.: Timeless Books (1987).

[391] ———. *The Tree of Yoga*. Oxford: Fine Line Books (1988).

[392] ———. "Chakras, Bandhas and Kriyas," *Iyengar Yoga Institute Review* 9 (1989): 1.

[393] ———. *The Art of Yoga*. New Delhi: HarperCollins (1993).

[394] ———. *Light on Pranayama*. New York: Crossroad Pub. Co. (1999).

[395] ———. In *Yogadhara*. Mombai: Light on Yoga Research Trust (2000).

[396] ———. *Astadala Yogamala*, vol. 1. New Delhi:

Allied Pub. (2000).

[398] ———. *Yoga: The Path to Holistic Health.* London: Dorling Kindersley (2001).

[399] ———. "The Meeting Point of Ancient Wisdom and Modern Science," in *Astadala Yogamala*, vol. 3. New Delhi: Allied Pub. (2002).

[400] ———. "Guidelines on Asanas for Teachers," in *Astadala Yogamala*, vol. 3. New Delhi: Allied Pub. (2002): 218.

[401] ———. *Light on the Yoga Sutras of Patanjali.* London: Thorsons (2002).

[402] ———. Personal communication to Rajvi Mehta (2003).

[403] ———. "Guruji on His First Public Classes in the West." *Yoga Rahasya* 12 (2005): 3.

[404] Iyengar, G. S. *Yoga, A Gem for Women.* Palo Alto: Timeless Books (1990).

[405] ———. "Effect of Inverted Yoga Postures on Menstruation and Pregnancy." *Yoga Rahasya* 4 (1997): 29.

[406] ———. "Clearing Doubts about Yoga Practice during Menstruation." *Yoga Rahasya* 10 (2003): 51.

[407] Iyengar, P. *Yoga Samachar.* (2005).

[408] ———. "A 'Class' after a Class." *Supplement to Yoga Rahasya.* (January 2000).

[409] ———. "Anatomy and Physiology through the Prism of Yoga" (audiotape). Iyengar Yoga Institute (2003).

[410] ———. "Shiva Svarodaya." *Yoga Rahasya* 12 (2005): 19.

[410a] Janisse, M. "Correcting Movement Imbalances with Yoga Therapy." *International Journal of Yoga Therapy* 11 (2001): 15.

[411] Jarvelainen, J., M. Schurmann, S. Avikainen, and R. Hari. "Stronger Reactivity of the Human Primary Motor Cortex During Observation of Live Rather Than Video Motor Acts." *Neuroimage* 23 (2004): 187.

[412] Jella, S. A., and D. S. Shannahoff-Khalsa. "The Effects of Unilateral Forced Nostril Breathing on Cognitive Performance." *International Journal of Neuroscience* 73 (1993): 61.

[413] Johnsen, L. "Breathing Secrets from the Shiva Svarodaya." *Yoga International* (Dec/Jan 2005): 64.

[414] Johnsen, S. "Transparent Animals." *Scientific American* (February 2000): 81.

[415] Johnson, B. E. *Adult Rheumatic Disease* (monograph, ed. 216, Home Study Self-Assessment Program). Kansas City, Missouri:

American Academy of Family Physicians (July 1997).

[416] Johnson, D. B., M. J. Tierney, and P. J. Sadighi. "Kapalbhati Pranayama: Breath of Fire Or Cause of Pneumothorax?: A Case Report." *Chest* 125 (2004): 1951.

[417] Johnson, E. "The Laughter Circuit." *Discover* (May 2002): 24.

[418] Johnson, S. "Fear." *Discover* (March 2003): 33.

[419] ———. "Laughter." *Discover* (April 2003): 62.

[420] Jones, N. "Soothing the Inflamed Brain." *Scientific American* (June 2000): 24.

[421] Jones, S. W., R. J. Hill, P. A. Krasney, B. O'Connor, N. Pierce, and P. L. Greenhaff. "Disuse Atrophy and Exercise Rehabilitation in Humans Profoundly Affects the Expression of Genes Associated with the Regulation of Skeletal Muscle Mass." *The Federation of Societies of Experimental Biology Journal.* 18 (2004): 1025.

[422] Juhan, D. *Job's Body: A Handbook for Bodywork.* Barrytown, NY: Station Hill Press (1987).

[423] Jung, C. G. *Collected Works, Vol. 17.* Princeton University Press (1954): 52.

[424] Kakigi, R., H. Nakano, K. Inui, N. Hiroe, O. Nagata, M. Honda, S. Tanaka, N. Sadato, and M. Kawakami. "Intracerebral Pain Processing in a Yoga Master Who Claims Not to Feel Pain during Meditation." *European Journal of Pain* 9 (2005): 581.

[425] Kamei, T., Y. Toriumi, H. Kimura, S. Ohno, H. Kumano, and K. Kimura. "Decrease in Serum Cortisol During Yoga Exercise Is Correlated with Alpha Wave Activation." *Perceptual and Motor Skills* 90 (2000): 1027.

[426] Kandel, E. "Small Systems of Neurons." *Scientific American* (September 1979): 67.

[427] Kandel, E. R., J. H. Schwartz, and T. M. Jessell. *Principles of Neural Science* (third ed.). Norwalk, Conn.: Appleton and Lange (1991).

[427a] Kandel, E. R. *In Search of Memory.* New York: W. W. Norton (2006).

[428] Kapandji, I. A. *The Physiology of the Joints: The Trunk and the Vertebral Column* (vol. III, second ed.) Edinburgh: Churchill, Livingstone (1974).

[429] ———. *The Physiology of the Joints: Upper Limb* (vol. I) Edinburgh: Churchill, Livingstone (1982).

[430] ———. *The Physiology of the Joints: Lower Limb* (vol. II, fifth ed.) Edinburgh: Churchill, Livingstone (1987).

[431] Kapit, W., and L. M. Elson. *The Anatomy*

Coloring Book. New York: HarperCollins (1977).

[432] Kapit, W., R. I. Macey, and E. Meisami. *The Physiology Coloring Book*. Menlo Park, CA: Addison Wesley (1987).

[433] Karandicar, S. V. *Yoga Therapy in Spinal Disorders*. Pune, India: private publication.

[434] Kasai, Y., K. Takegami, and A. Uchida. "Change of Barometric Pressure Influences on Low Back Patients with Vacuum Phenomenon within Lumbar Intervertebral Disc." *Journal of Spinal Disorders and Techniques* 15 (2002): 290.

[435] Kathotia, M. L. *Color Therapy for Common Diseases*. Delhi: Hind Pocket Books (1996).

[435a] Katz, S. "Rebuttal to a Surgeon's Warnings." *International Journal of Yoga Therapy* 13 (2003): 43.

[436] Keen, S. "Fear in the Belly." *Yoga Journal* (May/Jun 1999): 58.

[437] Keller, D. "Reconcilable Differences." *Yoga Journal* (Nov/Dec 1999): 104.

[438a] Keil, D. www.yoganatomy.com.

[439] Keizer, G. "Sound and Fury," in *The Best American Science and Nature Writing, 2002*, N. Angier (ed.). Boston: Houghton Mifflin (2002).

[440] Kennedy, B., M. G. Zeigler, and D. S. Shannahoff-Khalsa. "Alternating Lateralization of Plasma Catecholamines and Nasal Patency in Humans." *Life Sciences* 38 (1986): 1203.

[441] Kerrigan, D. C., M. K. Todd, and P. O. Riley. "Knee Osteoarthritis and High-Heeled Shoes." *Lancet* 351 (1998): 1399.

[442] Kiley, E. Private communication (2006) and www.scoliyogi.com.

[443] Kilham, C. "Nada Yoga: Sound Current Meditation." *Yoga Journal* (Sep/Oct 1981): 47.

[444] Kilmurray, A. "Studying with Dona Holleman." *Institute for Yoga Teacher Education* 3 (1982): 1.

[445] ———. "Gravity, Newton's Third Law and Asana." *American Yoga Newsletter* 1 (1983): 5.

[446] ———. "The Safe Practice of Inversions." *Yoga Journal* (Nov/Dec 1983): 24.

[447] ———. "Understanding Twists." *Yoga Journal* (Sep/Oct 1984): 31.

[448] ———. "Sarvangasana." *Yoga Journal* (Sep/Oct 1990): 33.

[449] ———. "Urdhva Dhanurasana." *Yoga Journal* (Nov/Dec 1990): 30.

[450] Kimball, J. www.ultranet.com

[451] Kimura, D. "The Asymmetry of the Human Brain." *Scientific American* 228 (1973): 70.

[452] King, R. *Michelangelo and the Pope's Ceiling*. New York: Walker (2003).

[453] Kingsland, J. "Colour-Coded Cures." *New Scientist* (June 2005): 42.

[453a] Kirsch, I., and D. Antonuccio. "Meaningful Advantages of Antidepressants Are Lacking." *Psychiatric Times* 19 (2002).

[455] Klein, A. C., and D. Sobel. *Backache Relief*. New York: Times Books (1985).

[456] Klein, R., and R. Armitage. "Rhythms in Human Performance: 1½ Hour Oscillations in Cognitive Style." *Science* 204 (1979): 1326.

[457] Kleiser, R., R. J. Seitz, and B. Krekelberg. "Neural Correlates of Saccadic Suppression in Humans." *Current Biology* 14 (2004): 386.

[458] Koch-Weser, J. "Sympathetic Activity in Essential Hypertension." *New England Journal of Medicine* 288 (1973): 627.

[459] Kolasinski, S. L., M. Garfinkel, A. G. Tsai, W. Matz, A. V. Dyke, and H. R. Schumacher. "Iyengar Yoga for Treating Symptoms of Osteoarthritis of the Knees: A Pilot Study." *Journal of Alternative and Complementary Medicine* 11 (2005): 689.

[460] Komisaruk, B. R., B. Whipple, A. Crawford, W. C. Liu, A. Kalnin, and K. Mosier. "Brain Activation During Vaginocervical Self-Stimulation and Orgasm in Women with Complete Spinal Cord Injury: fMRI Evidence of Mediation by the Vagus Nerves." *Brain Research* 1024 (2004): 77.

[461] Konar, D., R. Latha, and J. S. Bhuvaneswaran. "Cardiovascular Responses to Head-Down Body-Up Postural Exercise (Sarvangasana)." *Indian Journal of Physiology and Pharmacology* 44 (2000): 392.

[462] Kosinski, R. J. biae.clemson.edu.

[463] Kothari, L. K., and O. P. Gupta. "The Yogic Claim of Voluntary Control over the Heart Beat: An Unusual Demonstration." *American Heart Journal* 86 (1973): 282.

[464] Kozak, S. S. *Yoga International* (Jun/Jul 2001): 14.

[465] Kraft, M., and R. J. Martin. "Chronobiology and Chronotherapy in Medicine." *Disease of the Month* 41 (1995): 501.

[466] Kraft, U. "Unleashing Creativity." *Scientific American Mind* 16 (2005): 17.

[467] Kramer, J. *The Passionate Mind*. Millbrae, CA: Celestial Arts (1974).

[468] Krishna, G. *The Awakening of Kundalini*. New

York: Dutton (1975).

[469] Kumar, P. *Yoga International* (Sep/Oct 1993): 34.

[470] Kurian, G., N. K. Sharma, and K. Santhakumari. "Left Arm Dominance in Active Arm Positioning." *Perception and Motor Skills* 68 (1989): 1312.

[471] Kurz, T. *Stretching Scientifically*. Island Pond, Vermont.: Stadion (1994).

[472] Lacroix, J. M., and A. H. Gowen. "The Acquisition of Autonomic Control through Biofeedback: Some Tests of Discrimination Theory." *Psychophysiology* 18 (1981): 559.

[473] Lad, V. *Ayurveda, The Science of Self-Healing*. Wilmot, Wisconsin: Lotus Light (1984).

[474] Lamberg, L. "Dawn's Early Light to Twilight's Last Gleaming." *Journal of the American Medical Association* 280 (1998): 1556.

[475] Landsberg, H. E. *Weather and Health*. Garden City, NY: Doubleday (1969).

[476] Lane, D. "Dark Angel." *New Scientist* (December 2004): 38.

[477] Lasater, J. "Eka Pada Sarvangasana." *Yoga Journal* (Sep/Oct 1981): 48.

[478] ———. "Understanding the Neck." *Institute for Yoga Teacher Education* 1 (1981): 1.

[479] ———. "Yoga and the Pregnant Woman," *Institute for Yoga Teacher Education Review* 2 (1981): 7.

[480] ———. "Sarvangasana." *Yoga Journal* (Jan/Feb 1982): 49.

[481] ———. "Muscle Tension and Breech Presentation." *Institute for Yoga Teacher Education Review* 3 (1982): 15.

[482] ———. "Posture and its Effects." *Institute for Yoga Teacher Education Review* 3 (1982): 7.

[483] ———. "The Plough: Good or Bad?" *Yoga Journal* (Jan/Feb 1983): 7.

[484] ———. "Asana: Handstand." *Yoga Journal* (Jul/Aug 1983): 7.

[485] ———. "Salamba Sirsasana." *Yoga Journal* (Jul/Aug 1984): 15.

[486] ———. "Headstand, Part Two." *Yoga Journal* (Sep/Oct 1984): 13.

[487] ———. "Incorporating Backbends into Your Practice." *Yoga Journal* (Nov/Dec 1986): 41.

[488] ———. "Touching: The Essence of Non-Verbal Communication." *Institute for Yoga Teacher Education Review* (Summer 1989): 16.

[489] ———. "Healthy Backbends." *Yoga Journal* (May/Jun 1991): 14.

[490] Lasater, J. H. "Yoga for the Overly Flexible." *Yoga Journal* (Jan/Feb 1993): 6.

[491] Lasater, J. *Relax and Renew*. Berkeley: Rodmell Press (1995).

[491a] ———. "Restorative Yoga." *Journal of the International Association of Yoga Therapists* 7 (1997): 22.

[492] ———. "Stability Revisited: Realigning the Sacrum in Asana." *Yoga International* (Apr/May 1999): 43.

[493] ———. "Breathing Lessons." *Yoga Journal* (May/Jun 1999): 104.

[494] ———. "Heading Off Headaches." *Yoga International* (Aug/Sep 1999): 51.

[495] ———. "Saving Your Neck: The Cervical Spine in Yoga Poses." *Yoga International* (Oct/Nov 1999): 47.

[496] ———. "Inversions?" *Yoga International* (Jun/Jul 2000): 10.

[497] ———. "Sit Up and Take Note." *Yoga Journal* (Jul/Aug 2000): 74.

[498] ———. "Building Strength." *Yoga International* (Dec/Jan 2000): 56.

[499] ———. *Yoga Journal* (Jan/Feb 2003): 103.

[500] Lawton, G. "To Sleep, Perchance to Dream." *New Scientist* (June 28, 2003): 28.

[500a] ———. "Go For the Burn." *New Scientist* (June 3, 2006): 36.

[501] Leclerc, J., W. J. Doyle, and W. J. Karnavas. "The Relationship Between the Nasal Cycle and Axillary Sweat Production." *Rhinology* 25 (1987): 249.

[502] Lee, J. "Metabolic Powerhouse." *New Scientist* (Life Sci., No. 135, November 11, 2000): 1.

[503] Lee, S., and G. Walsh. "Let it Flow." *Yoga Journal* (May/Jun 2003): 14.

[504] Lemley, B. "Isn't She Lovely." *Discover* (February 2000): 42.

[505] Le Page, M. "Women's Orgasms Are a Turn Off for the Brain." *New Scientist* (June 25, 2005): 14.

[506] Lepicovska, V., C. Dostalek, and M. Kovarova. "Hathayogic Exercise Jalandharabandha in its Effect on Cardiovascular Response to Apnoea." *Activitas Nervosa Superior* 32 (1990): 99.

[507] Leskowitz, E. "The Third Eye: A Psychoendocrine Model of Hypnotizability." *American Journal of Clinical Hypnosis.* 30 (1988): 209.

[508] ———. "Seasonal Affective Disorder and the Yoga Paradigm: A Reconsideration of the Role

of the Pineal Gland." *Medical Hypotheses* 33 (1990): 155.

[509] Leslie, K. R., S. H. Johnson-Frey, and S. T. Grafton. "Functional Imaging of Face and Hand Imitation: Towards a Motor Theory of Empathy." *Neuroimage* 21 (2004): 601.

[510] Levi, F. "Biological Rhythms." *Annales Cardiologie et d'Angiologie* 46 (1997): 426.

[511] Levy, A. R. "A New Attitude about Asthma." *Yoga Journal* (Sep/Oct 2002): 35.

[512] Libby, P. "Atherosclerosis: The New View." *Scientific American Special* 14 (2004): 50.

[513] Liberman, J. *Light: Medicine of the Future.* Santa Fe, NM: Bear and Co. (1991).

[514] Lindsley, D. B., and W. H. Sassaman. "Autonomic Activity and Brain Potentials Associated with 'Voluntary' Control of the Pilomotors." *Journal of Neurophysiology* 1 (1938): 342.

[515] Lipinski, B. "Biological Significance of Piezoelectricity in Relation to Acupuncture, Hatha Yoga, Osteopathic Medicine and Action of Air Ions." *Medical Hypotheses* 3 (1977): 9.

[516] Lipson, E. "Yoga Works!" *Yoga Journal* (Winter 1999): 6.

[516a] Lisbet, B. *Mind Time: The Temporal Factor in Consciousness.* Boston: Harvard University Press (2004).

[517] Little, T. Personal communication (2002).

[518] ———. "Fluidity and Form." *Yoga International* (September 2003): 90.

[519] Logothetis, N. K. "Vision: A Window on Consciousness." *Scientific American* (November 1999): 69.

[520] Lorch, I. "Total Vision." *East West* (April 1990): 49.

[521] Lovett, R. "Beat the Clock." *New Scientist* (April 6, 2002): 30.

[522] ———. "Get Up, Get Out of Bed." *New Scientist* (August 20, 2005): 52.

[523] Lucentini, J. "Nod Yourself to Certainty." *Discover* (November 2003): 13.

[524] Lufkin, E. G., and M. Zilkoski. *Diagnosis and Management of Osteoporosis.* American Family Physician, Monograph No. 1 (1996).

[525] Luskin, F. M., K. A. Newell, M. Griffith, F. F. Marvasti, M. Hill, K. R. Pelletier, and W. L. Haskell. "A Review of Mind/Body Therapies in the Treatment of Musculoskeletal Disorders with Implications for the Elderly." *Alternative Therapies* 6 (2000): 46.

[526] Lutz, E. G. "Credit-Card Wallet Sciatica." *Journal of the American Medical Association* 240 (1978): 738.

[527] Lye, M. "Rhythm of Life and Vicissitudes of Old Age." *Lancet* 353 (1999): 1461.

[528] Macey, R. I. *Human Physiology.* Englewood Cliffs, NJ: Prentice-Hall (1968).

[529] Mackinnon, L. *Advances in Exercise Immunology.* Champaign, IL: Human Kinetics (1999).

[530] Macleod, M. "Why Red Is the Colour If Winning Is the Game." *New Scientist* (May 21, 2005): 16.

[531] MacMullen, J. "Yoga and the Menstrual Cycle." *Yoga Journal* (Jan/Feb 1990): 65.

[532] Malathi, A., and V. G. Parulkar. "Effect of Yogasanas on the Visual and Auditory Reaction Time." *Indian Journal of Physiology and Pharmacology* 33 (1989): 110.

[533] Manjunath, N. K., and S. Telles. "Factors Influencing Changes in Tweezer Dexterity Scores Following Yoga Training." *Indian Journal of Physiology and Pharmacology* 43 (1999): 225.

[533a] ———. "Improved Performance in the Tower of London Test Following Yoga." *Indian Journal of Physiology and Pharmacology* 45 (2001): 351.

[534] ———. "Effects of Sirsasana Practice on Autonomic and Respiratory Variables." *Indian Journal of Physiology and Pharmacology* 47 (2003): 34.

[535] Manjunatha, S., R. P. Vempati, D. Ghosh, and R. L. Bijlani. "An Investigation into the Acute and Long-Term Effects of Selected Yogic Postures on Fasting and Postprandial Glycemia and Insulinemia in Healthy Young Subjects." *Indian Journal of Physiology and Pharmacology* 49 (2005): 319.

[536] Maquet, P. "The Role of Sleep in Learning and Memory." *Science* 294 (2001): 1048.

[537] Marchant, J. "Reading Your Mind." *New Scientist* (August 12, 2000): 20.

[538] Margo, C. E., J. Rowda, and J. Barletta. "Bilateral Conjunctival Varix Thromboses Associated with Habitual Headstanding." *American Journal of Ophthalmology* 113 (1992): 726.

[539] Marieb, E. N. *Human Anatomy and Physiology.* New York: Benjamin/Cummings (1992).

[540] Marks, P. "Blast from the Past." *New Scientist* (February 19, 2000): 11.

[541] Martindale, D. "The Body Electric." *New*

Scientist (May 15, 2004): 38.

[542] Mason, B. "Sweet Smells Banish Pain." *New Scientist* (June 2002): 14.

[543] Massimini, M., F. Ferrarelli, R. Huber, S. K. Esser, H. Singh, and G. Tononi. "Breakdown of Cortical Effective Connectivity During Sleep." *Science* 309 (2005): 2228.

[544] Matthews, G. G. *Cellular Physiology of Nerve and Muscle* (third ed.). Oxford: Blackwell (1998).

[545] Matthews, R. "Death by Crucifixion." *New Scientist* (January 23, 2000).

[546] Mattio, T. G., T. Nishida, and M. M. Minieka. "Lotus Neuropathy: Report of a Case." *Neurology* 42 (1992): 1636.

[547] McCall, T. "Western Science vs. Eastern Wisdom." *Yoga Journal* (Jan/Feb 2003): 88.

[548] ———. "Upside Downside." *Yoga Journal* (Sep/Oct 2003): 34.

[549] McComas, A. J. *Skeletal Muscle: Form and Function*. Champaign, IL: Human Kinetics (1996).

[550] McCraty, R., M. Atkinson, and D. Tomasino. "Science of the Heart: Exploring the Role of the Heart in Human Performance." California: Heartmath Research Center (www. Heartmathstore.com)

[550a] McCraty, R. "The Energetic Heart: Bioelectrical Communication within and between People," in *Clinical Applications of Bioelectromagnetic Medicine*, P. J. Rosch and M. S. Markov (eds.). New York: Dekker (2004).

[551] McCrone, J. "Rebels with a Cause." *New Scientist* (January 22, 2000): 22.

[552] ———. "Not-So Total Recall." *New Scientist* (May 13, 2003): 26.

[553] McDonald, J. W. "Repairing the Damaged Spinal Cord." *Scientific American* (September 1999): 65.

[554] McDougal, H. "Wide-Angled Vision." *New Scientist* (May 17, 2003): 24.

[555] McDougal, J. in B. Baptiste and K. F. Mendola, "Rx for Runner's Cramps." *Yoga Journal* (Mar/Apr 1999): 36.

[556] McLanahan, S. A. *Yoga Journal* (Mar/Apr 2001): 17.

[557] Mehta, R. H. "Our Digestive System." *Yoga Rahasya* 2 (1995): 157.

[557a] ———. "Understanding Yoga Therapy." *International Joournal of Yoga Therapy* 12 (2002): 5.

[558] ———. Personal communication from B. K. S. Iyengar (2003).

[559] Mehta, S., M. Mehta, and S. Mehta. *Yoga the Iyengar Way*. New York: Knopf (1997).

[560] Melton, L. "Age Breakers." *Scientific American* (July 2000): 16.

[561] ———. "His Pain, Her Pain." *New Scientist* (January 19, 2002): 32.

[561a] ———. "Aching Atrophy." *Scientific American* (January 2004): 22.

[562] Melzack, R., and P. D. Wall. *The Challenge of Pain*. New York: Basic Books (1983).

[563] Mendenhall, K. Personal communication (2003).

[564] Menon, S. "The Way the Cortex Crumples." *Discover* (June 1997).

[565] *The Merck Manual of Diagnosis and Treatment*. Merck, Sharp and Dohme Res. Labs (1966).

[566] Meyers, B. "Sequence for Depression." *Iyengar Yoga Association of Greater New York Newsletter* (Spring 1994): 15.

[567] Michels, P. J. *Anxiety*. American Academy of Family Physicians, Monograph No. 212, Home Study Self-Assessment Program (January 1997).

[567a] Middlekauff, H. R., J. L. Yu, and K. Hui. "Acupuncture Effects on Reflex Responses to Mental Stress in Humans." *American Journal of Physical, Regulatory, Integrative and Comparative Physiology* 280 (2001): R1462.

[568] Milius, E. "Using One's Head." *Science News* 167 (2005): 389.

[569] Miller, A. I. "A Thing of Beauty." *New Scientist* (February 24, 2006): 50.

[570] Miller, E. B. "Yoga for Scoliosis." *Yoga Journal* (May/Jun 1990): 66.

[571] ———. "Yoga for Teens with Scoliosis." *Yoga Samachar* (vol. 7, no. 2, 2003): 11.

[572] ———. *Yoga for Scoliosis*. Self-published (2003).

[572a] ———. "Back to Back." *Yoga Journal* (May 2006): 74.

[573] Miller, G. "The Dark Side of Glia." *Science* 308 (2005): 778.

[574] Miller, J. *The Body in Question*. New York: Random House (1978).

[575] Miller, J. J., K. Fletcher, and J. Kabat-Zinn. "Three Year Follow-Up and Clinical Implications of a Mindfulness Meditation-Based Stress Reduction Intervention in the Treatment of Anxiety Disorders." *General Hospital Psychiatry* 17 (1995): 192.

[576] Miller, R. C. "The Psychophysiology of

Respiration: Eastern and Western Perspectives." *Journal of the International Association of Yoga Therapists* (vol. 2, no. 1, 1991).

[577] ———. "The Therapeutic Application of Yoga on Sciatica: A Case Study." *Journal of the International Association of Yoga Therapists* 3 (1992): 10.

[578] Minninger, J. *Total Recall.* New York: MJF Books (1984).

[579] Miyamura, M., K. Nishimura, K. Ishida, K. Katayama, M. Shimaoka, and S. Hiruta. "Is Man Able to Breathe Once a Minute for an Hour?: The Effect of Yoga Respiration on Blood Gases." *Japanese Journal of Physiology* 52 (2002): 313.

[579a] Mohan, M. "Nostril Dominance (Svara) and Bilateral Volar Galvanic Skin Response." *International Journal of Yoga Therapy* 9 (1999): 33.

[580] Monro, R., and L. Fitzgerald. "A Scientific Look at Yoga and Diabetes." *Yoga Biomedical Bulletin* 1 (1986): 71.

[581] Monro, R., R. Nagarathna, and H. R. Nagendra. "Yoga Therapy: The Eyes Have It." *Yoga International* (April 1998): 45.

[582] Montagna, W. *Comparative Anatomy.* New York: John Wiley (1959).

[583] Montagu, A. *Touching. The Human Significance of the Skin* (third ed.). New York: Harper and Row (1986).

[584] Moore-Ede, M. C., F. M. Sulzman, and C. A. Fuller. *The Clocks That Time Us.* Cambridge: Harvard Press (1982).

[585] Morris, K. "Meditating in Yogic Science." *Lancet* 351 (1998): 1038.

[586] Mossman, K. "Migraine, Not Sinus." *Scientific American Mind* 17 (2006): 6.

[587] Motiwala, S. N., and R. H. Mehta. "Treating Chronic Ailments with Yoga. Acidity." *Yoga Rahasya* 2 (1995): 28.

[588] ———. "Treating Chronic Ailments with Yoga II (Cervical Spondylosis)." *Yoga Rahasya* 3 (1996): 29.

[589] ———. "Treating Ailments with Yoga IV (Chronic Fatigue Syndrome)," *Yoga Rahasya* 4 (1997): 32.

[590] Motluk, A. "Dicing with Albert." *New Scientist* (March 18, 2000): 43.

[591] ———. "No, No, This Way: Why Men and Women Argue over Which Route to Take." *New Scientist* (March 25, 2000): 13.

[592] Motluk, A., and A. Raine. "Not Guilty." *New Scientist* (May 13, 2000): 42.

[593] Motluk, A. "Fingered." *New Scientist* (June 24, 2000): 32.

[594] ———. "Out of the Mouths of Babes." *New Scientist* (September 7, 2002): 21.

[595] ———. "Sleep with the Boss." *New Scientist* (June 1, 2002): 9.

[596] ———. "Doctor's Dilemma." *New Scientist* (July 10, 2004): 38.

[597] ———. "Seeing without Sight." *New Scientist* (January 29, 2005): 37.

[598] ———. "Particles of Faith." *New Scientist* (January 28, 2006): 34.

[598a] ———. "The Teen Gene." *New Scientist* (July 23, 2006): 34.

[599] Moyer, D. "Sarvangasana." *Yoga Journal* (Sep/Oct 1987): 30.

[600] Muir, H. *New Scientist* (February 23, 2002):15.

[601] Murphy, M., and R. A. White. *The Psychic Side of Sports.* Reading, MA: Addison-Wesley (1978).

[602] Murphy, M. *The Future of the Body.* New York: J. P. Tarcher (1992).

[602a] Murphy, M., and S. J. Ayan. "The Will to Win." *Scientific American Mind* 16 (2005): 64.

[603] Myers, T. W. *Anatomy Trains.* Edinburgh: Churchill, Livingstone (2001).

[604] Nagarathna, R., and H. R. Nagendra. "Yoga for Bronchial Asthma: A Controlled Study." *British Medical Journal* 291 (1985): 172.

[605] Nagarathna, R., H. R. Nagendra, and R. Monro. *Yoga for Common Ailments.* London: Gaia Books (1990).

[606] Nagler, W. "Vertebral Artery Obstruction by Hyperextension of the Neck: Report of Three Cases." *Archives of Physical and Medical Rehabilitation* 54 (1973): 237.

[607] Narendran, S., R. Nagarathna, V. Narendran, S. Gunasheela, and H. R. Nagendra. "Efficiency of Yoga on Pregnancy Outcome." *Journal of Alternative and Complementary Medicine* 11 (2005): 23.

[609] Nemeroff, C. B. "The Neurobiology of Depression." *Scientific American* (June 1998): 42.

[610] Nespor, K. "Psychosomatics of Back Pain and the Use of Yoga." *International Journal of Psychosomatics* 36 (1989): 72.

[611] Nesse, R. M., and G. C. Williams. "Evolution and the Origins of Disease." *Scientific American* (November 1998): 86.

[612] Nestler, E. J., and R. C. Malenka. "The Addicted Brain." *Scientific American* (March

2004): 78.

[613] Netter, F. H. *Atlas of Human Anatomy.* Summit, NJ: Ciba-Geigy Corp. (1989).

[614] Netting, J. "Wink of an Eye." *Scientific American* (May 1999): 26.

[615] Netz, Y., and R. Lidor. "Mood Alteration in Mindful versus Aerobic Exercise Modes." *Journal of Psychology* 137 (2003): 405.

[616] Neurolinguistic Programming website: http://www.nlp.de/research/

[617] Nicholic, M., D. Molnar-Dragojevic, D. Bobinack, S. Bajek, B. Jerkovic, and T Soic-Vranic. "Age Related Skeletal Muscle Atrophy in Humans: An Immunohistochemical and Morphometric Study." *Collegium Anthropologium* 25 (2001): 545.

[618] Nieman, D. C. *Fitness and Sports Medicine,* Palo Alto: Bull Publishing (1990).

[619] Norman, R. A., M. E. Norman, and R. Holtz. "Stress Thrombosis." *Osteopathic Medical News* (Apr 1990): 26.

[620] Noveen, K. V., R. Nagarathna, H. R. Nagendra, and S. Telles. "Yoga Breathing through a Particular Nostril Increases Spatial Memory Scores without Lateralizing Effects." *Psychological Reports* 81 (1997): 555.

[621] Novitt-Moreno, A. D. *How the Brain Works,* Emeryville, CA: Ziff-Davis (1955).

[622] Nowak, R. "Life in the Old Dog." *New Scientist* (July 22, 2000): 36.

[623] ———. "Men Behaving Sadly." *New Scientist* (March 2, 2002): 4.

[624] Nuernberger, P. "Effects of Breath Training on Personality Test Scores." *Research Bulletin of the Himalayan International Institute* 3 (1981): 9.

[625] ———. "Stress: A New Perspective." *Research Bulletin of the Himalayan International Institute* 3 (1981): 7.

[626] ———. *Freedom from Stress,* Honesdale, PA: Himalayan International Institute (1981).

[627] Oaklander, A. L., K. Romans, S. Horasek, A. Stokes, P. Hauer, and R. A. Meyer. "Unilateral Post-Therapeutic Neuralgia Is Associated with Bilateral Sensory Neuron Damage." *Annals of Neurology* (November 1998): 789.

[628] Oaklander, A. L., and J. M. Brown. "Unilateral Nerve Injury Produces Bilateral Loss of Distal Innervation." *Annals of Neurology* (May 2004): 639.

[629] O'Brien, C. "Vision Enhances Perception of Touch." *New Scientist* (September 9, 2002): 20.

[630] Ohlson, K. *New Scientist* (October 5, 2002): 44.

[631] Ohsawa, G., and W. Duffy. *You Are All Sanpaku.* New York: Citadel Press (2002).

[632] Olsen, A., and C. McHose. *Body Stories.* Barrytown, NY: Station Hill Press (1991).

[633] Omori, M. "Ask Discover." *Discover* (December 2003): 21.

[634] O'Neill, L. A. J. "Immunity's Early-Warning System." *Scientific American* (January 2005): 38.

[635] Ornstein, R. E. *The Psychology of Consciousness.* New York: Harcourt Brace, Jovanovitch (1977).

[636] Ornstein, R., and C. Swencionis (eds.). *The Healing Brain.* New York: Guilford Press (1990).

[637] Oschman, J. L. *Energy Medicine: The Scientific Basis.* Edinburgh: Churchill, Livingstone (2000).

[638] Ott, J. "Responses of Psychological and Physiological Functions to Environmental Light, Part I." *Journal of Learning Disabilities* 1 (1968): 18.

[639] Overeem, S. G., J. Lammers, and J. G. van Dijk. "Weak with Laughter." *Lancet* 354 (1999): 838.

[640] Pacheco, J. "Red Light, Green Light: Somatics and Yoga." *Yoga International* (Feb/Mar 1999): 17.

[641] Paddon-Jones, D., M. Leveritt, A. Lonergan, P. Abernathy. "Adaptation to Chronic Eccentric Exercise in Humans: The Influence of Contraction Velocity." *Journal of Applied Physiology* 85 (2001): 466.

[641a] Page, S. J., P. Levine, and A. Leonard. "Mental Practice in Chronic Stroke." *Stroke* (April 2007): 1293.

[642] Pain, S. "Dr. Coley's Famous Fever." *New Scientist* (November 12, 2002): 54.

[643] ———. "Super Sopranos." *New Scientist* (March 25, 2006): 52.

[644] Palkhivala, A. Personal communication (1999).

[645] ———. *Yoga Journal* (2002): 40.

[646] ———. "Asana: Parsva Sarvangasana," *Yoga Journal* (Jul/Aug 2003): 110.

[647] Parker Chiropractic Research Foundation. *Chart of Effects of Spinal Misalignment* (1975).

[648] Patel, C., and M. Marmot. "Can General Practitioners Use Training in Relaxation and Management of Stress to Reduce Mild Hypertension?" *British Medical Journal* 296 (1988): 21.

[649] Patterson, E. Personal communication (1999).

[650] Pelling, A. E., S. Sehati, E. B. Gralla, J.

S. Valentine, and J. K. Gimzewski. "Local Nanomechanical Motion of the Cell Wall of Saccharomyces Cerevisiae." *Science* 305 (2004): 1147.

[651] Penfield, W. G., and T. B. Rasmussen. *The Cerebral Cortex of Man: A Clinical Study of Localization of Function.* New York: Macmillan (1950).

[652] Perennou, D. A., B. Amblard, C. LeBlond, and J. Pelissier. "Biased Postural Vertical in Humans with Hemispheric Cerebral Lesions." *Neuroscience Letters* 252 (1998): 75.

[653] Perkowitz, S. "Feeling Is Believing." *New Scientist* (September 1999): 34.

[654] Pert, C. B. *Molecules of Emotion,* Touchstone, NY, 1997.

[655] Peterson, J. "Ten Reasons Why Warming Up Is Important." *Health and Fitness Journal,* (Jan/Feb 1999): 52.

[656] Petty, F. "SciAm Ask the Experts: Is There a Biochemical Test that Accurately Diagnoses Bipolar Disorder?" (no date)

[657] Phillips, H. "Perchance to Learn." *New Scientist* (September 25, 1999): 26.

[658] ———. "The Truth Is in There." *New Scientist* (November 15, 2003): 10.

[659] ———. "The Cell that Makes Us Human." *New Scientist* (June 19, 2004): 32.

[660] *Physicians' Desk Reference,* 51st ed. (1997).

[661] Pickering, T. G. "Why is Hypertension More Common in African Americans?" *Journal of Clinical Hypertension* 3 (2001): 50.

[662] Pierce, M. "Breathing for Modern Life." *Yoga Journal* (Sep/Oct 1998): 104.

[663] Pilkington, K., G. Kirkwood, H. Rampes, and J. Richardson. "Yoga for Depression: The Research Evidence." *Journal of Affective Disorders* 89 : 13.

[664] Pincus, D. J., T. R. Humiston, and R. J. Martin. "Further Studies on the Chronotherapy of Asthma with Inhaled Steroids: The Effect of Dosage Timing on Drug Efficacy." *Journal of Allergy and Clinical Immunology.* 100 (1997): 771.

[665] Pinker, S. *How the Mind Works.* New York: Morton (1997).

[666] ———. "The Blank Slate." *Discover* (October 2002): 33.

[667] Pirisi, A. "Yogis Score High on Happiness." *Yoga Journal* (May/Jun 2000): 33.

[667a] Pizzagalli, D. A., J. B. Nitschke, R. Oakes,

A. M. Hendrick, K. A. Horras, C. L. Larson, H. C. Abercrombie, S. M. Schaefer, J. V. Koger, R. M. Benca, R. D. Pascual-Marqui, and R. J. Davidson. "Brain Electrical Tomography in Depression: the Importance of Symptom Severity, Anxiety and Melancholic Features." *The World of Biological Psychiatry* 52 (2002): 73.

[668] Plocher, D. W. "The Auditory Response to Inverted Posture." *Archive Otolaryngolica.* 111 (1985): 135.

[669] Pohl, M., A. Rosler, I. Sunkeler, H.-J. Braune, W. H. Oertel, and S. Lautenbacher. "Insertion Pain in Needle Electromyography Can Be Reduced by Simultaneous Finger Slapping." *Neurology* 54 (2000): 1201.

[670] Pollack, A. A., and E. H. Wood. "Venous Pressure in the Saphenous Vein at the Ankle in Man During Exercise and Changes in Posture." *Journal of Applied Physiology* 1 (1949): 649.

[671] Ponte, D. J., G. J. Jensen, and B. E. Kent. "A Preliminary Report on the Use of the McKenzie Protocol versus Williams' Protocol in the Treatment of Low-Back Pain." *Journal of Orthopaedic and Sports Physical Therapy* 6 (1984): 130.

[671a] Poritsky, R. *Neuroanatomy: A Functional Atlas of Parts and Pathways.* Philadelphia: Hanley and Belfus (1992).

[672] Prakasha. "Science and Yoga." *Ascent* (Summer 2000): 16.

[673] Priplata, A., J. Niemi, M. Salen, J. Harry, L. A. Lipsitz, and J. J. Collins. "Noise-Enhanced Human Balance Control." *Physical Review Letters* 89 (2002): 238101.

[674] Priplata, A. A., J. B. Niemi, J. D. Harry, L. A. Lipsitz, and J. J. Collins. "Vibrating Insoles and Balance Control in Elderly People." *Lancet* 362 (2003): 1123.

[675] Priplata, A. A., B. L. Patritti, J. B. Niemi, R. Hughes, D. C. Gravelle, L. A. Lipsitz, A. Veves, J. Stein, P. Bonato, and J. J. Collins. "Noise-Enhanced Balance Control in Patients with Diabetes and Patients with Stroke." *Annals of Neurology* 59 (2006): 4.

[676] Provencher, M. T., D. C. Wester, B. L. Gillingham, M. E. Hoffer, and K. R. Gottshall. "Vestibular Dysfunction in Adolescent Idiopathic Scoliosis." *Spinal Connection* 20 (2004): 1.

[677] Rad, S. "Impact of Ethnic Habits on Defecographic Measurements." *Archives of Iranian Medicine* 5 (2002): 115.

[678] Radnot, M. "Effects of Testicular Extirpation upon Intraocular Pressure." *Annals of the New York Academy of Science* 117 (1964): 614.

[679] Raghuraj, P., R. Nagarathna, H. R. Nagendra, and S. Telles. "Pranayama Increases Grip Strength Without Lateralized Effects." *Indian Journal of Physiology and Pharmacology* 41 (1997): 129.

[680] Raghuraj, P., A. G. Ramakrishnan, H. R. Nagendra, and S. Telles. "Effect of Two Selected Yogic Breathing Techniques on Heart Rate Variability." *Indian Journal of Physiology and Pharmacology* 42 (1998): 467.

[680a] Raghuraj, P., and S. Telles. "Improvement in Spatial and Temporal Measures of Visual Perception Following Yoga Training." *Journal of Indian Psychology* 20 (2002): 24.

[681] ———. "Effect of Yoga-Based and Forced Uninostril Breathing on the Autonomic Nervous System." *Perception and Motor Skills* 96 (2003): 79.

[682] ———. "Right Uninostril Yoga Breathing Influences Ipsilateral Components of Middle Latency Auditory Evoked Potentials." *Neurological Sciences* 25 (2004): 274.

[683] Raloff, J. "Medicinal EMF's." *Science News* 156 (1999): 316.

[684] ———. "Step Up to Dense Bones," *Science News* 167 (2005): 270.

[684a] ———. "Light Impacts," *Science News* 169 (2006): 330.

[685] Rama, S., R. Ballentine, and S. Ajaya. *Yoga and Psychotherapy*. Honesdale, PA: Himalayan International Institute (1976).

[686] Rama, S. *Joints and Glands Exercises*. Honesdale, PA: Himalayan International Institute (1977).

[687] Rama, S., R. Ballentine, and A. Hymes. *Science of Breath*. Honesdale, PA: Himalayan International Institute (1979).

[688] Rama, S. "The Science of Prana: Basic Breathing Exercises." *Research Bulletin of the Himalayan International Institute* 2 (1980): 1.

[689] ———. "Pranayama." *Research Bulletin of the Himalayan International Institute* 3 (1981): 1.

[689a] Ramachandran, V. S., and E. M. Hubbard. "Hearing Colors, Tasting Shapes." *Scientific American Mind* 16 (2005): 17.

[690] Ramachandran, V. S., and D. Rogers-Ramachandran. "How Blind Are We?" *Scientific American Mind* 16 (2005): 96.

[691] ———. "Stability of the Visual World." *Scientific American Mind* 17 (2006): 14.

[691a] Ramachandran, V., and L. Oberman. "The Search for Steven." *New Scientist* (May 13, 2006): 48.

[692] Ramamurthi, B. "Yoga: An Explanation and Probable Neurophysiology." *Journal of the Indian Medical Association* 48 (1967): 167.

[693] Raman, K. "Migraine and Yoga." *Yoga Rahasya* 3 (1996): 57.

[694] ———. *A Matter of Health*. Madras: Eastwood Books (1998).

[695] Randerson, J. "Second Sight." *New Scientist* (December 8, 2001): 16.

[696] ———. "Hot Pants." *New Scientist* (April 13, 2002).

[697] ———. "It's the Brain Not the Body That Hits the Wall." *New Scientist* (July 31, 2004): 11.

[698] Rao, S. "Metabolic Cost of Headstand Posture." *Journal of Applied Physiology* 17 (1962): 117.

[699] ———. "Yoga and Autohypnotism." *British Journal of Medical Hypnotism* 17 (1965): 38.

[700] Rattenborg, N. C., S. L. Lima, and C. J. Amlaner. "Half-Awake to the Risk of Predation." *Nature* 397 (1999): 397.

[701] Renner, R. "Nietzsche's Toxicology." *Scientific American* (September 2003): 28.

[702] Restak, R., and D. Mahoney. *The Longevity Strategy: How to Live to 100 Using the Brain-Body Connection*. New York: Wiley (1999).

[703] Rice, R., and R. C. Allen. "Yoga in Glaucoma." *American Journal of Ophthalmology* 100 (1985): 738.

[704] Rist, C. "The Pain in the Brain." *Discover* (March 2000): 57.

[705] Robbins, J. "Wired for Sadness." *Discover* (April 2000): 77.

[706] Robbins, M. W. "Scientists See Yet Another Reason to Go to the Gym." *Discover* (January 2004): 42.

[707] Robb-Nicholson, C. "By the Way, Doctor." *Harvard Women's Health Watch* (vol. 12, July 2005): 8.

[708] Roberts, T. D. M. *Understanding Balance*. London: Chapman and Hall (1995).

[709] Robin, M. *A Physiological Handbook for Teachers of Yogasana* first ed. Tucson: Fenestra Books (2002).

[710] Robin, M. B. "Neuromuscular Transformations as Driven by Yogasana Practice." *Yoga Rahasya* 10

(2003): 86.

[711] Robin, M. "Reconciling Western Science and the Iyengar-Family Approach to Yogasana Practice." *Yoga Rahasya* 10 (2003): 59.

[712] Robin, M. B. Personal experience (1983).

[712a] Robin, M. B., "Gravity and You: Perfect Together," in Yogacharya Commemorative Volume, K. Busia, Ed., Santa Clara, CA, 2007, p. 145.

[713] Rode, G., C. Tiliket, and D. Boisson. "Predominance of Postural Imbalance in Left Hemiparetic Patients." *Scandinavian Journal of Rehabilitative Medicine* 29 (1997): 11.

[714] Rolf, I. P. *Rolfing*. Rochester, VT: Healing Arts Press (1977).

[715] Root-Bernstein, R., and M. Root-Bernstein. *Honey, Mud, Maggots and Other Medical Marvels.* New York: Houghton Mifflin (1998).

[716] Rose, K. J. *The Body in Time*, New York: Wiley (1988).

[717] Rose, M. C. "Can Human Aging Be Postponed?" *Scientific American Special* 14 (2004): 24.

[718] Rosen, C. J. "Restoring Aging Bones." *Scientific American Special* 14 (2004): 70.

[719] Rosen, R. "Imaginary Movements." *Yoga Journal* (Mar/Apr 1998): 79.

[720a] Ross, P. E. "The Expert Mind." *Scientific American* (August 2006): 64.

[721] Rossi, E. L. *The Psychobiology of Mind-Body Healing.* New York: Norton (1986).

[722] Roth, G. "The Quest to Find Consciousness." *Scientific American Mind* 14 (2004): 32.

[723] Rothenberg, B., and O. Rothenberg. *Touch Training for Strength.* Champaign, IL: Human Kinetics (1995).

[724] Rowland, T. G. Personal communication.

[725] Ruiz, F. P. "What Science Can Teach Us About Flexibility." *Yoga Journal* (Mar/Apr 2000): 92.

[726] ———. "Bodhi Building." *Yoga Journal* (Jul/Aug 2000): 84.

[727] ———. "Insight for Sore Eyes." *Yoga Journal* (Sep/Oct 2000): 74.

[728] ———. "Symbolic Gestures." *Yoga Journal* (December 2002): 116.

[729] Ruoslahti, E. "Stretching Is Good for a Cell." *Science* 276 (1997): 1345.

[730] Russell, W. R. "Yoga and the Vertebral Arteries." *British Medical Journal* (March 11, 1972): 685.

[731] Rychner, A. "Getting Out from Under: Asana for Relieving PMS." *Yoga International* (Mar/Apr 1995): 57.

[732] Sabina, A. B., A. L. Williams, H. K. Hill, S. Bansal, G. Chupp, and D. L. Katz. "Yoga Intervention for Adults with Mild-to-Moderate Asthma: A Pilot Study." *Annals of Allergy, Asthma and Immunology* 94 (2005): 543.

[733] Sample, I. "Ultrasound Scans May Disrupt Fetal Brain." *New Scientist* (December 10, 2001): 56.

[734] Samuel, E. "Walking on Shakey Shoes." *New Scientist* (November 12, 2002): 22.

[735] Samuels, N. "Chronotherapy and Traditional Chinese Medicine." *American Journal of Chinese Medicine* 28 (2000): 419.

[736] Sander, E. "Menopause: The Yoga Way." *Yoga Journal* (Jan/Feb 1996): 61.

[737] Saper, R. B., D. M. Eisenberg, R. B. Davis, L. Culpepper, and R. S. Phillips. "Prevalence and Patterns of Adult Yoga Use in the United States: Results of a National Survey." *Alternative Therapies in Health and Medicine* 10 (2004): 44.

[738] Sapolsky, R. M. "Stressed-Out Memories." *Scientific American Mind* 14 (2004): 28.

[739] Sapolsky, R. "Sick of Poverty." *Scientific American* (December 2005): 93.

[740] Sapolsky, R., and J. Cape. *Monkeyluv: And Other Lessons on Our Lives As Animals.* New York: Scribners (2005).

[741] Sarasohn, L. "Honoring the Belly." *Yoga Journal* (Jul/Aug 1993): 76.

[742] Saraswati, S. *The Effects of Yoga on Hypertension* (second ed.). Bihar, India: G. K. Kejriwal (1984).

[743] ———. *Health Benefits of Inverted Asanas* (second ed.). Bihar, India: G. K. Kejriwal (1992).

[744] ———. *Health Benefits of Backward Bending Asanas* (second ed.). Bihar, India: G. K. Kejriwal (1992).

[745] Sarno, J. E. *Healing Back Pain: the Mind-Body Connection.* New York: Warner Books, (1991).

[746] ———. "How to Say No to Back Pain." *Bottom Line/Personal* (June 15 1991): 13.

[747] Satyananda Saraswati, S. *Health Benefits of Forward Bending Asanas*, Bihar, India: Bihar School of Yoga (1992).

[748] Savic, I., and H. Berglund. "Right-Nostril Dominance in Discrimination of Unfamiliar, But Not Familiar Odours." *Chemical Senses* 25 (2000): 517.

[749] Schauss, A. G. "Tranquilizing Effect of Color Reduces Aggressive Behavior and Potential

Violence." *Journal of Orthomolecular Psychiatry* 8 (1979): 218.

[750] Schatz, M. P. "Inversions and Menstruation." *Yoga Journal* (Nov/Dec 1983): 30.

[751] Schatz, M. "Stress and Relaxation: Hypertension and Yoga," *Institute for Yoga Teacher Education Review* (1984): 7.

[752] ———. "Yoga, Circulation and Imagery." *Yoga Journal* (Jan/Feb 1987): 54.

[753] Schatz, M. P. "Yoga, the Mind and Immunity." *Yoga Journal* (Jul/Aug 1987): 42.

[754] ———. "You Can Have Healthy Bones." *Yoga Journal* (Mar/Apr 1988): 43.

[755] ———. "Yoga and Aging." *Yoga Journal* (May/Jun 1990): 58.

[756] ———. *Back Care Basics*. Berkeley: Rodmell Press (1992).

[757] ———. "In a Slump? Unrounding Your Lower Back." *Yoga International* (Oct/Nov 1998): 55.

[758] ———. "A Woman's Balance: Inversions and Menstruation." http://www.iyengar.ch/Deutsch/text_menstruation.htm (August 24, 2000).

[759] Schievink, W. I. "Spontaneous Dissection of the Carotid and Vertebral Arteries." *New England Journal of Medicine* 344 (2001): 898.

[760] Schiff, B. B., and S. A. Rump. "Asymmetrical Hemispheric Activation and Emotion: The Effects of Unilateral Forced Nasal Breathing." *Brain and Cognition* 29 (1995): 217.

[761] Schneider, V. "The Healing Power of Color." *Yoga Journal* (Jan/Feb 1987): 7.

[762] Schueller, G. H. "Thrill or Chill." *New Scientist* (April 29, 2000): 20.

[763] Schulman, P. "Snooze Button." *Discover* (January 1997).

[764] Schultz, R. L., and R. Feitis. *The Endless Web: Fascial Anatomy and Physical Reality*. Berkeley: North Atlantic (1996).

[765] Schumacher, J. "Preparing for Inversions." *Yoga Journal* (Jul/Aug 1990): 68.

[766] ———. "Preparing for Arm Balances." *Yoga Journal* (Jul/Aug 1989): 69.

[767] Scott, E. M., J. P. Greenwood, S. G. Gilbey, J. B. Stoker, and D. A. S. G. Mary. "Water Ingestion Increases Sympathetic Vasoconstrictor Discharge in Normal Human Subjects." *Clinical Science* 100 (2001): 335.

[768] Seibert, C. "The Chakras and Modern Science." *Yoga International* (Sep/Oct 1993): 5.

[769] Selim, J. "Useless Body Parts." *Discover* (June 2004): 42.

[770] Selvamurthy, W., U. S. Ray, K. S. Hegde, and R. P. Sharma. "Physiological Responses to Cold (10° C) in Men after Six Months' Practice of Yoga Exercise." *International Journal of Biometrology* 32 (1988): 188.

[771] Selvamurthy, W., K. Sridharan, U. S. Ray, R. S. Tiwari, K. S. Hegde, U. Radhakrishna, and K. C. Sinha. "A New Physiological Approach to Control of Essential Hypertension." *Indian Journal of Physiology and Pharmacology* 42 (1998): 205.

[772] Selye, H. *The Stress of Life*. New York: McGraw Hill (1956).

[773] Serber, E. "Yoga Cures for Headaches." *Yoga International* (Jan/Feb 1999): 42.

[774] Shankardevananda Saraswati, S. *The Practice of Yoga for the Digestive System*. Bihar, India: Bihar School of Yoga (1987).

[775] Shannahoff-Khalsa, D. S., and B. Kennedy. "The Effects of Unilateral Forced Breathing on the Heart." *International Journal of Neuroscience* 73 (1993): 47.

[776] Shannahoff-Khalsa, D. S., and L. R. Beckett. "Clinical Case Report: Efficacy of Yogic Techniques in the Treatment of Obsessive Compulsive Disorder." *International Journal of Neuroscience* 85 (1996): 1.

[777] Shannahoff-Khalsa, D. S., B. Kennedy, F. E. Yates, and M. G. Ziegler. "Ultradian Rhythms of Autonomic, Cardiovascular and Neuroendocrine Systems Are Related in Humans." *American Journal of Physiology* 270 (1996): R873.

[778] ———. "Low-Frequency Ultradian Insulin Rhythms Are Coupled to Cardiovascular, Autonomic, and Neuroendocrine Rhythms." *American Journal of Physiology* 272 (1997): R962.

[779] Shannahoff-Khalsa, D. S., J. C. Gillin, F. E. Yates, A. Schlosser, and E. M. Zawadzki. "Ultradian Rhythms of Alternating Cerebral Hemispheric EEG Dominance Are Coupled to Rapid Eye Movement and Non-Rapid Eye Movement Stage 4 Sleep in Humans." *Sleep Medicine* 2 (2001): 333.

[780] Shannahoff-Khalsa, D. S., B. B. Sramek, M. B. Kennel, and S. W. Jamieson. "Hemodynamic Observations on a Yogic Breathing Technique Claimed to Help Eliminate and Prevent Heart Attacks: A Pilot Study." *Alternative and Complementary Medicine* 10 (2004): 757.

[781] Shapiro, D., and K. Cline. "Mood Changes Associated with Iyengar Yoga Practice: A Pilot

Study." *International Journal of Yoga Therapy* 14 (2004): 35.

[782] Shepard, N. T. "Normal Operation of the Balance System in Daily Activities," in *The Consumer Handbook on Dizziness/Vertigo,* D. Poe, ed. (2003).

[783] Shepard, R. J. "Aging and Exercise," in *Encyclopedia of Sports Medicine and Science,* T. D. Fahey, ed. Internet Society for Sport Science (1998).

[784] Sherman, D. G., R. G. Hart, and J. D. Easton. "Abrupt Change in Head Position and Cerebral Infarction." *Stroke* 12 (1981): 2.

[785] Shermer, M. "Full of Holes: The Curious Case of Acupuncture." *Scientific American* (August 2005): 30.

[785a] Shimada, K., K. Kario, Y. Umeda, S. Hoshide, Y. Hoshide, and K. Eguchi. "Early Morning Surge in Blood Pressure." *Blood Pressure Monitoring* 6 (2001): 349.

[786] Shipley, T. "Rod-Cone Duplexity and Autonomic Action of Light." *Vision Research* 4 (1964): 155.

[787] Shyam Sundar Goswami. *Hatha-Yoga.* London: L. N. Fowler (1959).

[788] Sieg, K. W., and S. P. Adams. *Illustrated Essentials of Musculoskeletal Anatomy.* Gainsville, FL: Mega Books (1985).

[789] Siegel, J. M. "The REM Sleep-Memory Consolidation Hypothesis." *Science* 294 (2001): 1058.

[790] Sikirov, B. A. "Etiology and Pathogenesis of Diverticulosis Coli: A New Approach." *Medical Hypothyses* 26 (1988): 17.

[790a] Simcox, F. J. "Letter: Sit Well, Hear Better." *New Scientist* (April 13, 2002): 52.

[791] Simon, H. B. "Longevity: The Ultimate Gender Leap." *Scientific American Special* 14 (2004): 18.

[792] Simpson, S. "Pain, Pain, Go Away." *Science News* 155 (2000): 108.

[793] Singer, E. "Exercise Makes the Brain Faster but Not Smarter." *New Scientist* (November 15, 2003): 8.

[794] Singh, V., A. Wisniewski, J. Britton, and A. Tattersfield. "Effect of Yoga Breathing Exercises (Pranayama) on Airway Reactivity in Subjects with Asthma." *Lancet* 335 (1990): 1381.

[795] Sinha, B., U. S. Ray, A. Pathak, and W. Selvamurthy. "Energy Cost and Cardiorespiratory Changes During the Practice of Surya Namaskar." *Indian Journal of Physiology and Pharmacology* 48 (2004): 184.

[797] Sjoman, N. E. *The Yoga Tradition of the Mysore Palace.* New Delhi: Abhinav Press (1996).

[798] Slauenwhite, D., and T. Leslie. "Starry Eyes." *New Scientist* (March 18, 2000): 97.

[799] Slede, L., and R. Pomerantz. "Yoga and Psychotherapy: A Review of the Literature." *International Journal of Yoga Therapy* 11 (2001): 61.

[800] Smith, B. *Yoga for a New Age.* Englewood Cliffs, NJ: Prentice-Hall (1982).

[801] Smith, C. U. M. *The Brain: Towards an Understanding.* New York: Capricorn (1972).

[802] Smith, R. "The Timing of Birth." *Scientific American* (March 1999):68.

[803] Smolensky, M., and L. Lamberg. *The Body Clock Guide to Better Health.* New York: H. Holt (2000).

[804] Smolensky, M. H., and F. Portaluppi. "Chronopharmaology and Chronotherapy of Cardiovascular Medications: Relevance to Prevention and Treatment of Coronary Heart Disease." *American Heart Journal* 137 (1999): S14.

[805] Snyder, P. J. "Effects of Age on Testicular Function and Consequences of Testosterone Treatment." *Journal of Clinical Endocrinology and Metabolism* 86 (2001): 2369.

[806] Snyder, S. H. "The Molecular Basis of Communication Between Cells." *Scientific American* (October 1985): 132.

[807] Sobel, N., R. M. Khan, A. Saltman, E. V. Sullivan, and J. D. E. Gabrieli. "The World Smells Different to Each Nostril." *Nature* 402 (1999): 35.

[808] Sovik, R. "Keep Your Nose Clean." *Yoga International* (Feb/Mar 1998): 61.

[809] ———. "Energy Rising: How to Establish Sushumna." *Yoga International* (Feb/Mar 1999): 57.

[810] ———. "Breathing Through Emotions." *Yoga International* (Feb/Mar 2000): 61.

[811] ———. "Learning to Exhale: The 2-to-1 Breath." *Yoga International* (Feb/Mar 2003): 52.

[812] ———. "Simply Sitting." *Yoga International* (Dec/Jan 2003): 46.

[813] ———. "Cultivating a Joyous Mind" *Yoga International* (Apr/May 2005): 42.

[814] Sparrowe, L. "Menstrual Essentials." *Yoga Journal* (Sep/Oct 1999): 74.

[815] Spicuzza, L., A. Gabutti, C. Porta, and N. Montano. " Yoga and Chemoreflex Response to Hypoxia and Hypercapnia." *Lancet* 356 (2000): 1495.

[816] Spiessbach, K. "Exercising the Brain." *Discover* (January 1997).

[817] Spinney, L. "Thought Control." *New Scientist* (March 3, 2001): 36.

[818] ———. "Taken at Face Value." *New Scientist* (March 24, 2001): 56.

[819] ———. "Get It Off Your Chest." *New Scientist* (November 9, 2002): 34.

[820] ———. "Signaling Right from the Womb." *New Scientist* (July 24, 2004): 13.

[821] Stark, J. "Change Your Posture, Change Your Mood." *Yoga Journal* (Jul/Aug 2002): 78.

[822] Stark, S. D. *The Stark Reality of Stretching.* Self-published (1997).

[823] Stefanick, M. "Effects of Inverted Poses on Cardiovascular Physiology." *Institute for Yoga Teacher Education Review* 3 (1983): 1.

[824] Stein, D. *The Women's Book of Healing.* St. Paul, Minn.: Llewellyn (1996).

[825] Steinberg, L. *Iyengar Yoga Therapeutics: The Knee.* Urbana, Ill.: Parvati Productions, Ltd. (August 2000).

[826] Stephan, K., and G. Iyengar. "A Visit with Geeta Iyengar." *Iyengar Yoga Association of Greater New York and Massachusetts Newsletter* (Spring/Summer 1990): 1.

[827] Stephens. http://home.hia.no/~stephens/coolinks.htm

[829] Stevens, K. A., and J. M. Parrish. "Neck Posture and Feeding Habits of Two Jurassic Sauropod Dinosaurs." *Science* 284 (1999): 798.

[830] Stewart, J. D., E. Angus, and D. Gendron. "Sciatic Neuropathies." *British Medical Journal* 287 (1983): 1108.

[831] Stickgold, R., J. A. Hobson, R. Fosse, and M. Fosse. "Sleep, Learning and Dreams: Off-Line Memory and Reprocessing." *Science* 294 (2001): 1052.

[832] Stiles, M. *Structural Yoga Therapy.* Boston: Weiser (2001).

[833] Stiles, M. T. "Know Your Knees." *Yoga International* (reprint series, "Yoga Therapy for Knees and Shoulders," 1998): 3.

[834] ———. "Wings of the Heart: Working with the Shoulders." *Yoga International* (reprint series, "Yoga Therapy for Knees and Shoulders," 1998): 12.

[835] Stoerig, P. "Varieties of Vision: from Blind Responses to Conscious Recognition." *Topics In Neural Science* 19 (1996): 403.

[836] Stoppard, M. *Menopause.* London: Dorling Kindersley (1994).

[837] Struthers, A. D. "Impact of Aldosterone on Vascular Pathophysiology." *Congestive Heart Failure* (Jan/Feb 2002): 18.

[838] Suda, N. "Earth's Background Free Oscillations." *Science* 279 (1998): 2089.

[839] Sunderland, S. "The Relative Susceptibility to Injury of the Medial and Lateral Popliteal Divisions of the Sciatic Nerve." *British Journal of Surgery* 41 (1953): 300.

[840] Svitil, K. A. "Fire in the Brain." *Discover* (May 2002): 51.

[841] Svoboda, R. E. *Aghora II: Kundalini,* Albuquerque: Brotherhood of Life (1993).

[842] Swami Veda Bharati. "What Is the Opposite Sex? *Yoga International* (Sep/Oct 1993): 7.

[843] Swanson, L. W. "The Hypothalamus" in *Handbook of Chemical Neuroanatomy: Integrated Systems of the CNS,* A. Bjorkland, T. Hokfelt, and L. W. Swanson (eds.). Amsterdam: Elsevier (1987).

[844] Szalavitz, M. "Sweet Solace: 10 Mostly Pleasant Truths about Pain." *Psychology Today* (October 2005): 74.

[845] Tagart, R. E. B. "The Anal Canal and Rectum: Their Varying Relationship and Its Effect on Anal Continence." *Diseases of the Colon and Rectum* 9 (1966): 449.

[846] Tai, Y. F., C. Scherfler, D. J. Brooks, N. Sawamoto, and U. Castiello. "The Human Premotor Cortex Is 'Mirror' Only for Biological Actions." *Current Biology* 14 (2004): 117.

[847] Talbot, M. "The Placebo Prescription." *New York Times Magazine* (January 9, 2000): 34.

[848] Tart, C. T., *States of Consciousness.* New York: Dutton (1975).

[849] Tavernarakis, N. "Death by Misadventure," *New Scientist* (February 15 2003): 30.

[850] Taylor, C. "Death by Crucifixion." *New Scientist* (January 23, 2000).

[851] Telang, S. D. *Understanding Yoga through Body Knowledge.* Pune: Arun Jakhade (2003).

[851a] Telles, S., and T. Desiraju. "Autonomic Changes in Brahmakumaris Raja Yoga Meditation." *International Journal of Psychophysiology* 15 (1993): 147.

[852] Telles, S., R. Nagarathna, and H. R.

Nagendra. "Breathing through a Particular Nostril Can Alter Metabolism and Autonomic Activities." *Indian Journal of Physiology and Pharmacology* 38 (1994): 133.

[853] Telles, S., B. H. Hanumanthaiah, R. Nagarathna, and H. R. Nagendra. "Plasticity of Motor Control Systems Demonstrated by Yoga Training." *Indian Journal of Physiology and Pharmacology* 38 (1994): 143.

[854] Telles, S., R. Nagarathna, and H. R. Nagendra. "Autonomic Changes during 'OM' Meditation." *Indian Journal of Physiology and Pharmacology* 39 (1995): 418.

[855] ———. "Physiological Measures of Right Nostril Breathing." *Journal of Alternative and Complementary Medicine* 2 (1996): 479.

[856] ———. "Autonomic Changes While Mentally Repeating Two Syllables—One Meaningful and the Other Neutral." *Indian Journal of Physiology and Pharmacology* 42 (1998): 57.

[856a] Telles, S., S. K. Reddy, and H. R. Negendra. "Oxygen Consumption and Respiration Following Two Yoga Relaxation Techniques." *Applied Psychophysiology and Biofeedback* 25(2000): 221.

[857] Telles, S., M. Joshi, M. Dash, P. Raghuraj, K. V. Naveen, and H. R. Nagendra. "An Evaluation of the Ability to Voluntarily Reduce the Heart Rate after a Month of Yoga Practice." *Integrative Physiological and Behavioral Science* 39 (2004): 119.

[857a] Thomas, A. "Yoga and Fascia." *Journal of the International Association of Yoga Therapists* 3 (1992): 39.

[858] Thomas, J., and M. G. Mawhinney. *Synopsis of Endocrine Pharmacology.* Baltimore: University Park (1973).

[859] Thorpe, A. Personal communication (2004).

[860] Tigunait, P. R. "Psychology of Consciousness." *Research Bulletin of the Himalayan International Institute* 3 (1981): 1.

[861] Tigunait, R. "Mind Games: How We Make Ourselves Sick." *Yoga International* (Jun/Jul 2000): 25.

[862] Tomlinson, C. "20/20 Vision Quest." *Yoga Journal* (Mar/Apr 1999): 120.

[863] Tortora, G. J., and N. P. Anagnostakos. *Principles of Anatomy and Physiology* (5th ed.). Cambridge, MA: Harper Row (1987).

[864] Trachtenberg, B. Personal communication (1998).

[865] Travis, J. "Mom's Eggs Execute Dad's Mitochondria." *Science News* 157 (2000): 5.

[866] ———. "Boning Up." *Science News* 157 (2000): 41.

[867] ———. "Protein May Help the Eyes Tell Time." *Science News* 157 (2000): 120.

[868] Treffert, D. A., and G. L. Wallace. "Islands of Genius." *Scientific American Mind* 14 (2004): 14.

[869] Treffert, D. A., and D. D. Christensen. "Inside the Mind of a Savant." *Scientific American* (December 2005): 106.

[870] Tyrrell, P. J., M. D. Feher, and M. N. Rossor. "Sciatic Nerve Damage Due to Toilet Seat Entrapment: Another Saturday Night Palsy." *Journal of Neurology, Neurosurgery, and Psychiatry* 52 (1989): 1113.

[870a] Umilta, M. A., E. Kohler, V. Gallese, L. Fogassi, L. Fadiga, C. Keysers, and G. Rizzolatti. "I Know What You Are Doing: A Neurophysiological Study." *Neuron* 31 (2001): 155.

[871] Upledger, J. E. *Cranial Sacral Therapy I Study Guide.* UI Pub. (1991).

[871a] Vance, G. " It Came from Another Time Zone." *New Scientist* (September 2, 2006): 40.

[871b] Velakonja, D., D. S. Weiss, and W. C. Corning. "The Relationship of Cortical Activation to Alternating Autonomic Activity." *Electroencephalography and Clinical Neurophysiology* 87 (1993): 38.

[872] Vempati, R. P., and S. Telles. "Yoga-Based Isometric Relaxation versus Supine Rest: A Study of Oxygen Consumption, Breath Rate and Volume and Autonomic Measures." *Journal of Indian Psychology* 17 (1999): 46.

[873] ———. "Yoga-Based Guided Relaxation Reduces Sympathetic Activity Judged from Baseline Levels." *Psychology Reports* 90 (2002): 487.

[874] Vescovi, A., R. Galli, U. Borello, A Gritti, M. G. Minasi, and C. Bjornson. "Skeletal Myogenic Potential of Human and Mouse Neural Cells." *Nature Neuroscience* (October 3, 2000): 986.

[874a] Vince, G. "The Many Ages of Man." *New Scientist* (June 17, 2006): 50.

[875] Vogel, C. M., R. Albin, and J. W. Albers. "Lotus Footdrop: Sciatic Neuropathy in the Thigh." *Neurology* 41 (1991): 605.

[876] Vogel, S. *Cat's Paws and Catapults.* New York: Norton (1998).

[877] ———. *Prime Mover.* New York: Norton

(2001).

[878] Von Hippel, A. *Human Evolutionary Biology.* Anchorage: Stone Age Press (1994).

[879] Voss, L. D., and B. J. R. Bailey. "Diurnal Variation in Stature: Is Stretching the Answer?" *Archive of Disease in Childhood* 77 (1997): 319.

[880] Walden, P. "Asanas to Relieve Depression." *Yoga Journal* (Nov/Dec 1999): 45.

[881] Walker, M. "Pressure Gets to You." *New Scientist* (August 1999): 16.

[882] Walker, M., G. Meekins, and S. C. Hu. "Yoga Neuropathy: A Snoozer." *Neurologist* 11 (2005): 176.

[883] Wartentin, S., U. Passant, L. Minthon, S. Karlson, L. Edvinsson, R. Faldt, L. Gustafson, and J. Risberg. "Redistribution of Blood Flow in the Cerebral Cortex of Normal Subjects during Head-Up Postural Change." *Clinical Autonomic Research* (April 2, 1992): 119.

[884] Watkins, J. *Structure and Function of the Musculoskeletal System.* Champaign, IL: Human Kinetics (1999).

[885] Weil, A. "Activity and Rest." *Yoga International* (October 1998): 49.

[885a] Weinberger, N. M. "Music and the Brain." *Scientific American* (November 2004): 89.

[886] Weindruch, R. "Caloric Restrictions and Aging." *Scientific American* (January 1996): 46.

[887] Weiner, H. "When Nerves Break Down." *New Scientist* (June 15, 2004): 44.

[888] Weintraub, A. "The Natural Prozac." *Yoga Journal* (Nov/Dec 1999): 40.

[889] Weintraub, M. I. "Beauty Parlor Stroke Syndrome." *Journal of the American Medical Association* 269 (1993): 2085.

[890] Weis, J., L. Balazs, and G. Adam. "The Effect of Monocular Viewing on Heartbeat Discrimination." *Psychophysiology* 31 (1994): 370.

[891] Wenger, M. A., B. K. Bagchi, and B. K. Anand. "Experiments in India on 'Voluntary' Control of the Heart and Pulse." *Circulation* 24 (1961): 1319.

[892] Westphal, S. P. "Make Light of Jet Lag." *New Scientist* (February 16, 2002): 17.

[893] White, R. J. "Weightlessness and the Human Body." *Scientific American* (September 1998): 57.

[894] Wilde, A. D., J. A. Cook, and A. S. Jones. "The Nasal Response to Isometric Exercise." *Clinical Otolaryngology.* 20 (1995): 345.

[895] Wilde, A. D., and A. S. Jones. "The Nasal Response to Axillary Pressure." *Clinical Otolaryngology* 21 (1996): 442.

[896] Williams, C. "The 25-Hour Day," *New Scientist* (February 24, 2006): 34.

[897] Williams, K. A., J. Petronis, D. Smith, D. Goodrich, J. Wu, N. Ravi, E. J. Doyle, Jr., R. G. Juckett, M. Munoz Kolar, R. Gross, and L. Steinberg. "Effect of Iyengar Yoga Therapy for Chronic Low Back Pain." *Pain* 115 (2005): 107.

[897a] Williams, K., L. Steinberg, and J. Petronis. "Therapeutic Application of Iyengar Yoga for Healing Chronic Low Back Pain." *International Journal of Yoga Therapy* 13 (2003): 55.

[898] Williams, L. *New Scientist* (April 6, 2002): 51.

[899] Williams, M. M. "Secrets of Redheads." *Discover* (December 2005): 13.

[900] Wojtys, E. M., L. J. Huston, T. N. Lindenfeld, T. E. Hewett, and M. L. Greenfield. "Association between the Menstrual Cycle and Anterior Cruciate Ligament Injuries in Female Athletes." *American Journal of Sports Medicine* 26 (1998): 614.

[901] Wojtys, E. M., L. J. Huston, M. D. Boynton, K. P. Spindler, and T. N. Lindenfeld. "The Effect of the Menstrual Cycle on Anterior Cruciate Ligament Injuries in Women as Determined by Hormone Levels." *American Journal of Sports Medicine* 30 (2002): 182.

[902] Wolman, D. "On the Other Hand." *New Scientist* (November 5, 2005): 36.

[903] Woolery, A., H. Meyers, B. Sternlieb, and L. Zeltzer. "A Yoga Intervention for Young Adults with Elevated Symptoms of Depression." *Alternative Therapies in Health and Medicine* 10 (2004): 60.

[904] Wright, K. "The Last Word." *New Scientist* (December 14, 2002).

[905] ———. "Physical Chemistry." *Discover* (July 2003): 57.

[906] ———. "Times of Our Lives." *Scientific American Special* 14 (2004): 42.

[907] www. discover.com/science_news.html.

[908] www.discover.com/science_news/clock.html.

[909] www.ditti-online.org.

[910] www.shef.ac.uk/uni/projects/mc/cary1.html.

[911] www.naturesplatform.com

[912] Yee, R. Personal communication (2000).

[913] *Yoga Calendar.* Berkeley: Yoga Journal (1993).

[914] Yoshikawa, Y. "Everybody Up Side Down." *Yoga Journal* (Sep/Oct 2000): 94.

[915] Young, E. "Balancing Act." *New Scientist*

(January 12, 2001): 25.

[916] ———. "Doing the Twist." *New Scientist* (March 1, 2001): 49.

[917] ———. "Caffeine Key to Curing a Headache." *New Scientist* (October 29, 2001).

[918] ———. "Amphetamine-Like Chemical Linked to Exercise Mood Boosts." *New Scientist* (September 27, 2001): 46.

[919] ———. "Heart Deaths Peak on 'Unlucky' Days." *New Scientist* (December 21, 2001): 10.

[920] ———. "Controversial Dyslexia Treatment Works." *New Scientist* (November 5, 2002): 59.

[921] ———. "TV is a Switch-Off for Back Muscles." *New Scientist* (August 28, 2004): 10.

[922] ———. "Inside the Brain of an Alcoholic." *New Scientist* (February 4, 2006): 18.

[923] Young, M. W. "The Tick-Tock of the Biological Clock." *Scientific American* (March 2000): 64.

[924] Zandonella, C. "Pheromones Can Banish Premenstrual Syndrome." *New Scientist* (July 18, 2001)

[925] ———. "Blue Christmas." *New Scientist* (December 22, 2001): 30.

[926] Zandonella, C., and P. Marks. "Eyeball This." *New Scientist* (March 23, 2002): 24.

[927] Zimmer, C. "Circus Science." *Discover* 19 (1996): 56.

[928] ———. "Into the Night." *Discover* 19 (1998): 10.

[929] ———. "Crystal Balls." *Natural History* (April 2002): 32.

[930] ———. "The Neurobiology of the Self." *Scientific American* (November 2005): 90.

[931] Zubieta, J. K., J. A. Bueller, L. R. Jackson, D. J. Scott, Y. Xu, R. A. Koeppe, T. E. Nichols, and C. S. Stohler. "Placebo Effects Mediated by Endogenous Opioid Activity on mu-Opioid Receptors." *Journal of Neuroscience* 25 (2005): 7754.

Index

The indicial display is strictly alphabetic; in cases where abbreviations have been used, the entry's placement in the index is according to its first initial when spelled out fully. For example, keyword and subtopic references to "premenstrual syndrome" use the abbreviation "PMS," as in the table below. However, the listing for it as a keyword is made according to the spelling "Premenstrual." Also, the same applies to the placement of keywords and subtopics beginning with Greek letters. Thus the keyword "α-motor neuron" is positioned on the basis of the spelling of its first word, "alpha." When two or more subtopics with identical page numbers appear under a keyword, they are listed alphabetically as "subtopic 1/subtopic 2/subtopic 3/…, page number" under that keyword.[1]

Abbreviated Terms

1   Assembly of the index was aided greatly by Karin Eisen and Alice Robin, and I am happy to acknowledge their generous help in this.

nuchae/*sarvangasana*, *465*; skin, *503*

Elbow: *adho mukha svanasana*/bone-on-bone/
interosseous membrane/*sarvangasana*/tendons,
338–9; arthritis/pain, *519*; balancing, *882*; biceps
brachii/brachioradialis, *326, 368, 420, 424–5*;
bursitis, *407*; carrying angle/dropped/epicondyles/
humerus/radius/ulna/ulnar nerve, *329, 338–9*;
cracking noise, *247*; cubital joint/tunnel, *62, 329*;
hyperextension, *248, 338, 340, 351*; lymph nodes,
577; muscle-lever types, *427*; *pincha mayurasana*,
878; *virabhadrasana I*, *243*; see also Useless elbow

Electrical resistance: energy blockage, *497*

Electrocardiogram (ECG): aging, *121*; arousal/carotid
sinus/sleep, *582*; atrium/AVN/cardiac contraction
P/Q/R/S/T waves/refractory period/SAN, *547–8*;
ANS, *162, 629*; baroreceptors/power spectrum,
550; brain waves/mental functioning/Schumann
resonances, *149–54*; examples/heart attack/
inflammation/heart rate/ion currents/ischemia/
variability, *548–50*; Swami Rama, *192, 546–7*; see
also Brain waves

Electrocution: extensors/flexors, *368*; muscle
contraction, *377*

Electroencephalogram (EEG): aging, *121*; alertness/lie
detector, *102, 152–3, 174*; alpha-delta-theta waves/
thalamus, *149, 154, 190*; arousal/ANS/gamma
waves, *151, 190*; basal ganglia/interval timer, *770*;
beta waves, *150, 190*; carotid arteries, *582*; cerebral
laterality, *629*; conscious control/nasal-cerebral
laterality, *168, 629, 632*; cortisol/memory/reticular
formation/*savasana*/*yogasana* postures, *151, 154*;
waves, *150–1*; depression, *182*; forced unilateral
breathing/ultradian cycles, *629–32*; gaze/visual
stress, *673*; left prefrontal lobe, *102, 182, 754*;
nasal/oral breathing, *624, 628*; pacemaker, *149–50*;
PNS, *935–7*; right prefrontal lobes, *102, 182, 754*;
sleep, *795, 802*; synchronicity, *149, 163, 930, 946*

Electrolyte balance/imbalance: cramps, *474–5*;
kidneys, *729*

Electroshock/electroconvulsion therapy: depression/
right hemisphere, *761*

Elevation/limb: lymph edema/RICE/*viparita karani*,
479

Elimination/pressure points: *savasana*/*supta virasana*/
vajrasana, *716*

Elongation: cylinder disrotation, *295–7*; spinal, *274*;
tendon, *411*

Embolism/emboli: case histories/marijuana/*pranayama*,
838–41; clots/platelets, *559–60*; hypertension,
576; injury/thrombosis, *117, 559–60*; vertebral
arteries, *278*

Embryo/infant: asymmetry, *844*; connective tissue, *482*

Emotional axis: level mixing/transformation/tripartite
yoga, *15–7*

Emotional bonding: psychotherapy, *755–6*

Emotional distress/pain: anterior cingulate/pain, *523*;
balancing, *931*; flexional tonic reflex, *451*

Emotional hyperflexibility: bipolar disorder, *764*

Emotional memory: amygdala/anxiety, *132, 766*;
conscious-subconscious/limbic system/prefrontal
cortex/SNS, *132*; REM, *801*

Emotional stress/release: aggression/muscle tension/
pleasure/rage/sexual feelings/*yogasana* practice,
755–6; anger/fear, *753, 756*; anxiety, *765*;
autonomic balance, *183*; blood pressure/urination,
731; chanting, *695, 754*; energy blockage/massage,
497–8; heart attack, *556*; herniated disc, *523*;
laughter, *459*; pain, *516, 525, 756*; *savasana*/tears,
723

Emotion: abdominal breathing/RSA, *620, 624,
635*; aging, *123, 816*; amygdala, *82, 123, 132,
167, 754, 817*; anger, *82, 168, 196*; anterior
commissure, *104*; apocrine sweat, *725*; attitudes/
brain asymmetry/centers/prefrontal lobes, *754*;
ANS/thermoregulation, *727*; backbending/self-
regulation, *755–6*; balancing, *931*; baroreceptors,
585; blood pressure, *731*; breath/OCD, *767–8*;
catecholamines, *134, 193*; cerebral laterality, *102,
182*; cingulate cortex, *97–8, 132*; depression,
762; dopamine, *97*; estrogen-progesterone, *739*;
extremes/mania, *764*; eyes/self-comforting,
513, 662, 680, 723; facial expressions, *753–4,
758*; forced unilateral breathing/nasal laterality,
630, 635; γ-motor neurons/muscle spindles/
patellar knee reflex, *433, 449, 766*; GTOs,
439; good health, *619–20*; hypertension, *576*;
hypothalamus, *167–8, 214*; immunity, *646, 753,
762*; interoception, *445*; ischemia/muscle strength-
tone, *437–8, 467*; limbic system, *80–3, 104, 132,
756, 760*; pain, *516–7, 523*; PNS, *182*; placebos,
528–9; reflex/uptight feeling, *450–2, 753–4*;
right hemisphere, *102*; SAD, *686*; *savasana*, *723*;
schizophrenia, *767*; smoking, *621*; stomach acid,
707; stress/strain, *168, 193–201, 753*; SNS, *132,
174*; touching/tickling, *511, 514*; *yogasana* practice,
755; see also Positive emotions, Negative emotions,
and Moods

Emotions/brain centers: amygdala, *132, 754, 817*;
anxiety, *765–6*; asymmetry/Buddhist meditators/
prefrontal lobes/reflex, *754, 760*; ANS, *174*;
depression/grief, *451, 580, 757*; fear, *132, 754,
817*; gender, *123*; hypothalamus, *168*; limbic
system, *82*

Empathy: anterior cingulate cortex/pain, *517*;
asymmetric deformities, *843*; facial expressions,
195, 754, 758; mirror neurons, *143–4, 754*

Emphysema: alveoli, *603*; dead air, *626*

Endocrine system/glands: adrenal/locations/types/

CPSIA information can be obtained
at www.ICGtesting.com
Printed in the USA
BVOW09s2040070617
486259BV00001B/1/P